# Motion Preservation Surgery of the Spine
## Advanced Techniques and Controversies


**James J. Yue**
Associate Professor
Department of Orthopaedic Surgery
Co-Chief, Division of Spinal Surgery
Director, Yale Spine Fellowship
Yale University School of Medicine
New Haven, Connecticut

**Rudolf Bertagnoli**
Chairman
First European Center for Spine Arthroplasty and
Associated Nonfusion Technologies (ECSA)
Elisabeth Krankenhaus Straubing
KKH Bogen, Germany

**Paul C. McAfee**
Chief, Spinal Reconstructive Surgery
Orthopaedic Associates
St. Joseph's Hospital
Towson, Maryland

**Howard S. An**
The Morton International Professor for Spine Research
Department of Orthopaedic Surgery
Rush Medical College
Chicago, Illinois


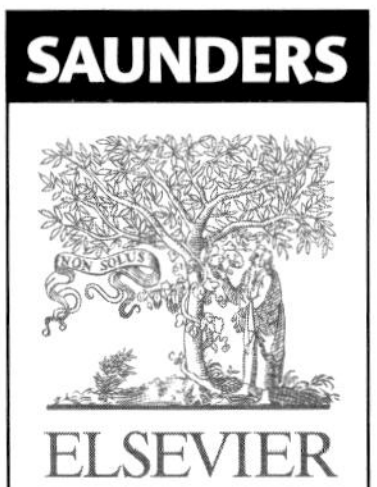

SAUNDERS
ELSEVIER

1600 John F. Kennedy Blvd.
Ste 1800
Philadelphia, PA 19103–2899

MOTION PRESERVATION SURGERY OF THE SPINE: ADVANCED TECHNIQUES AND CONTRVERSIES
ISBN: 978-1-4160-3994-5



**Notice**

Knowledge and best practice in this field are constantly changing. As new research and experience broaden our knowledge, changes in practice, treatment and drug therapy may become necessary or appropriate. Readers are advised to check the most current information provided (i) on procedures featured or (ii) by the manufacturer of each product to be administered, to verify the recommended dose or formula, the method and duration of administration, and contraindications. It is the responsibility of the practitioner, relying on their own experience and knowledge of the patient, to make diagnoses, to determine dosages and the best treatment for each individual patient, and to take all appropriate safety precautions. To the fullest extent of the law, neither the Publisher nor the Editors assumes any liability for any injury and/or damage to persons or property arising out or related to any use of the material contained in this book.

The Publisher

**Library of Congress Cataloging-in-Publication Data**

Motion preservation surgery of the spine : advanced techniques and controversies / edited by James J. Yue . . . [et al.]. –1st ed.
p. ; cm.
Includes bibliographical references.
ISBN 978-1-4160-3994-5
1. Intervertebral disk–Surgery. 2. Intervertebral disk prostheses. 3. Spine–Surgery.
4. Arthroplasty. I. Yue, James J. [DNLM: 1. Spine–surgery. 2. Arthroplasty, Replacement–methods.
3. Motion. 4. Spinal Diseases–surgery. WE 725 M888 2008]

RD771.I6M68 2008
617.5′6–dc22
2007027127

*Acquisitions Editor:* Kimberly Murphy
*Developmental Editor:* Adrianne Brigido
*Publishing Services Manager:* Joan Sinclair
*Design Direction:* Gene Harris



Printed in China

Last digit is the print number: 9 8 7 6 5 4 3 2 1

To my wife and children: Susan, Lauren, and Emily. My three 1 in a millions!

—James J. Yue

To my mentors, friends, colleagues, and entrepreneurs of these techniques—especially those in the SAS society and those who promote motion preservation.

To my wife and children.

—Rudolf Bertagnoli

I wish to acknowledge the most talented biomechanical engineers who have taught me enough to really make a positive impact in patient care—Manohar Panjabi, Fred Werner, Al Berstein, Helmut Link, and David Paul. I came into contact with each one of these internationally recognized giants at precisely the right time in my career, and I am grateful for their friendship.

—Paul C. McAfee

# Foreword

The human axial skeleton is composed of 24 mobile segments, with three articulations at each level. Although motion is not identical in degree at each level, it is also not the same in each of the 6 degrees of motion. There are specific range and quality at each anatomical region. Therefore, the preservation of motion is a daunting challenge for the scientists and surgeons.

Years of study, testing, and experimentation have gone into enhancing our knowledge of spinal motion and complex technologies are emerging. Biomaterials are evolving to enable properties that are essential for compatibility, safety, and efficacy. Biomechanics are thoroughly tested to mimic physiologic motion as closely as possible, yet being certain durability and wear characteristics are carefully monitored.

Animal studies meeting the (high) regulatory standards are done when necessary for tissue compatibility and, in some cases, for efficacy. No animals are like the human so the ultimate trial is pilots (small), then when safe, proceed to larger efficacy randomized control studies. This is difficult as what is needed for regulatory clearance is not necessarily the best control trial. However, diligent choices are often picked to get the best possible Level I studies and evidence.

Minimally invasive and yet maximally beneficial technologies are slowly coming to the fore. The biologics arena is abundant with theory, but with only early proof of concepts. What better motion preservation can there be than tissue engineering, with regenerative technologies, after early, appropriate diagnosis?

The editors have brought together between the covers of this first edition of *Motion Preservation Surgery of the Spine*, a comprehensive textbook covering the bulk of motion technologies. It includes (classic) contributions by several founding scientist surgeons. Even before this first edition has been completed, concepts and ideas for a second edition have been initiated by the editors due to the explosion of innovations in this area.

My congratulations to James J. Yue, Rudolf Bertagnoli, Paul C. McAfee, and Howard S. An for this huge task of love and dedication.

Hansen A. Yuan, MD
President, Spine Arthroplasty Society

# Preface

Vertebra, from Latin, from *vertere*, to turn

Some may say that current evolution of the treatment of degenerative disorders of the spine is, in many ways, a *revolution*. The essence of this apparent revolution is based on many factors including the realization that the pioneering work of Fernstrom and his advocates was not medical heresy but rather medical innovation. The eventual professional and personal persecution of these innovators that ensued was inappropriate and has predictably fueled today's scientific rapid development of motion-sparing technology. A first-hand account of the medical-socio-legal-political environment by Dr. Alvin McKenzie, a recipient of multi-level Fernstrom ball procedure, is meant to further elucidate the foundation of the recent evolving revolution in the treatment of spondylosis.

Whatever procedure a surgeon and his or her patient decide upon to remedy the debilitating effects of spondylosis, the choice should be based on the fundamental principal that the vertebrate spine is a "motion-protective" anatomical structure. An inherent duality exists in this motion-protective function. First, our spine is designed to allow positioning of our cranium and torso in our ever increasing multi-dimensional world, thereby permitting and enhancing our interactive and protective abilities and responsibilities. Coupled to this pro-motion functional adaptation is the intrinsic protection to the neural elements that our vertebrate spinal column provides. Herein lies the duality and balance of our motion-protective spinal column. Our vertebrate spinal column allows us to protect ourselves by allowing us to move and interact with our physical environment but it also protects the neurological elements that give our musculoskeletal and dermatomal systems the ability to perform these functions.

*Motion Preservation Surgery of the Spine: Advanced Techniques and Controversies* was written to provide a general understanding of the basic principles of nonfusion surgery as well as an advanced platform to approach the inevitable revision and/or additional procedures that may become necessary, as may occur with any surgical procedure. Inherent in each chapter are specific case examples that the authors have selflessly provided. In addition, clinical trial data are also provided to allow the reader to gain a sense of the potential place for a given technology in their practice. As one can ascertain from a review of the author list, we have chosen contributors based on their expertise in a given technology. Often this expertise was obtained from many parts of the globe. This multicultural and multi-national perspective is unique and truly invaluable to the reader given the long-term perspective that countries such as Germany and France have had using nonfusion technology.

Shortly after production of *Motion Preservation Surgery of the Spine: Advanced Techniques and Controversies* began, the Spine Arthroplasty Society requested that the text be included as one of the core teaching texts of their organization. In order to fulfill this honored request, multiple chapters dedicated to the concept of how to study motion-sparing technologies, both in the clinical as well as the laboratory setting, have been included. Future editions, both English and translated, will bring additional materials, learning supplements, and teaching aids.

The preparation of this textbook would not have been possible without the inspiration and diligent work of our contributing authors. We are deeply indebted and grateful to them for their tireless patience and determination in completing their chapters. We have also been fortunate to have benefited from the pioneering work of our mentors, including Henry Bohlman, Karin Büttner-Janz, Jürgen Harms, John Kostuik, John P. O'Brien, Robbie Robinson, Arthur Steffe, and Hansen Yuan to name just a few. Our support from our publisher, Elsevier, has been unequalled. Specifically, we would like to thank our Development Editor, Adrianne Brigido. Without her efforts, this book would not have been possible. We also sincerely thank Ms. Kimberly Murphy, Publishing Director, Global Medicine Elsevier, for her invaluable guidance. We believe you will find this textbook informative and a comprehensive platform and foundation for learning about motion-sparing technology of the spine.

James J. Yue

Rudolf Bertagnoli

Paul C. McAfee

Howard S. An

# Contributors

**Jean-Jacques Abitbol, MD**
Orthopaedic Spine Surgeon, California Spine Group, San Diego, California
*The CerviCore Cervical Intervertebral Disc Replacement*

**Michael Ahrens, MD**
University of Luebeck, Neustadt, Germany
*DASCOR*

**Todd F. Alamin, MD**
Assistant Professor, Department of Orthopaedic Surgery, Stanford University Medical Center, Stanford, California
*Invasive Diagnostic Tools*

**Todd J. Albert, MD**
James Edwards Professor and Chairman of Orthopaedic Surgery, Jefferson Medical College, Thomas Jefferson University, Philadelphia, Pennsylvania
*DISCOVER Artificial Cervical Disc*

**Jérome Allain**
Professor, University Paris XII, Paris, France
Professor, Hôpital Henri Dondor, Créteil, France
*Mobidisc Disc Prosthesis*

**Marc Ameil, MD**
Professor, Department of Orthopaedics, Polyclinique Saint-André, Reims, France
*Mobidisc Disc Prosthesis*

**Howard S. An**
The Morton International Professor for Spine Research, Department of Orthopaedic Surgery, Rush Medical College, Chicago, Illinois
*Animal Models for Human Disc Degeneration; Growth Factors for Intervertebral Disc Regeneration*

**Ravi Ananthan**
Theken Disc, LLC, Akron, Ohio
*Theken eDisc: A Second-Generation Lumbar Artificial Disc*

**Paul A. Anderson, MD**
Associate Professor of Orthopaedic Surgery, Department of Orthopaedics, University of Wisconsin, Madison, Madison, Wisconsin
*Preclinical Evaluation of Dynamic Spinal Stabilization: Animal Models and Basic Scientific Methods*

**S.A. Andrew**
*Scient'x IsoBar TTL Dynamic Rod Stabilization*

**Lucie Aubourg, PhD**
Clinical Research Manager, LDR Medical, Troyes, France
*Mobidisc Disc Prosthesis*

**Stephane Aunoble, MD**
Unité de Pathologie, Centre Hospitalier Pellegrin, Bordeaux, France
*Minimally Invasive Posterior Approaches to the Lumbar Spine*

**Jonathon R. Ball, BMed, BMedSC(Hons), FRACS**
Neurosurgical Registrar, Royal North Shore Hospital, New South Wales, Australia
*Cervical Arthroplasty with Myelopathy*

**Qi-Bin Bao, PhD**
Pioneer Surgical Technology, Marquette, Michigan
*Aquarelle Hydrogel Disc Nucleus; NUBAC Intradiscal Arthroplasty*

**Jacques Beaurain, MD**
Department of Neurosurgery, University Hospital, Dijon, France
*Mobi-C; Mobidisc Disc Prosthesis*

**Marco Bérard, MD**
Alice Hyde Orthopaedic and Sports Medicine Center, Alice Hyde Medical Center, Malone, New York
*Orthobiom: A Nonfusion Treatment for Pediatric Scoliosis*

**Ulrich Berelmann, MD**
M.E. Müller Institute for Surgical Technology and Biomechanics, University of Bern, Bern, Switzerland
*NuCore Injectable Nucleus: An In Situ Curing Nucleus Replacement*

**Pierre Bernard, MD**
Centre Aquitain du Dos, Clinique Saint-Martin, Pessac, France
*Mobi-C*

**Rudolf Bertagnoli, MD**
Chairman, First European Center for Spine Arthroplasty and Associated Nonfusion Technologies (ECSA), Elisabeth Krankenhaus Straubing, KKH Bogen, Germany
*Lateral Approaches to the Lumbar Spine: The Anterolateral Transpsoatic Approach; coflex Interspinous Implant for Stabilization of the Lumbar Spine; Hybrid Nonfusion Techniques; Autologous Chondrocyte Disc Transplant: Early Clinical Results; Multilevel Lumbar Disc Arthroplasty; Cervical Arthroplasty Adjacent to Fusion, Multiple-Level Cases, and Hybrid Applications*

**Robert S. Biscup, DO, MS, FAOAO**
Chairman, Biscup Spine Institute, Fort Lauderdale, Florida
*Satellite: Spherical Partial Disc Replacement*

**Jason D. Blain**
Chief Technology Officer, Spinal Elements, Carlsbad, California
*The Zyre Facet Replacement Device*

**Jon E. Block, PhD**
President, Jon E. Block, PhD, Inc., San Francisco, California
*The M6 Artificial Cervical Disc*

**Scott L. Blumenthal, MD**
Orthopaedic Spine Surgeon, Texas Back Institute, Plano, Texas
*CHARITÉ Artificial Disc; Simultaneous Lumbar Fusion and Total Disc Replacement*

**Nicholas R. Boeree, BSc, FRCS Orth, FRCS Ed**
Consultant Orthopaedic Surgeon, Southampton University Hospital Trust, Southampton, United Kingdom
*Wallis Dynamic Stabilization*

**Iohan Bogorin, MD**
Service de Chirurgie Orthopédique, du Rachis et de Traumatologie du Sport, Hôpitaux Universitaires de Strasbourg, Strasbourg, France
*Mobidisc Disc Prosthesis*

**David S. Bradford, MD**
Professor, University of California San Francisco
Professor and Chair Emeritus, University of California, San Francisco, California
*History and Evolution of Motion Preservation*

**Jacob M. Buchowski, MD, MS**
Assistant Professor of Orthopaedic and Neurologic Surgery, Washington University in St. Louis, St. Louis, Missouri
Chief, Degenerative and Minimally Invasive Spine Surgery, Washington University in St. Louis, St. Louis, Missouri
*Primary Indications and Disc Space Preparation for Cervical Disc Arthroplasty*

**Karin Büttner-Janz, MD, PhD**
Professor, Charité Universitätsmedizin, Berlin; Director of Orthopedic Clinic, Vivantes Klinikum im Friedrichshain, Berlin, Germany
*Classification of Spine Arthroplasty Devices*

**Andrew G. Cappuccino, MD**
Orthopaedic Spine Surgeon, Buffalo Spine Surgery, Lockport, New York
*Cervical Disc Replacement Revisions: Clinical and Biomechanical Considerations*

**Allen Carl, MD**
Professor, Orthopaedic Surgery and Pediatrics, Albany Medical College, Albany, New York
Attending Surgeon, Albany Medical Center, Albany, New York
*Anatomic Facet Replacement System (AFRS)*

**Antonio E. Castellvi, MD**
Spine Fellowship Director; Spine Surgeon, Florida Orthopaedic Institute, Tampa, Florida
*Scient'x IsoBar TTL Dynamic Rod Stabilization*

**Joseph C. Cauthen, MD**
Orthopaedic Spine Surgeon, Neurosurgical and Spine Associates, Gainesville, Florida
*Repair and Reconstruction of the Annulus Fibrosus with the Inclose Surgical Mesh System*

**Hervé Chataigner, MD**
Service de Chirurgie des Scolioses et Orthopedie Infantile, Hôpital St. Jacques, Besançon, France
*Mobidisc Disc Prosthesis*

**Boyle C. Cheng, PhD**
Assistant Professor, University of Pittsburgh, Pittsburgh, Pennsylvania
*Biomechanics of Nonfusion Devices: Novel Testing Techniques, Standards, and Implications for Future Devices*

**Robert J. Chomiak, MD**
Paradigm Spine, LLC, New York, New York
*coflex Interspinous Implant for Stabilization of the Lumbar Spine; Orthobiom: A Nonfusion Treatment for Pediatric Scoliosis*

**Christine Coillard, MD**
Research Centre, Sainte-Justine Hospital, Montreal, Quebec, Canada
*Orthobiom: A Nonfusion Treatment for Pediatric Scoliosis*

**Christopher Cole**
Engineer, Theken Disc, LLC, Akron, Ohio
*Theken eDisc: A Second-Generation Lumbar Artificial Disc*

**Dennis Colleran**
Vice President, Research and Development, IlluminOss Medical Inc., Tiverton, Rhode Island
*Innovative Spinal Technologies Dynamic Stabilization Device*

**Domagoj Coric, MD**
Chief of Neurosurgery, Carolinas Medical Center, Charlotte, North Carolina
Carolina Neurosurgery and Spine Associates, Charlotte, North Carolina
*Cervical Approaches: Anterior and Posterior; NUBAC Intradiscal Arthroplasty*

**G. Bryan Cornwall, PhD, PEng**
Vice President, Research and Clinical Resources, NuVasive, Inc., San Diego, California
*The NeoDisc Elastomeric Cervical Total Disc Replacement; Cerpass Cervical Total Disc Replacement*

**Etevaldo Coutinho, MD**
Spine Surgeon, Santa Rita Hospital, São Paulo, Brazil
*Lateral Lumbar Total Disc Replacement*

**Andrew H. Cragg, MD**
Interventional Radiologist, Minnesota Vascular Clinic, Suburban Radiologic Consultants, Edina, Minnesota
*TranS1 Percutaneous Nucleus Replacement*

**Bryan W. Cunningham, MSc**
Associate Professor, Department of Orthopaedic Surgery, Johns Hopkins University, Baltimore, Maryland
Director, Spinal Research, St. Joseph Medical Center, Towson, Maryland
*Preclinical Evaluation of Dynamic Spinal Stabilization: Animal Models and Basic Scientific Methods; Cervical Disc Replacement Revisions: Clinical and Biomechanical Considerations; Anatomic Facet Replacement System (AFRS)*

**David Cutter**
NuVasive Inc., San Diego, California
*Cerpass Cervical Total Disc Replacement*

**Frank Daday, MBBS, FANZCA**
Visiting Medical Officer, Allamanda Private Hospital, Gold Coast, Queensland, Australia
*Overall Revision Strategies: Lumbar*

**Reginald J. Davis, MD**
Assistant Professor, Neurosurgery, Johns Hospital Medical Institute; Clinical Instructor, Neurosurgery, University of Maryland Medical Center, Baltimore, Maryland
Division Head of Neurosurgery, Greater Baltimore Medical Center, Towson, Maryland
*PDN-SOLO and HydraFlex Nucleus Replacement; Dynesys Dynamic Stabilization System*

**Rick B. Delamarter, MD**
Associate Clinical Professor, University of California, Los Angeles, Los Angeles, California;
Fellowship Director, The Spine Institute, Santa Monica, California
*ProDisc-C Total Cervical Disc Replacement; ProDisc-L Total Disc Replacement*

**Joël Delécrin, MD, PhD**
Associate Professor, Department of Orthopedic Surgery, Nantes University, Nantes, France
*Mobidisc Disc Prosthesis*

**Malan DeVilliers, BEng (Mech), MEng, PhD (Eng)**
Managing Director, Southern Medical (PTY) LTD, Irene, Centurion, South Africa
*Kineflex*

**Roberto Díaz, MD**
Assistant Professor, Department of Neurosurgery, San Ignacio University Hospital, Javeriana School of Medicine, Bogota, Columbia
*Cervical Disc Replacement Revisions: Clinical Biomechanical Considerations; TranS1 Percutaneous Nucleus Replacement; TOPS: Total Posterior Facet Replacement and Dynamic Motion Segment Stabilization System*

**Juan M. Dipp, MD**
Chief, Orthopedic and Spine Surgery, Hospital del Prado, Tijuana, Mexico
Chief Spine Surgeon, Hospital Angeles, Tijuana, Tijuana, Mexico
*The PercuDyn System*

**Gary A. Dix, MD, FRCS(C)**
Medical Director of Spine Services, Anne Arundel Medical Center, Annapolis, Maryland
*Persistent Pain After Cervical Arthroplasty*

**Thomas B. Ducker, MD, FACS**
Johns Hopkins Medical School, Baltimore, Maryland
Anne Arundel Medical Center, Annapolis, Maryland
*Persistent Pain After Cervical Arthroplasty*

**Thierry Dufour, MD**
Neurosurgeon, Centre Hospitalier Regional, Orléans, France
*Mobi-C; Mobidisc Disc Prosthesis*

**Jacob Einhorn**
Vice President, Research and Development, Intrinsic Therapeutics, Inc., Woburn, Massachusetts
*The Intrinsic Therapeutics Barricaid Device*

**Lukas Eisermann, BS**
Director of Advanced Technology Development, NuVasive, Inc., San Diego, California
*The NeoDisc Elastomeric Cervical Total Disc Replacement; Cerpass Cervical Total Disc Replacement*

**Thomas J. Errico, MD**
Chief, Division of Spine Surgery, Department of Orthopaedic Surgery, New York University—Hospital for Joint Diseases; Associate Professor of Orthopaedics and Neurosurgery, New York University School of Medicine, New York, New York
*The FlexiCore Intervertebral Disc*

**Teddy Fagerstrom, MD**
Department of Orthopedics, Huddinge University Hospital, Stockholm, Sweden
*FENIX Facet Resurfacing Implant*

**Daniel R. Fassett, MD, MBA**
Assistant Professor, Department of Neurosurgery, University of Illinois College of Medicine Peoria, Peoria, Illinois
*Advanced Spinal Anatomy for Cervical and Lumbar Nonfusion Surgery*

**Jeffrey S. Fischgrund, MD**
Orthopaedic Spine Surgeon, William Beaumont Hospital, Royal Oak, Michigan
*The CerviCore Cervical Intervertebal Disc Replacement*

**Ricardo Flores, MD**
Chief of Neurosurgery, Departments of Neurology and Neurosurgery, Hospital Almater, Mexicali, Mexico
*The PercuDyn System*

**Jean-Marc Fuentes, MD**
Hôpital Pellegrin, Bordeaux, France
*Mobi-C*

**Josue Gabriel, MD**
Clinical Director, Biodynamics Laboratory, The Ohio State University, Columbus, Ohio
Clinical Assistant Professor, Department of Orthopaedic Surgery, The Ohio State University, Columbus, Ohio
*The Development of a Personalized Hybrid EMG-Assisted/Finite Element Biomechanical Model to Assess Surgical Options*

**Rolando García, MD, MPH**
Spinal Surgeon, Orthopedic Care Center, Aventura, Florida
*Activ-L Artificial Disc; Dynamic Pedicle-Screw Stabilization with Nucleus Replacement*

**Fred H. Geisler, MD, PhD**
Founder, Illinois Neuro-Spine Center at Rush-Copley Medical Center, Aurora, Illinois
*Statistical Outcome Interpretation of Randomized Clinical Trails; Simultaneous Lumbar Fusion and Total Disc Replacement*

**Ihab Gharzeddine, MD**
Spine Surgeon, Santa Rita Hospital, São Paulo, Brazil
*Cervical Disc Replacement Revisions: Clinical and Biomechanical Considerations; Lateral Lumbar Total Disc Replacement; Revision Strategies Following Lumbar Total Disc Replacement Complications*

**Vijay K. Goel, PhD**
Endowed Chair and McMaster-Gardner Professor of Orthopaedic Bioengineering; Co-Director, Engineering Center for Orthopaedic Research Excellence (E-CORE), Departments of Bioengineering and Orthopaedic Surgery, Colleges of Engineering and Medicine, University of Toledo, Toledo, Ohio
*Theken eDisc: A Second-Generation Lumbar Artificial Disc; Anatomic Facet Replacement System (AFRS)*

**Jeffrey A. Goldstein, MD**
Assistant Professor of Orthopaedic Surgery, New York University School of Medicine, New York, New York
Director of Spine Service, New York University—Hospital for Joint Diseases, New York, New York
*Persistent Pain After Lumbar Total Disc Replacement*

**Matthew F. Gornet, MD**
Staff Physician, The Orthopedic Center of St. Louis, St. Louis, Missouri
*Maverick Total Disc Replacement*

**Steven L. Griffith, PhD**
Vice President, Scientific Affairs, Anulex Technologies, Inc., Minnetonka, Minnesota
*Repair and Reconstruction of the Annulus Fibrosus with the Inclose Surgical Mesh System*

**Geneste Guilhaume**
Department of Orthopaedic Surgery, Clinique du Parc, Castelnau-le-Lez, France
*Can Lumbar Disc Replacement Be Used Adjacent to a Scoliotic Deformity?*

**Giancarlo Guizzardi, MD**
Neurosurgery Unit, Careggi Hospital, Florence, Tuscany, Italy
*DIAM Spinal Stabilization System*

**Richard D. Guyer, MD**
Spine Surgeon; Co-Director of the Spine Surgery Fellowship Program, Texas Back Institute, Plano, Texas
*Socioeconomic Impact of Motion Preservation Technology*

**Nader M. Habela, MD**
Orthopaedic Associates and Spine Center, St. Joseph Medical Center, Towson, Maryland
*Indications and Contraindications for Cervical Nonfusion Surgery: Patient Selection*

**Ulrich Reinhard Hähnle, MD**
Post-Graduate Studies, University of Witwatersrand, Johannesburg, Gauteng, South Africa
Orthopedic Surgeon, Nedcare Linksfield Hospital, Johannesburg, Gauteng, South Africa
*Kineflex*

**Horace Hale**
CEO, GerraSpine, St. Gallen, Switzerland
*FENIX Facet Resurfacing Implant*

**Nadim James Hallab, MS, PhD**
Associate Professor, Department of Orthopedic Surgery, Rush University Medical Center, Chicago, Illinois
*Material Properties and Wear Analysis*

**David Hannallah, MD, MS**
Staff Physician, The Cardinal Orthopaedic Institute, Columbus, Ohio
*Adjacent Segment Degeneration and Adjacent Segment Disease: Cervical and Lumbar*

**Matthew Hannibal, MD**
Director of Spine Research; Associate Director, San Francisco Orthopedic Research Program, Department of Orthopedic Surgery, San Francisco, California
*X-STOP Interspinous Process Decompression for Lumbar Spinal Stenosis*

**Victor M. Hayes, MD**
Trinity Spine Center, Tampa, Florida
*Lumbar Endoscopic Posterolateral (Transforaminal) Approach*

**Alan S. Hilibrand, MD**
Department of Orthopaedic Surgery, Thomas Jefferson University, Philadelphia, Pennsylvania
*Adjacent Segment Degeneration and Adjacent Segment Disease: Cervical and Lumbar*

**John A. Hipp, PhD**
Director, Spine Research Laboratory, Orthopedic Surgery, Baylor College of Medicine, Houston, Texas
Chief Scientist, Medical Metrics, Inc., Houston, Texas
*Quantitative Motion Analysis (QMA) of Motion-Preserving and Fusion Technologies for the Spine*

**Stephen H. Hochschuler, MD**
Spine Surgeon, Texas Back Institute, Plano, Texas
*The Future of Motion Preservation*

**Gordon Neil Holen, DO**
Spine Surgery, Department of Orthopedic Surgery, Mease Countryside Hospital, Safety Harbor, Florida
*Total Facet Arthroplasty System (TFAS)*

**Istvan Hovorka, MD**
Department of Orthopaedics and Sports Traumatology, University of Nice–Archet 2 Hospital, Nice, France
*Mobi-C*

**Robert W. Hoy, MEng**
Facet Solutions Inc., Logan, Utah
*Anatomic Facet Replacement System (AFRS)*

**Kenneth Y. Hsu, MD**
Co-Medical Director, Department of Orthopedics, St. Mary's Spine Center, San Francisco, California
*X-STOP Interspinous Process Decompression for Lumbar Spinal Stenosis*

**Jean Huppert, MD**
Clinique du Parc, Saint-Priest-en-Jarez, France
*Mobi-C*

**Cary Idler, MD**
Spine Fellow, St. Mary's Medical Center, San Francisco, California
*X-STOP Interspinous Process Decompression for Lumbar Spinal Stenosis*

**Andre Jackowski, MD, FRCS**
Department of Spinal Surgery, Royal Orthopaedic Hospital, Birmingham, United Kingdom
*The NeoDisc Elastomeric Cervical Total Disc Replacement*

**Joshua J. Jacobs, MD**
Associate Dean for Research Development, Department of Orthopaedic Surgery, Rush University Medical Center; Associate Dean for Academic Programs, Department of Orthopaedic Surgery, Rush University Medical Center; Inaugural Crown Family Professor of Orthopaedic Surgery, Department of Orthopaedic Surgery, Rush University Medical Center, Chicago, Illinois
*Material Properties and Wear Analysis*

**Jorge Jaramillo, MD**
Department of Orthopaedic Surgery and Rehabilitation, Yale University School of Medicine, New Haven, Connecticut
*Disc Space Preparation Techniques for Lumbar Disc Arthroplasty*

**Shiveindra B. Jeyamohan, MD**
Department of Neurosurgery, Thomas Jefferson University, Philadelphia, Pennsylvania
*Advanced Spinal Anatomy for Cervical and Lumbar Nonfusion Surgery*

**James D. Kang, MD**
Vice Chairman, Department of Orthopaedic Surgery; Professor, Departments of Orthopaedic and Neurological Surgery; Director, Ferguson Laboratory for Orthopaedic Spine Research, University of Pittsburgh School of Medicine, Pittsburgh, Pennsylvania
Professor, Departments of Orthopaedic Surgery and Neurological Surgery, University of Pittsburgh Medical Center, Pittsburgh, Pennsylvania
*Gene Therapy for Intervertebral Disc Repair and Regeneration*

**Larry T. Khoo, MD**
Assistant Professor, Department of Surgery, University of California, Los Angeles, Los Angeles, California
*TranS1 Percutaneous Nucleus Replacement (PNR);*
*TOPS: Total Posterior Facet Replacement and Dynamic Motion Segment Stabilization System*

**Seok Woo Kim, MD, PhD**
Associate Professor, Department of Orthopaedic Surgery; Chief, Spine Services, Hallym University, Seoul, South Korea
Director, International Spine Center, Hangang Sacred Heart Hospital, Hallym University Medical Center, Seoul, South Korea
*Cervical Disc Replacement Combined with Cervical Laminoplasty*

**Scott H. Kitchel, MD**
Orthopaedic Physician and Surgeon, Orthopaedic Spine Associates LLC, Eugene, Oregon
*Cerpass Cervical Total Disc Replacement; The Zyre Facet Replacement*

**Gregory G. Knapik, MS**
Senior Research Associate Engineer, The Ohio State University Biodynamics Laboratory, Columbus, Ohio
*The Development of a Personalized Hybrid EMG-Assisted/Finite Element Biomechanical Model to Assess Surgical Options*

**Manoj Krishna, MCh(Orth), FRCS**
Consultant Spinal Surgeon, University Hospital of North Tees, Stockton-on-Tees, United Kingdom
*Posterior Lumbar Arthroplasty*

**Greg Lambrecht**
President and CEO, Intrinsic Therapeutics, Inc., Woburn, Massachusetts
*The Intrinsic Therapeutics Barricald Device*

**Carl Lauryssen, MD**
Director, Research and Education, Olympia Medical Center, Beverly Hills, California
*The Zyre Facet Replacement Device*

**William Lavelle, MD**
Fellow, Cleveland Clinic Spine Institute, Cleveland Clinic, Cleveland, Ohio
*Anatomic Facet Replacement System (AFRS)*

**James P. Lawrence, MD**
Department of Orthopaedic Surgery and Rehabilitation, Yale University, New Haven, Connecticut
*Indications and Contraindications for Lumbar Nonfusion Surgery: Patient Selection*

**Jean-Charles Le Huec, MD, PhD**
Professor and Head, Orthopaedic Department; Chief, Spine Unit; Director, Surgical Research Lab, Bordeaux University Hospital, Bordeaux, France
*Minimally Invasive Posterior Approaches to the Lumbar Spine; DASCOR*

**Juliano Lhamby, MD**
Orthopedic Spine Surgeon, Santa Rita Hospital, São Paulo, Brazil
*Cervical Disc Replacement Revisions: Clinical and Biomechanical Considerations; Lateral Lumbar Total Disc Replacement; Revision Strategies Following Lumbar Total Disc Replacement Complications*

**Gary L. Lowery, MD, PhD**
Executive Vice President, Research and Technology, Paradigm Spine, LLC, New York, New York
*coflex Interspinous Implant for Stabilization of the Spine; Orthobiom: A Nonfusion Treatment for Pediatric Scoliosis*

**George Malcolmon**
Aphatec Spine, Inc., Carlsbad, California
*The Stabilimax NZ Posterior Lumbar Dynamic Stabilization System*

**Thierry Marnay, MD**
Department of Orthopaedic Surgery, Clinique du Parc, Castelnau-le-Lez, France
*Can Lumbar Disc Replacement Be Used Adjacent to a Scoliotic Deformity?*

**William S. Marras, MS, PhD**
Professor, College of Engineering; Professor, College of Medicine, The Ohio State University Biodynamics Laboratory, Columbus, Ohio
*The Development of a Personalized Hybrid EMG-Assisted/Finite Element Biomechanical Model to Assess Surgical Options*

**Larry Martin, Jr., MD**
Resident, Department of Orthopaedic Surgery, Indiana University School of Medicine, Indianapolis, Indiana
*The Bryan Artificial Disc*

**Joseph M. Marzluff, MD**
Neurosurgeon, Roper St. Francis Healthcare, Charleston, South Carolina
*SECURE-C Cervical Artificial Disc*

**Koichi Masuda, MD**
Professor, Department of Othropedic Surgery and Biochemistry, Rush Medical College at Rush University Medical Center, Chicago, Illinois
*Animal Models for Human Disc Degeneration; Growth Factors for Intervertebral Disc Regeneration*

**Paul C. McAfee, MD**
Associate Professor of Orthopedic Surgery and Neurosurgery, Johns Hopkins Hospital, Baltimore, Maryland
Chief of Spinal Surgery, St. Joseph's Hospital, Baltimore, Maryland
*Indications and Contraindications for Cervical Nonfusion Surgery: Patient Selection; Porous-Coated Motion (PCM) Cervical Arthroplasty; Complications of Anterior Cervical Approaches: Cervical Revision: Approach-Related Considerations; Cervical Disc Replacement Revisions: Clinical and Biomechanical Considerations; Cervical Disc Replacement Combined with Cervical Laminoplasty; Spinal Deformity in Motion-Sparing Technology*

**Jeffrey R. McConnell, MD**
Clinical Assistant Professor of Surgery, Pennsylvania State University College of Medicine, Hershey, Pennsylvania
*SECURE-C Cervical Artificial Disc*

**Alvin H. McKenzie, MD, MChOrth, FRCSC**
Senior Active Staff, Department of Orthopaedic Surgery, Royal Alexandra Hospital Edmonton, Alberta, Canada
*The Basis for Motion Preservation Surgery: Lessons Learned from the Past*

**Alan McLeod, PhD**
Group Director Research and Development: Embroidery Technology, NuVasive (UK) Ltd., Taunton, United Kingdom
*The NeoDisc Elastomeric Cervical Total Disc Replacement*

**Lionel N. Metz, MD**
Medical Student Research Fellow, University of California, San Francisco, School of Medicine, San Francisco, California
*History and Evolution of Motion Preservation*

**Richard Blondet Meyrat, MD**
Chief Resident, Department of Neurosurgery, Baylor College of Medicine, Houston, Texas
*Minimally Invasive Posterior Approaches to the Lumbar Spine*

**Scott Dean Miller, DO**
Orthopaedic Surgeon, Crystal Clinic Orthopaedic Group, Akron, Ohio
*Theken eDisc: A Second-Generation Lumbar Artificial Disc*

**Joji Mochida, MD, PhD**
Professor, Tokai University School of Medicine, Isehara, Kanagawa, Japan
Professor and Chairman, Department of Orthopaedic Surgery, Tokai University Hospital, Isehara, Kanagawa, Japan
*Cell Therapy for Intervertebral Disc Degeneration*

**Richard Navarro**
Vice President, Research and Development, Theken Disc, LLC, Akron, Ohio
*Theken eDisc: A Second-Generation Lumbar Artificial Disc*

**Hazem Nicola, MD**
Orthopedics Spine Surgeon, Department of Biomechanics, Universidad Simón Bolívar, Caracas, Venezuela
*TranS1 Percutaneous Nucleus Replacement (PNR)*

**Daniel M. Oberer, MD**
Attending Neurosurgeon, Department of Neurosurgery, Carolinas Medical Center, Charlotte, North Carolina
*Cervical Approaches: Anterior and Posterior*

**Donna D. Ohnmeiss, MD**
President, Texas Back Institute Research Foundation, Plano, Texas
*Socioeconomic Impact of Motion Preservation Technology; Simultaneous Lumbar Fusion and Total Disc Replacement; The Future of Motion Preservation*

**Carlos E. Oliveira, MD**
Head of Spine Sector of Orthopedic Department, Hospital de Servidor Publico Estadual, São Paulo, Brazil
*Anatomic Facet Replacement System (AFRS)*

**Douglas G. Orndorff, MD**
Resident, Department of Orthopaedic Surgery, University of Virginia Medical Center, Charlottesville, Virginia
*DISCOVER Artificial Cervical Disc*

**Brett A. Osborn, DO**
Orthopedic Care Center, Aventura, Florida
*Dynamic Pedicle-Screw Stabilization with Nucleus Replacement*

**Corey A. Pacek, MD**
Resident Physician, Department of Orthopaedic Surgery, University of Pittsburgh School of Medicine, Pittsburgh, Pennsylvania
Resident Physician, Department of Orthopaedic Surgery, University of Pittsburgh Medical Center, Pittsburgh, Pennsylvania
*Gene Therapy for Intervertebral Disc Repair and Regeneration*

**Charles Park, MD**
Division Chief, Neurosurgery, Harbor Hospital, Baltimore, Maryland
*Theken eDisc: A Second-Generation Lumbar Artificial Disc*

**Avinash G. Patwardhan, PhD**
Professor, Department of Orthopaedic Surgery and Rehabilitiation, Loyola University Stritch School of Medicine, Maywood, Illinois
Director, Musculoskeletal Biomechanics Laboratory, Edward Hines, Jr. VA Hospital, Hines, Illinois
*The M6 Artificial Cervical Disc*

**Carlos Fernando Arias Pesántez, MD**
Neurospine Surgeon, Santa Rita Hospital, São Paulo, Brazil
*Revision Strategies Following Lumbar Total Disc Replacement Complications*

**Piero Petrini, MD**
Department of Orthopaedics, City Hospital, Castle, Italy
*DIAM Spinal Stabilization System*

**Luiz Pimenta, MD, PhD**
Associate Professor, University of California, San Diego, San Diego, California; Assistant Professor, Department of Neurosurgery, Federal University, São Paulo, Brazil; Assistant Professor, Department of Neurosurgery, Faculdade de Jundiai, São Paulo, Brazil
Chief of Spine Surgery, Hospital Santa Rita, São Paulo, Brazil
*Cervical Disc Replacement Revisions: Clinical and Biomechanical Considerations; Lateral Lumbar Total Disc Replacement; Revision Strategies Following Lumbar Total Disc Replacement Complications; TranS1 Percutaneous Nucleus Replacement (PNR); NUBAC Intradiscal Arthroplasty; TOPS: Total Posterior Facet Replacement and Dynamic Motion Segment Stabilization System*

**Vinod K. Podichetty, MD, MS**
Director, Division of Research, Cleveland Clinic Florida, Weston, Florida
*Satellite: Spherical Partial Disc Replacement*

**Kornelis A. Poelstra, MD, PhD**
Assistant Professor of Orthopaedics, University of Maryland Medical Center, Baltimore, Maryland
*DISCOVER Artificial Cervical Disc*

**Ben B. Pradhan, MD, MSE**
Director of Clinical Research, The Spine Institute, Santa Monica, California
*ProDisc-C Total Cervical Disc Replacemet; ProDisc-L Total Disc Replacement*

**Ann Prewett, PhD**
President, Replication Medical, Inc., Cranbury, New Jersey
*NeuDisc Artificial Lumbar Nucleus Replacement*

**James P. Price**
Engineer, Theken Disc, LLC, Akron, Ohio
*Theken eDisc: A Second-Generation Lumbar Artificial Disc*

**James Robert Rappaport, MD**
Assistant Clinical Professor, University of Nevada, Reno, Reno, Nevada; Sierra Regional Spine Institute, St. Mary's Regional Medical Center, Reno, Nevada
*Kineflex|C Cervical Artificial Disc*

**Christopher Reah, PhD**
Manager of Embroidery Technology Development, NuVasive (UK) Ltd, Taunton, United Kingdom
*The NeoDisc Elastomeric Cervical Total Disc Replacement*

**Alejandro A. Reyes-Sánchez, MD**
Professor of Spine Surgery, Facultad de Medicina, Universidad Nacional Autonoma de México, Mexico, Distrito Federal, Head of Spinal Surgery Division, National Institute of Rehabilitation, Mexico, Distrito Federal
*The M6 Artificial Cervical Disc*

**Souad Rhalmi, MSc**
Department of Neurosurgery, Research Centre, Sainte-Justine Hospital, Montreal, Quebec, Canada
*Orthobiom: A Nonfusion Treatment for Pediatric Scoliosis*

**K. Daniel Riew, MD**
Professor, Washington University School of Medicine, St. Louis, Missouri
Mildred B. Simon Distinguished Professor of Orthopaedic Surgery; Professor of Neurological Surgery, Barnes-Jewish Hospital, St. Louis, Missouri
*Primary Indications and Disc Space Preparation for Cervical Disc Arthroplasty*

**Charles H. Rivard, MD**
Department of Neurosurgery, Research Centre, Sainte-Justine Hospital, Montreal, Quebec, Canada
*Orthobiom: A Nonfusion Treatment for Pediatric Scoliosis*

**German Rodríguez, MD**
Attending Physician, Emergency Department, Hospital Del Prado, Tijuana, Mexico
*The PercuDyn System*

**Thomas F. Roush, MD**
Orthopaedic Surgeon, Southeastern Spine Institute, Mount Pleasant, South Carolina
*Simultaneous Lumbar Fusion and Total Disc Replacement*

**Scott A. Rushton, MD**
Assistant Professor, Department of Orthopedic Surgery, University of Pennsylvania, Philadelphia, Pennsylvania
*SECURE-C Cervical Artificial Disc*

**Ashish Sahai, MD**
Clinical Instructor, Standford University Medical Center, Stanford, California
Staff Orthopedic Surgeon, VA Palo Alto Health Care System, Palo Alto, California
*Invasive Diagnostic Tools*

**Samer Saiedy, MD**
Department of Surgery, St. Joseph Hospital, Baltimore, Maryland
*Lumbar Anterior Revision: Preoperative Preparation and Approach Considerations*

**Daisuke Sakai, MD, PhD**
Assistant Professor, Tokai University School of Medicine, Isehara, Kanagawa, Japan
Assistant Professor and Attending Surgeon, Department of Orthopaedic Surgery, Tokai University Hospital, Isehara, Kanagawa, Japan
*Cell Therapy for Intervertebral Disc Degeneration*

**Rick Sasso, MD**
Associate Professor; Chief of Spine Surgery—Clinical Orthopaedic Surgery, Indiana University School of Medicine, Indianapolis, Indiana
Vice-Chairman, Department of Orthopaedic Surgery; Director, St. Vincent Spine Center, St. Vincent Hospital, Indianapolis, Indiana
*The Bryan Artificial Disc; TranS1 Percutaneous Nucleus Replacement (PNR)*

**Thomas Schaffa, MD**
General Surgeon, Santa Rita Hospital, São Paulo, Brazil
*Lateral Lumbar Total Disc Replacement; Revision Strategies Following Lumbar Total Disc Replacement Complications*

**Othmar Schwarzenbach, MD**
Spital Thun-Simmental AG, Thun, Switzerland
*NuCore Injectable Nucleus: An In Situ Curing Nucleus Replacement*

**Matthew Scott-Young, MBBS, FRACS, FAOrthA**
Associate Professor, Faculty of Health Sciences and Medicine, Bond University, Gold Coast, Queensland, Australia
Visiting Medical Officer, Allamanda Private Hospital, Southport, Queensland, Australia
*Overall Revision Strategies: Lumbar; Cervical Arthroplasty Adjacent to Fusion, Multiple-Level Cases, and Hybrid Applications*

**Lali H.S Sekhon, MD, PhD, FRACS, FACS**
Adjunct Associate Professor, Department of Physiology and Cell Biology, University of Nevada School of Medicine, Reno, Nevada
Co-Diector, SpineNevada, Reno, Nevada
*Cervical Arthroplasty with Myelopathy*

**Dilip K. Sengupta, MD**
Assistant Professor, Department of Orthopedics, Dartmouth College, Hanover, New Hampshire
Assistant Professor, Department of Orthopedics, Dartmouth-Hitchcock Medical Center, Lebanon, New Hampshire
*Dynamic Stabilization System*

**Rajiv K. Sethi, MD**
Associate Spinal Surgeon, Department of Neurosurgery, Virginia Mason Medical Center, Group Health Spinal Surgery, Department of Neurosurgery, Seattle, Washington
*History and Evolution of Motion Preservation*

**Farhan N. Siddiqi, MD**
Trinity Spine Center, Tampa, Florida
*Lumbar Endoscopic Posterolateral (Transforaminal) Approach*

**Kern Singh, MD**
Assistant Professor, Department of Orthopedic Surgery, Rush University Medical Center, Chicago, Illinois
*Animal Modes for Human Disc Degeneration*

**Matthew N. Songer, MD**
President and CEO, Pioneer Surgical Technology, Marquette, Michigan
*NUBAC Intradiscal Arthroplasty*

**Gwendolyn A. Sowa, MD, PhD**
Assistant Professor, Department of Physical Medicine and Rehabilitation; Assistant Professor, Department of Orthopaedic Surgery; Co-Director, Ferguson Laboratory for Orthopaedic Spine Research, University of Pittsburgh School of Medicine, Pittsburgh, Pennsylvania
Assistant Professor, Department of Physical Medicine and Rehabilitation; Assistant Professor, Department of Orthopaedic Surgery, University of Pittsburgh Medical Center, Pittsburgh, Pennsylvania
*Gene Therapy of Intervertebral Disc Repair and Regeneration*

**Kristina Spate, MD**
Department of Vascular Surgery, Yale University School of Medicine, New Haven, Connecticut
*Management of Complications of the Anterior Exposure of the Lumbar Spine*

**Jean Stecken, MD**
Neurosurgeon, Neurosurgical Department, Centre Hospitalier Regional, Orléans, France
*Mobidisc Disc Prosthesis*

**Jean-Paul Steib, MD**
Professor of Orthopaedic Surgery, Université Louis Pasteur, Faculté de Medicine, Strasbourg, France
Surgeon, University Hospital, Department of Orthopaedic Surgery Spine Unit, Strasbourg, France
*Mobi-C; Mobidisc Disc Prosthesis*

**Jonathan R. Steiber, MD**
Fellow, Division of Spine Surgery, New York University—Hospital for Joint Diseases, New York, New York
*The CerviCore Cervical Intervertebral Disc Replacement; The FlexiCore Intervertebral Disc; Persistent Pain After Lumbar Total Disc Replacement*

**Brian J. Sullivan, MD, FACS**
Director of Brain Services, Anne Arundel Medical Center, Annapolis, Maryland
*Persistent Pain After Cervical Arthroplasty*

**Bauer E. Sumpio, MD, PhD**
Professor of Surgery and Radiology, Yale University School of Medicine, New Haven, Connecticut
Chief, Vascular Surgery; Program Director, Vascular Surgery Fellowship Training Program, Yale-New Haven Medical Center, New Haven, Connecticut
*Technique of Anterior Exposure of the Lumbar Spine; Management of Complications of the Anterior Exposure of the Lumbar Spine*

**Andelle L. Teng, MD**
Fellow, Orthopaedic Spine Service, Orthopaedic Spine Surgery, UCLA Medical Center, Los Angeles, California
*NFlex*

**Randall Theken, MS**
Founder and CEO, The Theken Family of Companies, Akron, Ohio
*Theken eDisc: A Second-Generation Lumbar Artificial Disc*

**Jens Peter Timm**
Vice President, Research and Development, Aphatec Spine, Inc., Carlsbad, California
*The Stabilimax NZ Posterior Lumbar Dynamic Stabilization System*

**P. Justin Tortolani, MD**
Orthopaedic Spine Surgeon, Orthopaedic Associates, Towson, Maryland
*Lumbar Anterior Revision: Preoperative Preparation and Approach Considerations*

**Vincent C. Traynelis, MD**
Professor of Neurosurgery, University of Iowa, Iowa City, Iowa
*The Prestige Cervical Disc*

**Patrick Tropiano, MD**
Department of Orthopaedic Surgery, Hôpital CHU Nord, Marseille, France
*Can Lumbar Disc Replacement Be Used Adjacent to a Scoliotic Deformity?*

**Anthony Tsantrizos, MSc, PhD**
Disc Dynamics Inc., Eden Prairie, Minnesota
*DASCOR*

**Alexander W.L. Turner, PhD**
Research and Testing Associate Manager, NuVasive, Inc., San Diego, California
*The NeoDisc Elastomeric Cervical Total Disc Replacement; Cerpass Cervical Total Disc Replacement*

**Alexander R. Vaccaro, MD**
Professor, Department of Orthopaedic Surgery, Rothman Institute, Thomas Jefferson University, Philadelphia, Pennsylvania
*Advanced Spinal Anatomy for Cervical and Lumbar Nonfusion Surgery*

**Jean-Marc Vital, MD**
Spinal Disorders Unit, Bordeaux University Hospital, Unité des Pathologies Rachidiennes, Hôpital Pellegrin, Bordeaux, France
*Mobi-C*

**Archibald von Strempel, MD, DEng**
Professor, Medizinische Universität Junsbruck, Junsbruck, Austria
Chief of the Orthopedic Department, Landeskrankenhaus, Feldkirch, Austria
*Cosmic: Dynamic Stabilization of the Degenerated Lumbar Spine*

**Corey J. Wallach, MD**
Spine Fellow, Orthopaedic and Neurosurgery, UCLA Comprehensive Spine Center, Los Angeles, California
*NFlex*

**Jeffrey C. Wang, MD**
Chief, Orthopaedic Spine Service; Associate Professor of Orthopaedic and Neurosurgery, UCLA Comprehensive Spine Center, Los Angeles, California
*NFlex*

**Douglas Wardlaw, MB, ChB, ChM, FRCS(Edinburgh)**
Honorary Senior Lecturer, University of Aberdeen, Aberdeen, United Kingdom
Honorary Professor, The Robert Gordon University, Aberdeen, United Kingdom
Consultant Orthopaedic Spinal Surgeon, NHS Grampian, Aberdeen, United Kingdom
*BioDisc Nucleus Pulposus Replacement*

**Scott A. Webb, DO**
Surgical Director; Fellowship Director, Florida Spine Institute Clearwater, Florida Spine Surgery; Department of Orthopedic Surgery Mease Countryside Hospital, Safety Harbor, Florida
*Total Facet Arthroplasty System (TFAS)*

**Ian R. Weinberg, MD**
University of the Witwatersrand, Johannesburg, Gauteng, South Africa
*Kineflex*

**William C. Welch, MD**
Chief, Department of Neurological Surgery, University of Pittsburgh, Pittsburgh, Pennsylvania
*Biomechanics of Nonfusion Devices: Novel Testing Techniques, Standards, and Implications for Future Devices*

**Bradley J. Wessman**
TranS1, Inc., Wilmington, North Carolina
*TranS1 Percutaneous Nucleus Replacement (PNR)*

**Peter G. Whang, MD**
Assistant Professor, Department of Orthopaedics, Yale University School of Medicine, New Haven, Connecticut
*Advanced Spinal Anatomy for Cervical Lumbar Nonfusion Surgery*

**Nicholas D. Wharton, MS**
Senior Engineer, Medical Metrics, Inc., Houston, Texas
*Quantitative Motion Analysis (QMA) of Motion-Preserving and Fusion Technologies for the Spine*

**Andrew P. White, MD**
Instructor, Harvard Medical School, Boston, Massachusetts
Spinal Surgeon, Department of Orthopaedic Surgery, Beth Israel Deaconess Medical Center, Boston, Massachusetts
*Adjacent Segment Degeneration and Adjacent Segment Disease: Cervical and Lumbar*

**Thomas Wilson**
Spine Wave, Inc., Shelton, Connecticut
*NuCore Injectable Nucleus: An In Situ Curing Nucleus Replacement*

**Markus Wimmer, PhD**
Director, Tribology and Human Motions Laboratories, Department of Orthopaedic Surgery, Rush University Medical Center, Chicago, Illinois
*Material Properties and Wear Analysis*

**Oscar Yeh, PhD**
Director, Research and Testing, Intrinsic Therapeutics, Inc., Woburn, Massachusetts
*The Intrinsic Therapeutics Barricaid Device*

**Anthony T. Yeung, MD**
Voluntary Clinical Instructor, University of California, San Diego, Department of Orthopedic Surgery, La Jolla, California; Desert Institute for Spine Care, Phoenix, Arizona; Executive Director of Intradiscal Therapy Sociey (IITS), Belgium, Wisconsin
*Lumbar Endoscopic Posterolateral (Transforaminal) Approach; NeuDisc Artificial Lumbar Nucleus Replacement*

**Christopher A. Yeung, MD**
Voluntary Clinical Instructor, University of California, San Diego, Department of Orthopedic Surgery, La Jolla, California
*Lumbar Endoscopic Posterolateral (Transforaminal) Approach*

**Hansen A. Yuan, MD**
Professor, Department of Orthopaedic and Neurological Surgery, SUNY Upstate Medical University, Syracuse, New York
*Theken eDisc: A Second-Generation Lumbar Artificial Disc; Aquarelle Hydrogel Disc Nucleus; NUBAC Intradiscal Arthroplasty*

**James J. Yue, MD**
Associate Professor, Department of Orthopaedic Surgery; Co-Chief, Division of Spinal Surgery; Director, Yale Spine Fellowship, Yale University School of Medicine, New Haven, Connecticut
*Indications and Contraindications for Lumbar Nonfusion Surgery: Patient Selection; Disc Space Preparation Techniques for Lumbar Disc Arthroplasty; Activ-L Artificial Disc; NeuDisc Artificial Lumbar Nucleus Replacement; The Stabilimax NZ Posterior Lumbar Dynamic Stabilization System; Can Lumbar Disc Replacement Be Used Adjacent to a Scoliotic Deformity? Considerations for Spinal Arthoplasty in Elderly and Osteoporotic Patients*

**James F. Zucherman, MD**
Associate Staff Surgeon, St. Mary's Hospital and Medical Center, San Francisco, California
*X-STOP Interspinous Process Decompression for Lumbar Spinal Stenosis*

# Contents

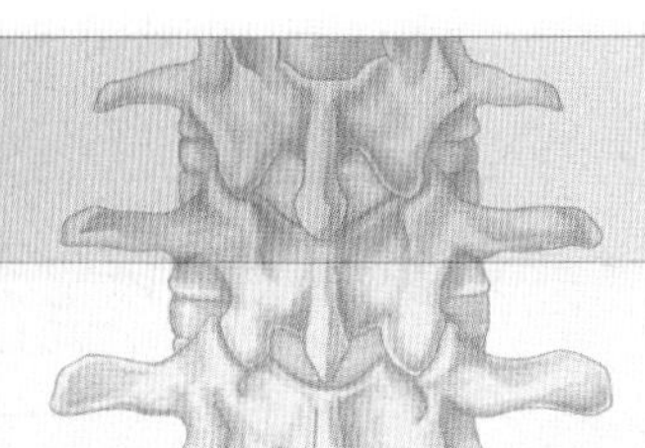

# PART I

# Introduction to Motion Preservation Surgery of the Spine

CHAPTER 1

# The Basis for Motion Preservation Surgery: Lessons Learned from the Past

**Alvin H. McKenzie**

"Structure is determined by need."
— Sir Harry Platt

"Structure is determined by function."
— John Hunter

"The purpose of man is action."
— Thomas Carlyle[1]

## KEY POINTS

- Mobility and stability are equal partners in the structure of the human spine as determined by our need, function, and purpose of action: to survive and excel. Even with all other properties intact, a spine cannot function at full purpose or in longevity by stability alone—it also requires mobility.
- The spinal column is articulated, but like its vertebral trabeculae, it has been structured like fractal end-pinned masts or columns that have been reinforced with flying buttresses, spreaders, stays, and shrouds. Its articulating discs permit stable mobility and contribute to the shock absorbency of the structure.
- The vertebral bodies, not the discs, are the main shock absorbers of the spine: The vertebral trabeculae bend, compress, and rebound; the discs' nucleus pulposus is the hard center of motion and the spherical piston of the segmental shock absorber that indents the adjacent vertebral bodies and stabilizes the loaded spine while the annulus, when taught, allows motion and provides stability to the unloaded spine.
- When other structures are intact, the ideal motion preservation device should probably adapt to the trabecular nature of the vertebrae; replicate the nucleus pulposus in size, shape, and incompressibility; and be inert, indestructible, and possibly self-lubricating.
- The main lesson from the past is that established concepts of structure and function may not have always been correct: Acceptance of new ideas occurs when there is need for change, when contingencies prove that the status quo should not prevail, when there is opportunity for new concepts and methods of treatment, and when an innovative choice can be made.

## INTRODUCTION

The upright spine has provided mankind with a *talisman* and occasionally with a *hoodoo.* The spine's structure and function (mobility, stability, and dynamic equilibrium) have helped engender the world's most successful species, even as its mastlike nature, altered by bows and many articulated segments, has had a bias for breakdown. The upright spine's ingenious *form* (shape, configuration, balance, articulations, and connectivity) and *substance* (strength, elasticity, compressibility, and consistency) that constitute its *structure* seem to have been determined by its possessor's *need, function,* and *purpose of action* to survive and gain pre-eminence in a treacherous world.

In health, the segmented spine's vital structures and vestments can perform like a multipinned ship's mast with power, agility, endurance, and grace to provide mobility with stability and (usually) freedom from pain. With damage to structure or rigging, it can still function after "bracing the mast" or "reefing the sails" and by careful, energetic sailing until it is "re-stepped by fixing" or fusion (mistakenly thought to produce stability). Since Mixter and Barr,[2] there has been an option for the spine's owner to take responsibility for excisional restepping or discectomy. When damage, disorder, or discectomy leaves excessive motion at one of the spine's segments, it often spawns the corrosion of facet arthritis at the same level with instability and breakdown at the next level or at levels beyond. When similar misadventure leaves loss of motion at one of the segments, the stiffness may stay the course in the short term but might ultimately forge the same superjacent and subjacent degenerative cascade that dogs instability or "successful" spinal fusion. The essential lesson to be learned from the past is that the spine cannot function at full purpose or in longevity without the essential duality of "*stability **and** motion*." At the end of the 20th century, this concept of duality had been ignored and even suppressed.

To paraphrase Shakespeare, "Whether 'tis nobler in the mind to suffer the slings and arrows of [spinal treatment learned from the past] or—by opposing end them: that is the question."[3] The answer may lie in those unheeded or rejected lessons from the past that deserve a second look.

## THE SPINAL COLUMN

We could first re-examine the structure, function, and needs of the spine, possibly the most complex organ we have. Pinned at the pelvis and sacrum like a fractal two-footed, keel-stepped, and single deck–stepped mobile mast, the conjoined spine then rises to the heavens with its spreaders, where its fractal, diverging condyles cup and double-pin the cranium: the receptor, modulator, transponder, and control center that contains and supersedes the lookout. The spine's dimensions accord remarkably well with a fir main mast of a ship (height = beam × 12 ÷ 5; diameter = 1 inch per 3 feet of height; critical load varies with the mast diameter by the power of three so that doubling the diameter would allow 8 times the load).[4] Critical load, determined by the Euler formula, also varies inversely with the square of the mast height, so that halving the height by bowing or other means could quadruple the maximum load. It has been suggested that bowing of a spine could increase its critical load from 2 N/mm$^2$ to 4 N/mm$^2$ or from about 300 psi to 600 psi. With the weight of the cranium and the effects of spine's many bony spreaders and tensioned muscular shrouds and ligamentous stays, the spine develops its three mobile curves or three bows that decrease mast height and, like other bows, store energy to initiate motion, aid balance, and prolong endurance.[5] The cervical spine remains mobile, stable, and capable of transport and relay of vital signals and elements. It provides suspension, motor power, circulation, and innervations for the body's mobile arms that aid balance but are primarily deployed for their myriad prehensile tasks. The thoracic spine also transports and transmits and is stabilized by the arrangement of its braced and cross-braced ribs and muscles that can be enhanced by generating the thoracic pressure cage.[5] While giving lodging to the body's wind-catcher and circulatory center, the thorax provides platforms and leverage to the upper limbs. Below stands the lumbar spine supported by its own investments and its muscular shrouds that deploy to the thorax, lower limbs, and abdominal wall and join with the sacral-pelvic complex to form the hold or hull. Reinforced by the abdominal pressure cage, the trunk is capable of stable mobility and of housing a share of the body's filters, transporters, transmitters, energy converters, and magazines.

The spine's bipedal and prehensile appendages synchronize with the spine for all manner and direction of motion and speed of propulsion or for feats of agility and strength. The healthy spine is expandable, contractile, resilient, rotatable, inclinable, flexible, lungeable, reboundable, deflectable, and stackable for stability and balance. It is articulated with flexible, firm discs and compressible and expandable bodies internally supplied with strong constantly remodeling trabeculae that bend or bow to transmit multidirectional forces along their axes and margins and give shelter to hemopoietic cells. Without this amazing spine, prehensile, bipedal self-sustaining human being with controlled positioning of limbs and body that can deliver power and agility where it is needed for flight, fight, work, or play with efficiency, endurance, and grace might not be the sceptered chieftain of the world but some extinct species of cephalopod or quadrapus. When it ails, we should aim not to diminish it or restrain it but to restore it.

### The Vertebral Body

The vertebral body is composed primarily of cancellous bone contained anteriorly and laterally by a thin mantle of cortical bone. At the back, it assumes a thicker cortex to support the pedicles and other posterior vertebral elements, and above and below, it has thicker peripheral vertebral plates that give rise to fibers of the annulus fibrosis. Posterocentrally in the nuclear recess lies the cribriform cartilage plate that accommodates a nucleus pulposus,[6] and is composed of chondral cartilage of notochord origin with no direct blood supply and no continuous underlying osseous plate. Instead, there are Y- and inverted Y-shaped, vertically directed, branching, or fractal[7] trabecular columns that blend into the cribriform plate on one side while fibers from the nucleus and the inner lamellae of the disc penetrate it on the other (Fig. 1–1). The trabecular columns form primary and secondary compression trabeculae: slender, compound, intermediate length masts that can bend and rebound not unlike a fresh wishbone. They fuse where they meet the transecting spreader-like tension trabeculae that prevent vertical buckling, and increase critical load. Paracentrally and posteriorly about the nuclear recess, the primary compression trabeculae are numerous and well developed, and in the central nuclear recess, they are less dense and weaker.[8] They

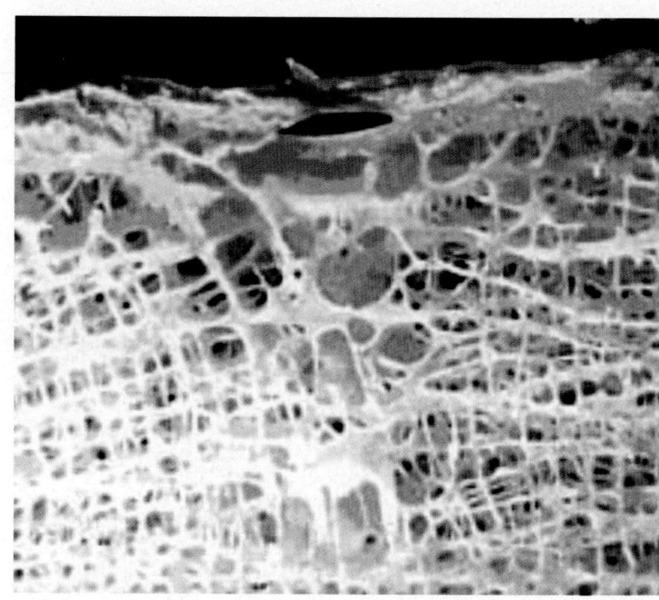

■ **FIGURE 1–1.** Fractal design of trabeculae in upper vertebral body at junction of cribriform plate and peripheral vertebral plate.

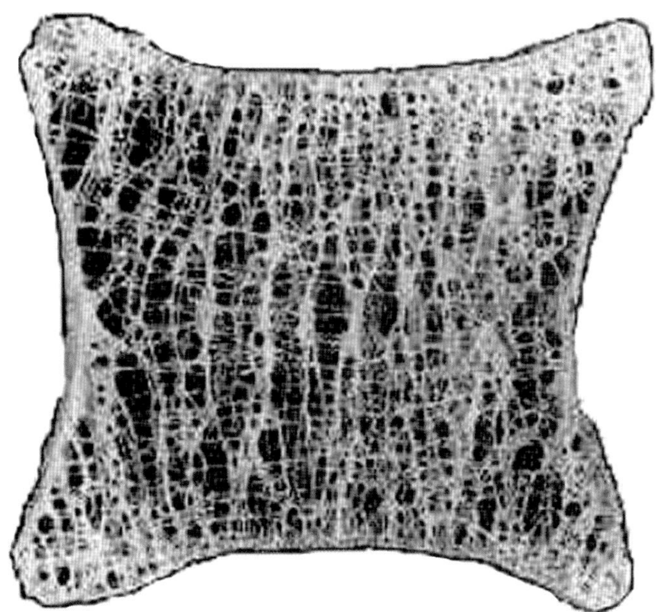

■ **FIGURE 1–2.** Primary (central) compression trabeculae bowing between cribriform plates: Secondary (peripheral) compression trabeculae running to vertebral walls. Both reinforced by primary horizontally bowed primary tension trabeculae.

increase their moment of inertia and critical load by expanding axially like barrel staves en route to the nuclear recess opposite (Fig. 1–2).[9] Secondary compression trabeculae from the bony vertebral plates run obliquely to the adjacent vertebral body walls. Primary tension trabeculae, which are more numerous close to the vertebral plates, run horizontal to the planes of the end plates, slightly bowed and at right angles to the primary compression trabeculae. Secondary tension trabeculae extend into the pedicles. Young's Modulus (the modulus of elasticity that corresponds to the critical load of the vertebral body) lies between that of wood and magnesium or aluminum.[4] Because trabecular bowing stores energy, and because the average healthy vertebral body can be compressed by one tenth of its height without trabecular fracture, a vertebra may be so compressed and rebound to its normal height (Fig. 1–3).[10] The vertebral body's strength varies with trabecular density in response to local stresses (Wolff's law).[11] The vertebral body column is also braced by its flying buttresses, the pedicles, laminae, and appendages. The side aisle of the buttresses, roofed with ligamentum flavum, becomes the halyard sleeve that guards the spinal cord, ganglia, and nerve roots; the articular facets permit guided and constrained spinal motion, and afford each segment two of its three points of stability; the spinous and transverse processes act as mast spreaders for muscular and ligamentous shrouds and stays that augment spinal shape, stability, and motion.

Possibly inspired by the fractal structure of the vertebral trabecular mesh that gives strength, compressibility, and rebound to the vertebral bodies, industry has created an airless metal tire, the Michelin *Tweel* (Fig. 1–4).[12]

## The Intervertebral Disc

The intervertebral discs, firmly bound to adjacent vertebral bodies, share their stresses and responsibility for controlled mobility through their *annulus fibrosis* and a *nucleus pulposus*, which also contribute to two (cephalad and caudal) cribriform end plates. Like the vertebral body, it derives blood from the anterior and lateral vertebral plexus that will drain to the Batson/azygos system of veins.[13]

***The annulus fibrosis*** is composed of laminated fibrocartilage with obliquely directed fibers that are anchored to the adjacent vertebral plates centrally and peripherally by extensions of trabecular fibers and peripherally by the periosteum and the overlying anterior and posterior longitudinal ligaments. Successive laminar layers of the annulus run obliquely in alternate directions and, therefore, become tight and rigid under tension of the normally positioned healthy nucleus pulposus.[6] The annulus may bulge when the nucleus pulposus, under vertical loading, indents the cribriform plates and causes the adjacent vertebral bodies to approach one another by up to 4 mm at each level.

***The nucleus pulposus*** is gelatinous and composed of "viscous proteoglycans imbedded with loose fibrous strands arranged in a felted mesh of undulating bundles that contain a profusion of fusiform cells resembling reticulocytes and vacuolar darkly nucleated chondrocytes."[6] The nucleus pulposus is hygroscopic and may

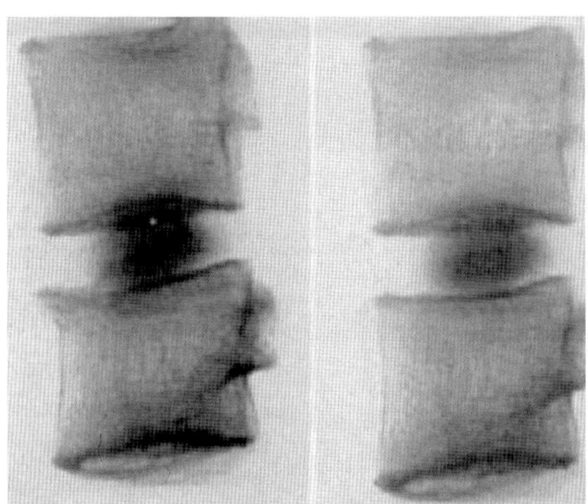

■ **FIGURE 1–3.** Discography with compression and rebound of vertebral bodies (Roaf).

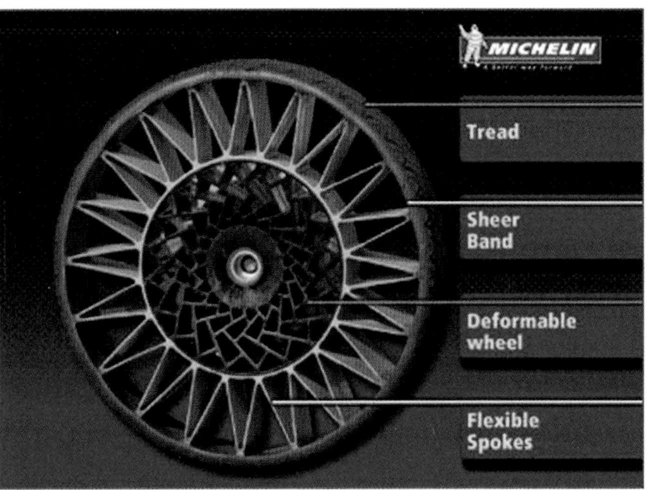


■ **FIGURE 1–4.** Michelin's fractal airless metal tire.

change internal tension by an ability to imbibe fluid.[14] In health, the nucleus pulposus lives and breathes by its contact with the cribriform cartilage plate. It exchanges metabolites and fluid in response to pressure gradients and osmalarity between the nucleus and the adjacent vertebral bodies. The healthy, in place, and intact nucleus pulposus, encased by multiple layers of annulus fibrosus, is not unlike the core of a classic golf ball (a round bag of latex compressed by layer after layer of elastic bands) that behaves like a hard sphere.[15] As Robert Roaf and others[10,16] have demonstrated, noncritical vertical loading of healthy vertebrae with an intact annulus and healthy nucleus pulposus and cribriform plate will cause the vertebral plates to spring inward while the nucleus pulposus retains its spherical shape (Fig. 1–5). As the rigid nucleus indents the adjacent vertebral bodies, it creates stability of the segment by friction of the nucleus with the indented body as the disc space narrows and only then will the annulus bulge. If the loading is relieved, the rebound of the vertebral body will return the nucleus pulposus to its place, tighten the annular fibers, restore shape of the annulus, and maintain stability. When the critical load is exceeded, the vertebral body will fracture, the nucleus pulposus will remain intact, and the segment can become unstable.[10]

*Notwithstanding any previous concepts or teachings about the roles of the vertebrae and the discs,* ***the vertebrae, not the discs, are the main shock absorbers of the spine.*** The annulus fibrosis is the check-ligament that permits limited universal intervertebral mobility. **With normal loading,** the healthy nucleus pulposus is transposed by vertebral body pressure to tighten the annulus and produce ligamentous intervertebral stability, and **with heavy loading,** the rigid, spherical nucleus obtains stable seating in the nuclear recesses, where it acts as a piston to depress the cribriform plates, bend the trabeculae. and produce contact stability. **With return of normal loading,** the vertebral body rebounds, the nucleus resumes its position, and the annulus tightens.

### Pathologic Changes in the Vertebral Body: Disc Complex

The post-traumatic, degenerative changes due to aging in the vertebral body, the intervertebral disc, and the nucleus pulposus probably begin with infraction of the cribriform cartilage plate[17] and nutrition failure of the nucleus pulposus succeeded by apoptosis and breakdown of nuclear tissue and biochemical changes in the disc. Interdiscal biologic irritants such as proteoglycans, prostaglandin $E_2$, inflammatory cytokines (tissue necrosis factor-$\alpha$ and interleukins) that can be activated by matrix metalloproteinases (extracellular kinases) create a medium with a low pH that invites inflammatory cells into the disc.[18,19] The granulation tissue forms scar tissue that promotes shrinkage of the nucleus and buckling of the annulus. With migration and dislocation of scar tissue and more breakdown of the fibrocartilage of the internal annulus, external annular buckling can lead to ruptures and possibly protrusions of degenerate discs (Fig. 1–6).[20]

The breakdown in the nucleus pulposus and annulus will ultimately cause alteration of the stresses affecting the adjacent vertebral bodies and their vertebral trabeculations. An irregular trabecular system may ultimately evolve (and observations suggest that initial changes occur in the horizontal trabeculae near the vertebral body plates[8]). Annular ruptures with or without protrusions may permit disc fluid to leak from the disc to generate backache, headache, or radicular pain without sensory or motor loss. Anterior ruptures of necrotic discs with low pH may cause abdominal pain to mimic abdominal catastrophes or pain of gynecologic origin.[21] Commonly, the degenerative disc becomes unstable and causes back pain of facet joint origin that can be accompanied by disc protrusions with the potential for neurologic impairment.[22]

Efforts by the patient to control pain from instability by hyperlordosing the spine and locking the facets can lead to posterior element hypertrophy with canal and foramenal stenosis.[23,24] The patient may or may not proceed from a state of good disc health to invalidism or follow any of a host of scenarios that may be slow, intermittent, or rapid. The degenerative disc may never become surgical by current criteria but can produce states of impairment

■ **FIGURE 1–5.** The vertebral body is compressed; the nucleus maintains its shape (Roaf).

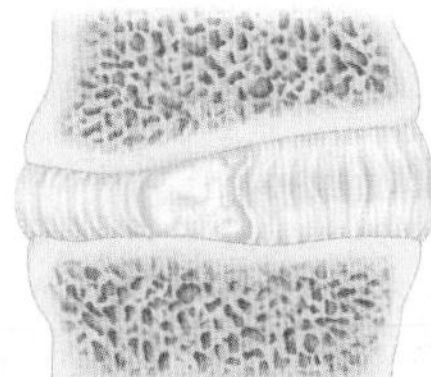

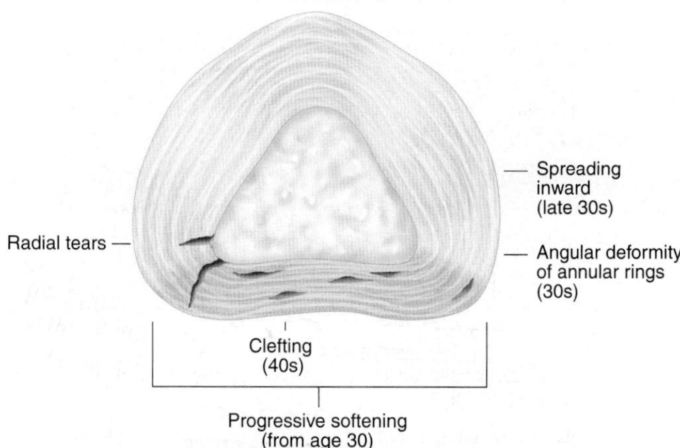


■ **FIGURE 1–6.** Fahrni's chronology of degenerative changes of the intervertebral disc.

that erode health, employability, well-being, social and economic equanimity, and happy pursuits. Motion preservation with stability and freedom from pain within reasonable parameters of safety should be one of the great medical missions of physicians and spinal surgeons of this new century, whatever the severity or stage of the spinal disorder.

## REQUIREMENTS FOR THE IDEAL MOTION PRESERVATION DEVICE

### Prerequisites

An effective motion preservation device (prosthesis) for the spine should expand the indications for spinal surgery. A cavalier attitude toward reconstructive spinal surgery is not being advocated, but there is a need of more and improved treatment choices for those who may fail to meet current guidelines for current treatment modalities but have unresolved chronic spinal pain of disc origin that impairs health and imposes significant social and economic hardship. A prosthesis may be used to maintain or restore discogenic instability and improve pain relief after discectomy or at sites of previous discectomy or to "top off" degenerative discs above or below levels requiring fusion for other reasons.[25] Patients selected for arthroplasty should be those with proven discogenic pain or instability, or both, with or without disc protrusion without advanced degenerative arthritis or structural annular or bony faults at the level of potential arthroplasty. Also, these patients have failed to respond to sustained comprehensive conservative treatment and have lost their ability to maintain well-being, productivity, strength, and agility. Other prerequisites would accord with the nature and extent of spinal pathology demonstrated by routine standing radiographs, magnetic resonance imaging (MRI) and discography, and observance of all the usual preoperative medical precautions.

### The Replacement Device or Prosthesis

An intervertebral prosthesis should ideally restore the deficiencies of the motion segment it is to occupy: It should restore to the segment its mobility, stability, and freedom from pain and enable it to function in longevity with power, agility, and endurance.

### Biomechanics

The prosthesis should maintain intersegmental ***stability*** and permit appropriate ***rotation*** *about the X, Y, and Z axes* (i.e., flexion X+ and extension X- ~10 degrees at L1–2 to 15 degrees at L5-S1; left rotation Y+ and right rotations Y- ~2 degrees average, and lateral bending right Z+ and lateral bending left Z- ~6 degrees average), as well as optimum ***translation*** *along the X, Y, and Z planes* (i.e., yaw left X+ or yaw right X- ~2 mm, elevate (ascend) Y+ or sink (descend) Y- ~2 mm, or shift fore Z+ or aft Z- ~2 mm) with ***coupling*** (the phenomenon of consistent association of one motion (rotation or translation) about or along one axis or plane with another motion about or along another axis or plane (Fig. 1–7).[8]

The prosthesis should permit those excursions required for normal spinal function but should also preserve segmental stability by limiting motion in accordance with the foregoing limits.

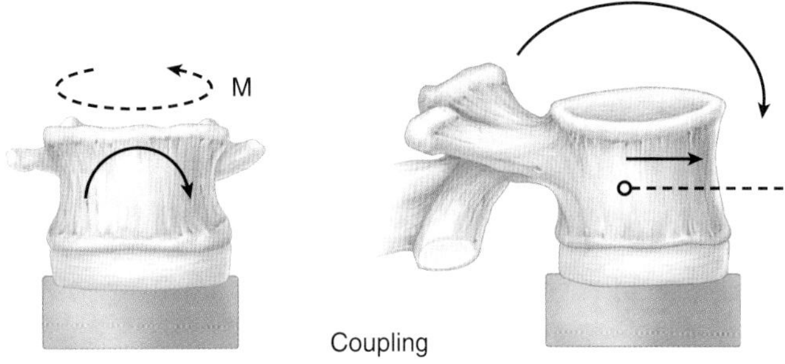


■ **FIGURE 1–7.** Coupling: the phenomenon of consistent association of rotation or translation about or along one axis or plane with another motion about or along a second axis or plane. *(White AA, Panjabi MM: Clinical Biomechanics of the Spine, 2nd ed. Philadelphia, JB Lippincott Company, 1990.)*

Integrity of the prosthesis and the segment in which the prosthesis resides will depend on the following factors:

- Comprehensive surgical management of all significant spinal pathology,
- Preparation of an adequate approach to the intervertebral space that is capable of or may be modified to become capable of providing safe entry for and biomechanically sound containment of an appropriate prosthesis,
- Presence of biomechanically sound opposing vertebral segments with reasonably compatible trabecular systems within the involved vertebral bodies,
- Subjacent and superjacent segmental health and reasonably normal annular, ligamentous, and neuromuscular controls, and
- Availability of a comprehensive selection of suitable, inert, indestructible, properly sized, self-lubricating, or self-incorporating prostheses.

### Lessons from the Past: The Logic of the Times (1950s and 1970s)

By mid-20th century, spinal problems were well recognized:

- ***Discectomy*** was frequently followed by disc space collapse, loss of mobility, recurrent protrusions, canal and foramenal stenosis, scarring with root entrapment, instability, and facet arthritis.
- ***Decompression,*** although seldom advocated or performed, could lead to recurrent stenosis, instability, perineural fibrosis, dural tears, failure of pain relief, and neurologic sequelae.
- ***Fusion*** was often attended by perioperative morbidity, pseudarthroses, stenosis, sacroiliitis, fixation failure, and adjacent level instability. Spinal fusion, with its shortcomings, became the gold standard of care for the failed spine.
- ***Stabilization*** of the spine after discectomy by Lucite pegs (Gardner, 1950s) and methyl acrylic (Cleveland, 1955; Hamby, 1957) had met with cool or no enthusiasm.[26]

Arthroplasty of the spine was considered to be a nasty phrase, as per the history of the specialists demonstrates:

- **Paul Harmon,** from 1959 to 1961, used vitallium balls through an anterior approach to stabilize vertebral segments to assist fusion. On nine out of 13 occasions, he found that they could work well as stand-alone stabilizers (the first disc arthroplast[27]) but had his California license suspended and spent 2 years in South America before his restoration.

- **Ulf Fernstrom,** from 1962 to 1972, favored steel ball arthroplasy of the spine over Hirsch's spinal wires to prevent and treat spinal instability. In 1966, he reported treating 105 patients by steel ball arthroplasty from a posterior approach with few complications, safe fixation, slow subsidence, retained stability, absence of spurring, and assisted mobility.[28] By 1972, he reported 195 total patients treated at 262 lumbar levels by posterior approach and 13 patients treated by anterior cervical approach, with excellent results in 65% of patients. Although 85% of his patients had been on total disability pension before surgery, 85% had returned to work after his surgery.[29] It was said by his detractors, "15% of his patients never worked again!" For his efforts, he was removed from his seat at the University of Udevalla to the village of Hudiksvaal, north of the Arctic Circle, with suppression of further opportunity to publish.
- **Reitz and Joubert,** (1964) had carried out steel ball, hemispherical, and Silastic top arthroplasties at 32 cervical and nine lumbar levels in South Africa before having their surgery suspended.[30]
- **Al McKenzie,** in 1971, reported short-term results of 40 steel ball arthroplasties carried out during 1969 and 1970.[31] Twenty-five years later, in 1995, the author was finally able to have published his report of 10- to 20-year (17-year average) results of re-examining 67 of 103 patients treated at 155 levels, whose age at surgery averaged 44 years.[32] Although obliged to suspend the procedures in 1974, the author reported excellent and good long-term results for 83% of patients in the discectomy and prosthesis group and 75% excellent and good results for the spondylosis and prosthesis group, with 95% of all patients having returned to work. One prosthesis became displaced and was exchanged, whereas another was removed for discitis. Disc space preservation had been excellent and good in 55%, fair in 28%, and poor in 17% (Fig. 1–8).

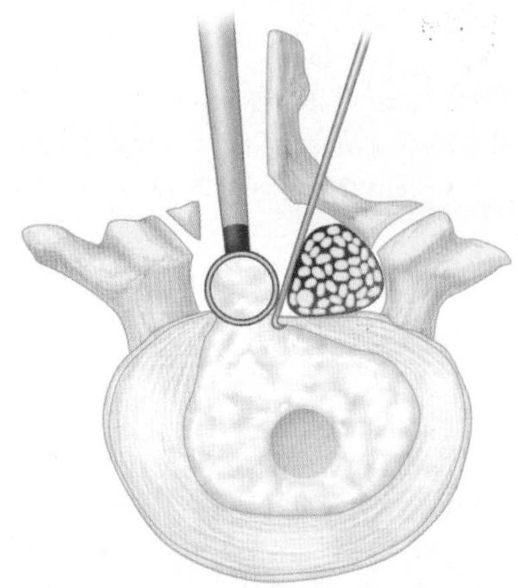

■ **FIGURE 1–9.** Need good exposure and thorough discectomy with accurate sizing, angulation, distraction, occasional intrusion on pedicle, protection of cauda and nerve, and accurate centering in nuclear recess.

### What About the Intervertebral Metal Ball Arthroplasty?

An inert, indestructible, properly sized, and correctly seated sphere appears to be an acceptable motion preservation device for use between vertebral bodies. In the lumbar spine, it can usually be inserted safely from a posterior approach (Fig. 1–9) and in the cervical spine from an anterior approach (Fig. 1–10). By its firmness, a carefully sized metal sphere can seat securely in a clean nuclear recess to restore intervertebral height, motion, and stability. When thus installed, it simulates the nuclear fulcrum to permit coupling in all planes and axes. Like the nucleus pulposus, the hardest part of the vertebral body/annulus/nucleus complex, it functions as the piston of the shock-absorbing mechanism of the intervertebral segment and achieves coaptation with the trabecular pattern already developed in the subjacent and superjacent vertebral bodies that

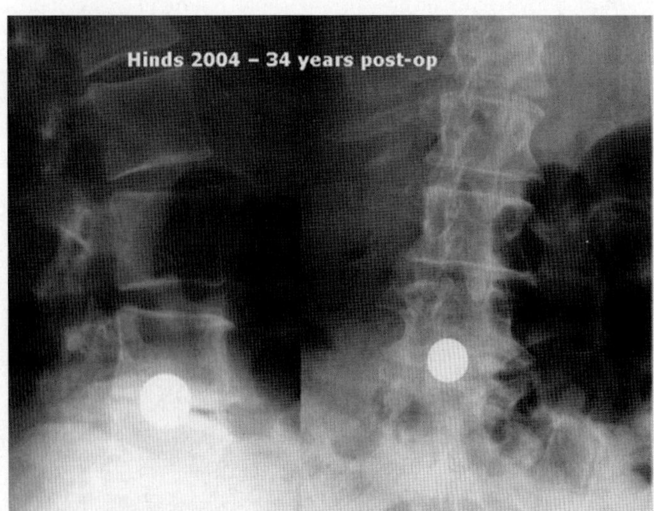


■ **FIGURE 1–8.** Fair preservation of disc space with minimal enthesopathy at target level: good preservation at superjacent level after 34 years.

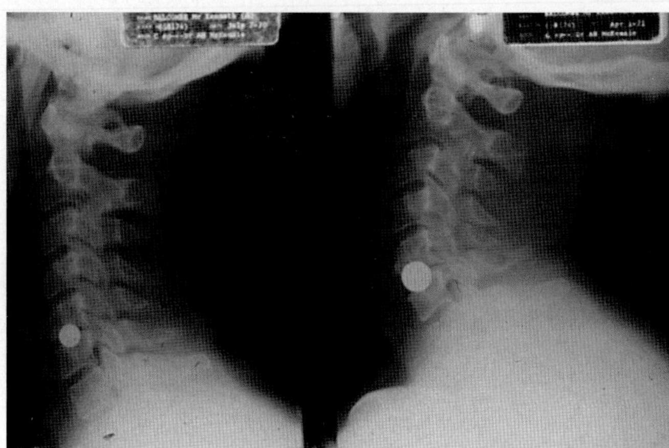

■ **FIGURE 1–10.** Anterior approach in cervical spine (rarely in lumbar spine). Should restore optimum lordosis. After larger prosthesis, this man returned to underwater research on Great Barrier Reef for the Australian government.

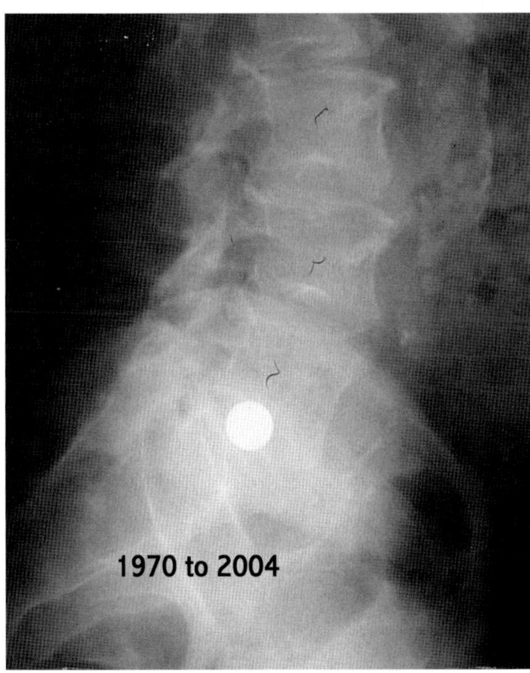


■ **FIGURE 1–11.** This patient has been able to pursue golf, weather permitting every snow-free day since he underwent surgery 34 years ago.

accord with Wolffe's law. An appropriately sized prosthesis of spherical shape is disinclined to initiate bone resorption, so that any subsidence of a sphere occurs only slowly while preventing instability at the level of placement and diminishing degenerative disc changes at levels above and below (Fig. 1-11).

If all of the foregoing were true, what happened? What logic shelved the procedure for more than 30 years? Speculation runs from inspired personal or political considerations to preservation of national image or the *mislogia* that Socrates[33] defined as the hatred of new ideas. The simple answer may be that spinal fusion had been designated as the gold standard of care in the belief that once it was perfected, all our spinal troubles would be over. In spite of an historical profusion of spinal tools, instruments (screws, hooks, rods, plates, and cages), and surgical approaches and the martialing of biologic agents, the comfort of the biopsychosocialists, and the outlawing of tobacco, the *need* for a gold standard remained unrequited. *Contingencies* continued to plague success. Surgeons once dedicated to the pursuit of better spinal fusions still looked for *opportunities* to deliver better spinal care. So far, the *choice* of arthroplasty has mostly been limited to those achieved by an anterior approach, with some of those surgeries producing new kinds of morbidity or being succeeded by prosthetic loosening.

## The Need for Change

Review of man's past history, errors, and oversights will reveal that mankind has developed a genetic resistance to new ideas and to change.[34] When tribal man bonded for protection, his little band grew into or was absorbed into a society.[35] Societies spawned self-appointed coteries (condo police) who supplied rules, myths, superstitions, and beliefs that regulated members for inclusion, hunting, defense, war, domesticity, agriculture, and industry. Surviving societies had strong establishments that could select the leader and control the loyal followers. Challenges to the order brought fight or flight, and harmony might bring a place in the choir.[36] Order bred habit, tradition, and sometimes prejudices, entrenched leadership, entrenched succession, and the status quo. Except in war, chaos, or catastrophe, there would usually be "no need" for change. Dror[37] wrote that either continuity of a status quo or acceptance of a new idea hung on the weighting of *need, contingencies, opportunity, and choice.* New ideas, unless conceived by the leaders, would fail unless there was a survival threatening *need* for it; unless failure to accept might result in a *contingency* that could prejudice their wisdom or authority; and unless there was *opportunity* for them to accept the "new" without loss of honor and especially when the *choice for change* could be made by the leaders. Tribal man may still be alive and well. If we are to see spinal arthroplasty supercede discectomy and spinal fusion as a favored option, we may need to persuade the sages that a need for change has occurred; that the contingencies might reflect unfavorably on those who embrace the status quo; that opportunities for change are at hand; and that worthy choices can be made (Fig. 1–12).

## Quo Vadis?

Those who elect to have **change** in the management of spinal disorders, who would propose motion preservation in the spine, must know their customer, the spinal column. They must understand its **needs**; anticipate the **contingencies**; determine where, when, and why the **opportunities** for motion preservation should be exercised; and what the **choice** of prosthesis should be. As one of Fernström's patients demonstrates (Fig. 1–13), long-term success is possible in spinal surgery.

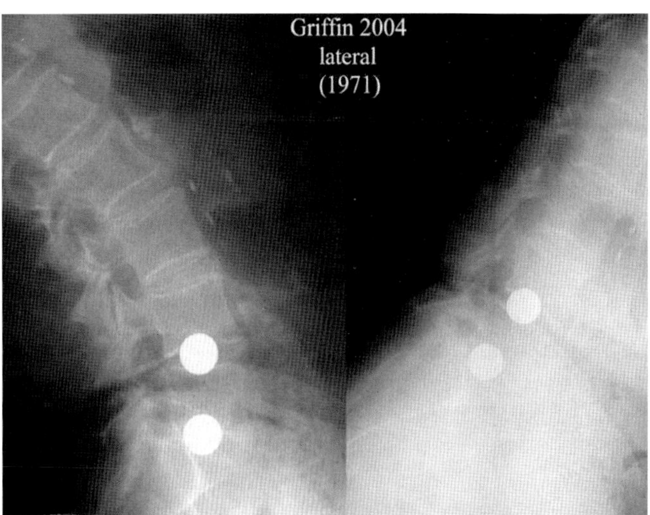


■ **FIGURE 1–12.** Large prostheses below appear to have preserved all levels of this lady's spine.

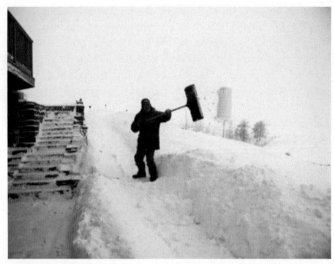

■ **FIGURE 1–13.** One of Fernstrom's patients in his 81st year, 38 years after disc replacement, clearing snow from his walk.

## REFERENCES


1. Carlyle T: On Heroes and Hero Worship and the Heroic in History. Project Guttenburg, 1841.
2. Mixter WJ, Barr JS: Rupture of the intervertebral disc with involvement of the spinal canal. New Eng J Med 211:210–215, 1934.
3. Shakespeare W: Hamlet. Second quarto, London, 1604. Printer, James Roberts for Nicolas Lang.
4. www.classicmarine.co.uk/Articles/masts.htm. Accessed December 5, 2006.
5. Gordon JE: Structures, or Why Things Don't Fall Down. London, Pelican Books, 1978.
6. Parke WW: Applied Anatomy of the Spine, Arthrology. *In* Rothman RH and Simeon FA (eds.): The Spine, 2nd ed. Philadelphia, WB Saunders, 1982, pp. 27–35.
7. Richardson MJ, Gillespy T III: Fractal Analysis of Trabecular Bone. University of Washington, Department of Radiology. *www.rad.washington.edu/exhibits/fractal.html*. Accessed December 10, 2006.
8. White AA, Panjabi MM: Clinical Biomechanics of the Spine, 2nd ed. Philadelphia, JB Lippincott Company, 1990.
9. Van Nostrand's Scientific Encyclopedia, 4th ed. Princeton, D. Van Nostrand Company, Inc., 1968, pp. 388–389.
10. Roaf R: A study of the mechanics of spine injuries. J Bone Joint Surg 42B:810–823, 1960.
11. Wolff J: Das Gesetz der Transformation de Knochen. Berlin, Hirschwald, 1892. (English translation: Maquet P, Furlong R: The law of bone remodeling. Berlin, Springer-Verlag, 1986.)
12. www.autoblog.com/2006/05/16/video-michelin-tweel-in-motion; www.michelin.com. Accessed December, 2006.
13. Piersol GA: Piersol's Human Anatomy. Philadelphia, JB Lippincott Company, 1930.
14. Charnley J: The imbibition of fluid as a cause of herniation of the nucleus pulposus. Lancet 1:124–127, 1952.
15. Armstrong JR: Lumbar Disc Lesions. London and Edinburgh, E & S Livingston, Ltd., 1952.
16. Lindahl O: Mechanical properties of dried defatted spongy bone. Acta Orthop Scand 47:11–19, 1976.
17. Schmorl G, Junghanns H: The Human Spine in Health and Disease, 2nd ed. New York, Grune & Stratton, 1971.
18. Herkowitz HN, Dvorak J, Bel G, et al: The Lumbar Spine, 3rd ed. Philadelphia, Lippincott Williams & Wilkins, 2004.
19. Mitchell PEG, Hendry NGC, Billewicz WZ: The chemical background of intervertebral disc prolapse, J Bone Joint Surg 43B:141–151, 1961.
20. Fahrni H: Age changes in lumbar intervertebral discs. Can J Surg 13:65–71, 1970.
21. Fernstrom U: Intervertebral disc degeneration with abdominal pain. Acta Chir Scand 113(6):436–437, 1957.
22. White AH: Lumbar Spine Surgery. Toronto, CV Mosby, 1987.
23. Kirkaldy-Willis WH: Lumbar spinal stenosis. Clin Orthop 99:30–50, 1974.
24. Kirkaldy-Willis WH: Spinal stenosis. Clin Orthop 115:2–3, 1976.
25. Steffe A: Personal communication, October 23, 2005.
26. Garcia R: Challenges to Spine Surgery Meeting. Puerto Rico, January 2002.
27. Harmon P: Personal communication, 1969.
28. Fernstrom U: Arthroplasty with intercorporal endoprosthesis in herniated disc and in painful disc. Acta Chir Scand 355 (suppl):154–159, 1966.
29. Fernstrom, U: Personal Communication.
30. Reitz H, Joubert MJ: Replacement of cervical intervertebral disc with a metal prosthesis. S Afr Med J 38:881–884, 1964.
31. McKenzie AH: Steel ball arthroplasty of lumbar discs. J Bone Joint Surg Br 54:266, 1972.
32. McKenzie AH: Fernstrom intervertebral disc arthroplasty: Long term evaluation. Orthopaedics Intl 3:313–324, 1995.
33. Plato: Dialogues of Plato. U.S.A., Pocket Books Inc., 1950.
34. Wells HG: The Outline of History. Doubleday Company, Garden City, NY, 1940.
35. Toynbee A: A Study of History. Oxford, UK, Oxford Press, 1972.
36. Keegan J: A History of Warfare. Vintage Books, Random House, Inc., 1993.
37. Dror Y: Submission to the United Nations Secretariat. New York, July 11, 1995.

CHAPTER 2

# History and Evolution of Motion Preservation

**Rajiv K. Sethi, Lionel N. Metz,** and **David S. Bradford**

## KEY POINTS

- This chapter focuses on various spirited and innovative approaches to motion preservation at the intervertebral disc.
- A device must be durable, biocompatible, and address the complex functions of the disc that provides both shock absorption and intervertebral motion.
- In many disc replacement designs, articular motion preservation is addressed at the expense of shock absorption.
- We have classified the described devices by their common design principles.
- The long-term outcomes of currently used disc replacements will influence future designs.

## INTRODUCTION

The intervertebral disc is an integral part of the triarticular vertebral motion segment. This joint lies between adjacent vertebral bodies and allows flexion and extension in the sagittal and coronal planes, rotation in the horizontal plane, and limits translation in the horizontal plane between two vertebral bodies. The disc has a viscoelastic nucleus pulposus that absorbs and redistributes axial load to the surrounding annulus fibrosus. Its elastic bandlike annulus fibrosus stores and returns energy from axial loads and constrains the mobility of the motion segment. The relative importance of these complex functions varies at different locations—cervical, thoracic, or lumbar—in the spine.

When considering the challenge of disc replacement, it is important to determine which of these functions and material properties are important to implement. This discussion reviews the evolution of a variety of conceptual designs in disc arthroplasty in the past several decades, with particular attention to the following core questions: Is it feasible to implant the device? Does the device offer a mechanical advantage over fusion? Will the device offer motion preservation that results in an outcome preferable to fusion and maintain the mechanics of the remaining healthy segments? How long will such a device function and will the failure rate be acceptable? And if there is a failure, can salvage be undertaken with little risk to the patient? Will the device function properly long enough to merit implantation? These key questions go into the design of the implant. Only long-term clinical studies will provide the definitive answers.

The precise events of intervertebral disc degeneration have been widely studied but not completely understood. However, it is known that when disc tissues become damaged or degenerated, pathologic joint mechanics as well as pathologic changes in innervation and nociception cause back pain, which is usually exacerbated by movement.[1] When this pain is persistent despite conservative treatment, operative management can be considered. Operative intervention for back pain such as a spinal fusion is itself fraught with complications and often has poor outcomes.[2]

One core principle of the orthopaedic approach to degenerative joint disease is that pathologic motion causes pain, and if that motion can be arrested, the patient will benefit. This concept of joint fusion guided the orthopaedic treatment of arthritis in the knee and hip for many years and continues to be the mainstay of spine surgery. The evolution toward arthroplasty to treat painful knees and hips has raised the important question of whether degenerative joint disease of the spine might be better treated by arthroplasty than by arthrodesis. Considering that fusion of a single lumbar motion segment for degenerative disease of the spine may result in pain relief in some patients, artificial disc replacement technology should at least replicate that or do better. Total joint replacement for end-stage arthritis of the hip and knee has revolutionized the field of orthopaedic surgery. Both primary total hip and knee replacement have resulted in high rates of patient satisfaction, and surgeons and patients have become accustomed to excellent long-term results. Surgeons hope to achieve similar benefits with disc arthroplasty.

In broad terms, the intervertebral disc serves two distinct roles: (1) facilitation of limited motion between two vertebral bodies, and (2) absorption of shock through viscoelastic properties of the nucleus pulposus/annulus fibrosis construct.[3] Thus, the application of arthroplasty to the degenerated intervertebral disc is more complex than that of the knee or hip. The efficacy of disc replacement is not only reliant on a mechanically sound replacement of the disc but also on the assurance that the disc is the primary source of pain. This would imply that the facet joints are not a contributory factor to the back pain. The innervation of the disc is also poorly understood, and therefore, disc replacement may not truly relieve the patient's symptoms.[4,5]

Early arthroplasty techniques attempted to use the abovementioned conceptual tenets and hypotheses. In 1955, David Cleveland published the first paper on disc arthroplasty utilizing methyl-acrylic in 14 patients. At 5 months after the operation, 100% of these patients had resolution of their back pain. To aid in the stabilization of the lumbar disc space, Paul Harmon devised a Vitallium sphere that he implanted through an anterior retroperitoneal approach in 13 patients from 1959 to 1961. In 1964, Ulf Fernstrom published his results of 105 lumbar cases in which he posteriorly implanted a stainless steel ball bearing device. The implant group had a 12% rate of low back pain following implantation versus 60% in the control group.

## RATIONALE FOR DISC ARTHROPLASTY

Arthrodesis at a single vertebral level is not associated with the same degree of functional loss as knee or hip arthrodesis.[6] Even patients with multiple fused levels adjust quite well to fusion and enjoy significantly improved quality of life at long-term follow-up.[7] Most surgeons would agree that simple motion preservation is not a good enough reason to pursue disc replacement. Although the loss of mobility in a single fused segment is small, it has a potentially large effect on the adjacent segments that compensate for the functional loss. This compensatory mechanism is implicated in the high rate of adjacent segment degeneration seen after short fusions.[8–10] Long-term studies confirming that disc arthroplasty is associated with a lower incidence of adjacent segment degeneration are needed to verify the value of this intervention.

## BIOMECHANICAL CHALLENGES

The vertebral column is a polyarticular structure that functions under the influence of a delicate balance of forces. Generally, the anterior structures, the vertebral bodies and discs, support 90% of the axial load, whereas the posterior elements, primarily the facet joints, support the remainder of the load in the lumbar spine. It is paramount that any disc replacement maintain the delicate load distribution and emulate the mechanics of the invertebral disc (IVD) as closely as possible to avoid facet arthrosis or adjacent segment degeneration. Disc arthroplasty can potentially avoid the compensatory motion in adjacent segments that occurs after short fusions, thus preventing adjacent segment disease. However, at present, there are no disc arthroplasty devices in common use that protect the spine by absorbing axial loads in addition to preserving articular motion.

Motion preservation in the posterior elements of the spine is arguably a simpler task than for the intervertebral disc. Dynamic stabilization systems such as Dynesys, as well as facet joint arthroplasty are in development. These systems are covered in later chapters of this volume. The remainder of this chapter focuses on various spirited and innovative approaches to motion preservation at the intervertebral disc. We have made extensive use of the thorough chronologic cataloguing of spine motion preservation patents performed by Szpalski et al in their 2002 review[11]; thus, we would like to make a special acknowledgement of their efforts.

## INTERVERTEBRAL DISC REPLACEMENT COMPREHENSIVE CLASSIFICATION SYSTEM

Ideas regarding disc replacement are not always the result of methodic review of previous patent designs and literature. Thus, newer patents often appear to be less sophisticated brethren of established designs. Therefore, rather than listing the patented inventions in chronologic order, the following discussion of disc replacement design describes the designs as derivations of prototypic designs. To this end we have attempted to classify these devices by the central mechanical principles. The 14 classifications used are as follows: ball bearing, ball and socket, fixed dome, articulating plates, hard plates/hard core, hard plates/soft core, screw-in dowel, spring and piston, complex mechanical/vertebral body replacement, fluid-filled bag, simple elastomer/polymer prostheses, spiral nucleoplasty, in situ polymerization, and biologic.

### Ball Bearing

The Fernstrom Ball, shown in Figure 2–1, is often credited with being one of the first substantial attempts at intervertebral disc arthroplasty.[12] The device is the prototypic simple ball bearing design. The ball is placed into the disc space after discectomy, allowing for movement in several planes. This device has an extremely low surface contact area on initial implantation, which leads to a predictable subsistence through the cancellous bone beneath. This subsistence was severe in many cases, often leading to pain, disc height loss, and eventually loss of motion and many times fusion at the implanted level. Subsequently, the use of the Fernstrom ball has been discontinued in the United States. Ultimately, the indications for use of the device have evolved to encompass fusion rather than motion.

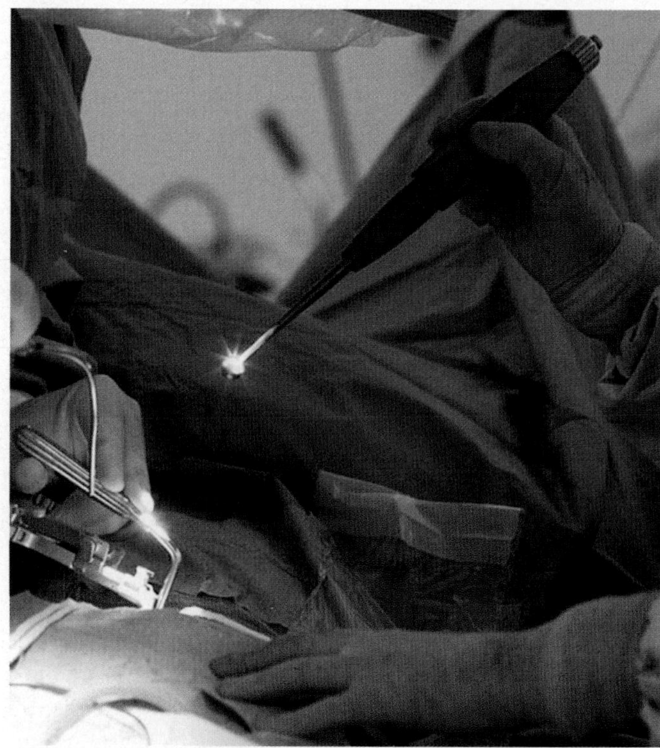

■ **FIGURE 2–1.** Fernstrom ball. http://jborden.org/etc/C2056846532/E20060723070512/index.html. Accessed January 23, 2007.

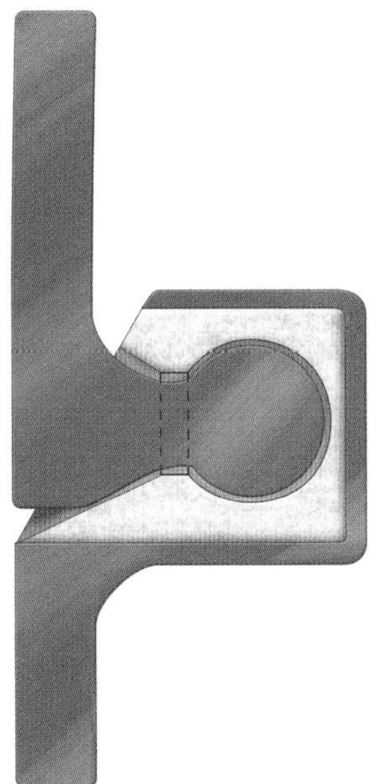

■ **FIGURE 2–2.** Ibo ball-and-socket prosthesis.

## Ball-and-Socket

The idea of using a ball-and-socket design is no doubt inspired by its successful application total hip arthroplasty.[13] This association is clearly demonstrated by Ibo's ball-and-socket implant (Fig. 2–2).[14] In contrast, the Graham prosthesis (Fig. 2–3) involves a cylindrical anchor that resides in each of two adjacent vertebral bodies and a ball-and-socket joint that lies in line with the axis of load.[15] The device also offers some compressive cushioning mediated by spacers around the ball joint. In 1994, Mazda put forth a similar device that incorporated an elastic annulus around his ball joint.[16] Xavier's design in 1998 added criss-crossed wires that would aid the stability of the construct.[17]

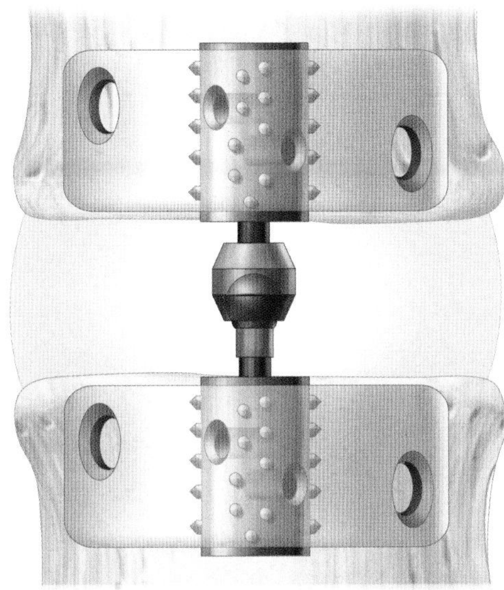

■ **FIGURE 2–3.** The Graham ball-and-socket device is designed with a ball-and-socket joint in-line with the cylindrical anchors, which are seated in the adjacent vertebral bodies.

## Fixed Dome

The Sabitzer and Fuss device (Fig. 2–4) is a prototype for the fixed dome concept.[18] In this device, the disc is replaced by a rigid dome that is firmly affixed to the inferior vertebral body and freely articulates with the inferior end plate of the superior vertebral body. The latter has a natural concavity that offers some restraint of movement as well as load repartition.[11] Kehr designed a cervical implant in which there is a mounting bracket resting on the inferior vertebral body with an arm that anchors into the side of the vertebral body.[19] A domed articulating prosthesis attaches to the bracket and articulates with the upper cartilaginous end plate.

## Articulating Plates

The articulating plate designs use hard materials with low friction coefficients to resurface the end plates, restore disc space height, and distribute the surface stress.[11] The concept involves one concave surface and one convex surface, resulting in a wide range of rotational and translational motions—up to 6 degrees of freedom like the native disc. These designs are derivations of the simple ball-and-socket designs used in hip arthroplasty. Although not the first example of this principle, Salib and Pettine's design (Fig. 2–5) had a small articulating surface and limited distribution of surface stresses.[20] Shinn and Tate describe a very similar design for their device.[21] Evolutions of this concept involve larger curved articulating surfaces, such as the device by Yuan (Fig. 2–6).[22]

Shelokov patented a similar device that uses two dome-shaped condyles, similar to the design of the leading total knee replacements.[23] Lesoin et al[24] designed an articulating plates device that screws into the vertebral bodies, much like the Salib and Pettine design.

Cauthen designed a slit-and-rib[11] implant (Fig. 2–7) that constrains rotational motion in the coronal and horizontal planes and allows for sagittal rocking chair–type motion and possibly some

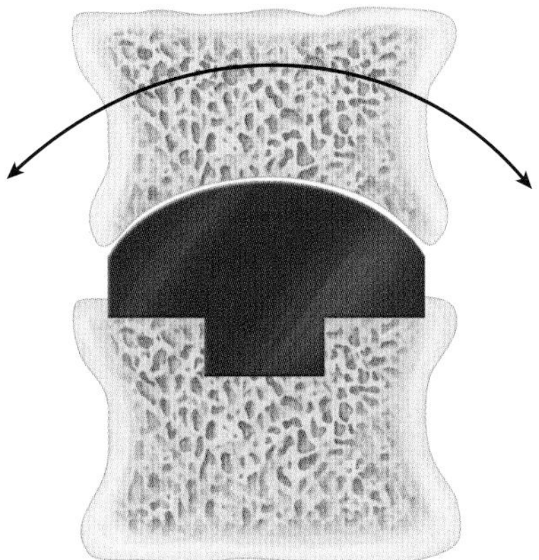

■ **FIGURE 2–4.** The Sabitzer and Fuss device involves a domed prosthesis that articulates with the upper end plate and anchors to the lower vertebral body.

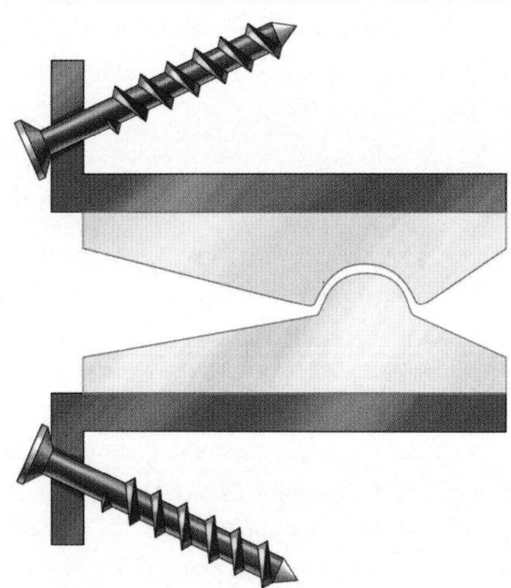

■ **FIGURE 2–5.** Salib and Pettine incorporate the ball-and-socket type of articulation into two plates, one concave and one convex.

anterior or posterior translation.[25] It would be easy to imagine a tremendous amount of stress at the base of the thin rib during side bending.

## Hard Plates/Hard Core

The previously discussed articulating plate designs have the limitation of high friction in cases in which metal on metal articulation is used. This predisposes them to problems with metallic wear debris, which may build up exponentially once wear is initiated. Both of these problems were addressed by the addition of a polymer core. In these designs, the core is either floating, unconstrained, between two concave end plates, such as in the Schellnack-Büttner Janz (SB) CHARITÉ[26] (Fig. 2–8), first implanted in 1984 by Karin Büttner Janz, or it is anchored to the flat surface of one endplate while it articulates to the concave surface of the other end plate, as in the semiconstrained ProDisc design,[27] first implanted in 1990 by Thierry Marnay. Both of these designs are discussed in detail in later chapters. Most designs use a polyethylene or other plastic type of core articulating with one or both metal end plates. In 1974, Hoffman-Daimler invented such a device that consisted of two metal plates with a complex plastic core.[28] The device was never implanted into humans.

In 1978, Weber patented a design slightly different from the prototype design, using two concave polyethylene surfaces and an ovoid ceramic core for use in the lumbar and cervical spine.[29,30] Various materials have been used for the core, such as metal,[31] fluoroplastic,[32] and ceramic. Ojima used hydroxyapatite-coated plates to allow for better bony incorporation of the implant,[33]

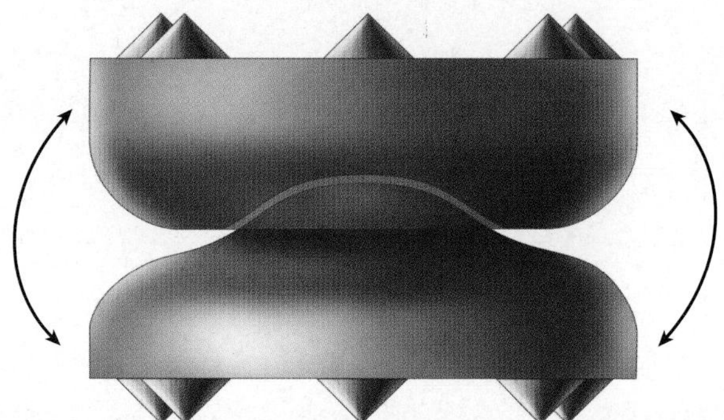

■ **FIGURE 2–6.** Yuan incorporated the articulating plate design into implants with large articulating surfaces.

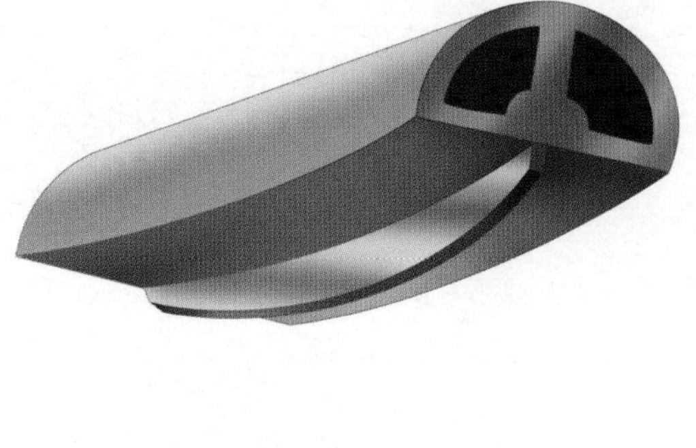

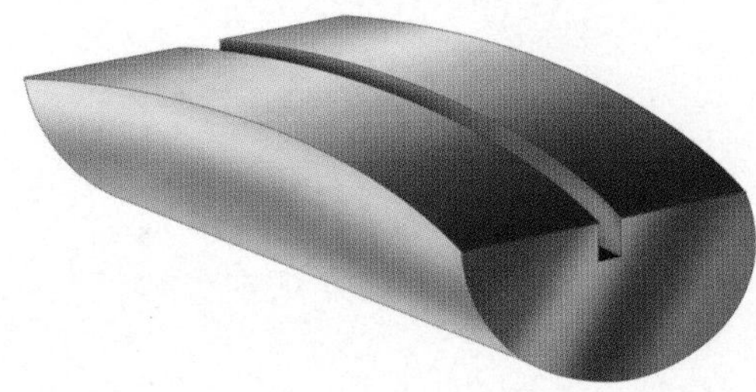

■ **FIGURE 2–7.** Cauthen's slit-and-rib design uses two articulating components, both convex at the articulating surfaces. It constrains rotational motion in the coronal and horizontal planes but allows for rocking motion in the sagittal plane.

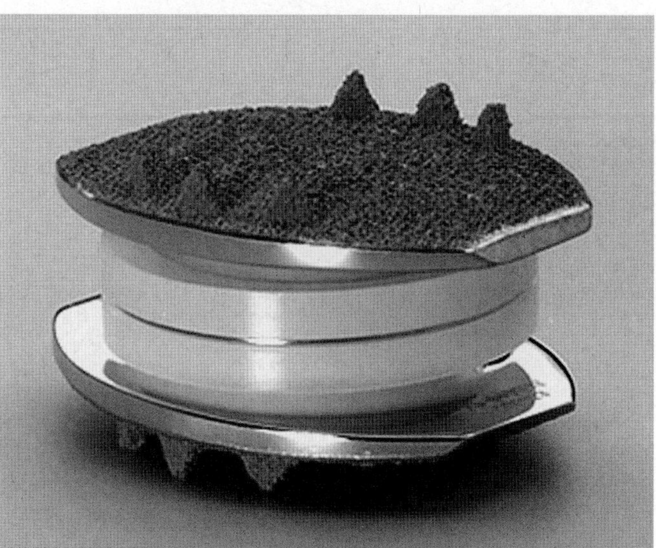

■ **FIGURE 2–8.** CHARITÉ Artificial Disc (DePuy Spine, Inc., Raynham, MA). *(Photograph Courtesy of DePuy Spine, Inc.)*

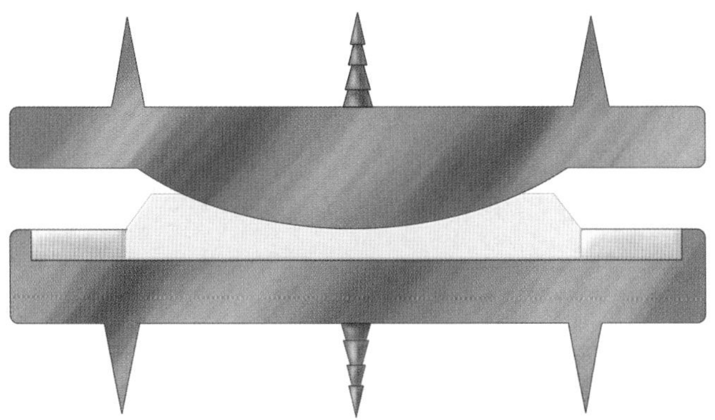

■ **FIGURE 2–9.** Erickson and Griffith device used a polymer core to decrease friction with the articulating superior end plate.

whereas others, Bryan and Kunzler,[34] used plate extensions that could be screwed into the anterior aspect of the superior and inferior vertebral bodies.

Variations on the hard plate/hard core theme involved a core secured to one of the plates. Gordon's[35] variation used a hemispheric bearing anchored to the inferior plate but articulating with the superior plate, similar to the ProDisc. Erickson and Griffith's design (Fig. 2–9) used a concave core. These designs offer rotational motion as well as some translational motion, depending on the difference between the radii of the convex and concave surfaces.[36] The Bullivant design appears to be very similar to the ProDisc II design, shown in Figure 2–10, with the core attached to the superior metal end plate instead of the inferior one.

### Hard Plates/Soft Core

Few of the above-mentioned designs adequately address axial shock absorption or try to re-create the indispensable viscoelastic properties of the IVD.[37] This is the limitation of the rigid materials used in the core of these designs. Several designs have used the concept of an articulating core and attempted shock absorption by using a compressible elastomer as the core material. Khvisuyk's[38] design is composed of a silicon cushion between two metallic plates. The Downey prosthesis[39] was similar and had two large bolts to screw it into the superior and inferior end plates.

Another example is the AcroFlex, by DePuy Spine (Raynham, MA), shown in Figure 2–11. It uses a silicone elastomer core bonded to two titanium plates.[40] It is designed for implantation in the lumbar spine.

Other designs involving a soft core secured to both plates were brought forth by Harms et al[41] and Oka et al.[47] Harms described a silicone rubber core that was sandwiched between two hard plastic plates. Oka's similar invention was composed of a composite body made of a polyvinyl alcohol hydrogel flanked by ceramic or metallic end plates. Zdeblick and McKay's[43] design called for rigid end plates separated by a core with properties similar to that of the nucleus pulposus.

Several similar designs followed by Graf.[44–46] Baumgartner and Takeda[47,48] used projecting rims on the inside of the end plate around the elastomeric core to constrain some of the translation and rotational motion as well as limit the extent of compression.[11] Some designs used capsule-like elastomer cores between hard plates with or without spikes.[49–51] Bainville et al[52] recognized the risk of core migration after several million cycles called for an antiexpulsion device around the core that would still allow for compression of the soft core. Viart and Marin's device (Fig. 2–12)[53] may have prevented core migration by using a doughnut-shaped core, but without a fulcrum in the center of the core, the device is likely to have limited sagittal and coronal rotational motion.

Graf envisioned a device that allowed for motion through asymmetric compression of the cushion, while providing shock absorption (Fig. 2–13). His blueprint used standard concave end plates and a hydrophilic gel core.

The mobile articulation hard plate/soft core designs have the additional consideration of an increased friction coefficient of many elastomeric materials compared with harder polymers. The nonarticulating soft core designs, such as the Graf device, undergo a tremendous amount of shear stress when resisting translation,[54] which is a concern for device longevity.

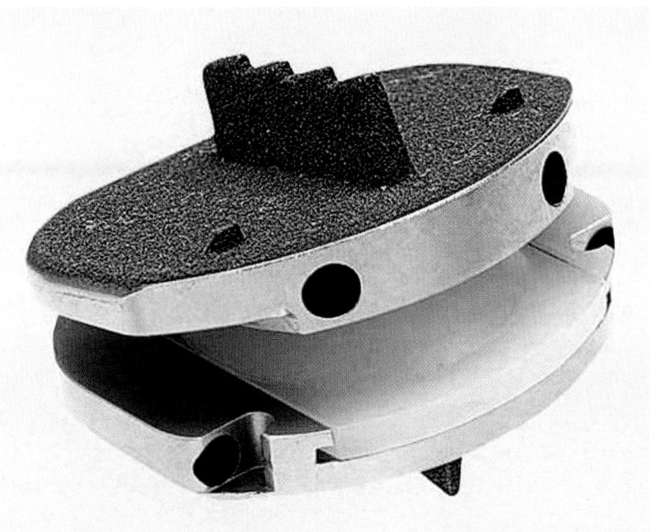

■ **FIGURE 2–10.** ProDisc II Lumbar Total Disc Replacement, courtesy of Synthes, Inc (West Chester, PA). The device has two metallic end plates separated by a polyethylene core that locks into the lower end plate.

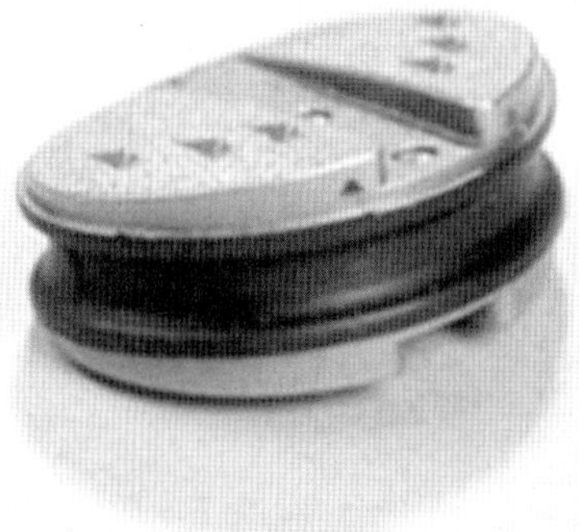

■ **FIGURE 2–11.** The second generation AcroFlex-100 consists of an HP-100 silicone elastomer core bonded to two titanium end plates (DePuy Spine, Inc., Raynham, MA). *(Courtesy of Spineuniverse.com.)*

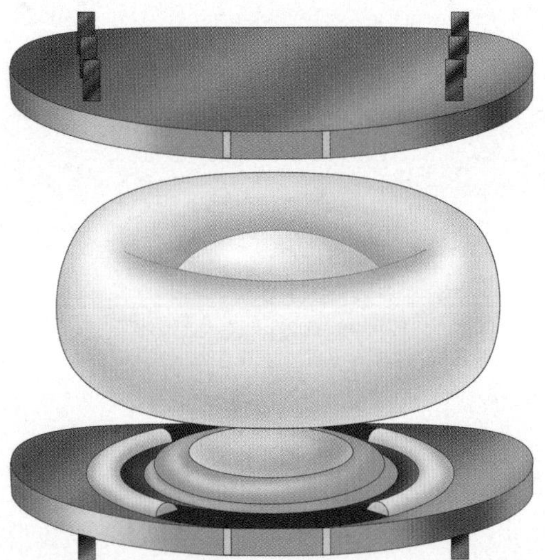

■ **FIGURE 2–12.** Viart and Marin's device uses a doughnut-shaped soft core designed to prevent core migration relative to the two hard plates.

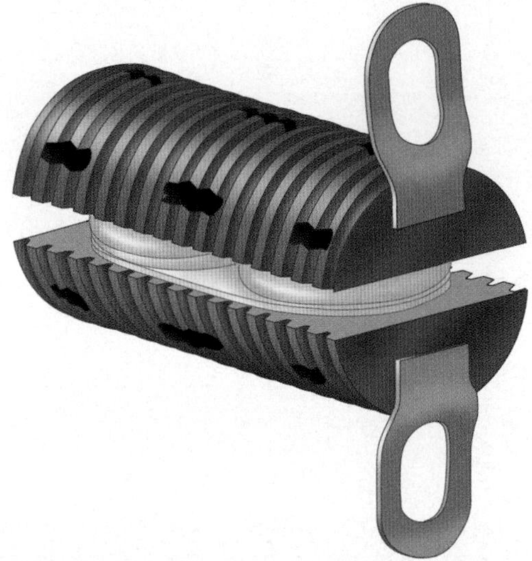

■ **FIGURE 2–14.** Bryan and Kunzler's cylindric implant is screwed into place and secured by anchoring brackets. The mobile elements, or "resilient bodies," reside in the center of the implant.

## Screw-In Dowel

The screw-in prostheses strongly resemble the BAK interbody fusion implants[55] manufactured by Zimmer. They are short-grooved cylinders bisected along the long axis to create hollow half cylinders. The functional components reside inside the half cylinders created by the bisection. One theoretic advantage of these devices is the ease of implantation. Bryan et al designed several of these devices; an example is shown in Figure 2–14, with varying motion-sparing or cushioning inner components.[56, 57] He refers to the inner components simply as "resilient bodies," which reflects the difficulty in predicting the ideal materials for this application. Also in 2000, Cauthen[58] designed an implant using two threaded, solid half cylinders separated by a ball bearing that was articulated with concavities in a flat surface (Fig. 2–15). The design was intended for use in the cervical spine. Mehdizadeh[59] used the concept of two threaded half cylinders but linked them with small springs to provide elasticity to the construct.

## Spring and Piston

The function of the healthy disc in absorbing axial shock[37] has led many inventors to investigate the role of small springs and pistons in IVD replacement. Patil's spring box (Fig. 2–16) is designated as our prototype for the spring-and-piston design.[60] It contained overlapping half boxes linked with several interposed springs.

Dumas et al also describe a spring-linked plate design.[61] Beer and Beer[62] patented a device very similar to the Patil device that includes screw plates for fixation to the anterior surface of the superior and inferior vertebral bodies. Butterman's complex design included pistons as shock absorbers.[63] The Pisharodi expandable device, shown in Figure 2–17, encapsulated the springs in a hollow bag and would be collapsible to a fraction of its expanded size to facilitate implantation.[64] The spring implant created by Hedman

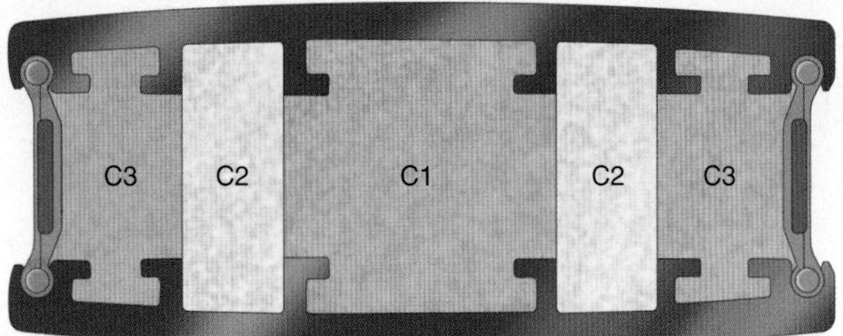


■ **FIGURE 2–13.** Graf's device constrained the soft core with interlocking teeth on the two hard plates, preventing core migration and presumably ascribing motion to differential compression rather than articulation.

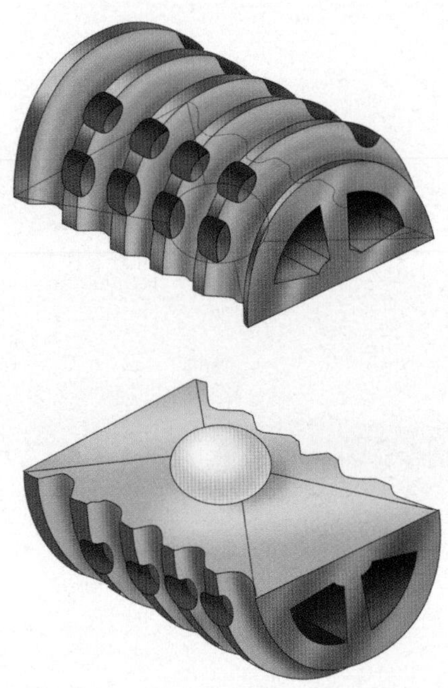

■ **FIGURE 2–15.** Cauthen's design incorporates the ease of a screw-in device with the simplicity of a ball-and-socket type of articulation.

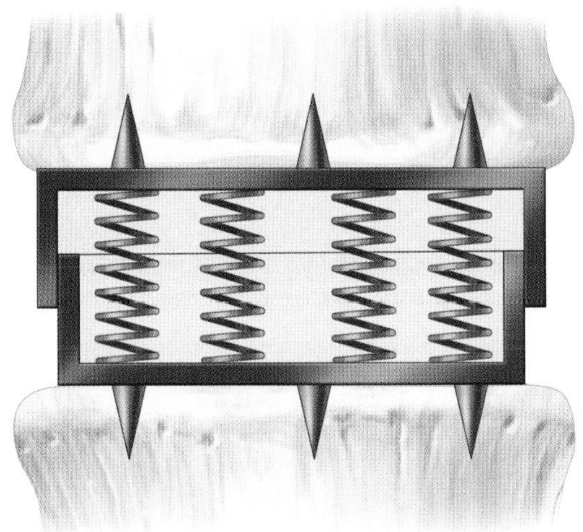

■ **FIGURE 2–16.** Patil's cervical interlocking plates are separated by springs, which impart a cushioning effect to the device.

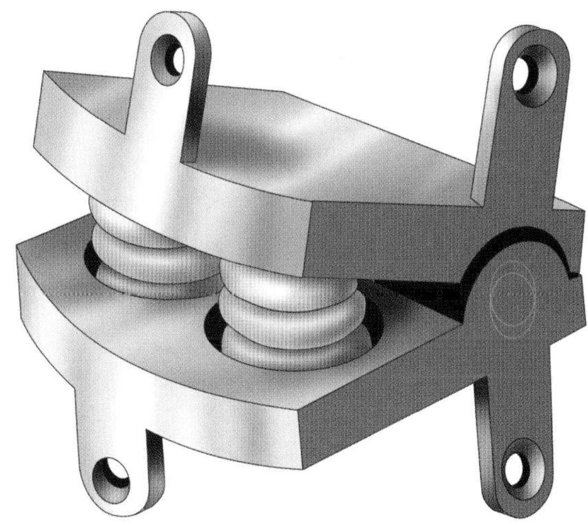

■ **FIGURE 2–18.** Kostuik's implant relied on two springs for compressive shock absorption and was wedge shaped to maintain lumbar lordosis.

et al of the Kostuik team[65] was implanted in large animal models, which is a more advanced stage of development than most of the previously described devices. The device involved two titanium plates, hinged posteriorly, and two springs to create an elastic construct (Fig. 2–18). The springs in this construct were said to have withstood more than 100 million cycles without failure and were implanted with some success in sheep models.[10] Overall, the success of hard plate/hard core prostheses has led to a decrease in the development of spring-containing designs.

## Complex Mechanical/Vertebral Body Replacement

There have been many proposed motion preservation devices for use in the lumbar spine that use complex designs that do not fit neatly into one category. These complex mechanical devices often have the burden of dozens of moving parts that may cause potential licensing companies to shy away. Simple devices often win out because production, quality control, and difficulty of implantation hinder the adaptation of complicated or clumsy devices. One clever device by Main et al (Fig. 2–19) used an expandable system capable of replacing the disc as well as a substantial amount of the adjacent vertebral bodies.[66] It incorporates an "elastomeric suspension medium" around each of the device's suspension plates at either end. Many other devices combine a multitude of mechanical principles and properties to re-create the disc's native properties and functions.

## Fluid-Filled Bag

Typically, these devices consist of a soft fillable bag with a specific shape and material properties that is filled with fluid of liquid or gaseous form. In 1975, Froning[67] designed a discoid bladder

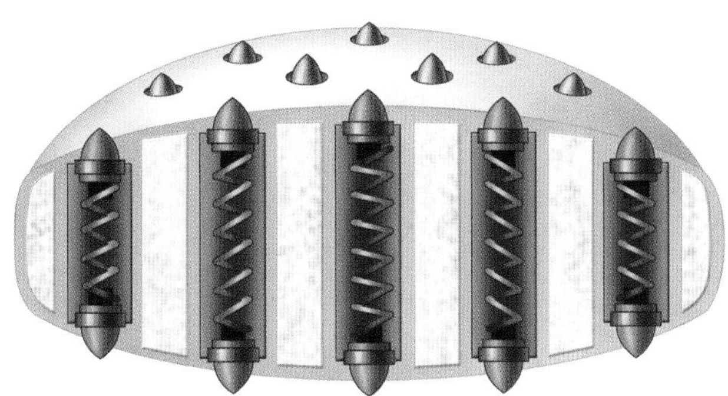

■ **FIGURE 2–17.** Pisharodi's expandable prosthesis uses springs to cushion axial loads and, more importantly, can be implanted in a collapsed state.

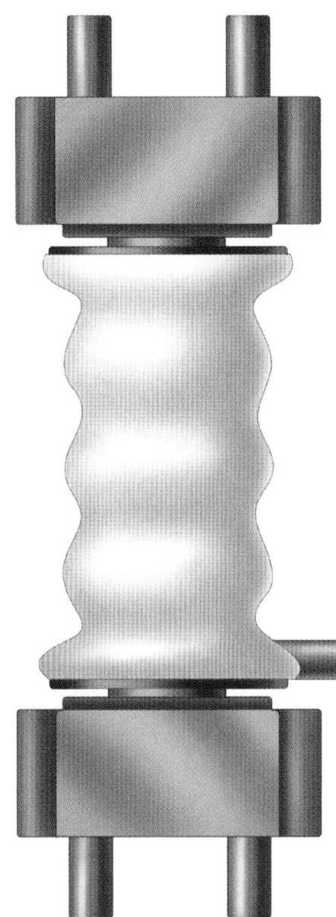

■ **FIGURE 2–19.** Main's device replaced the vertebral bodies as well as the disc. It has a mobile element in the center of its length that may allow for some degree of normal biomechanics at that level.

that was to be inserted into the disc space in deflated form and then filled with fluid once positioned in place. The disc bladder design has been one of the most popular forms of disc prosthesis because of its inherent shock absorption and small size before implantation. Several others made variations on the size, shape, material, and filling fluids used in these devices.[68–78]

### Simple Elastomer/Polymer Prostheses

The observation that some elastomers have similar viscoelastic properties to the IVD[79] led to the trial of several of these materials as simple disc replacements. Many of these designs were very crude, simply using a polymer cast in the shape of the nucleus. The prototype design by Nachemson, in the 1950s, sought to replace the degenerated nucleus pulposus with a resilient material, such as silicone.[80] Others also used silicone, but various similar materials have been used to achieve the desired amount of compressibility and friction.[81–83] A major distinction of these devices is that no artificial end plate is used as an articulating surface, so the native cartilaginous or bony end plates form the articular surfaces. There are many other notable designs.[84,85]

Although the physical properties of native nucleus pulposus (NP) and these materials may be similar, the remodeling potential of the NP allows these material properties to be maintained for several decades, whereas even the most resilient elastomer is likely to fall prey to wear over this time period. Kotani's woven disc prosthesis,[86] shown in Figure 2–20, might be less susceptible to shear forces but may be prone to a substantial foreign body reaction from microfiber degradation.[87]

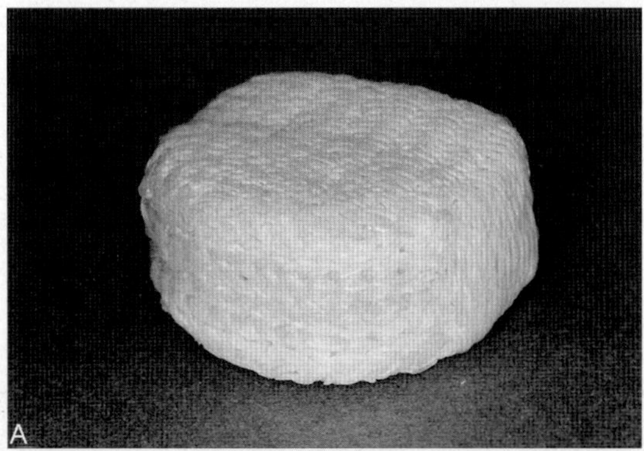


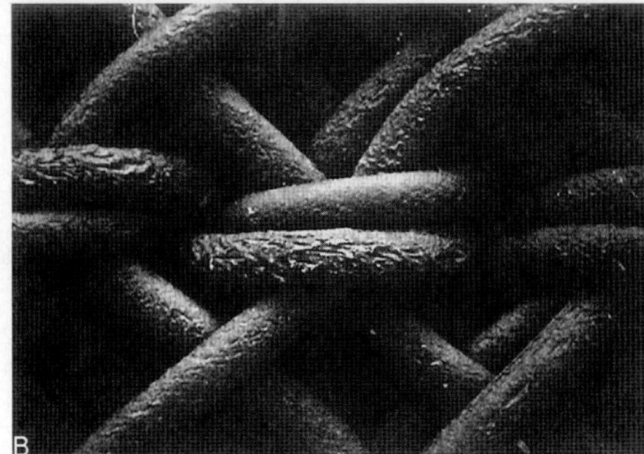


■ **FIGURE 2–20.** Kotani used advanced techniques in polymer design to weave a three-dimensional disk-shaped structure out of ultra-high-molecular-weight polyethylene fibers. Spray coated with ceramic granules, the implant was designed to incorporate into the surrounding structures.[86]

### Spiral Nucleoplasty

Most of these devices are similar to the above-mentioned elastomer prostheses. The novelty in this design is that the elastomer can be implanted through a much smaller annulotomy. This is one of the few device types that can be inserted through a minimally invasive posterior approach after removal of the nucleus. In 1975, Stubstad patented his coiled elastomer implant (Fig. 2–21),[88] spawning several similar designs, collectively referred to as spiral nucleoplasty devices.[89]

### In Situ Polymerization

Hydrogels and other biocompatible polymers have been investigated. This approach has appeal because it can potentially be performed through a posterior minimally invasive approach. Despite these benefits, the design lacks the ability to resist degradation. Challenges arising from polymer resorption and degradation, and precipitation of a foreign body reaction may hinder the efficacy of such systems.

### Biologic

Cells have the remarkable ability to produce impressively resilient tissues capable of being strong yet flexible. Both biologic tissues and synthetic materials with these properties are subject to wear and eventually failure. However, only living tissues have the unique ability to adapt and remodel, properties that allow tissues to retain or even increase their resiliency. Unfortunately, these properties can also lead to pathologic remodeling to the point where the native function of the tissue is lost as in degenerative disc disease.[90,91] Nonetheless, it is quite reasonable to assume that motion preservation of the spine would be best accomplished by a faithful restoration of the living tissues. Thus, many inventors have sought to find appropriate cells, carriers, and implantation techniques to biologically regenerate the intervertebral disc.[92,93]

Most of these designs seek to restore the desiccated nucleus pulposus in degenerative disc disease. Two cellular candidates have prevailed in these designs: (1) chondrocytes, which produce a large

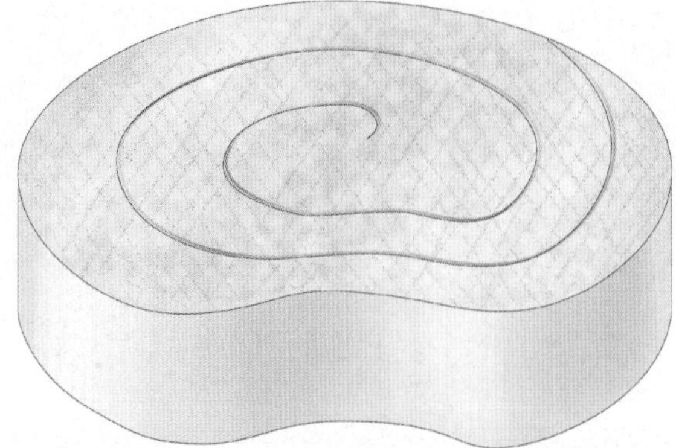

■ **FIGURE 2–21.** This spiraled variant of Stubstadt's elastomer implants might have been implanted minimally invasively.

amount of aggrecan, the substance that imbibes water in the nucleus and imparts viscoelastic properties to the disc, and (2) mesenchymal stem cells, which are capable of both proliferating and differentiating into nucleus pulposus–like cells. These technologies are areas of active research and are covered in more detail in later chapters.

## LESSONS LEARNED

Several lessons about spinal implants have been learned. The contact surface between the implant and the vertebral end plate must be maximized in order to prevent subsistence of the device.[11] This concept was demonstrated by the Fernstrom ball implants, which have a very small end plate contact surface. A larger contact surface allows for wider load repartition and less stress on the end plates; however, this factor mandates that disc arthroplasty with rigid materials will likely always require an anterior approach.

The complex role of the disc, providing both viscoelastic load distribution and articular motion, creates a difficult design challenge. Most designs used today, namely the CHARITÉ III and ProDisc II, have largely abandoned viscoelastic considerations and focused on motion preservation. Other designs using the viscoelastic properties of silicone, or elastic properties of springs or pistons, or both, put less importance on motion preservation, particularly in the transverse plane. Seldom has a device aimed to accurately reproduce both roles, and none has been very successful in completing this task. Indeed, experience has shown that materials best suited for millions of cycles of articular motion are hard and have low friction coefficients. These materials, such as metals, polyethylene, and ceramics, inherently lack additional viscoelastic properties.

## CONCLUSION

Each of the designs presented attempts to emulate one or more of the essential biomechanical properties of the intervertebral disc. Long-term clinical outcomes of the few disc replacements that have been evaluated in clinical trials continue to be measured; these outcomes will guide the next generation of disc arthroplasty designs. Surgeons must be increasingly circumspect when considering performing new procedures whose long-term efficacy is not established. The appropriately high treatment expectations of our patients will be properly addressed by prudent clinical judgment in selecting the best, as opposed to the newest, intervention.

## REFERENCES


1. Vernon-Roberts B, Pirie CJ: Degenerative changes in the intervertebral discs of the lumbar spine and their sequelae. Rheumatology 16:13–19, 1977.
2. Ibrahim T, Tleyjeh IM, Gabbar O: Surgical versus non-surgical treatment of chronic low back pain: a meta-analysis of randomised trials. Int Orthop Nov. 21, 2006, epub.
3. Lotz JC, Hsieh AH, Walsh AL, et al: Mechanobiology of the intervertebral disc. Biochem Soc Trans 30:853–858, 2002.
4. Aoki Y, Akeda K, An H, et al: Nerve fiber ingrowth into scar tissue formed following nucleus pulposus extrusion in the rabbit anular-puncture disc degeneration model: effects of depth of puncture. Spine 31:E774–E780, 2006.
5. McCarthy PW: Innervation of lumbar intervertebral disks—a review. J Peripher Nerv Syst 3:233–242, 1998.
6. Chow DH, Luk KD, Evens JH, Leong JC: Effects of short anterior lumbar interbody fusion on biomechanics of neighboring unfused segments. Spine 21:549–555, 1996.
7. Padua R, Padua S, Aulisa L, et al: Patient outcomes after Harrington instrumentation for idiopathic scoliosis: a 15- to 28-year evaluation. Spine 26:1268–1273, 2001.
8. Ghiselli G, Chen J, Kaou M, et al: Adjacent segment degeneration in the lumbar spine. J Bone Joint Surg 86:1497–1503, 2004.
9. Eck JC, Humphreys SC, Hodges SD: Adjacent-segment degeneration after lumbar fusion: a review of clinical, biomechanical, and radiologic studies. Am J Orthop 28:336–340, 1999.
10. Kostuik JP: Intervertebral disc replacement: Experimental study. Clin Orthop Rel Res 337:27–41, 1997.
11. Szpalski M, Gunzburg R, Mayer M: Spine arthroplasty: a historical review. Eur Spine J 11:65–84, 2002.
12. Fernstrom U: Arthroplasty with intercorporal endoprothesis in herniated disc and in painful disc. Acta Chir Scand Suppl 357:154–159, 1966.
13. Charnley J: The long-term results of low-friction arthroplasty of the hip performed as a primary intervention. J Bone Joint Surg Br 54:61–76, 1972.
14. Ibo I, Pierotto E, inventors: Prosthesis of the cervical intervertebralis disk. US patent 5,755,796, May 26, 1998.
15. Graham DV, inventor: Artificial disk. US patent 5,246,458, September 21, 1993.
16. Mazda, inventor: Prothèse discale intervertébrale, French Patent 2694882, 1994.
17. Xavier R, Xavier S, Xavier S, inventors: Vertebral body prosthesis. US patent 6,063,121, May 16, 2000.
18. Sabitzer and Fuss, Austrian Patent 405237B, 1997.
19. Kehr, European Patent 069926, 1996.
20. Salib RM, Pettine KA, inventors: Intervertebral disk arthroplasty. US patent 5,258,031, November 2, 1993.
21. Shinn GL, Tate JD, inventors: Artificial intervertebral disk prosthesis. US patent 5,683,465, November 4, 1997.
22. Yuan HA, inventor: Low wear artificial spinal disc. US patent 5,676,701, October 14, 1997.
23. Shelokov AP, inventor: Articulating spinal disc prosthesis. US patent 6,039,763, March 21, 2000.
24. Lesoin et al, French Patent 2718635, 1995.
25. Cauthen, JC, inventor: Articulating spinal implant. US patent 6,179,874, January 30, 2001.
26. Link HD: History, design and biomechanics of the LINK SB Charité artificial disc. Eur Spine J 11:98–105, 2002.
27. Rousseau MA, Bradford DS, Bertagnoli R, et al: Disc arthroplasty design influences intervertebral kinematics and facet forces. Spine J 6:258–266, 2006.
28. Hoffman-Daimler, German Patent 2263842, 1974.
29. Weber, Swiss Patent 624673, 1978.
30. Weber, Swiss Patent 640131, 1979.
31. Keller A, inventor: Surgical instrument set. US patent 4,997,432, March 5, 1991.
32. Savchenko et al, Russian Patent 2140229, 1999.
33. Ojima, European Patent 0317972, 1989.
34. Bryan V, Kunzler A, inventor: Human spinal disc prosthesis. US patent 5,865,846, February 2, 1999.
35. Gordon J, inventor: Intervertebral disc replacement prothesis. US Patent 20050234553, October 20, 2005.
36. Huang RC, Giardi FP, Commisa FP Jr, Wright TM: The implications of constraint in lumbar total disc replacement. J Spinal Discord Tech 16:412–417, 2003.
37. Vuono-Hawkins M, Langiana NA, Parsons JR, et al: Materials and design concepts for an intervertebral disc spacer. II. Multidurometer composite design. J Appl Biomater 6:117–123, 1995.
38. Khvisuyk, USSR Patent 895433, 1982.
39. Downey EL, inventor: Vertebra prosthesis. US patent 5,147,404, September 15, 1992.

40. Fraser RD, Ross ER, Lowery GL, et al: AcroFlex design and results. Spine J 4:245–251, 2004.
41. Harms et al, German Patent 3911610, 1990.
42. Oka M, Gen S, Ikada Y, Okimatsu H, inventors: Artificial intervertebral disc. US patent 5,458,643, October 17, 1995.
43. Zdeblick and McKay, World Patent 0074606, 2000.
44. Graf, French Patent 2772594, 1999.
45. Graf, French Patent 2775891, 1999.
46. Graf, French Patent 2801782, 1999.
47. Baumgartner, Europe Patent 0566810, 1992.
48. Takeda M, inventor: Display apparatus. US patent 5,270,697, December 14, 1993.
49. Grammon and Gauchet, French Patent 2723841, 1996.
50. Yves-Alain, inventor: Elastic disc prosthesis. US patent 5,676,702, October 14, 1997.
51. Bisserie M, inventor: Intervertebral disk prosthesis. US patent 5,702,450, December 30, 1997.
52. Bainville D, Laval F, Roy-Camille R, et al, inventors: Intervertebral disk prosthesis. US patent 5,674,294, October 7, 1997.
53. Viart and Marin, French Patent 2895985, 2001.
54. Bao QB, Yuan HA: Prosthetic disc replacement: the future. Clin Orthop Rel Res 394:139–145, 2002.
55. Nibu K, Panjabi MM, Oxland T, Cholewicki J: Multidirectional stabilizing potential of BAK interbody spinal fusion system for anterior surgery. J Spinal Disord 10:357–362, 1997.
56. Bryan V, Kunzler A, inventor: Human spinal disc prosthesis. US patent 5,865,846, February 2, 1999.
57. Bryan et al, World Patent 0013620, 2000.
58. Cauthen JC, inventor: Articulating spinal implant. US patent 6,019,792, February 1, 2000.
59. Mehdizadeh HM, inventor: Disc replacement prosthesis. US patent 6,231,609, May 15, 2001.
60. Patil AA, inventor: Artificial intervertebral disc. US patent 4,309,777, January 12, 1982.
61. Dumas et al, French Patent 2734148, 1996.
62. Beer JC, Beer JM, inventors: Synthetic intervertebral disc. US patent 5,458,642, October 17, 1995.
63. Butterman GR, inventor: Intervertebral prosthetic device. US patent 5,827,328, October 27, 1998.
64. Pisharodi M, inventor: Artificial spinal prosthesis. US patent 5,123,926, June 23, 1992.
65. Hedman TP, Kostuik JP, Fernie GR, Maki B, inventors: Artificial spinal disc. US patent 4,759,769, July 26, 1988.
66. Main JA, Wells ME, Keller TS, inventors: Vertebral prosthesis. US patent 4,932,975, June 12, 1990.
67. Froning EC, inventor: Intervertebral disc prosthesis and instruments for locating same. US patent 3,875,595, April 8, 1975.
68. Edeland HG: Suggestions for a total elasto-dynamic intervertebral disc prosthesis. Biomater Med Devices Artif Organs 9:65–72, 1981.
69. Monson GL, inventor: Synthetic intervertebral disc prosthesis. US patent 4,863,477, September 5, 1989.
70. Frey O, Koch R, Planck HMF, inventors: Joint endoprosthesis. US patent 4,932,969, June 12, 1990.
71. Strong MD, inventor: Method of determining the quality of a crimped electrical connection. US patent 5,197,186, March 30, 1993.
72. Baumgartner W, inventor: Intervertebral prosthesis. US patent 5,171,280, December 15, 1992.
73. Fuhrmann G, Gross U, Kaden B, et al, inventors: Intervertebral disk endoprosthesis. US patent 5,002,576, March 26, 1991.
74. Monteiro, Spanish Patent 2094077, 1997.
75. Krapiva PI, inventor: Disc replacement method and apparatus. US patent 5,645,597, July 8, 1997.
76. Gauchet, World Patent 0035387, 2000.
77. Minda and Schmidt, European Patent 1157675, 2001.
78. Weber and Da Silva, World Patent 0190786, 2001.
79. Kennedy JP: From thermoplastic elastomers to designed biomaterials. J Polymer Sci Part A: Polymer Chemistry 43:2951–2963, 2005.
80. Carl A, Ledet E, Yuan H, Sharan A: New developments in nucleus pulposus replacement technology. Spine J 4:325–329, 2004.
81. Schneider PG, Oyen R: Surgical replacement of the intervertebral disc. First communication: replacement of lumbar discs with silicon-rubber. Theoretical and experimental investigations (author's transl). Z Orthop Ihre Grenzgeb 112:1078–1086, 1974.
82. Schneider PG, Oyen R: Proceedings: Disk displacement. Experimental studies—clinical consequences. Z Orthop Ihre Grenzgeb 112:791–792, 1974.
83. Kuntz JD, inventor: Intervertebral disc prosthesis. US patent 4,349,921, September 21, 1982.
84. Marcolongo and Lowman, World Patent 0132100, 2001.
85. Banks, World Patent 0112107, 2001.
86. Kotani Y, Abumi K, Shikinami Y, et al: Artificial intervertebral disc replacement using bioactive three-dimensional fabric: design, development, and preliminary animal study. Spine 27:929–935, 2002.
87. Willert HG: Reactions of the articular capsule to wear products of artificial joint prostheses. J Biomed Mater Res 11:157–164, 1977.
88. Stubstad JA, Urbaniak JR, Kahn P, inventors: Prosthesis for spinal repair. US patent 3,867,728, February 25, 1975.
89. Studer and Schärer, European Patent 1157876, 2001.
90. Duance VC, Crean JK, Sims TJ, et al: Changes in collagen cross-linking in degenerative disc disease and scoliosis. Spine 23:2545–2551, 1998.
91. Crean JK, et al: Matrix metalloproteinases in the human intervertebral disc: role in disc degeneration and scoliosis. Spine 22:2877–2884, 1997.
92. Crevensten G, Walsh AJ, Ananthakrishnan E, et al: Intervertebral disc cell therapy for regeneration: mesenchymal stem cell implantation in rat intervertebral discs. Ann Biomed Eng 32:430–434, 2004.
93. Lotz JC, Kim AJ: Disc regeneration: why, when, and how. Neurosurg Clin N Am 16:657–663, vii, 2005.

CHAPTER 3

# Classification of Spine Arthroplasty Devices

**Karin Büttner-Janz**

## KEY POINTS

- Numerous devices for arthroplasty of the lumbar and cervical spine have been developed notably in the past 10 years, which are classified in this chapter according to main categories and subcategories.
- A definite classification of the devices following clinical indications is not possible yet because of missing data and clinical experience. However, the present knowledge about biomechanics and derived thereof of clinical effectiveness of devices is being critically carried together as a fundament for a classification based on indications.
- The five main categories of the classification are theoretically aimed at uniform topographic regions of the lumbar and cervical spine. The three categories for dorsal implantation so far pertain only to the lumbar spine, and for the cervical spine, nucleus replacement is used only to a small degree.
- Because clinical long-term objectives preferentially stand in the foreground, the main categories and subcategories of spine arthroplasty devices are listed according to the materials and material combinations, implant designs, biomechanical principles, and kinds of application with respect to the devices.
- By using this classification, all presently available and probably all future devices can be classified, although it will be need to be determined whether a sixth main category for the replacement of the complete functional spinal unit will have to be added.

## INTRODUCTION

The constantly increasing number of spine arthroplasty devices allows for no complete overview of implants and materials that are already being clinically applied for the preservation of spinal motion. In this chapter, the majority of the presently known devices are dwelled on as much such as to use and explain their major characteristics for the classification of the respective implant or material groups. For this chapter, we requested that 60 companies complete a questionnaire. Twenty-one of these companies responded. The author's personal experience with motion preservation devices over 25 years also aided in the evaluation of implants and materials as well as coherences.

## DEFINITION

The term spine arthroplasty refers to a replacement in the region of the spine, by which a motion is achieved ("arthro" = joint, "plasty" = replacement). The common criteria of all devices for spine arthroplasty are their respective implant design and material characteristic for a repair, preservation, or improvement of function of the cervical or lumbar functional spinal unit (FSU), including motion. The term implant is used for a replacement with a specific design, and the term material is used for substances including their characteristics. Device is the generic term for both. FSU is used synonymously for spinal motion segment.

## ANATOMY AND BIOMECHANICS

The intervertebral disc and the facet joints of the same motion segment together generate a three-joint complex. This functional unit of a spinal motion segment and its dependence on the biomechanical loads differs from the biomechanics of the hip or knee joint.

The intervertebral discs increase in height from cranial to caudal and are mostly higher ventrally than dorsally in the cervical and lumbar spine, thus resulting in a ventrally open intervertebral angle. During the load transfer within an intact intervertebral disc, the nucleus pulposus with its high internal pressure protects the annulus fibrosus against overloading. With its internal pressure, the nucleus pulposus on the one hand maintains the distance between the vertebral bodies, and on the other hand, it firmly holds them together because the pressure acting on the annulus fibrosus strains the lamellae of the fibrous ring going from vertebra to vertebra.[1] The nucleus pulposus thus secures the intervertebral distance and the height of the foramina intervertebralia, as well as part of the stability of the FSU.

The annulus fibrosus functions by limiting all segmental movement, including rotation; it also modulates range of motion. The annulus fibrosus thus has a strong influence on the quality of the segmental motion and the stability of the spinal motion segment. The facet joints and the ligaments of the spine (particularly the ventral and dorsal longitudinal ligament and the muscles) also have an influence on the stability.

During movement of adjacent vertebrae, the intact intervertebral disc adjusts to the change of the distance between vertebral bodies by mass movements within the nucleus pulposus, resulting in the intervertebral inclinations. Depending on the age of the person, the disposition for degeneration, the spinal topography, the functional loads, and other factors, the range of motion of different functional spinal units of the spine differ in magnitude. There are, however, mean values for the segmental extension, flexion, lateral bending, and axial rotation for the cervical as well as the lumbar spine.[2,3] These mean values for extension, flexion, lateral bending, and axial rotation vary up to 2.5-fold in the caudal motion segments of the cervical spine and up to 8.5-fold in the caudal motion segments of the lumbar spine.

The sagittal position of the facets differs for the cervical spine compared with the lumbar spine and has an effect on the extent of mobility, especially axial rotation. In the lumbar spine, the mean facet joint angle in the transversal plane increases from 25 to 53 degrees from L1-L2 to L5-S1[3] as evidence for the action of facet joints in resisting shear forces. At the same time, the position of the center of rotation changes.

Whereas the facet joints are real joints, the intervertebral discs do not have the typical anatomic structures of a joint despite their mobility. Phylogenetically, only a limited morphologic adaptation to the upright human gait took place. This can be seen in physiologic changes to the aging intervertebral discs and the high rate of morbidity of the cervical and lumbar spine worldwide. The closed functional interaction of an intervertebral disc with the facet joints of the same motion segment can be seen in corresponding degenerative changes of the facet joints as a result of degeneration of an intervertebral disc with the decreased height of the intervertebral space. Conversely, a resection of dorsally stabilizing spinal structures, including parts of the facet joints, leads to higher loads and in the long term degeneration of the intervertebral disc at the same level.

The physiologic curve of the spine from cervical to lumbosacral can produce damping, or shock absorption, for the spine during load transfer. However, in many cases with degenerative changes this function no longer exists because of the erect position of the lumbar or cervical spine. This reactive adaptation leads to the question of the importance of a damping function of the human spine. Relief of the strain of the facet joints by virtue of a craniocaudal damping caused by the intervertebral disc is not given and not necessary when the facet joints are in a vertical position, as is the case in the lumbar spine. Comparative consideration of the construction of intervertebral discs of quadrupeds also shows characteristics of damping, although there is no vertical spinal load.[4] Anatomically and phylogenetically, there is no relevance to the shock absorption function for a load relieving of facet joints of same level or of neighboring intervertebral discs and facet joints given. Therefore the integrated damping function of an intervertebral disc is rather to be seen as a prerequisite for intervertebral mobility. However, vibration loads may cause a malfunction in the region of the intervertebral disc in humans.[5] With respect to all 23 intervertebral discs of the human body, the loss of one shock absorber should not affect the vibration transferred into adjacent levels. Putz[6] writes that intervertebral discs absorb shock only to a limited degree.

## BACKGROUND OF MOTION PRESERVATION DEVICES

Motion preservation devices can directly influence the biomechanical function of the motion segment depending on their design, material, the region of the spine intended for the implantation, and the place of implantation into the FSU. The biomechanical functioning of the spinal motion segment may, in turn, have short- or long-term effects on the patient's symptoms and clinical progress. Depending on the effect on the FSU, the devices can also influence adjacent and other distant segments with respect to their own mechanics or material characteristics.[7]

Owing to the complex structure of the FSU, the high functional loads, the different degrees of degenerative changes with different, large pathologic significance, and numerous individual influences, motion preservation devices have been developed and implanted in patients for many years. The ideal case should lead to a normalization of the complete FSU, with positive effects on the adjacent segments. The complexity of the spinal motion segment, and the not finalized trial and probation of spinal devices can be seen not only in the different approaches within the FSU but also in the different methods for the treatment of degenerative spinal disorders. On the one hand, the still limited knowledge about the lumbar and cervical FSU in connection with motion preserving devices and, on the other hand, the lack of data on long-term outcomes after the insertion of the different implants and materials are reflected in this relationship.

## OVERVIEW OF MOTION PRESERVATION DEVICES

At present, there is no precise delineation of the groups of motion preservation devices according to anatomic, biomechanical, and clinical criteria. The objective of this chapter is to present a classification of known devices and those assessed as feasible, preferentially those that have already been used in humans.

The devices are classified according to

- The spinal region being treated;
- The morphologic structure within the spine that is being replaced;
- The material or materials from which the device is made;
- The type of mechanical construction, including the primary and secondary mechanism of fixation;
- The biomechanical effect of the device within the FSU;
- The approach to the spine by which the device is implanted; and
- The clinical indication for which the device is used.

Previously, motion preservation devices for the spine were categorized according to the type of replacement, such as

- Total disc replacement (TDR) of the cervical and lumbar spine;
- Nucleus replacement;
- Posterior dynamic stabilization;
- Facet joint replacement.

The classification of spine arthroplasty devices developed in this chapter is primarily categorized by

- The topographic structure of the FSU to be replaced;
- The extent of degenerative changes;
- Biomechanical principles; and
- The design and material composition of the device.

As far as is possible, specific subcategories will be developed for the main categories in the classification to increase the understanding of the devices and materials.

## Total Di

This cat ... al and lur ... te function ... ic- tion of t ... *us plates* in ... lso belongi ... tic plates o

Mot ... ing require

1. Physiologic mobility, in ... gic translation;
2. Re-creation and preservation of the distance within the intervertebral space, as in the adjacent intervertebral disc;
3. Stabilization, including prevention of micro-instabilities;
4. Damping of load transfer, so there is no hindrance of the three major tasks.

Physiologic mobility is different in its range of motion in the lumbar and cervical spine with respect to the mean extension, flexion, lateral bending, and axial rotation. During extremes of movement, there should be no nonphysiologic apposition of the adjacent vertebral bodies. The translation is greater in the cervical spine than in the lumbar spine.

Intervertebral height should be restored without hyperdistraction, and orientated at the height of the adjacent intervertebral space.

The facet joints as part of the "three-joint complex", have to be considered in all requirements of total disc replacements, including the physiologic range of motion and avoidance of hypermobilities and microinstabilities.

The increased load on the lumbar spine increases the risk that the initial height of the compressible elastic implants will degenerate, resulting in a decrease of the intervertebral height. In this situation, segmental hypermobility and destabilization may occur.

Under the main category of TDR, there are three subcategories: functional three-component prostheses, functional two-component prostheses, and functional one-component prostheses (Table 3–1).

### Functional Three-Component Prostheses

Functional three-component prostheses for total disc replacement have two articulation surfaces as their main characteristic. The CHARITÉ Artificial Disc (DePuy Spine, Inc., Raynham, MA) is the first prosthesis with the aim of the total replacement of the intervertebral disc. The device was developed in 1982 in Berlin/Germany.[8] The CHARITÉ prosthesis has a cranial and caudal symmetric articulation surface composed of the sliding core of a ball-and-socket type and two symmetric articulation surfaces of the prosthetic plates fixed to the two vertebral bodies. The prosthesis is specifically designed for implantation into the lumbar spine. The three components of the prosthesis with metal-polyethylene articulating surfaces allow a translation within the motion segment that is relatively well adapted to physiologic conditions. The prosthesis is constrained during extension and flexion, and during lateral bending, because the metal and polyethylene surfaces may come into contact. During axial rotation, it is unconstrained. The motion amplitudes in all planes are not in the physiologic extent, so that after a balanced implantation of the prosthesis, hypermobility with a higher stress on adjacent spinal structures, including the facet joints, may result, especially during axial rotation. There are indications that the facet joints will undergo postoperative degeneration at same level over the long term.[9] The very limited elastic characteristics of the polyethylene result in a minimal damping function of the prosthesis. In summary, the CHARITÉ prosthesis completely replaces the cartilaginous plates and the nucleus pulposus. However, the functions of the annulus fibrosus of a natural intervertebral disc are not reproduced by the device (Fig. 3–1).

**TABLE 3–1. Total Disc Replacement**

| |
|---|
| A. Functional three-component prostheses |
| B. Functional two-component prostheses |
| C. Functional one-component prostheses |

A modified CHARITÉ disc is in development with lateral anchoring spikes on the prosthetic plates. Other functional three-component prostheses such as the Mobidisc and Mobidisc C (LDR, Troyes, France), the Kineflex and Kineflex|C (Spinal Motion, Inc., Mountainview, CA), the Activ-L (Aesulap Spine, Tuttlingen, Germany), the Dynardi (Zimmer Spine, Minneapolis, MN), the Secure-C (Globus Medical, Inc., Audubon, PA), and the Baguera (International Center Cointrin, Geneva, Switzerland) also function according to the ball-and-socket principle and also partly replace a normal intervertebral disc, with numerous differences in design, in the multiplicity of components, in the material, the saving of the sliding core, and in mechanism for fixation of the prosthetic plates to the vertebral bodies. In some devices a metal-to-metal contact of prosthetic components may occur at maximal ranges of motion.

The Kineflex and the Kineflex|C have metal-metal bearing surfaces, with the mobile core being held by a retention ring of the prosthetic plates. All components are made of cobalt chrome. There is one core height for the lumbar spine and one core height for the cervical spine, but there are many different end plates. Lumbar lordosis is achieved by angled inferior plates (Figs. 3–2 and 3–3).

In the case of the Dynardi (Dynamic Artificial Disc), the osseous end plates of the vertebral bodies have to be adjusted to the partially convex shape of the prosthetic. The two symmetric sliding surfaces of the prosthesis consist of ball-and-socket articulation

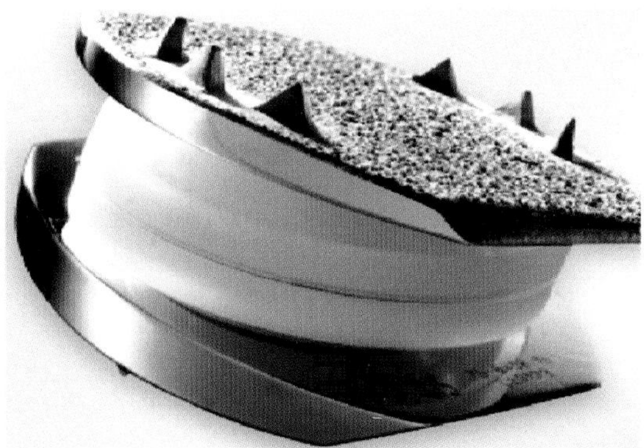

■ **FIGURE 3–1.** CHARITÉ Artificial Disc.

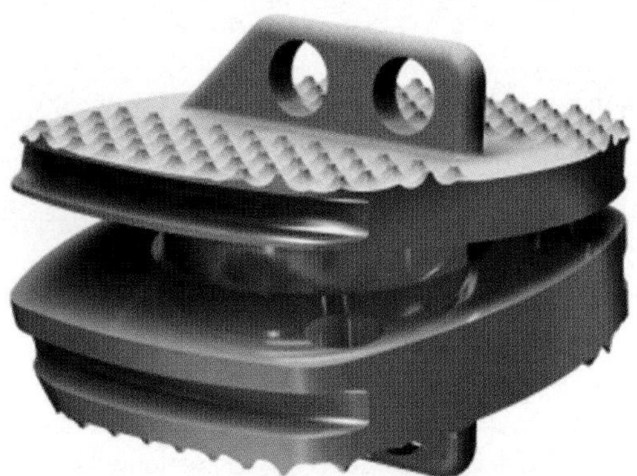

■ FIGURE 3–2. Kineflex|C.

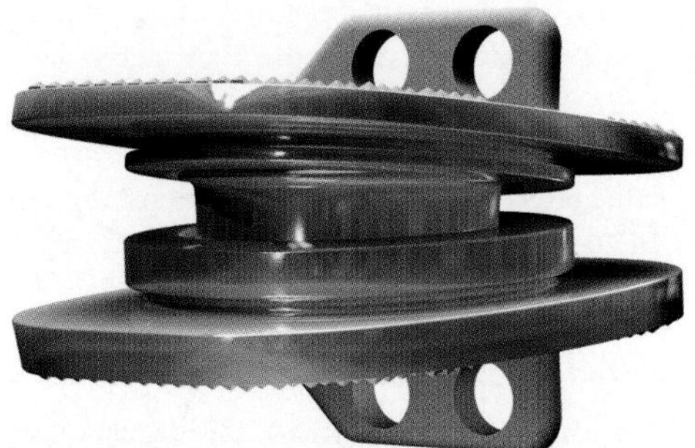

■ FIGURE 3–3. Kineflex.

surfaces. A central pin within the plates and corresponding holes in the sliding core prevent luxation of the insert. The kinetic center is dorsally displaced. The first implantation of this prosthesis was performed in 2006 (Fig. 3–4).

The Secure-C prosthesis differs from the biarticular ball-and-socket type; it allows a greater extension and flexion compared with lateral bending, because along with a cranial ball-and-socket sliding surface, a second sliding surface caudally is present in the shape of a cylindrical segment.

The sliding core of the Mobidisc shows, added to the ball-and-socket surface, an additional plane sliding surface that includes a limitation of axial rotation. However, it is not suited for a limitation of rotation of the prosthesis because the ball-and-socket surface allows an unlimited axial rotation. The same basic biomechanical principle also applies to the Baguera, where a damping is integrated. It results from a cavity between the PE-sliding core

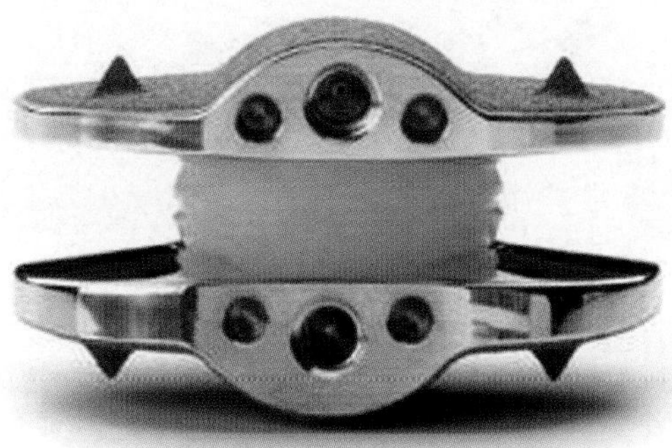

■ FIGURE 3–4. Dynardi.

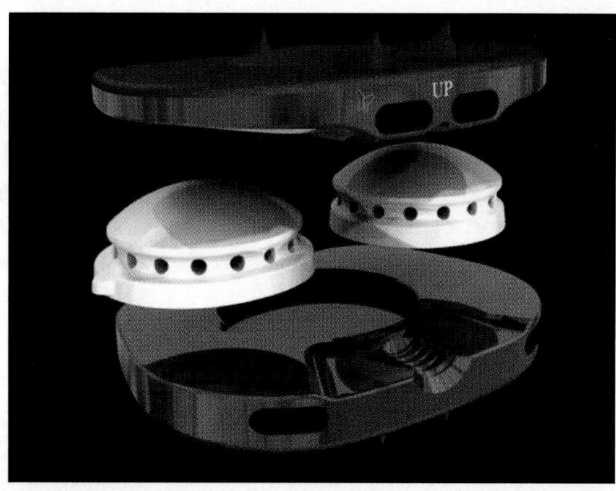


■ FIGURE 3–5. Baguera L (with two versions of the sliding core).

and the lower prosthetic plate as well as from the design of the sliding core itself. The prosthetic plates are composed of a TiAlV alloy (Figs. 3–5 and 3–6).

### Functional Two-Component Prostheses

Functional two-component prostheses have one articulation surface as their major characteristic. The first functional two-component prosthesis with the aim of a total replacement of the intervertebral disc is the ProDisc-L (Synthes, West Chester, PA) for the lumbar spine. The first model of this device was developed in the '80s after the CHARITÉ prosthesis. Approximately 15 years later, after modifications of the prosthesis, the ProDisc-C (Synthes, West Chester, PA) for the cervical spine was developed and the first implantation was performed in 2002. Both prostheses have a ball-and-socket articulation surface in the combination polyethylene-metal and a keel anchor of the plates (Figs. 3–7 and 3–8).

The major biomechanical difference between subcategory A prostheses and subcategory B prostheses is the constant center of rotation of subcategory B prostheses with its differing biomechanics, including segmental translation and load on facet joints. Only the results of long-term clinical studies can clarify whether the biomechanical differences will result in different treatment outcomes. Additional characteristics of the individual prostheses, such as differing radii of the ball-and-socket articulation surfaces or the position of the kinetic center of the prostheses, will also produce physiologic effects.

Other subcategory B prostheses are the Maverick (Medtronic Sofamor Danek, Inc., Memphis, TN), FlexiCore (SpineCore Inc.,

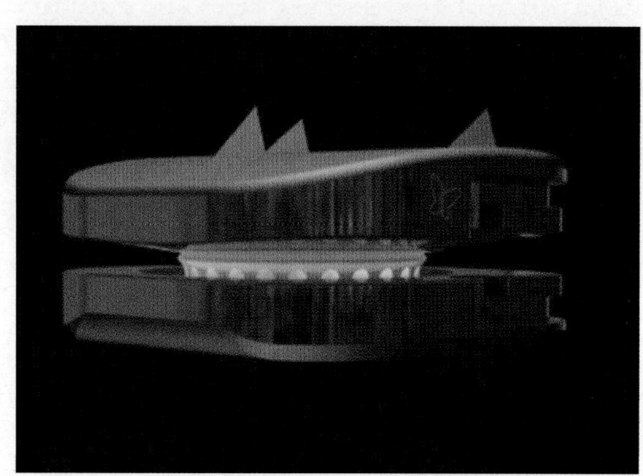

■ FIGURE 3–6. Baguera C.

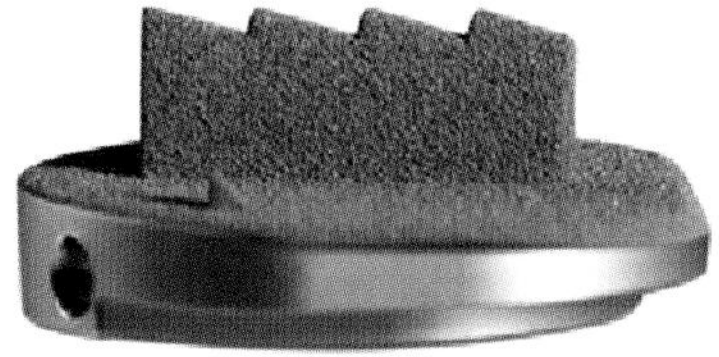

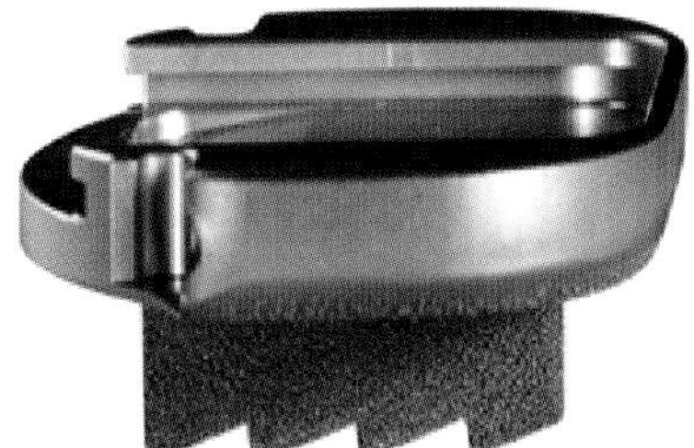

■ **FIGURE 3–7.** ProDisc-L.

Summit, NJ), Cervicore (Stryker Spine, Summit, NJ), PCM (Cervitech, Inc., Rockaway, NJ), DISCOVER (DePuy Spine, Raynham, MA), Prestige (Medtronic Sofamor Danek, Memphis, TN) and Discocerv (Scient'x USA, Inc., Maitland, FL). The Maverick device with the first metal-metal sliding partners in a TDR has a dorsal center of rotation, adapted to lumbar kinetics. The first two-component TDR with an integrated (stiff) limitation of rotation resulting from an internal stop of metallic prosthetic components is the FlexiCore. This prosthesis for the lumbar spine has no translation. The Prestige, which is used in the cervical spine, has an articulation principle that differs from the ball-and-socket principle. It has a ventrally extended socket to achieve a greater translation. The CerviCore, being a metal-metal prosthesis, completely differs from the partly spherical shape of the articulation partners, with the aim of

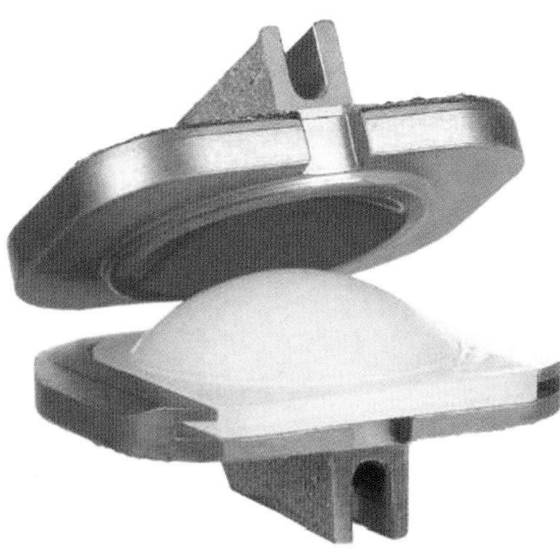

■ **FIGURE 3–8.** ProDisc-C.

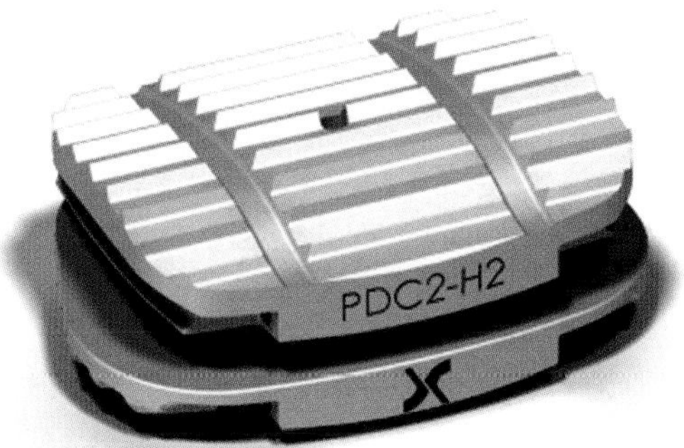


■ **FIGURE 3–9.** Discocerv.

approximating physiologic mobility. In addition to the sliding partner polyethylene-metal and metal-metal for the cervical spine, there are also ceramic-ceramic articulation surfaces. An example of a device with this type of articulation is the Discocerv, which was first implanted in 1999. The upper convex ceramic surface consists of alumina, and the lower cup consists of zirconia (Fig. 3–9).

In comparison with the ball-and-socket prostheses, different radii lead to different material loads in the finite element model.[10] For example, the DISCOVER device presents material innovations in TDRs with highly cross-linked ultra high-molecular-weight polyethylene (UHMWPE) for the core and the bioactively coated TiAlV plates that result in improved postoperative radiographic diagnostics (Fig. 3–10).

More material improvements as well as new materials, material combinations, and coatings, including poly-ether-ether-ketone (PEEK) and carbon, are being developed.

The biomechanics of presently known prostheses of subcategory B enables a partial replacement of a natural intervertebral disc, depending on different adaptations of the prosthesis for the simulation of the physiologic conditions. The development of modular prostheses started with the porous coated motion (PCM) disc. This prosthetic system includes a constrained version that eliminates translation.

All sliding surfaces of the prostheses of subcategories A and B are meant to function according to the low-friction principle of the joint components. The ball-and-socket type shows a long-term consistency when an adequate material combination and correct prosthetic implantation are used. This can be seen from the follow-up examinations for the CHARITÉ prosthesis.[11,12] Likewise, the tribological

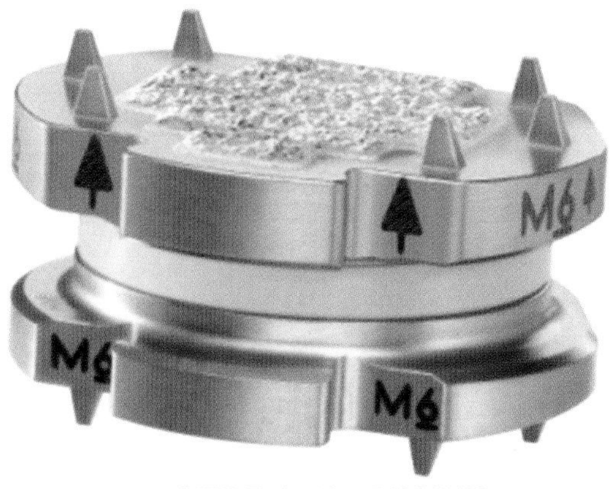


■ **FIGURE 3–10.** DISCOVER.

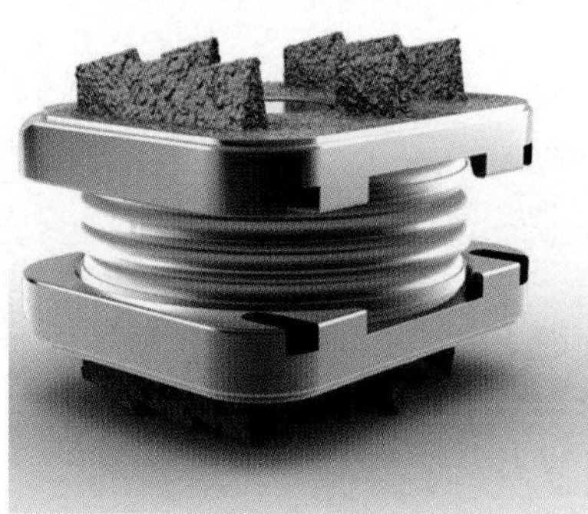

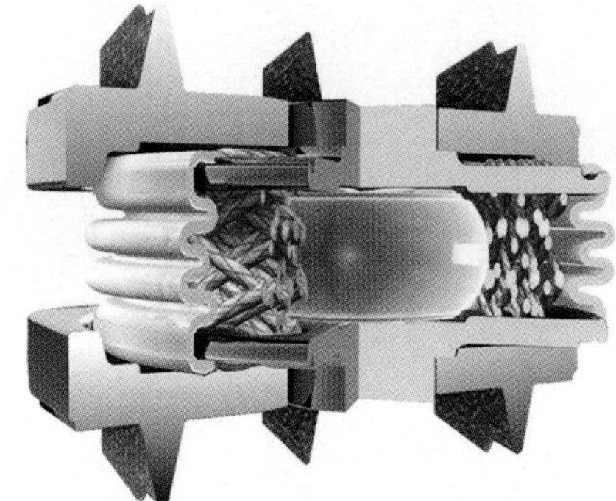

■ **FIGURE 3–11.** M6.

pairing Metasul (metal-metal) in total hip replacement has proven successful over the long term.[13] Compared with the sliding surfaces in total hip replacements, the Maverick and Kineflex have spiral-shaped grooves on the convex surfaces of their sliding partners.

In summary, the development of functional three- and two-component TDRs is not complete because despite a sufficient assortment of components and with the correct selection of components, exact implantation of prostheses with the existing prosthetic models, and depending on its design, a functional overload, such as hypermobility within the motion segment, may result in nonphysiologic stress on the facet joints. As a result, present long-term comparison studies of patients with fusion surgeries and patients with implanted prostheses are not definitely suited to prove the qualitative difference between these two treatment alternatives. It cannot even be ruled out that patients with implanted TDRs of present designs may profit less in the long term than patients with fusion surgeries. The time has come to develop and implant TDRs that have a natural mobility to mimic the intervertebral disc, so that the spinal motion segment will be physiologically replaced in the area of the intervertebral disc.

### Functional One-Component Prostheses

In this subcategory of prostheses, the device allows physiologic mobility including the damping function, that is, a total disc replacement. These are compact prostheses, so there are no articulation surfaces.

There is compressible material between two prosthetic plates. Polycarbonate polyurethane elastomere is used preferentially. The functions result from the material characteristics. If the material combination of each compact prosthesis is the same throughout, differing mean segmental ranges of motion for each direction as well as between cervical and lumbar spine cannot be achieved. Therefore, physiologic motion resulting from the material characteristics is not possible.

A forerunner of this type of prosthesis, with a low number of implantations in the 1980s, was the AcroFlex (DePuy Spine Inc., Raynham, MA) for the lumbar spine. Its development halted owing to problems with the material. These problems were dislocation of the material between the titanium plates and, thus, dislocation of the motion segment. Representative of subcategory C prostheses is the Bryan prosthesis (Medtronic Sofamor Danek, Memphis, TN) for the cervical spine, the construction of which allows function by virtue of the inclusion of polyurethane between two titanium plates. The *M6* (SpinalKinetics, Sunnyvale, CA) is also being applied for the cervical spine, with an elastomeric polymer made of polycarbonate polyurethane in the center and a soft limitation of motion including rotation through an additional peripheral mesh of UHMWPE woven fibers. A peripheral polymer gasket prevents tissue ingrowth and contains wear debris, which is also described for the Bryan prosthesis (Fig. 3–11).

The Physio-L (Nexgen Spine, Whippany, NJ) was developed for the lumbar spine. It consists of a multidurometer elastomeric core constructed using different grades of polycarbonate polyurethane between the two prosthetic plates of titanium (Fig. 3–12).

The Freedom Lumbar Disc (AxioMed Spine Corporation, Cleveland, OH) was also developed for the lumbar spine. A viscoelastic polymer core is positioned between the two titanium plates (Fig. 3–13).

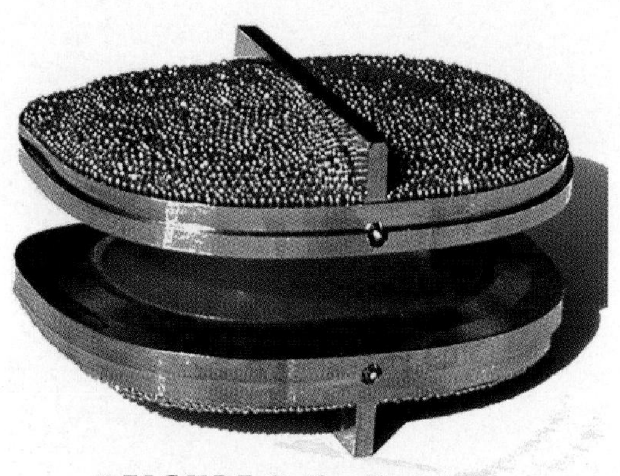

■ **FIGURE 3–12.** Physio-L.

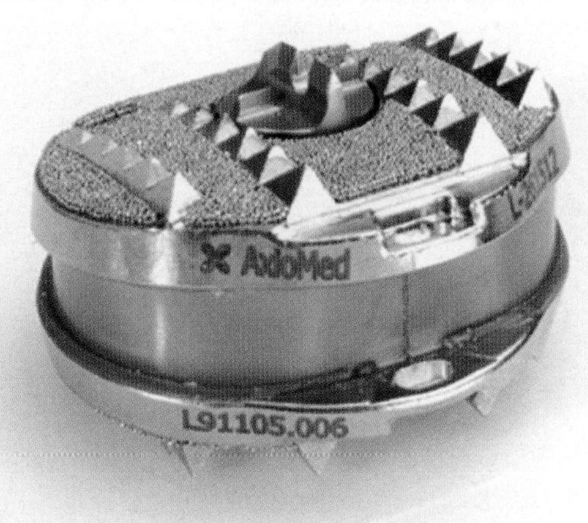


■ **FIGURE 3–13.** Freedom Lumbar Disc.

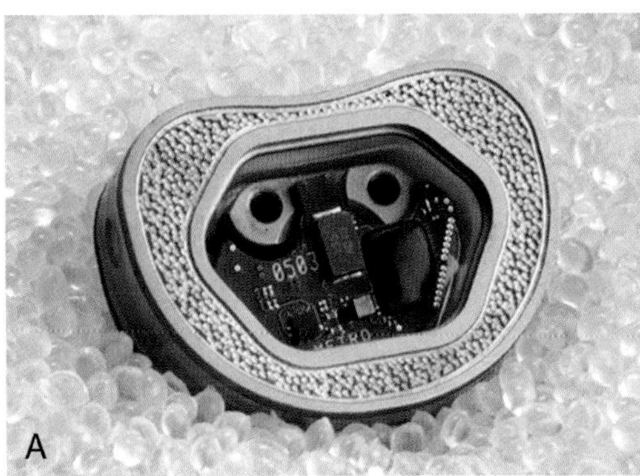
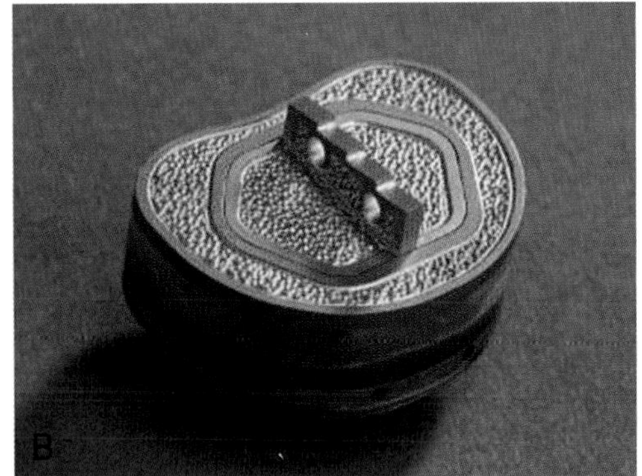

■ FIGURE 3–14. **A** and **B,** Theken eDisc.

The Theken eDisc (Theken Disc, Akron, OH) for the lumbar and cervical total disc replacement are also single-component discs, made of an elastomeric design between two titanium plates. The lumbar disc is additionally planned with electronics for the measurement of forces (Fig. 3–14A and B).

Further prostheses of subcategory C are the CAdisc-L (Ranier Technology Limited, Cambridge, England) and the CAdisc-C (Ranier Technology Limited, Cambridge, England) made of polycarbonate polyurethane as compact versions without metal plates. Short-term fixation should be achieved by the compliant nature of the device applying a force to the vertebrae under low preload conditions. For long-term stabilization, a combination of a macrotexture, a microtexture, and a CaP coating that works like hydroxyapatite is alleged (Fig. 3–15).

On the whole, the extent of elasticity in compact prostheses counteracts the stability and ultimately the intervertebral height, decisively depending on the biomechanical load on the spine. The subcategory C prostheses still have to prove their reliability in the clinical long term internally as implant material as well as in terms of the preservation of the height of the intervertebral space and of the segment stabilization.

The mechanism of fixation of all three main categories of prostheses for the total replacement of an intervertebral disc shows, for primary safe fixation, the two main versions—spikes and keel—in different expressions. Some prostheses have additional screws or special shaped prosthetic surfaces corresponding with the vertebral bodies, for example, ridges or convex rough-coated surfaces. The long-term fixation takes place through a bioactive coating with different chemical compositions.

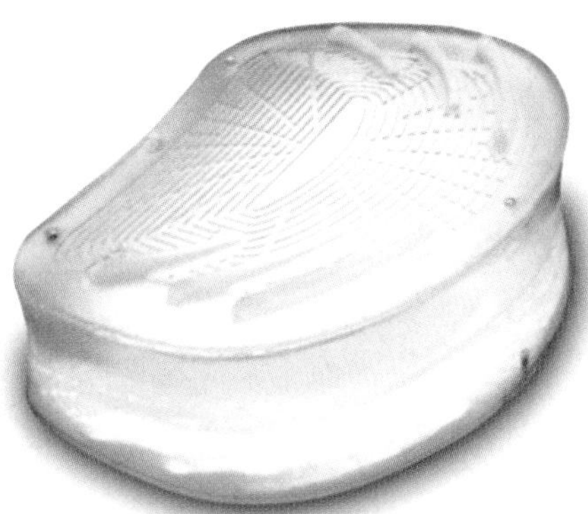

■ FIGURE 3–15. CAdisc-L.

All clinically approved TDRs displace fusion surgeries and have to be implanted via a ventral approach. The contraindications are always to be considered. After implantation, TDRs lead to pain reduction immediately postoperatively, thus bringing a great benefit to patients. The first prospective randomized comparative studies between different TDRs are being carried out (Kineflex in comparison to the CHARITÉ Artificial Disc).

To reduce potential complications, TDRs intended for a ventrolateral or lateral approach to the lumbar spine are being developed. The question arises for prostheses of a ball-and-socket type as to whether in the postoperative course a parallel positioning of adjacent vertebral body end plates in the anteroposterior view can be achieved if a small intervertebral space existed preoperatively, the extensive preparation only took place from one lateral side, and in addition, there was an intervertebral distraction.

Prostheses for a total replacement of the intervertebral disc of the lumbar spine intended for implantation from a dorsal approach are also being developed. In this case, it needs to be considered whether a potential complication caused through a ventral approach should be exchanged by a definitely arising approach morbidity resulting from a dorsal approach. A dorsal prosthetic implantation is not possible without extensive resection of muscles, bone, ligamentous structures, and possibly even parts of the facet joints, resulting in instability. Furthermore, there is a greater risk of postoperative subsidence of the implant as a result of a lesser surface area for load transfer of the dorsally introduced prostheses.

In summary, further developments are necessary for a TDR to completely replace the human intervertebral disc of the lumbar and cervical spine, as a physiologic partner within the three-joint complex.

## Nucleus Replacement

Spherical prostheses made of steel or vitalium were implanted approximately 40 to 50 years ago into the cervical and lumbar spine from the dorsal approach. Probably because of the approach, these prostheses were retrospectively described as nucleus replacements.

However, despite considerable design differences, there are no clear biomechanical differences among present total disc replacements. It was soon realized that the surface area for the load transfer of the spheres was too small, leading to a large degree of subsidence into the adjacent vertebrae.[14] Instilling soft materials such as polyurethane[15] and silicon[16] into intervertebral discs is regarded as the predecessor of the present nucleus replacements, although both of these treatment methods were abandoned by the end of the 1970s.

The nucleus pulposus takes about 30% to 50% of the whole area in the cross-section of an intervertebral disc. This surface area is completely replaced by a so-called TDR of the present generation and only partly replaced by various types of nucleus replacements, to different extents. The nucleus replacement of the smallest area can be achieved by injecting a fluid in the early degenerative stages of the intervertebral disc.[17] The fluid, acting as spare material, enters into cleavages within the nucleus pulposus tissue. After changing the consistency of the material, it is intended to reduce or eliminate pain and discomfort resulting from micro-instability.

There is not much time in the course of the painful degeneration of the intervertebral disc to perform optimal nucleus replacement, that is, with the annulus fibrosus still intact. Along with the loss of stability in the region of the nucleus pulposus, there are increased shear forces and higher biomechanical load in the annulus fibrosus, leading to wear and tear of the annulus fibrosus. However, the complete functions of the nucleus pulposus may only be ensured in cooperation with the annulus fibrosus. This leads to the conclusion that the annulus fibrosus should be intact for a nucleus replacement. However, because this is increasingly not the case in the course of intervertebral disc degeneration and TDR is regarded as the final treatment alternative (also because of the risk of the surgical approach), lumbar devices for nucleus replacement are being applied with increasing stiffness, depending on the degree of degeneration of the intervertebral disc, in an attempt to compensate for the lack of stability of the annulus fibrosus. As a result of this nucleus replacement, implants were developed, which show a transition to present TDRs, an example of this being the PEEK-on-PEEK articulating implant NUBAC (Pioneer Surgical Technology, Marquette, MI). However, the consequence of a stiffer nuclear implant is to increase the share of load acting on the central area of the vertebral end plate.

A nucleus replacement may result in adaptations as well as risks that apply to a total replacement of the intervertebral disc, for example, reactions of the vertebral end plates as well as intravertebral subsidence of the device. But there are also other influences that nucleus replacement may have on motion in other planes such as extension, flexion, lateral bending, and rotation. Because of the high biomechanical stress on the intervertebral disc, nucleus implants and replacement materials without specific fixation mechanisms are particularly at risk of postoperative horizontal or vertical dislocation. To reduce the risk of dislocation, developments of mechanism and chemical methods for an intradiscal fixation of the nucleus replacements have already been carried out; further developments with respect to material and implants are still necessary. A stable integration of a nucleus implant or material into the intervertebral space not only increases the indication span, but also increases the indication safety of surgeons clinical application.

The degree of nucleus replacement required depends on the degree of degeneration. However, it can be assumed that with less original nucleus tissue, an increasingly stable or quantitatively more extensive nucleus replacement will be required, also for the protection of the annulus fibrosus.

During the surgical introduction of a device for nucleus replacement, the function of the annulus is impaired depending on the size of the incision. In order to preserve the motion-modulating and motion-stabilizing function of the annulus fibrosus, the approach through the annulus and the incision should be small as possible. The risk of dislocation of a material or implant for nucleus replacement is usually also reduced with a small incision.

The following questions must be answered for a successful application of an implant or material for nucleus replacement:

- What is the indication? Is the procedure intended to restabilize the area, as in the case of an early intervertebral disc degeneration, or is it intended as a prophylactic measure against a postdiscectomy syndrome during microscopic discectomy?
- What is the condition of the annulus fibrosus? Is it suited for the planned device?
- Can the nucleus replacement be safely placed into the intervertebral space, so that it cannot dislocate dorsally toward the adjacent nerves?
- Is the risk of subsidence into the adjacent vertebral bodies so low that the nucleus replacement can be implanted?
- Is it a biocompatible material with strongly delayed resorption?
- Are wear debris from the implant or material itself that may be in contact with the surrounding tissue a concern?

A classification of nucleus replacement devices can be made following different criteria. The loading capacity and physiologic balance of the intervertebral disc within the motion segment are to be improved or normalized, with the expectation of reducing or eliminating the patient's pain. Because there has been no success to produce a complete and permanent conjunction between the implant or material and the surrounding nucleus and/or annulus tissue and the cartilaginous plates, the direct loading capacity of the implant or material is important in relation to the known intradiscal pressures. For the evaluation of the suitability of a material or an implant for nucleus replacement, the consistency of the device may not be considered in comparison to normal nucleus tissue outside any load. Because this is a nucleus replacement aimed at replacing a physiologic nucleus pulposus including the protective function for the present annulus fibrosus, the biomechanically effective consistency of the implant material that withstands the mean intradiscal pressure during everyday activities, or the mean external load that is needed to compress the disc of a functional spinal unit with a physiogically adapted nucleus replacement, is of importance. Based on this definition, a classification of the nucleus replacement is feasible. At present, however, no data are available.

The following subcategories of nucleus replacement are classified according to the kind of application, the protection of materials, substance groups, material characteristics, stiffness of the material, and mechanical criteria (Table 3–2).

The classification focuses on presently known devices for nucleus replacement and brings them into coherent order. Because of the large variety of nucleus replacements, other classifications are also feasible,

**TABLE 3–2. Nucleus Replacement**

A. Injectable, in situ curing materials
1. Uncontained
   a. Hydrogel adhesive (examples: NuCore, BioDisc)
   b. Nonhydrogel nonadhesive (example, Sinux)
2. Contained
   a. Hydrogel (no example at present)
   b. Nonhydrogel (examples: DASCOR, PNR, PDR)

B. Preformed implants
1. Nonarticulating
   a. Hydrogel (examples: PDN-SOLO), Hydraflex, NeuDisc, Aquarelle)
   b. Nonhydrogel (examples: Newcleus, NeoDisc, Regain)
2. Articulating
   a. Same material of components (example: NUBAC)
   b. Different materials of components (no example at present)

for example, according to the degree of degeneration of the motion segment with derived indication for a specific nucleus device. For this approach, spinal diagnostics are necessary with emphasis on the annulus fibrosus so that with the knowledge of its constitution including its stability as well as other factors, the appropriate device can be selected. Tests still need to be conducted on this measure. For an adapted therapy depending on the condition of the motion segment, the composition, load resistance, and other factors of the device must be examined to evaluate their suitability to the patient. If the intervertebral loads could be balanced with the implanted nucleus replacement to reduce or eliminate the patient's pain, a treatment algorithm within the group of different nucleus replacements could be developed.

Following the soft nucleus replacement materials, which were described in 1977 (polyurethane) and 1978 (silicone), the Prosthetic Disc Nucleus (PDN) (Raymedica, Inc., Minneapolis, MN) prosthesis was first implanted in 1996. It comprises a polymeric hydrogel encased in a high-tenacity polyethylene jacket that allows the device to absorb fluid and expand in height.[18] In the meantime, there has been an evolution from the stiff PDN to the PDN-SOLO (Raymedica, Inc., Minneapolis, MN) and lastly HydraFlex (Raymedica, Inc., Minneapolis, MN).

The present group of nucleus replacements varies widely. In the limited context of this chapter, only a few devices can be described. If only the field of spine arthroplasty materials and implants is considered, the treatment of early degeneration of the intervertebral disc begins with injections. The percutaneous computed tomography–guided injection of NuCore (Spine Wave, Inc., Shelton, CT) into the nucleus pulposus has been used.[19] The NuCore Injectable Nucleus is an adhesive, protein polymer that is curable in situ. The components are silk-elastin copolymer solution and diisocyanate cross-linker. NuCore is one of the least stiff materials used in nucleus replacement devices. Biomechanical testing in cadavers has shown that implantation of NuCore restores function and stability to the spine after a destabilizing discectomy procedure (Fig. 3–16).[20]

Another material in the group of injectable, in situ curing materials is the *DASCOR* Disc Arthroplasty Device (Disc Dynamics, Inc., Eden Prairie, MN). It involves the insertion of an in situ–polymerizing polyurethane, cured within a polyurethane balloon in the disc space. This device was first implanted in 2002 through an open procedure that required a 5-mm hole in the annulus (Fig. 3–17).

The NeoDisc (NuVasive, Inc., San Diego, CA) is an implant with a smooth transition to TDR, because it is meant to partially replace the annulus fibrosus and even the ventral longitudinal ligament in the cervical spine. NeoDisc consists of an elastomere core in a polyester annular jacket with anterior flanges for fixation to the anterior surface of adjacent vertebrae.

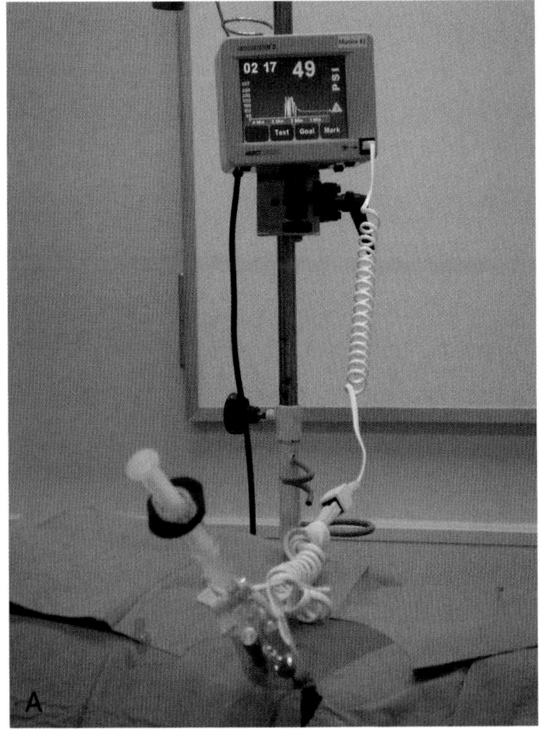


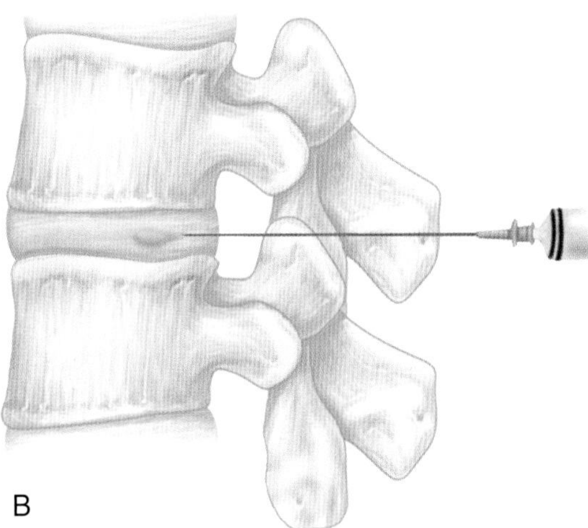


■ **FIGURE 3–16.** **A** and **B,** NuCore injection.

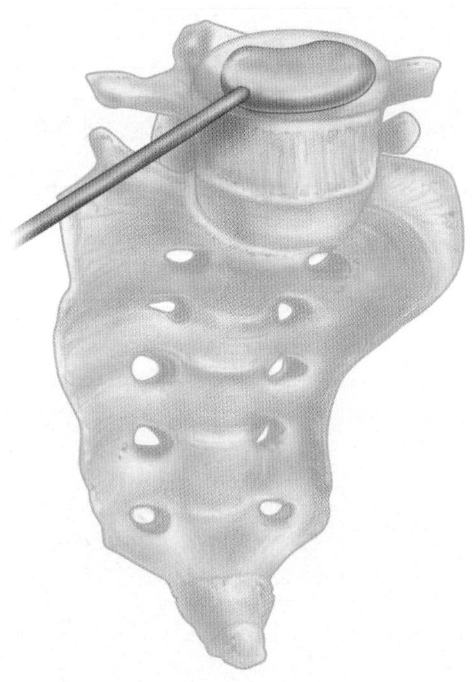

■ FIGURE 3–17. DASCOR.

The Percutaneous Nucleus Replacement (PNR) and Percutaneous Disc Reconstruction (PDR) devices (TranS1, Wilmington, NC) are introduced by the transsacral approach. When this device is implanted, there are vertical screw pistons in vertebral bodies L5 and S1 with an intervertebral disc replacement, including an enclosing balloon lying within the intervertebral space L5-S1.

## Posterior Dynamic Stabilization—Screws and Connectors

The basic principle for dorsal dynamic stabilization is mainly based on screw fixation in adjacent pedicles and vertebral bodies. Because the ventral sections of the spine carry out the segmental transfer of axial load up to about 80%, the replacement seems to be of less importance. In contrast to this, primarily dorsal procedures with the option of function-preserving stabilization may be indicated in cases of dorsal pathologies of the spine. Furthermore, a dorsal dynamic stabilization is particularly beneficial in older patients with a higher rate of morbidity with the anterior approach or decreased bone-loading capacity. In cases of intervertebral disc degeneration, the intervertebral disc remains a source of pain after implantation of dorsal dynamic implants. The implant–bone interface and the material stability are of particular interest because of the different elasticity modules between bone and implant and also because of the biomechanical dorsal strains, especially regarding shear forces. The design of the device influences the load of the implant–bone interface and the load of the implant itself. A balance between the extent of mobility of the implant to avoid an overload of the bone–implant interface and an effective stabilization of the spinal motion segment must be found.

**TABLE 3–3. Posterior Dynamic Stabilization—Screws and Connectors**

A. Mobile screw parts
B. Mobile connectors (beginning from retainer on the screw) and rods made of
   1. Plastic material
   2. Metal
   3. Combination of metal and plastic material
C. Combination of A und B

There are many ways in which dorsal mobility between adjacent vertebrae could be realized, partly under consideration of the COR. The Posterior Dynamic Stabilization classification is based on present knowledge (Table 3–3).

### Mobile Screw Parts

The heads of screws are mobile with respect to the screw piston through a special mechanism.

In the case of the Cosmic Posterior Dynamic System (Ulrich Gm bH & Co. KG, Ulm, Germany), the thread of the screw is connected by a hinge for a permanent movable connection between screw and rod. The complete system allows axial load distribution and prevents any rotation and translation. The device was first implanted in a patient in 2002 (Fig. 3–18).

### Mobile Connectors

#### From Retainer on the Screw—and Rods of Plastic Material

Implants that exclusively have plastic material between the pedicle screws are always less resistant to shear forces, which have to be absorbed up to 80% by the dorsal lumbar spine.

One of the earliest pedicle screw-based devices was the Graf Ligament System (Sem Co., Montrouge, France). This system used braided polyester bands looped around the screws instead of rods with the aim of providing stability while allowing motion. After the spine was exposed and pedicle screws inserted, the bands were connected under applied compressive force between the pedicle screws as a ligamentoplasty.

In 1994, Dynesys (Dynamic Neutralization System for the Spine; Zimmer Spine, Inc., Warsaw, IN) was implanted for the first time as a dorsal dynamic instrumentation, which has cords

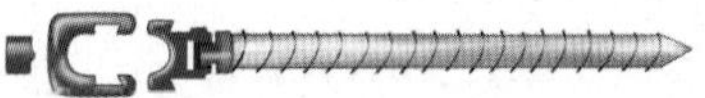
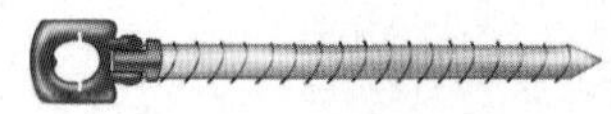
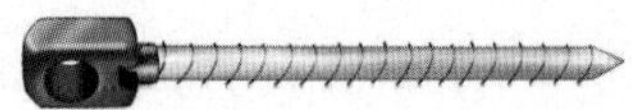

Cosmic screws

■ FIGURE 3–18. Cosmic screws.

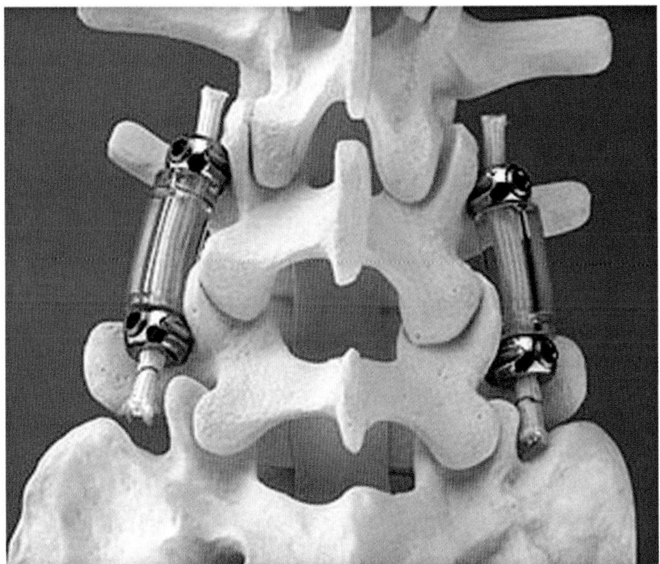

■ **FIGURE 3–19.** Dynesys.

of polyethylene terephthalate with a tube made from polycarbonate urethane slid over them and fixed to two adjacent pedicle screws with nuts. The screws are made of a titanium alloy and are coated with hydroxyapatite if required (Fig. 3–19).

The pedicle-based CD HORIZON LEGACY PEEK Rod (Medtronic Sofamor Danek, Memphis, TN) has been developed as a new generation of rods made of the semi-crystalline thermoplastic polymer PEEK as a semi-rigid alternative to titanium rods. PEEK has a modulus of elasticity between that of cortical and cancellous bone, and it is radiolucent.

#### From Retainer on the Screw—and Rods of Metal

On the one hand, these are rods made of "soft" metal, so that axial deformations of the rods are possible. Furthermore, this group includes rods that have outside notches, such as in a screw thread, and which are therefore shapeable. An example is the semi-rigid AccuFlex system with a double helical cut made within a standard 6.5-mm rod. AccuFlex (Globus Medical, Inc., Audubon, PA) is 50% as stiff as solid rods; it is stiff in anterior shear and rotation but allows motion primarily in the flexion extension mode.

Systems with integrated loop are also counted to this group, for example, the BioFlex System (Bio-Spine Corp., Seoul, Korea).[21] It is based on Nitinol, which is an alloy of nickel and titanium and has various characteristics such as high elasticity and high tensile force, and flexibility or rigidity according to temperature change.

#### From Retainers on the Screw—and Rods as Combination of Metal and Plastic Material

NFlex (N Spine, Inc., San Diego, CA) is a dynamic stabilization system, used with polyaxial titanium pedicle screws and titanium and polycarbonate urethane rods. The system allows an elongation of the posterior elements during spinal flexion and compression during extension. There is a layer of polycarbonate urethane between the titanium core and the pedicle screw attachment that allows a small translation perpendicular to the long axis of the rod. A rotational stop is provided by the titanium core within the piston. The first devices were implanted in 2006 (Fig. 3–20).

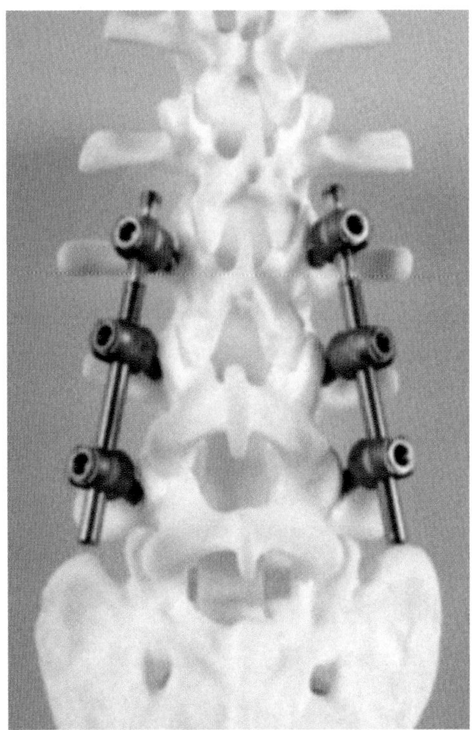

■ **FIGURE 3–20.** NFlex.

The Isobar TTL Dynamic Rod (Scient'x, Maitland, FL) is made of TiAlV alloy, and a dampener is fixed between monoaxial or polyaxial pedicle screws. Stacked washers within the dampening element provide dynamism. The rod allows extension, flexion, and dampening (Fig. 3–21).

The rod of the CD HORIZON AGILE Dynamic Stabilization Device (Medtronic Sofamor Danek, Memphis, TN) is made of a thin rod of TiAlV alloy within a pure titanium rod and a bumper of polycarbonate polyurethane surrounding the thin rod. It is used as single level and adjacent to fusion motion–retaining implant with two different sizes of the kinetic center (Fig. 3–22).

The AXIENT Dynamic Fixation System (Innovative Spinal Technologies, Mansfield, MA) has pedicle screws with polyaxial screw heads and articulating CoCr sliding rods with a component for damping during extension, made of polycarbonate urethane. The implant allows segmental movement with integral stops to avoid excessive motion in extension, flexion, axial rotation, and sagittal translation. This system is described as semiconstrained, and the AXIENT TOTAL Dynamic Fixation System with a greater range of motion is described as unconstrained,

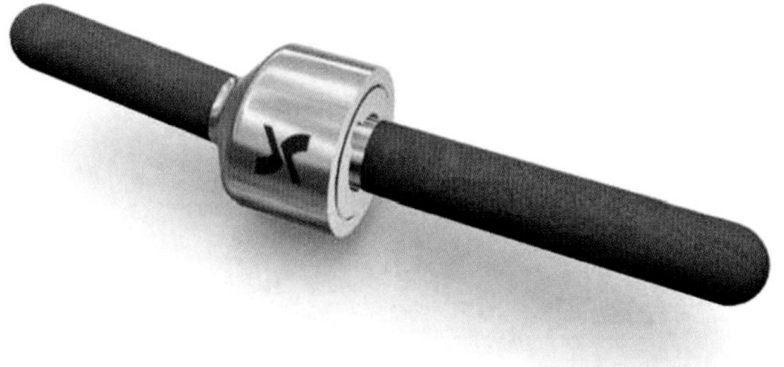

■ **FIGURE 3–21.** Isobar TTL dynamic rod.

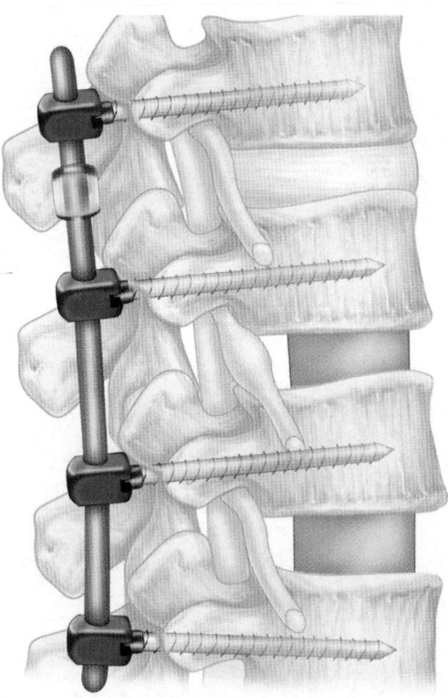

■ **FIGURE 3–22.** CD HORIZON AGILE Dynamic Stabilization Device.

where there is no integral stop of the segmental motion. With the incorporation of rotary bearings in the implants, stress and strain to the bone-screw interface should be reduced (Fig. 3–23).

The Stabilimax NZ (Applied Spine Technologies, New Haven, CT) has a mobility beginning from the retainer of the pedicle screws, described for this region as a ball and socket. The implant uses two independent concentric springs on each side that allow motion in all directions as well as a damping function. The springs are incorporated into the system through connecting rods.

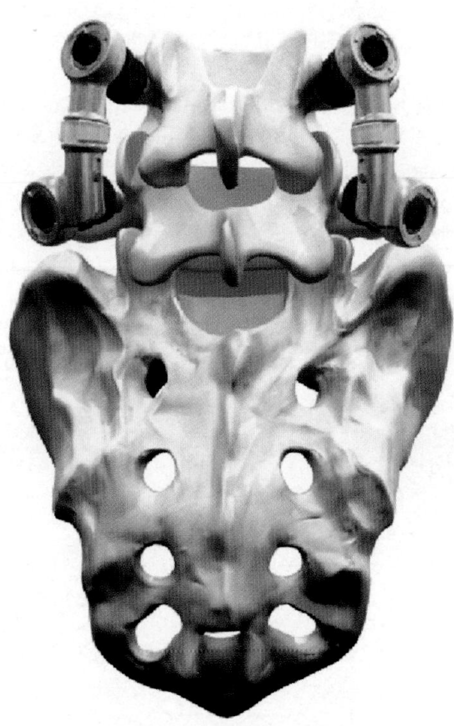

■ **FIGURE 3–23.** AXIENT Dynamic Fixation System.

The Stabilimax NZ is already being classified as a total facet replacement by Khoueir et al.[22]

## Posterior Dynamic Stabilization—Facet Arthroplasty

The function-retaining replacement of the facet joints needs to be viewed critically because the arthritis of these joints usually results from a degeneration of the intervertebral disc. In this case, a sole replacement of the facet joints leaves the intervertebral disc as a pain generator and in a combined total disc and facet joint replacement, the replaced facet joints could be exposed to threshold loads or overloads as the result of nonphysiologic motion amplitudes of currently available TDRs. Depending on the design of the facet joint replacements, a hypermobility of the whole FSU could also result, including an irritation of nerval structures or a subluxation within the FSU. In elderly patients with a severe narrowed spinal canal, the removal of facet joints can be necessary. It must be determined whether these patients would benefit from stabilization with motion preservation or rigid stabilization.

The following classification in subcategories is feasible (Table 3–4).

### Partial Facet Replacement

The smallest device is a replacement with only one component between both facets of a facet joint, which is fixed by a cord through both facets. These devices can be implanted with little resection of body tissue and with little effort. The challenge lies in the constancy of position of this implant, made of metal, between the two facets during extensive segmental motion.

### Total Facet Replacement

#### Metal

The Total Facet Arthroplasty System (TFAS) implant (Archus Orthopedics, Inc., Redmond, WA) totally replaces the facet joints of a motion segment. The system consists of two stems that are fixed in the pedicles and concave discs connected to them, which allow two spherical parts (one on each side) to move on their surfaces. The two spherical parts are connected to the stems in the pedicles of the adjacent vertebra. Because the implant is completely made of metal, there are metal-metal articulating surfaces. The stems have no threading; they are cemented. For the implantation, a full laminectomy including facet resection is necessary.

#### Metal and Plastic Material

The Total Posterior Arthroplasty (TOPS) System (Impliant Spine, Princeton, NJ) is a pedicle screw–based system with a

**TABLE 3–4. Posterior Dynamic Stabilization—Facet Arthroplasty**

A. Partial facet replacement
   1. Plastic material
   2. Metal
   3. Combination of metal and plastic material
B. Total facet replacement
   1. Plastic material
   2. Metal
   3. Combination of metal and plastic material

**TABLE 3–5. Posterior Dynamic Stabilization—Interspinous Implants**

A. Implant with function by itself
   1. Primarily design dependent
   2. Primarily material dependent
B. Spacer without own function
   1. Plastic material
   2. Metal
   3. Combination of metal and plastic material

metal-on-polymer articulation to cushion against hard stops. TOPS is designed for the treatment of spinal stenosis combined with severe facet arthritis. It has been determined that TOPS allows a nearly physiologic range of motion, including sagittal translation.

## Posterior Dynamic Stabilization—Interspinous Implants

The interspinal implants are to serve for foraminal distraction, the off-loading of facets, and the dorsal disc unloading in extension. There are two basic types of interspinous implants: (1) implants whose function results from the design or the material characteristics, and (2) implants that solely act as interspinal spacers without a specific function. Those in the second group are not defined as spine arthroplasty devices. However, there is still a certain segmental motion after implantation even in stiff materials because of the mainly axial load transfer through the intervertebral disc, away from the implant positioning (Table 3–5).

### Implant with Function by Itself

#### Primarily Design Dependent

A major representative of this type of device is the coflex implant (Paradigm Spine, LLC, New York, NY). coflex is a functionally dynamic interspinous implant for levels L1-L5, which is compressible in extension, allows flexion, and has slight rotational stabilization. It is made of a TiAlV alloy. The implant wings can be crimped to achieve sufficient fixation to the spinous processes (Fig. 3–24).

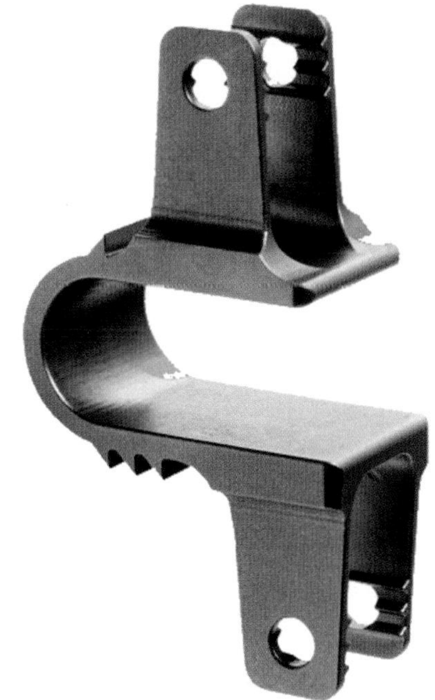

■ **FIGURE 3–24.** coflex.

#### Primarily Material Dependent

The Device for Intervertebral Assisted Motion (DIAM) (Medtronic Sofamor Danek, Memphis, TN) is an H-shaped polyester-covered silicone bumper that is placed between the spinous processes with a mesh band and is sutured to hold it in place.

### Spacer Without Own Function

#### Plastic Material

The Wallis system (Abbott Spine, Inc., Austin, TX) is a rigid interspinous spacer which consists of PEEK and two woven polyester bands, through which the fixation to the spinous processes is achieved. The spacer is suited for a limitation of the extension and flexion, without influence on rotation and lateral bending. The first implantation of the device was performed in 1987; since 2002, a second generation of the implant has been produced (Fig. 3–25).

#### Metal

The X-STOP Interspinous Process Decompression Device (Kyphon, Inc., Sunnyvale, CA) is a two-component titanium implant that fits between the spinous processes of the lumbar spine to limit extension. The first component is implanted next to and under the spinous process, and the second component is placed on the opposite side of the spinous process and is then attached to the first. The supraspinous ligament is retained.

The Superion Spacer (VertiFlex Inc., San Clemente, CA) consists of a titanium alloy and is implanted percutaneously directly from dorsal between two adjacent spinous processes. The stabilization takes place by enfolding of the two wings surrounding the upper and lower spinous process (Fig. 3–26).

#### Combination of Metal and Plastic Material

The In-Space Interspinous Distraction Device (Synthes, West Chester, PA) can be implanted from L1-S1 percutaneously laterally or through the unilateral posterior approach. It is a cylindrical distance holder made from PEEK with wings made from TiAlV alloy for fixation to the spinous processes. The device prevents extension and allows flexion, lateral bending, and rotation. The device was first implanted in 2006 (Fig. 3–27).

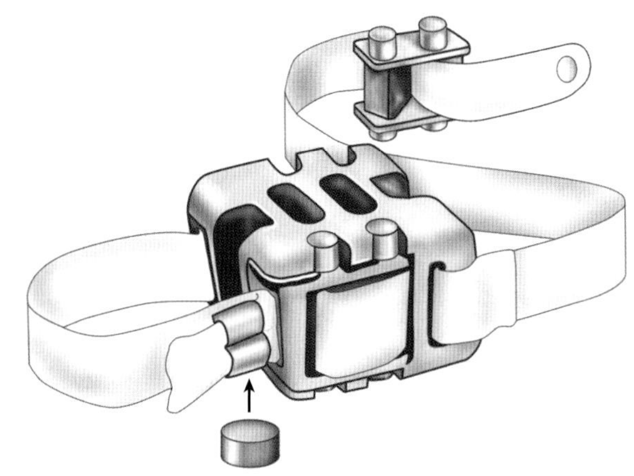

■ **FIGURE 3–25.** Wallis.

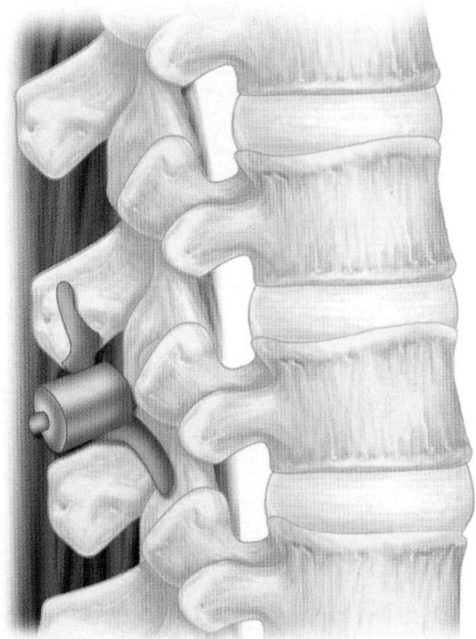

■ **FIGURE 3–26.** Superion spacer.

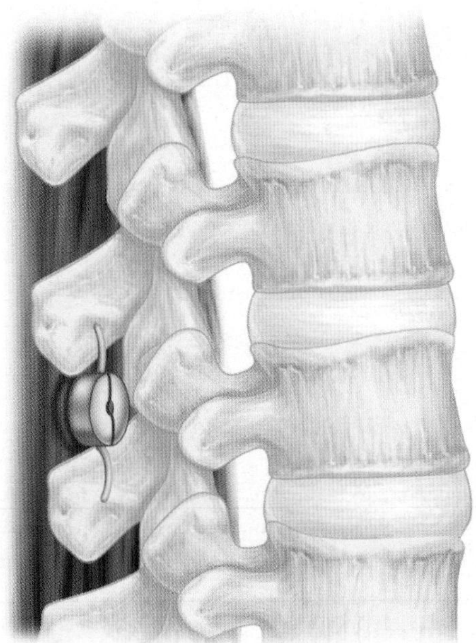

■ **FIGURE 3–27.** In-Space.

## FINAL REMARKS

This is the first classification of all available spine arthroplasty devices. Concepts for replacement of the complete functional spinal unit have already been presented. These concepts have not been clinically tested and are therefore not considered in this chapter. For anatomic and biomechanical reasons, a total replacement of the annulus fibrosus also is not included. A partial replacement of the annulus fibrosus could close a gap in the annulus caused by surgery, but it remains to be proven whether the biomechanics of the complete annulus would be restored.

An algorithm for the degree of degeneration of the FSU and for the device derived therefrom cannot be compiled at this time owing to a lack of basic science data as well as all-embracing clinical knowledge. As an orientation, the implant or material should always be selected, with which the individual physiologic condition of the respective patient can be preserved or repaired most precisely, with the least risk and effort for the patient, and with the best expected long-term effect. Therefore, it is necessary to exactly analyze in which topographic region the pathology is located to reconstruct a biomechanical regular three-joint complex as a precondition for a reduction of the patient's pain.

## ACKNOWLEDGMENTS

I would like to express my sincere gratitude to the companies who responded to my questionnaire. Implants and materials of these companies were preferentially explained and illustrated. My special thanks is given to Mr. Andrew J. Carter, PhD (Spine Wave, Inc. Shelton, CT), with whom I had the opportunity to discuss theoretical basics. At the beginning of the research, Mr. Bruno Paton, HIPPOCRAFT, LLC, and Ms. April C. Bright, Marketing Manager of KNOWLEDGE Enterprises, INC., supplied an overview of the companies with motion-preservation devices.

## REFERENCES

1. Junghanns H: Die Wirbelsäule in der Arbeitsmedizin. Teil I. Biomechanische und biochemische Probleme der Wirbelsäulenbelastung. Hippokrates, Stuttgart, Die Wirbelsäule in Forschung und Praxis 78, 1979.
2. White AA, Panjabi MM: Clinical Biomechanics of the Spine. Philadelphia, JB Lippincott Co., 1978.
3. White AA, Panjabi MM: Clinical Biomechanics of the Spine, 2nd ed. Philadelphia, JB Lippincott Co., 1990.
4. Johnson EF, Caldwell RW, Berryman HE, et al: Elastic fibers in the annulus fibrosus of the dog intervertebral disc. Acta Anat (Basel) 118:238–242, 1984.
5. Pope MH, Magnusson M, Wilder DG: Low back pain and whole body vibration. Clin Orthop Rel Res 354:241–248, 1998.
6. Putz R: Function-related morphology of the intervertebral disks. Radiologe 33:563–566, 1993.
7. Panjabi M, Malcolmson G, Teng E, et al: Hybrid Testing of Lumbar CHARITÉ versus Fusions. Spine 32:959–966, 2007.
8. Büttner-Janz K: The Development of the Artificial Disc SB CHARITÉ. Dallas, Texas, Hundley & Associates, Inc., 1992.
9. Harms J: Motion preservation in spine surgery—dream or reality. 7th Annual Meeting of Spine Arthroplasty Society, May 1–4, Berlin, Germany, 2007.
10. Moumene M, Harms J, Albert TJ: The implication of the implant core radius in cervical total disc replacement, 7th Annual Meeting of Spine Arthroplasty Society, May 1–4, Berlin, Germany, 2007.
11. Lemaire J-P, Carrier H, Sari Ali E-H, et al: Clinical and radiological outcomes with the Charité™ artificial disc. A 10-year minimum follow-up. J Spinal Disord Tech 18:353–359, 2005.
12. David T: Long-term results of one-level lumbar arthroplasty: Minimum 10-year follow-up of the CHARITÉ artificial disc in 106 patients. Spine 32:661–666, 2007.
13. Boaten K, Schmidt G, Büttner-Janz K: Metal-on-Metal: Results of a Prospective Study after 10 years, 25th Anniversary of Alloclassic™ Zweymüller™ Stem, June 17–19, Vienna, Austria, 2004.
14. Fernström U: Der Bandscheibenersatz mit Erhaltung der Beweglichkeit. In: Zukunftsaufgaben für die Erforschung und Behandlung der Wirbelsäulenleiden (Erdmann H). In Junghanns H (ed): Die Wirbelsäule in Forschung und Praxis. Stuttgart, Germany, Hippokrates, 55, 1972, pp. 125–130.

15. Schulman Ch M: Metod kombinirowannogo chirurgitscheskogo letschenija kompressionnych form pojasnitschnogo osteochondrosa s alloprotesirowaniem porashennych meshposwonkowych diskow. Z Vopr Neirokhir 2:17–23, 1977.
16. Fassio B, Ginestié J-F: Prothèse discale en silicone. Etude expérimentale et premières observations cliniques. La Nouvelle Presse Médicale 7:207, 1978.
17. Pfirrmann CWA, Metzdorf A, Zanetti M, et al: Magnetic resonance classification of lumbar intervertebral disc degeneration. Spine 26:1873–1878, 2001.
18. Ray CD: Spinal fusion alternative: Device expands, fills disc space. Orthop Today Int 1:32–38, 1998.
19. Büttner-Janz K: Percutaneous application of nucleus replacements. BIOSPINE 2, Leipzig, Germany, September 20–22, 2007.
20. Boyd LM, Carter AJ: Injectable biomaterials and vertebral endplate treatment for repair and regeneration of the intervertebral disc. Eur Spine J 15(Suppl 3):S414–S421, 2006.
21. Kim Y-S, Zhang H-Y, Moon B-J, et al: Nitinol spring rod dynamic stabilization system and Nitinol memory loops in surgical treatment for lumbar disc disorders: short-term follow-up. Neurosurg Focus 22:1–9, 2007.
22. Khoueir P, Kim KA, Wang MY: Classification of posterior dynamic stabilization devices. Neurosurg Focus 22:1–8, 2007.

CHAPTER 4

# Advanced Spinal Anatomy for Cervical and Lumbar Nonfusion Surgery

**Daniel R. Fassett, Shiveindra B. Jeyamohan, Alexander R. Vaccaro,** and **Peter G. Whang**

## KEY POINTS

- An in-depth understanding of the surrounding anatomy and vertebral anatomy is needed to accurately place motion-preserving spinal devices.
- Poor alignment of motion-preserving spinal implants can adversely affect the biomechanics of the spine.
- The functional spinal unit, which is composed of two adjacent vertebrae articulating at the intervertebral disc and facet joints, has unique features in cervical and lumbar regions of the spine that contribute to the biomechanical properties of these areas.
- In the cervical spine, the uncovertebral joints, in addition to often being the source of neural compressive pathology, contribute significantly to segmental stability.
- In the lumbar spine, placement and development of motion-sparing technologies should consider the larger vertebral size and end plate structure, the relatively narrow angulation between the axial center of rotation and the facets, the importance of ligamentous structures in stability, and the complexity of surrounding anatomy in surgical approaches to this area of the spine. Motion-sparing strategies are being developed and employed as an alternative to fusion procedures for the treatment of degenerative spinal conditions such as axial pain syndromes, radiculopathy, and occasionally myelopathy. Cervical and lumbar total disc arthroplasty procedures have been performed in Europe for more than a decade. A series of clinical trials on lumbar disc replacements have been completed in the United States, and a number of cervical clinical trials are under way. In addition, new technologies such as nucleus pulposus replacement and posterior motion-sparing devices are now being studied.
- The main argument for motion-sparing surgery is to reduce adjacent-segment degeneration, which has been thought to occur after fusion procedures due to increased stress on adjacent segments. Although adjacent-segment degeneration is likely multifactorial, there is some credible evidence that a fusion accelerates spondylosis at adjacent segments. In addition, motion-sparing technologies potentially avoid the morbidity associated with fusion such as bone graft harvesting and pseudoarthrosis.

To recognize the potential benefit of restoring normal biomechanics and preventing adjacent-segment stresses, it is imperative that motion-sparing devices be placed precisely and that the technologies work harmoniously with surrounding anatomy in a biomechanically sound manner. A keen understanding of the surrounding anatomy, disc space anatomy, and radiographic anatomy are needed for accurate placement of motion-sparing devices.

## ANATOMY OF THE FUNCTIONAL SPINAL UNIT

The functional spinal unit is created by the articulation of two adjacent vertebrae, the intervening intervertebral disc (IVD) anteriorly and facet complex posteriorly (Fig. 4–1). The IVD is a complex structure composed of an inner nucleus pulposus that is surrounded by a dense annulus fibrosis and is bounded superiorly and inferiorly by the cartilaginous end plates of the adjacent vertebral bodies. The central nucleus pulposus has a very sparse cell population and is composed largely of an extracellular matrix of hydrophilic proteoglycans and type II collagen. The hydrophilic nature of a healthy nucleus pulposus draws water into the nucleus to maintain hydrostatic pressure within the disc space and tense the surrounding annulus fibrosis and ligamentous structures. The annulus fibrosis is composed predominantly of layers of type I collagen fibers that are arranged in an alternating lamellar pattern (Fig. 4–2). Within a single lamellar layer of the annulus, all of the collagen fibers are aligned in the same direction at an approximate 30-degree orientation with the horizontal vertebral end plates. Consecutive annular layers are oriented in an alternating pattern with one layer oriented obliquely to the right and the next layer oriented obliquely to the left. This alternating lamellar pattern of the annulus has been compared with a radial tire with excellent tensile strength to resist shear and prevent disruption. The combination of nucleus pulposus and annulus fibrosus of the intervertebral disc work together to provide biomechanical stability at each spinal segment, with the nucleus supporting compressive loads and the annulus, together with the facet joints and ligaments, resisting shear forces.

The cartilaginous end plates that form the cephalad and caudal borders of the IVD are initially composed of hyaline cartilage, which calcifies with aging. Beneath the cartilaginous end plates is subchondral bone that can vary in thickness depending on its level in the spine and location within the disc space. The vertebral end

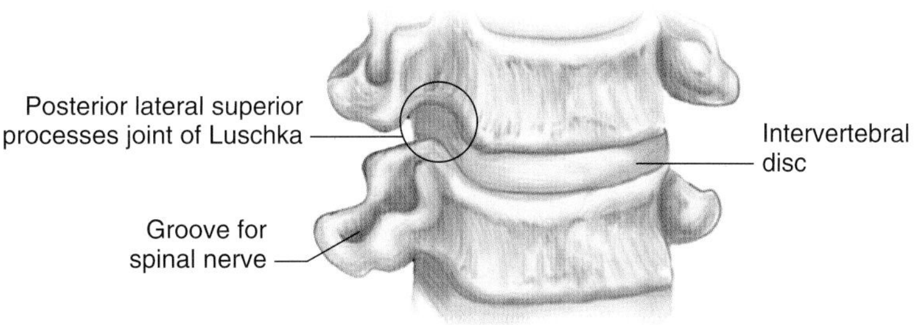


■ **FIGURE 4–1.** A functional spinal unit is composed of an anterior intervertebral disc and posterior facets that act together to allow motion between adjacent vertebrae while providing stability to maintain spinal alignment and protect the neural elements. *(Adapted from Vaccaro AR, Papadopoulos S, Traynelis VC, et al: Spinal Arthroplasty: The Preservation of Motion. Philadelphia, WB Saunders, 2007.)*

plates are very important anatomic structures for anterior motion-sparing technologies because end plate subsidence has been noted with some anterior motion-sparing devices. In the lumbar spine, the vertebral end plates are the strongest at the outer margins of the disc space and weakest in the central portion. In the cervical spine, the superior end plates are strongest at the dorsal margins and the inferior end plates are strongest at the ventral margins. The end plates are also the source of nutrition to the adjacent avascular disc space and may be the limiting factor in disc regeneration strategies to preserve motion.

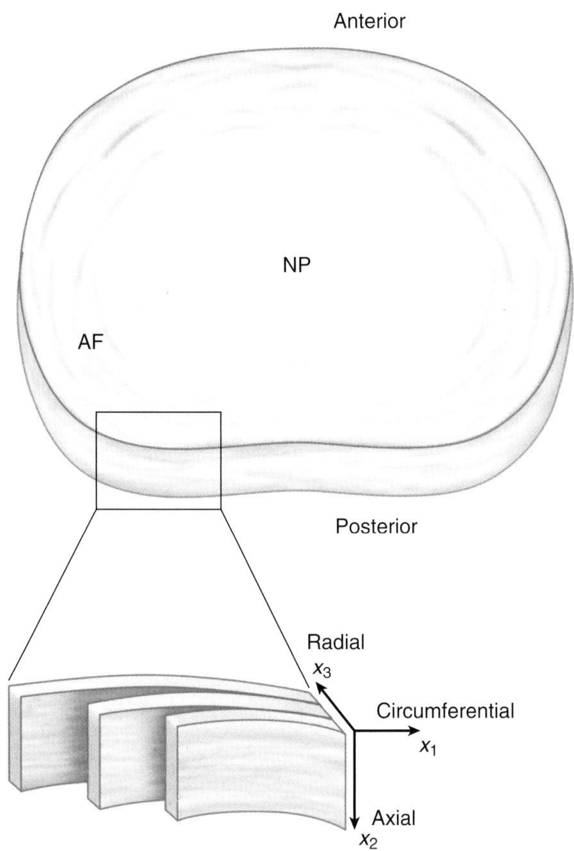


■ **FIGURE 4–2.** The intervertebral disc is composed of a central gelatinous core, the nucleus pulposus (NP), surrounded laterally by dense annulus fibrosis (AF). The lamellar architecture of the annulus with an alternating pattern of collagen fibers provides excellent tensile strength to resist shear force.

The facets complete the functional spinal unit, and the size and orientation of the facets are dependent on their location within the spine. In the cervical spine, the facets have a more vertical orientation in the coronal plane and the facet-to-disc-surface area ratio is larger in the cervical spine in comparison to the lumbar spine. In addition, the cervical facets are based at a wider angle from the axial center of rotation (larger arc of influence) than in the lumbar spine, and, therefore, have a greater contribution to axial stability (Fig. 4–3). As a result of all these factors, the cervical facets are thought to contribute more to rotational stability, and, for this reason, it has been reported that a cervical disc replacement may be more biomechanically sound in comparison to lumbar disc replacement.[1]

The ligaments of the spine are also important stabilizing structures and should be considered in the application of motion-sparing technologies. The anterior longitudinal ligament (ALL), posterior longitudinal ligament (PLL), ligamentum flavum (LF), facet capsular ligaments, and interspinous ligaments contribute to spinal stability (Fig. 4–4A). The ALL runs along the anterior aspect of the vertebral column beginning at the anterior margin of the foramen magnum and extending to the anterior surface of the sacrum. The ALL gets wider and stronger as it descends into the lumbar spine, and it is the thickest over the intervertebral disc spaces. At the disc spaces, the deep fibers of the ALL travel only

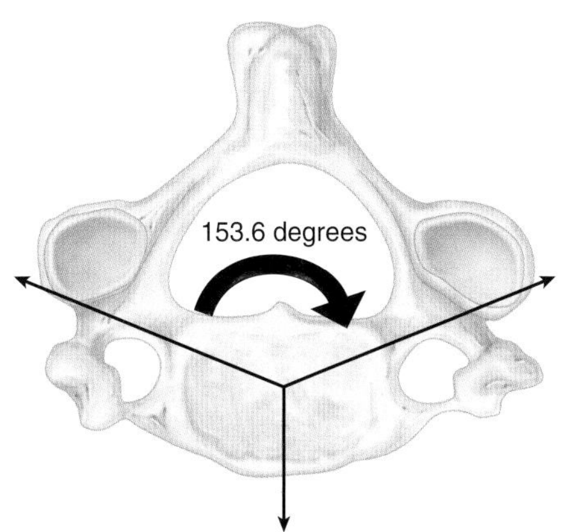


■ **FIGURE 4–3.** The arc of influence (AOI) is the angle formed between the axial center of rotation and the posterior facets. In the cervical spine, the facets are wider in relation to the axial center of rotation (larger AOI) and provide more stability against axial shear.

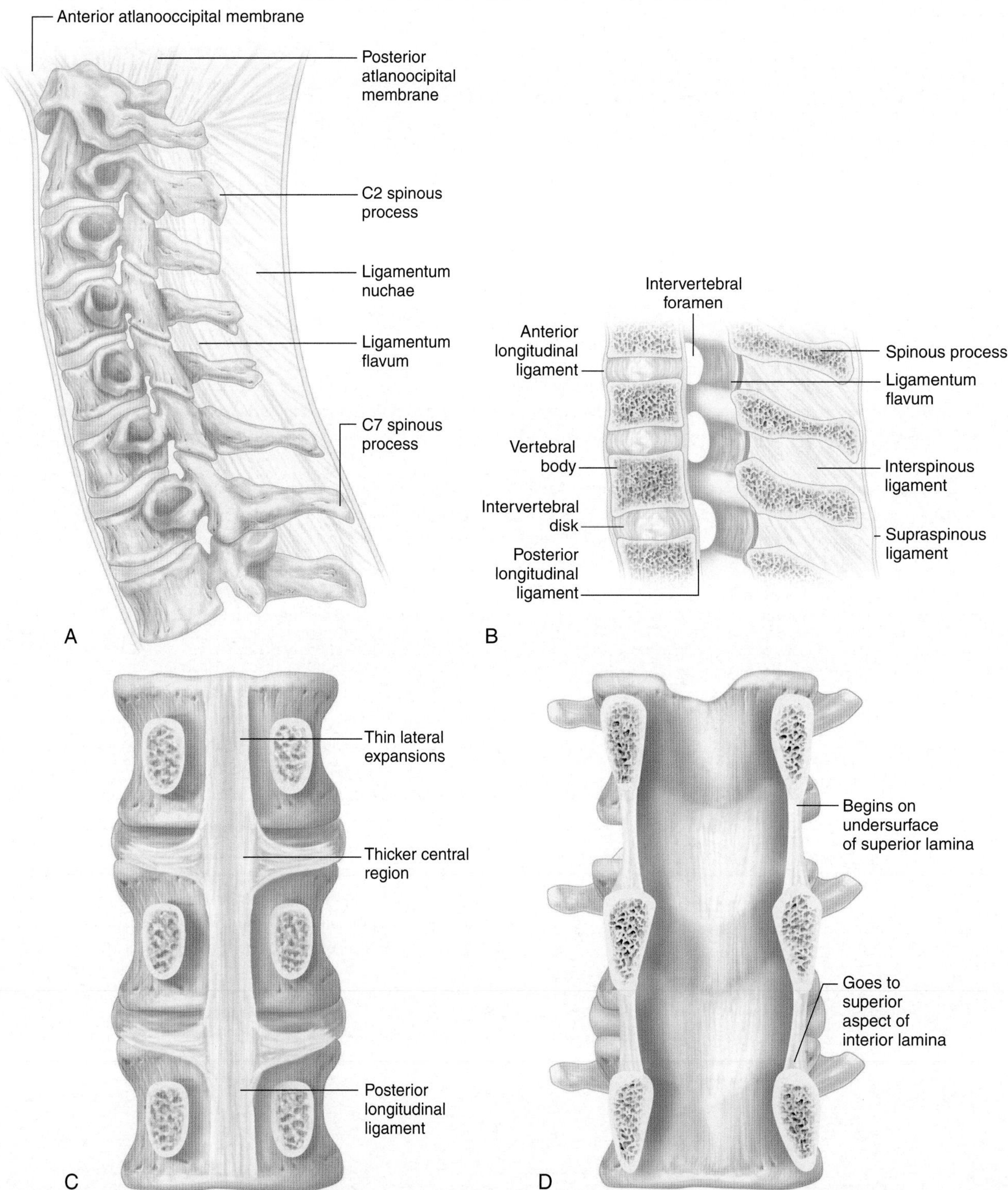


■ **FIGURE 4–4.** The spinal ligaments contribute substantially to spinal stability. **A** and **B,** The anterior longitudinal ligament (ALL), posterior longitudinal ligament (PLL), ligamentum flavum (LF), facet capsular ligaments (FCLs), interspinous ligaments (ISLs), and supraspinous ligaments are shown. **C,** The posterior longitudinal ligament has a very thick middle portion that extends laterally over the disc spaces for additional stability. **D,** The LF runs along the ventral aspect of the lamina, extending from the undersurface of the lamina above to top of the lamina below.

one interspace and anchor the adjacent vertebral bodies together. The PLL also runs along the entire spinal column along the posterior surface of the vertebral bodies. The PLL is narrow and very thick in the midline over the vertebral bodies and extends laterally over the disc spaces for additional support (Fig. 4–4B). The LF (yellow ligament) runs between adjacent lamina extending from the undersurface of the inferior aspect lamina above to the top of the lamina below (Fig. 4–4C).

In the lumbar spine, the ALL and PLL have the highest tensile strength, whereas in the cervical spine, the capsular ligaments and

LF have higher tensile strength than the ALL and PLL. Destruction of one of these ligaments during a motion-sparing procedure can have adverse impact on the biomechanics of the functional spinal unit. It has been speculated that cutting the ALL during lumbar arthroplasty may contribute to rotational deformities that have occurred with some lumbar disc replacements.[1]

## ANTERIOR CERVICAL SPINE ANATOMY

### Surrounding Anatomy

The anterior approach to the cervical spine is one of the most commonly performed approaches in spinal surgery and can expose the ventral spine from C2 to T2. The dissection plane is carried down along the medial border of the sternocleidomastoid muscle (Fig. 4–5). The carotid artery can easily be palpated and retracted laterally with the contents of the carotid sheath (carotid artery, internal jugular vein, and vagus nerve). The trachea and esophagus are gently retracted medially, and the ventral surface of the spine can be palpated. The prevertebral fascia can be opened with a combination of sharp and blunt dissection techniques. Structures at risk for injury on this dissection include the contents of the carotid sheath, esophagus, sympathetic chain, recurrent laryngeal nerve, and superior laryngeal nerve, with dysphagia and laryngeal nerve palsies being the most common complications in anterior cervical spine surgery. With the use of careful blunt dissection and palpation of the carotid with lateral retraction, injury to the carotid sheath structures should be avoided. With lateral retraction of the carotid sheath, the inferior and superior thyroid vessels may bridge from lateral to medial and obstruct the surgical exposure. These vessels can be ligated, but care should be taken to avoid neural structures in this area because the superior laryngeal nerve can course with these vessels. The esophagus may be traumatized during the initial dissection, but it is more likely to be injured at the time of decompression when it can protrude around the medial-lateral retractor blades and be wound in the shaft of a high-speed drill. The sympathetic trunks pass along the ventral surface of the longus coli muscles and can be traumatized with excessive elevation or cutting of the longus coli muscles.

The superior laryngeal nerve (SLN) arises from the vagus nerve just as it exits the skull and descends in the neck just medial to the carotid arteries. At the level of the hyoid bone, the SLN turns medially and divides into the internal (sensory) and external (motor) branches. Injury to the SLN can cause changes in the pitch of the voice (external branch injury) and have significant aspiration risk owing to loss of sensation above the vocal cords (internal branch injury). The SLN is at greatest risk on upper cervical approaches (C3-C4 and higher), and, thus, is likely an uncommon complication of arthroplasty procedures, which are most commonly performed in the middle and lower cervical spine.

The recurrent laryngeal nerves (RLN) have a more complex course and are more vulnerable to injury in lower cervical spine surgeries in comparison to the SLN. On the left side of the body, the RLN, after arising from the vagus nerve, passes beneath the aorta at the level of the ligamentum arteriosum before ascending to the laryngeal structures in the neck. The left RLN has a more vertical and predictable course within the tracheoesophageal groove

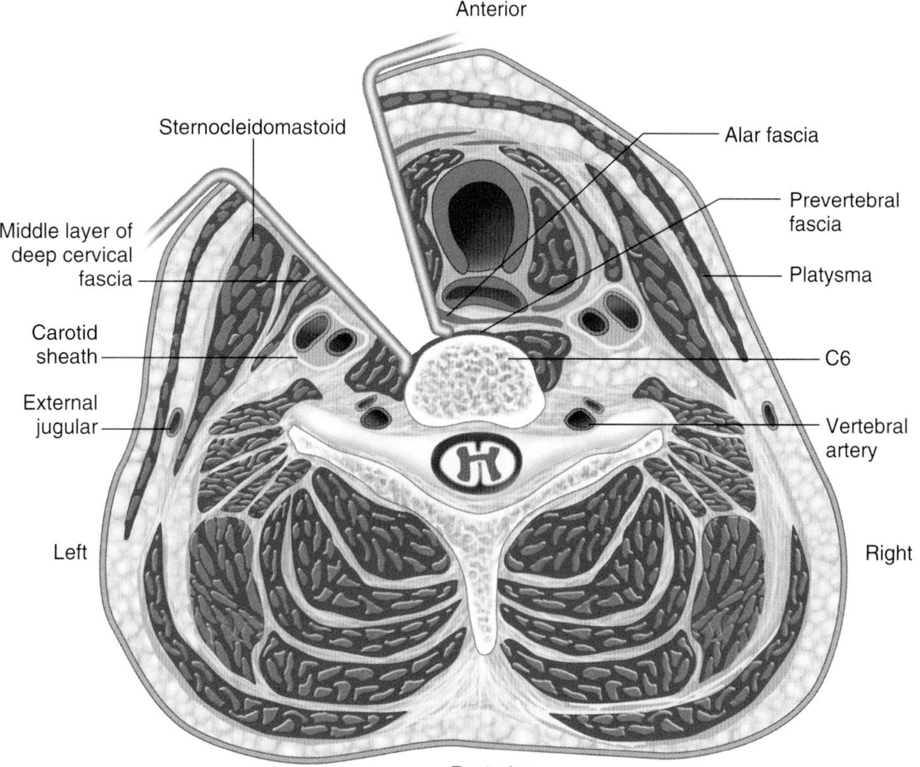


■ **FIGURE 4–5.** The anterior cervical approach to the spine uses soft tissue planes medial to the sternocleidomastoid muscle. The carotid sheath structures are retracted laterally, and the esophagus and trachea are retracted medially to expose the ventral surface of the spine. *(Adapted from Albert T, Balderston R, Northrup B: Surgical Approaches to the Spine, Philadelphia, WB Saunders, 1997, p. 10.)*

in comparison to the right RLN. The right RLN takes a more oblique course in its ascent after passing beneath the right subclavian artery and is in a more vulnerable location outside of the tracheoesophageal groove throughout a large portion of its course. In addition, a variant called a nonrecurrent laryngeal nerve, which arises from the mid-cervical vagus nerve and passes directly to the laryngeal structures, is occasionally (<2% of people) found on the right side. This nonrecurrent nerve is more prone to injury than typical recurrent laryngeal nerves. For these reasons, some anatomists and surgeons have theorized that a left-sided approach is lower risk for RLN injury, but conflicting results exist in the surgical literature. A right-sided approach is more ergonomic for a right-handed surgeon in terms of easily manipulating instruments and performing microsurgery. For disc arthroplasty, the surgeon should choose the side he or she is most comfortable working with to allow for precise placement of the arthroplasty device.

## CERVICAL VERTEBRAL ANATOMY

The subaxial cervical vertebrae (C3-C7) are composed of vertebral bodies, transverse processes, pedicles, lateral masses, articular processes (upper and lower or superior and inferior), lamina, and spinous processes (Fig. 4–6A). The vertebral bodies and intervertebral discs make up the anterior column of the spine and support much of the loads carried through the spine. The vertebral bodies are relatively small in relation to the vertebral canal and remainder of the spine.

The uncovertebral joints are a unique feature of the cervical spine intervertebral disc articulation. The lateral and upper portion of the C3-C7 vertebral bodies have uncinate processes that extend up from the vertebral body. The superior end plates of these vertebral bodies are concave and cup the inferior end plate of the supra-adjacent vertebrae, which has a convex shape (Fig. 4–6B). In normal adults, the uncinate process may articulate with up to one third of the lateral surface of the supra-adjacent vertebrae and is an important stabilizing mechanism of the adult cervical spine. The uncovertebral joints can serve as a reliable landmark to assess the midline in arthroplasty procedures. With both uncovertebral joints exposed, the surgeon can estimate the midline between these two lateral structures.

The enlargement of the posterior uncovertebral joints are often the source of foraminal stenosis and nerve root irritation. Posterior bone spurs from the uncovertebral joints are often resected during anterior decompression procedures. In instrumented arthrodesis procedures, a large portion of the uncinate process can be removed without significant impact on stability owing to the rigidity of the instrumentation. However, in motion preservation procedures,

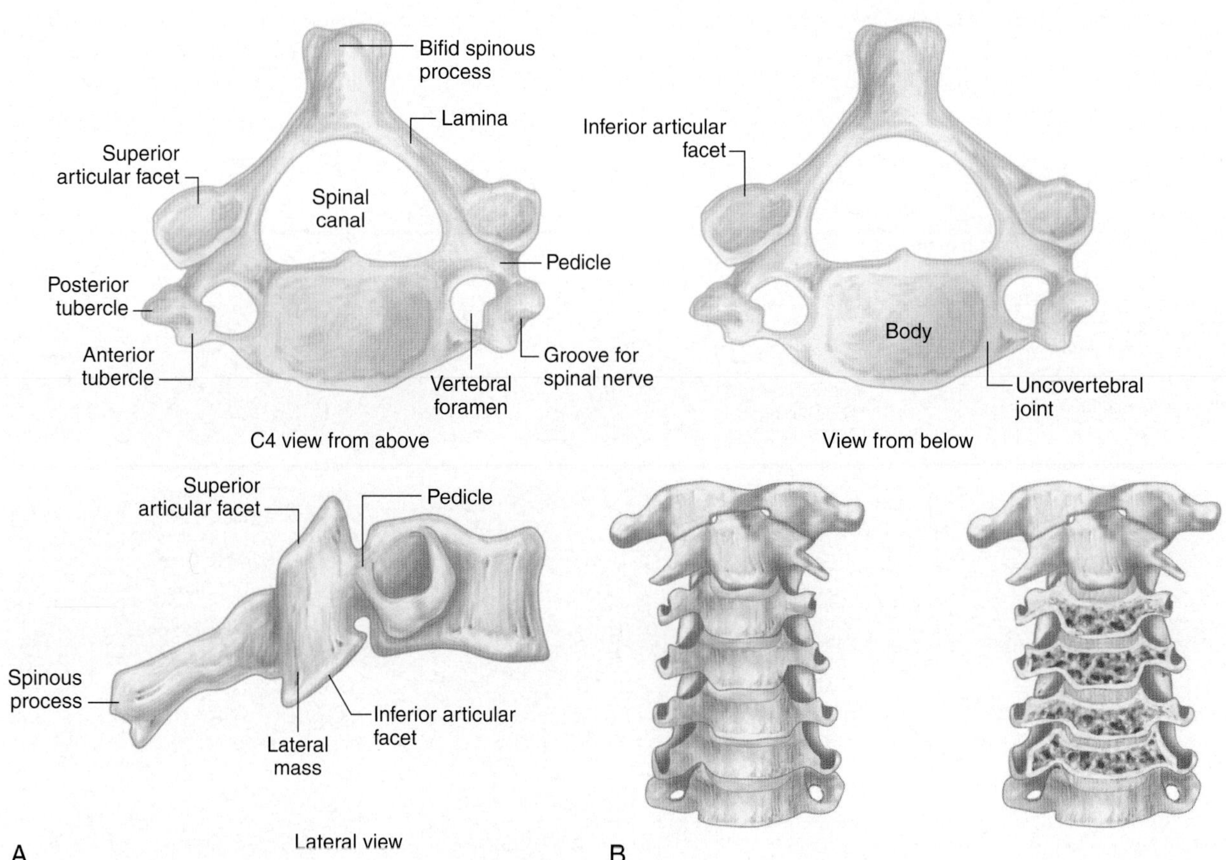


■ **FIGURE 4–6.** **A,** Subaxial cervical vertebrae are composed of a body, transverse processes, pedicle, lateral masses with superior and inferior articular processes, lamina, and spinous processes. **B,** The uncovertebral joints arise on the lateral aspect of the subaxial intervertebral disc space. *(Adapted from Vaccaro AR: Core Knowledge in Orthopaedics—Spine, Philadelphia, Elsevier-Mosby, 2005, p. 4.)*

removal of the uncovertebral joints may result in nonphysiologic amounts of intervertebral motion and possible instability.[1] At the same time, a meticulous decompression of the posterior uncinate should be performed to remove all nerve compressive pathology because the combination of continued motion and nerve compression will likely result in persistent radiculopathy.

In the normal adult spine, the height of the cervical vertebral bodies, as measured in the midline, is typically between 12 and 15 mm, and increases slightly with descent into the lower cervical spine. At the lateral aspect of the vertebral bodies, the height is 2 to 3 mm greater owing to the extension of the uncinate processes. Midline disc space height is typically between 1 and 7 mm (mean approximately 4 mm) and is dependent on patient gender (slightly larger in men) and the amount of degenerative changes present (more disc collapse with severe degeneration). The width of the cervical vertebral bodies can vary from 17 to 34 mm, with a mean width around 25 mm. Vertebral body width is usually larger in the lower cervical spine in comparison to the upper cervical spine and larger in men in comparison to women. The depth of the vertebral bodies in the sagittal plane can vary from 10 to 24 mm and is typically deeper at the end plates than at the midportion of the vertebral bodies.[2,3]

Understanding the location of the vertebral arteries and nerve roots in relation to the vertebral bodies is essential to avoiding complications in anterior cervical spine surgery. The vertebral arteries usually enter the transverse foramen of the C6 vertebral bodies and ascend along the lateral aspects of the vertebral bodies in close proximity to the uncinate processes (Fig. 4–7). The distance from the tip of the uncinate to the vertebral artery ranges from 0 to 6 mm and is usually closer in the upper cervical spine.[3] The exiting nerve roots lie dorsal to the vertebral arteries at the intervertebral foramen, and the length of exiting nerve root proximal to the vertebral artery increases from approximately 3 mm at C3 to 8 mm at C7.[4] Close evaluation of the preoperative axial computed tomography and magnetic resonance images can help assess vertebral body width and avoid complications such as vertebral artery injury or implantation of an oversized implant.

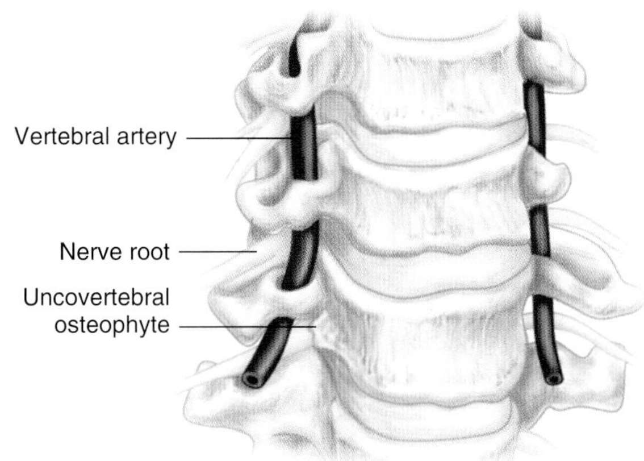


■ **FIGURE 4–7.** The vertebral arteries and exiting nerve roots lie in close proximity to the uncinate processes and may be injured during decompression of the neural foramen.

## ANTERIOR LUMBAR SPINE ANATOMY

### Surrounding Anatomy

A number of surrounding structures can be injured during retroperitoneal and transperitoneal approaches to access the anterior lumbar spine including the bowel, bladder, ureter, sympathetic chain, the hypogastric plexus, lumbar nerve roots, and the pelvic vessels. In the more commonly performed retroperitoneal approach, the peritoneal structures and ureter are swept medially with dissection in the retroperitoneal plane (Fig. 4–8). This exposes the psoas muscles, ventral surface of the spine, and the great vessels in the pelvis. The great vessels are the greatest challenge to obtaining good exposure to the ventral aspect of the spine (Fig. 4–9). The abdominal aorta descends on the left of the inferior vena cava on the ventral surface of the spine and divides into the common iliac arteries around L4. The arteries are typically easier to manipulate, in comparison to veins, because they have thicker vessel walls and are more easily mobilized with blunt dissection. The veins are typically more troublesome during anterior lumbar approaches, with the iliocaval junction and the left common iliac vein most commonly causing obstruction to either the L4-L5 or L5-S1 disc spaces, respectively. The iliocaval junction is most commonly present over the L5 vertebral body but may occur anywhere from the lower aspect of the L4 body to the upper aspect of the sacrum. Venous obstruction of a lower lumbar disc space exposure has been reported to occur in up to 40% of cases.[5,6] Careful assessment of the iliolumbar (ascending lumbar vein) should be performed when approaching the L4-L5 disc space for interbody procedures. One should also note the location of the left L5 nerve root directly posterior to the ascending lumbar vein.

The hypogastric nerve plexus is an important structure for sexual function and typically overlies the ventral spine in the lower lumbar region below the bifurcation of the great vessels. This plexus, if injured, can result in impotence in males secondary to retrograde ejaculation. Blunt dissection with a sweeping of the soft tissues away from the disc spaces and avoidance of monopolar cautery has been recommended to prevent this complication. The sympathetic chain also runs along the psoas muscle just lateral to the spine. Although injury to the sympathetic chain is typically well tolerated, this injury may be avoided with blunt dissection and an awareness of surrounding anatomy.

In addition to direct anterior approaches to the ventral lumbar spine, lateral (trans-psoas) approaches to the lumbar disc spaces have been developed for fusion techniques and are being considered for motion-sparing technologies for both initial implantation and revision (Fig. 4–10). The major benefit of the trans-psoas approach in motion-sparing surgery is that it would avoid damage to the anterior longitudinal ligament, which is very important to rotational stability in the lumbar spine. In addition, this approach avoids the great vessels and thus can be very important in the revision of motion-sparing devices with the scarring associated with a previous retroperitoneal approach. With a trans-psoas approach, a retroperitoneal dissection is performed from a direct lateral position on the patient. A muscle-splitting dissection is carried through the psoas muscle to the lateral aspect of the disc space. This approach puts the exiting nerve roots at risk for injury, and for this reason, it is typically performed with continuous

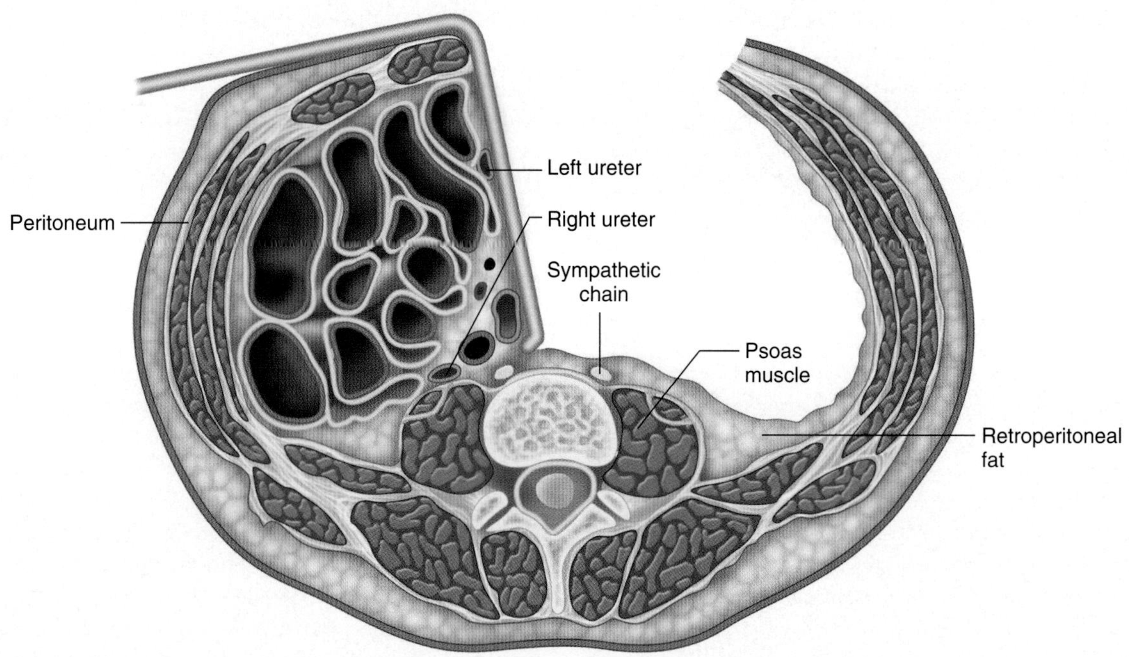


■ **FIGURE 4–8.** Retroperitoneal approach to the anterior lumbar spine. *(Adapted from Albert T, Balderston R, Northrup B: Surgical Approaches to the Spine, Philadelphia, WB Saunders, 1997.)*

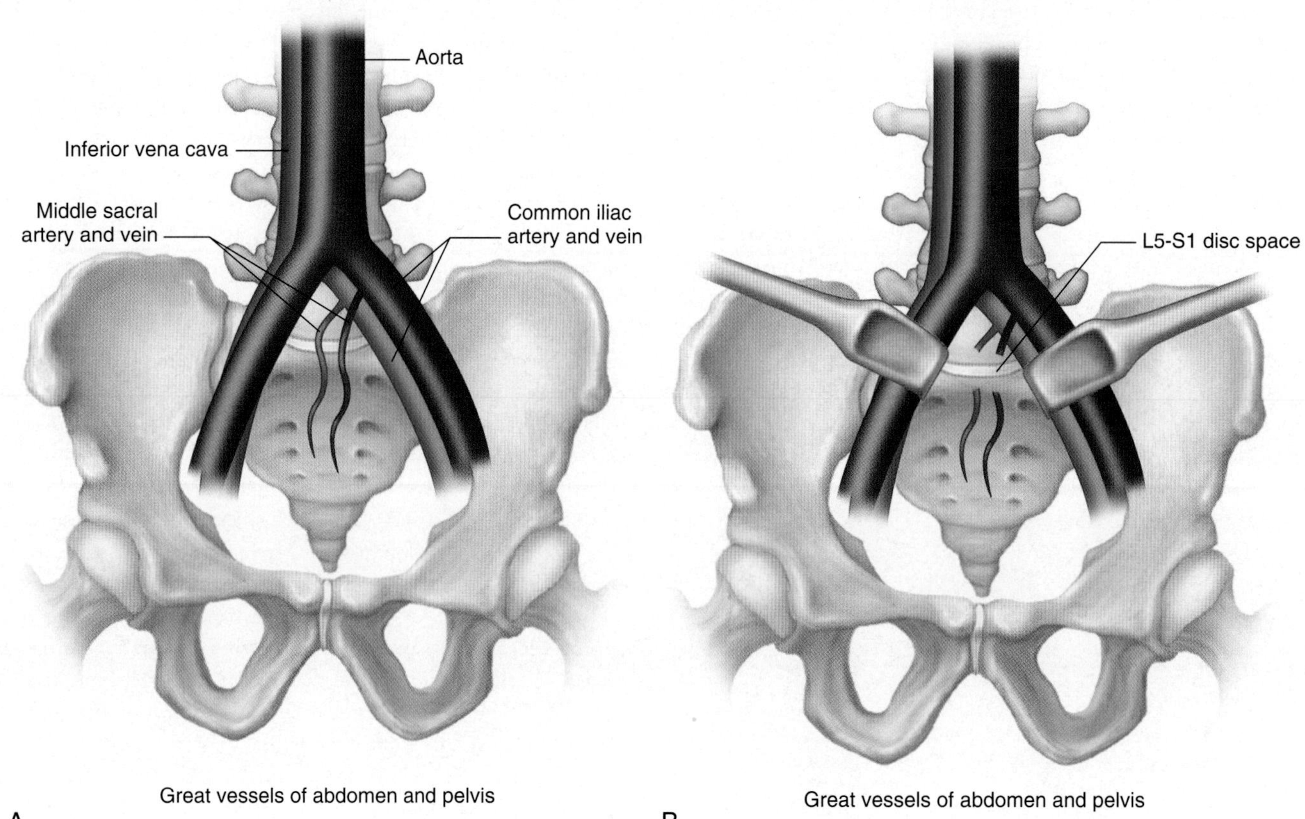


■ **FIGURE 4–9.** **A** and **B,** The great vessels of the abdomen and pelvis often obstruct the ventral aspect of the vertebral bodies. With careful blunt dissection, these vessels may be mobilized for improved exposure to the disc space of interest. The L5/S1 disc space is exposed in this image, with middle sacral vein extending over the middle aspect of the disc space. *(Adapted from Vaccaro AR, Papadopoulos S, Traynelis VC, et al: Spinal Arthroplasty: The Preservation of Motion. Philadelphia, WB Saunders, 2007.)*

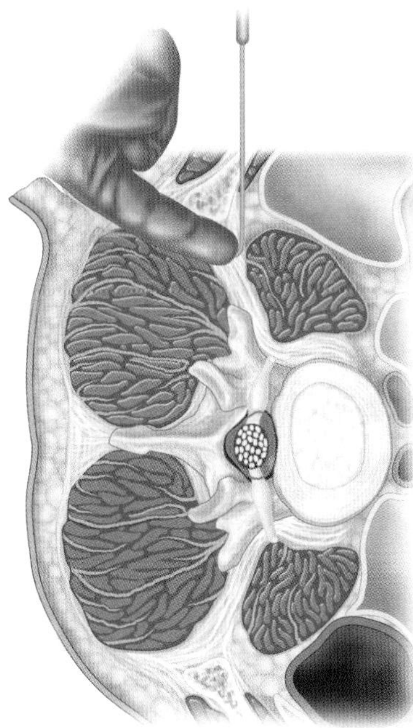

■ **FIGURE 4–10.** A trans-psoas approach to the lumbar disc space has been proposed for use with some motion-sparing technologies. The benefit of this approach is that it preserves natural biomechanical stability of the anterior longitudinal ligament.

neuromonitoring for electromyographic activity. The exiting nerve roots typically run in the dorsal one third of the psoas muscle, and, therefore, blunt dissection is usually performed in the ventral one half of the psoas muscle. It should be noted that the nerve roots exit more ventrally in the lower lumbar region, and great care is required in this area.[7]

## LUMBAR VERTEBRAL ANATOMY

The vertebrae of the lumbar spine are much larger than those of the cervical spine because the lumbar spine must withstand substantial loads. The vertebral bodies are wider transversely than they are deep and tall (Fig. 4–11). The pedicles are short and wide, and join with the pars interarticularis. A superior articular process extends up from the pars, and the inferior articular process extends down. The facet orientation is in the sagittal plane for most of the lumbar vertebrae and resists axial torsion predominantly. The L5/S1 facet is the exception because it is more coronally oriented to resist translation at this level.

The width of lumbar vertebral bodies can range from 32 to 67 mm (mean 48 mm) and is typically wider in men and in the lower lumbar areas. The vertebral body depth ranges from 24 to 38 mm (mean 35 mm) and again is deeper in men. The vertebral body height is longer ventrally than dorsally, which helps create the lordosis of the lumbar segment. The mean anterior vertebral

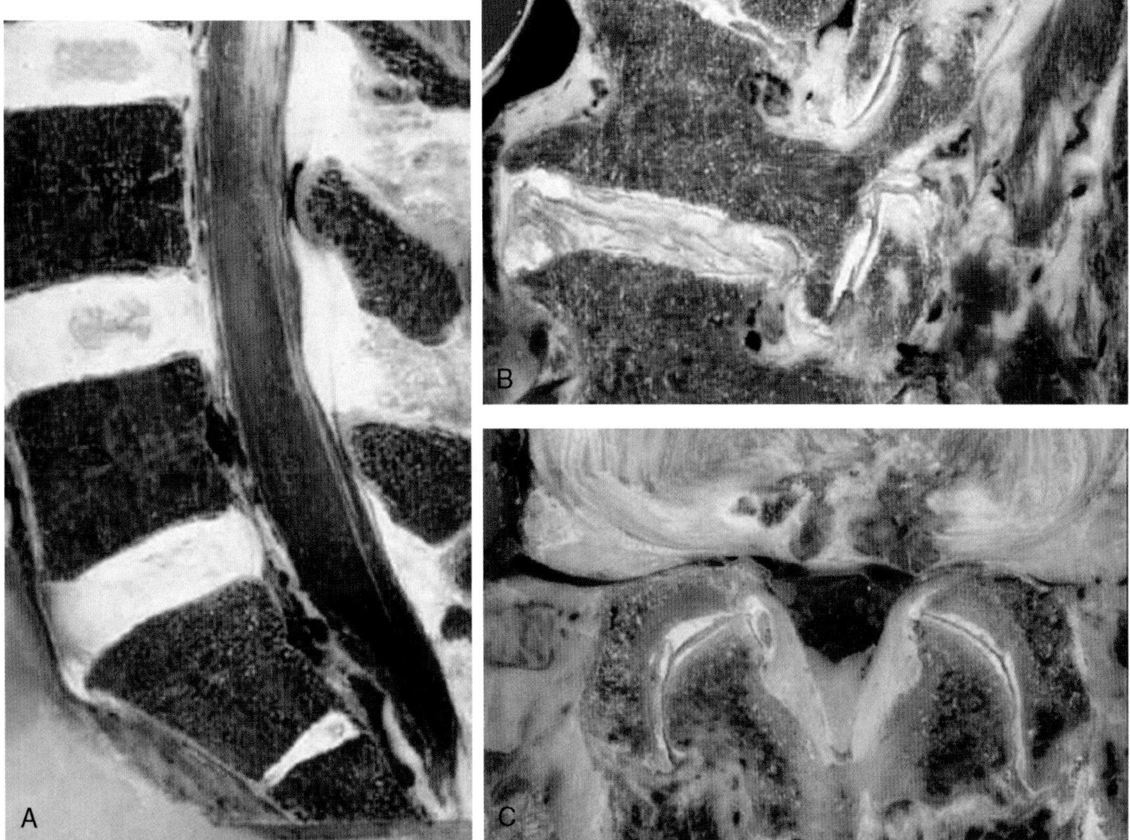


■ **FIGURE 4–11.** **A** to **E,** The lumbar vertebrae are larger to withstand the significant loads that must be carried by the lower spine. The vertebral bodies are wider with a larger surface area to distribute these forces. The facets are oriented in a sagittal plane for better resistance to axial torsion. *(Reprinted with permission of Wolfganga Raushning, MD, PhD, 2000.)*

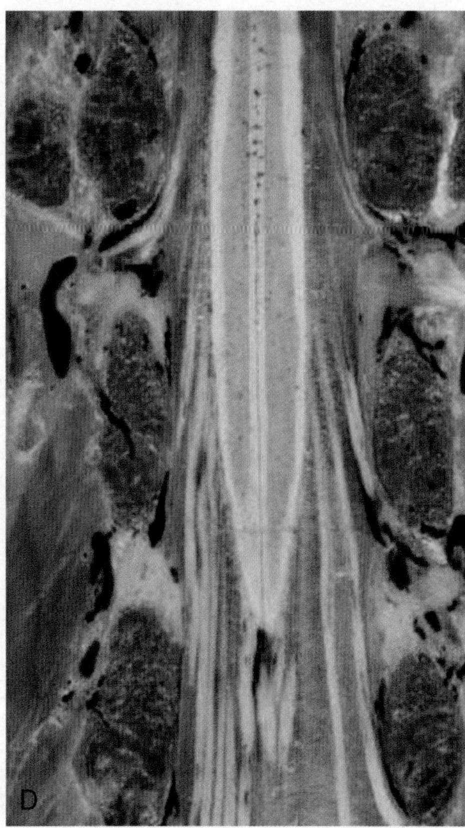


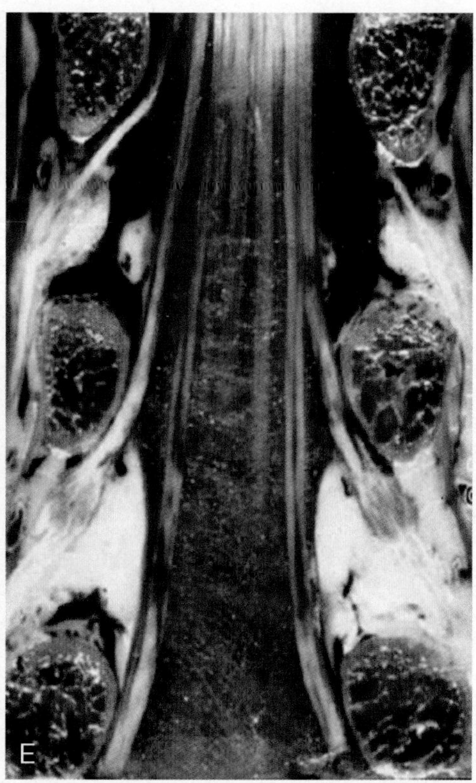


■ **FIGURE 4–11 Cont'd.**

body height has been reported at 30 mm (range 23 to 38 mm) for lumbar vertebrae, with a mean posterior body height of approximately 28 mm (range 21 to 37 mm). Normal disc heights can range from 5 to 16 mm (mean 10 mm) and are typically larger in men in comparison to women and smaller at the L5/S1 level.[8] Given the significant range in anterior vertebral dimensions, a thorough preoperative evaluation of the imaging is recommended to confirm that the adequate size is available for motion-sparing prosthesis.

## CONCLUSIONS

Motion-preserving techniques are being developed as an alternative to fusion procedures in the treatment of various spine pathologies. The hope of these new technologies is to restore normal biomechanics to a degenerative spinal level and preserve motion to prevent adjacent-segment changes. To fully restore normal biomechanics, these devices need to be placed precisely, and thus an in-depth knowledge of spinal anatomy is required for these procedures.

## REFERENCES


1. McAfee PC, Cunningham BW, Hayes V, et al: Biomechanical analysis of rotational motions after disc arthroplasty: implications for patients with adult deformities. Spine 31(19):S152–S160, 2006.
2. Kwon BK, Song F, Morrison WB, et al: Morphologic evaluation of cervical spine anatomy with computed tomography: anterior cervical plate fixation considerations. J Spinal Disord Tech 17:102–107, 2004.
3. Pait TG, Killefer JA, Arnautovic KI: Surgical anatomy of the anterior cervical spine: the disc space, vertebral artery, and associated bony structures. Neurosurgery 39:769–776, 1996.
4. Ebraheim NA, Lu J, Biyani A, et al: Anatomic considerations for uncovertebral involvement in cervical spondylosis. Clin Orthop Relat Res 334:200–206, 1997.
5. Cho DS, Kim SJ, Seo IH, et al: Quantitative anatomical and morphological classification of the iliac vessels anterior to the lumbosacral vertebrae. J Neurosurg Spine 3:371–374, 2005.
6. Capellades J, McCarthy ID, McGregor AH, et al: Magnetic resonance anatomic study of iliocava junction and left iliac vein positions related to L5-S1 disc. Spine 25:1695–1700, 2000.
7. Bertagnoli R, Vazquez RJ: The Anterolateral TransPsoatic Approach (ALPA): a new technique for implanting prosthetic disc-nucleus devices. J Spinal Disord Tech 16:398–404, 2003.
8. Zhou SH, Pellisé F, Rovira A, et al: Geometrical dimensions of the lower lumbar vertebrae—analysis of data from digitised CT images. Eur Spine J 9:242–248, 2000.

CHAPTER 5

# Biomechanics of Nonfusion Devices: Novel Testing Techniques, Standards, and Implications for Future Devices

**Boyle C. Cheng** and **William C. Welch**

## KEY POINTS

- Laboratory biomechanical testing results are most similar to perioperative results but may not represent the long-term stability of a particular construct.
- Biomechanical testing parameters are based on estimates of the clinical situation.
- Safety parameters of motion preservation devices include wear–debris generation and maintenance of mechanical integrity.
- Current biomechanical measures of device performance have been based primarily on fusion constructs.
- Future methods for biomechanical evaluation will need to include criteria for evaluating the quality of motion, for example, axis of rotation, neutral zone effects, and transitions in stiffness.

A broad spectrum of specialized spinal instrumentation and techniques are currently available and entirely at the surgeons' discretion as to which will be considered optimal for patient care. The study of spinal biomechanics may assist clinicians in understanding certain functional aspects of the spine as well as facilitate clinicians in selecting appropriate instrumentation to correct specific pathologies. Moreover, biomechanics should be used to predict how a given treatment will affect the spinal structures that have been compromised by disease.

Indications that have historically required surgical attention include congenital, developmental, degenerative, and traumatic conditions. Scoliotic deformities, degenerative discs with gross instability, and traumatic burst fractures are clinical indications potentially requiring surgical intervention and the use of spinal instrumentation. Rigid fixation, for example, posterior lumbar pedicle screws and rods, were originally designed to provide immediate stabilization and fixation. In order to determine the efficacy of device design, biomechanical testing has been used to evaluate the rigidity of instrumented functional spinal units (FSUs). As such, the history behind biomechanical spine testing has been relevant to motion segments and the effect of rigid instrumentation. Consequently, concepts that are most familiar are descriptions of test machines, methods of analysis, and report parameters that have been commonly found in fixation and fusion literature.[1–7]

Clinical studies have hypothesized that the biomechanical stiffness of a device contributes to successful clinical outcomes in the lumbar spine. Correspondingly, implants that significantly reduce the range of motion (ROM) of a spinal motion segment, that is, fixation devices, have increased in terms of mechanism and interface strength. However, the stiffness of devices and the subsequent stiffening of the FSUs may potentially lead to additional complications.

Although the presence of adjacent-level disease due to hardware instrumentation remains controversial,[8,9] it is important to recognize kinematic differences that occur both locally and globally due to instrumented FSUs. Through rigid instrumentation and fusion, the increased stiffness of the index level is believed to lead to increased or abnormal loading at other levels.[10–12] Ultimately, the adjacent levels are subjected to a combination of nonphysiologic motion and loading that may contribute to or accelerate degeneration at the juxtaposed levels. The basis for motion preservation devices and techniques is based on the stabilization at a symptomatic level, with considerable attention given to adjacent motion segments. Thus, motion preservation devices must provide a safe and efficacious solution for spinal pathologies while allowing physiologic motion and loading. In order to validate the current generation of spinal implants, biomechanical testing of these devices will be necessary as part of the overall burden of proof.

## INTRODUCTION TO BIOMECHANICS

Clinically relevant biomechanical studies involving the spine have been in the literature for more than decades. An early study by Virgin[13] described various biomechanical aspects of the intervertebral disc, including the effects of compressive loading and the observation of hysteresis during loading and unloading. Likewise,

Hirsch and Nachemson[14] reported on the influence of spine motion and the associated disc pressures. The study of FSUs under controlled loading has provided biomechanical insight into clinically relevant issues including instability of the spine. The FSU and the goals of spinal instrumentation have been verified based on similar biomechanical studies involving controlled loading and accurate measurements. Devices are developed with theoretical clinical and biomechanical end goals, and for motion preservation devices, the ability to achieve FSU stability while allowing physiologic motion is the primary biomechanical objective.

Biomechanical evaluation protocols for rigid spinal instrumentation as an adjunct to fusion have been thoroughly documented.[15–19] Furthermore, certain biomechanical findings have been clinically validated through randomized, prospective clinical trials and retrospective studies. Recently, biomechanical techniques and methodologies have been carried over to motion preservation devices despite the difference in the clinical end goal between rigid fusion and motion preservation implants. A specific aim of this chapter is to provide an overview of current test methods and the biomechanical impact of motion preservation devices. A second aim is to examine physiologic test methodologies and future directions for new test parameters.

### Biomechanics of the Instrumented Functional Spinal Units for Spinal Instability

Instability has various definitions as it relates to biomechanics of the spine. A kinematic response for an FSU under a given physiologic load in excess of the response found in the normal healthy condition, for example, inordinate ROM in a lumbar FSU, has been used to characterize the instability of a motion segment. Surgical intervention has the potential to treat pathologies of the spine concomitantly with biomechanical instability. Should the clinical conditions be appropriate for surgical intervention, a repeatable kinematic response of the FSU should be predictable and well described.

Biomechanical loading and displacement protocols for benchtop testing have been developed for spinal treatment comparisons. Historically, test methodologies have been designed primarily for the detection of changes in rigidity as a measure of stability in arthrodesis and deformity correction treatments.[20] In conjunction, precision-measuring devices have also been necessary in order to measure the relative motion between vertebral bodies. The combination has led to a conventional wisdom suggesting that effectiveness of an implant is governed solely by ROM alone. Thus, few parameters describing the quality of motion have been consistently reported. Furthermore, parameters in standardizing test methods and reporting the quality of motion must have consensus from clinicians and biomechanicians. References in the literature relevant to fusion parameters have provided a basis for spine biomechanical tests, and further guidance in study design have been found in animal models,[21] standard and alternative flexibility studies,[22–24] and computer modeling and simulation.[25–27] Panjabi was one of the first to describe the fundamentals of spine biomechanical testing.[5] In a recent article, Goel et al[28] provided further guidelines through broad-based agreement for biomechanical testing involving the spine.

As the design and commercialization of motion preservation devices begin to mature, American Society for Testing and Materials (ASTM) guidelines, biomechanical testing, and the techniques to evaluate the devices also need further development. For example, in a motion-preserving device, the ROM measured for a FSU may be a resultant of device motion in combination with the motion between the implant and the vertebral body interface. With a torque rotation plot, as shown in Figure 5–1, a description indicating the maximum and minimum angular displacement, for example, the standard ROM measurement, does not fully describe the source of motion, that is, originating from the device or from implant slip. The ROM parameters that were suitable for rigid fixation devices may require fuller descriptions for the new generation of spinal implants.

Subsequent interpretation of the data becomes more significant if there are clinical conclusions that can be derived from in vitro biomechanical testing. The clinical relevance of biomechanical testing is difficult to correlate perfectly, particularly for the diseased state. Human cadaveric studies only represent the condition immediately postoperatively. Long-term animal studies potentially provide information at key clinical follow-up periods but can be overly optimistic owing to the relative disease-free condition of a majority of the test subjects. The variables associated with the physical test apparatus, the biologic specimen, and the potential quagmires found in patient assessment all combine for difficulty in repeating studies in either the clinical or laboratory setting. Regardless of patient compliance, biologic variability, and artifacts of biomechanical studies, the fundamental basis of measurement parameters should be understood and taken into consideration along with the clinical factors in order to fully appreciate a patient's condition and the ramifications of surgical intervention.

## STANDARDIZED MATERIALS AND CONSTRUCT TESTING

The complex nature of the human spine has often led to difficulties in simulating normal physiologic loading and evaluating treatments for the spine. Although accurately controlled physiologic loads and moments can be applied along the primary axis, capturing the three-dimensional kinematic response is cumbersome but essential in understanding the biomechanics of the intact FSU and subsequent treatments. Simple situations, including single-axis strength testing in the laboratory environment, rarely result in single-axis kinematic response from cadaveric FSU testing. Motions in the spine are coupled motions. For example, with a lordotic lumbar section during segmental testing, axial loading has the potential to result in both a coupled flexion extension response due to facet orientation and an axial displacement in the normal intact condition. In order to minimize variability, standardized protocols have required repeatable methods for testing, that is, the reduction of inconsistency attributed to biologic sample irregularity.

Standardized testing, such as ASTM test protocols, has theoretically allowed comparison from different test laboratories and the ability to compare techniques and treatments. Determining strength, fatigue, and long-term survivability are important for spine implant studies and are more applicable with measures and parameters that are repeatable. Extrapolation of this information or data presents a broader challenge. More clinically relevant data can be found in experiments that replicate physiologic loading on

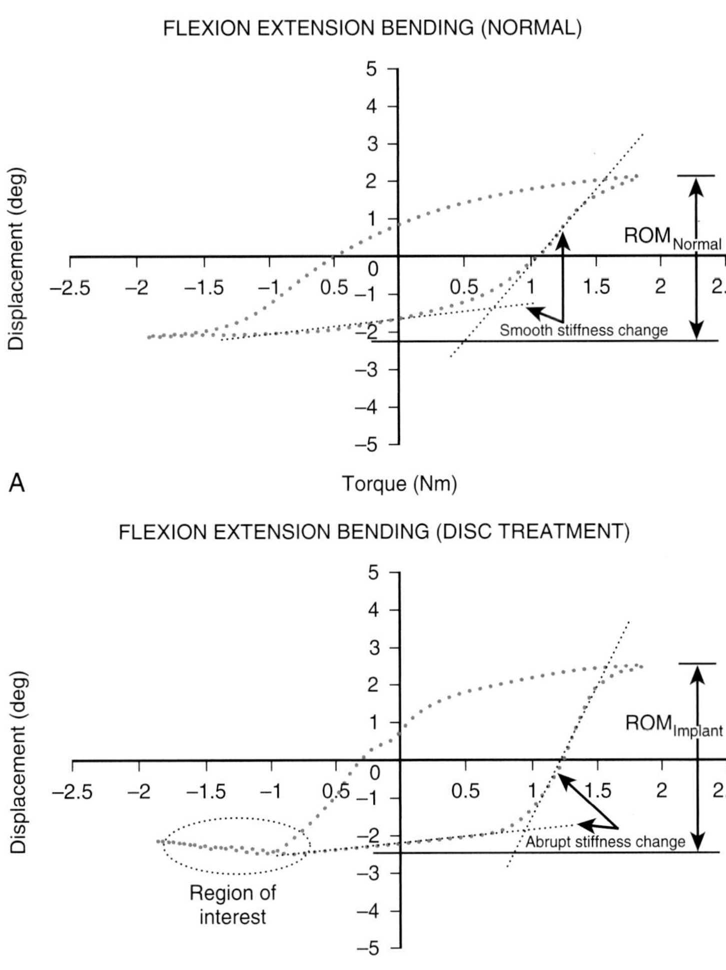


■ **FIGURE 5–1.** **A,** Representative load displacement graph for a complete bending cycle in a human cadaveric spine. **B,** Representative load displacement graph for a complete bending cycle in a human cadaveric spine with a motion preservation device. New parameters would need to report additional parameters for the quality of motion. Note the hysteresis within both plots.

anatomically correct specimens. However, for implant characterization and repeatable measures, standardized testing provides the ideal data set for comparative purposes.

The ASTM testing protocols for spinal implants are designed and published primarily for standardization purposes. Test protocols and guidelines may address strength, fatigue, wear, and function. Testing of standard fixation instrumentation including pedicle screws and anterior cervical plating are well defined, and all systems commercialized for the U.S. market are subjected to ASTM F1717-04 Standard Test Methods for Spinal Implant Constructs in a Vertebrectomy Model. However, motion preservation standards are currently only in draft form and may require considerable time and revision before consensus can be reached. Draft documents currently being discussed for motion preservation devices include a standard for implants outside the interbody space, which would include pedicle screw–based dynamic stabilization devices for the lumbar spine. Also, draft documents for the characterization of facet replacements, nucleus implants, and annular repair devices have been proposed.

Test procedures are important in understanding the response of the implant under controlled loading. Construct properties, for example, run-out fatigue loads, screw plate interface strength, and rod screw slippage, are measurable and should be reported. Standards for excessive load conditions or combined loading effects found in physiologic conditions have not been agreed upon for rigid fixation instrumentation. Also, challenges arise with newer technologies including motion preservation devices because test procedures or guidelines take time to develop, establish consensus, and implement. Figure 5–2 is an example of a method to test facet replacement devices and is currently able to satisfy the proposed standard guide which is in draft form.

Currently, devices commercialized worldwide are subjected to varying policies and procedures established by governments and responsible agencies. In the United States, the Food and Drug

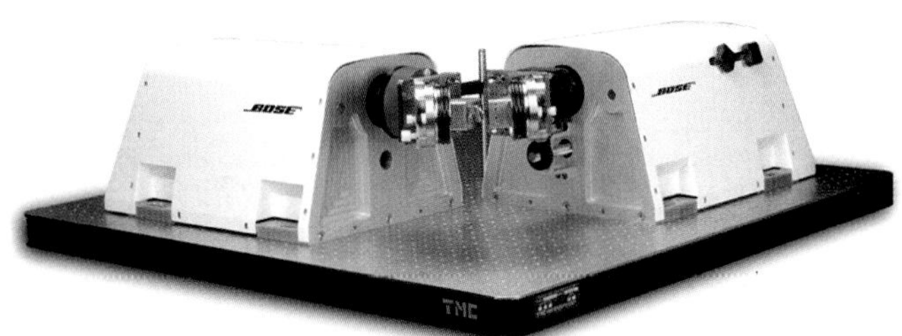

■ **FIGURE 5–2.** Proposed test apparatus for facet replacement technologies. The action will simulate physiologic complex loading patterns on facet implants.

Administration (FDA) regulates medical implants and the equipment to support spine procedures. In Europe, spinal implants must have Conformité Européaene Marking (CE Marking) while in Japan, the Ministry of Health, Labour, and Welfare determines the policies for device approval.

In the United States, the FDA has accepted test data from ASTM standards in approving specific classes of implants for commercialization. The standards for predicate fixation devices, that is, devices that were marketed before May 28, 1976, and approved by the FDA through a 510(k) clearance, are well established and repeatable from test facility to test facility. Devices that do not have an approved predicate before 1976 are subjected to premarket approval requirements and typically require additional data. These tests are designed to prove safety and efficacy of the device under review for FDA approval. However, research that is clinically relevant, including biomechanical stability, should be a prerequisite for clinical use.

Applying physiologic loads in order to mimic the clinical setting is important for understanding the efficacy of fixation devices. Although the ASTM F1717-04 test requires rough approximations of the vertebral bodies, the constructs are designed to represent the corpectomy condition. Owing to the high loads and moments that may potentially be generated from this method of testing, the condition represents the worst case scenario. For more frequently seen clinically relevant conditions for a FSU, biomechanical tests involving cadaveric tissue and specific spine testing equipment, for example, flexion extension bending motors, have been reported in the literature. However, variability in the data has prevented widespread acceptance and, thus, standardization for test protocols and guidelines remains focused on the implant constructs and disregards the bone implant interface.

## Methods of Spine Testing in Experimental Designs

Spine biomechanical research, including in the area of spinal implant testing of cadaveric FSUs, is an evolving discipline. Biomechanical test outcomes should be independent of location and laboratory, and repeatable from experiment to experiment. Ultimately, the goal is to build consensus among spine researchers on the biomechanical effect for a given spine device or technique. A number of authors have defined the necessary components to standardization including Panjabi and his article on a conceptual framework. Biomechanical test guidelines are the basis for consistent test methods, and important concepts have been widely implemented since description.[5,29] More recently, the criteria have been modernized to accommodate new concepts beyond fixation.[28] The need to carefully apply and measure both load and displacement are essential for spine stability testing.

Six independent motions can completely describe the kinematic motion for a given vertebral body, that is, three translations and three rotations. Displacements must be defined according to three orthogonal axes and are commonly defined relative to adjacent vertebrae, and when both vertebrae and associated soft tissue are tested, the response is commonly referred to as FSU motion. A clear understanding of the clinical biomechanics of the spine is based on the three-dimensional kinematic response of the FSU. Additionally, other testing paradigms used for spinal biomechanics have been described including ultimate vertebral body strength, annulus strain, facet loading, disc pressure, and so on. Spine biomechanical parameters used for comparative purposes, however, have predominantly based on kinematic responses as opposed to material properties. Often studies report the effects of treatments based on FSU ROM, which is a kinematic response. Although rare, reported material properties–based parameters include end plate and cancellous bone failure strength.

Ideally, a physiologic load applied to a FSU responds with a ROM limited in magnitude by the intact osteoligamentous structures and the kinematically stabilizing surgical treatment. As illustrated in Figure 5–1, treatments need to be compared and many metrics, including reductions in ROM and neutral zone (NZ), have been used to evaluate the stability of spine following fixation instrumentation.[3,28,30,31] For the sake of completeness, the spine testing configuration must be explained to describe basic assumptions made and to justify the kinematic response. Instant fixation devices provide excellent rigidity, but long-term survivability and positive patient outcome depend to some degree on arthrodesis. It should be noted that between fixation and the normal healthy condition, a continuum with a trade-off between rigidity and mobility exists. The region between rigid fixation and arthrodesis and normal motion shown in Figure 5–3 should be established as a stability target following surgical intervention involving the use of a motion preservation device. However, the quality of motion parameter for this stability spectrum has yet to be fully defined and ratified.

## Spine Test Configurations

Spine testers are designed to apply load in a physiologic manner to anatomic models for which questions of stability and treatments of instability may be measured and compared. Many methods have been documented for FSU testing. They range from reporting the kinematic response of a single axis test to validation of finite element models to sophisticated axial loading routines.[4,32–34] However, owing to wide variability that exists in biologic specimen, data are most useful for comparison testing and absolute parameters have been difficult to validate clinically.

Single-axis materials testers require certain features for biologic testing. Many have been retrofitted to accommodate bending grips and linear slides for biomechanical spine testing. Currently, standard spine fixtures capable of applying flexion extension and lateral bending moments are readily available. Sophisticated automated computer controls, high-grade bearing seals, and axial torsion capabilities are some of the manufacturers' features provided on standard spine testing equipment. Figure 5–4 represents a

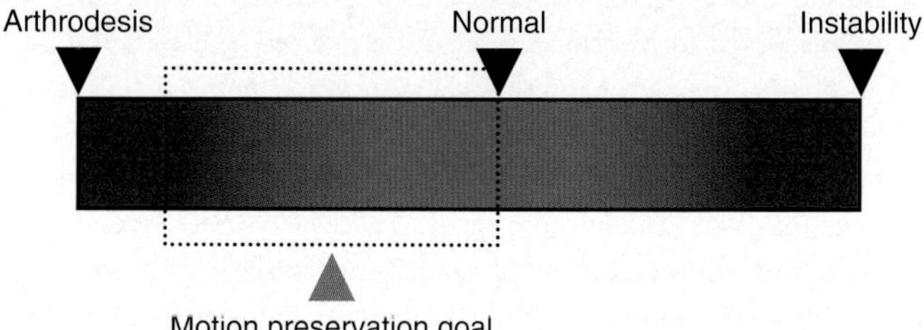


■ **FIGURE 5–3.** Continuous spectrum of stability. Motion preservation devices are expected to fall within the region defined by the rectangular plot.

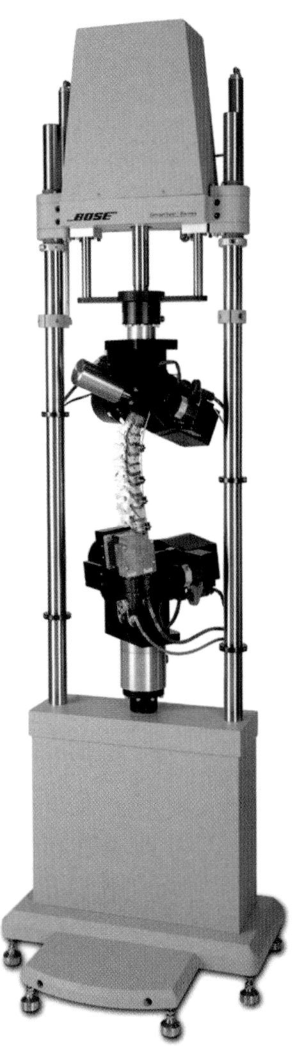

■ **FIGURE 5–4.** Spine tester with automated follower load capability. *(Courtesy of Welch Neurosurgical Research Laboratory, University of Pittsburgh, Pittsburgh, PA.)*

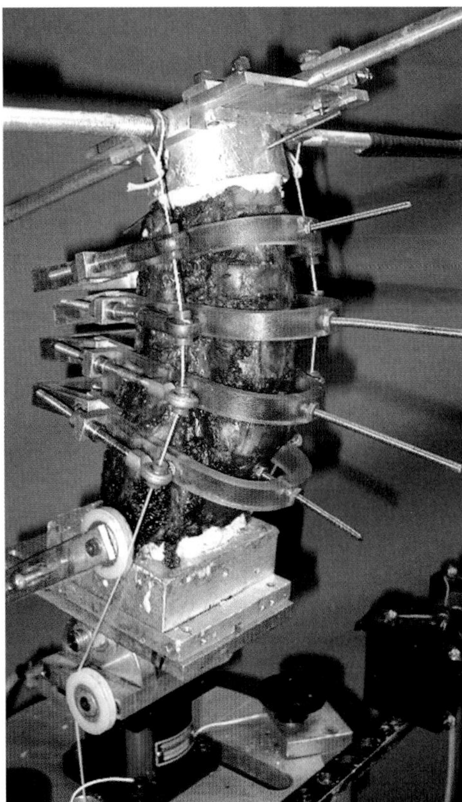

■ **FIGURE 5–5.** Spine tester using a transfer pump system to apply bending moments and a weight system to apply a follower load. *(Courtesy of Musculoskeletal Biomechanics Laboratory, Edward Hines Jr, VA Hospital, Hines, IL.)*

commercially available state-of-the-art standard spine tester capable of loading six axes with automated follower load capability.

Generally, spine testers apply a controlled load, and a measured response is recorded. Alternatively, displacements can be controlled and the corresponding load can be recorded. Finally, a third algorithm incorporating both load and displacement control at various stages in the protocol is possible, which are often referred to as hybrid control algorithms. Test configurations are important to understand because each configuration comes with a set of underlying assumptions and rationale on the method in which the load is applied. The assumptions are important in understanding artifacts from testing as opposed to treatment effects on a FSU. Turnkey solutions based on materials testers have been available for biomechanical spine testing. It is important to note that other credible custom apparatus for flexibility comparison testing of FSUs have been designed and developed by various investigators. An example of an alternative method of applying a moment has been reported, along with physiologic axial compression, as shown in Figure 5–5.

One of the first automated flexion-extension bending coupled motors that applied pure moments was described by Kunz et al[35] in the literature. Mounted on a materials tester capable of axial compression and axial torsion, the system was retrofitted for a matched set of stepper motors applying counteracting torques or displacements at each end. This method of pure moment application has been well documented.[36–39] Cunningham et al describes a similar custom-designed spine simulator with 6 degrees of freedom (6DOF-SS) that has been the source of many studies and cited in peer-reviewed journals.[1,4,22,31] Three independent stepper motors, harmonic drives, and electromagnetic clutches provide controllable loads in several independent degrees of freedom for a given spine test specimen. Additionally, artificial shear forces can be negated in this test arrangement through the use of linear bearing guide rails. The primary actuator provides an axial compressive capability to the system, which provides an additional degree of freedom.

Many spine test configurations have been documented for stability testing. Each of these configurations can replicate standardized load protocols for compression, torsion, and bending. Alternative test setups have also been described along with nonstandardized parameters. However, continued collaborative studies are needed in order to fully appreciate the differences. Because physiologic loading has been in ever-increasing demand, the relationship between standard loading versus physiologic loading must be further established and ultimately correlated to clinical implications.

### Standard Measurement Parameters

Descriptions of motion are important for a number of clinical reasons. The many methods of performing in vitro testing on constructs have provided insight into the nature of the performance of the instrumented spine. Each system has demonstrated carefully controlled loading methods. Whether the load is applied as a pure moment through a stepper motor or through a system of weights and pulleys, the response of the spine can be accurately measured.

The FSU response may be described in a load displacement curve, as shown in Figure 5–1. For any given FSU testing, there are six different types of independent loads and moments that can be applied and response in various contributions along the six degrees of freedoms that can be measured. The resulting three-dimensional kinematic outcome, whether in a single axis, single plane, or expressed as coupled motion in multiple planes is important, depending on the type of information that is necessary in understanding spinal instability.

An example of a one-dimensional physiologic response is load sharing in which axial compression is applied along the axial direction of the FSU. In order to deduce the amount of load transferred through the anterior and middle columns versus the load transferred through the posterior column, displacements are measured from axial compression tests. Assumptions made for cervical load–sharing protocols include elastic displacement and load distribution between columns. Rapoff et al[40] calculated the load-sharing properties of a cervical plate by axially compressing a spine with one and two times standard transmitted head weights, 45N and 90N, respectively, in a load-sharing biomechanical study. Axial test protocols have been used since to determine instrumented FSU characteristics for static and dynamic cervical implant design.[41] Load displacement data have been used to identify load percentages between functional anatomy, interbody spacer, and that of the fixation hardware.

Typically, the most clinically relevant response has often been reported as ROM. Two-dimensional planar parameters are common for a clinical measurement of flexion extension stability. Fusion treatments require a stable environment for arthrodesis, and it has been shown that the stiffer systems promote better clinical outcomes. Thus, a reduction in normalized two-dimensional sagittal ROM has often been linked to stability that promotes better clinical outcomes.[42] The same conditions can potentially cause nonphysiologic loading and displacements at alternate levels within the same segment. However, more sophisticated analysis and standardization are needed in reporting of coupled motion responses. Similar correlations between increased motion for FSUs and clinical outcomes are needed for combined loading or three-dimensional effects.

Regardless of the method of testing and the attempts at standardizing FSU test configurations, the results for stability measurements should be reported and discussed with the relevant parameters. Often, the trend has been to normalize to the intact control and to use ROM displacements relative to local coordinates.[5,29,43] Methods and results have been published and continue to evolve.[28] As new test methods evolve and surgical paradigms change, consistent reporting of the test configuration, along with standardized results, will allow quick adaptation of sophisticated test algorithms.

Currently, test configurations have referenced strain and load rates associated with osteoligamentous protocols previously described in joint biomechanics and testing. For cervical testing, 2.5 Nm torque has been justified, and for lumbar bending, 7.5 Nm has been documented. Load and displacement limits are often empirically derived. The condition of the cadaveric test specimen often dictates the load limits of testing and, thus, may not fully test the efficacy of treatment devices. Nonetheless, reporting of several important biomechanical parameters for implanted FSUs including the following has been consistent, frequently analyzed, and discussed in the literature[29]:

- NZ
- ROM
- Elastic zone
- Neutral zone stiffness
- Elastic zone stiffness

The parameters are essential to the understanding of the native intact condition as well as the various treatments of the spinal column for most test configurations. Until recently, the methods of reporting have been independent of the method of testing. ROM can be reported whether load is applied through pure moments, a follower load, or alternative methods.

A three-dimensional kinematic motion is a response for a vertebral body relative to the adjacent vertebrae and, ideally, a measure of the three-dimensional kinematic FSU response. Such results are the basis for comparison between treatments and the foundation for understanding the biomechanical effects on the clinical FSU. Parameters for motion preservation devices should include parameters for the quality of motion. Examples may potentially include smoothness criteria from flexion to extension bending, quantifying implant interface micromotion, and viscoelastic properties for the FSU. Parameters that have been proposed and are gaining acceptance include helical screw axis presented as instantaneous axis of rotation and disc pressure at adjacent levels.

The data most often generated and reported for biomechanical FSU testing are the resultant FSU ROM data. For fixation studies, the criteria are relatively simple when evaluating the biomechanical data that include ROM, that is, the smaller the ROM, the better the fixation result. Although ROM alone is not sufficient to describe the biomechanical characteristics of a FSU subjected to a motion preservation device treatment, it has been a key biomechanical parameter in assessing and predicting stability, particularly for the case immediately postoperatively. Therefore, ROM can be extrapolated to the clinical decision-making process. However, for newer technologies and implants, additional parameters may become more important, although currently, the motion parameters and clinical impact of quality of motion remain unclear.

## CONCLUSIONS FOR INSTRUMENTED SPINAL STABILITY

Biomechanical effects on a FSU, based on the described measurement methodologies, are important for a number of different reasons. Primarily for motion preservation techniques and devices, surgical intervention can relieve pain and restore function given the appropriate implant design. As devices are developed that allow motion and provide stability to the entire FSU, clinicians still require a means to biomechanically evaluate the potential for such treatments at the index and adjacent levels. Biomechanical stability testing is one facet that may help in the decision-making process for the clinical management of pathologies involving the spine.

## REFERENCES


1. Cunningham BW, Kotani Y, McNulty PS, et al: The effect of spinal destabilization and instrumentation on lumbar intradiscal pressure: an in vitro biomechanical analysis. Spine 22:2655–2663, 1997.
2. Harris BM, Hilibrand AS, Savas PE, et al: Transforaminal lumbar interbody fusion: the effect of various instrumentation techniques on the flexibility of the lumbar spine. Spine 29:E65–E70, 2004.
3. Heller JG, Zdeblick TA, Kunz DA, et al: Spinal instrumentation for metastatic disease: in vitro biomechanical analysis. J Spinal Disord 6:17–22, 1993.
4. Kanayama M, Ng JT, Cunningham BW, et al: Biomechanical analysis of anterior versus circumferential spinal reconstruction for various anatomic stages of tumor lesions. Spine 24:445–450, 1999.
5. Panjabi MM: Biomechanical evaluation of spinal fixation devices: I. A conceptual framework. Spine 13:1129–1134, 1988.
6. Patwardhan AG, Carandang G, Ghanayem AJ, et al: Compressive preload improves the stability of anterior lumbar interbody fusion cage constructs. J Bone Joint Surg Am 85-A:1749–1756, 2003.
7. Truumees E, Demetropoulos CK, Yang KH, Herkowitz HN: Effects of a cervical compression plate on graft forces in an anterior cervical discectomy model. Spine 28:1097–1102, 2003.
8. Hilibrand AS, Carlson GD, Palumbo MA, et al: Radiculopathy and myelopathy at segments adjacent to the site of a previous anterior cervical arthrodesis. J Bone Joint Surg Am 81:519–528, 1999.
9. Lee CK: Accelerated degeneration of the segment adjacent to a lumbar fusion. Spine 13:375–377, 1988.
10. Eck JC, Humphreys SC, Lim TH, et al: Biomechanical study on the effect of cervical spine fusion on adjacent-level intradiscal pressure and segmental motion. Spine 27:2431–2434, 2002.
11. Matsunaga S, Kabayama S, Yamamoto T, et al: Strain on intervertebral discs after anterior cervical decompression and fusion. Spine 24:670–675, 1999.
12. Pickett GE, Rouleau JP, Duggal N: Kinematic analysis of the cervical spine following implantation of an artificial cervical disc. Spine 30:1949–1954, 2005.
13. Virgin WJ: Experimental investigations into the physical properties of the intervertebral disc. J Bone Joint Surg Br 33-B:607–611, 1951.
14. Hirsch C, Nachemson A: New observations on the mechanical behavior of lumbar discs. Acta Orthop Scand 23:254–283, 1954.
15. Dick JC, Zdeblick TA, Bartel BD, Kunz DN: Mechanical evaluation of cross-link designs in rigid pedicle screw systems. Spine 22:370–375, 1997.
16. Hitchon PW, Goel VK, Rogge T, et al: Biomechanical studies on two anterior thoracolumbar implants in cadaveric spines. Spine 24:213–218, 1999.
17. Korovessis P, Papazisis Z, Koureas G, Lambiris E: Rigid, semirigid versus dynamic instrumentation for degenerative lumbar spinal stenosis: a correlative radiological and clinical analysis of short-term results. Spine 29:735–742, 2004.
18. Lund T, Nydegger T, Rathonyi G, et al: Three-dimensional stabilization provided by the external spinal fixator compared to two internal fixation devices: a biomechanical in vitro flexibility study. Eur Spine J 12:474–479, 2003.
19. Zdeblick TA, Wilson D, Cooke ME, et al: Anterior cervical discectomy and fusion. A comparison of techniques in an animal model. Spine 17:S418–S426, 1992.
20. McNally DS: The objectives for the mechanical evaluation of spinal instrumentation have changed. Eur Spine J 11(suppl 2):S179–S185, 2002.
21. Wilke HJ, Kettler A, Claes LE: Are sheep spines a valid biomechanical model for human spines? Spine 22:2365–2374, 1997.
22. Cunningham BW, Gordon JD, Dmitriev AE, et al: Biomechanical evaluation of total disc replacement arthroplasty: an in vitro human cadaveric model. Spine 28:S110–S117, 2003.
23. DiAngelo DJ, Foley KT: An improved biomechanical testing protocol for evaluating spinal arthroplasty and motion preservation devices in a multilevel human cadaveric cervical model. Neurosurg Focus 17:E4, 2004.
24. Patwardhan AG, Havey RM, Meade KP, et al: A follower load increases the load-carrying capacity of the lumbar spine in compression. Spine 24:1003–1009, 1999.
25. Goel VK, Clausen JD: Prediction of load sharing among spinal components of a C5-C6 motion segment using the finite element approach. Spine 23:684–691, 1998.
26. Puttlitz CM, Goel VK, Traynelis VC, Clark CR: A finite element investigation of upper cervical instrumentation. Spine 26:2449–2455, 2001.
27. Tschirhart CE, Nagpurkar A, Whyne CM: Effects of tumor location, shape and surface serration on burst fracture risk in the metastatic spine. J Biomech 37:653–660, 2004.
28. Goel VK, Panjabi MM, Patwardhan AG, et al: Test protocols for evaluation of spinal implants. J Bone Joint Surg Am 88(suppl 2): 103–109, 2006.
29. Wilke HJ, Wenger K, Claes L: Testing criteria for spinal implants: recommendations for the standardization of in vitro stability testing of spinal implants. Eur Spine J 7:148–154, 1998.
30. Akamaru T, Kawahara N, Sakamoto J, et al: The transmission of stress to grafted bone inside a titanium mesh cage used in anterior column reconstruction after total spondylectomy: a finite-element analysis. Spine 30:2783–2787, 2005.
31. Oda I, Cunningham BW, Abumi K, et al: The stability of reconstruction methods after thoracolumbar total spondylectomy. An in vitro investigation. Spine 24:1634–1638, 1999.
32. Dimar JR II, Voor MJ, Zhang YM, Glassman SD: A human cadaver model for determination of pathologic fracture threshold resulting from tumorous destruction of the vertebral body. Spine 23:1209–1214, 1998.
33. Shannon FJ, DiResta GR, Ottaviano D, et al: Biomechanical analysis of anterior poly-methyl-methacrylate reconstruction following total spondylectomy for metastatic disease. Spine 29:2096–2102, 2004.
34. Tschirhart C, Finkelstein J, Whyne C: Metastatic burst fracture risk assessment based on complex loading of the thoracic spine. Ann Biomed Eng 34:494–505, 2006.
35. Kunz DN, McCabe RP, Zdeblick TA, Vanderby R Jr: A multi-degree of freedom system for biomechanical testing. J Biomech Eng 116:371–373, 1994.
36. Deguchi M, Cheng BC, Sato K, et al: Biomechanical evaluation of translaminar facet joint fixation. A comparative study of poly-L-lactide pins, screws, and pedicle fixation. Spine 23:1307–1312, discussion 1313, 1998.
37. Mihara H, Cheng BC, David SM, et al: Biomechanical comparison of posterior cervical fixation. Spine 26:1662–1667, 2001.
38. Mihara H, Onari K, Cheng BC, et al: The biomechanical effects of spondylolysis and its treatment. Spine 28:235–238, 2003.
39. Rohlmann A, Neller S, Claes L, et al: Influence of a follower load on intradiscal pressure and intersegmental rotation of the lumbar spine. Spine 26:E557–E561, 2001.
40. Rapoff AJ, O'Brien TJ, Ghanayem AJ, et al: Anterior cervical graft and plate load sharing. J Spinal Disord 12:45–49, 1999.
41. Rapoff AJ, Conrad BP, Johnson WM, et al: Load sharing in Premier and Zephir anterior cervical plates. Spine 28:2648–2650, discussion 2651, 2003.
42. Zdeblick TA: A prospective, randomized study of lumbar fusion: Preliminary results. Spine 18:983–991, 1993.
43. Goel VK, Goyal S, Clark C, et al: Kinematics of the whole lumbar spine. Effect of discectomy. Spine 10:543–554, 1985.

CHAPTER 6

# Material Properties and Wear Analysis

**Nadim James Hallab, Markus Wimmer,** and **Joshua J. Jacobs**

## KEY POINTS

- Material properties central to orthopaedics are strength, toughness (fracture toughness, fatigue resistance), corrosion resistance, wear resistance, ductility, and modulus (of elasticity). Biocompatibility is the ability of a biomaterial to demonstrate host and material response appropriate to its intended application and thus changes with each application; that is, it is not inherent to a material and is not a material property.
- Implant debris is generated by both wear and corrosion.
- Corrosion resistance is the resistance to electrochemical degradation. Metal implant corrosion is controlled by (1) the extent of the thermodynamic driving forces, which cause corrosion (oxidation/reduction reactions), and (2) physical barriers, which limit the kinetics of corrosion (the protective oxide layer that forms on the surface of all metals).
- Wear resistance is currently extolled as paramount for reducing the debris of bearing surfaces in orthopaedics. Wear resistance is the property of a material to resist the loss of surface material as a consequence of a relative motion between two surfaces.
- Generally, **polymers** are relatively compliant (soft, low modulus), low-friction surfaces used for articulating bearings, with inert (less chemically reactive) debris or as fixative materials that can cure in situ (e.g., polymethyl methacrylate [PMMA]). **Ceramics** are valued for their high wear resistance and high strength. **Metals** offer a compromise of material properties such as high strength, ductility, fracture toughness, and hardness necessary for long-term use in high-cyclic, load-bearing roles required in fracture fixation and joint arthroplasty, and thus, metals remain the central material of orthopaedic implants even though they corrode (chemically degrade over time).

The material properties of biomaterials determine why a particular type of material is chosen for a particular orthopaedic application. Orthopaedic biomaterials are generally limited to those materials that withstand cyclic load-bearing applications, and include all three major types of materials: (1) metals, (2) polymers, and (3)ceramics. Material properties critical to fracture fixation and total joint arthroplasty (TJA) include high strength, ductility, fracture toughness, wear resistance, and corrosion resistance. Wear resistance is currently extolled as paramount for reducing the debris of bearing surfaces in TJA. That is, wear debris is currently considered the primary factor affecting the long-term performance of joint replacement prostheses, and the primary source of orthopaedic biomaterial debris (based on overall implant mass or volume lost). Implant debris is generated by both wear and corrosion, and results in the formation of an inflammatory reaction. This reaction eventually promotes a foreign-body granulation tissue response that has the ability to invade the bone–implant interface. This response commonly results in progressive local bone loss that threatens the fixation of both cemented and cementless devices alike.[1] Thus corrosion and wear resistance of spinal implant materials are discussed in detail in this chapter.

The first part of this chapter covers the basic material properties of metals, ceramics, and polymers that are important for orthopaedic implants (with greater focus on corrosion). The second part of the chapter discusses how implant materials used for orthopaedic applications were chosen based on these material properties. The third part of this chapter covers how analysis of wear is conducted to determine whether or not components meet acceptable levels of wear.

## MATERIAL PROPERTIES

It is the properties of polymers, ceramics, and metals that make each material suitable for different roles in orthopaedic implants, including all those implants covered in the later chapters of this textbook. The first part of this section addresses questions such as what are these important material properties, and how are these properties defined? The latter portion of this section covers which materials embody a maximal amount of these properties and for which applications they are typically used.

Although it is an overgeneralization, the material properties of each category of material are determined by the chemical bonds associated with that type of material (Table 6–1).

Although these chemical bonds determine beneficial material properties, they are also responsible for shortcomings associated with each material as well; for example, polymers have low strength, ceramics have low fracture toughness, and metals are chemically reactive (prone to corrosion). Furthermore, it is the material properties within each type of material that determine which of the many types of polymers, ceramics, and metals are best suited for use as orthopaedic implants. These "more" important properties for each type of material are generally (1) strength and wear resistance for polymers, (2) fracture toughness and wear

TABLE 6–1. Material Properties

| Material | Molecular Bonds | General Properties |
|---|---|---|
| Polymers | Carbon to carbon covalently bonded chains, weak secondary bonds | Chemically inert, ductile, deformable, low modulus |
| Ceramics | Ionic bonds | Chemically inert, hard, wear resistant |
| Metals | Metallic bond | Chemically noninert, ductile, strong, tough |

resistance for ceramics, and (3) strength, corrosion resistance, and wear resistance for metals.

Some material properties such as density are important, but they are not typically used as critical design criteria in orthopaedic implants and are not discussed here. Other material properties such as cost and machinability that are not inherent to the material (i.e., they change with human technologic innovation) are extremely important to implant manufacturers but are not theoretically important to the orthopaedic surgeons or scientists who seek to improve implants. Generally, the material properties that are most central to orthopaedic designs are listed below, followed by a more extensive discussion:

- Strength
- Toughness (fracture toughness, fatigue resistance)
- Corrosion resistance
- Wear resistance
- Ductility
- Modulus (of elasticity)

## Strength

Strength is the property that enables any material to resist deformation under load. There are various measures of strength, but all are related to the point at which an applied load begins to permanently deform the material, that is, begins to irreversibly affect the materials' bonds/microstructure. Figure 6–1 shows the strength properties of a material as measured with a stress versus strain curve, in which stress is a load per unit area and strain is the amount of stretch. The ultimate strength is the highest stress a material can withstand. Tensile strength is a measurement of the resistance to being pulled apart when placed in a tension load. Fatigue strength is the ability of material to resist various kinds of rapidly changing stresses and is expressed by the magnitude of alternating stress for a specified number of cycles. Impact strength is the ability of a metal to resist suddenly applied loads and is measured in foot-pounds of force.

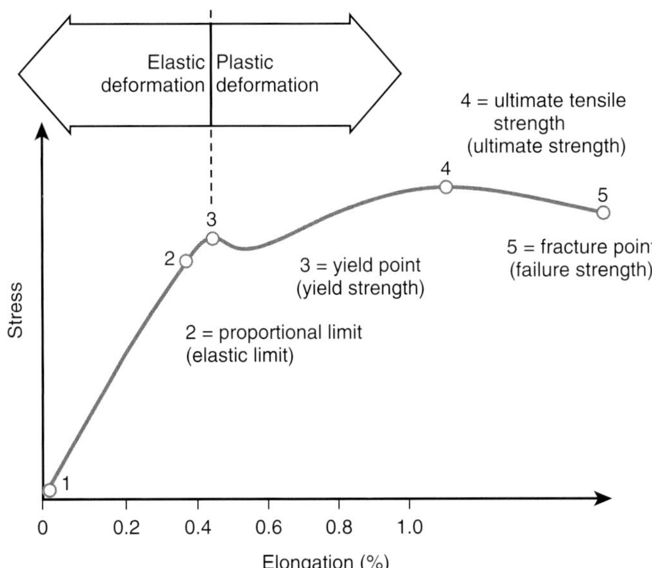


■ FIGURE 6–1. Generic stress-strain curve showing the different material property measures of strength.

## Toughness (Fracture Toughness, Fatigue Resistance)

Toughness is the property that enables a material to withstand shock and to be deformed without rupturing. Toughness may be considered a combination of strength and plasticity and is defined as the area underneath the stress versus strain curve, that is, the total work to failure (Fig. 6–2). Fatigue resistance generally varies with toughness and ductility, and is the ability of a material to resist fracture under a repeated load.

## Corrosion Resistance

Corrosion resistance is the resistance to electrochemical degradation. Electrochemical processes include generalized corrosion uniformly affecting an entire surface, and localized corrosion affecting either areas of a device relatively shielded from the environment (crevice corrosion), or seemingly random sites on the surface (pitting corrosion). All metals corrode, even gold and platinum, which do it at very low rates.

## Wear Resistance

Wear resistance is the property of a material to resist the loss of surface material as a consequence of a relative motion between two surfaces. Two materials placed together under load will only contact over a small area of the higher peaks or asperities. Electrorepulsive and atomic binding interactions occur at the individual contacts, and when the two surfaces slide relative to one another, these interactions are disrupted. There are primarily three processes that can cause wear: (1) abrasion, by which a harder surface "plows" grooves in the softer material; (2) adhesion, by which a softer material is smeared onto a harder counter surface, forming a transfer film;

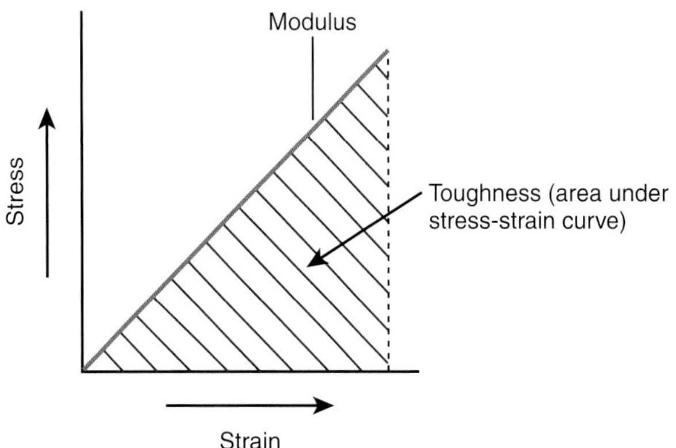


■ FIGURE 6–2. Toughness is defined as the area under the stress-strain curve of a given material.

and (3) fatigue, by which alternating episodes of loading and unloading result in the formation of subsurface cracks, which propagate to form particles that are shed from the surface. This feature is covered in more detail in the second section of this chapter.

## Ductility

Ductility is the ability of a material to deform (e.g., stretch, bend, or twist) without cracking or breaking (Fig. 6–3).

## Modulus (of Elasticity)

The elasticity of a material is the degree to which a load stretches, compresses, or twists (deforms) a material. The modulus of elasticity is generally defined as the change in length (strain) over a given change in applied load (stress) or the linear slope of the stress versus strain curve.

Biocompatibility is often talked about as a "material property"; however, technically it is not. Biocompatibility is officially described as "the ability of a biomaterial to demonstrate host and material response appropriate to its intended application." Thus, the biocompatibility of a material changes with each application and cannot be inherent to a material in the same way the above-mentioned properties are. Biocompatibility is discussed only briefly in this chapter.

Today, the biocompatibility of an implant is largely focused on the ability of a material to resist degradation. Although tissue reaction to wear debris is currently extolled as the primary factor limiting the longevity of joint replacement prostheses, much is unknown regarding which type of debris is more pathogenic. Thus, the biocompatibility of a particular material is currently more narrowly defined as what type of reactivity will result from the kind of debris produced when employed in a particular application.

## Corrosion of Implant Metals

Corrosion resistance is the primary material property responsible for limiting the choice of available metal alloys to the relatively few available for use in orthopaedics. However, it is not a simple property to understand; thus, the following discussion will attempt to summarize why metals corrode and how implant metals resist this tendency. Metal implant corrosion is controlled by (1) the extent of the thermodynamic driving forces that cause corrosion (oxidation/reduction reactions) and (2) physical barriers that limit the kinetics of corrosion. In practice, these two factors that mediate the corrosion of orthopaedic biomaterials can be broken down into a number of parameters: geometric variables (e.g., taper geometry in modular component hip prostheses), metallurgical variables (e.g., surface microstructure, oxide structure and composition), mechanical variables (e.g., stress and/or relative motion), and solution variables (e.g., pH, solution proteins, enzymes).

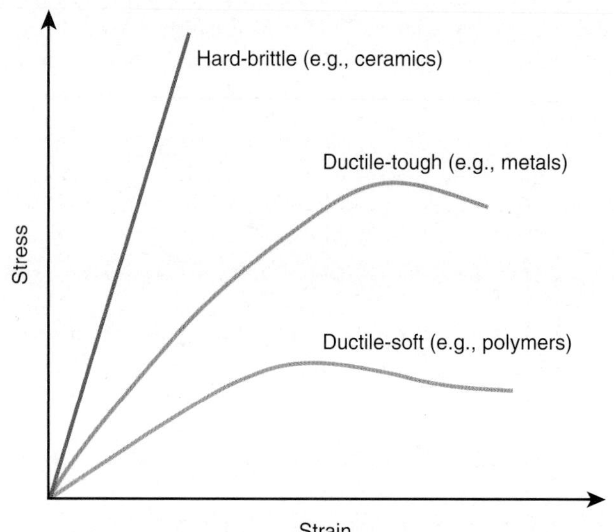


■ **FIGURE 6–3.** Different stress-strain curves representing generic behavior differences between metals, ceramics, and polymers.

### Thermodynamic Considerations: How and Why Metals Corrode

The basic reaction that occurs during corrosion is the increase of the valence state (i.e., loss of electrons) of the metal atom.

$$M \rightarrow M^{z+} + z_{e^-} \text{ (oxidation)} \quad \textbf{6-1}$$

This oxidation event (loss of electrons and increase in valence) may result in the release of free ions from the metal surface into solution (which can then migrate away from the metal surface), or may result in many other reactions such as the formation of metal oxides, metal chlorides, organometallic compounds, or other species. These "end" products may also be soluble in solution or may precipitate to form solid phases. Solid oxidation products may be subdivided into those that form adherent compact oxide films, and those that form nonadherent oxide (or other) particles that can migrate away from the metal surface.

For corrosion to occur at all, it must be chemically desirable (i.e., have a thermodynamic driving force for the reduction of metal atoms). Gold and platinum are examples of metals that have little or no driving force for oxidation in aqueous solutions, and thus, they tend to corrode very little in the human body. However, most orthopaedic metals have very negative potentials, indicating that, from a chemical driving force perspective, they are much more likely to corrode. For example, Ti has a very large negative potential, −1.6V, indicating that there is a large chemical driving force for corrosion (oxidation). If surface oxide formation (or passivation) did not intervene, pure Ti would react with its surroundings (typically oxygen, water, or other oxidizing species) and corrode vigorously. But it does not, thanks to the formation of chemically stable metal oxides.

### Kinetic Barriers to Corrosion: Oxide Film Formation

The second primary factor that governs the corrosion process of metallic biomaterials is the formation of stable surface barriers or limitations to the kinetics of corrosion. These barriers prevent corrosion by physically limiting the rate at which oxidation or reduction processes can take place. The formation of a metal-oxide passive film on a metal surface is one example of a kinetic limitation to corrosion. The general reaction that governs this formation is as follows:

$$M^{z+} + \frac{z}{2}H_2O \rightarrow \frac{z}{2}MO + zH + z_{e^-} \quad \textbf{6-2}$$

In general, kinetic barriers to corrosion prevent either the migration of metallic ions from the metal to the solution, the migration of anions from solution to metal, or the migration of electrons across the metal-solution interface. Passive oxide films are the most well known forms of kinetic barriers in corrosion, but other kinetic barriers exist, including manufactured polymeric coatings.

Orthopaedic alloys rely almost entirely on the formation of passive films to prevent significant oxidation (corrosion) from taking place. These films consist of metal oxides (ceramic films) that form spontaneously on the surface of the metal in such a way that they prevent further transport of metallic ions and electrons across the film. To be effective barriers, the films must be compact and fully cover the metal surface; they must have an atomic structure that limits the migration of ions and/or electrons across the metal-oxide-solution interface; and they must be able to remain on the surface of these alloys even with mechanical stressing or abrasion, which is expected with orthopaedic devices.

Passivating oxide films spontaneously grow on the surface of metals. These oxide films are very thin (on the order of 5 to 70 Å) and may be amorphous or crystalline, which depends on the potential across the interface as well as solution variables like pH.[2] When an oxide film is detached from the metal substrate, unoxidized metal is exposed to solution. These films tend to reform or repassivate, and the magnitude of the repassivation currents may be large. This is due to the normally large driving forces that are present for the oxidation process, which, when the kinetic barrier is removed, can operate to cause oxidation. However, the extent and duration of the oxidation currents will depend on the repassivation kinetics for oxide film formation. Hence, the mechanical stability of the oxide films, as well as the driving force associated with their formation, is central to the performance of oxide films in orthopaedic applications.

## MATERIALS WITH ACCEPTABLE PROPERTIES FOR ORTHOPAEDICS

Of the many polymers, ceramics, and metals usually chosen for orthopaedic applications, a relative few dominate as implant materials. These are listed below:

Polymers: Ultra-high-molecular-weight polyethylene (UHMWPE), polymethyl methacrylate (PMMA), polyetheretherketone (PEEK)*, and polyurethane (PU)*

Ceramics: Alumina, zirconia

Metals: Cobalt-chromium-molybdenum alloy, Ti alloy, pure Ti, stainless steel, zirconium and tantalum

Why is it that among the many polymers, ceramics, and metals, only a relative few dominate orthopaedics and are used in spinal implants? First, there are distinct advantages of each kind of material (polymer versus metal; see Figure 6–3). Second, within each material type, there are generally only a few winning candidates that have an optimal mix of desired properties that have endured the test of time, for example, titanium (Ti) and cobalt (Co) alloys.

Desirable properties of all orthopaedic implants include high strength, high wear resistance, low modulus (close to bone or cartilage), high ductility, high fracture toughness, and high corrosion resistance. Of course, some of these properties remain mutually exclusive, such that a low modulus, highly ductile (e.g., polymeric) material is not currently capable of simultaneously processing high strength like a metal and high wear resistance like a ceramic. Because no material excels in all property categories and because not all implant components require that the same material property be the most important, implant components are often made of different materials based on which material best suits the design criteria for that "section" of the implant.

Generally, polymers are compliant (soft), low-friction surfaces for articulating bearings, with inert (less chemically reactive) debris or as fixative materials that can cure in situ (e.g., PMMA). Ceramics are valued for their wear resistance and high strength. Metals provide the best mix of material properties (high strength, ductility, fracture toughness, hardness, formability, and high-energy osteophilic surfaces-biocompatible) necessary for long-term use in high-cyclic load-bearing roles required in fracture fixation and joint arthroplasty, and thus metals, remain the central material of orthopaedic implants even though they corrode.

### Polymers

Polymers are most commonly used in orthopaedics as low friction and compliant (low modulus) articulating bearing surfaces of joint replacements and as an interpositional cementing material between the implant surface and bone. They are the lowest-strength materials used in orthopaedic implants but are highly ductile and compliant (Table 6–2). Material properties such as creep (the ability of a material to flow under load) and viscoelasticity (the ability of a material to change its stress versus strain response when the rate at which a load is applied changes) are unique concerns of polymeric implant materials. Of these two properties, it is only creep that is critical to implant design, as discussed later in this section. Polymers used as articulating surfaces must have low coefficients of friction and low wear rates when in articulating contact with an opposing surface, which is usually made of metal. Initially, John Charnley used Teflon (PTFE) for the acetabular component of his total hip arthroplasty. However, its accelerated creep and poor strength caused it to fail in vivo, requiring replacement with UHMWPE. Polymers used for fixation as a structural interface between the implant component and bone tissue require appropriate mechanical properties of a polymer, which can be molded into shape and cured in vivo. The first type to be used, PMMA, was again popularized by Charnley. He adapted PMMA as a "grouting material" to fix both the stem of the femoral component and the acetabular component in place, and thus distribute the loads more uniformly from the implants to the bone interface. Because high interfacial stresses result from the accommodation of a high-modulus prosthesis within the much lower modulus bone, the use of a lower modulus interpositional material has been a goal of alternative polymers seeking to improve upon PMMA fixation. Thus, polymers such as polysulfone have been tried as porous coatings on the implant's metallic core to permit mechanical interlocking through bone and soft tissue ingrowth into the pores. However, to date, PMMA remains the method of choice for orthopaedic surgeons. This requires that polymers have surfaces that resist creep under the stresses found in clinical situations and have high enough yield strengths to minimize plastic deformation. As indicated earlier, the important mechanical properties of orthopaedic polymers are yield stress, creep resistance, and wear

*Newer implant materials in use or development.

TABLE 6–2. Mechanical Properties of Dominant Orthopedic Biomaterials[12]

| Orthopaedic Biomaterial | ASTM Standard | Elastic Modulus (Young's Modulus) | Yield Strength (Elastic Limit) | Ultimate Strength | Fatigue Strength (Endurance Limit) | Hardness | Elongation at Fracture |
|---|---|---|---|---|---|---|---|
| | | (GPa) | (MPa) | (MPa) | (MPa) | HVN | (%) |
| Cortical Bone* | | | | | | | |
| low strain | — | 15.2 | 114t | 150c/90t | 30–45 | — | — |
| high strain | — | 40.8 | — | 400c–270t | — | — | — |
| CERAMICS | | | | | | | |
| Alumina | ASTM F60310 | 366 | 310t 3,790c | 310t 3,790c | 4 MPa/mL/2 | 22 GPa | — |
| Zirconia | ASTM F-1873-98 | 201 | 420t 7,500c | 420t 7,500c | 6 MPa/mL/2 | 12 GPa | — |
| POLYMERS | | | | | | | |
| UHMWPE | ASTM F648 | 0.5–1.3 | 20–30 | 30–40t 30–40c | 13–20 | 60–90 (MPa) | 130–500 |
| PEEK | ASTM F2026-02 | 3.6–13 | 12–60 | 70–208t 80–120c | 33–36 | 100–120 MPa | 25–80 |
| Polyurethane | ASTM F624-98a | 0.0018–0.009 | 28–40 | 28–40t 33–50c | 21–30 | 50–120 (MPa) | 600–720 |
| PMMA | ASTM F451-99 | 1.8–3.3 | 35–70 | 38–80t 45–107c | 19–39 | 100–200 (MPa) | 2.5–6 |
| METALS | | | | | | | |
| Stainless Steel | ASTM F138 | 190 | 792 | 930t | 241–820 | 130–180 | 43–45 |
| *Co-Cr Alloys* | ASTM F75 | 210–253 | 448–841 | 655–1,277t | 207–950 | 300–400 | 4–14 |
| | ASTM F90 | 210 | 448–1,606 | 1,896t | 586–1,220 | 300–400 | 10–22 |
| | ASTM F562 | 200–230 | 300–2,000 | 800–2,068t | 340–520 | 8–50 (RC) | 10–40 |
| | ASTM 1537 | 200–300 | 960 | 1,300t | 200–300 | 41 (RC) | 20 |
| Ti Alloys | | | | | | | |
| CPTi | ASTM F67 | 110 | 485 | 760t | 300 | 120–200 | 14–18 |
| Ti-6A1-4V | ASTM 136 | 116 | 897–1,034 | 965–1,103t | 620–689 | 310 | 8 |
| Tantalum | ASTM F-560-05 | 186 | 325–690 | 900 | 230 | 873 MPa | — |
| Zirconium | ASTM F2384-05 | 95 | 230 | 330 | — | 150 | 32 |

ASTM, American Society for Testing and Materials; c, compression; Co, cobalt; Cr, chromium; HVN, Vickers Hardness Number, kg/mm; PEEK, polyether-ether-ketone; PMMA, polymethylmethacylate; RC, Rockwell Hardness Scale; t, tension; Ti, titanium; UHMWPE, ultra-high-molecular-weight polyethylene.
*Cortical bone is both anisotropic and viscoelastic thus mechanical properties listed are overly generalized to low strain rates and isotropic averages.

rate. These factors are controlled by such parameters as molecular chain structure, molecular weight, and degree of branching or (conversely) of chain linearity.

### Ultra-High-Molecular-Weight Polyethylene

One of the more prevalent polymers used in orthopaedics today is a highly cross-linked-UHMWPE, which is typically used in TJA as a load-bearing articulating surface, designed to provide low-friction load-bearing articulation. This material, which has gained popularity in hip arthroplasty, is gaining acceptance in knee arthroplasty as well where concerns of delamination and lower fracture toughness of the harder, more wear-resistant material are being tested. Polyethylene is available commercially in three different grades: low density, high density, and UHMWPE. The better packing of linear chains within UHMWPE results in increased crystallinity and provides improved mechanical properties required for orthopaedic use, even though there is a decrease in both ductility and fracture toughness.

UHMWPE has a molecular weight of 2 to 10 million g/mol.[3] Wear of polyethylene in total hip arthroplasty (THA) applications produces billions of wear particles annually (predominantly in the <1 micron range). Extra cross-linking of polyethylene, using chemical and radiation techniques, has only recently improved this wear/abrasion resistance in joint arthroplasty applications. The wear resistance of UHMWPE is improved by cross-linking with gamma irradiation at 2.5 to 5.0 Mrad; however, this can negatively affect physical properties such as tensile strength and fracture toughness. Usually, manufactured components of UHMWPE are sterilized by $\gamma$-irradiation, because UHMWPE is heat sensitive, and both intrastructural or dimensional changes of the material occur under the influence of heat. Thus, most manufacturers use machining processes to form the ultimate implant shape after treatments such as extra cross-linking.[4]

For spinal applications, UHMWPE artificial discs require high wear resistance as well as resistance to cold flow. Although loading is similar to other joint prostheses (e.g., total knee arthroplasty), the relative motion of bearing surfaces is approximately an order of magnitude less. Past reports by Lee and Pienkowski[5] indicate that creep occurs in the amorphous regions of the UHMWPE (rather than in the crystalline regions), and recovery occurs within the same regions. Therefore, it is more advantageous to retain a high degree of more typical crystalline structure in non-highly cross-linked UHMWPEs. This is because polyethylene (PE) crystallinity can be reduced by ~15%[6] by cross-linking. Consequently, extra cross-linking may not be worth the advantages for UHMWPE when used as bearing material in artificial discs.

The cold flow limit of UHMWPE is 22 N/mm. Thus, an inadequate thickness of UHMWPE components can adversely affect mechanical properties. Total knee replacements have demonstrated that polyethylene components should have a minimal thickness of 6 to 8 mm. This advice is listed in a European Standard (EN 12564, 19998) and a Food and Drug Administration (FDA) Guidance document (Draft Guidance for the Preparation of Premarket Notifications, for cemented and semi-constrained total knee prosthesis, 1993). This is particularly important when small-sized implants or nonparallel components for large lordotic angles are used when the load limit per cubic millimeter may be exceeded, resulting in significant creep, thinning, and, ultimately, fracture.

## Ceramics

Over the past decade, ceramics and glass ceramics have played an increasingly important role in implants as bearing surfaces. The primary reason for the introduction of this alternative bearing surface is the superior wear resistance of ceramics when compared with metal–metal or metal–polymer bearing surfaces. This and other improved properties such as resistance to further oxidation (implying inertness within the body), high stiffness, and low friction require the use of full-density, controlled, small, uniform grain size (usually less than 5 μm) ceramic materials. The small grain size and full density are important because these are the two principal bulk parameters controlling the ceramic's mechanical properties. Any voids within the ceramic's body will increase stress, degrading the mechanical properties. Grain size controls the magnitude of the internal stresses produced by thermal contraction during cooling. In ceramics, such thermal contraction stresses are critical because they cannot be dissipated as they can in ductile materials through plastic deformation.

Alumina ($Al_2O_3$) and zirconia ($ZrO_2$) ceramics have been used in orthopaedic THA for the past 30 years. The first ceramic couple (alumina/alumina) was implanted in 1970 by Pierre Boutin. Since the outset, the theoretical advantage of hard-on-hard articulating surfaces was low wear. Ceramics, because of their ionic bonds and chemical stability, are also relatively biocompatible. Initial concerns about fracture toughness and wear have been addressed by lowering grain size, increasing purity, lowering porosity, and improving manufacturing techniques (e.g., hot isostatic pressing [HIP]). Early failures of these couples were plagued with both material-related and surgical errors. The very low wear rates combined with steadily decreasing rates of fracture (now estimated to occur 1/2,000 over 10 years) have resulted in the growing popularity of all ceramic bearings.

Zirconia was introduced in 1985 as a material alternative to alumina for ceramic femoral heads, and has been gaining market share because of its demonstrable enhanced mechanical properties in the laboratory when compared with alumina. Femoral heads of zirconia can typically withstand 250 kN (or 25 tons), a value generally exceeding that possible with alumina or metal femoral heads. However, mechanical integrity of all ceramic components is extremely dependent on manufacturing quality controls, as evidenced in the recent recall of thousands of zirconia-ceramic femoral heads by their manufacturer, St. Gobain Desmarquest on August 14, 2001. This was because of in vivo fracture of some components due to an unlikely and unintended variation in the manufacturing sintering process caused when the company upgraded to a high-throughput assembly line–type oven. In general, ceramic particulate debris is chemically stable and more biocompatible than metallic debris because it is less reactive to cells.

## Metals

Current implant alloys were originally developed for the maritime and aviation industries over half a century ago, in which mechanical properties such as high strength and corrosion resistance are paramount. There are three principal metal alloys used in orthopaedics and particularly in TJA: (1) Ti-based alloys, (2) Co-based alloys, and (3) stainless steel alloys (Table 6–3).[7] Alloy-specific differences in strength, ductility, and hardness generally determine which of these three alloys is used for a particular application or implant component (see Table 6–2). However, it is the high corrosion resistance of all three alloys, more than anything, that has led to their widespread use as load-bearing implant materials (Table 6–4).[8]

Metals remain the central material component of state-of-the-art total hip arthroplasties. Metals provide appropriate material properties such as high strength, ductility, fracture toughness, hardness, corrosion resistance, formability, and biocompatibility necessary for use in load-bearing roles required in fracture fixation and TJA. These material properties of metals (see Table 6–2) are due to the miraculous nature of the metallic bond, molecular microstructure, and elemental composition of metals.

### Stainless Steel Alloys

All stainless steels are composed of iron, carbon, chromium, nickel, and molybdenum (see Table 6–3). The form of stainless steel most commonly used in orthopaedic practice is designated 316LV (American Society for Testing and Materials F-138, ASTM F-138): 316 classifies the material as austenitic, the L denotes the low carbon content, and V the vacuum under which it is formed. The carbon content must be kept at a low level to prevent carbide (chromium-carbon) accumulation at the grain boundaries. This carbide formation weakens the material by allowing a combination of corrosion and stress to degrade the material at its grain boundaries.

**TABLE 6–3. Approximate Weight Percent of Different Metals Within Popular Orthopaedic Alloys**

| Alloy | Ni | N | Co | Cr | Ti | Mo | Al | Fe | Mn | Cu | W | C | Si | V |
|---|---|---|---|---|---|---|---|---|---|---|---|---|---|---|
| **Stainless Steel** | | | | | | | | | | | | | | |
| (ASTM F138) | 10–15.5 | <0.5 | * | 17–19 | * | 2–4 | * | 61–68 | * | <0.5 | <2.0 | <0.06 | <1.0 | * |
| **CoCrMo Alloys** | | | | | | | | | | | | | | |
| (ASTM F75) | <2.0 | * | 61–66 | 27–30 | * | 4.5–7.0 | * | <1.5 | <1.0 | * | * | <0.35 | <1.0 | * |
| (ASTM F90) | 9–11 | * | 46–51 | 19–20 | * | * | * | <3.0 | <2.5 | * | 14–16 | <0.15 | <1.0 | * |
| (ASTM F562) | 33–37 | * | 35 | 19–21 | <1 | 9.0–11 | * | <1 | <0.15 | * | * | * | <0.15 | * |
| **Ti Alloys** | | | | | | | | | | | | | | |
| CPTi (ASTM F67) | * | * | * | * | 99 | * | * | 0.2–0.5 | * | * | * | <0.1 | * | * |
| Ti-6A1–4V (ASTM F136) | * | * | * | * | 89–91 | * | 5.5–6.5 | * | * | * | * | <0.08 | * | 3.5–4.5 |
| 45TiNi | 55 | * | * | * | 45 | * | * | * | * | * | * | * | * | * |

Al, aluminum; ASTM, American Society for Testing and Materials; C, carbon; Co, cobalt; Cr, chromium; Cu, copper; Fe, iron; Mn, manganese; Mo, molybdenum; Ni, nickel; N, nitrogen; Si, silicon; Ti, titanium; V, vanadium; W, tungsten.

*Indicates less than 0.05%

Note: Alloy compositions are standardized by the American Society for Testing and Materials (ASTM vol. 13.01).

TABLE 6–4. Electrochemical Properties of Implant Metals (Corrosion Resistance) in 0.1 M NaCl at pH=7 (Except Where Indicated)*

| Alloy | ASTM Standard | Density | Corrosion Potential (versus Calomel) OCP | Passive Current Density ($I_p$) | Breakdown Potential ($E_b$) | Polarization Current (i) and Polarization Resistance (Rc) at 37°C | | Repassivation Time in 0.3 M NaCl (0.9%) (mseconds) | |
|---|---|---|---|---|---|---|---|---|---|
| | | g/cm³ | mVolts | μAmps/cm² | mVolts | i μA/cm² | Rc kΩ/cm² | −500 mV | +500 mV |
| **Stainless Steel** | ASTM F138 | 8.0 | −400 | 0.56 | 200–770 | 0.006 | 1,670 | 72,000 | 35 |
| **Co-Cr-Mo Alloys** | ASTM F75 | 8.3 | −390 | 1.36 | 420 | 0.004 | 2,500 | 44 | 36 |
| **Ti Alloys** | | | | | | | | | |
| *cpTi* | ASTM F67 | 4.5 | −90 to −630 | 0.72–9.0 | >2,400 | 0.010 | 1,000 | 43 | 44 |
| *Ti-6Al-4V* | ASTM 136 | 4.43 | −180 to −510 | 0.9–2.0 | >1,500 | 0.008 | 1,250 | 37 | 41 |
| *Ti5Al2.5Fe* | ‡ | 4.45 | −530 | 0.68 | >1,500 | † | † | 110–130 | 120–160 |
| *Ti 45Ni* | ‡ | 6.4–6.5 | −430 | 0.44 | 890 | † | † | † | † |

ASTM, American Society for Testing and Materials; Co, cobalt; Cr, chromium; Fe, Iron; Mo, molybdenum; Ni, nickel; Ti, titanium.
*The Corrosion Potential represents the open circuit potential (OCP) between the metal and a calomel electrode. The more negative the OCP, the more chemically reactive and thus the less corrosion resistance. Generally low current density indicates greater corrosion resistance. The higher the breakdown potential the better, (i.e., the more elevated the breakdown potential, the more stable the protective layer).
†Data not available.
‡No current ASTM designation.

Molybdenum is added to enhance the corrosion resistance of the grain boundaries, whereas chromium dissipated evenly within the microstructure allows the formation of chromium oxide ($Cr_2O_3$) on the surface of the metal. Stainless steels and other implant alloys are surface treated (e.g., in nitric acid) to promote the growth and thickening of this passive oxide layer. Although the mechanical properties of stainless steels are generally less desirable than those of the other implant alloys, stainless steels do possess greater ductility indicated quantitatively by a threefold greater "percentage of elongation at fracture" when compared with other implant metals (see Table 6–2). This aspect of stainless steel has allowed it to remain as a popular material for cable fixation components in TKA. However, the superior mechanical properties of Co- and Ti-based alloys have led to their dominance in TJA stem and head components.[9–11]

Although stainless steel has been used widely in spinal instrumentation (Harrington rods, hooks, pedicle screws, and so on), today's trend toward Ti implants is largely due to clinical history of enhanced biocompatibility in TJA applications. Additionally, Ti produces fewer artifacts in magnetic resonance imaging (MRI) and computerized tomography.[12] However, the cost-effectiveness of stainless steel has led to its worldwide popularity for temporary implants (screws, nails, bone plates, and so on).[6]

### Cobalt-Chromium Alloys

The two basic constituents of all cobalt-chromium (CoCr) alloys are Co (approximately 65%) and Cr (approximately 35%). Molybdenum is added to decrease the grain size and thus improve mechanical properties. Cobalt-chromium implant alloys fall into one of two categories: those with nickel and other alloying elements, and those without. Of the many CoCr alloys available, there are two most commonly used as implant alloys (see Table 6–3): 1) cobalt-chromium-molybdenum (CoCrMo), which is designated ASTM F-75 and F-76; and 2) cobalt-nickel-chromium-molybdenum (CoNiCrMo) designated as ASTM F-562. CoNiCrMo alloys which contain large percentages of Ni (25–37%), promise increased corrosion resistance yet raise concerns of possible toxicity and immunogenic reactivity (discussed later) from released Ni. The dominant implant alloy used for total joint components is CoCrMo (ASTM F-75). The corrosion resistance of CoCrMo alloys is primarily due to the Cr content within the metal which results in the formation of a protective passive layer of Cr oxide on the surface of the metal. Although CoCrMo alloys are among the strongest, hardest, and most fatigue-resistant of the metals used for joint replacement components, care must be taken to maintain these properties because the use of finishing treatments can also function to reduce these same properties (see Table 6–2). For example, sintering of porous coatings onto components can decrease the fatigue strength of the alloy to 150 Mpa. This is a concern for total disc replacement (TDR), in which sintered porous Ti coatings are essentially an industry standard and the available thickness of TDR end plates is restricted.[13]

### Titanium Alloys

Ti alloys were developed in the mid-1940s for the aviation industry and were first used in orthopaedics around the same time. Two post–World War II alloys, commercially pure Ti (CPTi) and Ti alloy (6% aluminum and 4% vanadium [Ti-6Al-4V]), remain the two dominant Ti alloys used in TJA implants. Commercially pure Ti (CPTi, ASTM F-67) is 98% to 99.6% pure Ti. The crystal structure of CPTi is hexagonal close packed, yet it can be cold worked for further improvement in mechanical properties. Although CPTi is most commonly used in dental applications, the stability of the oxide layer formed on CPTi (and consequently its high corrosion resistance) and its relatively higher ductility (i.e., the ability to be cold worked) compared with Ti-6Al-4V have led to its use in porous coatings (e.g., fiber metal) of TJA components. Generally, Ti-6Al-4V (ASTM F-136) is used for joint replacement components because of its superior mechanical properties in comparison to CPTi (see Table 6–2). Ti alloys are particularly good implant materials because of their high corrosion resistance compared with stainless steel and CoCrMo alloys. A stable passive oxide film (primarily of $TiO_2$) protects both Ti-6Al-4V and CPTi components. This stable and adherent passive oxide film protects Ti alloys from pitting corrosion, intergranular corrosion, and crevice corrosion attack, and in large part is the reason for Ti alloys' superior biocompatibility. Generally, the strength of Ti-6Al-4V exceeds that of stainless steel, with a flexural rigidity roughly half of stainless steel and CoCrMo alloys. Therefore, the torsional and the axial stiffness (moduli) of Ti alloys are closer to bone and theoretically provide less stress shielding than do Co alloys and stainless steel. However, Ti alloys are notch sensitive. This reduces the effective strength of a component by increasing the material's susceptibility to crack initiation and propagation, which is a concern for thin TDR load-bearing components. Generally, a material's "hardness" (resistance to indentation) correlates with resistance to wear; however, this is not a direct correlation or always true. Ti-6Al-4V alloy is an example of a material that can be approximately 15% softer than CoCrMo alloys, yet when used in orthopaedic-bearing applications, results in more than 15% greater wear than CoCrMo. Thus, Ti alloys are seldom used as materials when resistance to wear is the primary concern.[7,9,10,14,15]

### New Alloys and Surface Coatings

There are a number of new metal alloys with improved biocompatibility and mechanical properties that may be appropriate for use in TDR once established as implant materials. The use of Ti alloys, CoCrMo alloys, or stainless steels in a specific application generally involves tradeoffs of one desirable property for another. These so-called new alloys are usually slight compositional variations of the implant metals previously described.

#### New Titanium Alloys

One new group of Ti alloys proposed for orthopaedic applications is the so-called beta-Ti's. These Ti alloys promise increased fatigue strength and 20% reduction in the elastic modulus, which is closer to bone, minimizing the potential for stress shielding. Other attempts at improving traditional Ti-6Al-4V alloys seek to improve biocompatibility and mechanical properties by the substitution of V (a relatively toxic metal) with other less toxic metals. Two such Ti alloys include Ti-5Al-2.5Fe and Ti-6Al-17Nb. These alloys have higher fatigue strength and a lower modulus, compared with Ti-6AL-4V, thus enhancing bone to implant load transfer (see Table 6–2).

#### New Stainless Steels

New alloys such as BioDur 108 (Carpenter Technology Corp.) attempt to solve increased corrosion resistance with an essentially nickel-free austenitic stainless alloy. This steel contains a high nitrogen content to maintain its austenitic structure and boasts improved levels of tensile yield strength, fatigue strength, and improved resistance to pitting corrosion and crevice corrosion as compared with nickel-containing alloys such as Type 316L (ASTM F-138).

#### Tantalum Alloys

Tantalum (Ta), although difficult to manufacture, is highly corrosion resistant and is gaining popularity as osteophilic bone subtrates, which can undergo large deformations without fracturing.

#### Zirconium

Zirconium implant alloy (ASTM F-2384-05, OxiniumTM, Smith and Nephew) is composed of 97.5% zirconium (Zr) and 2.5% niobium (Nb), and is now widely available for use in hip and knee arthroplasty. It is an expensive material that boasts higher wear resistance and corrosion resistance than Co alloys typically used in bearing applications. Both zirconium (Zr) and Ta are characterized as refractory metals (others include molybdenum and tungsten) because of their relative chemical stability (passive oxide layer) and high melting points. Zr and Ta alloys are currently in use and may be gaining popularity as orthopaedic metals. Because of the surface oxide layer stability, Zr and Ta (like Ti) are highly corrosion resistant. Additionally, these refractory metals generally possess high levels of hardness (12 Gpa) and wear resistance (approximately 10-fold that of Co and Ti alloys, using abrasion testing), which makes them well suited for bearing surface applications. The thickness of the surface oxide layer (approximately 5 μm) and ability to extend ceramic-like material properties (i.e., hardness) into the material through techniques such as oxygen enrichment are the primary reasons for Zr's enhanced properties (e.g., Oxidized Zirconium or Oxinium™). As difficulties associated with forming and machining these metals are overcome (i.e., costs are decreased), the use of these materials is expected to grow. Corrosion resistance generally correlates with biocompatibility (although not always) because more stable metal alloys tend to be less chemically active and less participatory in biologic reactions. This makes metals such as Zr valuable for people who are overly sensitive to the degradation products of metal alloys, as people who exhibit strong histories of metal allergy.

## WEAR ANALYSIS

In the long term, wear debris from spinal implants such as total discs replacements will likely be the limiting factor similar to hip and knee replacements. Wear debris in total hip and knee replacements has been related to osteolysis and subsequent loosening of the implant. Understanding general mechanics of wear and preclinical wear testing has also become a requirement for artificial spinal joints. In the subsequent paragraphs, a systemic approach toward wear and wear analysis is reviewed.

### Systemic Approach of Wear Analysis

Wear has been defined as material loss from the bodies in contact due to mechanical action; thus, a pure dimensional change as it occurs during creep or plastic deformation is not a form of wear because it does not produce wear debris. Also, corrosion is not necessarily related to wear because it can take place without mechanical activation.

It is reasonable to analyze wear as a system property rather than as a material property to take multiple and interrelated factors into account.[16] The analysis of the structure of the tribologic system and the type of dynamic interaction between its elements should be the first step of a focused and successful strategy to reduce wear at any artificial joint. As shown in Figure 6–4, body and counterbody comprise the artificial articulation. They may be equal or differ with regard to material, geometric shape, and surface roughness parameters. Most likely, the bodies undergo different movement patterns because they are attached to different vertebrae of the spinal column. Knowledge of the specific movement patterns, that is, motion amplitudes within the sagittal, frontal, and transverse planes, their specific shape (e.g., sinusoidal), as well as occurring phase differences, is as important as a

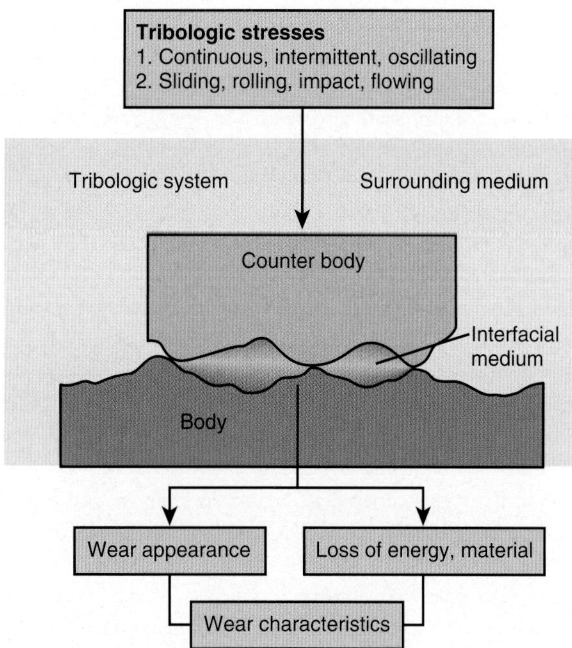


■ **FIGURE 6–4.** Basic structure of a tribologic system. *(Courtesy of BioEngineering Solutions Inc.)*

precise understanding of the applicable loads. Today, there is only limited understanding of the segmental motions and loads during the daily activities of life. Motion and load, however, comprise important input parameters to the wear system and characterize the tribologic stresses, namely, relative speed, load, loading time, and temperature.

The interfacial medium, as depicted in Figure 6–4, describes the lubricant of the system and is currently matter of scientific debate. The artificial disc articulates in a nonsynovial space that supposedly contains fewer proteins when compared with the pseudosynovial fluid of artificial knees and hips. Although the ISO/DIS 18192 standard recommends a protein concentration of 30 g/L, which has been adapted from general practice of hip and knee wear testing, the protein content of healthy cerebrospinal fluid is typically less than 2 g/L. However, the exact conditions under which an artificial disc operates are still unknown and a matter of ongoing research.

The consideration of potential third bodies, which can be intrinsic (e.g., wear debris, corrosion products) or extrinsic (e.g., bone cement, bone chips), is another important aspect for the longevity of artificial discs. Third bodies are attributed to the interfacial medium in the systemic approach in Figure 6–4. Last but not least, the surrounding environment of the artificial joint should be taken into account. The latter defines important parameters like ambient temperature and oxygen content of the tribologicsystem, which are defined by the human body.

## Wear Modes, Wear Appearances, and Wear Mechanisms

In order to describe wear phenomena completely, one needs to distinguish between *wear modes*, *wear appearances*, and *wear mechanism.*[17]

"The *wear mode*—also referred to as 'type of wear'"—defines the general mechanical conditions under which the bearing is functioning when wear occurs. Wear modes are defined by the macroscopic structure of the tribologicsystem and the kinematic interaction of its elements. For the artificial disc, it will be typically sliding wear. However, if movements of the disc are small, that is, smaller than the actual contact area, fretting wear may prevail. It should be noted that the wear mode is not a steady-state condition and can transform from one to another. For example, implant flattening running-in could limit the motion of the implant and turn the problem of sliding wear into a fretting-related phenomenon. Depending on the circumstances, this may call for completely different counteractions to reduce wear.

The *wear appearances* describe the visible changes of the surface as a consequence of wear. Wear pattern or wear damage is a synonym that can also be found in the literature. Wear appearances are characteristic signs of the occurring wear mechanisms. Only if in vivo wear mechanisms are replicated in in vitro experiments, can the test results be meaningful and allow extrapolations to the human system. A sole replication of wear rates is not sufficient in most cases. This is the reason why a thorough analysis of retrieved components is of enormous importance. Long-term multi-institutional analysis of total disc arthroplasty will enable correlation of in vivo results with simulator data. Current TDA designs have not been used in the United States long enough to enable such investigations, but many underpowered short-term studies are currently under way.

The wear mechanisms describe the mechanical, physical, and chemical interaction of the elements of a tribologicsystem. Today, four major wear mechanisms are distinguished: adhesion, abrasion, surface fatigue, and tribochemical reactions (Fig. 6–5):

*Adhesion* leads to the formation of local junctions between the surfaces, which may be adhesive or cohesive (in case of self-mating materials). Fragments of one surface are pulled out and adhere to the other. Later, these fragments may be detached and form loose wear particles or adhere back to the original surface. Typical wear appearances are craters and material transfers. Because the surfaces become rougher and harder after material transfers, adhesion is often accompanied by abrasion.

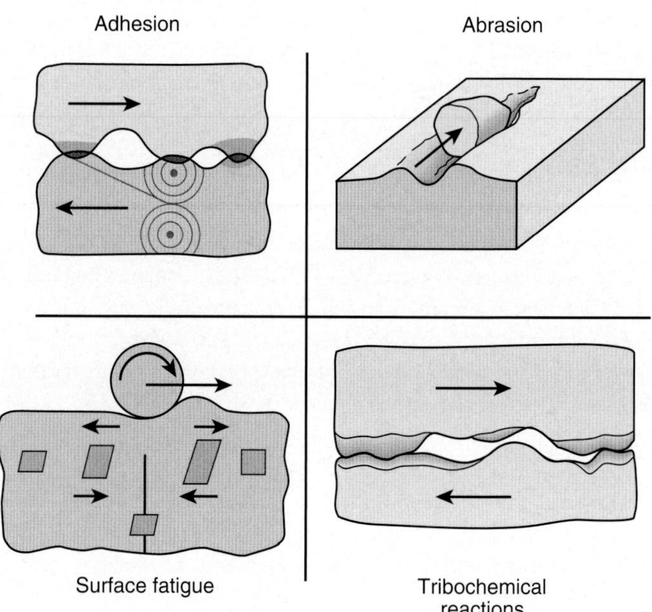


■ **FIGURE 6–5.** The four major wear mechanisms. *(Zum Gahr, K-H: Microstructure and Wear of Materials, Tribology Series Vol.10, Elsevier, Amsterdam, The Netherlands, 1987.)*

*Abrasion* occurs when a rough, hard surface (or a soft surface containing hard protuberances) slides on a soft surface and ploughs or cuts into it. The material removed from the grooves forms the particulate debris. Thus, grooves and scratches are typical wear appearances of abrasion.

*Surface fatigue* wear is observed during repeated rolling or sliding over a wear track. The repeated loading and unloading cycles to which the material is exposed may induce the formation of surface or subsurface cracks. Eventually, this will result in the loss of large material fragments due to pitting and delamination.

*Tribochemical reactions* are caused by mechanically induced chemical reactions of body and counterbody with the interfacial material and the environment. Wear particles are then released owing to the continual removal and new formation of chemical reaction products at the surfaces. It should be noted that tribochemical reactions are not necessarily bad for the tribologicsystem, but hinder adhesion owing to the nonmetallic characteristics of the reaction products.

## Wear Countermeasures

The wear process itself can be very complex. On many occasions, more than one mechanism is acting at a time. Then it becomes challenging to disentangle the complex situation and find the primary reason for wear. However, the key to any solution of a tribologic problem (friction-lubrication and wear) is linked to the knowledge of the primary acting wear mechanism. It is known that even for the same wear mode, different design or material modifications are appropriate. For example, the parameters of the wear mode, three-body abrasion of a metal-on-metal bearing with incorporated mineral particles can change in such a way that either the mechanism adhesion (cold welding of surface spots by plastic deformation of surface asperities), abrasion (grooving of surfaces by plastic flow), or surface fatigue (predominantly cyclic elastic deformation) apply. Depending on the principally acting mechanism, wear countermeasures may comprise a reduction of the normal force and improvement in lubrication (adhesion), an increase in surface hardness (adhesion/abrasion), or an increase in the ductility and cold working capability of the metal (surface fatigue). Thus, a successful plan to improve the wear characteristics of the materials in contact demands an exact understanding of the structure of the tribologicsystem and the interaction of its elements.

## Wear Testing

Wear testing has become a requirement for spinal artificial joints, even though little is known about the appropriate spine simulator input values, although input parameters have been recently specified in a newly produced ASTM F2423-05 guidance document (Standard Guide for Functional, Kinematic, and WEAR Assessment of Total Disc Prostheses) as well as an ISO standard ISO/DIS 18192 (Implants for surgery—Wear of total intervertebral spinal disc prostheses—Part 1: Loading and displacement parameters for wear testing and corresponding environmental conditions for test., ISO 18192 2006). Current thought is that "without a substantial clinical retrieval history of IVD prostheses, actual loading profiles and patterns cannot be delineated at the time" [ASTM F2423-05]. This is an important statement because the specified motion conditions do not necessarily reflect those occurring in vivo. For this reason, different wear rates may be realized than what is occurring during routine activities of daily life of a typical patient.

The importance of knowing "correct" simulator input has been recently demonstrated by Nechtow et al,[18] who generated drastically different wear rates dependent on simulator input. In their study, two temperature-controlled, eight-station spine simulators were mounted with artificial discs representing Co-Cr/polyethylene bearing couples. Two different implant designs were tested, namely a semi-constrained and an unconstrained design. Simulator 1 employed a frequency shifted "cross-shear" motion profile, whereas simulator 2 employed a curvilinear motion profile with the same magnitudes of the loading and motion profiles of simulator 1, except that lateral bending was not input and all inputs were in phase at 1 Hz.

The wear rates of the two artificial disc designs were similar for each input scenario. However, wear between the two input scenarios differed drastically. The application of cross-shear motion caused an increase in wear resulting in 50-fold higher wear rates, reaching 20 mg per million cycles. Considering that spinal implants are loaded every step compared with artificial hip/knee joints, which are loaded only every second step, actual wear rates may be closer to the range of artificial hips with conventional (non-cross-linked) polyethylene. Wear rates of the latter fall between 30 and 100 mg per million cycles.

As previously indicated, these particulates are recognized as a major factor limiting the longevity of joint reconstruction and the overall success of TJA procedures. Although it is well established that particulate debris in hip and knee joints have been associated with osteolysis that can lead to periprosthetic bone loss and aseptic loosening of the implant, the degree to which wear debris play a role in disc arthroplasty performance and peri-implant osteolysis has yet to be determined by prospective longitudinal investigation.

Until a consensus of motion and input parameters for simulators is reached, wear testing of disc arthroplasty may be conservatively conducted under extreme (worst case) conditions involving all three axes of movement and cross-shear at the surface. Figure 6–6 depicts the relevant movement axes and loads for

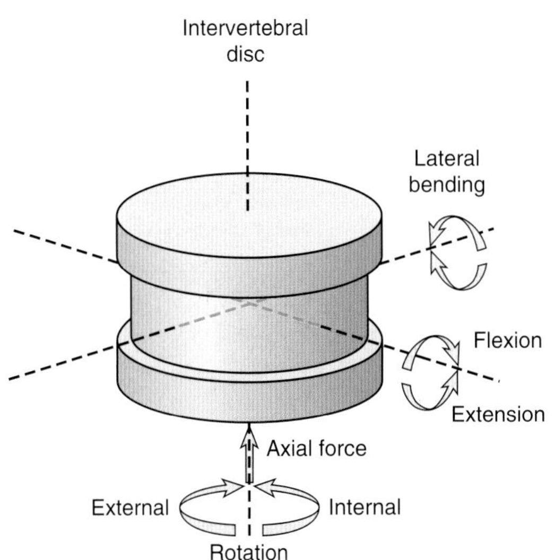


■ **FIGURE 6–6.** Axes of movement for consideration in spinal implant simulator testing.

spinal implant testing. Unidirectional testing may underestimate actual wear and may not be sufficient. Currently, standards suggest that simulators should employ maximum motions (displacements) typical of the implant site. This may not necessarily be the worst case condition. Minimal motion generating a fretting-type phenomenon could cause serious problems as well. Therefore, it is important to continue tracking and defining the segmental motions of the spine after implantation with an artificial disc. This motion analysis should include the various activities of daily life including walking, sitting, lifting, and so on.

## CONCLUSIONS

Current orthopaedic materials are chosen for their material properties. Although polymers and ceramics are emerging as materials for use in spinal implants, it is the metals (Ti alloys, Co alloys, stainless steels) that have been the four dominant materials, with greater than 50-year track records. Polymers offer compliant low-friction surfaces for articulation, disc replacement and in situ curing for fixation cement. Ceramics offer low wear and inert surfaces and debris. Metals, which are relatively less inert than polymers or ceramics (i.e., they corrode), have been used successfully for many years as spinal implants because they have high strength, high wear resistance, acceptable corrosion resistance, and toughness. Although newer alloys (such as zirconium) may be better able to address some design criteria and may represent biomaterial enhancement to TJA design, the critical environment of the spine requires material properties such as high strength, high corrosion resistance, high toughness (fatigue resistance), and low modulus. The local systemic and biologic effects of long-term use of metal alloys and polymeric materials remain largely uncharacterized for newer spinal implants such as total disc arthroplasty. However, it is important to note that when evaluating the biocompatibility of a particular metal component, the results do not necessarily apply to all implants made of the same material. Biocompatibility is defined as the ability of a material to demonstrate host and material response appropriate to its intended application and is thus a product of its material properties. Reasons for poor implant performance can be attributed to many factors, which include manufacturing errors, mechanical design errors, surgical errors, and inappropriate choice of material for a given application. Wise material selection cannot compensate for poor implant design or surgical error. It must be emphasized that currently there is no universal "best" material for all implant applications. That many different materials are used by competing manufacturers for the same device (e.g., a THA acetabular cup) illustrates the difficulty in asserting the superiority of one material over another even when confined to the comparison of a single component of a single device. However, a working knowledge of what material properties are important to spinal implants is prerequisite to understanding why different materials are used in different implant designs.

## REFERENCES


1. Jacobs JJ: Particulate wear. JAMA 273:1950–1956, 1995.
2. Lacombe P: Corrosion and oxidation of Ti and Ti alloys. In Williams JC, Belor AF (eds): Ti and Ti alloys, New York, Plenum Press, 1982, pp. 847–880.
3. Büttner-Janz K, Hahn S, Schikora K: Principles for Successful application of the Link® SB CHARITÈ artificial disc. Orthopäde 31:441–453, 2002.
4. Kurtz SM. Advances in the processing, sterilization, and crosslinking of ultra-high molecular weight polyethylene for total joint arthroplasty. Biomater 20:1659–1688, 1999.
5. Lee KY, Pienkowski D: Viscoelastic recovery of creep deformed ultra-high molecular weight polyethylene (UHMWPE) characterization and properties of ultra-high molecular weight polyethylene. ASTM STP;1307, 1998.
6. Wright TLS: eg. Biomaterials. ASTM Special Technical Publication 1307, American Academy of Orthopaedic Surgeons, Rosemont, IL, 2000.
7. Black J: Biomaterials, 2nd ed. New York, Marcel Dekker, Inc., 1992.
8. Black J: Orthopaedic Biomaterials in Research and Practice. New York, Churchill Livingstone, 1988.
9. Park JB: Biomaterials Science and Engineering. New York, Plenum Press, 1984.
10. Silver FH, Christiansen DL: Biomaterials Science and Biocompatibility. New York, Springer, 1999.
11. Jacobs JJ, Gilbert JL, Urban RM: Corrosion of metal orthopaedic implants. J Bone Joint Surg [Am] 80:268–282, 1998.
12. Bertagnoli RKS: Indications for full prosthetic disc arthroplasty: a correlation of clinical outcome against a variety of indications. Eur Spine J 11:131–136, 2002.
13. McKellop HA, Sarmiento A, Brien W, Park SH: Interface corrosion of a modular head total hip prosthesis. J Arthroplasty 7:291–294, 1992.
14. Breme J, Biehl V: Metallic biomaterials. In Black J, Hastings G (eds): Handbook of Biomaterial Properties. London, Chapman and Hall, 2001, pp. 135–214.
15. Black J: Prosthetic Materials. New York, VCH Publishers, Inc., 1996.
16. Czichos H: Tribology—A systems approach to the science and technology of friction, lubrication and wear. Amsterdam:Elsevier, 1978.
17. ZumGahr KH: Microstructure and Wear of Materials. Tribology Series Vol. 10. Amsterdam:Elsevier, 1987.
18. Nechtow W, Hintner M, Bushelow M, Kaddick C: IVD replacement mechanical performance depends strongly on input parameters. Chicago, IL, Trans 52nd Annual Meeting of the Orthopaedic Research Society, 2006.

CHAPTER 7

# Preclinical Evaluation of Dynamic Spinal Stabilization: Animal Models and Basic Scientific Methods

**Bryan W. Cunningham** and **Paul A. Anderson**

## KEY POINTS

- The use of in vivo animal models to assess device safety and efficacy are essential for preclinical testing of innovative methods for spinal arthrodesis and arthroplasty. Modeling allows for control of individual variables and quantification of predetermined experimental endpoints.
- The current chapter addresses the animal models and experimental endpoints used to address the three most commonly asked basic science questions with regard to dynamic spinal stabilization:
  1. What are the biomechanical motion-preserving properties of dynamic spinal instrumentation?
  2. Do these implants osseo-integrate, and what are the mechanisms and patterns of this process at the prosthetic–bone interface?
  3. Does metallic and polymeric particulate wear debris from dynamic spinal stabilization systems affect the surrounding tissue and potentially compromise long-term biologic device performance?

## INTRODUCTION

Dynamic spinal stabilization represents a new paradigm in the surgical management of spinal pathology. Preclinical animal modeling and basic scientific methods to assess the in vivo performance of dynamic stabilization systems remain at the forefront of basic science research endeavors. As an alternative to conventional methods of spinal arthrodesis, dynamic spinal stabilization serves to replace the symptomatic degenerative structures, restore the functional biomechanical properties of the motion segment, and protect neurovascular structures. As we move from an era of arthrodesis to one in which segmental motion is preserved, this promising new technology offers a variety of clinical and research challenges.

To this end, the implanted device should reestablish near-normal kinematics to the functional spinal unit, encourage or at least not inhibit osseointegration at the bone–metal interface, minimize particulate wear debris, and promote an anterior/posterior column load-sharing environment. The current chapter provides insight into the animal models and experimental endpoints used to address the three most commonly asked basic science questions with regard to dynamic spinal stabilization.

First and foremost are the biomechanical motion preserving properties of the device. Assuming proper surgical technique and implant positioning are achieved, the initial biomechanical stability and motion preserving kinematics are of primary concern. Second, what are the mechanisms and patterns of osseointegration at the prosthetic-bone interface? As with total joint replacement arthroplasty, histologic osseointegration at the prosthetic-bone interface of total disc replacements is necessary for long-term implant survivorship and function. Having achieved adequate postoperative segmental range of motion and the absence of radiolucent lines at the prosthetic interface, the local and systemic histopathologic response to particulate wear debris resulting from bearing surfaces and third-body wear remains a clinical concern.

## VERTEBRATE MODELS—DYNAMIC SPINAL STABILIZATION

### Animal Research Permission

The use of in vivo animal models for experimental studies is required by law to be conducted in strict accordance with federal regulations as outlined in the Animal Welfare Act.[1] The Institutional Animal Care and Use Committee (IACUC) at each center performing these studies granted approval for the investigations before the initiation of the study. Surgery, perioperative care, housing, sanitation practices, husbandry, and veterinary care followed the recommendations of the *NIH Guide for the Care and Use of Laboratory Animals* (HHS, NIH Pub. No. 85–23, 1985).

### Experimental Animal Models

The use of in vivo animal models to assess device safety and efficacy is essential for preclinical testing of innovative methods for spinal arthrodesis and arthroplasty. Modeling allows for control of individual variables and quantification of predetermined experimental endpoints. These preclinical experiments, designed to evaluate device feasibility and efficacy, are generally studied in a systematic progression from lower to higher order vertebrate models, constructing a foundation of basic science evidence to substantiate the "burden of proof" necessary for device approval.

Animal models reported in the literature for spinal arthrodesis are variable and range from mice,[2] Guinea pigs,[3] rats,[4] rabbits,[5] canine,[6] sheep,[7] pigs,[8] goats,[9] non-human primates[10,11] (rhesus monkeys and baboons) to horses.[12] Of interesting note, both the mouse (posterior fusion) and thoroughbred racehorse (interbody fusion) were used to assess spinal arthrodesis. In contrast, there are far fewer models reported in dynamic spinal stabilization studies, which are limited to canines,[13] sheep,[14] chimpanzees,[15] goats,[16,17] and baboons.[18,19]

In contrast to arthrodesis models, motion preservation devices necessitate a more technically exacting operation, with further consideration given to the in vivo anatomic and kinematic properties of the operative motion segments. To this end, the experimental models must offer suitable intervertebral discs and transpedicular morphometry for proper device implantation, without the need to down-size or otherwise modify the implants. The models chosen and most widely reported on include the caprine (goat) and chimpanzee for cervical disc arthroplasty and non-human primate baboon for lumbar nucleoplasty, total disc arthroplasty, and posterior motion preservation.

## Experimental Endpoints

Of equal importance to the selection of animal model are the experimental endpoints (assays) performed and postoperative time intervals. The assays typically include, but are not limited to, radiography, biomechanics, and histopathology. The radiographic analysis may include plain film radiographs, magnetic resonance imaging, and computed tomography obtained at different time intervals based on endpoints (e.g., intradiscal signal intensity following nucleoplasty).

Biomechanical evaluation of the operative and adjacent segment highlights the comparative kinematics of the motion preserving implants, with comparison to the intact spine and conventional methods of spinal arthrodesis. Multidirectional flexibility testing is typically performed using a six-degree-of-freedom spine simulator, permitting pure moment load application with subsequent calculation of the functional spinal unit range of motion (ROM) and neutral zones.

Histopathologic analyses can be divided into local tissue, systemic tissues and undecalcified vertebral assays. Samples of local tissue and the spinal cord directly overlying the operative site highlights macrophage and proinflammatory cytokine (interleukin-1 [IL-1], interleukin-2 [IL-2], interleukin-6 [IL-6], interleukin-8 [IL-8], tumor necrosis factor-$\alpha$ [TNF-$\alpha$] and tumor necrosis factor-$\beta$ [TNF-$\beta$]) reactivity to the implanted device, whereas systemic/reticuloendothelial tissues characterize the dissemination, if any, of particulate wear debris and systemic effects. In consideration of the Food and Drug Administration's concerns of unintended particulate wear debris from motion preserving implants, these types of assays should be considered. The undecalcified vertebral bone histology highlights facet and intervertebral disc morphology, and permits histomorphometric quantification of tissue areas and trabecular apposition at the implant–bone interface. Comprehensive blood serum chemistry profiles and urinalysis at different time intervals are of interest for new implant materials and particulate wear studies; however, these tests present challenges due to animal handling issues.

## Cervical Spine Models: Anatomic and Kinematic Considerations

Mature Nubian or Spanish goats (*Capra aegagrus*) have been used for cervical arthroplasty, with postoperative follow-up periods extending to twelve months. From a kinematic standpoint, White and Panjabi[20] outlined the normal load-displacement properties of the human lower cervical spine, the restoration of which is the goal of cervical arthroplasty. The normal cervical ROM can be listed at C5-C6 and C6-C7 as total ROM. The normal ROM for axial rotation, flexion-extension, and lateral bending are: 7, 10, and 6.5 degrees, respectively. The comparable kinematics of the lower cervical spine is one of the criteria used in selecting the goat as the animal model for cervical disc arthroplasty. The caprine (goat) model has been used to test a variety of brands and models of cervical disc replacements due to similarity of the following criteria: (1) anatomic dimensions between the caprine C3-C4 intervertebral disc and human C5-C6 and C6-C7 discs; and (2) kinematic properties in axial rotation and flexion-extension loading conditions.

In the caprine model, the normal cervical ROM at the C3-C4 intervertebral disc is axial rotation (6 degrees), flexion-extension (14 degrees), and lateral bending (15 degrees). The center of intervertebral rotation at C3-C4 is located in the lower vertebral end plate, similar to the human cervical spine (Fig. 7–1). The intervertebral disc displays more of a dome-like shape than the human cervical disc. With caprine anteroposterior and mediolateral disc dimensions of 20 and 25 mm, respectively, and intervertebral heights of 6 mm, human-sized cervical disc replacements can be implanted at C3-C4. From a surgical standpoint, the anterior Smith-Robinson approach to the cervical spine can be easily adapted through a left-sided longitudinal incision. Once the anterior cervical vertebral elements are exposed, the C3-C4 intervertebral disc is radiographically identified, and a standard anterior cervical discectomy and decompression of the spinal canal can be performed. In standard fashion, the overlying end plate fibrocartilage should be removed using curettage and a high-speed burr to obtain planar geometry of the vertebral end plates, ensuring proper implant positioning. However, the caprine model absolutely represents a worst case scenario with regard to evaluating the durability of the cervical prosthesis. The goats are ambulatory without a brace several hours after the surgery. They engage in head butting, and occasionally leap over 5-foot stockade fences becoming completely airborne.

## PCM Arthroplasty–Goat Model

To investigate the biomechanical, porous ingrowth and histopathologic characteristics of the porous-coated motion cervical disc replacement (PCM) (Cervitech, Inc., Rockaway, NJ), 12 mature Nubian goats were divided into two groups based on postoperative survival periods of six ($n = 6$) and 12 months ($n = 6$).[16] Using an anterior surgical approach, a complete discectomy was performed at C3-C4, followed by implantation of the PCM device. The device is composed of two cobalt-chrome alloy end plates, ultra-high-molecular-weight polyethylene (UHMWPE) core and a unique bioactive titanium/calcium phosphate (TiCaP) hydroxyapatite coating.

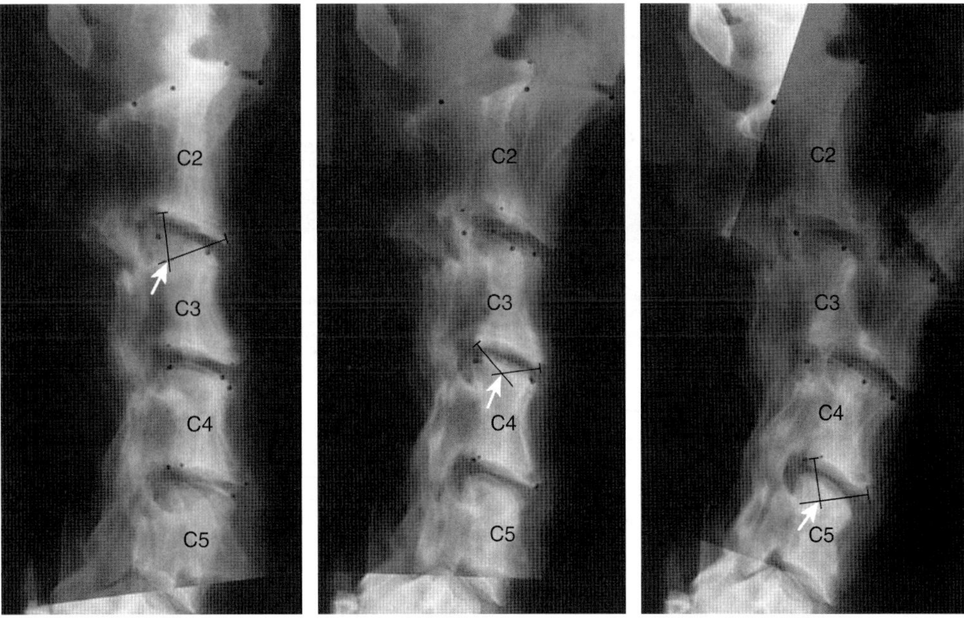


■ **FIGURE 7–1.** Lateral plain film radiographs of the caprine cervical spine. Full flexion and extension views are superimposed on each to define the center of intervertebral rotation occurring at the C2-C3, C3-C4, and C4-C5 intervertebral levels. Similar to the human spine, the center of intervertebral rotation at C3-C4 is located in the superior vertebral end plate of C4.

Functional outcomes of the disc prosthesis were based on plain film radiography, multidirectional flexibility testing, undecalcified vertebral histology, histomorphometry, and immunocytochemical analyses. There was no evidence of neurologic, vascular, or infectious complications throughout the 6- and 12-month survival periods. Plain film radiographic analysis of the 6- and 12-month lateral bending and flexion-extension radiographs demonstrated no incidence of implant migration, subsidence, or end plate radiolucencies (Fig. 7–2). Multidirectional flexibility testing of the operative functional spinal units under axial rotation and lateral bending indicated no differences in full range of intervertebral motion between the disc prosthesis and nonoperative controls at either time period ($P > 0.05$). However, at both 6- and 12-months intervals, flexion-extension loading indicated diminished range of motion compared with the intact condition ($P < 0.05$) (Fig. 7–3).

Histopathologic interpretation of the slide-mounted undecalcified specimens indicated no evidence of significant pathologic changes in tissues within or surrounding any of the 12 operative specimens. Based on plain and polarized light microscopic review of the undecalcified histologic slide-mounted vertebral specimens, there was evidence of an interpositional fibrous/collagenous tissue interface in some regions of the prosthesis–bone interface at 6 months, which was supplanted by mature trabecular bone by the 12-month postoperative time interval (Fig. 7–4). Histomorphometric analysis at the metal–bone interface indicated the mean trabecular ingrowth of 40.5 ± 24.4% and 58.65 ± 28.04% for the 6- and 12-month treatments, respectively. Moreover, review of the spinal cord at the operative levels indicated no evidence of cord lesions, inflammatory reaction, wear particles, or significant pathologic changes in any treatment.

## Lumbar Spine Models: Anatomic and Kinematic Considerations

The nonhuman primate baboon (*papio cynocephalus*) offers a semi-upright spine and is the preferred model for nucleoplasty, lumbar disc arthroplasty, and posterior motion preserving devices. The animals exhibit anatomic and kinematic features suitable for motion preserving implants. From a kinematic standpoint, the average range of motion for the human L4-L5 and L5/S1 levels is as follows: axial rotation (3 degrees), flexion-extension (15 degrees), and lateral bending (9 degrees).[20] The comparable kinematics of the baboon L5-L6 level—axial rotation (2 degrees), flexion-extension (8 degrees), and lateral bending (13 degrees)—was one criteria used in selecting this animal model for lumbar arthroplasty. Moreover, the disc space dimensions (8-mm height, 25-mm depth, and 30-mm width) are more accommodating to the smaller human-sized prosthetic implants, with minimal end plate resection required compared with other animal models, such as sheep, goats, and canines (Fig. 7–5).[21]

These models can also be used for defining the anatomic feasibility of the surgical approach and instrument design strategies. From a surgical standpoint, an anterior transperitoneal approach is used to access the L5-L6 level for lumbar nucleoplasty or disc arthroplasty procedures. The peritoneum is far too thin for successful retroperitoneal access. A posterior muscle preserving Wiltse approach is recommended for posterior instrumentation procedures because it preserves the paraspinal musculoligamentous complexes and prevents deinnervation of the operative levels. In similarity to the caprine model, the baboon is biomechanically challenging because the animals are not braced or immobilized postoperatively, rapid to ambulate, and perform their natural gymnastics, trapeze utilization, and cage rocking within the first postoperative week.

### Lumbar Nucleoplasty—Baboon Model

This nucleoplasty study was designed to evaluate the mechanical behavior and elicited histopathologic response of a nucleus pulposus implant (DASCOR Device; Disc Dynamics, Inc., Eden Prairie, MN) and its component materials following long-term implantation in a functional animal (baboon) model. Analyses were based on

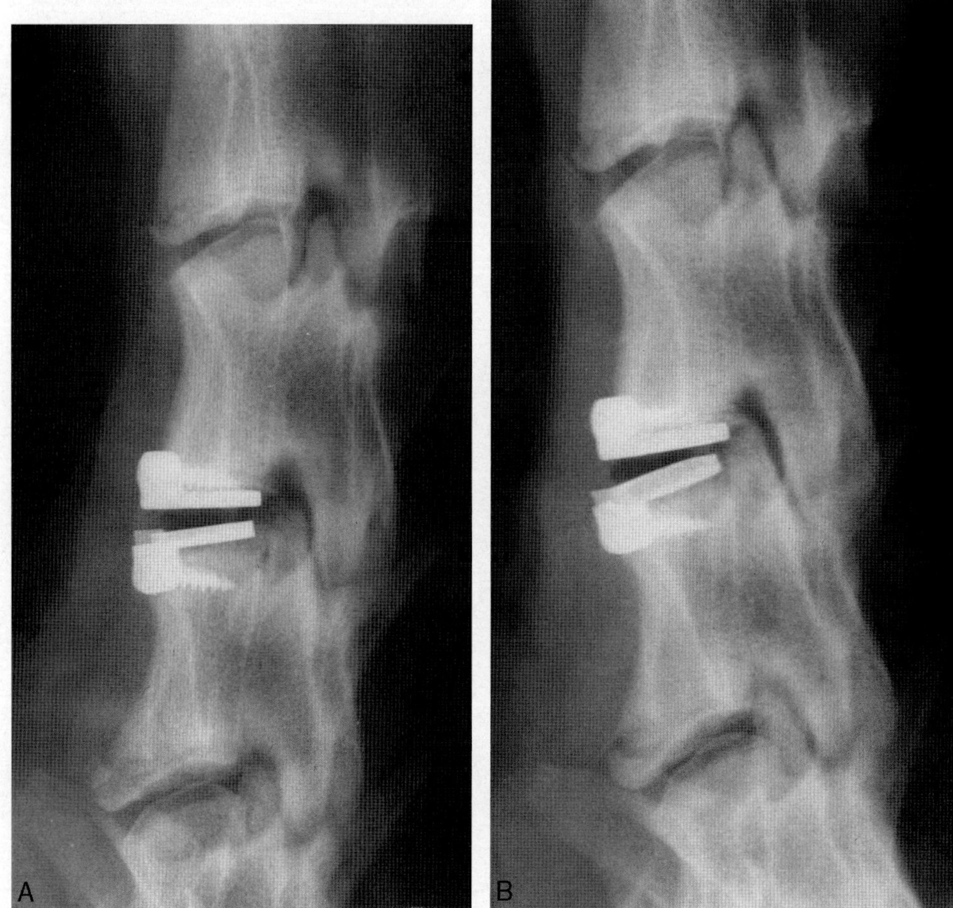


■ **FIGURE 7–2.** Twelve-month postoperative flexion **(A)** and extension **(B)** plain film radiographs demonstrating physiologic range of segmental motion without evidence of implant migration or end plate radiolucencies.

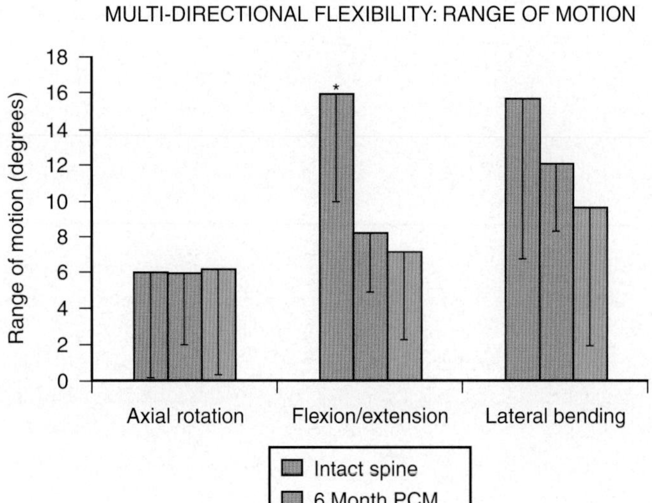

MULTI-DIRECTIONAL FLEXIBILITY: RANGE OF MOTION

Range of motion (degrees)

18
16
14
12
10
8
6
4
2
0

Axial rotation
Flexion/extension
Lateral bending

Intact spine
6 Month PCM
12 Month PCM

* $P < 0.05$ vs. 6- and 12-month PCM

■ **FIGURE 7–3.** Multidirectional flexibility: range of motion. A bar chart comparing the intact spine to the PCM device at 6 and 12 months postoperatively under three loading modalities. Significance is indicated between the intact spine and PCM treatment under flexion-extension loading at both time intervals (*$P < 0.05$).

magnetic resonance imaging (MRI), multidirectional flexibility testing, and biocompatibility assays (local and systemic histology) performed at the 6- and 12-month postoperative time points. A total of 14 mature male baboons *(Papio cynocephalus)* were randomized into two postoperative time periods of 6 months ($n = 7$) and 12 months ($n = 7$), postoperatively. Each animal underwent a lateral transperitoneal surgical approach, followed by a complete nucleotomy at L3-L4 and L5-L6 levels. The inferior L5-L6 level was reconstructed using the DASCOR Device—an in situ cured polyurethane device with an elastic modulus similar to that of the natural disc, and L3-L4 served as a surgical (nucleotomy) control for each case.

Postmortem analyses included MRI assessment of implant position, Modic Type end plate changes (Grade 0 to 3), multidirectional flexibility testing with comparisons to non-operative intact spines, systemic histopathology and undecalcified histology. All animals survived the operative procedure and postoperative intervals without significant intra- or perioperative complications. Based on MRI radiography, two nucleus implants migrated laterally out of the intervertebral disc (6 months $n = 1$; 12 months $n = 1$). Postmortem MRI analysis exhibited significant Modic Type I end plate changes in five out of seven nucleus replacement (L5-L6) levels versus zero out of seven controls (L3-L4), which were identified as

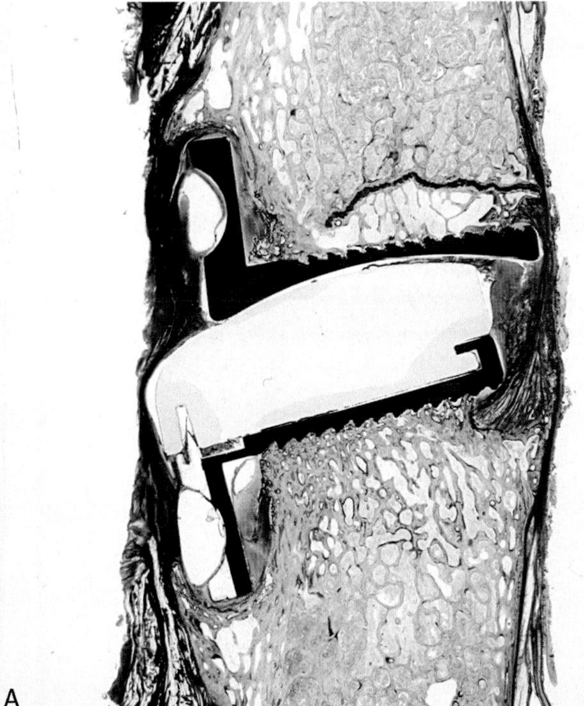


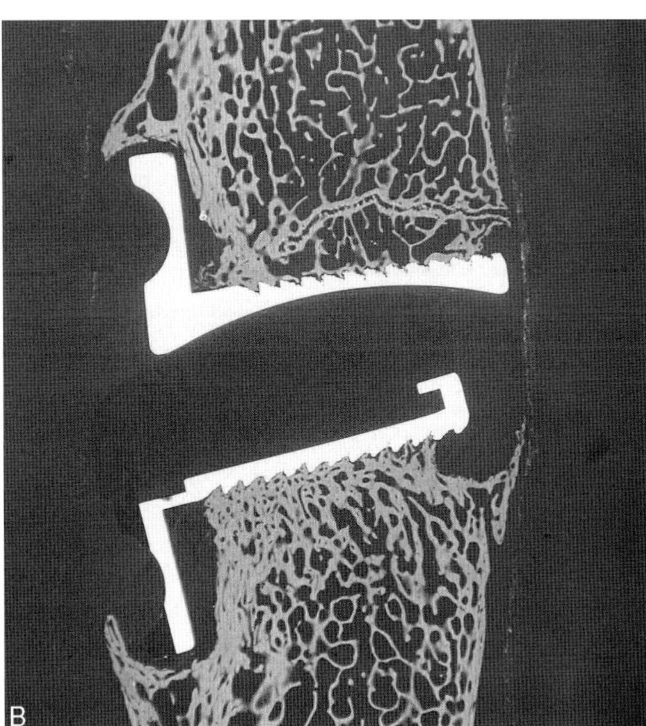


■ **FIGURE 7–4.** Representative undecalcified histologic specimen of the PCM device following a 12-month postoperative period. A midsagittal histologic specimen is shown **(A)** and corresponding microradiograph **(B)**. The trabecular bone in direct contact with the end plates was lamellar in structure, without evidence of sclerosis. Interstitial marrow cavities, devoid of fibrosis, account for the remainder of the implant–bone interface. (Osteochrome Villanueva bone stain.)

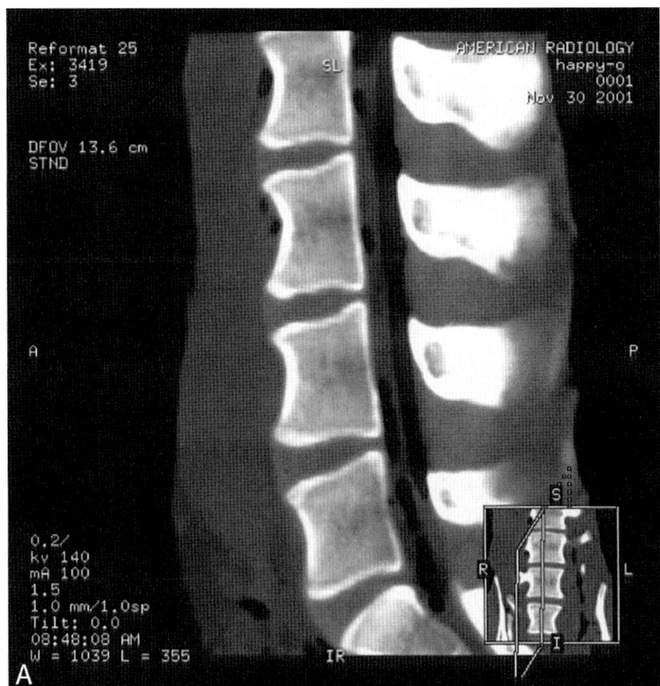


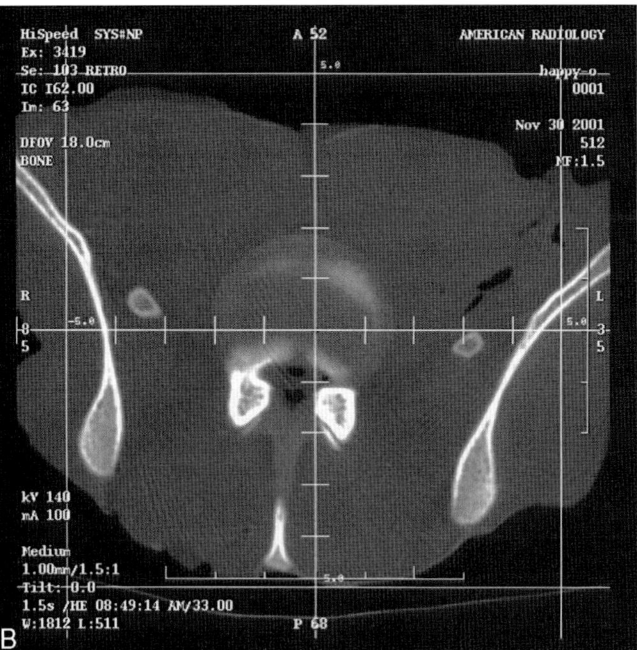


■ **FIGURE 7–5.** Computed tomography images of the baboon lumbar spine demonstrating disc space geometry and dimensions in the sagittal **(A)** and axial **(B)** planes.

Modic Type 0. For the 12-month group, Type I changes were identified in three out of seven nucleus replacement (L5-L6) levels versus zero out of seven controls (L3-L4). Intervertebral hydration signals at the operative and control surgical levels were markedly reduced at both time intervals (Fig. 7–6).

Multidirectional flexibility testing indicated no difference in axial rotation ($P > 0.05$) for the 6- and 12-month groups, comparing the intact spine with surgical motion segments. Flexion-extension and lateral bending exhibited reduced segmental motion for the nucleus replacement and operative control levels at 6 months versus the nonoperative intact spine ($P < 0.05$). By 12 months, flexion-extension motion at the nucleus replacement level was restored to intact condition ($P > 0.05$).

Histopathologic analysis of the nucleus replacement treatments exhibited increased densification of trabeculae along the end plate periphery, which corroborated the Modic Type I changes observed radiographically. No change in densification or end plate sclerosis was observed at the L3-L4 surgical control levels (Fig. 7–7). Using a non-human primate model, this study investigated the in vivo response to nucleus pulposus replacement following nucleotomy. MRI Modic Type changes were observed to a greater extent at the operative versus control levels; however, these changes appeared to reduce from the six- to twelve-month intervals. Multidirectional flexibility testing indicated restoration of segmental motion for the nucleus replacement under flexion-extension by the twelve-month time interval. The observed implant migrations are considered secondary to the harsh biomechanical environment produced by the experimental model. Most importantly, the histopathology—both vertebral and systemic—indicated no evidence of significant histopathological changes secondary to the implanted device. This study serves as a basic scientific basis for ongoing clinical investigations into the use and efficacy of the DASCOR Device for replacement of the intervertebral nucleus pulposus.

## Lumbar Disc Arthroplasty—Baboon Model

Using an in vivo nonhuman primate model, Cunningham and McAfee et al[22] investigated the biomechanical, histochemical, and biologic ingrowth characteristics of three different lumbar disc prostheses—AcroFlex and CHARITÉ (DePuy Spine, Inc., Raynham, MA), and the Three-Dimensional Fabricube (3DF) device (Takiron, Inc., Osaka, Japan)—for total disc arthroplasty. In this comprehensive analysis, a total of 43 mature baboons ($n = 43$, *Papio cynocephalus*) underwent L5-L6 total disc arthroplasty procedures using one of three devices: (1) the AcroFlex device ($n = 10$ levels), which consists of sintered titanium beaded ingrowth surfaces bound together by a hexene-based polyolefin rubber core; (2) the CHARITÉ ($n = 17$ levels) device, which contains prosthetic vertebral cobalt chrome end plates, covered by two layers of thin titanium with an electrochemically bonded hydroxyapatite coating and an UHMWPE core; (3) the 3DF Device ($n = 16$ levels), which is manufactured using a triaxial three-dimensional fabric woven with a UHMWPE fiber and spray-coated using bioactive ceramics (Fig. 7–8).

Following a 6-month survival period, the ROM of the CHARITÉ and intact nonoperative controls under axial rotation and flexion-extension showed no statistical difference ($P > 0.05$). However, both exhibited greater ROM compared with the AcroFlex and 3FD Device treatments under flexion-extension and lateral bending loading modes ($P < 0.05$) (Table 7–1). Plain film radiographic analysis showed no radiolucencies or loosening of the metallic prosthetic vertebral end plates.

Gross histopathologic analysis of the AcroFlex and CHARITÉ prosthesis demonstrated excellent ingrowth at the level of the implant–bone interface, without evidence of fibrous tissue or synovium (Figs. 7–9 and 7–10). Light microscopic analysis of the 3DF Device demonstrated relatively low patterns of osseointegration at the level of the implant–bone interface, with the extent of fibrous tissue surrounding the implant exceeding the area of trabecular bone contact (Fig. 7–11). In all specimens reviewed, there was no evidence of local or systemic accumulation of particulate wear debris, giant cell reaction/inflammatory response, or other significant histopathologic changes. Porous ingrowth calculations showed the mean ingrowth (linear apposition) ranging from 47.9% ± 9.12 for the CHARITÉ device to 54.59% ± 13.24 for the AcroFlex device (Fig. 7–12).

The porous ingrowth coverage at the bone–metal interface was more favorable for total disc replacement compared with that reported for cementless total joint components in the appendicular skeleton (range 10% to 30%). The reason for the improved degree of porous ingrowth in total disc replacement prostheses is probably due to ligamentotaxis causing sustained compression across the metal–bone interface. This project serves as the first comprehensive in vivo investigation comparing three different types of unconstrained disc prostheses with alternate ingrowth surfaces and establishes an excellent research model in the evaluation of total disc replacement arthroplasty.

## Lumbar Dynamic Posterior Fixation—Baboon Model

The baboon also serves as an excellent model for evaluation of posterior dynamic fixation. In a study reported by Cunningham and coworkers,[23] the safety and efficacy of the Dynesys (Zimmer Spine, Inc., Warsaw, IN) dynamic posterior spinal stabilization system was evaluated. Success criteria were based on postmortem radiographic, biomechanical, and immunohistochemical analyses. In this study, eight mature baboons ($n = 8$, *Papio cynocephalus*) were randomized into two groups based on postoperative survival periods of 6 ($n = 6$) and 12 ($n = 2$) months. Using a Wiltse muscle-preserving approach to the posterior lumbar spine, a dynamic spinal stabilization system was implanted from L3 through L5. The device itself consists of titanium pedicle screws, polycarbonate urethane spacers, and polyethylene terephthalate cords, which are collectively tensioned to 300 Newtons intraoperatively (Fig. 7–13).

Following animal sacrifice, status of the operative specimens was evaluated using radiography, biomechanical testing (L3-L5), facet joint histology, and immunocytochemistry of local and systemic tissues. Biomechanical analysis of the in vivo specimens was first tested with the instrumentation intact and then removed (In vivo Dynesys). Data were compared with nonoperative intact and instrumented control spines (Acute Dynesys) to determine the effect of in vivo loading on device performance. All baboons survived the surgery without incidence of neurologic, vascular, or infectious complications.

Radiography indicated no evidence of pedicle screw radiolucencies or implant loosening at the 6-month interval; however, the 12-month specimens had a 25% incidence of radiolucency (Fig. 7–14). Biomechanical testing in axial rotation demonstrated

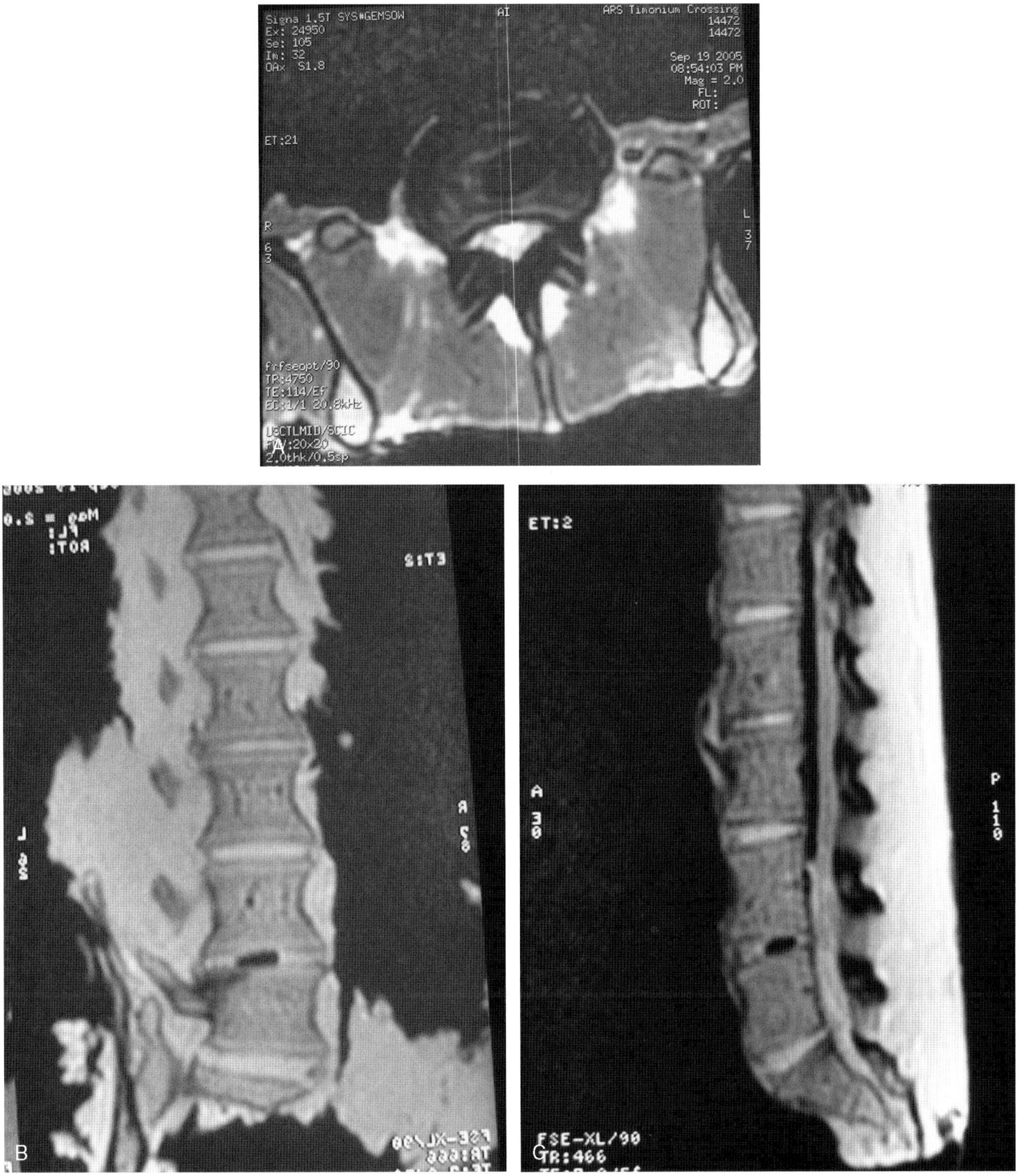

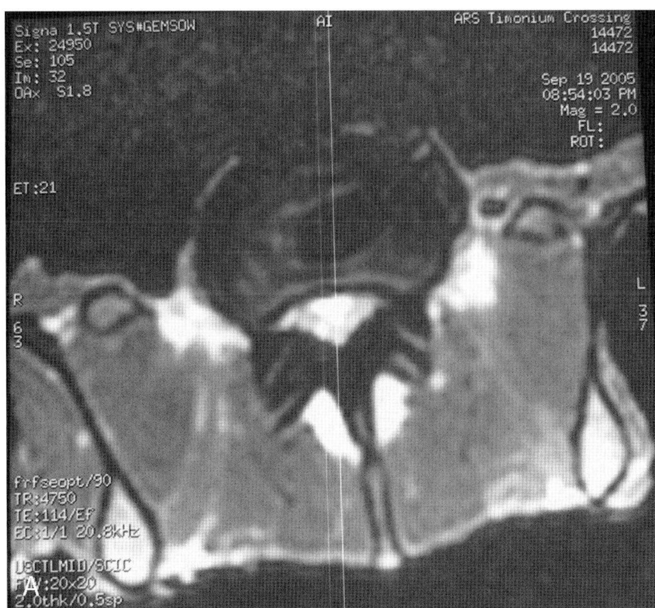


■ **FIGURE 7–6.** Magnetic resonance images of the baboon lumbar spine 12 months after implantation of an in situ cured polyurethane device (DASCOR Device; Disc Dynamics, Inc., Eden Prairie, MN). Type I Modic changes were identified in 3 of 7 nucleus replacement (L5-L6) levels versus 0 of 7 control (L3-L4) at the 12-month interval. **A,** Axial image. **B,** Coronal image. **C,** Sagittal image.

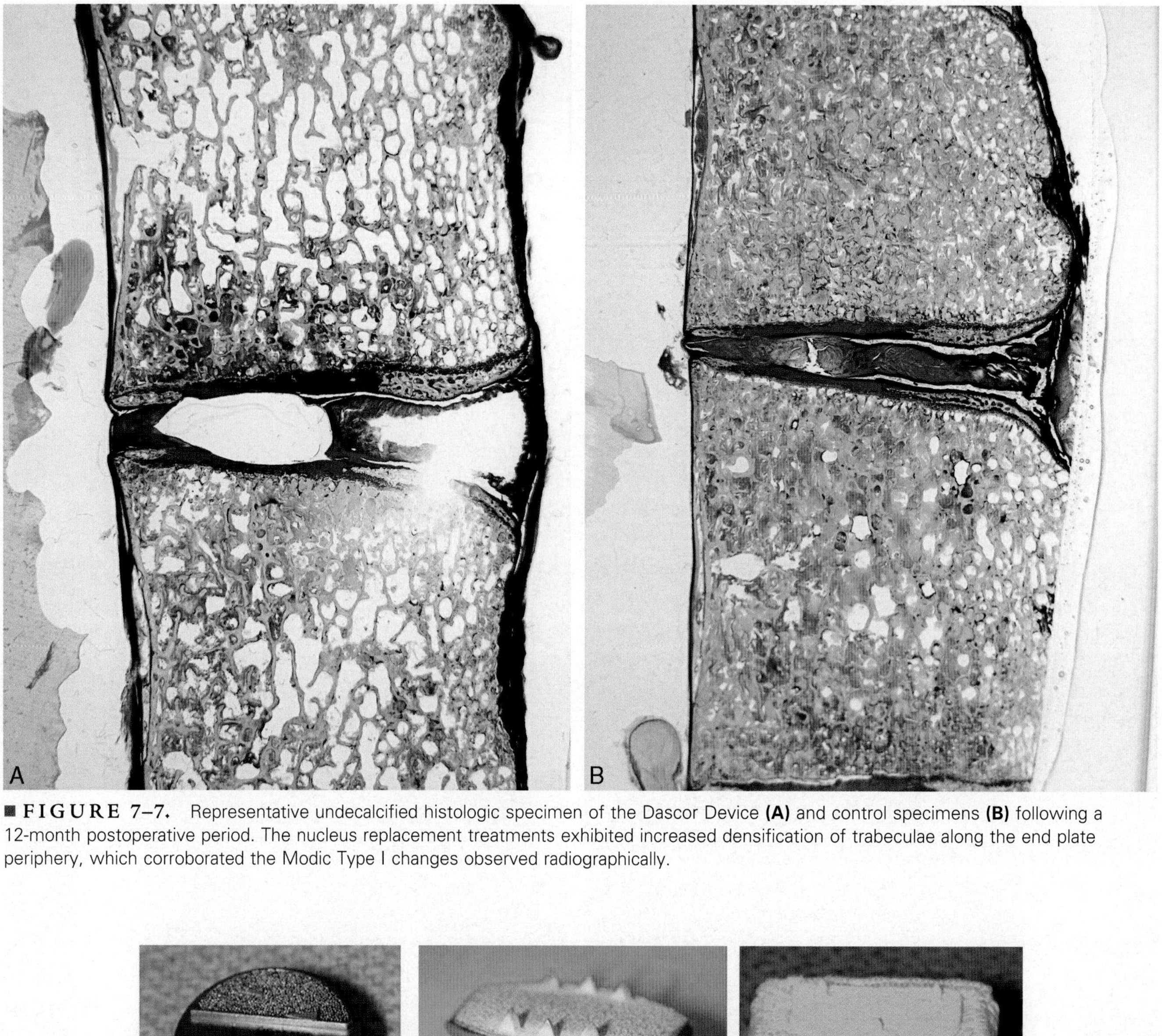

■ **FIGURE 7–7.** Representative undecalcified histologic specimen of the Dascor Device **(A)** and control specimens **(B)** following a 12-month postoperative period. The nucleus replacement treatments exhibited increased densification of trabeculae along the end plate periphery, which corroborated the Modic Type I changes observed radiographically.

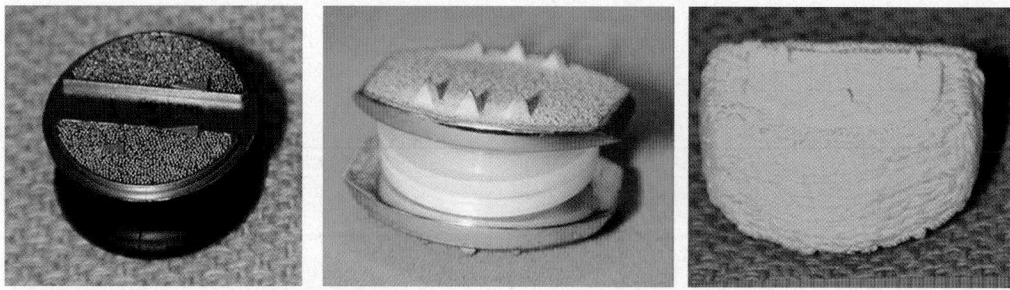

■ **FIGURE 7–8.** Three lumbar disc arthroplasty implants were included in the baboon studies. AcroFlex Device *(left)*, CHARITÉ *(middle)*, and Three-Dimensional Fabricube device *(right)*.

**TABLE 7–1. Multidirectional Flexibility Testing Data**

| Treatment Group | Axial Rotation | | Flexion-Extension | | Lateral Bending | |
|---|---|---|---|---|---|---|
| | Mean | SD | Mean | SD | Mean | SD |
| Intact spine | 2.442 | 1.3 | 6.928* | 2.899 | 14.12* | 4.82 |
| 3DF | 2.337 | 1.084 | 4.267 | 2.042 | 2.898 | 1.111 |
| AcroFlex | 1.673 | 0.696 | 3.856 | 1.505 | 3.79 | 1.06 |
| CHARITÉ | 3.87* | 1.216 | 7.714* | 3.298 | 10.044† | 3.95 |

3DF, Three-Dimensional Fabricube; SD, standard deviation.
*,†Indicates difference from all other treatment groups at $P < 0.05$.

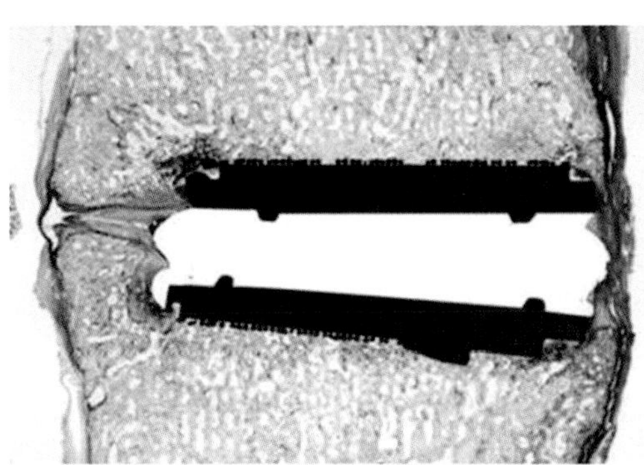
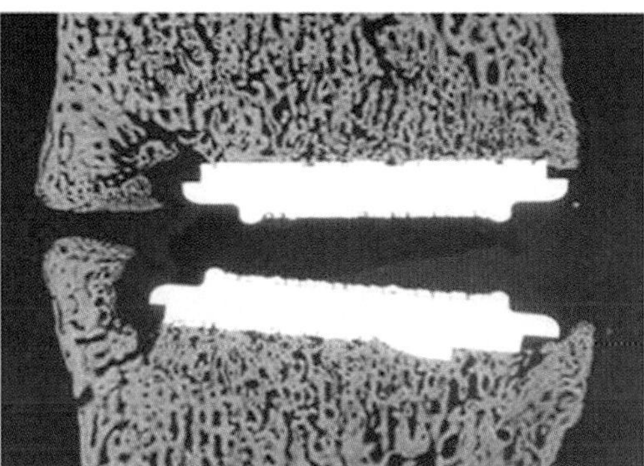

■ **FIGURE 7–9.** Representative undecalcified histologic specimen of the AcroFlex device *(left)* and corresponding microradiograph *(right)* following a 6-month postoperative period. (Villanueva bone stain, magnification ×2.5.)

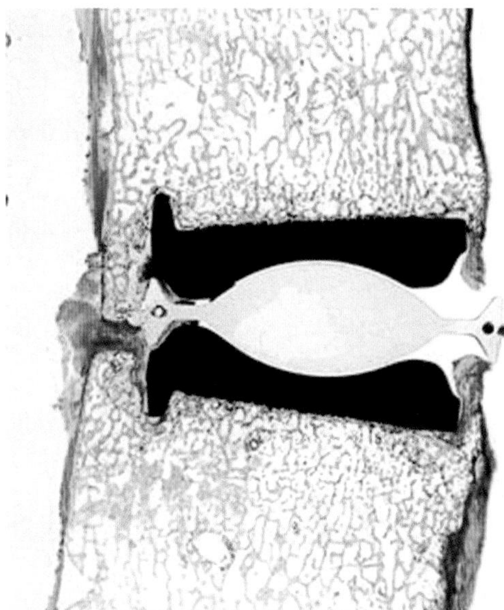
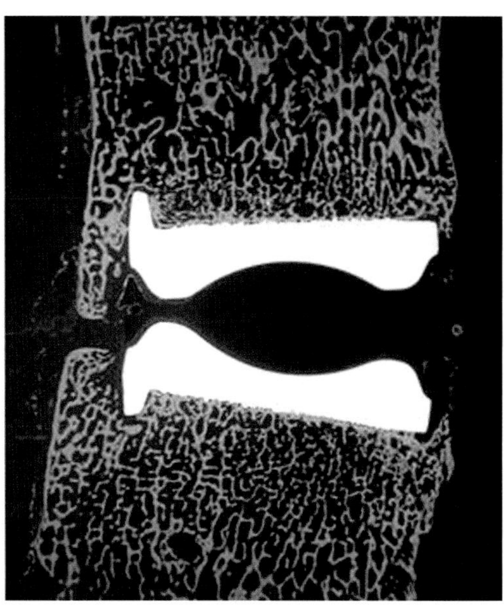

■ **FIGURE 7–10.** Representative undecalcified histologic specimen of the CHARITÉ device *(left)* and corresponding microradiograph *(right)* following a 6-month postoperative period. (Villanueva bone stain, magnification ×2.5.)

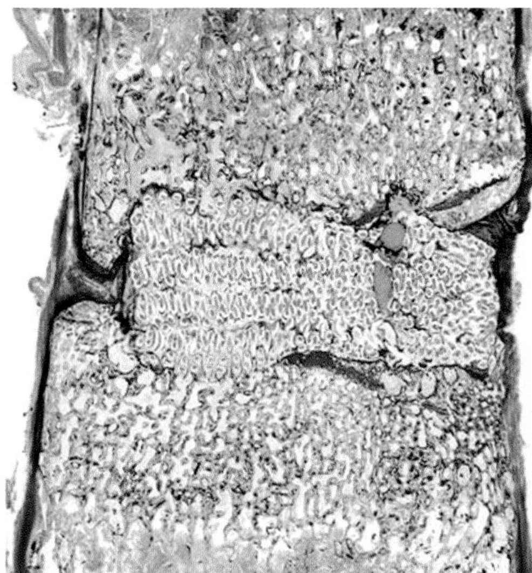
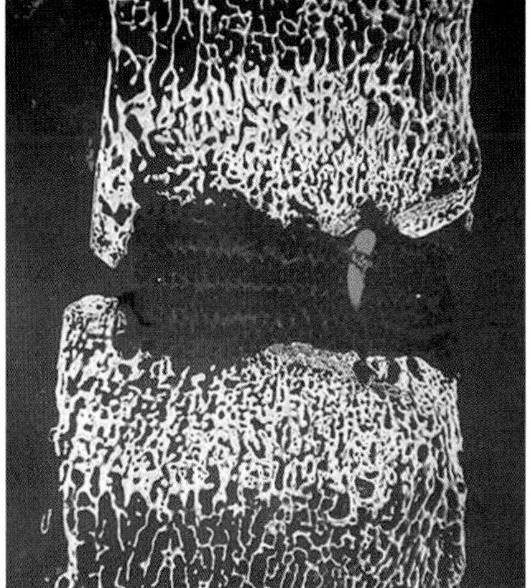

■ **FIGURE 7–11.** Representative undecalcified histologic specimen of the Three-Dimensional Fabricube (3DF) device specimen *(left)* and corresponding microradiograph *(right)* following a 6-month postoperative period. (Villanueva bone stain, magnification ×2.5.)

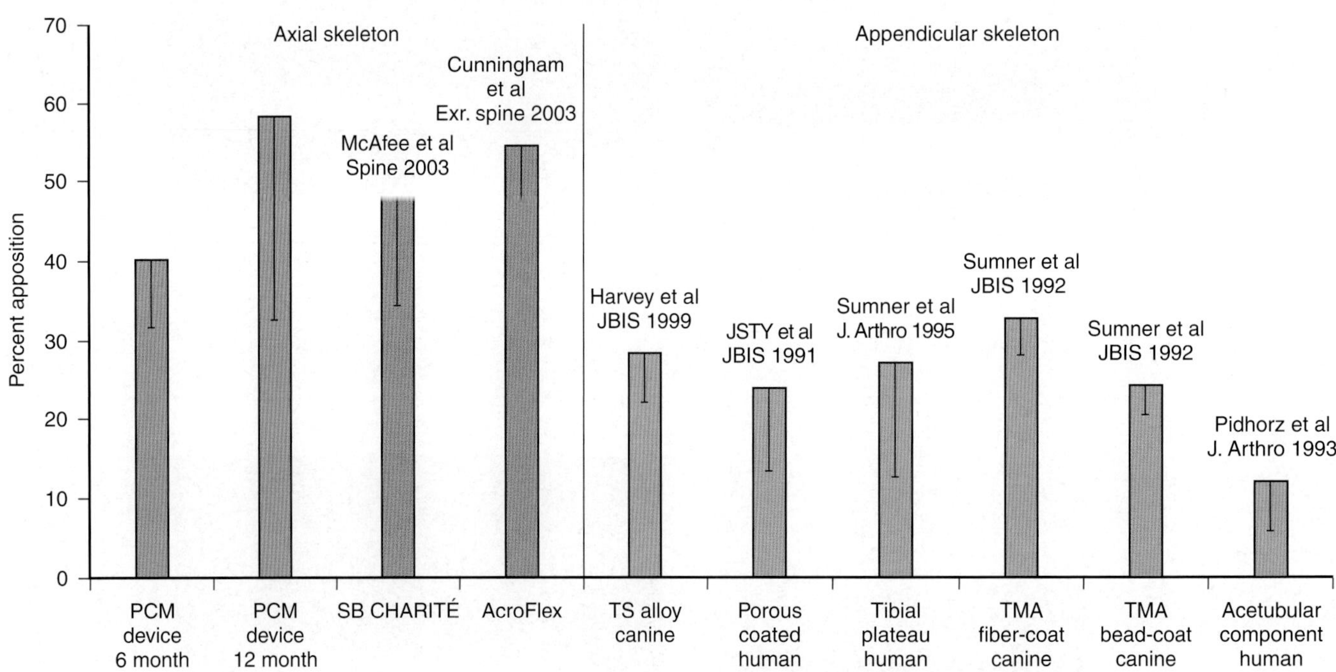


■ **FIGURE 7–12.** A bar chart comparing the percent linear bone apposition of cervical and lumbar total disc arthroplasty versus that reported for total joint arthroplasty in the appendicular skeleton. Osseointegration in the axial skeleton (~4%) exceeds that observed in historical controls for the appendicular skeleton (~25%), which is probably secondary to the ligamentotaxis causing sustained compression across the metal–bone interface. Bar values indicate sample mean, and error bars indicate one standard deviation.

no statistical differences between any groups ($P > 0.05$). Flexion-extension testing indicated that the acute instrumented Dynesys produced 30% of the intact motion. Following 6 months in vivo, this value increased to 50%, and 64% by the 12-month time interval ($P < 0.05$). Lateral bending testing indicated the acute instrumented Dynesys afforded 15% of the intact motion. Following 6 months in vivo, this value increased to 27%, and 49% by the 12-month time interval ($P < 0.05$).

Facet joint histology at the operative or adjacent levels demonstrated no evidence of facet arthrosis. However, based on immunohistochemistry, there was evidence of polymeric particulate wear debris and proinflammatory cytokines (macrophage activity) at the implant interconnection mechanisms, leading to an upregulation in IL-1 and TNF-β in local tissues at the 6-month treatments. In vivo loading of the Dynesys System led to implant stress relaxation with functional restoration in flexion-extension (64% of intact) and lateral bending (49% of intact) segmental kinematics. However, there was evidence of polymeric particulate wear debris, proinflammatory cytokines, and macrophage activity at the implant interconnection mechanisms. Using a nonhuman primate model, this study demonstrated the in vivo motion preserving properties of a dynamic posterior spinal stabilization system and serves as a basic science foundation for the results obtained in ongoing clinical investigations.

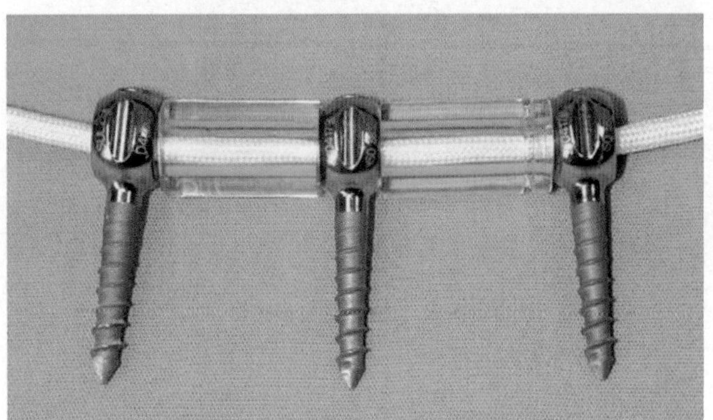

■ **FIGURE 7–13.** Image of the Dynesys configuration used in the baboon in vivo studies. The construct imaged represents a unilateral construct (three screws, two polycarbonate urethane spacers, and polyethylene terephthalate [PET] cord). Each baboon specimen was reconstructed bilaterally.

## Neurotoxicity Rabbit Model—Particulate Wear Debris

The effect of particulate wear debris from the bearing surfaces of motion-preserving spinal implants remains a clinical concern. Using an in vivo rabbit model, Cunningham and co-workers[24] investigated the neural and systemic tissue histopathologic response following epidural application of ten different types of particulate wear debris used in motion-preserving spinal implants. One hundred New Zealand White rabbits were included in this study and equally randomized into 10 groups ($n = 10$ groups) based on treatment material: (1) sham (control group), (2) stainless steel (316LVM), (3) titanium alloy (Ti-6AL-4V), (4) cobalt chrome alloy, (5) UHMWPE, (6) polycarbonate urethane, (7) polyetheretherketone (PEEK), (8) polyvinyl alcohol, (9) polyester, and (10) ceramic. The surgical procedure consisted of a midline posterior approach, followed by resection of the L6 spinous process and ligamentum flavum at L5-L6, permitting interlaminar exposure of the

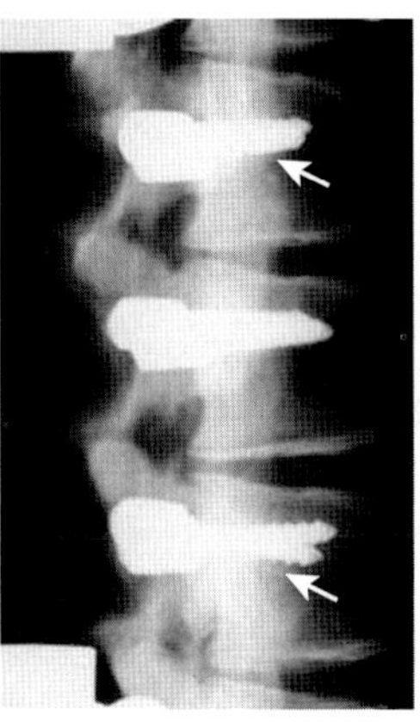
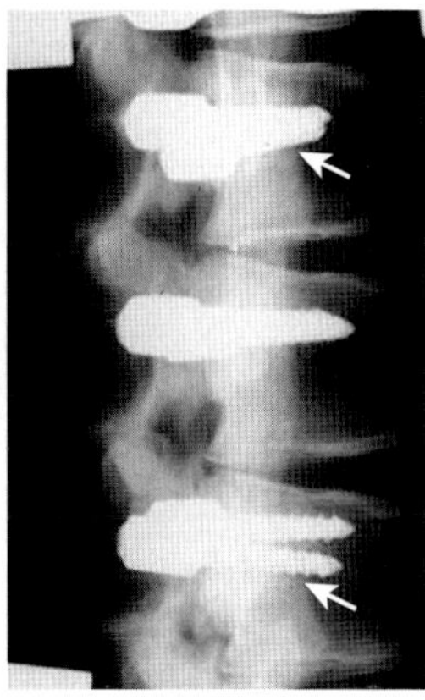
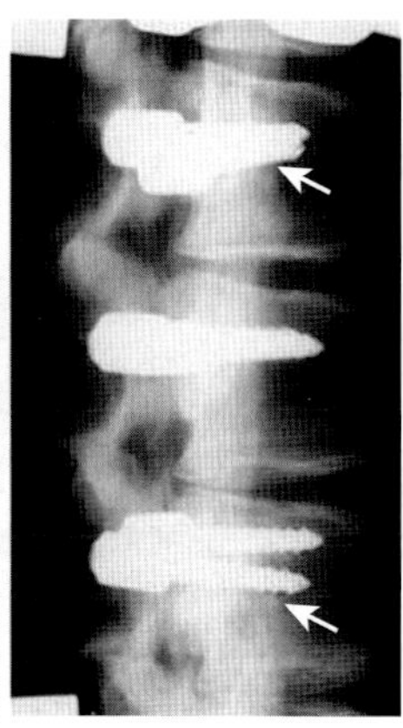

**FIGURE 7–14.** Plain film radiographs analysis demonstrated no incidence of implant migration. However, based on anteroposterior, lateral *(left two images)* and flexion-extension films *(right two images)*, there was a 25% (3 of 12 screws) incidence of radiolucency at the bone–screw interface.

dural sac. Four milligrams of the appropriate treatment material was then implanted in dry, sterile format (Fig. 7–15). The sham procedure consisted of epidural exposure alone. All particles (size range 0.3 to 50 μ diameter; dosage 300 to 600 million particles) were verified to be endotoxin free before implantation.

Five animals from each treatment group were sacrificed at 3 months and five at 6 months postoperatively. Postmortem analyses included cultures from the epidural site, cytology, and histopathologic assessment of local and systemic tissues. Immunocytochemical analysis of the spinal cord and overlying fibrosis quantified the extent of macrophage activity, proinflammatory cytokines (TNF-α, TNF-β, IL-1α, IL-1β, IL-6, IL-8), and histiocytosis. All animals survived the procedures without evidence of neurologic or infectious complications. Postmortem blood chemistry profiles were within normal limits for all treatment groups, and epidural cultures were negative for nearly all cases. There was no evidence of particulate debris or pathology in the distant systemic or reticuloendothelial tissues. Gross histopathology demonstrated increased levels of epidural fibrosis in the experimental treatments versus operative controls. Plain and polarized light microscopic evaluation of the epidural fibrous tissues (H&E and macrophage stains) indicated definitive evidence of histiocytic reaction containing phagocytized particles and foci of local inflammatory changes in all treatments. Immunohistochemistry of the spinal cord and epidural tissue demonstrated a transient upregulation in IL-6 for the stainless steel, titanium, and UHMWPE groups versus the control group at 3 months ($P < 0.05$). The spinal cord demonstrated no evidence of significant lesions or neuropathology in all treatment groups. However, multiple treatments from the metallic groups indicated a chronic macrophage response to particulate debris ($P < 0.05$) with elevated histiocytes versus sham controls ($P < 0.05$). In many cases, the macrophages diffused intrathecally to the innermost spinal meninx and spinal cord itself (Fig. 7–16). Direct epidural application of particulate wear debris produced a chronic histiocytic reaction localized within the epidural fibrous layers. Wear particles have the capacity to diffuse intrathecally, eliciting a macrophage/cytokine response within the epidural tissues and spinal cord. Overall, based on the postoperative time periods evaluated, there was no evidence of an acute neural or systemic histopathologic response to the 10 implant materials included in the current study.

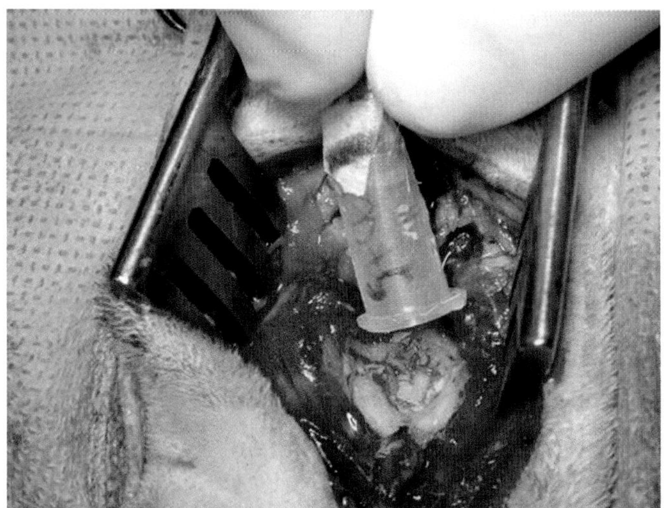

**FIGURE 7–15.** Intraoperative posterior view demonstrating epidural application of the stainless steel particulate wear debris. The experimental treatments were then implanted directly on the dura as a sterile, dry material.

## DISCUSSION

Preclinical animal modeling and basic scientific methods to assess functionality and in vivo performance of dynamic spinal stabilization remains at the forefront of basic science and clinical research endeavors. The current review provides a methodologic basis to investigate dynamic spinal stabilization devices in terms of the multidirectional flexibility properties, patterns of histologic osseointegration, and neurohistopathologic effects of particulate wear debris using in vitro and in vivo animal models. The implementation of dynamic spinal instrumentation systems for fusionless correction of spinal deformity, dynamic posterior stabilization, and total disc replacement arthroplasty necessitates improved understanding in terms of the biomechanical stabilizing properties of these devices, patterns of implant osseointegration, if any, and the neurohistopathologic

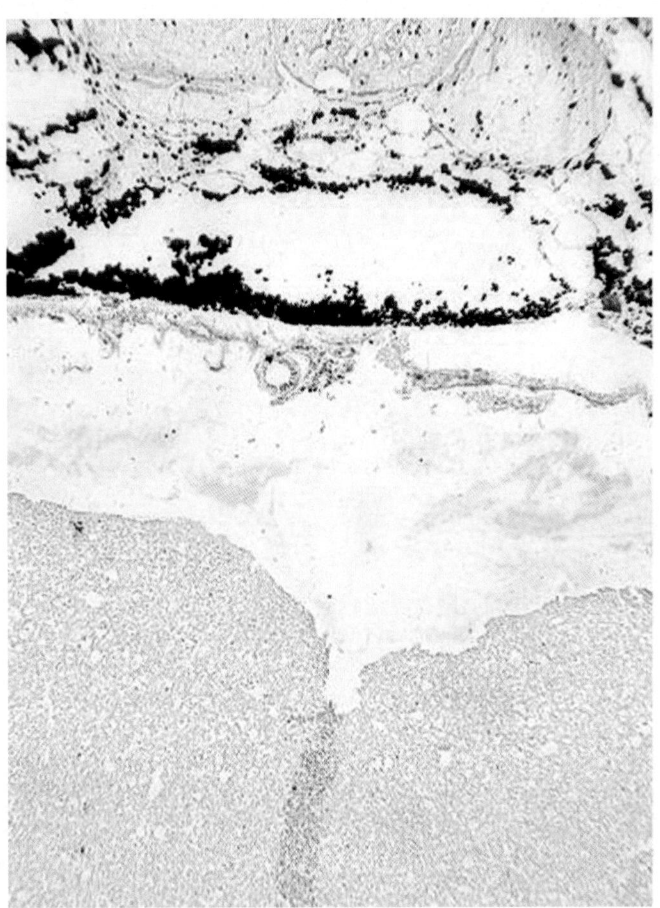

■ **FIGURE 7–16.** Cobalt chrome–treated spinal cord. Plain light microscopy demonstrating a histologic cross-section from a 6-month cobalt chrome specimen. Note the epidural layer of particulate debris and intrathecal dissemination to within the spinal cord itself. This diffusion process was coupled with histiocytic macrophage response consistent with a localized, chronic inflammatory reaction (macrophages; red-staining regions) (HAM-56 macrophage stain, magnification ×10).

response to particulate wear debris. Future research directions should focus on optimizing surgical implant techniques to re-establish near-normal intervertebral kinematics, maximizing implant osseointegration while preserving segmental motion and the minimization of particulate debris generation through judicious selection of implant materials and bearing surfaces. Diligence in these areas, coupled with well-characterized clinical experience will likely result in optimized long-term biomechanical and biologic clinical performance of dynamic spinal stabilization systems.

## REFERENCES


1. The Complete Animal Welfare Act including all amendments (1970, 1976, 1985, 1990) following the 1966 enactment. United States Code, Title 7, Sections 2131 to 2156.
2. Rao RD, Bagaria VB, Cooley BC: Posterolateral intertransverse lumbar fusion in a mouse model: surgical anatomy and operative technique. Spine J 7:61–67, 2007. Epub 2006 Nov.
3. Thomas I, Kirkaldy-Willis WH, Singh S, Paine KW: Experimental spinal fusion in guinea pigs and dogs: the effect of immobilization. Clin Orthop Relat Res 112:363–375, 1975.
4. Lu SS, Zhang X, Soo C, et al: The osteoinductive properties of Nell-1 in a rat spinal fusion model. Spine J 7:50–60, 2007. Epub 2006 Nov 17.
5. Boden SD: Biology of lumbar spine fusion and use of bone graft substitutes: present, future, and next generation. Tissue Eng 6:383–699, 2000.
6. McAfee PC, Farey ID, Sutterlin CE, et al: 1989 Volvo Award in basic science. Device-related osteoporosis with spinal instrumentation. Spine 14:919–926, 1989.
7. Nagel DA, Kramers PC, Rahn BA, et al: A paradigm of delayed union and nonunion in the lumbosacral joint. A study of motion and bone grafting of the lumbosacral spine in sheep. Spine 16:553–559, 1991.
8. Li H, Zou X, Springer M, et al: Instrumented anterior lumbar interbody fusion with equine bone protein extract. Spine 32:E126–E129, 2007.
9. Smit TH, Krijnen MR, van Dijk M, Wuisman PI: Application of polylactides in spinal cages: studies in a goat model. J Mater Sci Mater Med 17:1237–1244, 2006.
10. Wang T, Dang G, Guo Z, Yang M: Evaluation of autologous bone marrow mesenchymal stem cell-calcium phosphate ceramic composite for lumbar fusion in rhesus monkey interbody fusion model. Tissue Eng 11:1159–1167, 2005.
11. Grobler LJ, Gaines RW, Kempff PG: Comparing Mersilene tape and stainless steel wire as sublaminar spinal fixation in the Chagma baboon (Papio ursinus). Iowa Orthop J 17:20–31, 1997.
12. Bagby GW: Arthrodesis by the distraction-compression method using a stainless steel implant. Orthopedics 11:931–934, 1988.
13. Vuono-Hawkins M, Zimmerman MC, Lee CK, et al: Mechanical evaluation of a canine intervertebral disc spacer: in situ and in vivo studies. J Orthop Res 12:119–127, 1994.
14. Kotani Y, Abumi K, Shikinami Y, et al: Two-year observation of artificial intervertebral disc replacement: results after supplemental ultra-high strength bioresorbable spinal stabilization. J Neurosurg 100(4):337–342, 2004.
15. Jensen WK, Anderson PA, Nel L, Rouleau JP: Bone ingrowth in retrieved Bryan Cervical Disc prostheses. Spine 30:2497–2502, 2005.
16. Hu N, Cunningham BW, McAfee PC, et al: Porous coated motion cervical disc replacement: a biomechanical, histomorphometric, and biologic wear analysis in a caprine model. Spine 31:1666–1673.
17. Anderson PA, Sasso RC, Rouleau JP, et al: The Bryan Cervical Disc: wear properties and early clinical results. Spine J 4(6):303S–309S, 2004.
18. Cunningham BW, Dmitriev AE, Hu N, McAfee PC: General principles of total disc replacement arthroplasty: seventeen cases in a non-human primate model. Spine 28:S118–S124, 2003.
19. Cunningham BW, Lowery GL, Serhan HA, et al: Total disc replacement arthroplasty using the AcroFlex lumbar disc: a non-human primate model. Eur Spine J 11(2):S115–S123, Epub 2002 Aug 20.
20. White AA, Panjabi MM: Kinematics of the spine. In: Clinical Biomechanics of the Spine, Philadelphia, PA, J.B. Lippincott, 1990, pp. 86–125.
21. Kotani Y, Abumi K, Shikinami Y, et al: Artificial intervertebral disc replacement using bioactive three-dimensional fabric: design, development, and preliminary animal study. Spine 27:929–935, 2002; discussion 935–936.
22. Cunningham BW, Dmitriev AE, Hu N, McAfee PC: General principles of total disc replacement arthroplasty: Seventeen cases in a non-human primate model. Spine 28:S118–S124, 2003.
23. Cunningham BW, Dawson J, Dmitriev AE, et al: Pre-clinical evaluation of a dynamic posterior spinal stabilization system (Dynesys$^{TM}$): a non-human primate model. Spine 200. (In Press).
24. Cunningham BW, Hallab NJ, Dmitriev AE, et al: Epidural application of spinal instrumentation particulate wear debris: an in-vivo animal model. Presented at the Annual Meeting of the Scoliosis Research Society 38:58, 2003.

CHAPTER 8

# Indications and Contraindications for Lumbar Nonfusion Surgery: Patient Selection

James J. Yue and James P. Lawrence

## KEY POINTS

- A "red flag" and non-spine-related history must be obtained.
- A standing physical and radiographic examination are mandatory.
- Unilateral back pain must be carefully scrutinized.
- Both computed tomography (CT) and magnetic resonance imaging (MRI) are essential in evaluating the patient for nonfusion surgery.
- Bone density should be evaluated in women older than 40 years, men older than 50 years, and in all smokers of any age or sex.
- Discography and spinal injections should be considered adjuncts to diagnosis.
- Reasonable expectations should be discussed with all patients, and the evolutionary nature of spinal spondylosis should be explained to the patient considering any motion-sparing technology.

## INTRODUCTION

Elements of a successful surgical outcome include, but are not limited to, proper surgical technique, appropriate implant selection, and of paramount importance, proper patient selection. This chapter explores the essentials of patient selection in reference to motion-sparing technology. The premise for any effective treatment modality is the formulation and correlation of an accurate diagnosis. Obtaining an accurate diagnosis is, at best, a daunting clinical challenge owing to the fluctuating and evolving nature of lumbar spondylopathies. Fortunately, the majority of cases of symptomatic lumbar spondylosis can be successfully treated without surgery. With failure of conservative treatment, including the usage of non-steroidal anti-inflammatory agents, physiotherapy, and the usage of injections, surgical intervention can become a consideration for the appropriate patient.

### Goals of Motion-Preserving Surgery

In comparison to fusion, lumbar disc arthroplasty and other motion-sparing technologies approach the patient with degenerative disc disease from an alternative perspective. The goals of arthroplasty focus on removal of the presumed pain generator and a preservation or re-creation of the biomechanics of the functional spinal unit. Arthroplasty aims to eliminate a potentially painful disc while restoring and maintaining motion of the functional spinal unit, re-creating the height of the normal disc, and preserving the relationship with the facet joints. The development of lumbar disc arthroplasty and other motion-sparing techniques has, therefore, relied upon an understanding of the normal, native functional spinal unit. The complex relationship between two vertebrae, including the intervening disc, the paired facet joints, and the related ligaments, dictates the functional anatomy of the spinal unit and, therefore, the goals of any motion-sparing surgical intervention.

## PATIENT EVALUATION

### OVERVIEW

Perhaps the most important aspect of the implementation of new technology in the clinical setting is patient selection. Patient selection encompasses several domains, from the recognition of the reason for the patient's arrival in the office of the physician (elimination of secondary gain issues) to the formation of the relationship of the history to examination and diagnostic imaging findings, and finally, to the formation of a targeted treatment plan that may involve surgical intervention.

### History

Evaluation of the patient with lumbar spondylosis constitutes a complex appreciation of a multitude of factors. The beginning of the evaluation is the history, which should allow the examiner to understand the patient's pain, activities that exacerbate the pain, the motion-related aspects of pain (flexion type or extension type), and any concomitant neurologic symptoms. A thorough review of symptoms should always be performed to identify occult causes of back pain, such as oncologic, gynecologic, vascular, intraperitoneal, or other "red flag" sources of pain. History of malignancy or prior surgical procedures (abdominal approaches) should be reviewed. Previous therapeutic modalities such as use of medication, physical therapy, and injections (facet, nerve root, or epidural) should be noted to help form an estimation of the patient's likelihood of a positive result with surgical intervention, as well as the possibility of patient adherence to other prescribed modalities such as physiotherapy. An exploration of the psychosocial factors contributing to the disease process, a history of psychiatric illness, and use of medication for anxiety, depression, and psychosis should be performed. As with any patient, a true understanding of the overall functional status and a discussion of reasonable expectations is critically important.

Patients with leg pain should be closely interviewed to identify those patients with isolated radicular complaints versus those patients with neurogenic claudication and spinal stenosis. Patients whose leg symptoms are improved with sitting and forward flexion should be closely evaluated for spinal stenosis rather than a discogenic source of low back pain with associated radiculopathy. Depending on the approach needed to apply a given surgical technique, a thorough review of previous surgical procedures should be obtained. For example, an interview for a possible total disc arthroplasty, previous abdominal–pelvic procedures, and a history of pelvic inflammatory disease should be elicited.

### Examination

A thorough physical and neurologic examination should be performed, with care taken to best identify area of the pain, assess the existing range of motion in the lumbar spine, form an understanding of the anatomic structures involved, and to identify any areas of neurologic deficit (motor, sensory, exam of the upper and lower reflexes) that could indicate ongoing radiculopathy, myelopathy, or neuromuscular dysfunction.

All patients should be placed in an examination gown. Observation of the patient sitting, standing, and walking should be performed. With the patient in the standing position, direct observation of the spinal contour should be performed in the neutral, flexion, and extension positions. The patient must be asked to identify the location of the pain. Localization of the pain in a *diffuse* pattern across the lower lumbar area is more indicative of a discogenic source of pain. Localization of the pain in a unilateral fashion may indicate facet degeneration (Fig. 8–1), sacroiliac disease, an L5 transverse process pseudoarticulation (Fig. 8–2), primary hip osteoarthritis, or other non-spine-related disease. Other important areas of assessment include the patient's height and weight (body mass index [BMI]) and general health (pulmonary, cardiovascular). Furthermore, if the patient becomes a candidate for intervention, a full medical and cardiac evaluation is important to assess the risks of general anesthesia and the operative procedure.

## DIAGNOSTIC EVALUATION

### Plain Radiographs

Standing plain radiographs are the first step in the evaluation of the patient with back pain who has not responded to conservative measures. Although authors differ on the universal use of radiographs, plain films serve to define the anatomy, the anatomic alignment (lordosis or kyphosis), measurement of the disc height, and the presence of observable pathology (such as a resting or dynamic spondylolisthesis) and vertebral body osteophytes or Modic changes suggestive of chronic discal degeneration. Oblique radiographs, although a useful screening tool for osteoarthritis of the facet joints, offer poor specificity in comparison with CT scans.

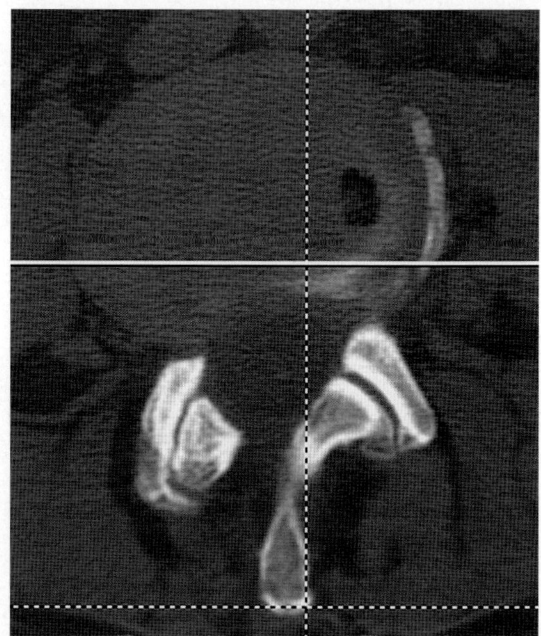

■ **FIGURE 8–1.** Unilateral facet degeneration in patient with right-sided low back pain.

Vertebral end plate morphology should be assessed for posterior and anterior sloping, central concavities, or a mixture of end plate dysmorphisms that could impede or negate the application of a particular surgical course of treatment. A recent end plate classification devised by the senior author has been recently evaluated and validated, and is illustrated in Figure 8–3.

### Flexion-Extension Radiographs

Standing flexion-extension radiographs are most useful to identify instability in patients with risk factors for instability, such as

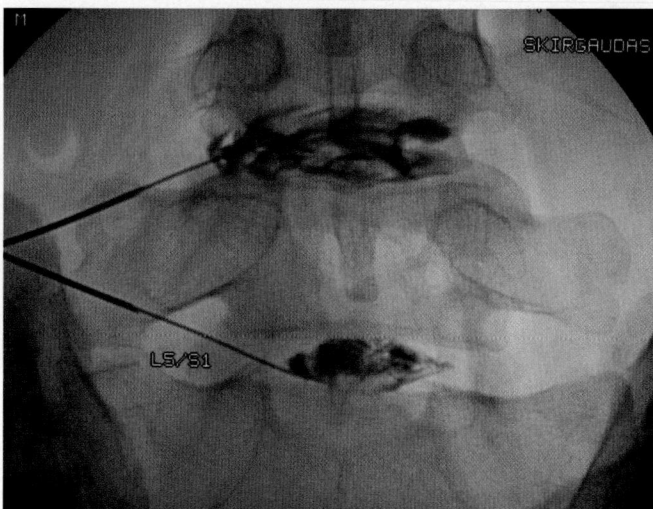


■ **FIGURE 8–2.** Right-sided L5 transverse process pseudoarticulation with sacrum and positive L4-5 discogram.

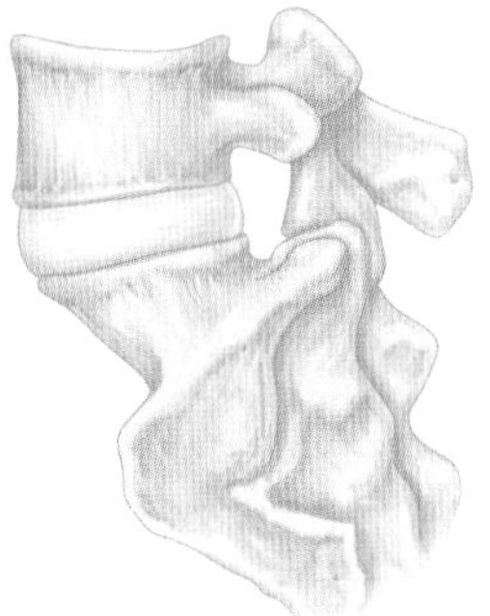

Type I - Flat end plates

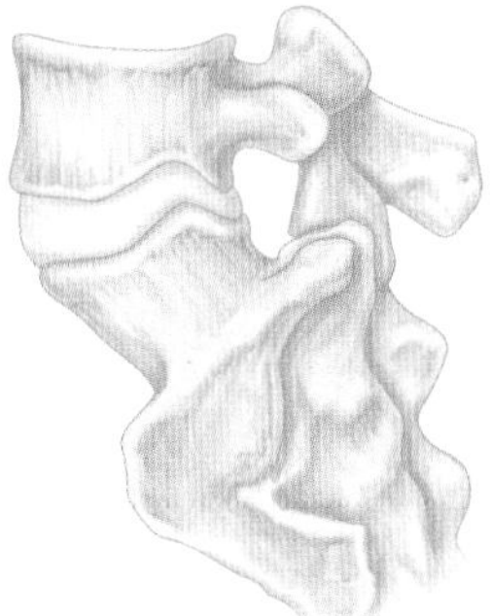

Type II - Hooked end plates

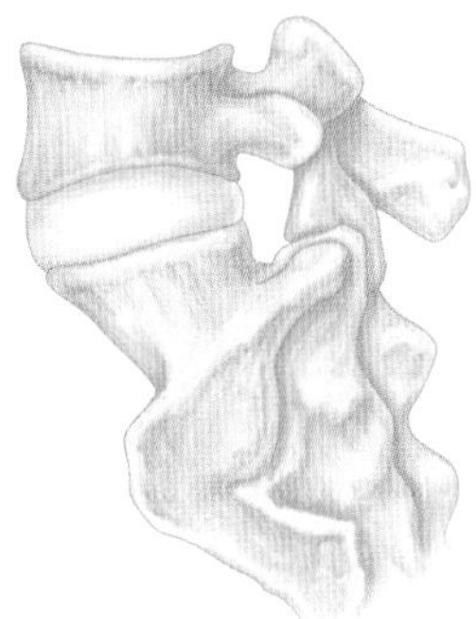

Type III - Concave end plates

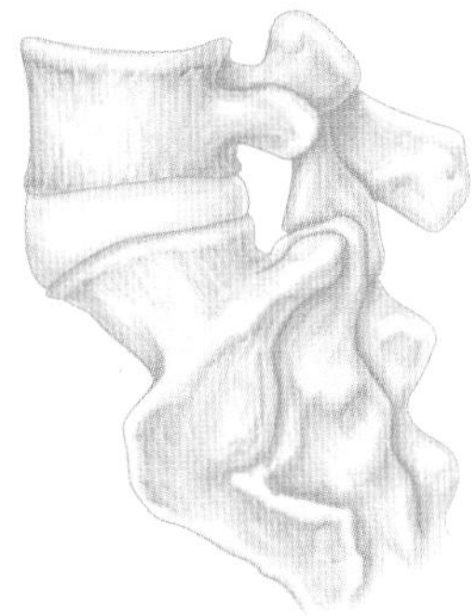

Type IV - Convex end plates

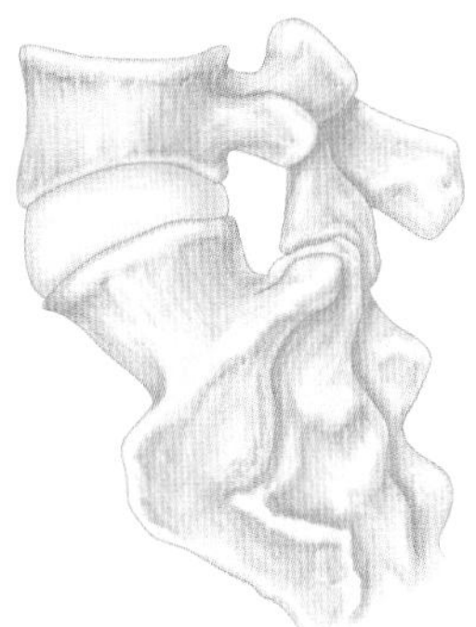

Type V - Combined end plates

■ **FIGURE 8–3.** The Yue-Bertagnoli vertebral end plate classification.

previous trauma, previous lumbar surgery (laminectomy), congenital anomalies, and autoinflammatory conditions. In addition, flexion-extension films can be useful in assessing motion occurring at each level throughout the lumbar spine.

## Computed Tomography Scans

CT scans are used to exclude osteoarthritis of the zygapophyseal joints, fractures of the pars interarticularis (spondylolysis), Baastrup's disease (kissing spines), and other sources of low back pain. Facet joint arthrosis may be graded based on the CT scan using the grading system as described by Fugiwara et al.[1] As a part of preoperative planning, CT scan is also useful in obtaining measurements of the vertebral body size parameters in preparation for arthroplasty.

## Magnetic Resonance Imaging

MRI provides great detail regarding the hydration of the intervertebral disc, the presence or absence of herniation, bulge, or extrusion, and provides great detail regarding the degenerative spine. It is important to note the commonality of MRI findings in the asymptomatic population. Numerous series have been reported that demonstrate the common presence of abnormalities of the intervertebral disc and the questionable correlation with the development of discogenic back pain. However, MRI may be most beneficial in the staging of the degree of disc degeneration and the identification of risk factors for disease progression.[2] MRI also allows for the detection of disc dehydration and bone marrow edema in the case of activated spondylochondrosis.

## Bone Scintigraphy

If osteoporosis or osteopenia is suspected, an osteodensitometry evaluation of the lumbar spine should be performed. Traditional methods include: dual-energy x-ray absorptiometry (DEXA) scanning, dual photon absorptiometry (DPA), ultrasound, and quantitative CT. The DEXA scan uses the least amount of radiation, is the least expensive, and most accurate. All women older than age 40, men older than age 50, and smokers should be evaluated with an osteodensitometry evaluation.

## Discography

The use of discography is advised in multilevel degeneration, cases with other potential sources of pain, and in patients in whom a chronic midline annular defect is thought to be present and producing discogenic back pain. The current literature on the use of discography has been focused on the use of fusion as a treatment modality.[3–13] The senior author uses discography in evaluating potential candidates for lumbar arthroplasty in most instances except in those patients with single-level degenerative disc disease in which there is clear evidence of disc height loss as compared with normal adjacent discs. Discography should be viewed as an adjunct to diagnosis. It does not define the need for or against surgical intervention. Discographic findings should complement MRI findings. Discography may be falsely negative in instances when intradiscal pressures cannot be achieved due to complete annular disruption. Further research is indicated in the use of traditional and more novel forms of discography such as functional anesthetic discography.

### Injection Diagnostics

The use of diagnostic injections should be tailored accordingly. For example, unilateral low back pain should be evaluated with facet and/or sacroiliac injections. Relief of low back pain with a facet block may indicate primary facet arthropathy, or it may indicate a secondary pain generator as a result of an incompetent disc complex that may ultimately be relieved by a lumbar total disc arthroplasty.

### Total Lumbar Disc Arthroplasty

The indication for total lumbar disc arthroplasty is severe discogenic low back pain in patients who have failed a protracted course of nonsurgical treatment. Lumbar inclusion criteria are the following:

- Men or women with Visual Analog Score (VAS) <4, Oswestry score >40%
- Age 18 to 60 years, optimally younger than age 50 years
- Symptomatic degenerative disc disease or lumbar spondylosis with objective evidence of degenerative disc disease by CT or MRI. Specific radiographic findings include
  1. Vacuum disc sign
  2. High-intensity zone signal
  3. Modic changes
  4. Contained herniated nucleus pulposus
  5. Paucity of facet joint degeneration changes
  6. Decrease of intervertebral disc height of at least 4 mm, and
  7. Scarring/thickening of annulus fibrosis with osteophytes indicating osteoarthritis.

There are many contraindications to the use of this new technology. Contraindications specific to the spine focus on pre-existing degenerative conditions, such as spondylolisthesis, spondylolysis, posterior element disease (facet joint arthritis or previous facet joint resection), central or lateral recess stenosis, fixed deformity, infection, osteoporosis, or herniated nucleus pulposus with radiculopathy that cannot be decompressed by way of anterior approach. Relative contraindications include general medical conditions such as obesity and psychosocial pathology. Many of these contraindications are common in patients with degenerative disc disease. A review of 100 consecutive patients undergoing lumbar spine surgery for degenerative spinal disease demonstrated the prevalence of at least one contraindication to Total Disc Replacement (TDR) was 95%. In the 56 patients in this series who underwent fusion, 100% had at least one contraindication to TDR. Few patients will be without at least one relative or absolute contraindication to lumbar arthroplasty, if these contraindications remain as are currently constituted.[14]

As with all procedures, consideration of the patient history, the physical examination, and the findings on noninvasive and invasive imaging are paramount. In the consideration of axial or discogenic back pain, the correlation of these factors remains complex.

The European experience with total disc replacement underscores the need for a clearer understanding of the potential indications and, more important, the contraindications for the use of these devices. A key concept is the recognition of the lumbar motion segment as a three-joint complex. Particular attention should be paid to the presence of facet joint degenerative changes, because this has been associated with poor clinical outcomes after arthroplasty. As noted by Bertagnoli and Kumar,[15] an accurate assessment of the status of the facet joints is an essential part of the preoperative evaluation of a patient considered for total lumbar disc replacement.

### Interspinous Spacer Devices

Interspinous devices are indicated for patients (age 50 and older in the United States) who have neurogenic intermittent claudication; leg/buttock/groin pain that is relieved when the spine is flexed such as when sitting in a chair due to central and lateral-recess lumbar spinal stenosis. Other indications include:

1. Spondylolisthesis up to grade 1.5 (of 4) (~35%), with neurogenic intermittent claudication.
2. Baastrup's syndrome/"kissing spine."
3. Axial load–induced back pain.
4. Facet syndrome.
5. Degenerative and iatrogenic (postdiscectomy) disc syndrome.
6. Contained Herniated Nucleus Replacement (HNP).
7. Unloading of disc adjacent to a lumbar fusion procedure, primary or secondary.

Contraindications include:

1. An allergy to titanium or titanium alloy.

Spinal anatomy or disease that would prevent implantation of the device or cause the device to be unstable in the body, such as:

1. Significant instability of the lumbar spine.
2. An ankylosed segment at the affected level(s).
3. Acute fracture of the spinous process or pars interarticularis.
4. Significant scoliosis.
5. Neural compression causing neurogenic bowel or bladder dysfunction.
6. Diagnosis of severe osteoporosis.
7. Active systemic infection or infection localized to the site of implantation.

### Nucleus Replacement, Posterior Dynamic Stabilizing, Facet Replacement, and Total Posterior Arthroplasty Devices

Given the relatively recent introduction of these and other devices, the indications and contraindications will be discussed further in subsequent chapters.

## CONCLUSIONS

Achieving an optimal result in the care of the patient with a lumbar spondylopathy amendable to motion-sparing technology is reliant on multiple factors. Accurately diagnosing and applying the principles of motion-sparing technology will optimize surgical outcomes. A complete understanding of the indications and contraindications for any proposed procedure is also essential in achieving a successful clinical outcome. It is essential to perform an erect examination as well as erect dynamic x-ray imaging. Unilateral back pain should be carefully scrutinized. The author recommends that both MRI and CT scans be obtained in all patients in which any motion-sparing surgery is contemplated to accurately assess the five-joint complex that comprises the functional spinal unit. Any female patient older than 40 years, any male patient older than 50 years, and all smokers should obtain bone densitometry evaluation. Reasonable expectations should be discussed with all patients, and the evolutionary nature of spinal spondylosis should be explained to the patient considering any motion-sparing technology.

## REFERENCES


1. Fujiwara A, Lim TH, An HS, et al: The effect of disc degeneration and facet joint osteoarthritis on the segmental flexibility of the lumbar spine. Spine 25:3036–3044, 2000.
2. Elfering A, Semmer N, Birkhofer D, et al: Risk factors for lumbar disc degeneration: a 5-year prospective MRI study in asymptomatic individuals. Spine 27:125–134, 2002.
3. Carragee EJ: Is lumbar discography a determinate of discogenic low back pain: provocative discography reconsidered. Curr Rev Pain 4:301–308, 2000.
4. Carragee EJ: Psychological and functional profiles in select subjects with low back pain. Spine J 1:198–204, 2001.
5. Carragee EJ, Alamin TF: Discography: a review. Spine J 1:364–372, 2001.
6. Carragee EJ, Alamin TF, Carragee JM: Low-pressure positive discography in subjects asymptomatic of significant low back pain illness. Spine 31:505–509, 2006.
7. Carragee EJ, Alamin TF, Miller J, et al: Provocative discography in volunteer subjects with mild persistent low back pain. Spine J 2:25–34, 2002.
8. Carragee EJ, Alamin TF, Miller JL, et al: Discographic, MRI and psychosocial determinants of low back pain disability and remission: a prospective study in subjects with benign persistent back pain. Spine J 5:24–35, 2005.
9. Carragee EJ, Hannibal M: Diagnostic evaluation of low back pain. Orthop Clin North Am 35:7–16, 2004.
10. Carragee EJ, Lincoln T, Parmar VS, et al: A gold standard evaluation of the "discogenic pain" diagnosis as determined by provocative discography. Spine 31:2115–2123, 2006.
11. Carragee EJ, Paragioudakis SJ, Khurana S: 2000 Volvo Award winner in clinical studies: Lumbar high-intensity zone and discography in subjects without low back problems. Spine 25:2987–2992, 2000.
12. Carragee EJ, Tanner CM, Khurana S, et al The rates of false-positive lumbar discography in select patients without low back symptoms. Spine 25:1373–1380; discussion 1381, 2000.
13. Carragee EJ, Tanner CM, Yang B, et al: False-positive findings on lumbar discography Reliability of subjective concordance assessment during provocative disc injection. Spine 24:2542–2547, 1999.
14. Huang RC, Lim MR, Girardi FP, et al: The prevalence of contraindications to total disc replacement in a cohort of lumbar surgical patients. Spine 29:2538–2541, 2004.
15. Bertagnoli R, Kumar S: Indications for full prosthetic disc arthroplasty: a correlation of clinical outcome against a variety of indications. Eur Spine J 11(2):S131–S136, 2002.

CHAPTER 9

# Indications and Contraindications for Cervical Nonfusion Surgery: Patient Selection

**Nader M. Habela** and **Paul C. McAfee**

**KEY POINTS**

- A careful history that reveals evidence of degenerative disk disease, radiculopathy, myelopathy, or myeloradiculopathy is the first step in patient selection for cervical disc replacement.
- Plain radiographs and MRI are the two most useful tools in confirming the diagnosis.
- The indications for cervical disc replacement are similar to anterior fusion surgery.
- Evaluation of the inclusion and exclusion criteria of each cervical disk replacement investigational study is the final step in patient selection prior to study participation.
- Unlike lumbar disc arthroplasty, where isolated discogenic low back pain is the main indication for surgery, cervical disc arthroplasty should be done for radiculopathy or myelopathy.

## INTRODUCTION

Cervical spondylosis or chronic disc degeneration and associated facet arthropathy, herniated nucleus pulposus, and isolated degenerative disc disease may result in a constellation of symptoms that includes axial neck pain, radiculopathy, myelopathy, or any combination of the above-mentioned problems.

Anatomically, the functional spinal unit, which consists of two vertebral bodies and the intervertebral disc, has been the primary focus of attention for relief of pain and restoration of function. The intervertebral disc and facet joints, believed to be the major pain generators, have been the center of extensive medical and surgical management.

Nonsurgical management of cervical spondylosis, herniated nucleus pulposus, and isolated degenerative disc disease includes the use of nonsteroidal and steroidal anti-inflammatory agents, isometric exercises and physical therapy, the judicious use of narcotic pain medications and muscle relaxants, and the administration of relatively more novel nerve-stabilizing medications.

Surgically, the elimination of motion at the functional spinal unit has been the mainstay of treatment for the past 40 years. Anterior cervical decompression and fusion have become the standard of care for relief of pain and stabilization associated with radiculopathy[1] and myelopathy,[2] with excellent long-term results.

The incredible success of total joint arthroplasty in the hip, knee, and shoulder to relieve pain and restore functional motion has been followed by similar efforts in the cervical and lumbar spines. The advent of modern artificial total disc arthroplasty in the cervical and lumbar spine has renewed interest in the potential for motion preservation, without the complications inherent to fusion surgery including pseudoarthrosis,[3] donor site morbidity, postoperative immobilization, and adjacent segment degeneration.[4]

This chapter discusses the importance of patient selection for cervical disc replacement surgery and highlights the indications and contraindications for the procedure. Patient selection, rather than the nuances of specific devices, plays the most important role in the clinical success of cervical disc replacement surgery. A careful history, physical examination, and appropriate diagnostic studies are the most important tools in successful patient selection. Although the indications and contraindications are similar to those for anterior cervical decompression and fusion, inclusion and exclusion criteria may vary among cervical disc replacement study protocols.

## PATIENT HISTORY

The clinical manifestations of neck pain, radiculopathy, and myelopathy are best considered by evaluating the underlying structural abnormalities caused by cervical spondylosis, herniated nucleus pulposus, and degenerative disc disease (Fig. 9–1). Such structural abnormalities may be amenable to surgical treatment if nonsurgical management fails to provide the patient with adequate relief.

Isolated degenerative disc disease may cause neck pain, occipital headache, periscapular pain, and shoulder pain as a result of irritated nerve fibers that innervate the intervertebral disc and facet joints. Mechanical stress, range of motion, or axial loading may further aggravate pain caused by isolated degenerative disc disease.

Radiculopathy, or nerve root compression, usually manifests as shoulder, arm, or hand pain. Continued nerve root compression may lead to numbness in the fingers, hands, or arms, which may be followed by the gradual loss of muscle strength.

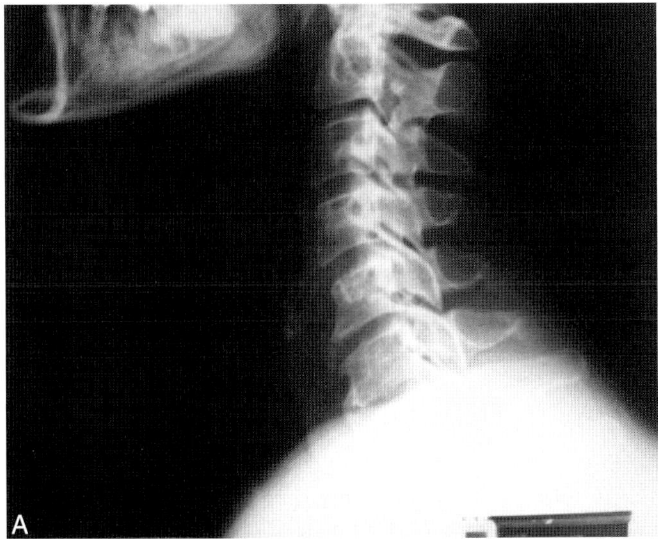


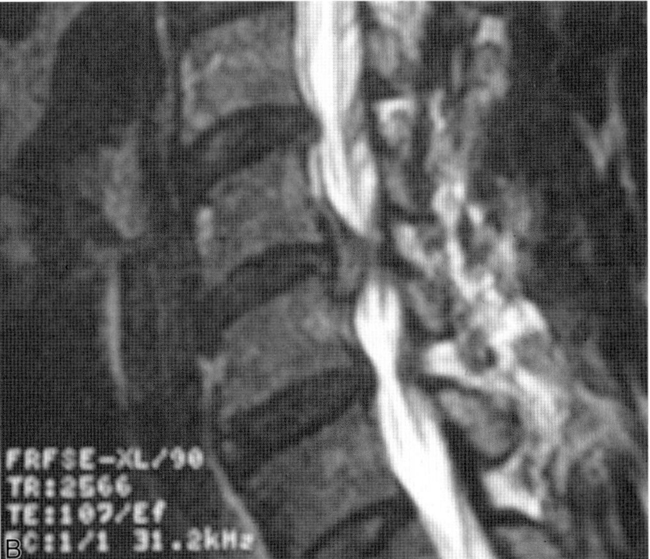


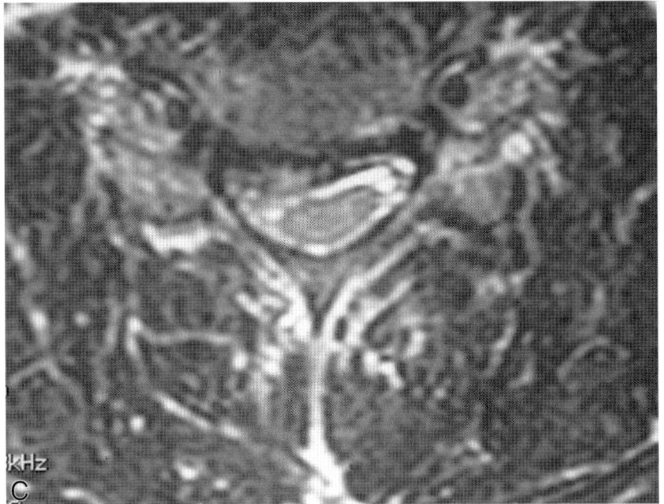


■ **FIGURE 9–1.** This is an ideal patient to consider for indication for anterior cervical arthroplasty. This is 45-year-old white man who presented with grade 4/5 left triceps weakness, lower extremity hyperreflexia, presence of Hoffman's sign bilaterally, tingling in his left hand, and uncontrolled jumping of his left leg. **A,** The plain lateral radiograph shows predisposing cervical spondylosis at C5–6. **B,** His sagittal magnetic resonance imaging (MRI) scan demonstrates a large disc herniation at C5–C6. **C,** The axial MRI demonstrates spinal cord compression and the cause of the myelopathy. In the U.S. studies, cervical arthroplasty is excluded if there is MRI evidence of myelomalacia.

Myelopathy, or spinal cord dysfunction, usually refers to upper motor neuron problems caused by continued mechanical and vascular compression of nerves located in the central nervous system. Although pain may be a complaint, decreased fine motor skills, ataxic gait, and upper extremity weakness are more commonly the primary focus of the patient's presenting symptoms.

These clinical presentations, from axial neck pain to frank upper extremity dysfunction, may be viewed along a spectrum of neurologic dysfunction. On one end of the spectrum lies degenerative disc disease, which causes pain related to sensory nerve irritation of the intervertebral disc. On the other end of the spectrum lies significant motor dysfunction, which is the result of continued neural compression. Although this wide spectrum helps in understanding the severity of specific patient complaints, often the clinical history may be associated with any combination of the above problems. A thorough understanding of the timing of the patient's complaints, the extent of their pain and dysfunction, a history of trauma or malignancy, and inciting as well as relieving events are all important in understanding the underlying anatomic abnormality.

Whereas a thorough history should be obtained from all patients, specific considerations for cervical disc replacement that may exclude patients from participation in current studies may include prior cervical spine infection, prior trauma, osteoporosis, prior surgery at or above the level to be treated, systemic diseases such as acquired immunodeficiency syndrome, human immunodeficiency virus, or hepatitis, morbid obesity, and a current or recent history of substance abuse.

## PHYSICAL EXAMINATION

A thorough neurologic examination of the spine and extremities is an indispensable aid in helping to lead the clinician to the correct diagnosis. Inspection, palpation, range of motion, functional motor and sensory examinations, reflex testing, and provocative maneuvers are all essential tools in the diagnostic work-up.[5]

Axial neck pain may be exacerbated by range of motion, especially rotation and side bending. Spurling's tests, axial loading of the head with lateral bending, may be positive in patients with intervertebral disc disease or facet arthritis.[6]

**TABLE 9–1. A Brief Overview of the Physical Examination of the Cervical Spine**

| | Neurologic Level | | | | |
|---|---|---|---|---|---|
| | C5 | C6 | C7 | C8 | T1 |
| Sensory deficit | Upper lateral arm, elbow | Lateral forearm, thumb, index finger | Middle finger | Ring finger, little finger, ulnar border of palm | Medial aspect of elbow |
| Motor weakness | Deltoid, biceps | Biceps, wrist extensors | Triceps, wrist flexors, finger extensors | Interossei, finger flexors | Interossei |
| Reflex | Biceps | Brachioradialis | Triceps | None | None |

From Hoppenfeld S, Hutton R: Physical Examination of the Spine and Extremities. New York, Appleton-Century-Crofts, 1976.

Radiculopathy is the result of nerve root compression and manifests as pain, paresthesias, or neurologic deficit in an anatomic distribution. Sensory, motor, and reflex changes may all result from continued nerve root irritation. A thorough musculoskeletal examination helps to localize the site of nerve root compression (Table 9–1). Diminished deep tendon reflexes are an indication of chronic nerve root compression and radiculopathy.

Myelopathy or dysfunction of the central spinal cord may be the result of disc protrusion, osteophyte formation, tumor, or other pathologic conditions including poliomyelitis, multiple sclerosis, and amyotrophic lateral sclerosis. Broad-based, ataxic gait is perhaps one of the most reliable indicators of cervical myelopathy. Functional gait examinations such as toe and heel walking as well as rising from a squatting position or stair climbing are good measures of the patient's functional neuromuscular strength.

Upper motor neurons inhibit the efferent output, which is part of a simple or polysynaptic reflex reaction. As a result of their dysfunction, hyperreflexia can be a reliable indicator of myelopathy. Provocative maneuvers such as Hoffman's sign, inverted brachioradialis reflex, small finger escape sign, Lhermitte's sign, and clonus may provide information about the health of the central cord and upper motor neuron function.

## DIAGNOSTIC STUDIES

Plain films may demonstrate loss of disc height, uncovertebral spurring, posterior osteophyte formation, and a host of bony abnormalities that may help in making the diagnosis of isolated degenerative disc disease, cervical spondylosis, and myelopathy. A good screening tool and initial evaluation, plain films are useful in only definitively evaluating bony anatomy.

Magnetic resonance imaging (MRI) has become the study of choice for soft tissue abnormalities, including loss of normal disc height and hydration in isolated degenerative disc disease, radicular pain caused by anatomic abnormalities, and cord compression resulting in myelopathy. It is important, however, that the MRI be used in conjunction with a good physical examination because MRI abnormalities of the cervical spine have been noted in up to 60% of asymptomatic individuals older than 60 years of age.[7] When MRI cannot be used due to the presence of a cardiac pacemaker or artifact as a result of existing hardware, a computed tomographic (CT) myelogram is the study of choice.

Additional studies such as flexion and extension cervical spine films as well as anteroposterior side-bending x-ray studies may be part of the protocol for certain cervical disc replacement studies. Some studies also require a dual-energy x-ray absorptiometry (DEXA) scan to evaluate overall bone-mineral density.

In patients with isolated degenerative disc disease who are considered for cervical disc replacement, discography may be considered if all other studies are either negative or inconclusive.

### Indications

Neurologic deficit caused by an anatomic lesion compressing the central cord or nerve roots that fails conservative management requires surgical decompression. Indications for cervical disc replacements, similar to those for anterior cervical decompression and fusion, include radiculopathy, myelopathy, myeloradiculopathy, and degenerative disc disease at a single level or at two levels between C3 and C7 that have not responded to the conservative treatment options mentioned earlier. Direct decompression of the spinal cord and nerve roots is achieved by the removal of disc material and posterior osteophytes. Indirect decompression by restoration of intervertebral disc and foraminal height prevents recurrence of neurologic symptoms. Indirect decompression may be achieved by fusion, which helps to stabilize the decompressed segment, or intervertebral disc replacement, which helps to restore motion.[8]

Inclusion criteria for all cervical disc replacement studies include cervical degenerative disc disease with signs or symptoms of radiculopathy, myelopathy, or both (Table 9–2). Age between approximately 18 and 65 years is necessary for study inclusion.

Degenerative disc disease with isolated axial neck pain, confirmed on MRI, CT, or discogram, is an inclusion criterion for some studies and an exclusion criterion for others.[9,10]

## CONTRAINDICATIONS

In general, contraindications to cervical disc replacement include ankylosing spondylitis, rheumatoid arthritis, insulin-dependent

**TABLE 9–2. General Inclusion Criteria for Most Cervical Disc Replacement Study Protocols**

- Age 18–65 years
- Clinical signs and symptoms of radiculopathy, myelopathy, or myeloradiculopathy symptomatic at 1–2 levels
- Radiographic evidence consistent with clinical diagnosis of radiculopathy, myelopathy, or myeloradiculopathy
- Failure of 6 weeks to 6 months of nonoperative management

**TABLE 9–3. General Exclusion Criteria for Most Cervical Disc Replacement Study Protocols**

| |
|---|
| Prior infection at site of surgery |
| Systemic disease including AIDS, HIV, hepatitis |
| Insulin-dependent diabetes mellitus |
| Tumor as source of symptoms |
| Osteoporosis with DEXA hip T-score <−2.5 |
| Pregnancy |
| Morbid obesity, defined as body mass index >40 |
| Prior fusion surgery at the level to be treated |
| Metabolic bone diseases including gout and Paget's disease |
| Absence of motion less than 2 degrees |
| Pregnancy |
| Known metal allergy |
| Bridging osteophytes |
| Any condition that would interfere with patient self-assessment |

AIDS, acquired immunodeficiency syndrome; DEXA, dual-energy x-ray absorptiometry; HIV, human immunodeficiency virus.

diabetes mellitus, a history of cervical infection, morbid obesity (body mass index [BMI] >40), ossification of posterior longitudinal ligament, and diffuse idiopathic skeletal hyperostosis[8] (Table 9–3).

Although many exclusion criteria do overlap, they are somewhat more distinct than inclusion criteria among studies. For example, in some studies, isolated axial neck pain without radicular symptoms is a criterion for exclusion. In others, prior fusion adjacent to the vertebral level being treated excludes patients from study participation. Although there is a significant amount of overlap among studies, a careful review of each cervical disc replacement inclusion and exclusion criteria is warranted before participation (Figs. 9–2 to 9–5).

## CONCLUSION

Appropriate patient selection is the cornerstone of any successful surgery. A careful history that reveals evidence of degenerative disc disease, radiculopathy, myelopathy, or myeloradiculopathy is the first step in patient selection for cervical disc replacement. Plain radiographs and MRI are the two most useful tools in confirming the diagnosis.

Although there are no long-term studies on cervical disc replacements that compare with those of anterior cervical decompression and fusion, provided the surgical indications remain the

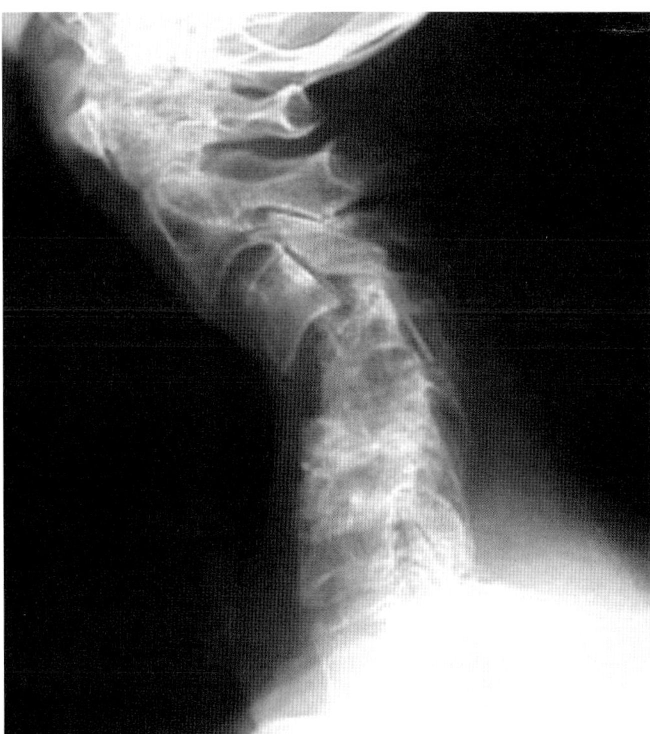

■ FIGURE 9–3. Patients with fixed cervical kyphosis, particularly with 3.5 mm or more cervical subluxation, should not be considered for current versions of cervical disc replacements.

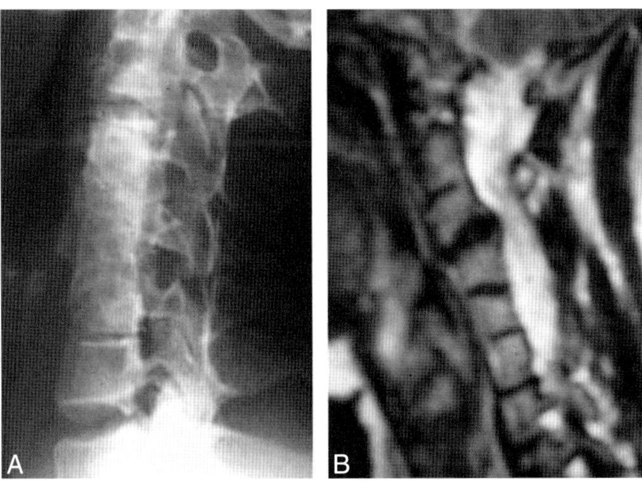


■ FIGURE 9–2. Contraindications for cervical arthroplasty are cases with extensive cervical spine immobility including congenital fusions, redundant posterior longitudinal ligament, multiple prior anterior cervical decompression and fusion, dural ectasia, and Klippel-Feil syndrome. The above lateral plain film **(A)** and sagittal MRI **(B)** reveal such extensive cervical spine immobility.

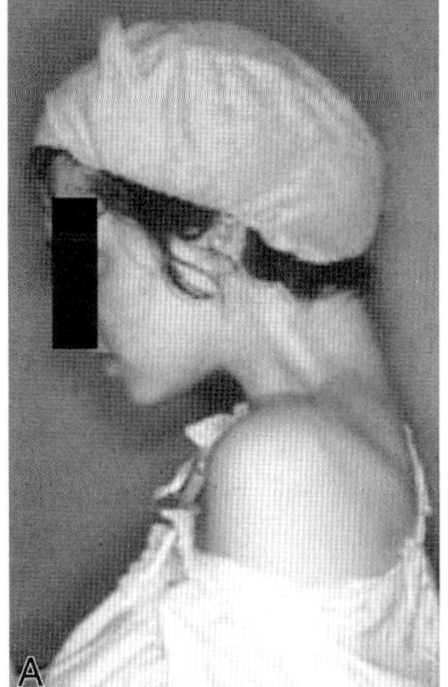


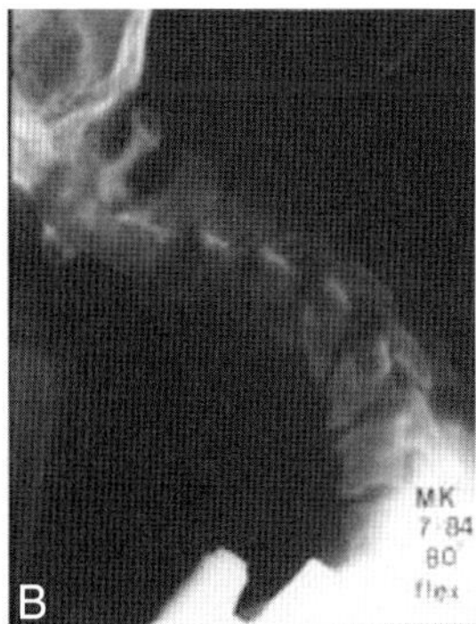


■ FIGURE 9–4. Post-traumatic kyphosis **(A)** and patients with posterior ligamentous disruption cannot be considered for cervical arthroplasty. The main stabilizing ligaments after cervical total disc replacement are the two zygoapophyseal capsular ligaments, so they need to be functioning well for a stable construct. This lateral radiograph **(B)** reveals significant kyphosis, a contraindication for cervical arthroplasty.

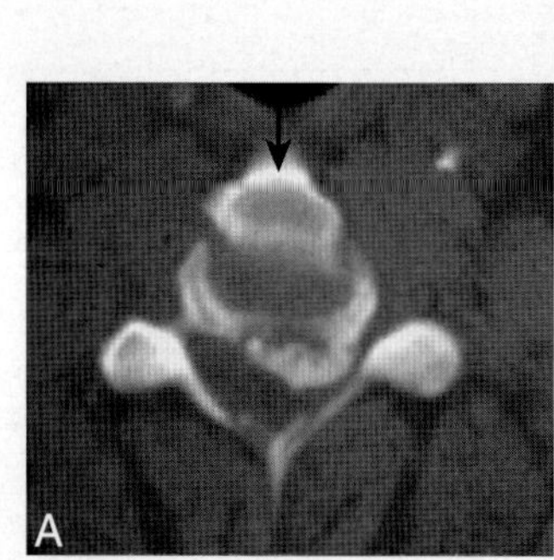

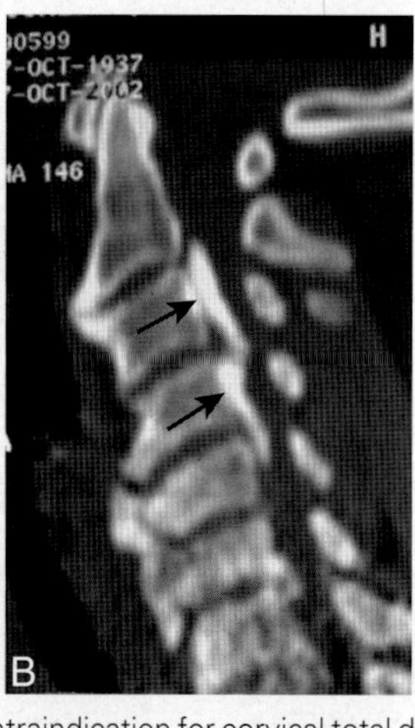

■ **FIGURE 9–5.** An absolute contraindication for cervical total disc replacement is ossification of the posterior longitudinal ligament (OPLL), the dura is ossified and cannot be mobilized. The ossification will recur and prevent motion. Furthermore, anterior decompression has a high incidence of cerebrospinal fluid leakage. The site of neurologic compression is behind the vertebral body **(A)** instead of at the level of the disc, so adequate decompression often requires a full corpectomy, resecting the bone required **(B)** for anchorage of the prosthesis.

same, it is hoped that results will also predictably improve patient pain and overall function.

Careful evaluation of the inclusion and exclusion criteria of each cervical disc replacement investigational study is the final step in patient selection before study participation.

## REFERENCES


1. Bohlman HH, Emery SE, Goodfellow DB, Jones PK: Robinson anterior cervical discectomy and arthrodesis for cervical radiculopathy. Long-term follow-up of one hundred and twenty-two patients. J Bone Joint Surg Am 75:1298–1307, 1993.
2. Emery SE, Bohlman HH, Bolesta MJ, Jones PK: Anterior cervical decompression and arthrodesis for the treatment of cervical spondylotic myelopathy. Two to seventeen year follow up. J Bone Joint Surg Am 80:941–951, 1998.
3. Zdeblick TA, Hughes SS, Riew KD, Bohlman HH: Failed anterior cervical discectomy and arthrodesis. Analysis and treatment of thirty-five patients. J Bone Joint Surg Am 79:523–532, 1997.
4. Hilibrand AS, Carlson GD, Palumbo MA, et al: Radiculopathy and myelopathy at segments adjacent to the site of a previous anterior cervical arthrodesis. J Bone Joint Surg Am 81:519–528, 1999.
5. Hoppenfeld S, Hutton R: Physical Examination of the Spine and Extremities. New York, Appleton-Century-Crofts, 1976.
6. Evans RC: Illustrated Orthopedic Physical Assessment, 2nd ed. St. Louis, Mosby, 2001.
7. Boden SD, McCowin PR, Davis DO, et al: Abnormal magnetic-resonance scans of the cervical spine in asymptomatic subjects. A prospective investigation. J Bone Joint Surg Am 72:1178–1184, 1990.
8. McAfee PC: The indications for lumbar and cervical disc replacement. Spine J 4(6):177S–181S, 2004.
9. Goffin J, Van Calenbergh F, van Loon J, et al: Intermediate follow-up after treatment of degenerative disc disease with the Bryan Cervical Disc Prosthesis: single-level and bi-level. Spine 28:2673–2678, 2003.
10. Pimenta L, McAfee PC, Cappuccino A, et al: Clinical experience with the new artificial cervical PCM (Cervitech) disc. Spine J 4(6): 315S–321S, 2004.

CHAPTER 10

# Quantitative Motion Analysis (QMA) of Motion-Preserving and Fusion Technologies for the Spine*

**John A. Hipp** and **Nicholas D. Wharton**

## KEY POINTS

- Widely used computer assisted methods are available to measure intervertebral motion in research studies, and these methods are validated to provide more accurate and reproducible measurements than obtainable with manual methods.
- The true fusion or pseudoarthrosis rates, the true type and frequency of adjacent segment changes, and the actual range of motion provided by motion-preserving technologies will only be known if maximal patient effort and high-quality imaging studies are used.
- Intervertebral motion can be measured by the quantity of rotation or translation, and by the quality of the motion as assessed by parameters such as the center of rotation.
- Many research studies have provided data to help define success criteria for interpreting intervertebral motion measurements. These studies are summarized in this chapter.
- More advanced methods for assessing the quality of intervertebral motion, including multiplanar assessment techniques, are being developed and will lead to a more comprehensive understanding of motion-preserving technologies.

Dynamic imaging studies are frequently used in research and clinical practice. Accurate and reproducible measurements of intervertebral motion obtained from these studies are critical to proving that motion-preserving treatments provide the intended motion, as well as for assessing fusions, the preoperative condition of the spine, and any postoperative changes adjacent to the treated level(s). Many of the methods that have been used in clinical practice and in research studies to quantify intervertebral motion are now known to have limitations in accuracy and reproducibility. These limitations can compromise the identification of pre- or postoperative abnormalities and the detection of differences between treatments. New computer-assisted methods have been proven to provide accurate and reliable measurements. These methods have been used in many studies, and are achieving standardization in laboratory and clinical research. However, even with accurate image assessment methods, the actual amount and type of motion that an implant provides can only be determined if the dynamic imaging is done with repeatable acquisition methods and sufficient gross motion through the spine. In addition, the true pseudoarthrosis rate with fusion surgery and the true incidence of adjacent segment disease will only be known with good quality control in the imaging studies. Recommended quality control guidelines to achieve this are provided in this chapter. These guidelines are important for reliably measuring both the quantity and quality of motion in the spine. Recommended guidelines for interpreting measurements related to both the quantity and quality of motion in the spine are also provided in this chapter.

## REQUIREMENTS FOR ACCURACY AND REPRODUCIBILITY OF INTERVERTEBRAL MOTION MEASUREMENTS

With many treatments for spinal disorders, it is important to know if pretreatment intervertebral motion is abnormal; in particular if excess (or insufficient) motion exists that must be addressed with treatment. This requirement necessitates a diagnostic test for intervertebral motion that can reliably detect the presence of motion abnormalities. Once the diagnosis is established, different treatment options can entail somewhat different requirements for intervertebral motion measurements. In particular, motion-preserving devices require a somewhat different emphasis on measurement technique and interpretation than with fusion devices. The critical question with respect to the functional definition of fusion has always been: "Is motion stopped?" There has been less concern about the magnitude of the motion than about the *presence or absence* of motion. Traditionally, motion has been measured only in the sagittal plane, since it is generally assumed that if motion is stopped in this plane, it is also stopped in other planes.

A pseudoarthrosis is functionally defined as motion between vertebrae in excess of a specific threshold used to define a solid fusion. This threshold has been typically assigned based on the accuracy limits of the measurement technology and the estimated

*There are more than one hundred peer-reviewed publications containing valuable information supporting the topics covered in this chapter, but not all could be included due to space limitations.

amount of deformation that would be consistent with a solid fusion. The reported fusion rate in a research study will depend on the threshold chosen to define fusion.[1,2] This threshold can have a dramatic effect on published fusion rates. The measurement techniques and thresholds used in many previous studies for assessing fusion were generally too inaccurate to detect most failed fusions, with the exception of gross failures.[3] General concerns over measurement error and reproducibility have caused most investigators to select a high threshold of motion to avoid misclassifying a successful fusion as a failure. A threshold of 4 to 5 degrees of motion has been commonly selected to define a failed fusion even though many experts recommend a lower threshold.[4] For a test to have a high true positive rate for failed fusion, the threshold of motion must be greater than the error in the measurements. This ensures that the test is sensitive for detecting failed fusions, but this approach makes the test nonspecific in that many failed fusions will be incorrectly classified as successful. In clinical practice, given the limited reliability of conventional measurement techniques, intervertebral motion measurements have been generally combined with subjective assessment of bridging bone to classify each level as fused or not fused. There is some evidence that the reproducibility, sensitivity, and specificity of diagnostic tests for spine fusion success can be substantially improved with computer-assisted analysis of flexion/extension x-rays.[3,5,6] However, until recently, most assessments were made with less reliable manual techniques, such as the Cobb method.[4]

In contrast to fusion technology, the success of a motion-preserving technology is defined in part by the quantity of motion the technology provides. The goal of some devices may be to provide for normal motion, while the goal for other devices may be to provide for "stable" or "safe" or "sufficient" motion. To determine if a motion-preserving device provides for normal motion, it is important to answer the question: "What is the quantity of motion?" The quantity of motion can also be important when establishing equivalence of a new device to a previously approved device.

Several motion parameters exist to describe quantity of motion. These parameters most commonly include: angular motion, translational motion, change in disc height, and change in functional spine unit (FSU) height.[7] The measurements are usually produced from flexion-extension or lateral bending x-rays or both. With special techniques, these parameters can also be measured from dynamic magnetic resonance imaging (MRI) studies. In many cases, these measurements are produced at multiple levels of the spine, both at the treated and at the adjacent levels. Results are frequently reported in degrees and millimeters. Normalization of the displacement and translation data is often used to eliminate the effect of variable magnification in the x-rays, as well as anthropometric variations, thereby facilitating comparisons across patients and across studies. Many studies report the total amount of motion from flexion to extension, or from left to right lateral bending. However, it may also be important to evaluate quantity of motion using neutral as a reference point. Component motion (e.g., neutral to flexion and neutral to extension) can be important for expressing the *balance of motion* between flexion and extension. If, for example, an implant places the level in hyperlordosis, then this component analysis would likely show limited motion in neutral to extension. Failure to reproduce the normal ratio of neutral to extension versus neutral to flexion may also be a risk factor for abnormal loading of the posterior or anterior structures of the spine, both at the implanted and adjacent levels. However, this analysis of the balance between flexion and extension is confounded by the variability in neutral posture between individuals.

A second, and potentially more important question is: "What is the quality of motion with a motion-preserving device?" The design objective of many motion-preserving devices is to replicate the natural kinematics of the intact disc or motion segment. Such kinematics may not be adequately described by simple measurements of intervertebral rotation and translation alone. More sophisticated measurement techniques can describe and characterize complex patterns of motion and can identify more subtle abnormalities that may result in longer-term complications. Several parameters exist to describe quality of motion. These parameters include: center of rotation (COR), the ratio between translation and rotation, helical axis of motion (HAM), load-displacement curves, and the neutral zone (NZ). Load-displacement curves and the NZ are important factors for understanding intervertebral motion and for evaluating quality of motion in laboratory studies, but are difficult to measure in patients because of the need to know the applied loads across a motion segment. Quality of motion parameters can be monitored on a continuous or instantaneous basis, or at multiple points in the motion cycle. Evaluating motion on a continuous basis may yield more significant information than can be obtained from analyzing the extremes of motion alone. Video fluoroscopy is excellent for this purpose, although image quality may be sacrificed when imaging the lumbar spine. Continuous motion assessment can detect discontinuities in motion or abnormal motion paths that might not be detected by analysis of x-rays taken at the end range of motion.[8] For example, it has been shown that the instantaneous axis of rotation moves slightly during flexion-extension.[9] However, evidence-based guidelines supporting a positive risk/benefit ratio for continuous motion assessment have yet to be established, and the clinical significance of discontinuities in motion has yet to be established.

With respect to patient selection criteria and for assessing changes adjacent to implanted levels, relationships have been documented between quantity and quality of motion parameters and forces in the spine, damage to soft tissues, and the state of degeneration in the spine. The quantity and quality of motion, when evaluated in combination, are important indicators of the normal balance of forces in the spine. Abnormal intervertebral motion measured from a flexion-extension study may indicate an inability of the spine to support normal forces and moments. Abnormal motion may also be associated with pain, neurologic symptoms, degeneration, and a worsening of the instability (see Schneider et al[10] for a representative study and a list of supporting references in the lumbar spine, and Amevo et al[11] and Ng et al[12] for cervical spine references). A spinal motion segment is composed of a complex combination of joints, ligaments, muscles, and other structures that provide complementary and redundant motion constraints and together serve to modulate motion. Disruption of any one component of this complex system may alter kinematics in subtle ways that may be difficult to detect acutely, but may affect the longevity of the segment. Measuring complex interactions in this system and the effect on intervertebral motion, especially in devices designed to mimic natural motion, requires sensitive and precise measurements, as well as data to facilitate interpretation of these measurements.

## ACCURACY AND REPRODUCIBILITY OF MANUAL METHODS FOR MEASURING INTERVERTEBRAL MOTION

This chapter focuses on measurements made from x-rays and other noninvasive imaging modalities that can be applied to large scale clinical studies. It is possible to measure intervertebral motion by other methods, such as by using pins percutaneously implanted into vertebrae, by analysis of multiplanar x-rays taken after implanting metal markers into vertebrae, or by inferring motion from measurements of the orientation of the skin overlying the spine. However, these techniques are limited in accuracy or their applicability to large-scale clinical studies. The accuracy and reproducibility of any measurement of intervertebral motion made from x-rays, MRI, or computed tomography (CT) will depend on image quality. With x-rays in particular, image quality is dependent on the specific imaging technique used by the technologist (which can be strongly influenced by the physician that requests the test). Important variables include the exposure settings (kVp, mas), the amount of out-of-plane motion of the patient, distortion in the images caused by the parallax effect, and post-processing of the images. Typical out-of-plane motion includes lateral bending or left-right twisting during a sagittal plane flexion-extension study. Parallax occurs in images formed by x-rays originating from a point source and projecting through the patient onto a large x-ray film. This creates a difference in the apparent relative position between vertebrae that can occur only because the position of the vertebrae with respect to the center of the x-ray film has changed. Consistent attention to imaging technique will improve the quality of clinical radiographs and thereby improve the accuracy and reproducibility of measurements produced from them.

Even with excellent image quality, the accuracy and reproducibility of measurements made from the images depend on the specific measurement technique. Conventional radiographic measurements have been most commonly based on manual line-drawing techniques and/or landmark selection methods. In general, an observer draws lines through the perceived plane of each end plate or along the perceived posterior wall of each vertebra.[13] The angle measured between lines on each radiograph describes the relative position between adjacent vertebrae, and the change in these angles between flexion and extension is a measure of angular motion between two vertebrae. There are many variations on this theme. For example, specific anatomic landmarks can be identified on a series of radiographic images, and the change in position of these landmarks can be used to describe disc heights and translations.

The Cobb method and the posterior tangent method, sometimes supplemented by superimposition of images, are common methods used in clinical practice to measure intervertebral rotation based on drawing lines either through the vertebral end plates or through the posterior aspect of the vertebral bodies. These methods have been documented to have limited accuracy and reproducibility.[13–15] These techniques are dependent on the ability of the observer to select a series of landmarks in one image and reproducibly select the identical series of landmarks in the next image. Irregularity of the vertebral end plates and variations in quality between images confounds this process. Poor visualization of the bony anatomy due to out-of-plane effects, parallax effects, overlapping tissues, exposure settings, surgery, or the presence of implants makes it difficult to achieve optimal reproducibility. The reliability of these methods may be improved by superimposing the x-rays, which helps to visualize changes in the relative position of adjacent vertebrae and provides additional visual cues to aid in landmark selection.[16]

Several investigators have reported on the errors in assessing sagittal plane intervertebral rotation in motion-preserving devices using methods that require the observer to draw lines along features of the implants. A recent reproducibility study measuring rotation between the superior and inferior components of a motion-preserving device found maximum errors of 5 to 13 degrees and average errors of 1.8 to 3.3 degrees (standard deviation: 2.2 to 4.2 degrees) depending on the specific implant feature used.[17] Another study reported 95% confidence intervals for errors to be between ±2 degrees and ±4.3 degrees for intra- and inter-observer errors.[18] The geometrically regular features and high-contrast of artificial discs should theoretically improve the reproducibility of standard measurement techniques.[17,18] As long as there is no relative motion between the implant and bone, the rotation between vertebrae at an implant site will be the same as the rotation between superior and inferior components of the implant. To be certain that motion has occurred across an implant, the motion must be greater than the error in the measurement technique. It is therefore essential to select geometric features of the device that maximize reproducibility and ensure that the method is as sensitive to small motions as possible.[17]

## ACCURACY AND REPRODUCIBILITY OF COMPUTER-ASSISTED TECHNIQUES

Most modern techniques in radiographic image analysis use region of interest (ROI) methods to track the motion of spinal vertebrae. These methods include geometric templating and pattern matching.[13,15,16,19,20] These methods are, by necessity, computerized and have been proven to enhance the accuracy and reproducibility of motion measurements.[15,16,21] Unlike manual techniques, which require selecting a number of reference points to assess motion, these methods typically match contours or patterns of vertebrae on radiographs using all of the information about a vertebra, including its size, shape, and density variation. The process is to define a template, or model, of a vertebral pattern in one image (e.g., flexion), and then search for its corresponding pattern in a target image (e.g., extension). The search is conducted by digitally superimposing the model on the target image and transposing it until a best-fit match is found. The model may contain the anterior body and posterior elements, or it may contain the anterior body alone. The process produces a mathematical transformation matrix that describes the spatial relationship between a vertebral pattern in one image and its corresponding pattern in another image. This process is repeated for multiple vertebrae, and it may be aided with automated algorithms or computer-assisted techniques.

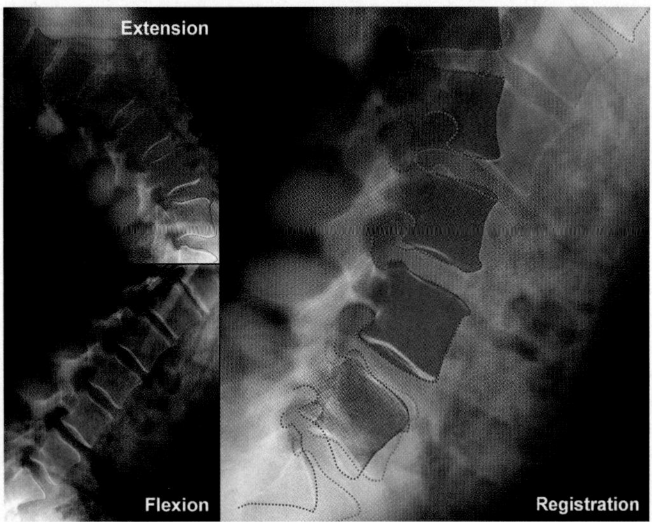


■ **FIGURE 10–1.** Digital registration of two images through superimposition.

Using the motion information obtained from the image analysis, radiographic images may be digitally superimposed and registered such that a particular vertebra occupies the same relative position in multiple images (Fig. 10–1). This process is conceptually similar to overlaying plain films on a light box until a specific vertebra is aligned in both images. Registration makes it possible to detect subtle differences in the position and orientation of adjacent or overlapping structures between two images. One published technique involves alternately displaying the registered images onscreen so that the registered vertebra appears to hold a constant position while the adjacent structures move relevant to it.[6,15,22] This technique, known as Feature Stabilization, makes it easier to visualize relative motion between vertebrae. Feature Stabilization also provides a visual feedback mechanism for evaluating the accuracy of the registration and, if necessary, correcting it. Imperfect stabilization may suggest that an adjustment is required to fine-tune the registration. If so, the direction and magnitude of the adjustment can be visualized. This ability to objectively identify error in the analysis, and correct it, is an important element of computer-assisted techniques.

The transformation matrix that describes how the position of a particular vertebra changes from one image to the next may be used to calculate the motion of selected anatomic landmarks. Based on matrix math, the position of landmarks selected in the first image may be recalculated in subsequent images. Calculating the position of the landmarks avoids the reproducibility errors commonly associated with manual techniques. The assumption of rigid body motion also assures that the relative position of vertebral landmarks remains constant between images. Radiographic projections of vertebrae rarely remain constant from image to image, which can compromise the accuracy of the calculated landmark positions. To ensure accuracy, computer-assisted techniques often minimize out-of-plane effects by tracking regions of bone, such as the spinous processes, that are least sensitive to these effects. Poor contrast may be improved by applying contrast enhancement filters, and magnification effects may be addressed with digital resizing methods.

Several published studies have been conducted to assess the accuracy and reproducibility of these computer-assisted techniques. Few studies provide definitive accuracy assessments because they require "gold standard" reference measurements, and the accuracy of some of these techniques is close to, or may surpass, the accuracy of available "gold standards." For this reason, some accuracy studies use frozen spines imaged in different positions. In these studies, any intervertebral motion reported by the method represents error in the measurements. Reported average accuracies range from 0.4 to 2.8 degrees for rotations and 0.5 to 1.5 mm for translations.[15,21,23] The reported average reproducibility of these measurements ranges from 0.4 to 2.6 degrees as measured by inter- and intra-observer variations.[16,20,24] The 95% confidence intervals for these methods range from 0.8 to approximately 3 degrees.[16,20,24] The accuracy and reproducibility of these methods may be reduced by poor quality images or vertebrae that or rotated or tilted out of the plane of imaging.

There are multiple different computer-assisted methods that have been described and used for measuring intervertebral motion.[13,15,16,19–21,24] When selecting a computer-assisted technique, it is important to critically assess the validation of the technique, since some methods are more thoroughly validated than others. Because no current computer-assisted method is fully automated, some operator intervention is needed with all published methods. It is therefore also preferable to ensure that the method has been validated by observers who have been blinded to the experimental design and experimental hypothesis, which minimizes sources of potential bias.

## PATIENT POSITIONING TECHNIQUES AND PATIENT EFFORT

Dynamic imaging studies must be performed with repeatable patient positioning and excellent patient effort. Whether a level is unstable or degenerating preoperatively, or whether motion is preserved or eliminated postoperatively, can only be determined and compared to other studies if the imaging is done with consistent patient positioning and a committed effort by the patient to maximally flex and extend. It has been shown that sequential recruitment of spinal levels occurs during flexion-extension, and certain levels eventually contribute more than others to the total motion.[25–27] This has been referred to as a phase lag in spinal motion.[26] With insufficient patient effort, motion may be non-existent at levels that are in fact capable of providing motion, and the relative proportion of motion measured at any particular level may inadequately describe the amount of motion that can be provided by that level.

Several studies have documented that the true amount of intervertebral motion that occurs at a treatment level when a patient is highly motivated to maximally flex and extend will be missed if the patient only makes a modest effort to flex and extend during the imaging. Miyasaka et al showed that maximal effort resulted in over twice as much intervertebral motion at the lower levels of the lumbar spine when patients were coached to flex and extend maximally versus being uncoached.[25] Measurements made with inadequate effort would have underreported the true motion of the spine, particularly at the lower levels. Miyasaka also showed that with maximal effort, the standard deviations were half what they were with modest effort. Dvorak et al also found greater motion and smaller variance in flexion extension studies of the cervical spine with methods that encouraged gross motion through the head and neck.[28] The smaller variations suggest that the physiologic restraints to motion in the spine may be fairly similar between individuals and that much of the variability reported in data describing motion in asymptomatic people is due to variability in subject effort. The obvious implication to clinical practice and research studies is that true instability in the spine, and the true extent of motion provided by an implant will remain unknown without assuring sufficient patient effort. In addition, the smaller standard deviations achievable with excellent patient effort will require fewer patients to show differences (or the lack thereof) between treatments.

Quality control (QC) criteria for assessing whether there is enough gross motion through the spine in a flexion-extension study to reliably assess intervertebral motion at specific levels have not been established but are clearly needed and can be estimated from existing scientific literature. Damage to the soft-tissue structures that normally control intervertebral motion will intuitively not be evident unless intervertebral motion is at least to the level where these structures normally begin to restrict motion. In the laboratory, this can be demonstrated by studying the neutral zone. The neutral zone is the range of motion between vertebrae that can be created with application of minimal loads. Damage to the soft tissues is evident as an enlargement of the neutral zone. The neutral zone and the proportion of the total range of motion included in the neutral zone are powerful parameters for understanding the biomechanics of the spine and spinal treatments. However, direct and objective assessment of the neutral zone, and the load-displacement behavior of the motion segment outside the neutral zone, requires knowledge of the loads being applied to the segment, which is generally difficult to obtain in clinical practice. Nevertheless, the size of the neutral zone has been described in several publications, and this provides guidelines for assessing motion from clinical x-rays. Based on the data from Panjabi et al,[29] the average neutral zone for the mid to lower cervical spine is approximately 3 degrees between flexion and extension. Intervertebral rotation would have to be at least one degree greater than the neutral zone at most levels to begin stressing the soft-tissue restraints, and also to be above measurement error in most computer-assisted measurement techniques. An alternative QC guideline is to require the total amount of motion through the spinal region to be within the 95% confidence interval for asymptomatic people (approximately 30 degrees from C2 to C7 or 30 degrees from L1 to S1). However, this criteria may be inappropriate in the presence of a multi-level fusion, motion limiting treatment, or preoperatively, since one or more levels may not be contributing normally to total motion.

Additional support for QC criteria can be derived from the observation of White and Panjabi that in the cervical spine, it is rare to have more than 11 degrees difference between adjacent levels in the angle between end plates defining the intervertebral disc spaces.[7] This measurement is made from a neutral or flexion x-ray and is part of the widely used American Medical Association (AMA) disability assessment guidelines for evidence of structural impairment to the spine.[30] Consistent with this observation, further analysis of data from the study by Reitman et al[22] revealed that less than 5% of asymptomatic people had intervertebral rotation from flexion to extension at any one level that was 11 degrees or more greater than at an adjacent level. It would clearly not be possible to apply these observations clinically unless there were at least 11 degrees of motion in at least one level in the cervical spine. This amount of rotation is only a modest requirement since it is below the average for most levels in the cervical spine (see Table 10–1). Based on these rationalizations, a reasonable and minimal QC guideline for intervertebral rotation in cervical flexion-extension x-rays is to require intervertebral motion to be at least 11 degrees at two non-fused levels, **and** at least greater than 4 degrees at an adjacent, non-fused level. Ninety-five percent of flexion/extension studies of 140 asymptomatic volunteers[22] satisfied these guidelines, based on a reanalysis of the original data. In that study of asymptomatic volunteers, subjects were coached to flex and extend as much as they could. In contrast, 33% of 457 cervical flexion-extension x-rays from a typical clinical practice that did not use any specific quality control protocol failed these guidelines (unpublished retrospective study).

Criteria for determining if a lumbar flexion-extension study has enough gross motion to be of diagnostic quality can also be justified based on the amount of motion seen between vertebrae in the asymptomatic population and on published data describing the lumbar neutral zone. Based on data from Panjabi et al,[31] the average neutral zone in the lumbar spine is approximately 5 degrees. Rotation would need to be at least 6 degrees to be certain soft tissue restraints are being tensioned and to account for measurement error. In an ongoing study of asymptomatic volunteers by the authors of this chapter, there were at least 9 degrees of intervertebral rotation in at least two lumbar levels in 95% of 75 volunteers, and less than 5% of the volunteers had greater than 9 degrees more rotation at one level compared to adjacent levels. Data from Harada et al[27] suggests that during flexion, motion first starts at the upper levels, with lower levels contributing to overall motion as flexion proceeds. At the point where motion was 9 degrees at any one level, their data suggest that all levels were contributing to motion. Thus, rational and minimal QC criteria for lumbar flexion-extension studies would be to require at least 9 degrees of intervertebral rotation in at least two levels and at least 6 degrees of rotation at an adjacent level. A drawback of these cervical and lumbar QC criteria in routine clinical practice is the need to first accurately analyze flexion-extension x-rays to determine if they are of sufficient quality. Nevertheless, these QC criteria can be easily applied to flexion-extension studies from clinical trials or research studies to avoid inclusion of data that are unreliable due to insufficient patient effort.

To minimize the number of unsatisfactory flexion-extension studies, it is very important that the physician stress to their patients that: 1) it is safe to maximally flex and extend their spine, and 2) it is important that they do this since the true condition of their spine can only be assessed with this effort. Many patients either are concerned that they may cause damage to their spine if they move too much, or are seeking empathy from the technologist performing the study by demonstrating how difficult it is for them to move. Both of these psychological restrictions to motion in the spine can be mitigated by reassurance and instructions from their physician. Rehearsing the motion with the patient can help assure that the patient understands what is required of them, but also allows the physician to order dynamic imaging studies only for those patients where they will obtain reliable information.

The patient positioning technique used during a flexion-extension study can also change the amount (and possibly quality) of motion that is measured between vertebrae. For both the cervical and lumbar spine, a variety of methods for patient positioning have been described in published studies. In selecting a method, it is important to consider how consistently the expected patient population will tolerate the method, whether rigorous reference data are available for the specific method, how good the method is at minimizing out-of-plane motion, and, most importantly, whether the test results will describe the true performance of the treatment.

In the cervical spine, flexion and extension can be performed with the patient standing or seated, with no known difference between these positions. To ensure maximum effort in flexion, patients should be coached to bring their chin to their chest without tilting or twisting their head to the left or right. Maximum extension can be obtained by coaching the patient to point their chin as far up toward the ceiling as they can, again without tilting or twisting their head to the left or right. Reitman et al[22] provided normative data for flexion-extension cervical range of motion using this technique. These data are summarized in Table 10–1.

Lumbar flexion-extension studies have been performed using a wide variety of patient positioning techniques including standing, seated, and lateral decubitus. There are pros and cons of each method. A version of the standing technique may currently be one of the most commonly used techniques in clinical practice, although this is difficult to document. Standing flexion-extension imaging occurs using a variety of techniques (including from a free-standing position, with the pelvis stabilized by a variety of mechanical systems, or with the patient leaning against a table). Standing flexion-extension using pelvis stabilization methods has been described in many research studies but is generally not performed in clinical practice. For sites that use an unsupported, free-standing protocol (Fig. 10–2A), Miyasaka et al[25] proved the advantage of one technique to ensure maximum patient effort. Miyasaka showed that patients who were coached to bring their hands as close to the floor as possible in flexion, and to extend as far back as they possibly could in extension, had 30% more motion at L1-L2 and 136% more motion at L5-S1. This was compared to patients who were asked to bend forward and backwards as is normally done in clinical practice without coaching.[25]

One previously reported positioning technique[32] that is now being utilized in a large study of intervertebral motion in the lumbar spine of asymptomatic people involves a simple seated technique (Fig. 10–2B). A stable, four-leg, low back chair is used with a specially designed cushion (model 583990, Infab Corp, Camarillo, CA) that facilitates maximum extension and prevents the pelvis from being tucked under the body. Patients are asked to bend forward and grab the front legs of the chair as far down as they can for flexion, and then to extend back over the cushion for extension (Fig. 10–2B). This seated technique is tolerated by patients, is easy to implement, and improves range of motion while minimizing out-of-plane effects. Normative data describing intervertebral motion and 95% confidence intervals in asymptomatic patients using this technique are provided in Table 10–2.

**TABLE 10–1. Intervertebral Motion Data for 129 Asymptomatic Individuals**

| Rotation (degree) | | | | | |
|---|---|---|---|---|---|
| **Level** | ***N*** | **Mean** | **Std. Dev.** | **LL** | **UL** |
| C2-C3 | 129 | 9.4 | 2.9 | 3.7 | 15.0 |
| C3-C4 | 129 | 14.6 | 3.7 | 7.5 | 21.8 |
| C4-C5 | 126 | 16.6 | 3.9 | 8.9 | 24.3 |
| C5-C6 | 121 | 16.5 | 5.0 | 6.7 | 26.3 |
| C6-C7 | 78 | 13.7 | 5.1 | 3.8 | 23.7 |
| **Rotation (% sum of rotation for all visualized levels)** | | | | | |
| **Level** | ***N*** | **Mean** | **Std. Dev.** | **LL** | **UL** |
| C2-C3 | 129 | 15.8 | 7.2 | 1.7 | 29.9 |
| C3-C4 | 129 | 23.7 | 6.5 | 10.9 | 36.6 |
| C4-C5 | 126 | 26.1 | 5.2 | 15.9 | 36.3 |
| C5-C6 | 121 | 24.8 | 5.5 | 14.1 | 35.5 |
| C6-C7 | 78 | 18.7 | 5.9 | 7.1 | 30.2 |
| **Translation (% AP End Plate Width)—Motion of the Posterior-Inferior Corner of the Superior Vertebra in a Direction Parallel to the Superior End Plate of the Inferior Vertebra.** | | | | | |
| **Level** | ***N*** | **Mean** | **Std. Dev.** | **LL** | **UL** |
| C2-C3 | 129 | 12.4 | 5.2 | 2.2 | 22.6 |
| C3-C4 | 129 | 15.9 | 5.2 | 5.6 | 26.1 |
| C4-C5 | 126 | 17.2 | 5.4 | 6.5 | 27.8 |
| C5-C6 | 121 | 13.7 | 5.4 | 3.2 | 24.3 |
| C6-C7 | 78 | 7.5 | 3.5 | 0.5 | 14.4 |
| **Center of Rotation—AP (% AP End Plate Width) Reported Relative to the Midpoint of the Superior End Plate of the Inferior Vertebra. Negative Values are Posterior to the Midpoint.** | | | | | |
| **Level** | ***N*** | **Mean** | **Std. Dev.** | **LL** | **UL** |
| C2-C3 | 127 | −9.7 | 9.6 | −28.4 | 9.1 |
| C3-C4 | 129 | −9.6 | 6.5 | −22.4 | 3.2 |
| C4-C5 | 125 | −7.4 | 6.1 | −19.3 | 4.6 |
| C5-C6 | 121 | −6.7 | 5.6 | −17.6 | 4.2 |
| C6-C7 | 76 | −7.9 | 6.2 | −20.0 | 4.2 |
| **Center of Rotation—Cranial-Caudal (% AP End Plate Width) Reported Relative to the Superior End Plate of the Inferior Vertebra. Negative Values are Inferior to the End Plate.** | | | | | |
| **Level** | ***N*** | **Mean** | **Std. Dev.** | **LL** | **UL** |
| C2-C3 | 127 | −49.0 | 20.3 | −88.9 | −9.2 |
| C3-C4 | 129 | −37.4 | 14.9 | −66.6 | −8.1 |
| C4-C5 | 125 | −35.0 | 12.7 | −59.9 | −10.0 |
| C5-C6 | 121 | −24.9 | 12.1 | −48.6 | −1.2 |
| C6-C7 | 76 | −8.9 | 11.6 | −31.7 | 13.9 |

These volunteers were selected from an original population of 140 subjects. Levels with moderate to severe degeneration or volunteers with multiple degenerated levels were excluded. The 129 volunteers included 55 males and 74 females (average age 39 for both sexes). C6-C7 and sometimes C5-C6 could not be visualized in some subjects.
LL and UL, lower and upper limits of the 95% confidence interval.

## REFERENCE DATA FOR INTERVERTEBRAL MOTION

Exactly how much motion should be provided by motion-preserving treatments has not been definitively determined and will be different depending on the goals of the specific treatment. For example, a total disc replacement may have the goal of restoring normal motion, a dynamic posterior stabilization device may have the goals of stabilizing the spine while providing enough motion to prevent adjacent level degeneration, and fusion treatments may have the goal of stopping measurable intervertebral motion. If

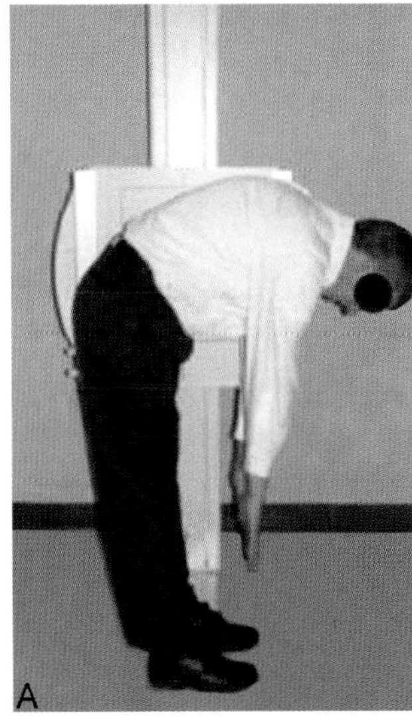

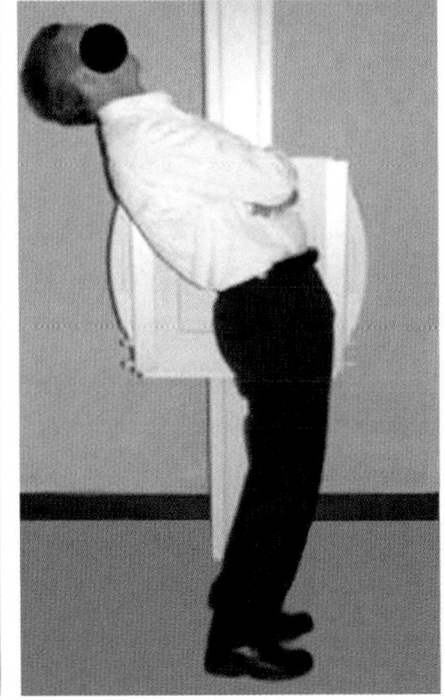
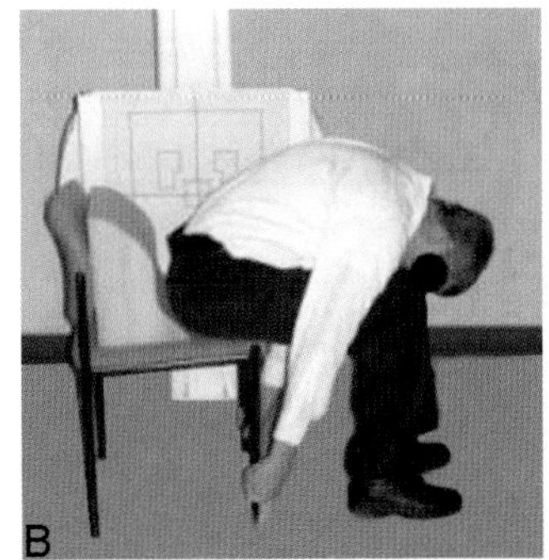

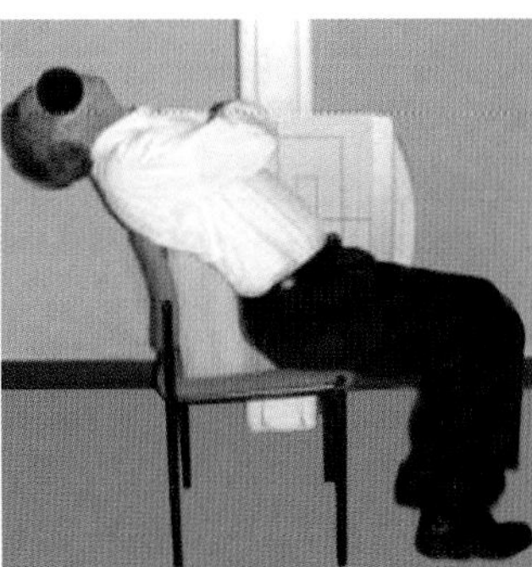

■ **FIGURE 10–2.** **A** and **B,** Protocol diagrams illustrating good sitting and standing techniques with adequate patient effort.

the goal is to provide normal motion at the implanted level, several studies provide data that can be used as guidelines for minimum and maximum allowable motion. Assessing whether motion is normal involves evaluating not only whether range of motion is within normal limits at each level (quantity of motion) but also whether the device preserves the natural kinematics and hence the natural balance of forces in the spine (quality of motion). Assessing whether the quantity of motion is normal includes both a lower and an upper limit of normal. A device could fail the intended goal by not providing enough motion, or it could fail by providing too much motion. An alternative goal for motion-preserving devices could be to retain the same motion as was measured preoperatively. However, preoperative range of motion is at least theoretically not a good reference since patients were symptomatic preoperatively. Their symptoms and underlying spinal disorder(s) may have compromised motion (due to instability, pain guarding, muscle spasms, etc.). Another goal may be to ensure that treated and adjacent non-treated levels contribute proportionally to motion through the spine and that a difference in motion across adjacent levels is within a normal range.

Dynamic stabilization devices require different criteria. The goals for these devices are primarily to provide stability to the treated level, but also to provide for some motion. Success criteria for the motion these devices provide may be based on the goals of preventing additional degenerative changes at the treated level and reducing adjacent level degeneration, with a possible additional goal of preventing fusion at the treated level.

Table 10–1 provides the mean, standard deviations, and 95% confidence intervals for intervertebral rotation and translations in the cervical spine of asymptomatic volunteers. The data in this table are from one specific study, but the data are not statistically different from data published by Frobin et al,[21] and there is good consistency with other published studies that provide intervertebral motion data for the asymptomatic cervical spine.[21,33,34] The data in Table 10–1 were originally published[22] after an adjustment was made to control for the effect of patient effort on the intervertebral rotations. The data in table 10–1 do not include this adjustment for patient effort, since this adjustment is generally not practiced in clinical studies. There is a highly ($P < 0.0001$) significant difference between levels, with motion being greatest at the C4-C5 level. Based on analysis of data from both Reitman et al[22] and Frobin et al,[21] there is also significantly greater intervertebral rotations at the C3-C4, C4-C5, and C5-C6 levels in females compared to males ($P < 0.05$). This observation could be used to obtain an even more precise discrimination between normal and abnormal motion. Table 10–1 also provides the rotation data expressed as a percent of the total rotation for all visualized levels between C2 and C7, since this may reduce the influence of patient effort and generally reduces scatter in the data (the standard deviations are a smaller percent of the means). It should be noted that intervertebral rotations, translations, and changes in disc height are generally interrelated by the biomechanics of the spine, and also tend to be statistically correlated with each other.[21,22,28,33]

Descriptive statistics for center of rotation (COR) were not originally reported in the study by Reitman et al,[22] but are presented in this chapter from the same subjects in the original study. Table 10–2 provides the means, standard deviations, and 95% confidence intervals for COR. The reference frame for this data is located at the midpoint of the superior end plate of the inferior vertebra. The x-axis is coincident with the end plate, and the y-axis is perpendicular to the end plate. The data are plotted in Figure 10–3A. The reference data reported in Table 10–2 are normalized to the anterior-posterior dimension of the superior end plate of the inferior vertebra. These data are consistent with data published by Amevo et al[35] after adjusting for differences in the normalization scheme and reference frame used in the two studies. When interpreting data for COR, it is important to pay careful attention to the coordinate system used to report COR. Different published studies may report equivalent data in different coordinate systems, which may confound comparisons of the data. Similar attention should be paid to the method used to normalize the data.

COR can be sensitive to technical errors in the technique used to compute it.[36] It is important that COR be calculated using

**TABLE 10–2. Intervertebral Motion Data for 63 Asymptomatic Individuals From an Original Study Population of 75**

| Rotation (degrees) | | | | | |
|---|---|---|---|---|---|
| **Level** | ***N*** | **Mean** | **Std. Dev.** | **LL** | **UL** |
| L1-L2 | 63 | 10.5 | 3.0 | 4.6 | 16.5 |
| L2-L3 | 63 | 12.0 | 2.5 | 7.0 | 17.0 |
| L3-L4 | 63 | 13.0 | 2.8 | 7.5 | 18.5 |
| L4-L5 | 63 | 14.1 | 3.9 | 6.5 | 21.7 |
| L5-S1 | 57 | 11.1 | 5.8 | 0.0 | 22.5 |
| **Rotation (% L1-S1 rotation)** | | | | | |
| **Level** | ***N*** | **Mean** | **Std. Dev.** | **LL** | **UL** |
| L1-L2 | 56 | 17.4 | 4.2 | 9.1 | 25.6 |
| L2-L3 | 56 | 20.0 | 3.8 | 12.5 | 27.4 |
| L3-L4 | 56 | 21.6 | 3.1 | 15.6 | 27.6 |
| L4-L5 | 56 | 23.5 | 4.2 | 15.3 | 31.7 |
| L5-S1 | 56 | 17.5 | 7.9 | 2.0 | 33.1 |
| **Translation (% AP End Plate Width)—Motion of the Posterior-Inferior Corner of the Superior Vertebra in a Direction Parallel to the Superior End Plate of the Inferior Vertebra.** | | | | | |
| **Level** | ***N*** | **Mean** | **Std. Dev.** | **LL** | **UL** |
| L1-L2 | 63 | 4.8 | 1.6 | 1.6 | 8.0 |
| L2-L3 | 63 | 6.3 | 1.9 | 2.5 | 10.1 |
| L3-L4 | 63 | 7.2 | 1.9 | 3.5 | 10.9 |
| L4-L5 | 63 | 7.1 | 2.6 | 2.0 | 12.2 |
| L5-S1 | 57 | 1.3 | 2.3 | -3.3 | 5.8 |
| **Center of Rotation—AP (% AP End Plate Width) Reported Relative to the Midpoint of the Superior End Plate of the Inferior Vertebra. Negative Values are Posterior to the Midpoint.** | | | | | |
| **Level** | ***N*** | **Mean** | **Std. Dev.** | **LL** | **UL** |
| L1-L2 | 63 | −5.4 | 6.2 | −17.5 | 6.6 |
| L2-L3 | 63 | −6.5 | 5.0 | −16.4 | 3.3 |
| L3-L4 | 63 | −6.7 | 5.6 | −17.7 | 4.2 |
| L4-L5 | 63 | −6.8 | 4.7 | −15.9 | 2.3 |
| L5-S1 | 45 | −12.5 | 5.7 | −23.7 | −1.4 |
| **Center of Rotation—Cranial-Caudal (% AP End Plate Width) Reported Relative to the Superior End Plate of the Inferior Vertebra. Negative Values are Inferior to the End Plate.** | | | | | |
| **Level** | ***N*** | **Mean** | **Std. Dev.** | **LL** | **UL** |
| L1-L2 | 63 | −5.4 | 7.5 | −20.0 | 9.3 |
| L2-L3 | 63 | −6.7 | 6.6 | −19.6 | 6.1 |
| L3-L4 | 63 | −7.8 | 6.0 | −19.6 | 3.9 |
| L4-L5 | 63 | −3.6 | 7.0 | −17.3 | 10.1 |
| L5-S1 | 45 | 10.9 | 10.3 | −9.4 | 31.1 |

Moderately to severely degenerated levels, and individuals with multiple degenerated levels in this asymptomatic population were excluded. There were 37 females and 26 males. There were 37 subjects under the age of 45 years, 21 in the 45- to 63-year age group, and 5 that were over 64 years old. The percent L1-S1 rotation could not be calculated in some subjects because L1 or S1 could not be visualized.

LL and UL, lower and upper limits of the 95% confidence interval.

validated and consistent methods, and that reproducibility be tested for various ranges of motion. The COR is unreliable when there is little actual rotation between vertebrae.[37] In this situation, small measurement errors may lead to large differences in the computed location of the COR. Depending on the technique used to compute COR, a minimum of 2 to 5 degrees of intervertebral motion is required to obtain reliable results. However, once this minimum threshold has been achieved, the position of the COR becomes generally insensitive to the degree of overall motion in the spine. Based on a re-analysis of previously published[22] data, intervertebral rotation at a specific level was highly dependent on the overall motion in the spine ($P < 0.001$), whereas the position of the COR was not ($P > 0.6$).

In most radiographic studies, the center of rotation is measured in the sagittal plane between the extremes of motion using maximum flexion and extension images. The center of rotation may also be measured continuously at intermediate stages of motion to assess the "instantaneous" center of rotation (ICR). Some investigators refer to an analogous measurement called the instantaneous axis of rotation (IAR). An *axis* of rotation is the axis perpendicular to the plane of motion along which every point of a moving body, or hypothetical extension of it, is stationary.[7] The *center* of rotation is the intersection of this axis with the plane of motion. Radiographically, the center of rotation is a point on an x-ray, while the axis is perpendicular to the x-ray. To calculate the center of rotation reliably, the motion must be in the plane of the x-ray. Since flexion-extension motion takes place predominately in a single plane that is (ideally) coincident with the imaging plane, COR can adequately describe this intervertebral motion. Although COR is typically reported in the sagittal plane for flexion-extension motion, it is important to recognize that the position of the COR may be different for maneuvers in other planes. For example, in the mid to lower cervical spine, in which coupled motion is not as severe as in the upper cervical spine, attempts at estimating the gross position of the COR in left-right bending have suggested that the COR may be located within or superior to the disc space in lateral bending while inferior to the disc space for flexion-extension.[38] This observation must be interpreted as an approximation since left-right bending motions are coupled with out-of-plane motions, such as axial rotation. Nevertheless, three-dimensional marker studies in cadavers have shown similar results.[39]

For coupled, multiplanar motions (representing the most common activities of daily living) a more general method to describe three-dimensional motion is called the helical axis of motion (HAM).[7] The HAM is a unique axis in space that completely defines the three-dimensional motion of a rigid body. It may be described conceptually as a three-dimensional IAR. The HAM cannot be assessed from radiographic images, which are limited to two-dimensional representations of three-dimensional motion. Instead, three-dimensional kinematic analyses using marker-based methods or dynamic MRI may be the best way to evaluate complex motion patterns of the spine. Data related to the use of the HAM to evaluate spinal kinematics is beginning to emerge, especially with respect to motion-preserving devices.[40]

Table 10–2 provides the means, standard deviations, and 95% confidence intervals for intervertebral motion in the lumbar spine of 75 asymptomatic subjects from one ongoing study by the authors of this chapter. Intervertebral motion was measured from flexion-extension radiographs obtained using the sitting method previously described. All volunteers had never sought medical treatment for back-related symptoms. Levels showing moderate to severe degeneration, and patients with multiple degenerated levels were excluded from the analysis. The intervertebral rotation data in Table 10–2 are statistically equivalent to data from Dvorak et al where intervertebral motion was measured from

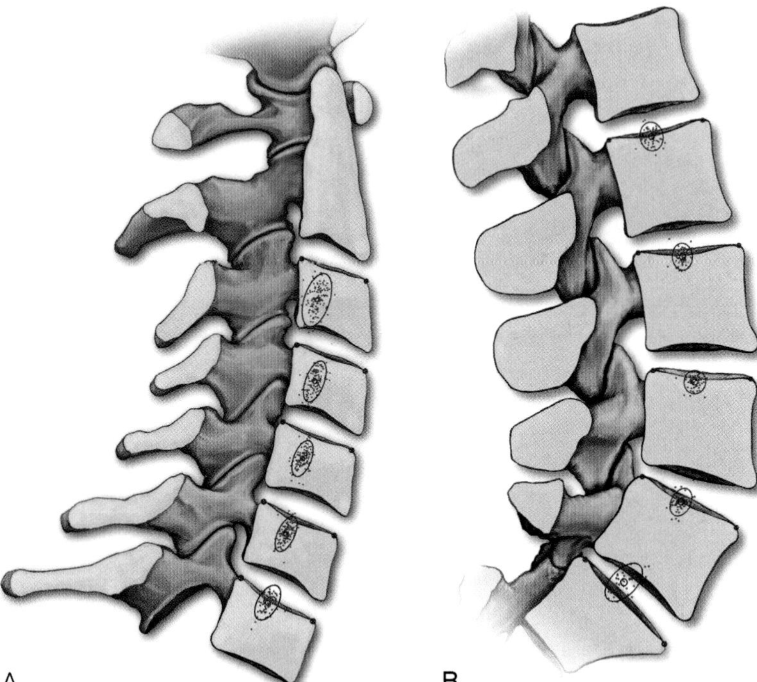


■ **FIGURE 10–3.** Illustrations of idealized cervical **(A)** and lumbar **(B)** spine segments with means and 95% confidence intervals for center of rotation. The individual data points for each asymptomatic subject are shown as red dots. The dark red ellipses depict the 95% confidence interval for the data while the dark red circle in the center of the ellipse depicts the average coordinates of the COR. The COR data were expressed normalized to the AP width of the superior end plate of the inferior vertebra for each level. Since not all individuals have the same ratio of vertebral width to height, the cranial-caudal position of the COR may be somewhat different than depicted for patients with shorter or taller vertebrae than illustrated in these figures. The COR data are referenced to a specific anatomic coordinate system, and the landmarks used to define the coordinate system at each level are also marked by dark red circles on the anterior- and posterior-most aspects of the superior end plate of the inferior vertebra at each level in these figures.

flexion-extension x-rays of asymptomatic volunteers in a standing position.[41] In the Dvorak study, the x-rays were taken as the investigators pulled (for extension) or pushed (for flexion) on the volunteer's shoulders to obtain maximum flexion and extension. The position of the COR provided in Table 10–2 and plotted in Figure 10–3B is consistent data with data from several previously published studies.[9,10] The same coordinate system was used as for the cervical data in Table 10–1. COR results for levels exhibiting less than 3 degrees of intervertebral motion were excluded.

For lateral bending studies of the cervical and lumbar spine, Table 10–3 provides the means, standard deviations, and 95% confidence intervals after combining data from two published studies of intervertebral motion in the cervical spine[38,42] and data from two studies of the lumbar spine.[43,44]

**TABLE 10–3. Summary of Published Data for Intervertebral Rotation Measured in the Coronal Plane During Lateral Bending in the Cervical[38,42] and Lumbar Spine[43,44]**

| Cervical | | | | | |
|---|---|---|---|---|---|
| **Level** | ***N*** | **Mean** | **Std. Dev.** | **LL** | **UL** |
| C2-C3 | 12 | 7.4 | 4.0 | 0.0 | 15.2 |
| C3-C4 | 12 | 7.0 | 2.8 | 1.5 | 12.5 |
| C4-C5 | 22 | 8.4 | 3.1 | 2.4 | 14.4 |
| C5-C6 | 24 | 9.5 | 2.6 | 4.5 | 14.6 |
| C6-C7 | 24 | 12.1 | 3.3 | 5.5 | 18.6 |
| **Lumbar** | | | | | |
| **Level** | ***N*** | **Mean** | **Std. Dev.** | **LL** | **UL** |
| L1-L2 | 14 | 9.9 | 2.8 | 7 | 15 |
| L2-L3 | 14 | 11.1 | 4.2 | 7 | 18 |
| L3-L4 | 30 | 11.2 | 4.8 | 5 | 12 |
| L4-L5 | 14 | 7.1 | 3.4 | 1 | 9 |
| L5-S1 | 10 | 3.0 | 3.8 | 1 | 6 |

The data from the published studies are pooled together in this table to the extent possible. Data from Plamondon et al[44] and Ishii et al[42] were published for one side bending only and were doubled for pooling with data from Wharton and Hipp.[38] Wharton and Hipp only provided data for C4-C5 to C6-C7. The lower limits (LL) and upper limits (UL) for the lumbar spine are the minimum and maximum values reported by Pearcy et al.[43]

## ENDPOINTS AND SUCCESS CRITERIA FOR THE QUANTITY AND QUALITY OF INTERVERTEBRAL MOTION

The radiographic endpoints and success criteria selected for a clinical study will depend on the intended goal of the treatment being studied. Preoperatively, excessive intervertebral motion could be identified as motion greater than the 95% confidence intervals in Tables 10–1 and 10–2. This motion could be abnormal with respect to intervertebral rotation, intervertebral translation, or the position of the center of rotation. Clinically, the presence of intervertebral motion greater than that measured in asymptomatic subjects is only of immediate clinical relevance if the motion correlates to patient symptoms. It is again important to note that the lack of excessive motion in the spine measured from a flexion-extension study can only be used to rule out excessive motion if there was sufficient patient effort. In particular, a patient who has motion limitations from muscle spasms and/or pain guarding can have gross instability that may not be evident from x-rays if the patient does not, or cannot, make a sufficient flexion-extension effort. In addition to excessive motion, hypomobility may also be important, as long as it is not due to insufficient patient effort. Hypomobility is characteristic of the advanced stages of degeneration, and may also occur with perched facets, severe facet disease, severe osteophytes, ossified ligaments, or muscle spasms, and may thereby provide clinically relevant information.

Post operatively, the success and failure criteria that can be applied to quantitative measurements of intervertebral motion depend on the goal of the treatment. In many clinical investigations of motion-preserving devices, fusion is the treatment control. For fusion, where the goal is to minimize motion and achieve solid bridging bone, the success criteria will be motion that is no more than allowed by elastic deformation of bone that has formed between vertebrae (assuming accurate measurements). The postoperative time to apply this success criteria remains unclear and depends on the type of fusion surgery, the healing potential of the individual, and other factors that are beyond the scope of this chapter. However, once a follow-up time has been established for the final fusion assessment, specific intervertebral motion criteria must be applied to assess the mechanical success of the fusion procedure. These criteria must account for potential deformation that may occur through the bone bridging between vertebrae or through the posterior elements in cases of anterior fusion. The other important factor in selecting fusion success criteria is the error in the measurement technique. With manual methods used in many previous studies, the inter- or intra-observer error in the measurement technique has been high, so the motion criteria for failure have been high. With respect to establishing pseudoarthrosis rates, these high success criteria minimize the possibility that a successful fusion will be missed. However, failed fusions will be missed where motion at the fusion site is below the threshold. Some fusion failures may also be missed because the patient did not move enough between flexion and extension to generate detectable motion at the fusion site. Intervertebral rotation is generally more reliable than intervertebral translations, since the scaling factor in the image does not have to be determined, and because with methods that use pattern-matching technology, the rotations do not require identification of specific landmarks. With accurate computer-assisted motion analysis techniques, the accuracy is generally under 1 degree[6,15] and the observer error is typically around 0.5 degree. Assuming the worst case of accuracy and observer error combined with a small amount of motion that could occur by elastic deformation of bridging bone, a threshold level of 2.0 degrees is a reasonable threshold to use in clinical studies. It may be necessary to combine this quantitative assessment of motion with subjective, visual assessments of bony bridging to confirm the final status of fusion.

The success criteria for motion-preserving or dynamic stabilization devices depend on the specific goal of the treatment. If the goal of the treatment is to provide for normal motion, then success criteria based on the lower and upper limits established for an asymptomatic population are appropriate. Assuming that comparable protocols were followed and patient effort was sufficient, the data in Tables 10–1 and 10–2 provide appropriate success criteria for sagittal-plane motion during flexion and extension. Intervertebral rotation, translations, and center of rotation are all important. In addition, a comprehensive assessment would also include quantitative analysis of lateral bending.

In general, quantitative assessments of intervertebral motion should show that motion is within the 95% confidence intervals for the normal patient population after accounting for measurement error. This includes determining if each individual level has motion within the 95% confidence interval for that specific level, but also identifying levels that are moving disproportionately more than the adjacent levels. In the cervical spine, there should not be more than an 11 degree difference in the range of motion between adjacent levels, based on a reanalysis of previously published data for 140 asymptomatic individuals.[22] Eleven degrees is also the difference in intervertebral angles between adjacent levels in the cervical spine that the AMA uses as evidence of a "loss of structural integrity" in the cervical spine.[30] In the lumbar spine, there should not be more than a 9-degree difference in the range of motion between adjacent levels, based on the analysis of intervertebral motion in the lumbar spine of 75 asymptomatic individuals (from an ongoing study by the authors of this chapter). Tables 10–1 and 10–2 provide the 95% confidence intervals for the proportion of total motion that should be provided by each level in the cervical and lumbar spine. This last criterion is only strictly valid in the absence of any fused levels. It must also be noted that the data in Tables 10–1 and 10–2 are for a population of people who have never had any significant spine-related symptoms that required medical treatment. Consistent with many other scientific studies, there were cases in these asymptomatic populations where there were radiographic abnormalities. Preliminary analysis of data from an ongoing study of the lumbar spine suggests that if only radiographically pristine levels are included, the standard deviations are substantially less than reported in Tables 10–1 and 10–2.

Not all motion-preserving treatments have the goal of providing for normal intervertebral motion. Some devices are intended to provide stability to an unstable segment while providing for enough motion to help minimize consequences to adjacent segments. For these devices, the success criteria are less clear. With respect to the goal of providing stability, this implies motion within normal limits, and these limits can be obtained from Tables 10–1 and 10–2. However, there are no data to conclusively define the lower limit of "sufficient" motion. Some amount of motion may be needed to prevent a spontaneous fusion, but the amount of motion required for this goal has not been scientifically proven. Since the asymptomatic subjects who have been studied in the cervical[22] and ongoing lumbar studies clearly have not fused any level, the lower limit of the 95% confidence intervals described in Tables 10–1 and 10–2 provide a reasonable estimate of sufficient motion. Some amount of motion is also hypothesized to be needed to minimize the effects on adjacent levels, but, again, the range of motion is not known. Once again, the lower limits for the 95% confidence intervals in Tables 10–1 and 10–2 provide a reasonable estimate of the motion required to avoid adjacent level effects. In addition to the quantity of motion criteria, it is also assumed that the quality of motion must be preserved. The most commonly used measure of motion quality is the center of rotation, and the 95% confidence intervals for the location of the center of rotation between flexion and extension are provided in Tables 10–1 and 10–2.

Finally, a comprehensive assessment of intervertebral motion should also include assessment of measurements typically made from x-rays of the spine in a neutral position. Currently, a range of criteria are used in research studies. Typical examples that would be applied at each intervertebral level would be requiring that the disc angle (lordosis or kyphosis) changes less than 10 degrees from pre- to postoperative, and requiring that post-operative changes in disc height remain less than 33% of the height of an adjacent normal disc. However, it is important to note that these criteria have not been validated to be predictive of clinical outcomes. Migration over time of a motion-preserving device relative to the vertebrae, subsidence of a device into a vertebra, and screw loosening with posterior stabilization systems are additional measurements made from neutral x-rays that can complement intervertebral motion measurements. Validated success criteria for these measurements have not been established.

## CONCLUSIONS

The technology to accurately and reliably measure both the quantity and quality of intervertebral motion from imaging studies of the spine is readily available and gaining widespread acceptance in research studies. Comparison of results between studies will be greatly facilitated by consistent use of validated methods. Even with accurate and reliable intervertebral motion measurements, the true fusion or pseudoarthrosis rates, the true type and frequency of adjacent segment changes, and the actual range of motion provided by motion-preserving technologies will only be known if high-quality imaging studies are used. Sufficient patient effort is essential. Substantial data are available in the literature to assess the quantity and quality of intervertebral motion, both pre- and postoperatively. With adoption of quality control standards and validated measurement technologies, Quantitative Motion Analysis (QMA) of the spine can be a valuable tool in research studies and clinical investigations. In particular, high-quality imaging studies will be essential to proving whether motion-preserving technology can reduce adjacent segment changes. The true value of QMA in routine clinical practice will likely be established once treatment algorithms are validated that require these measurements.

## REFERENCES


1. Hipp JA, Reitman CA, Wharton N: Defining pseudoarthrosis in the cervical spine with differing motion thresholds. Spine 30(2):209–210, 2005.
2. Santos ER, Goss DG, Morcom RK, Fraser RD: Radiologic assessment of interbody fusion using carbon fiber cages. Spine 28 (10):997–1001, 2003.
3. Ghiselli G, Jatana S, Wong D, Wharton N: Pseudarthrosis in the cervical spine: What is the gold standard? CT scan vs. flexion extension quantitative motion analysis with intraoperative correlation. Spine J 6:60S–61S, 2006.
4. McAfee PC, Boden SD, Brantigan JW, et al: Symposium: A critical discrepancy—a criteria of successful arthrodesis following interbody spinal fusions. Spine 26(3):20–34, 2001.
5. Fassett DR, Apfelbaum RI, Hipp JA: Comparison of fusion assessment techniques: Computer-assisted versus manual measurement. Cervical Spine Research Society Proceedings of the 33rd Annual Meeting, 162, 2005.
6. Reitman CA, Hipp JA, Nguyen L, Esses SI: Changes in segmental intervertebral motion adjacent to cervical arthrodesis: A prospective study. Spine 29(11):E211–E226, 2004.
7. White AA III, Panjabi MM: Clinical Biomechanics of the spine, 2nd ed. Philadelphia, J.B. Lippincott, 1990.
8. Takayanagi K, Takahashi K, Yamagata M: Using cineradiography for continuous dynamic-motion analysis of the lumbar spine. Spine 26 (17):858–865, 2001.
9. Pearcy MJ, Bogduk N: Instantaneous axes of rotation of the lumbar intervertebral joints. Spine 13(9):33–41, 1988.
10. Schneider G, Pearcy MJ, Bogduk N: Abnormal motion in spondylolytic spondylolisthesis. Spine 30(10):159–164, 2005.
11. Amevo B, Aprill C, Bogduk N: Abnormal instantaneous axes of rotation in patients with neck pain. Spine 17(7):48–56, 1992.
12. Ng HW, Teo EC, Lee KK, Qiu TX: Finite element analysis of cervical spinal instability under physiologic loading. J Spinal Disord Tech 16:15–65, 2003.
13. Herrmann AM, Geisler FH: A new computer-aided technique for analysis of lateral cervical radiographs in post-operative patients with degenerative disease. Spine 29(16):795–803, 2004.
14. Harvey SB, Hukins DW: Measurement of lumbar spinal flexion-extension kinematics from lateral radiographs: Simulation of the effects of out-of-plane movement and errors in reference point placement. Med Eng Phys 20:603–609, 1998.
15. Zhao KD, Yang C, Zhao C, et al: Assessment of noninvasive intervertebral motion measurements in the lumbar spine. J Biomechanics 38(9):943–946, 2005.
16. Penning L, Irwan R, Oudkerk M: Measurement of angular and linear segmental lumbar spine flexion-extension motion by means of image registration. Eur Spine J 14(2):63–70, 2005.
17. Lim MR, Girardi FP, Zhang K, et al: Measurement of total disc replacement radiographic range of motion: a comparison of two techniques. J Spinal Disord Tech 18(3):52–56, 2005.
18. Cakir B, Richter M, Puhl W, Schmidt R: Reliability of motion measurements after total disc replacement: The spike and the fin method. Eur Spine J 15(2):165–173, 2006.
19. Breen AC, Muggleton JM, Mellor FE: An objective spinal motion imaging assessment (OSMIA): Reliability, accuracy and exposure data. BMC Musculoskeletal Disorders 7(7):1–10, 2006.
20. Teyhen DS, Flynn TW, Bovik AC, Abraham LD: A new technique for digital fluoroscopic video assessment of sagittal plane lumbar spine motion. Spine 30(14):E406–E413, 2005.
21. Frobin W, Leivseth G, Biggemann M, Brinckmann P: Sagittal plane segmental motion of the cervical spine: A new precision measurement protocol and normal motion data of healthy adults. Clin Biomech 17(1):1–31, 2002.
22. Reitman CA, Mauro KM, Nguyen L: Intervertebral motion between flexion and extension in asymptomatic individuals. Spine 24:2832–2843, 2004.
23. Dvorak J, Panjabi MM, Grob D, et al: Clinical validation of functional flexion/extension radiographs of the cervical spine. Spine 18(1):20–27, 1993.
24. Champain S, Benchikh K, Nogier A, et al: Validation of new clinical quantitative analysis software applicable in spine orthopaedic studies. Eur Spine J 15(6):82–91, 2006.

25. Miyasaka K, Ohmori K, Suzuki K, Inoue H: Radiographic analysis of lumbar motion in relation to lumbosacral stability: Investigation of moderate and maximum motion. Spine 25(6):32–37, 2000.
26. Kanayama M, Abumi K, Kaneda K, et al: Phase lag of the intersegmental motion in flexion-extension of the lumbar and lumbosacral spine: An in vivo study. Spine 21(12):416–422, 1996.
27. Harada M, Abumi K, Ito M, Kaneda K: Cineradiographic motion analysis of normal lumbar spine during forward and backward flexion. Spine 25(15):932–937, 2000.
28. Dvorak J, Froehlich D, Penning L, et al: Functional radiographic diagnosis of the cervical spine: Flexion/extension. Spine 13(7):48–55, 1988.
29. Panjabi MM, Crisco JJ, Vasavada A, et al: Mechanical properties of the human cervical spine as shown by three-dimensional load-displacement curves. Spine 26(24):692–700, 2001.
30. Andersson BGJ, Cocchiarella L: Guides to the Evaluation of Permanent Impairment, 5th ed. Chicago: American Medical Association, 2002.
31. Panjabi M, Oxland T, Yamamoto I, Crisco J: Mechanical behavior of the human lumbar and lumbosacral spine as shown by three-dimensional load-displacement curves. J Bone Joint Surg 76-A:413–423, 1994.
32. McGregor AH, Anderton L, Gedroyc WM, et al: The use of interventional open MRI to assess the kinematics of the lumbar spine in patients with spondylolisthesis. Spine 27(14):582–586, 2002.
33. Lin RM, Tsai KH, Chu LP, Chang PQ: Characteristics of sagittal vertebral alignment in flexion determined by dynamic radiographs of the cervical spine. Spine 1:26(3):56–61, 2001.
34. Holmes A, Wang C, Han ZH, Dang GT: The range and nature of flexion-extension motion in the cervical spine. Spine 19(22):505–510, 1994.
35. Amevo B, Worth D, Bogduk N: Instantaneous axes of rotation of the typical cervical motion segments:—A study in normal volunteers. Clin Biomech 6(2):11–17, 1991.
36. Amevo B, Worth D, Bogduk N: Instantaneous axes of rotation of the typical cervical motion segments, 2: Optimization of technical errors. Clin Biomech 6(1):8–46, 1991.
37. Panjabi MM, Goel VK, Walter SD, Schick S: Errors in the center and angle of rotation of a joint: An experimental study. Journal of Biomechanical Engineering 104(3):32–37, 1982.
38. Wharton ND, Hipp JA: Intervertebral motion in the asymptomatic cervical spine during lateral bending. Spine Arthroplasty Society, Annual Meeting, 2006.
39. Crawford NR, Brantley AGU, Baek S: Three-Dimensional Cervical Axis of Rotation During Lateral Bending. Spine Arthroplasty Society Annual Meeting, 2007.
40. Kettler A, Marin F, Sattelmayer G, et al: Finite helical axes of motion are a useful tool to describe the three-dimensional in vitro kinematics of the intact, injured and stabilised spine. Eur Spine J 13(6):53–59, 2004.
41. Dvorak J, Panjabi MM, Chang DG, et al: Functional radiographic diagnosis of the lumbar spine: Flexion-extension and lateral bending. Spine 16(5):62–71, 1991.
42. Ishii T, Mukai Y, Hosono N, et al: Kinematics of the cervical spine in lateral bending: In vivo three-dimensional analysis. Spine 31 (2):55–60, 2006.
43. Pearcy MJ, Tibrewal SB: Axial rotation and lateral bending in the normal lumbar spine measured by three-dimensional radiography. Spine 9(6):82–87, 1984.
44. Plamondon A, Gagnon M, Maurais G: Application of a stereoradiographic method for the study of intervertebral motion. Spine 13 (9):27–32, 1988.

CHAPTER 11

# Invasive Diagnostic Tools

**Ashish Sahai** and **Todd Alamin**

## KEY POINTS

- Invasive diagnostic tests are designed to gain physiologic information about pain that is lacking at the conclusion of an anatomic work-up.
- The key goal of an invasive diagnostic test is to link a patient's complaint of pain with a specific anatomic lesion.
- A diagnostic tool is useful to the extent that its use improves patient outcomes.
- Invasive diagnostic tests in the spine are difficult to analyze because they are typically directed at disease processes for which a gold standard for diagnosis does not exist.
- It is hoped that improvements in our ability as spinal clinicians to confirm diagnoses with certainty will result in both improved outcomes of treatment and a better ability to differentiate among newer treatment modalities for these conditions.

## INTRODUCTION

As the options for treatment of spinal disease continue to expand, the importance of knowing with precision the origin of pain or the location of the "pain generator" becomes increasingly important. In a healthy patient without other complicating medical or psychosocial issues who develops an acute complaint of leg pain in a specific dermatome with associated motor loss, a sensory deficit, and minimal back pain, the diagnostic connection with the disc herniation seen on the magnetic resonance imaging (MRI) scan is typically clear. The diagnosis is much less clear when confounding factors are present: complex medical issues, such as chronic pain, secondary pain issues, and psychological comorbidities. The chief complaint itself can also be much less specific as well: axial back pain, pelvic pain, or isolated buttock pain. In such common clinical scenarios, it may be extremely difficult to know with certainty the diagnostic significance of the anatomic lesions noted on imaging studies, and the clinician is often left wanting reassurance that a causal relationship between the imaging finding and the clinical complaint truly exists.

The ability to interpret the clinical significance of an anatomic lesion noted on an imaging study in the face of a relatively nonspecific clinical complaint hinges on an understanding of the prevalence of the finding in an asymptomatic population with similar demographic features to the patient of concern. Such an understanding rests upon studies of imaging including the spine performed for clinical concerns other than spinal pathology (e.g., KUB films in patients with abdominal pain, or chest x-ray studies in patients with pulmonary issues), or alternatively on imaging studies in asymptomatic subjects. In a study examining CT scans in asymptomatic patients, Wiesel et al found disc herniations identified in 19.5% of the patients under 40 years old. In the group older than 40 years of age, there was an average of 50% abnormal findings, with diagnoses of disc herniation, facet degeneration, and stenosis occurring most frequently.[1] Boden's classic articles evaluating cervical and lumbar spine MRI scans demonstrated that degenerative findings are common in asymptomatic subjects, and become increasingly more common as the subject's age increases (Table 11–1 and Fig. 11–1).

To further understand and confirm the causal relationship between the anatomic lesions seen on imaging studies and the patient's clinical complaint, many different invasive diagnostic tools have been developed. These tools have been studied, but in many cases, they have been used to address clinical problems for which a gold standard for the diagnosis does not exist. The most notable and prevalent of these conditions is axial spinal pain. This fact has made it impossible to establish with certainty the specificity and sensitivity of these diagnostic tests in these conditions, and has led to much controversy surrounding them. Furthermore, these tools involve a subjective response on the part of the patient, but also involve in many cases a physiologic response as well; it is this interconnection with the subjective experience of pain and with physiology that makes these studies typically compelling to the involved clinician and patient, and hard to examine objectively. This inherent subjectivity may also make these tests problematic or less compelling from the point of view of the external reviewer.

With regard to the cause of axial back pain, it is easiest to group these causes anatomically. Based on several large studies, many authors have concluded that most chronic axial pain complaints originate at least in part in either the intervertebral disc (IVD) or the facet joints. There are some clues to the origin of pain on history and physical examination, but the sensitivity and specificity of these findings are not known. Classically, in helping to differentiate the source of pain by history, flexion increases

TABLE 11–1. Abnormal Cervical Disc MRI Findings in Asymptomatic Subjects

| Age | Any Major Abnormality (%) | Herniated Disc (%) | Bulging Disc (%) | Degenerated Disc (%) |
|---|---|---|---|---|
| < 40 | 14 | 10 | 0 | 25 |
| > 40 | 28 | 5 | 3 | 60 |

MRI, magnetic resonance imaging. Modified from Boden SD, McCowin PR, Davis DO, et al: Abnormal MRI scans of the cervical spine in asymptomatic subjects. A prospective investigation. J Bone Joint Surg Am 72:1178–1184, 1990.

loads on the disc, and therefore pain with flexion typically correlates with pain that arises in the disc. Extension loads the facet joints, and so pain that predominantly occurs with extension implicates the facet joints as a causative factor. Several studies have attempted to estimate the sensitivity and specificity of physical findings in predicting the origin of the complaint. These studies, however, have found only weak correlation between lateral flexion and rotation and back pain.[2–4]

### Intervertebral Disc

The IVD has been the major focus of back pain research for decades. Specifically in the degenerative spine, disc degeneration is believed to precede all other degenerative changes. The disc is the major anterior load-bearing element in axial compression and flexion. The primary load transmission in the normal disc is through the hydrostatic couple of the nucleus pulposus and the annulus. Axial load is transmitted from the end plate of the vertebra above to the nucleus, which is contained by the annulus. As the nucleus is loaded, it generates a radially directed force onto the annulus. Hoop stresses are generated and resisted in tension by the fibers of the annulus; this resistance allows the annulus/nucleus complex to support the axial loads borne by it. The annulus is well suited to resisting torsion as well by the alternating 30-degree lamellar arrangement of its fibers. The annulus (specifically, the outer third) is the most innervated aspect of the disc. The innervation is primarily the sinovertebral nerve from the dorsal primary ramus.[5,6] The second portion that is innervated and likely involved in pain perception in the painful degenerated disc is the end plate. Recent work has demonstrated that the end plate is innervated by the sinovertebral nerve; this pathway is thought to be a major source of nociceptive afferent flow from the disc.[7]

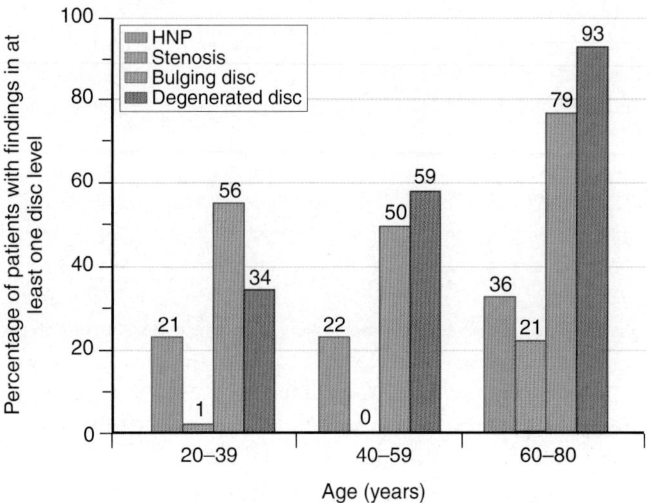


■ FIGURE 11–1. Abnormal magnetic resonance imaging scans of the lumbar spine in asymptomatic subjects. *(Adapted from Boden SD, Davis DO, Dina TS, et al: Abnormal MRI scans of the lumbar spine in asymptomatic subjects. A prospective investigation. J Bone Joint Surg Am 72:403–408, 1990.)*

### Facet

Facet joint-mediated pain is a significant problem in patients with chronic low back pain. Its prevalence has been estimated at 15% in younger patients with chronic back pain, and at 53% of older patients.[8–10] It has been well known that facet joints can be a significant source of pain as evident by isolated fractures, infections, and localized disease process affecting the facets. Each facet joint receives dual innervation from the medial branches of the primary dorsal ramus from the same level and segment above. The medial branch runs caudally and dorsally, lying against the bone where the transverse and superior articular processes join. The load on the facets varies between 3% and 25% of the total axial load.[11] This load increases significantly with degenerative condition of the spine, including disc space narrowing and facet arthritis, to 80%. The clinical complaints associated with facet joint pain are nonspecific. Patients typically present with a deep, aching pain in the low back and buttock with occasional radiation into the posterior thighs. The pain is often nondermatomal in distribution as well.[12]

## MECHANISM OF DIAGNOSTIC INJECTIONS

Invasive diagnostic techniques work in two potential ways. The first is provocation, in which the testing method aims to reproduce the patient's primary complaint through a localized stimulus. The classic example of this is provocative discography. The logic of a provocative test is as follows: If a precisely localized stimulus can reliably reproduce a patient's symptoms, then it is much more likely that the locus of the stimulus is the site of the origin of the patient's pain. The provocation technique relies upon the ability of the patient to reliably recognize and differentiate amongst different potential sources of pain, and also upon the ability of the stimulus to re-create the patient's pain in a non-physiologic manner. The second is anesthetic, in which the effect of the localized infusion of anesthetic on the patient's primary complaint is assessed. This anesthetic technique depends on the ability of the clinician to both accurately place and contain the anesthetic, and on the patient's ability to reliably elicit his typical pain (both before and after the infusion of anesthetic so that the response can be assessed). The typical concern involving provocative tests regards the specificity of this sort of test; anesthetic tests are more commonly criticized with regard to their sensitivity (their specificity may also be called into doubt if the anesthetic is not contained).

## Selective Nerve Root Block

The selective nerve root block (SNRB) is a useful invasive diagnostic test that can be used in situations in which the source of a patient's radiating pain is not clear but is believed to be radicular in origin. There are many different potential causes of pain radiating into the extremities, including radicular pain, large joint arthritis, sacroiliac pain, and facet-mediated pain. In the face of an equivocal clinical examination and history with moderate compressive findings on noninvasive imaging studies such as MRI, the clinician may be uncertain about the relationship of the spinal imaging findings and the patient's clinical complaint of pain. In such cases, a test to further confirm the significance of the imaging findings can be extremely useful.

The terms SNRB and transforaminal block are often used interchangeably, but in the strictest sense, the two differ in two major ways that make the SNRB more of a diagnostic procedure.[13,14] The SNRB is distal to the root sleeve, limiting the amount of injectate that may flow into the epidural space. The second is that only local anesthetic is used (no corticosteroid) and in limited quantity, usually less than 1 mL. More than this amount may result in spread to the epidural space, limiting the diagnostic accuracy of the injection. A transforaminal block is placed in the foramen proper, proximal to the end of the root sleeve, and thus often involves epidural spread of injectate (Fig. 11–2).[13] Steroid is often also used in a transforaminal block.

However, SNRBs remain an invaluable tool both diagnostically and therapeutically. Imaging studies can accurately demonstrate neural compression whether they are in the neural foramen or the thecal sac in the central canal. However, these studies cannot differentiate symptomatic from asymptomatic compression; this is particularly an issue when there are multiple sites and levels of compression that may be symptomatic. SNRBs help to localize pain to a specific nerve root, and can also aid in the nonoperative management of radicular pain.

### Indications

As mentioned earlier, SNRBs have many uses from the diagnostic to the therapeutic. They can aid in the evaluation of atypical extremity pain as well as in evaluating the significance of multiple potential sites of symptomatic compression.

### Technique

Either a single- or double-needle technique is used to access the intertransverse foramen. Previously, the "safe triangle" of Pauza and Bogduk (Fig. 11–3) was thought to be an ideal location for needle placement[15]; however, recently this has been brought into question.[16] A combination of steroid and anesthetic is subsequently injected.

Newer techniques have been developed including direct nerve root stimulation. In this technique, needles are placed into the affected foramen, and into the one above and below. The nerve roots are sequentially electrically stimulated, and provocative responses are noted for concordancy. Local anesthetic is then delivered to the concordant level to assess the anesthetic response, and then steroid is delivered to the root.[17]

### Injection Location

The location of injection has led to significant variability within the practicing community and has been reflected in the many

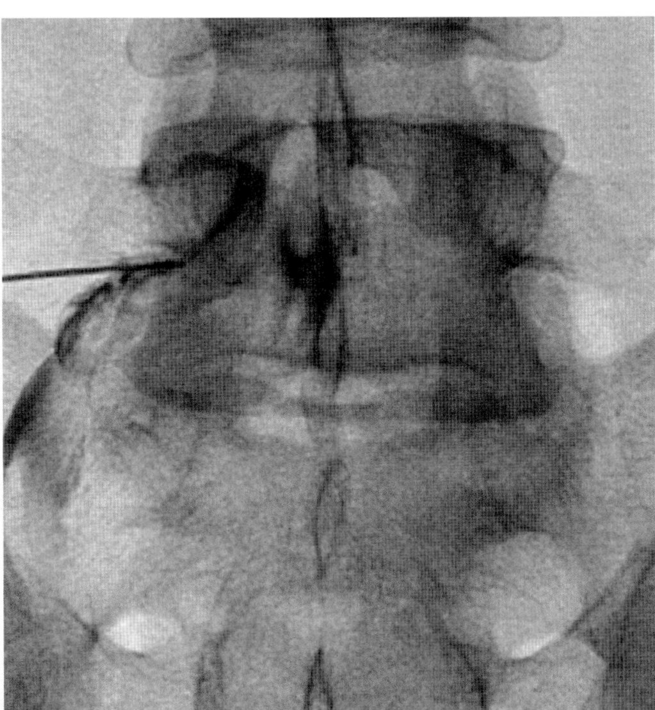

■ **FIGURE 11–2.** Example of a transforaminal block; note epidural spread of contrast.

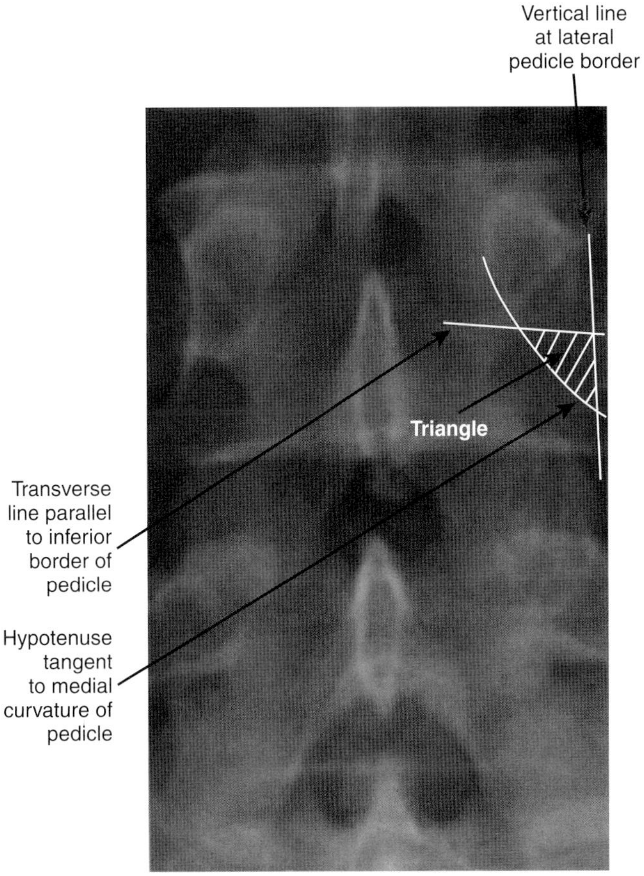

■ **FIGURE 11–3.** "Safe triangle" described by Pauza and Bogduk.

approaches to injections and the literature supporting it. Most recently, a retrospective study of more than 1,700 injections hypothesized that needle placement within or adjacent to the intervertebral foramen would result in similar immediate pain reduction to the theoretical "ideal" position or "safe triangle" of Pauza and Bogduk.[15] The presumed ideal position is the safest position next to the nerve root. The foramen was divided into quadrants in both the anteroposterior (AP) and lateral views, and multiple needle positions in the quadrants were determined. The results demonstrated that the needle tip position did not significantly affect immediate pain reduction.[16]

### Diagnostic Value

SNRBs can also be beneficial in predicting the outcome of surgery especially in combination with an imaging test. A comparison of surgical outcomes between MRI and SNRB 1 year postoperatively was conducted for cervical or lumbar radiculopathy. Ninety-one percent of patients with a positive SNRB had good surgical outcomes, whereas 60% with a negative SNRB had good outcomes. This was differentiated from those in which a positive MRI revealed 87% good surgical outcomes, and a negative MRI had surprisingly similar outcomes of 85%. A positive MRI was considered one in which there was clear evidence of neural impingement or severe central/lateral recess/foraminal stenosis, whereas a negative MRI had only mild-to-moderate stenosis, no clear evidence of impingement or equivocal findings. When the findings differed between selective nerve root injection (SNI) and MRI, surgery at a level consistent with the SNI was more strongly associated with a good surgical outcome. Of the patients with a poor surgical outcome, surgery was most often performed at a level inconsistent with the SNI finding. The authors went on to state the SNI was found to be most helpful when the MRI results were unclear or unequivocal.[18]

A recent systematic review graded all the recent studies on selective nerve root blocks based on strength of evidence as well as methodologic quality evaluation. Datta et al[19] reviewed the current literature to assess the accuracy of SNRBs in diagnosing spinal pain. Of the initial 336 studies, they narrowed down the studies using the Agency for Healthcare Research and Quality (AHRQ) and Quality Assessment Studies of Diagnostic Accuracy (QUADAS) criteria. Studies were graded and evidence classified into five levels: conclusive, strong, moderate, limited, and indeterminate, and could be either prospective or retrospective. The conclusion of the study was that there is still limited evidence on the effectiveness of selective nerve root injections as a diagnostic tool for spinal pain. The major concern regarded the potential for significant epidural spread despite careful imaging; this likely limits its diagnostic utility.[19] Castro et al showed epidural spread in 48% and spread to an adjacent nerve root in 27% of cases with their lowest injected volume (i.e., 0.5 mL).[20] Wolff et al used a combination of fluoroscopy and electrostimulation to perform the selective nerve root block, but still found epidural spread in 47% of L4 and 28% of L5 blocks and spread to adjacent nerve roots in 5%.[21] The authors went on to state that with the available literature there is moderate evidence for the use of SNRBs in the preoperative evaluation of patients with negative or inconclusive imaging studies.[21]

Schutz et al[22] reported finding a corroborative lesion at the time of surgery in 87% of patients with a positive diagnostic block. Dooley et al[23] reported a specificity of 94%. Van Akkerveeken[24] attempted to establish the diagnostic value of selective nerve root injections by comparing 37 patients with confirmed lumbar radiculopathy to nine patients with pain due to metastases. With these small numbers, the calculated sensitivity for determining pain of spinal neural origin was 100%.[24] The specificity was studied by comparison to a normal level on imaging and examination with an SNRB, and it was 90%.[24] Of the 37 patients with lumbar radiculopathy, some declined surgery. The predictive value for a good outcome was determined with, and without, patients who did not want surgery. If all patients who declined surgery were included in the analysis as surgical failures, the positive predictive value of a good surgical outcome with a positive SNRB was 70%. The positive predictive value was 95% when patients who had surgery were the only ones included in the analysis. In this study, the authors concluded that SNRBs were a highly sensitive, specific test with high predictive value for surgical outcome.[24] In a study in 2006, Anderberg et al[25] concluded that for a block to be truly selective enough for diagnostic investigations, only 0.6 mL of total injectate is acceptable. However, these high levels of specificity and sensitivity have to be interpreted with caution because they have not been repeated in controlled trials. These results were compared with evidence shown by North et al in a prospective, randomized single-blinded study that nerve root blocks have sensitivities between 9% and 42% and a specificity of 24%.[26]

### Therapeutic Value

Not only do SNRBs have a role in determining whether a patient is a surgical candidate, but for certain types of pathology, they can also be therapeutic. Riew et al[27] in a prospective, randomized, controlled, double-blinded study looked at the effect of nerve root blocks on the need for operative treatment of lumbar radicular pain. They examined operative candidates who avoided surgery for a minimum of 5 years after receiving an SNRB with either bupivacaine or combination of steroid and bupivacaine. Of the 55 patients, 29 avoided an operation in the original study at a follow-up of 13 to 28 months. Twenty-one of 29 patients were re-evaluated, and 17 of the 21 still did not have surgery at 5 years. There was no difference between the groups treated with steroid or those treated with bupivacaine and steroid despite the initial belief that steroid provided a better effect at the initial study with a minimum 1-year follow-up. In a disease process that has a favorable natural history, an intervention that affords relief for some period of time may allow the patient to tolerate their pathology until the natural history of spontaneous improvement occurs.

### Complications

Complication rates were reviewed in a large study of more than 2,000 injections. The similar needle tip positions were determined using the similar quadrant method described earlier in the needle location section. An overall 5.5% complication rate of minor transient complications, such as transient increased pain, transient leg weakness, light-headedness, vasovagal response, dural puncture and injection into the subarachnoid space that usually abated in 24 hours, was reported. However, the authors did not find that multiple injections rendered a higher complication rate than did single injections.[28]

## Facet Blocks

No independent gold standard exists to confirm a diagnosis of facet pain. The symptoms associated with facet pain are relatively nonspecific. In an attempt to better map pain-referral patterns, a map of facet-referred pain was developed by injection of hypertonic saline into facet joints of normal research subjects by Mooney and others. Wide overlap was demonstrated between the referral patterns of lumbar facet joints.[12] A larger study demonstrated a wide range of referred pain with no consistent pattern of referral. These results have been reproduced in several subsequent studies (Fig. 11–4).[12,29,30] The facet joints capsules are densely innervated with nociceptors that fire when the capsule is stretched or subjected to compressive force. In both patients with pain and volunteers, chemical or mechanical stimulation of the facets has been shown to elicit back and/or leg pain.[29–31]

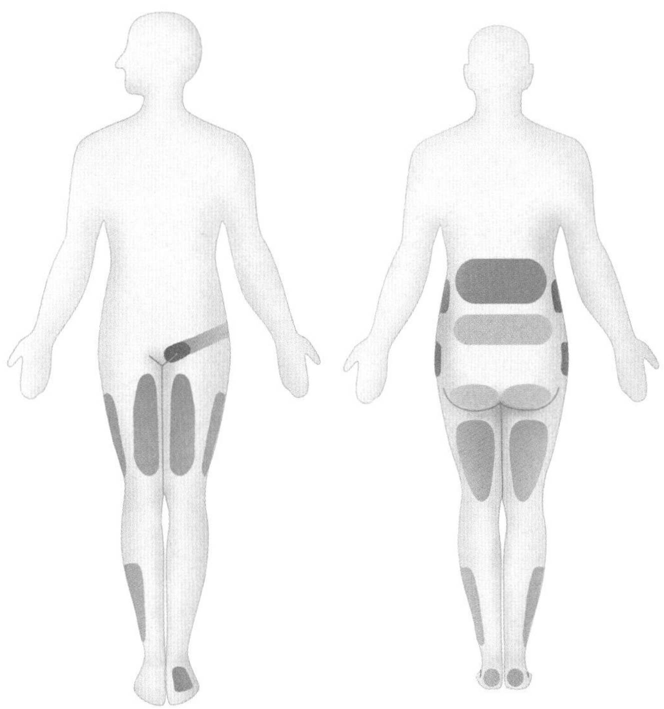


**FIGURE 11–4.** Pain referral patterns from the lumbar facet joints. In descending order, the most common referral patterns extend from the *darkest* (low back) to the *lightest* regions (flank and foot). The key at the bottom of the figure legend is listed in order of affected frequency (i.e., low back to foot). The facet levels next to each location represent the zygapophyseal joints associated with pain in each region. Low back: L5-S1, L4-L5, L3-L4; Buttock: L5-S1, L4-L5, L3-L4; Lateral thigh: L5-S1, L4-L5, L3-L4, L2-L3; Posterior thigh: L5-S1, L4-L5, L3-L4; Greater trochanter:L5-S1, L4-L5, L3-L4, L2-L3; Groin: L5-S1, L4-L5, L3-L4, L2-L3, L1-L2; Anterior thigh: L5-S1, L4-L5, L3-L4; Lateral lower leg: L5-S1, L4-L5, L3-L4; Upper back: L3-L4, L2-L3, L1-L2; Flank: L1-L2, L2-L3; Foot: L5-S1, L4-L5. *(Data adapted from McCall et al., Marks, and Fukui et al. Adapted from Cohen SP, Raja SN: Pathogenesis, diagnosis, and treatment of lumbar zygapophysial (facet) joint pain. Anesthesiology 106:591–614, 2007.)*

The ability to correlate a diagnostic facet block to specific findings on clinical history and physical examination is limited. In 1988, Helbig and Lee[32] coined the term lumbar facet syndrome based on a retrospective study. Patients who responded to intra-articular facet injections (the full parameters of the injection were not included) were more likely to have back pain associated with groin/thigh pain, paraspinal tenderness. and reproduction of pain during extension-rotation maneuvers. Pain radiating distal to the knee was not associated with a positive response to facet blocks. However, since the early description, multiple larger studies have been unable to reproduce the consistent associations found in this study.

### Technique

The two commonly accepted techniques for performing a facet joint block are the facet intra-articular block and the medial branch block (MBB). Several studies have demonstrated that both blocks have similar efficacy rates.[33,34] However, each has its particular problems.

An intra-articular block would appear to be the more logical choice in diagnosing facet joint pain. From a technical standpoint, an intra-articular facet block involves advancing a needle into the facet joint, confirming the position via fluoroscopy and an injection of contrast, followed by injection of either anesthetic or a combination of anesthetic and steroid. Unfortunately, owing to its small size and complex anatomy, the joint is often difficult to enter; once accessed, it is difficult to ensure that the injected anesthetic stays within the joint. An injection of between 1 and 2 mL into the facet often causes the capsule to rupture, allowing the injectate to extravasate and potentially anesthetize adjacent structures.

The other approach to anesthetizing a facet joint involves anesthetizing the nociceptive afferents of the joint. The MBB has the potential to achieve this; however, it, too, has significant limitations. To perform this block, it is essential to understand the anatomy of the innervation to the lumbar zygapophyseal (l-z) joint. For example, the L4-L5 l-z joint is innervated by the medial branches of both L4 and L3. Each medial branch traverses the transverse process of the vertebra below. Therefore, the L4 medial branch will cross the L5 transverse process. An MBB is further complicated by the fact that a small amount of local anesthetic has the potential to anesthetize not only the immediate facet by blocking the medial branch but also the intermediate and lateral branches of the nerve arising from the primary dorsal ramus. This could result in a false-positive response through a block of the nociceptive afferents of the surrounding paraspinal musculature, fascia, periosteum of the neural arch, and the overlying skin.

The actual block is performed by advancing the needle to the upper third of the groove formed by the superior articular process and the transverse process (Fig. 11–5). In order to anesthetize one joint, both medial branches that innervate it must be blocked. Radiographically, the target point is the upper part of the "eye of the scotty dog," which is seen with the patient in an oblique/prone position. Each nerve is infiltrated with the preferred anesthetic/steroid combination. The injection is performed slowly over approximately 30 seconds.

There are only two studies comparing MBB to intra-articular blocks with regard to their therapeutic effectiveness. Marks et al[30] randomly assigned 86 axial low back pain (LBP) patients to receive either

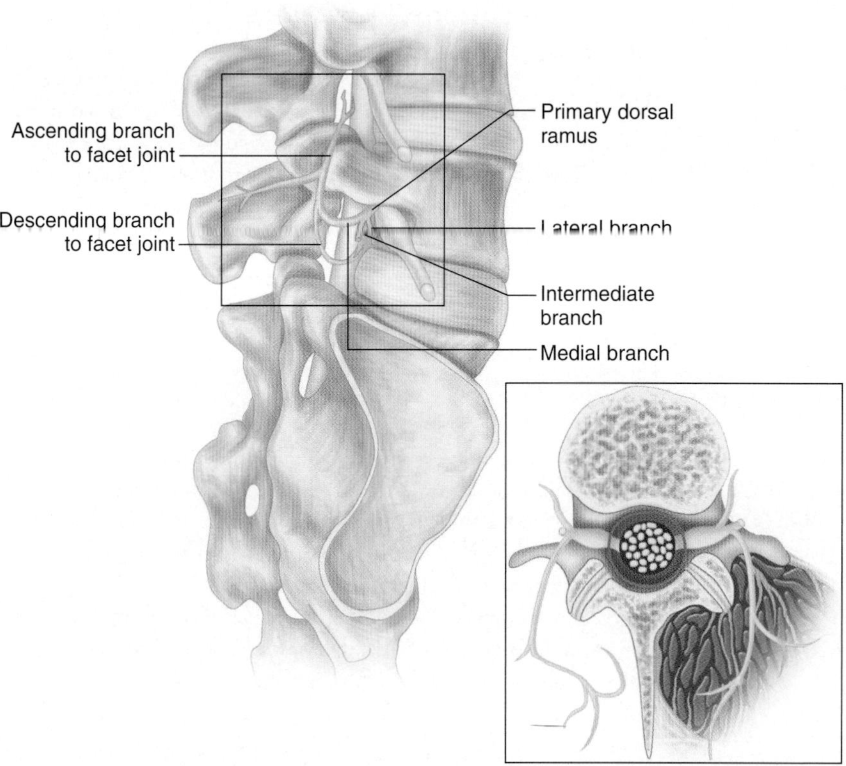


■ **FIGURE 11–5.** Right lateral oblique of vertebral body and dorsal rami. *(Adapted from Cohen SP, Raja SN: Pathogenesis, diagnosis, and treatment of lumbar zygapophyseal [facet] joint pain. Anesthesiology 106:591–614, 2007.)*

intra-articular injections or MBBs. The authors found no difference in the immediate response between the two groups, although the intra-articular group experienced better pain relief at their 1-month follow-up but not the 3-month follow-up. Nash conducted a prospective study in 67 patients with axial LBP who were randomly assigned to receive either MBB or intra-articular injections. In the 26 pairs who completed the study, the MBB was shown to be more beneficial in 12 at the 1-month follow-up: 11 reported the intra-articular injection to be better, and three reported no difference between the two.[35]

Unfortunately, radiologic imaging has also not been conclusively shown to predict a response to diagnostic l-z joint blocks, but it has been conflicting at best. Some studies have found a positive correlation between CT, MRI, or other imaging studies and response to l-z joint blocks; however, a similar number have not. The largest study, which was conducted by Jackson et al, found no relation between radiographic evidence of l-z joint degeneration and the response to single intra-articular facet injections in 390 patients.[36] In contrast, Carrera and Williams found that 73% of chronic LBP patients demonstrating CT evidence of lumbar facet disease experienced pain relief after large-volume (2–4 mL) facet blocks compared with only 13% in whom CT scans showed no pathology.[37]

### False-Negative Blocks

When performing these injections, care has to be taken to recognize that the needle is in the correct position and that the possibility of aberrant anatomy can lead to a misleading conclusion. In 18 asymptomatic volunteers, Kaplan et al found that properly performed MBBs result in failure to anesthetize the corresponding facet joint 11% of the time (as assessed by pain provoked by secondary intra-articular injections of contrast), even with the avoidance of venous uptake.[38] They also found that inadvertent venous uptake occurred during 33% of nerve blocks. When the needle was repositioned to avoid venous uptake, analgesia was achieved only 50% of the time.[38] The authors concluded that when venous uptake occurs, it may be advantageous to repeat the procedure on a separate occasion rather than redirect the needle to avoid false-negative results.

### False-Positive Blocks

Numerous studies have documented a high false-positive rate for lumbar facet blocks, ranging from 20% to 40% using comparative blocks or saline controls despite the type of block used (intra-articular or MBB).[39,40] The reasons for false-positive facet blocks are multiple including the concern of spread of injectate to pain-generating structures other than those targeted, a placebo response to diagnostic facet interventions, and the concomitant use of other pain-altering interventions—either opioids or local/topical anesthetic.

## DISCOGRAPHY

Pain originating from degenerated or injured discs may be the most commonly implicated cause of disabling chronic low back pain. Discography was described nearly 60 years ago as a method to radiographically demonstrate intervertebral disc herniations. Lindblom[41] and Hirsch[31] reported this method of identifying herniated discs in the lumbar spine through an intradiscal injection of contrast, with subsequent radiographs demonstrating the contrast extending around disc material into the epidural space. The authors noted in the report that a reproduction of the patient's typical low back pain was common during the injection. After this initial note of back pain as a side effect of the disc injection, reproduction of the patient's complaint of back pain rapidly became the predominant goal of the test. Discography has since become a standard method of attempting to correlate degenerative imaging findings with pain. It is used most commonly in the lumbar spine, but it is also in the cervical and occasionally in the thoracic spine. It is hoped that when discography is used, it can better determine that the disc is the predominant source of pain, and as such is sufficient to account for most of the patient's clinical complaints of pain. The extent to which provocative discography achieves these diagnostic goals determines the extent to which it is a clinically useful tool.

This is, in the end, a heavy burden that is carried by a presurgical diagnostic test, as interventional treatment strategies are often based on its results. If the results of the test are not reliable, then even a 100% effective therapy that is based on the test is likely to fail at a rate that is *at best* the false-positive rate of the method of diagnosis (in this case, provocative discography), minus any nonspecific or placebo effects. It may be that at this stage of our ability to treat discogenic pain that precision in the presurgical diagnosis may affect overall patient outcomes more than variations in the surgical treatment strategy (e.g., fusion versus disc replacement).

## Indications

The most common indication for discography is to further confirm an intradiscal source of pain in a patient in whom an invasive procedure is being considered. In 1995, the North American Spine Society (NASS) issued a position statement on discography recommending a minimum of 4 months' duration of symptoms before consideration of the procedure.[42]

## Technique (Cervical Spine)

The cervical disc is accessed from a right anterior approach to avoid the esophagus while the trachea and esophagus are pressed left of midline to keep them from being injured. A double-needle technique is used with an outer 18- or 20-gauge needle and inner 22- or 25-gauge needle to access the disc itself. Contrast is injected with pressure recorded on initial dye flow, and then during the subsequent injection of contrast. The patient's pain intensity, location, and character are recorded throughout the process. When significant pain is elicited by the injection, the patient is asked to assess the degree of concordancy of the pain experienced during the injection with the patient's usual pain. A rating of "similar" or "exact" is typically believed to be significant. One or two discs around the suspected painful disc are usually injected to help serve as the "control."

## Technique (Lumbar Spine)

The first reported approach for lumbar discography by Lindblom[41] and Hirsch[31] was an interlaminar, transdural approach to the disc. Over time. an oblique, extrapedicular approach was developed that minimized the concurrent damage to neural elements. With this approach, the exiting nerve root is the structure most often irritated—if significant leg pain is encountered during insertion of the needle, it is repositioned. The double-needle technique similar to that of the cervical spine is used. In the lumbar spine, the approach is posterolateral instead of the anterolateral approach used to access discs of the cervical spine. Again, a control disc is typically analyzed as well.

## Criteria for a Positive Result

After performing the test, there are several different elements that are used to interpret the result. The first is an assessment of the technique of the study: dye was injected into the nucleus and not the annulus, the patient was not overly sedated, and no other technical difficulties were noted. The second is whether by imaging studies done after contrast injection, there is some anatomic evidence of an annular disruption. The third element used to interpret the results of the study is the patient's response to the injection—the pressure at which the pain is noted, its rating on a VAS scale for pain, and its character. This response is an inherently subjective one; it is assessed by whether or not the criteria for a positive test are satisfied. Some evidence of pain behavior (grimacing, verbalization) is also important. The criteria for a positive test are not universally accepted; the most widely accepted criteria are

1. Low-pressure injection (<20 psi above the opening pressure or <50 psi) causing painful response
2. Pain of intensity greater than or equal to 6/10
3. Pain familiar to patient in quality and location (concordancy)
4. Evidence of annular disruption

These criteria may be divided into primary, or "major," criteria for a positive provocative discogram, and several other "minor" criteria which have been suggested to improve the specificity of the test (Table 11–2).[43,44]

An alternative set of criteria by which to interpret provocative discography has been developed by the International Spinal Injection Society (ISIS); the results of the test are grouped into one of four categories:

1. Unequivocal Discogenic Pain—stimulation of the target disc reproduces concordant pain at a level of 7/10 or greater at a pressure of less than 15 psi above opening pressures and stimulation of two adjacent discs produces no pain at all
2. Definite Discogenic Pain—stimulation of the target disc reproduces concordant pain at a level of 7/10 or greater and
   a. pain is reproduced <15psi above opening pressure and stimulation of one adjacent disc produces no pain *or*
   b. pain is reproduced at a pressure <50 psi above opening pressure and stimulation of two adjacent discs does not reproduce pain at all

**TABLE 11–2. Proposed Major and Minor Criteria for a Positive Provocative Discogram (Carragee and Alamin, 2001)[43]**

| |
|---|
| **Major criteria** |
| Injection produces significant pain (>5/10 pain) |
| Pain elicited familiar in quality and location to usual Pain |
| **Minor criteria** |
| Negative control disc |
| Annular penetration of the dye |
| Relative or very low pressure injection |
| Single painful disc only |

3. Probable Discogenic Pain—stimulation of target disc reproduces concordant pain at least 7/10 at a pressure of <50 psi above opening pressure and stimulation of one adjacent disc reproduces no pain at all, whereas another adjacent disc produces pain >50 psi but not concordant
4. Indeterminate Disc—does not meet all the above criteria yet still produces pain

In an attempt to better quantify the results of individual provocative discography tests, ISIS has further proposed a matrix with which the results can be tabulated to facilitate interpretation. It involves a relatively complicated algorithm in which injection pressure, degree of pain, concordancy, and control injections are incorporated (Table 11–3).

## Diagnostic Validity

Discography has been used by some as the default gold standard for diagnostic confirmation of axial back pain of discogenic origin. The validity of the study is a critical issue; this cannot be assessed without an understanding of its specificity and sensitivity. Most of the clinical worries regarding provocative discography center on its specificity: A false-positive result leads directly to a surgery, which is unlikely to be successful. The issue of specificity of provocative discography in the absence of a gold standard for diagnosis has been a difficult one to directly address.

**TABLE 11–3. Evaluation of Discs with Concordant or Nonconcordant Pain**

1. For each disc studied (see columns), enter the appropriate score for each of the variables indicated (rows).
   For discs with CONCORDANT PAIN,
   Enter 30 if the concordant pain is produced
   Enter 5 if the pain produced is greater than 5/10
   Enter another 5 if the pain produced is also greater than 7/10
   Enter 10 if the pressure at which pain occurred is anything less than 50 psi
   Enter another 10 if the pressure is also less than 15 psi
   For discs at CONTROL LEVELS, that is, nonconcordant pain,
   Enter +30 if the disc was painless
   Enter −10 if pain occurred at a pressure less than 50 psi
   Enter another −10 if pain occurred at a pressure also less than 15 psi
2. For the CONCORDANT DISCS, add up the scores in each row and record the sum of each row in the column labeled Sum of Rows.
3. Add up the sums of the rows for all concordant discs, that is, all scores above the double line. Divide this total by the number of concordant discs, and record the quotient in the cell indicated, immediately below the double line, in the column labeled Sum of Rows.
4. For the NONCONCORDANT DISCS, add up the scores in the rows, taking heed of any negative numbers, and record the sum of each row in the column labeled Sum of Rows.
5. Add up the total of the Sums column below the double line, taking care to heed negative numbers.
6. Interpretation: >70 points = POSITIVE
   40–60 points = INDETERMINATE
   <40 points = NEGATIVE

| | L3/L4 | L4/L5 | L5/S1 | Sum of Rows |
|---|---|---|---|---|
| Concordant Pain | | | | |
| Control Levels | | | | |
| Nonconcordant Pain | | | | |
| **Total** | | | | |

Authors have attempted to address the specificity of provocative discography by answering a series of different questions:

1. Does the production of significant pain by a disc injection allow the clinician to conclude that the disc in question is not only degenerated but also painful?
   This question was initially addressed by Holt[44] in 1964, who reported on a group of 50 asymptomatic prison "volunteers" without neck pain who underwent provocative cervical discography. His findings of significant pain reproduction in all subjects at every level (3 levels per patient) on the injection of Hypaque (50% sodium diatrizoate). The pressure of injection was not recorded in this study. The author believed that his experience condemned the use of provocative discography in the cervical spine; methodologically, issues with the study have led many to disregard the results of this study as misleading.
   Walsh et al[45] in 1990 performed a carefully controlled set of discograms in 10 paid asymptomatic young male volunteers and 7 patients with low back pain. Of the 30 discs injected in the asymptomatic group, 1 patient (3.3%) had "bad" pain. The pain, on a scale of five, was rated as a 3/5. As their criteria for a positive injection included a minimum pain rating of 4/5, this study has been referenced as reporting a 0% false-positve rate. In this series of injections, a pain behavior sign was elicited in 3 of 30 (10%).
   Carragee et al[46] reported on the results of provocative discography in a group of 30 asymptomatic subjects with no history of back pain, using a similar protocol to that used by Walsh et al.[46] In asymptomatic subjects with demonstrable annular disruption but no psychological distress or chronic pain behavior, the rate of painful injections was significant but low (10%). With increasing psychological distress, compensation issues, and chronic pain behavior, the rates of positive injections in these asymptomatic subjects became proportionately highter (40% to 80%).
   Derby et al[47] performed provocative discography on five asymptomatic subjects and nine asymptomatic physicians. Fifty-six percent of disc injections were not painful, and 44% of disc injections were painful. Painful injections were typically mildly painful, and usually so at high pressures. The authors concluded that with attention to injection pressure and the degree of pain reported, the risk of false-positive responses was less than 10%. Small subject numbers and the lack of blinding to the purposes of the study perhaps limit the validity of this conclusion.
2. Is the reproduction of pain through provocative discography significant in the face of specific anatomic abnormalities?
   In a separate study of 20 subjects with normal psychometric features who had previously undergone a limited discectomy with an excellent result and no residual back pain, Carragee et al[48] reported a high risk of painful injections (40%). This study casts doubt on the specificity of provocative discography performed at previously operated segments. A study regarding the likelihood of provocative discography provoking pain at disc levels with high-intensity zones (HIZ) assessed the prevalence of HIZ in a symptomatic and an asymptomatic group. The prevalence was higher in the symptomatic group

(59% versus 24%), but on provocative discography, there was no difference in the rate of painful injections (73% versus 70%) at these levels with an HIZ present.[49]

3. How reliable is the concordancy criterion?

A case series of patients with positive provocative discograms who ultimately were found to have clearly remote and distinct causes for their chief complaint of pain (fracture nonunion, deep infection, tumor) was reported by Carragee et al, and initially called into question the specificity of the concordancy criterion used in the interpretation of discography. A small experimental trial with iliac crest pain in which subjects without low back pain but with pain related to a recent iliac crest graft harvest underwent provocative discography; the findings of a concordant pain response in 64% ("similar" or "exact") suggested that clear discrimination of pain from among different deep structures about the spine was unlikely.[50]

4. Does provocative discography clearly identify clinically relevant spinal pathology?

This question was addressed in a study reported on by Carragee et al,[51] in which 25 subjects with mild persistent low backache (who were not receiving or seeking medical treatment for low back pain, taking no medications for backache, had no activity restrictions due to backache, and had normal psychometric scores) were evaluated by provocative discography. The criteria of Walsh et al[45] were used to analyze the results of discography. Thirty-six percent of the subjects had positive provocative discograms with negative control disc injections; this result in the absence of clinically significant low back pain was believed to challenge the specificity of provocative discography in identifying clinically relevant spinal pathology.

Provocative discography continues to be used by many as an important diagnostic tool. Worrisome issues exist, however, regarding its use in the clinically relevant circumstance of evaluating patients with pre-existing psychosocial risk factors that may render the test highly nonspecific. Such risk factors clearly exist in patients coming to surgical consideration for discogenic pain; it is in these patients that the validity of the diagnostic test is perhaps most critical.

## TEMPORARY EXTERNAL TRANSPEDICULAR FIXATION

Temporary segmental immobilization of the spine would seem to be a logical, if invasive, method of predicting the success of a lumbar fusion. This technique was first described by Olerud et al[52] in 1986 as a method of alleviating spinal pain due to instability, but it was suggested in the report that it might be a useful method of diagnosis. Subsequent studies have reported on its use as a diagnostic measure.

### Indications

The indications for temporary external transpedicular fixation (TETF) are similar to those for any diagnostic study targeted toward discogenic pain: patients who are considering surgical management with chronic low back pain believed to be discogenic in origin by history, physical examination, and imaging studies.

### Technique

The approach for the placement of external transpedicular fixation is identical to that used for percutaneous pedicle screw placement. Pedicle screws are either 5- or 6-mm Schanz pins inserted percutaneously under fluoroscopic guidance, with care being taken to avoid adjacent facet joints. Anesthesia can be either sedation with local anesthetic or general anesthesia, depending on the institution and surgeon. The construct is then configured with a bar rigidly connecting the screws across the desired motion segments. It is typically fixed in a neutral postion without compression or distraction. In the later modified "dynamized state," the fixator bars are fixed alternately either segmentally (horizontally) or intersegmentally (vertically) (Fig. 11–6). In this manner, the clinician is able to alternately allow motion or abolish it across the instrumented level while blinding the patient to the configuration. This addition to the technique allows for a placebo response to be analyzed in determining the results of the test.

### Results

There have been several reported studies regarding the effectiveness of TEFT in predicting the results of surgery with variable results.

Bednar[53] in 2001 reviewed his experience with the technique. Of his patients with chronic low back pain coming to evaluation for potential surgical management, TETF provided pain relief in 60%. Of those patients who went on to have subsequent anatomically successful fusion with bone grafting and posterior instrumentation, only 55% with sufficient follow-up had definitive benefit. In the group not on disability insurance, 10 of 13 (77%) patients who had relief with TETF had pain relief after the arthrodesis. There was no control group in the study and no placebo trial of nonfixation. After investigating his results, the author stopped using TETF as a diagnostic tool.

Elmans et al[54] reported on a prospective study of 330 patients evaluated preoperatively with TETF. A positive test was described as one in which the patient reported pain relief in the fixed position subtracted from that reported in the unfixed position was greater than 30 on a 100-point scale. Eighty-eight of the 125

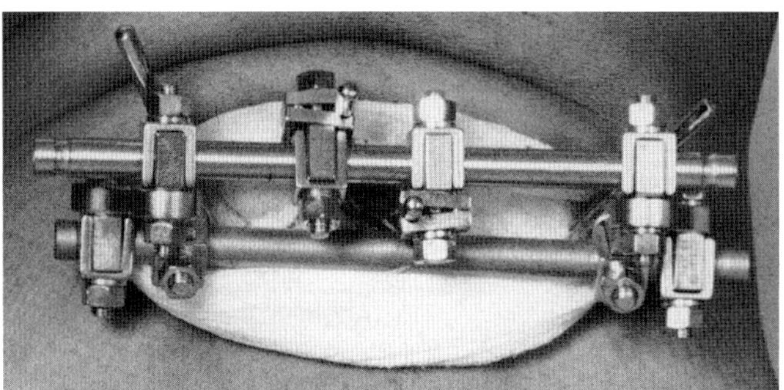

■ **FIGURE 11–6.** Clinical picture of external fixation in place. *(From Bednar, D. Failure of External Fixation to Improve Predictability of Lumbar Arthrodesis. J Bone Joint Surg Am 83:1656–1659, 2001.)*

patients (70%) with a positive TETF were fused; 35 of 176 patients (20%) with a negative test underwent fusion. The authors found that the improvement in VAS scores and the improvement in working capacity seen in the 123 fusion patients were not significantly better in the positive TETF group than in the negative TETF group, and in both groups, this improvement was low. The authors believed that TETF did not appear to be of value in selecting suitable candidates for spinal fusion. The heterogeneous nature of the patient group and the large variability in the rate of surgery in the two groups likely limit the extent to which this conclusion can be deemed valid.

Good overall results using this technique were reported by van der Schaaf et al[55] in their clinical follow-up of 133 patients with chronic low back pain who underwent a trial of TETF. In this trial, patients were evaluated with the segment both immobilized and not, and patients with significant pain relief only in the immobilized state were offered fusion. In the 55 patients treated surgically, improved VAS scores were noted (preoperatively 77, postoperatively 40), along with improved patient satisfaction compared with the conservatively treated group. The authors emphasized the importance of a placebo trial (unimmobilized state) because 37 of 78 patients with negative test results had pain relief in both the immobilized and unimmobilized states. These patients would have been considered positive if a placebo trial had not been included.

A recent article reported on the results of lumbar fusion for axial spinal pain in a series of patients who were evaluated preoperatively with provocative discography and by temporary external transpedicular fixation. In this series, the decision for surgery was made based on the results of TETF (provocative discography was not used in the decision), and the investigators wished to determine if the clinical result was affected by whether the disc adjacent to the fusion was painful on provocative discography. Data were available for 197 patients out of the original 209; 82 patients underwent fusion based on this diagnostic work-up. The authors defined clinical success as achieving at least a 30% reduction in the VAS score for back pain at follow-up, and with this metric there was no difference in the likelihood of clinical success with an adjacent level painful disc (45%) or a painless disc (45%). The authors' conclusions were that the presence or absence of a concordant pain response did not affect the clinical results of fusion for symptomatic degenerative disc pathology diagnosed by TETF, but the poor overall clinical results in their series perhaps limit the ability to generalize on this conclusion.[40]

### Complications

The major limiting feature of this test is its invasiveness. Patients are typically hospitalized for 7 to 10 days after the placement of the external fixator. Misplacement of the screws causing nerve root irritation is reported at a rate of 0% to 9%. No permanent neurologic deficits have been reported. Pin tract infections are fairly common occurrences with this technique, with reported rates of 2% to 18%.[53–56]

## THE FUNCTIONAL ANESTHETIC DISCOGRAM

In an attempt to address problems with the diagnosis of discogenic low back pain, the senior author (T.F.A.) has developed a novel test, the functional anesthetic discogram (FAD).[57] Similar to clinically useful anesthetic tests used elsewhere in the body for the localization of pain (such as intra-articular hip and knee injections, and subacromial injections for rotator cuff pathology), it seems logical to attempt to apply this sort of diagnostic technique to discogenic pain. Anesthetic discography has been used in the past, and reported on for the evaluation of cervical discogenic pain.[58,59] In these reports, the authors reported 93% good-to-excellent results in 71 patients treated with anterior cervical fusions (Roth), and 81% good-to-excellent surgical results in 32 patients (Osler).

Problems with the simple injection of anesthetic into the disc do exist, however. In a setting in which the patient is in a position that is not typically painful (the prone position), and has recently been injected with contrast as part of a provocative discography, it is difficult to determine the significance of a response in which pain is relieved, or not relieved. If a long-acting local anesthetic is used and significant time is allowed to elapse before the evaluation of pain in ordinarily painful activities, the examiner can be less confident of the location of the local anesthetic; if a significant amount has migrated out of the disc during this period of time, then the specificity of the injection could be called into doubt. Thus, a technique is needed to allow for the injection of short-acting local anesthetic while the patient is performing an activity or assuming a position that is ordinarily painful so that more physiologic information may be obtained.

### Technique

This test involves first a standard provocative discogram using a 2-needle technique (outer needle, 18 g; inner needle, 22 or 25 g). Once candidate painful discs are noted on provocative discography, the next step involves the placement of a catheter into the relevant lumbar discs that were either painful on injection or radiographically highly suggestive of a being a possible pain generator.

In the early experience with the technique, the outer 18-g needle was then inserted into the center of the involved disc, with care being taken to avoid irritation of the exiting nerve root at this level. An epidural catheter (20 g) was then modified via removal of the distal portion of the catheter including the side ports. The catheter was then carefully threaded into the involved disc, and then the outer 18-g needle was removed while attempting to maintain the catheter position inside the nucleus. A Tuohy-Borst adapter was then attached to the proximal end of the catheter and contrast introduced to ensure that the tip of the catheter was still intradiscal. The contrast was then flushed out of the catheter with injectible normal saline. The catheter was then attached to the patient's skin in a sterile fashion, and the patient was then allowed to recover from the procedure in the PACU (Fig. 11–7). A dedicated FAD catheter (Kyphon, Inc., Sunnyvale, CA) has recently been approved by the FDA and is commercially available; it is inserted over a guidewire and has a balloon anchor at its tip, which prevents migration of the catheter out of the disc during functional testing.

The patient is then allowed to recover from sedation and assume a position or begin an activity that would ordinarily be painful for him or her. It is critical that the patient be able to reliably elicit his or her pain with a particular position or activity; if this is not the case, the findings of the procedure will be difficult

■ **FIGURE 11–7.** Functional anesthetic discogram catheter with balloon anchor deployed.

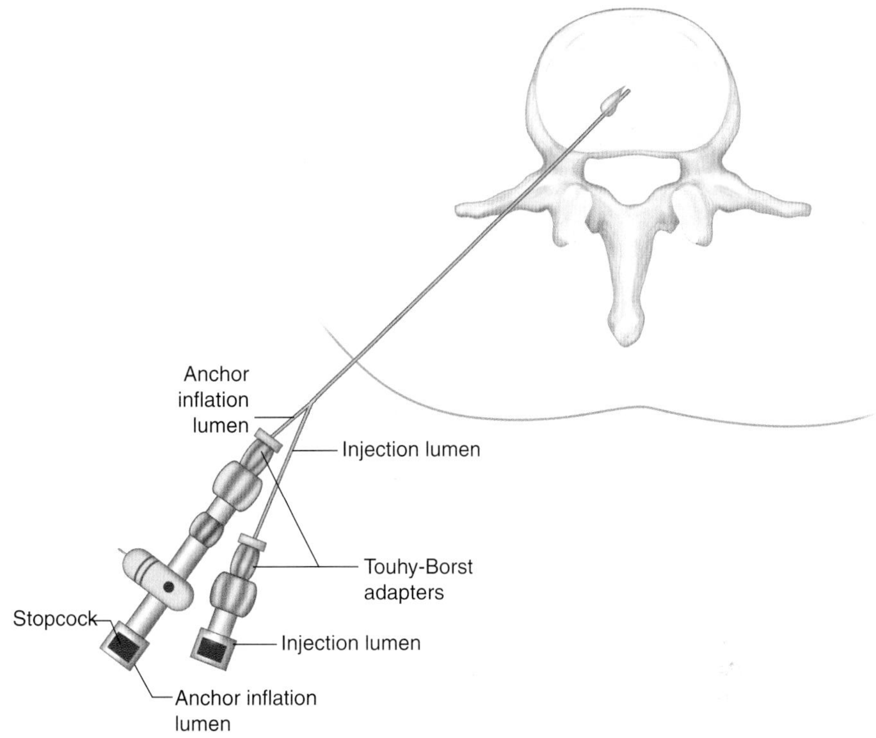


to interpret. The seated position is the most common provocative position used for the procedure. An injection of a small volume (0.6 mL) of short-acting local anesthetic (4% lidocaine) or placebo control (normal saline) is then delivered into the disc, and the response of the patient to the anesthetic or placebo is recorded (Fig. 11–8). A volume of 0.6 mL for the injection was chosen because this is a volume typically well below the volume of disc injection at which extravasation into the epidural space is noted on fluoroscopy during discography (1 to 1.5 mL in degenerated discs), and as such minimizes the likelihood of the anesthetic effect being due to an epidural effect.

The initial injection of anesthetic into a disc selected by provocative discography typically causes an exacerbation of the patient's typical low back pain, followed by, in positive cases, the onset of the effect of the 4% lidocaine in approximately 2 to 5 minutes. The effect of the 4% lidocaine typically lasts 25 to 30 minutes, and then the injection can be repeated as necessary to confirm the diagnosis. We have designated a positive result as one in which the patient reports that the intradiscal delivery of the local anesthetic causes a decrease in the VAS score of 2 points or greater during the provocative position or activity, and reports that the pain is significantly less than is typical for them. At the conclusion of the test, 0.7 mL of 0.75% bupivacaine is injected into the disc as a confirmatory measure; the patient is instructed to keep a pain diary during the remainder of the day. In positive cases, the typical duration of effect of the 0.75% bupivacaine is approximately 6 to 8 hours.

Care must be taken to ensure that the insertion site is medial and inferior in Kambin's safe triangle (formed by the traversing nerve root medially, the exiting nerve root laterally, and the inferior end plate inferiorly) to minimize the risk of irritation of the exiting nerve root during subsequent functional testing. If the exiting nerve root is irritated by the presence of the catheter, the interpretation of the test is more difficult; the usual strategy is to deliver local anesthetic into the disc followed immediately by removal of the catheter. The patient is then instructed to compare the pain level during the provocative maneuver or position to the typical pain level. It should be remembered that the medial border of the exiting nerve root often abuts the lateral border of the inferior pedicle of the segment, and thus, the appropriate spot on the

**Functional Anesthetic Discogram Data Sheet**

Patient:

Provocative Discography Findings:

FAD Findings:

Level:

Pre-injection VAS:

Injection substance:

During injection VAS:

5 minutes post:

10 minutes post:

20 minutes post:

■ **FIGURE 11–8.** Functional anesthetic discogram data sheet. VAS, Visual Analog Scale.

posteroanterior (PA) radiograph for the outer needle to dock on the posterolateral margin of the annulus is in line and proximal to the inferior pedicle (Fig. 11–9). In the setting of facet joint hypertrophy, this may require that a bend be applied to the outer needle to allow it to pass lateral to the facet joint and yet still dock on the annulus in line with the pedicle.

## Results

It is important to remember that this is a new technique, and so there are as yet no reported large series of patients with discogenic low back pain investigated by FAD with clinical follow-up. Two reports have been submitted for publication at this stage: one comparing the results of pressure-controlled provocative discography with that of FAD in a group of patients with chronic low back pain, and a second study examining the early results of lumbar fusion in patients selected in this manner.

In the study comparing the results of the FAD analysis with that of provocative discography, different results were obtained in 49% of the 43 patients: in 28% of cases, the provocative discogram was positive and the FAD test was negative; in 16% the provocative discogram was positive at two levels, and the FAD was positive at a single level only; and in 5% of cases, the provocative discogram was negative and the FAD test was positive. Sixteen of the patients who had positive results on the FAD have undergone surgery and have had minimum 6-month follow-up. The mean Oswestry Disability Index (ODI) in this group improved from a preoperative mean of 55 to a postoperative mean of 25. The mean preoperative VAS score for back pain was 6.9; the postoperative mean was 2.6. These results are encouraging but clearly early and preliminary.[60]

Two more studies are also under way: a multicenter pilot study and a multicenter prospective, randomized study in which patients are assigned to undergo treatment based on the results of clinical examination, imaging findings, and provocative discography or alternatively treatment based on the results of clinical examination, imaging findings, and the FAD. It is hoped that either this new diagnostic technique or another such technique will allow increased precision of diagnosis of discogenic low back pain, which will translate into improved overall clinical outcomes. Better diagnostic methods should also allow spinal clinicians to better evaluate different treatment strategies and techniques because the outcome "scatter" effect due to lack of precision in diagnosis is minimized.

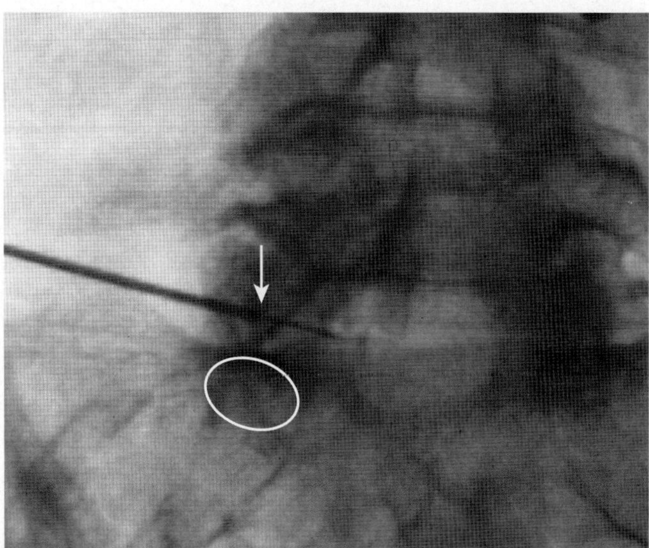

■ **FIGURE 11–9.** Appropriate docking site on posterior annulus *(arrow)* immediately superior to pedicle *(oval)*.

## Complications

FAD is a newly described technique, but it should likely have similar complications to those associated with provocative discography. The presence of the transcutaneous catheter likely increases the potential for infection; use of strict sterile technique and preoperative antibiotics is imperative.

## REFERENCES


1. Wiesel SW, Tsourmas N, Fetter HL, et al: A study of computer-assisted tomography, I: The incidence of positive CAT scans in an asymptomatic group of patients. Spine 9:549–551, 1984.

   In order to study the type and number of computed tomographic (CT) scan abnormalities of the lumbar spine that occur in asymptomatic people, 52 studies from a control population with no history of back trouble were mixed randomly with six scans from patients with surgically proven spinal disease, and all were interpreted by three neuroradiologists in a blinded fashion. Irrespective of age, 35.4% (26.6%, 51.0%, and 31.3%) were found to be abnormal. Spinal disease was identified in an average of 19.5% (23.8%, 22.7%, and 12.5%) of the under 40-year-olds, and it was a herniated nucleus pulposus in every instance. In the over 40-year-old age group, there was an average of 50% (29.2%, 81.5%, and 48.1%) abnormal findings, with diagnoses of herniated disc, facet degeneration, and stenosis occurring most frequently.

2. Michel A, Kohlmann T, Raspe H, et al: The association between clinical findings on physical examination and self-reported severity in back pain: Results of a population-based study. Spine 22:296–303; discussion 303–304, 1997.

   **Study Design**
   A cross-sectional population-based study of back pain.

   **Objective**
   To evaluate the association between clinical findings on physical examination and subjective severity in nonspecific back pain.

   **Sumary of Background Data**
   Assessment of severity of back pain always has been controversial. Most studies evaluating the role of clinical findings in back pain have been hospital-or-clinic based, often representing a highly select population. This selection is avoided in the population-based approach of the present study.

   **Methods**
   Approximately 4,000 German inhabitants of Lubeck, age 25 to 74, were selected randomly from the local population registry and received a postal questionnaire. Those who reported "back pain today" ($n$ = 1,200) or "back pain within the past 12 months but no back pain before" ($n$ = 75) were invited to come in for a clinical examination. Thirty-four physical measurements were taken. They were divided into four groups: static measurements, dynamic measurements, neurologic findings, and non-organic physical signs. Self-reported severity of back pain was measured by a pain questionnaire and a 12-item activities of daily living list to assess functional disability.

**Results**

Within each of the four groups of physical measurements, those that corresponded best with the subjective severity of back pain could be identified (e.g., rotation, lateral flexion, and fingertip-to-floor distance, scoliosis, the position of the side plumb line, and pain on percussion of the spine pseudo-Lasegue and hand-muscle strength). Those that corresponded best could be differentiated statistically from less correlative measurements such as kyphosis and lordosis; flexion of the lumbar, thoracic, or cervical spine; abdominal muscle strength; and axial loading. The agreement between the classification of back pain severity based on clinical findings and the classification based on self-reports was moderate (kappa = 0.47).

**Conclusions**

Assessment of severity in back pain can be only partly based on the clinical findings of a physical examination. There is a relatively weak agreement between the results of physical examination and the subjective reporting of pain and disability.

3. Mellin G: Chronic low back pain in men 54–63 years of age: Correlations of physical measurements with the degree of trouble and progress after treatment. Spine 11:421–426, 1986.

Conservative treatment for chronic low back pain was given to 151 men aged 54 to 63 years. Pretreatment for back trouble and progress were assessed by subjective ratings in questionnaires before the treatment and at 2-, 6-, and 12-month follow-up examinations. Physical measurements were made before the treatment and at the 2-month follow-up. Pretreatment low back trouble correlated significantly and positively with lumbar disc degeneration and negatively with spinal lateral flexion and rotation, hip flexion and extension, capacity for dynamic exercises, trunk isometric extension and flexion strength, and intraindividual trunk extension/flexion strength ratio. Progress was significantly associated with follow-up increases of spinal lateral flexion and rotation, hip flexion and lateral rotation, and trunk extension and flexion strength. Combinations of variables did not substantially improve their correlative power as indicators of low back trouble and progress.

4. Mellin G: Correlations of spinal mobility with degree of chronic low back pain after correction for age and anthropometric factors. Spine 12:464–468, 1987.

Correlations of age, height, weight, lordosis, and kyphosis with noninvasive spinal mobility measurements were studied in 301 men and 175 women, aged 35 to 55 years, who suffered from chronic or recurrent low back pain (LBP). Correlations of the different spinal movements with the degree of LBP were analyzed, with corrections for these relationships. Age had significant indirect correlations with most of the mobility measurements, but the effect of height was minor. Weight had considerable negative correlations with the mobility measurements except lateral flexion. Lordosis and kyphosis had significant relationships with mobility in the sagittal and frontal planes. Correction for the factors analyzed only slightly reduced the correlations between spinal mobility and LPB. Thoracolumbar mobility had higher correlations with LBP than mobility of the lumbar spine. Thoracal spinal mobility alone also correlated with LBP. Lateral flexion and rotation, except for rotation in women, had stronger relationships than forward flexion and extension with LBP.

5. Bogduk N: The anatomy of the lumbar intervertebral disc syndrome. Med J Aust 1:878–881, 1976.

Four elements of the nervous system may be involved in the production of the lumbar intervertebral disc syndrome. These are the lumbosacral nerve roots, the spinal nerves, the dorsal rami, and the sinuvertebral nerves. Each nerve is associated with a particular group of pathological conditions which may irritate the nerve and produce symptoms. The anatomy of each nerve determines which particular conditions may irritate it. Moreover, one or both of two mechanisms may be involved in symptom production. The type of nerve irritated determines which mechanism is involved. In the first mechanism, low back pain and referred lower limb symptoms are produced when afferent fibres from dorsal and ventral rami are stimulated where they pass in common through spinal nerves or nerve roots. In the second mechanism, dorsal rami or sinuvertebral nerves are stimulated. This directly produces low back pain, but referred pain is produced by reflex mechanisms in the spinal cord.

6. Bogduk N, Tynan W, Wilson AS: The nerve supply to the human lumbar intervertebral discs. J Anat 132(Pt 1):39–56, 1981.

The lumbar intervertebral discs are supplied by a variety of nerves. The posterior aspects of the discs and the posterior longitudinal ligament are innervated by the sinuvertebral nerves. The posterolateral aspects of the discs receive branches from adjacent ventral primary rami and from the grey rami communicantes near their junction with the ventral primary rami. The lateral aspects of the discs receive other branches from the rami communicantes. Some rami communicantes cross intervertebral discs and are embedded in the connective tissue of the disc deep to the origin of psoas. Such paradiscal rami are likely to be another source of innervation to the discs. The anterior longitudinal ligament is innervated by recurrent branches of rami communicantes.

7. Fagan A, Moore R, Vernon Roberts B, et al: ISSLS prize winner: The innervation of the intervertebral disc: A quantitative analysis. Spine 28:2570–2576, 2003.

**Objective**

The first quantitative analysis of the innervation of the lumbar intervertebral disc is presented.

**Methods**

A sheep model was used allowing evaluation of the whole motion segment. Four sheep spines were used. One was processed for protein gene product (PGP) 9.5 immunofluorescence, and three were processed for PGP 9.5 immunoperoxidase histochemistry. A count was made of the densities of innervation of the end plate and annulus, and these were compared.

**Results**

There is no significant difference between end plate and annulus innervation densities. The end plate innervation is concentrated centrally adjoining the nucleus. The richest area of innervation is in the periannular connective tissue.

**Discussion**

The lumbar intervertebral disc has a meager innervation. This is concentrated in the periannular connective tissue and the central end plate. Although receptor threshold is more closely related to nociceptive function than innervation density, these findings have important implications for any treatment of discogenic pain.

8. Manchikanti L: Transforaminal lumbar epidural steroid injections. Pain Physician 3:374–398, 2000.

Low back pain is an important medical, social, and economic problem involving approximately 15% to 39% of the population. Of the numerous therapeutic interventions available for treatment of chronic low back pain, including surgery, epidural administration of corticosteroids is one such intervention commonly used. Several approaches available to access the lumbar epidural space are the caudal, interlaminar, and transforaminal, also known as nerve root or selective epidural injection. The objective of an epidural steroid injection is to deliver corticosteroid close to the site of pathology, presumably onto an inflamed nerve root. This objective can be achieved by the transforaminal route rather than the caudal or interlaminar routes. Reports of the effectiveness of epidural corticosteroids have varied from 18% to 90%. However, reports of the effectiveness of transforaminal epidural steroids have shown it to be superior, with outcome data indicating cost-effectiveness as well as safety. This review describes various aspects of transforaminal epidural steroid injections in managing chronic low back pain.

9. Manchikanti L, Pampati V, Bahkit CE, et al: Effectiveness of lumbar facet joint nerve blocks in chronic low back pain: a randomized clinical trial. Pain Physician 4:101–117, 2001.

This randomized clinical trial was designed to determine the effectiveness of therapeutic lumbar facet joint nerve blocks. Two hundred patients were evaluated with controlled diagnostic blocks for the presence of facet joint mediated pain. Eighty-four patients, or 42%, were determined to have lumbar facet joint–mediated pain. These patients were randomly allocated into two groups: Group I receiving therapeutic injections with local anesthetic and Sarapin, and Group II receiving therapeutic injections with a mixture of local anesthetic, Sarapin, and methyl prednisolone. A total of 73 patients were treated with medial branch blocks under fluoroscopy. Results showed that patients underwent multiple procedures over a period of 2½ years. The mean number of procedures or interventions was 2.5 ± 0.09 from 1 to 3 months, whereas it was 4 ± 0.13 for 4 to 6 months, 6.1 ± 0.21 for 7 to 12 months, and 8.4 ± 0.31 for 13 to 32 months. Cumulative significant relief with one to three injections was 100% up to 1 to 3 months, 82% for 4 to 6 months, 21% for 7 to 12 months, and 10% after 12 months, with a mean relief of 6.5 ± 0.76 months. There was significant improvement noted in overall health status, with improvement not only in pain relief but also with physical, functional, and psychological status, as well as return-to-work status. In conclusion, the results of this study demonstrate that medial branch blocks with local anesthetic and Sarapin, with or without steroids, are a cost-effective modality of treatment, resulting in improvement in pain status, physical status, psychological status, functional status and return to work.

10. Schwarzer AC, Wang SC, Bogduk N, et al: Prevalence and clinical features of lumbar zygapophysial joint pain: A study in an Australian population with chronic low back pain. Ann Rheum Dis 54:100–106, 1995.

**Objectives**

To determine the prevalence of pain arising from the zygapophyseal joint in patients with chronic low back pain and to determine whether any clinical features could distinguish patients with and without such pain.

**Methods**

Sixty-three patients with chronic low back pain were studied prospectively. All patients underwent a detailed history and physical examination, as well as a series of intra-articular zygapophysial joint injections of 0.5% bupivacaine starting at the symptomatic level to a maximum of three levels or until the pain was abolished. They also received injections of normal saline into paraspinal muscles to act as controls.

**Results**

All patients proceeded with the injections. Twenty (32%; 95% confidence interval [CI] 20 to 44%) obtained greater than 50% relief of their pain following the administration of saline. Fifty-seven patients completed the study; 23 of them (40%; 95% CI 27 to 53%) failed to obtain relief following the injection of saline but obtained relief following one or more intra-articular injections of local anesthetic. None of the historical features or clinical tests could discriminate those patients with and those without zygapophysial joint pain.

**Conclusion**

Pain originating from the zygapophyseal joint is not uncommon, but this study failed to find any clinical predictors in patients with such pain.

11. Yang KH, King AI: Mechanism of facet load transmission as a hypothesis for low-back pain. Spine 9:557–565, 1984.

Low-back pain has a complex and multifaceted etiology. The articular facets have been shown to be load-bearing structures and may be a site for low-back pain. The aim of this paper is to establish the mechanism for the transmission of axial load across a facet joint and to propose a facet-related hypothesis for low-back pain. The mechanism of load transmission was studied by two methods. Lumbar segments were instrumented with an intervertebral load cell (IVLC) to measure disc load so that facet load could be deduced. The applied load was moved 10 mm anteriorly and 12.5 mm posteriorly from the center of the vertebral body. The facets then were separated from the body and loaded axially to determine their stiffness in tension and compression and to observe the failure mode of the joint. It was shown optically that compressive loading of the isolated facet joints was equivalent to spinal extension and tensile loading to spinal flexion. Last, a finite element model of a lumbar motion segment was developed to simulate the transmission of facet load and to study the effects of disc degeneration on facet loads. Results of the study on six lumbar segments revealed that the normal facets carried 3% to 25%. If the facet joint was arthritic, the load could be as high as 47%. Experiments on isolated facet joints revealed that they behaved as a stiffening spring in compression and were weak in tension.

12. Mooney V, Robertson J: The facet syndrome. Clin Orthop Relat Res 115:149–156, 1976.

Injection of irritant fluid precisely into the facet joint causes referred pain patterns indistinguishable from the pain complaints frequently associated with the "disc syndrome." Even straight leg raising and diminished reflex signs can be obliterated by precise local anesthetic injection into the facet joint. The use of radiographically localized injection of steroids and local anesthetic into the facet joint has been presented as a diagnostic-therapeutic procedure. Clinical experience with a group of 100 consecutive patients suggests that this treatment alone can achieve long-term relief in one fifth of the patients with lumbago and sciatica, and partial relief in another one third of these patients. This information suggests that the structures related to the facet joint can be a persistent contributor to the chronic pain complaints of individuals with low back and leg pain.

13. Bogduk N: Lumbar spinal nerve blocks. *In* Practice Guidelines for Spinal Diagnostic and Treatment Procedures, 1st edition. International Spine Intervention Society, 2004, pp 3–19.
14. Gajraj NM: Selective nerve root blocks for low back pain and radiculopathy. Reg Anesth Pain Med 29:243–256, 2004.
15. Pauza K, Bogduk N: Lumbar transforaminal injection of corticosteroids. Int Spine Injection Soc Newsl 4:4–20, 2003.
16. Crall TS, Gilula LA, Kim YJ, et al: The diagnostic effect of various needle tip positions in selective lumbar nerve blocks: An analysis of 1,202 injections. Spine 31:920–922, 2006.

**Study Design**

Retrospective chart review.

**Objective**

To determine the effect of various needle tip positions on immediate postinjection pain in selective lumbar nerve blocks.

**Sumary of Background Data**

To our knowledge, no large study has examined the effect of various needle tip positions within or adjacent to the intervertebral foramen on immediate pain outcome.

**Methods**

A total of 1,774 cases of intervertebral lumbar nerve blocks performed by our radiology staff between April 7, 1997, and May 31, 2002, were reviewed. Of the 1,774 cases, 1,202 met the study criteria (i.e., a single-level injection in an adult). The position of the needle tip and degree of immediate postinjection pain relief were examined.

**Results**

The blocks resulted in an average pain reduction of 4.14 U, as graded on a 0 to 10 ordinate scale (95% confidence interval, 3.98 to 4.30). The degree of pain reduction was not associated with the needle tip position.

**Conclusions**

Our results suggest that precise needle tip position within or adjacent to the intervertebral foramen made no difference on immediate pain reduction. These findings allow the practitioner more freedom in performing an injection. This study does not evaluate the long-term effects of various needle tip positions in selective lumbar nerve blocks.

17. Haynsworth RF Jr: Selective nerve root blocks: A new technique using electrical stimulation. Pain Physician 6:517–520, 2003.

Selective nerve root blocks (SNRB) have been used for many years as a diagnostic tool in patients with low back pain with radicular symptoms. However, the accuracy, specificity, and sensitivity of these blocks have been questioned as a screening tool for spine surgery. The use of current SNRB techniques relies primarily on the relief of pain when local anesthetic is injected. However, patient responses are often nonspecific, and pain relief after injecting local anesthetic is often difficult to interpret. A new technique for performing SNRB using electrical stimulation is described in this article. The technique has been developed in order to reproduce radicular pain by stimulation with electrical current rather than to rely on a response to local anesthetic injection. The technique decreases the reliance on spread of local anesthetic for interpretation, and, therefore, can reduce false-positive results from too much anesthetic (epidural spread affecting more than one nerve root) or not enough anesthetic (block peripheral to the area of inflammation or the "pain generator"). By stimulating several nerve roots in random order in a blind fashion to the patient, the technique can also eliminate placebo responders.

Sixteen patients from the study have undergone fusion and have been followed for at least 6 months (6 to 24 mo). The mean preoperative Oswestry score was 55; mean 6-month postoperative score was 25. Mean preoperative Visual Analog Scale (VAS) score for back pain was 6.9; the mean 6-month postoperative score was 2.6.

**Discussion**

This is the first description of a novel technique, which through future study and evaluation, may prove a useful method of establishing the diagnosis of discogenic low back pain. In 49% of the patients reported here, the results of the Functional Anesthetic Discogram (FAD) test altered the treatment plan that would have been developed with the results of provocative discography. Early postoperative results of patients selected in this manner treated with fusion are very promising; with larger numbers of patients, we will be able to both refine the technique and more definitively report on the predictive value of the test in evaluating patients with chronic low back pain as surgical candidates. A secure method of diagnosis in the evaluation of patient with putative discogenic low back pain should allow us to significantly improve the outcomes of patients being treated for this clinical problem.

18. Sasso RC, Macadaeg K, Nordman D, Smith M: Selective nerve root injections can predict surgical outcome for lumbar and cervical radiculopathy: Comparison to magnetic resonance imaging. J Spinal Disord Tech 18:471–478, 2005.

**Objective**

Diagnostic selective nerve root injection (SNI) results were analyzed in 101 patients who underwent lumbar or cervical decompression for radiculopathy and compared with surgical outcome 1 year postoperatively. A comparison of surgical outcomes was also examined between magnetic resonance imaging (MRI) and SNI results.

**Results**

Of the 101 patients, 91 (90%) had positive and 10 had negative SNI results at the level operated. Ninety-one percent of the patients with a positive SNI had good surgical outcomes, whereas 60% of the patients with a negative SNI had good outcomes. Of the patients with a positive MRI result, 87% had good surgical outcomes, whereas a similar percentage of the patients with a negative MRI (85%) had good surgical outcomes. When findings between SNI and MRI differed ($n = 20$), surgery at a level consistent with the SNI was more strongly associated with a good surgical outcome. Of the patients with a poor surgical outcome, surgery was most often performed at a level inconsistent with the SNI finding.

**Conclusions**

Our study found that a diagnostic SNI can safely and accurately discern the presence or absence of cervical or lumbar radiculopathy. The diagnostic SNI can persuade surgeons from operating on an initially suspicious, but incorrect, level of radiculopathy. In cases in which MRI findings are equivocal, multilevel, or do not agree with the patient's symptoms, the result of a negative diagnostic SNI (i.e., lack of presence of radiculopathy) becomes superior in predicting the absence of an offending lesion.

19. Datta S, Everett CR, Trescot AM, et al: An updated systematic review of the diagnostic utility of selective nerve root blocks. Pain Physician 10:113–128, 2007.

**Background**

Selective nerve root blocks or transforaminal epidural injections are used for diagnosis and treatment of different spinal disorders. A clear consensus on the use of selective nerve root injections as a diagnostic tool does not currently exist. Additionally, the effectiveness of this procedure as a diagnostic tool is not clear. A systematic review of diagnostic utility of selective nerve root blocks was performed and published in January 2005, which concluded that selective nerve root injections may be helpful as a diagnostic tool in evaluating spinal pain with radicular features, but its role needs to be further clarified.

**Objective**

To evaluate and update the accuracy of selective nerve root injections in diagnosing spinal disorders.

**Study Design**

A systematic review of selective nerve root blocks for the diagnosis of spinal pain.

**Methods**

A systematic review of the literature for clinical studies was performed to assess the accuracy of selective nerve root injections in diagnosing spinal pain. Methodologic quality evaluation was performed using Agency for Healthcare Research and Quality (AHRQ) and Quality Assessment Studies of Diagnostic Accuracy (QUADAS) criteria. Studies were graded and evidence classified into five levels: conclusive, strong, moderate, limited, or indeterminate. An extensive literature search was performed utilizing resources from the library at Vanderbilt University Medical Center, PubMed, EMBASE, BioMed, and Cochrane Reviews. Manual searches of bibliographies of known primary and review articles, and abstracts from scientific meetings within the last 2 years were also reviewed.

**Results**

There is limited evidence on the effectiveness of selective nerve root injections as a diagnostic tool for spinal pain. There is insufficient research for stronger support, but the available literature is supportive of selective nerve root injections as a diagnostic test for equivocal radicular pain. There is moderate evidence for use in the preoperative evaluation of patients with negative or inconclusive imaging studies. The positive predictive value of diagnostic selective nerve root blocks is low, but they have a useful negative predictive value.

**Conclusion**

Selective nerve root injections may be helpful as a diagnostic tool in evaluating spinal pain with radicular features. However, their role needs to be further clarified by additional research and consensus.

20. Castro WMH, Gronemeyer D, Jerosoh J, et al: How reliable is lumbar nerve root sheath infiltration. Eur Spine J 3:255–257, 1994.
21. Wolff AP, Groen GJ, Wilder-Smith OH: Influence of needle-position on lumbar segmental nerve root block selectivity. Reg Anesth Pain Med 31:523–530, 2006.
22. Schutz H, Lougheed WM, Wortzman G, Awerbuck BG: Intervertebral nerve-root in the investigation of chronic lumbar disc disease. Can J Surg 16:217–221, 1973.
23. Dooley JF, McBroom RJ, Taguchi T, Macnab I: Nerve root infiltration in the diagnosis of radicular pain. Spine 13:79–83, 1988.

Clinical and standard radiographic evaluation of patients with lumbosacral radicular symptoms may, on occasion, fail to delineate a cause. This study retrospectively reviews 62 patients who had undergone nerve root infiltration (NRI) and assesses the accuracy and indications for this diagnostic study. Surgical exploration of patients with a Group 1 response (typical pain reproduced by needle placement and then relieved by NRI) confirmed local root pathology in all. Exclusive of patients with arachnoiditis, a Group 1 response showed 85% accuracy in identifying a single symptomatic root. A Group 2 response (typical pain reproduced by needle placement but not relieved by local anesthesia) indicated multiple root involvement. Patients with a Group 3 or Group 4 response (typical pain not reproduced by needle insertion, with or without relief of pain by local anesthesia) were seldom relieved of radicular pain. NRI was most useful in investigation of patients with radicular symptoms in whom other investigations were (1) normal, (2) showed multiple level involvement, or (3) were difficult to interpret because of previous surgery.

24. van Akkerveeken PF: The diagnostic value of nerve root sheath infiltration. Acta Orthop Scand Suppl 251:61–63, 1993.
25. Anderberg L, Annertz M, Rydholm U, et al: Selective diagnostic nerve root block for the evaluation of radicular pain in the multilevel degenerated cervical spine. Eur Spine J 15:794–801, 2006.

    In patients with radiculopathy due to degenerative disease in the cervical spine, surgical outcome is still presenting with moderate results. The preoperative investigations consist of clinical investigation, careful history and most often magnetic resonance imaging (MRI) of the cervical spine. When MRI shows multilevel degeneration, different strategies are used for indicating which nerve root/roots are affected. Some authors use selective diagnostic nerve root blocks (SNRBs) for segregating pain mediating nerve roots from nonpain mediators in such patients. The aim of the present study is to assess the ability of transforaminal SNRBs to correlate clinical symptoms with MRI findings in patients with cervical radiculopathy and a two-level MRI degeneration, on the same side as the radicular pain. Thirty consecutive patients with cervical radiculopathy and two levels of MRI pathology on the same side as the radicular pain were studied with SNRBs at both levels. All patients underwent clinical investigation and neck and arm pain assessment with Visual Analog Scales (VASs) before and after the blocks. The results from the SNRBs were compared with the clinical findings from neurologic investigation as well as the MRI pathology and treatment results. Correlation between SNRB results and the level with most severe degree of MRI degeneration was 60%, and correlation between SNRB results and levels decided by neurologic deficits/dermatome radicular pain distribution was 28%. Twenty-two of the 30 patients underwent treatment guided by the SNRB results, and 18 reported good or excellent outcome results. We conclude that the degree of MRI pathology, neurologic investigation, and the pain distribution in the arm are not reliable parameters enough when deciding the affected nerve root or roots in patients with cervical radiculopathy and a two-level degenerative disease in the cervical spine. SNRB might be a helpful tool together with clinical findings/history and MRI of the cervical spine when performing preoperative investigations in patients with two or more levels of degeneration presenting with radicular pain that can be attributed to the degenerative findings.

26. North RB, Kidd DH, Zahurak M, Piantadosi S: Specificity of diagnostic nerve blocks: a prospective, randomized study of sciatica due to lumbosacral spine disease. Pain 65:77–85, 1996.
27. Riew KD, Park JB, Cho YS, et al: Nerve root blocks in the treatment of lumbar radicular pain: A minimum five-year follow-up. J Bone Joint Surg Am 88:1722–1725, 2006.

    **Background**
    In a previous prospective, randomized, controlled, double-blinded study on the effect of nerve root blocks on the need for operative treatment of lumbar radicular pain, we found that injections of corticosteroids were more effective than bupivacaine for up to 13 to 28 months. We performed a minimum 5-year follow-up of those patients who had avoided surgery.

    **Methods**
    All of the patients were considered to be operative candidates by the treating surgeon, and all had initially requested operative intervention. They had then been randomized to be treated with a selective nerve root block with either bupivacaine or bupivacaine and betamethasone. Both the treating physician and the patient were blinded to the type of medication. Of 55 randomized patients, 29 avoided an operation in the original study. Twenty-one of those 29 patients were reevaluated with a follow-up questionnaire at a minimum of 5 years after the initial block.

    **Results**
    Seventeen of the 21 patients still had not had operative intervention. There was no difference between the group treated with bupivacaine alone and the group treated with bupivacaine and betamethasone with regard to the avoidance of surgery for 5 years. At the 5-year follow-up evaluation, all of the patients who had avoided operative treatment had significant decreases in neurologic symptoms and back pain compared with the baseline values.

    **Conclusions**
    The majority of patients with lumbar radicular pain who avoid an operation for at least 1 year after receiving a nerve root injection with bupivacaine alone or in combination with betamethasone will continue to avoid operative intervention for a minimum of 5 years.

28. Stalcup ST, Crall TS, Gilula L, Riew KD: Influence of needle-tip position on the incidence of immediate complications in 2,217 selective lumbar nerve root blocks. Spine J 6:170–176, 2006.

    **Background**
    Selective lumbar nerve blocks (SLNBs) are a popular, minimally invasive treatment and diagnostic tool for lumbar radiculopathy. Therefore, it is relevant to determine the complication rate for SLNBs, as well as examine the association between needle-tip position and complication rates in order to improve safety.

    **Purpose**
    The purposes of the present study are to determine the overall rate of immediate postprocedural complications in a large cohort of patients who received SLNBs and if certain needle-tip positions are less likely to cause complications. To our knowledge, this is the first paper to examine the relationship between needle-tip position and complications.

    **Study Design**
    A large retrospective cohort was assembled from patients who had undergone a SLNB. We determined the overall immediate complication rate for all injections. In addition, all patients who received only a single injection were compiled into another cohort, and needle-tip position was determined. The complication rate was determined for each needle-tip position.

    **Patient Sample**
    All adult patients who underwent a SLNB in a single radiology department from April 1, 1997, to May 31, 2002.

    **Outcome Measures**
    Patients were observed for 15 to 30 minutes after their procedure, then interviewed about any self-reported weakness, light-headedness, increase in pain from the preprocedural levels, or development of new pain. Their postprocedural pain was then rated on the Visual Analog Scale. The radiologic notes from each examination were reviewed for incidence of these, or any other, complications.

    **Methods**
    SLNBs were performed as they would be in the normal course of care, using fluoroscopic guidance and methodology established by a single radiologist overseeing the procedures. The radiologist's record of each visit was examined for note of immediate postprocedural complications. The radiographs from the patients who received a single injection during their visit were examined to determine the position of the needle tip during the procedure. The needle-tip positions from the "Complications" and "No Complications" single-injection cohorts were compared to determine if certain needle tip positions cause less complications than others.

    **Results**
    Minor complications were encountered in 98 of the 1,777 total patient visits, for an overall complication rate of 5.5%. All complications were transient, and no patient suffered lasting harm. There were 1,232 procedures in which the patient received a single injection, and a minor complication was encountered in 62 of these visits. The complication rate approached 5% for all needle-tip positions, which is not statistically different from the overall complication rate. However, there was an

increased likelihood of complications in patients undergoing a multiple-injection procedure versus those who had only one injection.

**Conclusions**

Our results suggest that SLNBs performed with fluoroscopic guidance have a low incidence of complications. All of the complications in our study were minor. The specific needle tip position within or adjacent to the lumbar neural foramen does not appear to be associated with the incidence of complications.

29. McCall IW, Park WM, O'Brien JP, et al: Induced pain referral from posterior lumbar elements in normal subjects. Spine 4:441–446, 1979.

Patterns of pain referral, induced from the posterior elements, have been studied in normal volunteer subjects. A series of intracapsular and pericapsular injections were performed at the L1-2 and L4-5 levels. The areas of pain referral indicate overlap between the upper and lower lumbar spine. It is also shown that the pericapsular and intrafacetal pain referral areas are similar and that the upper lumbar spine is more sensitive than the lower.

30. Marks RC, Houston T, Thulbourne T, et al: Facet joint injection and facet nerve block: A randomised comparison in 86 patients with chronic low back pain. Pain 49:325–328, 1992.

Eighty-six patients with refractory chronic low back pain were randomly assigned to receive either facet joint injection or facet nerve block, using local anesthetic and steroid. There was no significant difference in the immediate response. The duration of response after facet joint injection was marginally longer than after facet nerve block ($P<0.05$ 1 month after infiltration), but for both groups, the response was usually short lived; by 3 months, only two patients continued to report complete pain relief. Patients who had complained of pain for more than 7 years were more likely to report good or excellent pain relief than those with a shorter history ($P<0.005$), but no other clinical feature was of value in predicting the response to infiltration. Facet joint injections and facet nerve blocks may be of equal value as diagnostic tests, but neither is a satisfactory treatment for chronic back pain.

31. Hirsch C, Ingelmark BE, Miller M, et al: The anatomical basis for low back pain: Studies on the presence of sensory nerve endings in ligamentous, capsular and intervertebral disc structures in the human lumbar spine. Acta Orthop Scand 33:1–17, 1963.
32. Helbig T, Lee CK: The lumbar facet syndrome. Spine 13(7):61–64, 1988.
33. Dreyfuss PH, Dreyer SJ, Herring S: Lumbar zygapophysial (facet) joint injections. Spine 20(18):2040–2047, 1995.
34. Dreyer SJ, Dreyfuss PH: Low back pain and the zygapophysial (facet) joints. Arch Phys Med Rehabil 77(3):290–300, 1996.
35. Nash TP: Facet joints: intra-articular steroids or nerve block? Pain Clin 3:77–82, 1990.
36. Jackson RP, Jacobs RR, Montesano PX: 1988 Volvo award in clinical sciences. Facet joint injection in low-back pain. A prospective statistical study. Spine 13(9):966–971, 1988.
37. Carrera GF, Williams AL: Current concepts in evaluation of the lumbar facet joints. Crit Rev Diagn Imaging 21(2):85–104, 1984.
38. Kaplan M, Dreyfuss PH, Halbook B, Bogduk N: The ability of lumbar medial branch blocks to anesthetize the zygapophysial joint. A physiologic challenge. Spine 23(17):1847–1852, 1998.
39. Schwarzer AC, Aprill CN, Derby R, et al: The false-positive rate of uncontrolled diagnostic blocks of the lumbar zygapophysial joints. Pain 58:195–200, 1994.

One hundred and seventy-six consecutive patients with chronic low back pain and no history of previous lumbar surgery were studied to determine the false-positive rate of single diagnostic blocks of the lumbar zygapophysial joints. All patients underwent diagnostic blocks using lignocaine. Those patients who obtained definite or complete relief from these blocks subsequently underwent confirmatory blocks using bupivacaine. Eighty-three patients (47%) had a definite or greater response to the initial, lignocaine injection at one or more levels, but only 26 (15%) had a 50% or greater response to a confirmatory injection of 0.5% bupivacaine. Using the response to confirmatory blocks as the criterion standard, the false-positive rate of uncontrolled diagnostic blocks was 38% and the positive predictive value of these blocks was only 31%. Because the positive predictive value of a test is lower when the pretest probability (prevalence) is low, and because the prevalence of lumbar zygapophysial joint pain is likely to be less than 50%, uncontrolled diagnostic blocks will always be associated with an unacceptably low positive predictive value. These features render uncontrolled diagnostic blocks unreliable for the diagnosis of lumbar zygapophysial joint pain, not only in epidemiologic studies but also in any given patient.

40. Dreyfuss PH, Dreyer SJ: Lumbar zygapophysial (facet) joint injections. Spine J 3:50S–59S, 2003.
41. Lindblom K: Technique and results of diagnostic disc puncture and injection (discography) in the lumbar region. Acta Orthop Scand 20:315–326, 1951.
42. Guyer RD, Ohnmeiss DD: Lumbar discography: Position statement from the North American Spine Society Diagnostic and Therapeutic Committee. Spine 20:2048–2059, 1995.

**Texas Back Institute, Plano, Texas, and the Institute for Spine and Biomedical Research, Plano**

**Study Design**

A comprehensive review of the literature dealing with lumbar discography was conducted.

**Objective**

The purpose of the review was to generate a position statement addressing criticisms of lumbar discography, identify indications for its use, and describe a technique for its performance.

**Summary of Background Data**

Lumbar discography remains a controversial diagnostic procedure. There are concerns about its safety and clinical value, although others support its use in specific applications.

**Methods**

Articles dealing with lumbar discography were reviewed and summarized in this report.

**Results**

Most of the recent literature supports the use of discography in select patients. Although not to be taken lightly, many of the serious and high complication rates were reported before 1970 and have decreased since because of improvement in injection technique, imaging, and contrast materials.

**Conclusions**

Most of the current literature supports the use of discography in select situations. Particular applications include patients with persistent pain in whom disc abnormality is suspect, but noninvasive tests have not provided sufficient diagnostic information or the images need to be correlated with clinical symptoms. Another application is assessment of discs in patients in whom fusion is being considered. Discography's role in such cases is to determine if discs within the proposed fusion segment are symptomatic and if the adjacent discs are normal. Discography appears to be helpful in patients who have previously undergone surgery but continue to experience significant pain. In such cases, it can be used to differentiate between postoperative scar and recurrent disc herniation and to investigate the condition of a disc within, or adjacent to, a fused spinal segment to better delineate the source of symptoms. When minimally invasive discectomy is being considered, discography can be used to confirm a contained disc herniation, which is generally an indication for such surgical procedures. Lumbar discography should be performed by those well experienced with the procedure and in sterile conditions with a double-needle technique and fluoroscopic imaging for proper needle placement. Information assessed and recorded should include the volume of contrast injected, pain response with particular emphasis on its location and similarity to clinical symptoms, and the pattern of dye distribution. Frequently, discography is followed by axial computed tomography scanning to obtain more information about the condition of the disc.

43. Carragee EJ, Alamin TF: Discography: A review. Spine J 1:364–372, 2001.
44. Holt EPJ: Fallacy of cervical discography: Report of 50 cases in normal subjects. JAMA 188:799–801, 1964.
45. Walsh TR, Weinstein JN, Spratt KF, et al: Lumbar discography in normal subjects: A controlled, prospective study. J Bone Joint Surg Am 72:1081–1088, 1990.

**Department of Orthopaedic Surgery, University of Iowa Hospitals and Clinics, Iowa City**

Major advances in the techniques of discography since 1968, in conjunction with major strides in the evaluation of pain in recent years prompted a study in which Holt's work on the specificity of discography was replicated and extended. For the present study, seven patients who had low back pain and 10 volunteers, who had been carefully screened, with a questionnaire and a physical examination to ensure that they had no history of problems with the back, had an injection at three levels, and all sessions were videotaped. After each injection, the participant was interviewed about the pattern and intensity of the pain, and then the discs were imaged with computed tomography. Five raters, who were blind to the condition of the participant, graded each disc as normal or abnormal on the basis of findings on magnetic resonance images that had been made before the injection and computed tomography (discography) were done. There was only one disagreement between the ratings that were made on the basis of the magnetic resonance images and those that were made on the basis of the discograms. Each participant's pain-related response was evaluated independently by two raters who viewed the videotapes of the discography. Inter-rater reliability was 0.99, 0.93, and 0.88 for the evaluation of intensity of the pain, pain-related behavior, and similarity of the pain to pain that the subject had had before the injection. In the asymptomatic individuals, the discogram was interpreted as abnormal for 17% (five) of the 30 discs and for five of the 10 subjects.

46. Carragee EJ, Alamin TF, Miller J, Grafe M: Provocative discography in volunteer subjects with mild persistent low back pain. Spine J 2:25–34, 2002.

**Background Context**

Whether discographic injections would be positive in subjects with benign persistent "backache" who are not seeking treatment is unknown. This information is important, because benign backache undoubtedly coexists in patients with chronic low back pain (CLBP) illness that is not discogenic in origin. If these subjects had a high rate of positive discography, the high background incidence of common backache would allow many positive tests in patients in whom discogenic processes were unrelated to their severe CLBP illness. Conversely, if subjects with benign low back pain rarely, if ever, had significant concordant pain reproduction on disc injections, the basic tenet of discographic diagnosis would be strengthened.

**Purpose**

To compare, using a strict experimental design, the relative pain and concordancy response to provocative discography in subjects with clinically insignificant "backache" and clinical subjects with CLBP illness considering surgical treatment.

**Study Design**

Comparison of experimental disc injections in subjects with mild persistent backache and those with CLBP illness.

**Patient Sample**

Twenty-five subjects with mild persistent low back pain (LBP) were recruited for an experimental discography study. Subjects were recruited from a clinical study of patients having had cervical spine surgery. Inclusion criteria required that subjects not be receiving or seeking medical treatment for LBP, be taking no medications for backache, have no activity restrictions because of LBP, and have normal psychometric scores. To more closely approximate the pain behavior in CLBP illness, 50% (12) of the "backache" group were recruited with a chronic painful condition (neck/shoulder) unrelated to the low back. CLBP subjects, patients coming to discography for consideration of surgical treatment, were used as control subjects.

**Outcome Measures**

Results of discography were determined using the criteria of Walsh et al pain response of 3 or greater, two or more pain behaviors, a negative "control" discographic injection, and a similar or exact concordancy rating.

**Methods**

Discography was performed on experimental subjects and control patients. Experienced raters, who were blinded to control versus experimental status of the subjects, scored the magnetic resonance image, discogram, psychometric tests, and discography videotapes of the subjects' pain behavior.

**Results**

Thirteen of 25 volunteer subjects had pain rated as "bad" or worse with disc injection. There were 12 painful and fully concordant disc injections in nine of these 25 "backache" subjects (36%). These injections met all the Walsh et al criteria for a positive diagnosis of discogenic pain. All positive discs had annular disruption to or through the outer annulus. Of the nine subjects with positive discograms, three had no chronic pain states and six did. All subjects with positive injections had negative control discs. In comparison, in 52 subjects with CLBP illness, 38 (73%) had at least one positive disc injection.

**Conclusions**

In a group of volunteer subjects with persistent "backache," 36% were found to have significant pain on disc injection, which is reported to be concordant with their usual pain. The presence of positive concordant pain responses and negative control discs in 33% of subjects without CLBP illness seriously challenges the specificity of provocative discography in identifying a clinically relevant spinal pathology.

47. Derby R, Lee SH, et al: Pressure-controlled lumbar discography in volunteers without low back symptoms. Pain Med 6:213–221, 2005.
48. Carragee EJ, Chen Y, Tanner CM, et al: Provocative discography in patients after limited lumbar discectomy: A controlled, randomized study of pain response in symptomatic and asymptomatic subjects. Spine 25:3065–3071, 2000.

**Study Design**

This was a prospective observational study of patients with low back pain and those without after laminotomy and discectomy.

**Objectives**

To determine, using a strict experimental design, the relative pain intensity response to provocative discography in symptomatic and asymptomatic subjects after lumbar discectomy for intervertebral disc herniation.

**Background**

Provocative discography frequently is used to evaluate persistent or recurrent low back pain syndromes in patients who have undergone posterior discectomy. The validity of interpreting painful injections during this procedure has not been critically assessed. The prevalence of significantly painful disc injections in a group with good outcomes after surgery is not known. Knowing the rates of significantly painful injections in asymptomatic patients after lumbar discectomy may clarify the meaning of painful injections in symptomatic patients.

**Methods**

From a cohort of 240 patients who had undergone single-level limited discectomy for sciatica, 20 asymptomatic volunteers were recruited for experimental three-level lumbar discography. Inclusion criteria required nearly perfect scores on standardized back pain rating instruments, no other spinal pathology, and normal psychometric screening.

A control group of 27 symptomatic patients, after single-level discectomy with intractable low back pain syndrome and without other spinal pathology, underwent discography. Seven patients in the control group had normal psychometric tests. Experienced raters who were blinded to control versus experimental status of the subjects scored the magnetic resonance imaging, discogram, psychometric tests, and discography videotapes of the subjects' pain behavior.

**Results**

There were eight of 20 (40%) positive injections of discs that had previous surgery in the asymptomatic group and 17 of 27 (63%) positive injections in the symptomatic group. Specifically with regard to the symptomatic group, there were three of seven (43%) positive injections (all concordant) in patients with normal psychometric scores, as compared with 14 of 20 (70%) positive injections (12 concordant) in patients with abnormal psychometric scores. Injections of discs that had previous surgery resulted in a mean pain score of 2.1 of 5 in the asymptomatic group, 2.1 in the symptomatic group with normal psychometric scores, and 3.4 in the symptomatic group with abnormal psychometric scores. Of the discs not treated with surgery, two were positive in the asymptomatic group (10%), three in two symptomatic subjects with normal psychological testing (29), and 18 in 13 symptomatic subjects with abnormal psychometric testing (76%).

**Conclusions**

A high percentage of asymptomatic patients with normal psychometric testing who previously have undergone lumbar discectomy will have significant pain on injection of their discs that had previous surgery (40%). This is not significantly different from the experience of symptomatic patients with normal psychometric testing undergoing discography on discs that had previous surgery. Patients with abnormal psychological profiles have significantly higher rates of positive disc injections than either asymptomatic volunteers or symptomatic subjects with normal psychological screening.

49. Carragee EJ, Paragioudakis SJ, Khuana S, et al: 2000 Volvo Award winner in clinical studies: Lumbar high-intensity zone and discography in subjects without low back problems. Spine 25:2987–2992, 2000.

**Study Design**

A prospective observational study of patients with low back pain and those without was performed.

**Objective**

To investigate the prevalence and significance of a high-intensity zone in a group of patients asymptomatic for low back pain, but who had known risk factors for lumbar disc degeneration. This asymptomatic group was compared with a symptomatic group of patients with respect to the presence of annular high-intensity zone and the pain response with discography.

**Summary of Background Data**

Some authors have estimated the prevalence of a high-intensity zone in a group of symptomatic patients to be 86%. They have reported a strong correlation between a high-intensity zone and positive discography in patients with low back pain. Other investigators have reported evidence either supporting or discounting these findings.

**Methods**

Patients with low back pain and those without underwent physical examination, psychometric testing, plain radiograph, magnetic resonance imaging, and discography. The presence of a high-intensity zone, annular disruption, and positive discographic pain was then compared between the two groups. There were strict inclusion criteria for both groups. A total of 109 discs in 42 patients were evaluated in the symptomatic group and compared with 143 discs in 54 patients in the asymptomatic group. The presence of a high-intensity zone was determined by a standardized criteria on T2-weighted magnetic resonance images. Psychometric testing also was administered to each patient before discography. Standard discography was performed on all the patients, and the pain response was recorded using a visual analog scale according to the Walsh et al criteria.

**Results**

The prevalence of a high-intensity zone in the patient populations was 59% in the symptomatic group and 24% in the asymptomatic group. In the symptomatic group, 33 (30.2%) of 109 discs were found to have a high-intensity zone. In the asymptomatic group, 13 of 143 discs were found to have a high-intensity zone. In the symptomatic group, 72.7% of the discs with a high-intensity zone were positive on discography, whereas 38.2% of the discs without a high-intensity zone were positive. In the asymptomatic group, 69.2% of the discs with a high-intensity zone were positive on discography, whereas 10% of the discs without a high-intensity zone were positive. In the patients with normal psychometric testing, 50% of the discs with a high-intensity zone were positive on discography, as compared with 100% positive discography results in patients with abnormal psychometric testing or chronic pain.

**Conclusions**

The presence of a high-intensity zone does not reliably indicate the presence of symptomatic internal disc disruption. Although higher in symptomatic patients, the prevalence of a high-intensity zone in asymptomatic individuals with degenerative disc disease (25%) is too high for meaningful clinical use. When injected during discography, the same percentage of asymptomatic and symptomatic discs with a high-intensity zone was shown to be painful.

50. Carragee EJ, Tanner CM, Yang B, et al: False-positive findings on lumbar discography: Reliability of subjective concordance assessment. Spine 24:2542–2547, 1999.

**Stanford University School of Medicine, California**

**Study Design**

Experimental disc injections in subjects with no history of low back symptoms.

**Objective**

To determine in an experimental model the reliability of patients' subjective interpretation of pain concordancy during provocative disc injection.

**Background**

Discography in the evaluation of low back pain relies on a patient's subjective assessment of pain magnitude and quality during disc injection. Reproduction of significant pain on disc injection, which is similar to patients' usual pain, is believed to prove that the disc injected is the source of the patient's low back pain. In the current study, this hypothesis was tested in a controlled setting on patients with known nonspinal pain in a common referral area of discogenic pain.

**Methods**

Patients with no history of low back pain were recruited to participate in a study of discography. Patients scheduled to undergo posterior iliac crest bone graft harvesting for nonthoracolumbar procedures were evaluated with lumbar radiography, magnetic resonance imaging, and psychometric testing. Two to 4 months after bone graft harvesting, patients underwent lumbar discography by strict blinded protocol. Patients were asked to compare the sensations elicited at discography to their usual back/buttock pain since bone graft harvesting. Pain was rated as 0 to 5 on a pain thermometer, and concordancy was rated as none, dissimilar, similar, or exact.

**Results**

Eight subjects completed the study, and 24 discs were injected. Of the 14 disc injections causing some pain response, five were believed to be "different" (nonconcordant) pains (35.7%), seven were "similar" (50.0%), and two were "exact" pain reproductions (14.3%). The presence of annular disruption predicted concordant pain reproduction ($P<0.05$). Of 10 discs with annular tears, injection of five elicited pain that was similar to or an exact reproduction of pain at the iliac crest bone graft harvest sites. By the usual criteria for positive discography, four of the eight patients (50%) would have been classified as positive. In these patients, the pain on a single disc injection was very painful, and the pain quality was noted to be exact or similar to the usual discomfort. All subjects had a negative control disc.

**Conclusions**

The findings of this study demonstrate that patients with no history of low back pain who had undergone posterior iliac bone graft harvesting for nonlumbar procedures often experienced a concordant painful sensation on lumbar discography with their usual gluteal area pain. Thus, the ability of a patient to separate spinal from nonspinal sources of pain on discography is questioned, and a response of concordant pain on discography may be less meaningful than often assumed.

51. Carragee EJ, Alamin TF, Carragee JM: Low-pressure positive discography in subjects asymptomatic of significant low back pain illness. Spine 31(5):505–509, 2006.
52. Olerud S, Hamberg M: External fixation as a test for instability after spinal fusion L4-S1. A case report. Orthopedics 9(4):547–549, 1986.
53. Bednar DA: Failure of external spinal skeletal fixation to improve predictability of lumbar arthrodesis. J Bone Joint Surg Am 83-A:1656–1659, 2001.

**Background**

Whether lumbar arthrodesis can relieve isolated low back pain in the absence of focal neurological findings or instability is unclear. The results of published studies are also inconsistent with regard to whether temporary back pain relief with external spinal skeletal fixation can predict lasting back pain relief after arthrodesis. This report presents the results, with regard to clinical benefit and complications, of more than 100 external spinal skeletal fixation procedures undertaken as a prelude to lumbar arthrodesis.

**Methods**

The records of all patients who underwent external spinal skeletal fixation between 1989 and 1999 were reviewed with attention to perioperative complications, pain relief from the test procedure, the clinical benefit from a subsequent arthrodesis, and the functional status after the arthrodesis. Analyzed data included the frequency of neurological complications and infections and the benefit (Prolo score) after staged spinal arthrodesis in patients who underwent arthrodesis after temporarily experiencing pain relief with the test procedure.

**Results**

A total of 103 external spinal skeletal fixation procedures were undertaken. Neurological complications occurred in two procedures (2%); one resulted in permanent sciatica. Infections occurred in five patients (5%). Sixty patients experienced pain relief during the external fixation test, but only 27 of 49 patients who went on to have an arthrodesis and had sufficient follow-up reported that they were doing well at a minimum of one year later. In no case did the external spinal skeletal fixation procedure cause a permanent increase in low back pain.

**Conclusions**

On the basis of this analysis, external spinal skeletal fixation should not be used as a predictor of pain relief after lumbar arthrodesis.

54. Elmans L, Willems PC, Anderson PG, et al: Temporary external transpedicular fixation of the lumbosacral spine: a prospective, longitudinal study in 330 patients. Spine 30:2813–2816, 2005.

**Study Design**

In this study, 330 patients with incapacitating low back pain underwent temporary external transpedicular fixation (TETF) of the lumbosacral spine in a prospective trial.

**Objective**

To evaluate TETF as a test for selecting suitable candidates for segmental spinal fusion.

**Summary of Background Data**

Few studies regarding TETF have been published, and contradictory results concerning predictive value and morbidity were reported.

**Methods**

All patients were tested with the external fixator in two different positions: fixation and nonfixation. Before and during the test and at follow-up examination, pain was assessed on a Visual Analog Scale (VAS). The TETF test was considered to be positive if the VAS score in the fixation state was 30 or more points lower than in the nonfixation state. Hence, a positive test would imply the decision to perform segmental lumbosacral fusion. When the reduction was less than 30 points, the test was negative. Individual pain reduction and working capacity were taken as measure of outcome.

**Results**

Most of the patients in this study (62%) underwent spinal surgery previously. The positive and negative TETF groups were quite similar, but a large within-group variation was found. Within the fusion group of 123 patients, improvement in VAS scores and improvement in working capacity were not significantly better for the positive TETF group in comparison with the negative TETF group.

**Conclusion**

In this heterogeneous group of chronic patients with low back pain, TETF of the spine (including a placebo trial) does not appear to be of value in selecting suitable candidates for spinal fusion.

55. van der Schaaf DB, van Limbeek J, Pavlov PW: Temporary external transpedicular fixation of the lumbosacral spine. Spine 24:481–484; discussion 484–485, 1999.

**Study Design**

In this study, 133 patients with incapacitating low back pain underwent temporary external transpedicular fixation of the lumbosacral spine in a prospective trial. Of these patients, 67% had undergone one or more spinal procedures in the past. On the basis of temporary external transpedicular fixation, 55 of 133 patients were treated conservatively. With an average follow-up period of 37 months, the clinical results were analyzed.

**Objective**

To evaluate temporary external transpedicular fixation as a test for selecting suitable candidates for fusion of the lumbosacral spine.

**Summary of Background Data**

The few reports regarding this test are contradictory in terms of predictive value and morbidity. Only three reports include a placebo trial.

**Methods**

All patients were tested with the external fixator in three different positions: neutral fixation, slight distraction, and nonfixation (bars disconnected). The patient was unaware of the exact position of the external fixator and thus served as his or her own control. Before and during the test and at follow-up examination, pain was assessed on a Visual Analog Scale (VAS).

**Results**

In the group that eventually underwent spinal fusion, the average preoperation VAS score was 77. During test fixation, the average score was 26; in nonfixation, 69; and at follow-up after surgery, 40. In the control group, these figures were 75, 53, 44, and 71, respectively. As statistical analysis showed, the only factors that could be associated with the improved pain score were the performance of the spinal fusion ($P = 0.0001$) and the duration of low back pain before the test ($P = 0.04$).

**Conclusion**

In selecting suitable candidates for spinal fusion, temporary external transpedicular fixation (including a placebo trial) can be a valuable test.

56. Soini J, Slätis P, Kannisto M, Sandelin J: External transpedicular fixation test of the lumbar spine correlates with the outcome of subsequent lumbar fusion. Clin Orthop Relat Res 293:89–96, 1993.

External transpedicular fixation was applied to the lower lumbar spine in a prospective study on 42 patients with chronic low back pain combined with suspected instability of the lumbar segments; the diagnosis was failed disc surgery, spondylolisthesis, and degenerative disc disease. The aim was to realign the involved segments, to restore disc height, and to record changes in pain and performance during the external fixation test. Pain was recorded on a Visual Analog Scale (VAS), and performance was assessed using the Oswestry Disability Score. An independent observer assessed the test and treatment results. Twenty-nine patients experienced relief of pain and performed better in the fixator; they were subjected to anterior interbody fusion, the external frame being kept as a stabilizing device for an additional 4 months. Twenty-two patients have had follow-up evaluations for 2 years. One and 2 years after successful lumbar fusion, significantly ($P$<0.02) better pain and performance scores were recorded; the results of lumbar fusion corresponded to the preoperative fixation test. A temporary external fixation test may be a useful procedure in patients considered for subsequent spondylodesis.

57. Alamin TF, Malek F: The functional anaesthetic discogram: Description of a novel diagnostic technique and report of three cases. 2006 (in press).

**Background Context**

The diagnostic evaluation of patients with presumed discogenic low back pain is controversial; recent studies have brought the specificity of the traditional technique, provocative lumbar discography, into question. One of the explanations for the relative lack of predictability in treatment outcomes for patients with discogenic low back pain may be a corresponding lack of certainty in the diagnosis.

**Purpose**

A new diagnostic technique is described for the evaluation of patients with presumptive discogenic low back pain; three patients in whom the technique was used are presented.

**Study Design/Setting**

Case series/University practice

**Methods**

A technique is described in which an anesthetic catheter is placed into putative symptomatic lumbar discs, the patient elicits his or her typical pain through a position or activity, and anesthetic or placebo is delivered to the disc. The effect of the injected substance on the patient's pain is then noted.

**Results**

In one patient, the new test was confirmatory of the results of the provocative discogram; in two patients, the test results were divergent.

**Conclusions**

These case studies and technical description are presented as a first step in examining this method of preoperative assessment. Further study of the technique will allow us to make more definitive recommendations with regard to its validity and utility.

58. Roth DA: Cervical analgesic discography: A new test for the definitive diagnosis of the painful-disk syndrome. JAMA 235:1713–1714, 1976.

The cervical discogenic (painful disc) syndrome consists of scapular pain radiating into the head, shoulder, and upper arm, often associated with paresthesias but without neurologic deficit. Plain roentgenograms or myelograms are normal or show degenerative changes. Positive-contrast discography has been useful but is subject to a high percentage of false-positive results roentgenographically and nonspecific pain patterns clinically. Analgesic discography more precisely confirms the diagnosis and more accurately locates the pain-producing disc. Injection of a local anesthetic into a painful disc produces transient symptomatic relief and full neck mobility. Its use during a 2-year period in 71 consecutive discogenic patients followed by anterior cervical fusion resulted in a 93% excellent or good recovery rate. Analgesic discography is the most effective test for diagnosis and location in the painful-disc syndrome.

59. Osler GEL: Cervical analgesic discography: A test for diagnosis of the painful disc syndrome. S Afr Med J 71:363, 1987.

The cervical discogenic (painful disc) syndrome consists of scapular pain radiating to the head, shoulder, and upper arm, often associated with paraesthesiae but without neurological deficit. Analgesic discography confirms the diagnosis and more accurately locates the pain-producing disc. In this series of patients, analgesic discography followed by anterior cervical fusion with or without discectomy resulted in an 81% excellent or good result. Analgesic discography is the most effective test for location of the lesion in the painful disc syndrome.

60. Alamin TF, Argarwal V, et al: FAD vs. Provocative Discography: Comparative results and postoperative clinical outcomes. NASS Proceedings, 2007.

**Functional Anesthetic Discogram Versus Provocative Discography: Comparative Results and Postoperative Clinical Outcomes**

**Introduction**

To address problems with the diagnosis of discogenic low back pain, we have designed a new test, the functional anesthetic discogram (FAD). This test involves the performance of a standard provocative discogram, followed by the placement of a catheter into the putative disc or discs found to be concordantly painful on injection. The patient then assumes a position that would ordinarily cause him or her pain. Anesthetic is then delivered into the disc, and pain relief in that position is recorded.

**Study**

We performed this study to determine the results of the FAD in 31 patients with chronic low back pain and compared these with the results of standard provocative discography in this group of patients.

**Study Design/Setting**

This study was an IRB-approved, prospective clinical trial of a novel technique performed in a university practice.

**Patient Sample**

Forty patients (21 women, 20 men) with chronic low back pain referred on for surgical consultation.

**Outcomes Measures**

Prestudy Visual Analog Scale (VAS), Oswestry, and DRAM scales were recorded; during the test, VAS scales, pain concordancy, and pressurization data were recorded. Postoperative VAS and Oswestry scores, along with pain medication use and activity level, were recorded, with minimum 6-month postoperative follow-up reported here.

**Methods**

The FAD was performed as described earlier. Patients with positive test results underwent instrumented lumbar fusions at the levels selected in this manner.

**Results**

Seven of the 41 (17%) patients had two-level findings on provocative discography that were reduced to one-level findings on the FAD test. Eleven patients (27%) had positive provocative discograms that were negative on FAD testing. Two patients (5%) had a negative provocative discogram, and yet pain relief on the FAD. Twenty-one patients (51%) had confirmatory findings on the FAD test. DRAM profile of DD or DS was a significant predictor of negative findings on the FAD test.

CHAPTER 12

# Adjacent Segment Degeneration and Adjacent Segment Disease: Cervical and Lumbar

**Andrew P. White, David Hannallah,** and **Alan S. Hilibrand**

### KEY POINTS

- Altered biomechanics after spinal fusion and the perceived associated risk of adjacent segment disease is one rationale for the development of arthroplasty as an alternative to fusion.
- The causal relationship between fusion and adjacent segment disease remains controversial.
- The role of arthroplasty in preventing exacerbation of neighboring joint degeneration is not yet well established.

## INTRODUCTION

Although generally successful in treating degenerative spinal conditions associated with instability, there are real and perceived shortcomings of spinal fusion. In the lumbar spine, the poor predictability of fusion outcomes has been one limitation. In both the lumbar and the cervical spine, potential untoward consequences of spinal fusion include pseudarthrosis, bone graft harvest morbidity, and adjacent segment disease. Because of these concerns, motion-preserving treatments, including total disc arthroplasty, have gained popularity as an alternative method of treating degenerative conditions in the cervical and lumbar spine.

Most surgeons believe that a surgical alteration in spinal anatomy through spinal fusion will result in an alteration in spinal biomechanics. For example, a segmental fusion has been shown to increase adjacent disc pressures[1,2] and adjacent vertebral motion.[3,4] Many surgeons also intuitively believe that these altered biomechanics will cause a change in the natural history of degeneration at that level. The causal relationship between these events, however, and their clinical significance is the subject of an important debate.

This debate is complex because much of the biomechanical and clinical evidence regarding the cause of adjacent segment disease is anecdotal and inconsistent. This chapter presents the evidence related to the development of adjacent segment changes in the cervical and lumbar spine. In addition, potential causal relationships between surgical alterations in anatomy (including fusion and arthroplasty) and adjacent level changes are considered.

For the purposes of this chapter, we define adjacent segment degeneration as the radiographic findings of arthrosis at vertebral motion segments adjacent to a fused or surgically altered segment. The use of this phrase does not connote anything in the way of clinical disease related to these changes. The term adjacent segment disease, however, will be used to refer to the symptoms that may be associated with these radiographic changes. This distinction is made because radiographic degeneration frequently does not correlate with the symptoms of adjacent segment disease in either the cervical[5,6] or lumbar[7] spine.

## SPINAL BIOMECHANICS AND THE ADJACENT LEVEL

One implicit goal of spinal arthroplasty is to re-create normal intervertebral mechanics and allow long-term motion, which may preclude or delay the development of adjacent segment changes. The normal intervertebral disc, however, is a highly complex and elegant structure, and it is unclear how closely an implant must mimic the normal intervertebral kinematics to achieve this goal.

If adjacent segment disease is related to abnormal mechanics, and if arthroplasty aims to prevent it by restoring normal motion, then a detailed comprehension of intervertebral kinematics is essential. The complex relationship between two vertebrae, including the intervening disc, paired facet joints, and related ligaments, dictates the mechanical goals of disc replacement. The intervertebral linkage is subjected to complex loading conditions. Motion in one plane is always coupled with motion in another plane. For example, axial rotation is characteristically coupled with lateral bending (Figs. 12–1 and 12–2). Early anatomic investigations first established this connection by considering the anatomic relationships among the bony and ligamentous structures.[8] More recently, the normal parameters of coupled motion have been accurately measured in vivo in both the cervical[9,10] and lumbar[11] spine. If an arthroplasty is to re-create normal physiologic motion in the effort of preventing adjacent segment changes, it may need to re-create this complex coupled motion.

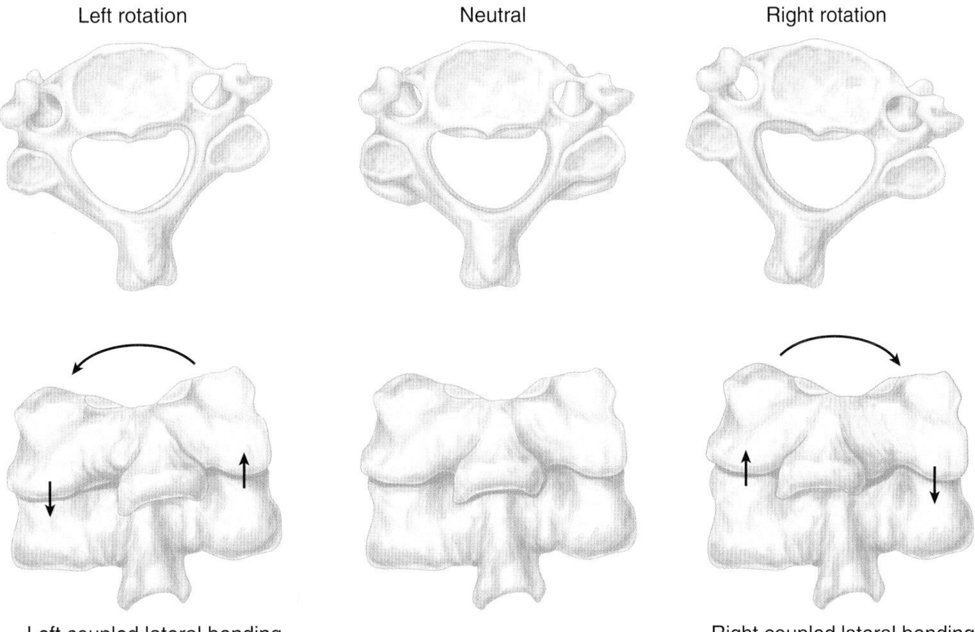


■ **FIGURE 12–1.** Depiction of coupled motion in the cervical spine. Here, the normal coupling between axial rotation and lateral bending is demonstrated.

To achieve coupled motion, the center of rotation (COR) between vertebrae must remain mobile. The path of the instantaneous COR can be used to describe the characteristic coupled motions of the normal spine.[12] For example, with a normal lumbar flexion-extension motion arc, the instantaneous COR moves along an elliptic pathway (Fig. 12–3) because flexion-extension is necessarily coupled to translation.[13] In the cervical spine, the flexion-extension COR traces a path in the subjacent vertebral body.[14] The character of coupled motion is level dependent in the human spinal column and changes with the facet joint orientation.[15] In the cervical spine, the facets are oriented in a relatively coronal plane, and provide limited resistance to flexion-extension and lateral bending. In the lumbar spine, however, the facet joints are oriented in a more sagittal plane and, therefore, restrict rotational motion.

One of the benefits of spinal fusion is the control over alignment. An anatomic relationship is surgically determined and becomes permanent once the goal of bony fusion is met. If the postoperative alignment is not correct, however, fusion may more dramatically change the forces imparted upon the adjacent motion segments. But if anatomic alignment is achieved, spinal fusion may alleviate the dilemma of balancing forces in the three-joint complex. Because fusion involves eliminating motion at the level being addressed, consideration of facet load at that level and the preservation of coupled motion both become immaterial.

## FUSION BIOMECHANICS: CERVICAL

In vitro studies suggest that cervical fusion alters the kinematics of the adjacent segments when compared with unfused intact specimens and with cervical arthroplasty devices. A cadaver study has established that the motion lost at a fused level is compensated by an increase in motion at the adjacent levels.[3] Additionally, an increase in flexion intradiscal pressures of 73% and 45%,

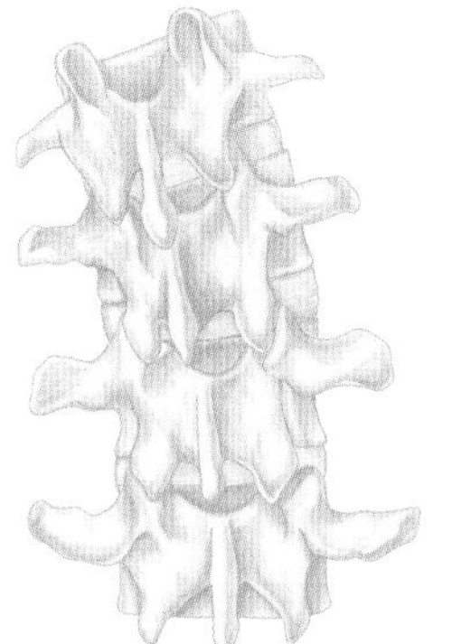
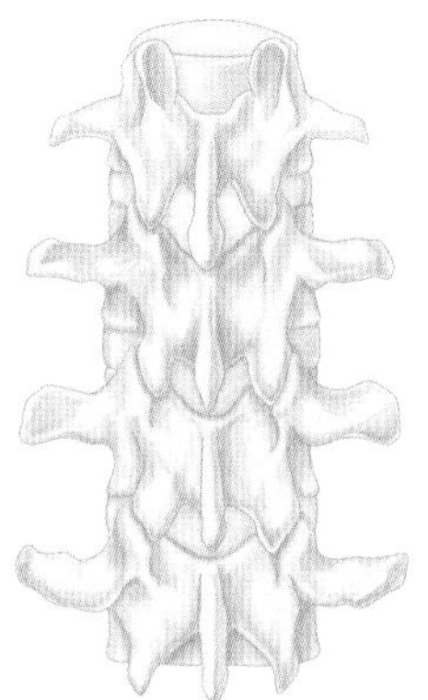
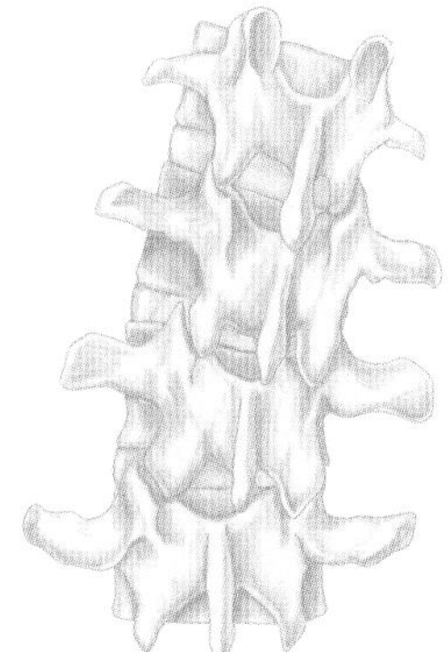

■ **FIGURE 12–2.** Lumbar coupled motion is depicted; with intervertebral rotation, lateral bending is induced.

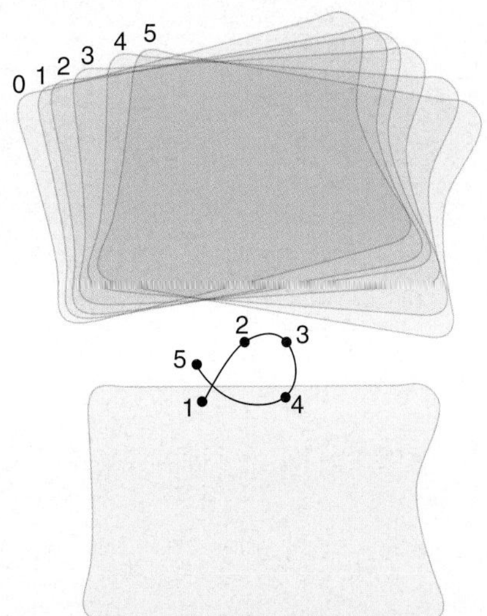


■ **FIGURE 12–3.** Changes in the instantaneous center of rotation (COR) with flexion and extension in the lumbar spine. In the normal disc, the changes in the COR create an elliptic pathway as flexion and extension occur.

respectively, has been recorded at the two levels adjacent to an instrumented C5-C6 segment.[16] These biomechanical alterations have been attributed to the longer lever arm of a fusion. Longer fusions, however, have not been found to be associated with higher rates of adjacent segment disease in the cervical spine.[17] Surgical techniques used during cervical fusion may also have an influence on the adjacent segment. Anterior plate impingement upon an adjacent disc is likely to accelerate adjacent level changes. An association between adjacent level ossification and the plate-to-disc distance was recently established in a retrospective review of 118 anterior cervical discectomy and fusion (ACDF) patients.[18] Postoperative malalignment after cervical fusion has also been identified as a risk factor for the degeneration of adjacent levels. Katsura and colleagues reported a statistically significant difference in the incidence of radiographic adjacent segment degeneration in patients with kyphosis at an average of 9.8 years after ACDF.[19]

## FUSION BIOMECHANICS: LUMBAR

Lumbar spinal fusion causes an alteration in the loads transferred to the boundaries of the fused segments. Cadaveric studies have demonstrated that lumbosacral fusions increase motion at the nonfused adjacent levels and that this transfer of motion appears to be greatest with the use of instrumentation.[4] A sheep model of spinal fusion demonstrated that kyphosis after fusion particularly influences the mechanical characteristics of the adjacent segment, with increased posterior ligamentous and lamina strain under flexion-extension loading.[20] It has also been reported that lumbar fusion increases the intradiscal pressure at adjacent levels and that elevated pressures correlate with the number of levels fused.[21] Alterations in intradiscal pressure and motion were also found at the adjacent levels following a single-level ALIF procedure in a calf model.[22] Like in the cervical spine, however, longer fusions in the lumbar spine have not been associated with higher rates of adjacent segment disease.[23]

## CERVICAL ADJACENT SEGMENT DEGENERATION

Primary anterior cervical fusion has been established as a reliable treatment for conditions including traumatic, neoplastic, infectious, deformity, and particularly degenerative spondylotic myelopathy[24] and radiculopathy.[25] With its wider acceptance, anterior cervical fusions are increasingly performed for younger patients at higher rates.[26] This has generated concerns regarding the long-term consequences, including the potential risk of adjacent segment disease (Fig. 12–4).

Several retrospective reviews of cervical fusion patients have reported postoperative progression of adjacent degenerative changes[27,28,29,30] (Table 12–1). Progressive cervical stenosis was observed by Baba et al in 25% of patients at an average of 8.5 years following ACDF for spondylotic myeloradiculopathy.[31] At a minimum of 5-year follow-up, Goffin and colleagues reported degenerative changes at levels adjacent to the fused level in 92% of 180 patients who underwent ACDF for a variety of conditions. The reoperation rate for clinically significant adjacent segment disease was limited, however, to 6%.[32] Bohlman and colleagues[25] reported a similar incidence of clinically significant adjacent segment disease requiring additional surgery in 9% of 122 patients evaluated at a mean of 6 years after undergoing ACDF.

These studies, and others, have established a high prevalence of radiographic degeneration at the motion segments adjacent to a cervical fusion. They have not, however, established a cause and effect relationship between fusion and adjacent segment disease. Regarding this potential relationship, it is important to consider the high incidence of spondylosis in the normal population. Degenerative changes can be found at one or more cervical levels in a majority of the population by age 50.[5,33,34] One study reported that 89%

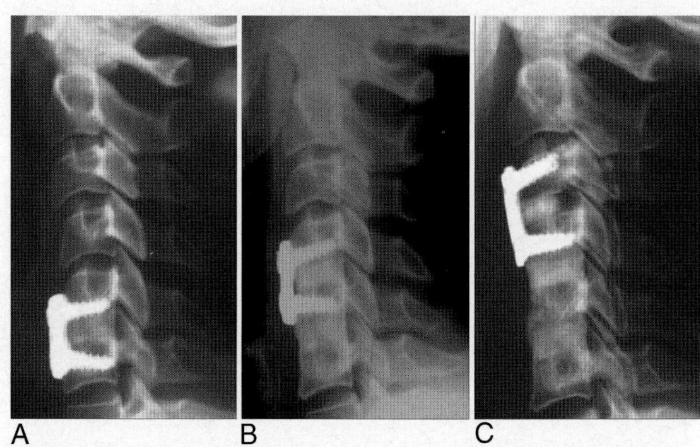


■ **FIGURE 12–4.** These lateral radiographs depict a case of "ascending" adjacent segment disease in the cervical spine. **A,** This patient initially underwent anterior cervical decompression and fusion (ACDF) at C5-C6. **B,** Spondylosis subsequently developed at the next most cranial level causing neurological compression, and the patient underwent ACDF at C4-C5 with removal of the plate at C5-C6. **C,** Next, symptomatic degeneration of the C3-C4 disc occurred. This was also treated with ACDF with removal of the C4-C5 plate.

**TABLE 12–1. Articles Reporting Incidence of Radiographic (R) Adjacent Segment Degeneration or Symptomatic (S) Adjacent Segment Disease After Anterior Cervical Spinal Fusion**

| Study | Patients | Criteria | Follow-up | Incidence (%) |
|---|---|---|---|---|
| Goffin et al, 2004[32] | 180 | R | 60 months | 92 |
| Goffin et al, 2004[32] | 180 | S | 60 months | 6 |
| Hilibrand 1999[17] | 374 | S | 120 months | 26 |
| Gore and Sepic, 1998[37] | 50 | S | 252 months | 14 |
| Wu et al, 1996[28] | 68 | R; MRI | 37 months | 28 |
| McGrory and Klassen, 1994[29] | 31 | R | 212 months | 29 |
| Shinomiya et al, 1993[30] | 443 | S | 72 months | 2.3 |
| Bohlman et al, 1993[25] | 122 | S | 72 months | 9 |
| Baba et al, 1993[31] | 106 | R | 102 months | 25 |
| Dohler et al, 1985[27] | 21 | R | 27 months | 52 |
| Gore and Sepic, 1984[6] | 121 | R | 60 months | 25 |
| Lunsford 1980[63] | 253 | S | 84 months | 7 |

MRI, magnetic resonance imaging.

of asymptomatic patients over 60 years of age have MRI evidence of degenerative disk disease.[35] Additionally, the prevalence of spondylosis is level dependent, with several sub-axial levels (C5-C6, C6-C7, C4-C5) comprising the large majority. For example, a patient that has developed cervical spondylosis at the most common level (C5-C6) may be predisposed to develop degeneration at an adjacent level (C6-C7 or C4-C5), based on natural history of the disease, whether or not a fusion is performed at the incident level.

While these previous studies cannot confirm or deny the potential causal relationship between cervical fusion and adjacent segment disease, there have been reports that do help address this issue. Gore and Sepic observed the onset of adjacent segment degeneration in 25% of 121 patients as well as the progression of existent disease in 25% of patients who had prior ACDF with a mean follow-up of 5 years.[36] Interestingly, they found no correlation between the radiographic findings and clinical symptoms. It was hypothesized that this degeneration may be related to natural history alone. These authors published an additional report on 50 patients that revealed that 14% of patients had additional surgery for adjacent level disease after ACDF.[37]

An investigation by Hilibrand et al [17] also explored the potential causal relationship between cervical fusion and the development of adjacent segment disease. They reported on 409 ACDF cases performed for radiculopathy or myelopathy. They reported a similar rate of additional surgery (14%) as Gore and Sepic, and reported a 3% annual incidence of adjacent segment disease. Using Kaplan-Meier survivorship statistics, they described a risk of developing adjacent segment disease following ACDF of 13.6% at 5 years and 25.6% at 10 years of follow-up. The authors noted, however, that fusions of longer length had a lower risk of adjacent segment disease. This inverse relationship between length of moment arm and risk of degeneration suggested that longer fusions may have circumvented the natural progression of degeneration at these levels by including them in the fusion, rather than increasing the risk of mechanically related degeneration at these levels adjacent to the fusion. This paper suggested that the development of adjacent segment disease may be related to the natural history of cervical spondylosis.

Other risk factors for the development of adjacent segment changes have been reported. The presence of pre-existing degenerative changes at adjacent segments before the time of ACDF is one of the most consistent predisposing factors for adjacent segment disease in several series.[17,31,38] The lower cervical levels are at highest risk, with degenerative changes most pronounced at C5-C6, followed by C6-C7, and then C4-C5.[39] Hilibrand and colleagues also reported that the prevalence of adjacent segment disease was related to the level: C2-C3, 1.2%; C3-C4, 7.6%; C4-C5, 9.3%; C5-C6, 13.8%; and C6-C7, 13.0%.[17] This level-related prevalence correlates with the levels of those most typically undergoing operative treatment.[36] Brodke reported cervical spondylosis surgery to be most common at C5-C6 (55%), followed by C6-C7 (28%), C4-C5 (13%), and C3-C4 (4%).[40]

Surgical technique, as discussed above, may also influence the progression of adjacent segment disease. Inaccurate anterior plate instrumentation[18] and postoperative saggital malalignment[19] have both been identified as risk factors for degeneration of the adjacent discs. Age may also be considered a predisposing factor for the development of adjacent segment disease. Characteristic spondylotic patients are typically over 50 years old, and degenerative changes measured by MRI have been reported to be age-related.[5,17,41]

Cervical total disc replacement may be associated with a reduction in the risk of adjacent segment changes. In a non-randomized, cohort evaluation of the Bryan cervical disc replacement (74 patients) compared to anterior cervical fusion (158 patients), radiographic and SF-36 outcomes were made at 2-year follow-up. This analysis compared arthroplasty and fusion patients from two previous trials, one evaluating the Affinity anterior cervical cage system, and the other evaluating the Bryan artificial cervical disc. An increase in the radiographic degeneration (anterior osteophyte formation, narrowing of the interspace, or calcification of the anterior longitudinal ligament) was observed in the fusion group at the adjacent level. Additionally, the incidence of symptomatic adjacent level disease was statistically greater in the fusion group than in the artificial disc group.[42] Since these two cohorts of ACDF and disc replacement patients were drawn from different studies with different inclusion criteria, however, the two groups should not be directly compared.

## LUMBAR ADJACENT SEGMENT DEGENERATION

The results of lumbar spine fusion for the treatment of degenerative disc disease are not universally satisfactory. There has been a poor correlation between successful fusion and good clinical outcome. Despite achieving a high rate of spinal fusion by modern techniques (>90–95%), clinical outcomes of the same magnitude have not been achieved.[43] Inappropriate indications, imprecise diagnoses, and psychosocial factors have each been blamed for this variability in pain reduction following spinal arthrodesis. Even for those patients that undergo an uncomplicated lumbar arthrodesis and enjoy an excellent reduction of pain, many surgeons remain concerned about the potential for development of radiographic and clinically symptomatic adjacent level changes.

The risk of fusion-related adjacent segment degeneration is difficult to accurately assess in published series because of variations in surgical indications, length of follow-up, and patient age. Additionally the prevalence of adjacent level degeneration may vary with the intervertebral level and the method of the fusion (anterior, posterior, both, etc). Surgical technique, particularly with pedicle screw instrumentation neighboring the preserved facet joints, may influence the risk of the development of adjacent segment disease. Regardless of its cause, however, the prevalence of radiographic adjacent segment degeneration after fusion is significant in long-term follow-up[44,45,46,47] (Table 12–2).

The rate of clinically significant adjacent segment disease following lumbar arthrodesis has been reported to be between 20% and 27% of patients requiring additional surgery in retrospective studies over varying periods of time.[48,49] Although the majority of reported cases involve a segment directly adjacent to the arthrodesis, selection bias must still be considered. It is likely that a patient with one degenerative disc is more likely to develop another degenerative disc than a patient without degenerative disc disease, regardless of whether a fusion was performed. In fact, a study by Ghiselli et al found no correlation between the rate of reoperation for adjacent segment disease and the length of fusion in 215 patients following posterior lumbar fusion. These authors reported that segments that were adjacent to a single-level fusion had a three times higher risk for the development of disease than did those that were adjacent to a multiple-level fusion.[23]

Clinically, however, the consequences of fusion on the adjacent segment remain unclear. Many authors have presented cohort studies evaluating the relationship between lumbar arthrodesis and the rate of adjacent segment degeneration, with conflicting results. Rahm and Hall reported a 5-year follow-up of 49 patients who underwent posterior instrumented lumbar fusion. The authors reported a 35% rate of adjacent segment degeneration and found that the degenerated patients had poorer clinical outcomes.[50] In support of a causal relationship between fusion and adjacent segment disease, the authors reported that their patients who developed pseudarthrosis were less likely to develop adjacent segment degeneration. Lehmann et al[51] presented a cohort of 62 lumbar arthrodesis patients with mean follow-up of 33 years. Although 45% of patients had developed radiographic degeneration at the segment caudal to the arthrodesis, and while there was a correlation between segmental degeneration and stenosis, there was no correlation between these radiographic findings and the patients' clinical symptoms.

Several other studies present data that does not support the proposed causal relationship between lumbar fusion and adjacent segment disease. A study by Penta et al reported a 10-year follow-up on 81 patients that underwent interbody fusion at the lumbosacral junction; they found no difference in the rate of adjacent segment disease as compared to matched control patients who did not undergo surgery.[52] Additionally, longer fusions were not associated with worse degeneration in their study.

Throckmorton et al also evaluated the association of adjacent level degeneration and outcomes of posterior lumbar fusion.[53] Patients that were fused adjacent to a normal disc were compared to patients that were fused adjacent to a degenerative disc. Those patients fused adjacent to a degenerative disc scored better on the SF-36, and there was no difference found between the two groups in the need for further surgery. This study indicated that the risk of developing clinically symptomatic adjacent segment disease was not increased by ending a fusion adjacent to a degenerated disc.

Ghiselli et al reported similar results in a cohort of 32 patients who had undergone isolate L4-L5 fusion. At an average of 7.3 years after fusion, they found that 97% of their patients had no evidence of symptomatic degeneration at L5-S1 requiring additional decompression or fusion. They did, however, report a trend of progression of the arthritic grade at L5-S1 from preoperative to postoperative examination, and found no correlation between preoperative arthritic grade and further degeneration. These authors concluded that the L5-S1 segment does not need to be included when performing a posterior lumbar fusion for patients with

**TABLE 12–2. Articles Reporting Incidence of Radiographic (R) Adjacent Segment Degeneration or Symptomatic (S) Adjacent Segment Disease After Lumbar Spinal Fusion**

| Study | Patients | Criteria | Follow-up | Incidence (%) |
|---|---|---|---|---|
| Wai et al, 2006[56] | 39 | R; MRI | 240 months | 23% |
| Ghiselli et al, 2004[23] | 215 | S | 80 months | 27% |
| Gillet, 2003[48] | 149 | R | 60 months | 41% |
| Gillet, 2003[48] | 149 | S | 60 months | 20% |
| Ghiselli et al, 2003[54] | 32 | S | 88 months | 3% |
| Kanayama et al, 2001[45] | 27 | S | 60 months | 18% |
| Kumar et al, 2001[47] | 28 | R | 360 months | 36% |
| Kuslich et al, 2000[46] | 196 | S | 48 months | 6% |
| Rahm and Hall, 1996[50] | 49 | R | 60 months | 35% |
| Penta et al, 1995[52] | 81 | R; MRI | 120 months | 32% |
| Lee, 1988[49] | 67 | S | 102 months | 27% |
| Lehmann et al, 1987[51] | 62 | R | 396 months | 45% |
| Frymoyer et al, 1979[44] | 96 | S | 164 months | 5% |

MRI, magnetic resonance imaging.

instability or stenosis at L4-L5 if no symptoms are attributed to the lumbosacral level.[54]

Other studies, however, have suggested that maintaining motion may reduce the risk of adjacent segment degeneration. Huang and colleagues retrospectively examined the follow-up radiographs of 42 patients 8.7 years after lumbar total disc arthroplasty.[55] The majority of the patients had the ProDisc device (Synthes, West Chester, PA) implanted at the L4-L5 or L5-S1 level (55 of 61). They evaluated the potential association between the preservation of motion and the development of adjacent level radiographic degeneration in these patients. Adjacent level degeneration was observed in 24% (10 of 42) of their patients. Patients demonstrating adjacent segment degeneration had a mean motion at the arthroplasty levels of 1.6 +/− 1.3 degrees, while those that did not demonstrated a mean motion of 4.7+/− 4.5 degrees. This difference was statistically significant. While there were no differences in clinical outcome, the authors concluded that preservation of motion after lumbar arthroplasty may reduce the risk of radiographic adjacent segment degeneration.

A 20-year follow-up of 39 ALIF patients has recently provided a long-term evaluation of lumbar adjacent segment degeneration.[56] This series of patients who had normal preoperative discogram at the adjacent levels underwent MRI to evaluate degeneration. Twenty-nine (74.3%) patients had MRI evidence of degeneration. Nine (23.1%) patients had advanced degeneration isolated to the adjacent level, and 7 (17.9%) patients had evidence of advanced degeneration with preservation at the level adjacent to the fusion. This prevalence of degenerative changes is similar to other studies involving normal asymptomatic subjects. The authors found no association between function and radiographic degeneration. Since the majority of degenerative changes occurred at multiple levels or at levels not adjacent to the fusion, the authors suggested that degeneration may be more likely related to natural history as opposed to the increased stresses focused at the adjacent level, arising from the original fusion.

## LUMBAR SAME SEGMENT DEGENERATION

With lumbar fusion procedures, the risk of "same segment" disease is limited to the patients who may develop a pseudarthrosis. With motion preservation treatments, however, patients may have an increased risk of new disease at the same level, which we term "same segment disease." This may occur at the facet joints, within the ligamentum flavum, or even at the intervertebral disc in the case of a nuclear replacement or a posterior stabilization. Consequently, while a surgical alteration in spinal biomechanics by fusion may alter the natural history of degeneration at the adjacent level, the surgical alteration in spinal biomechanics by motion-preserving technologies may alter the natural history of the degeneration at the operative level.

For example, while many of the disc arthroplasty designs currently under human investigation endeavor to mimic the natural linkage between vertebral bodies, none can precisely match the well defined motion characteristics of the natural intervertebral disc. The imperfections in implants, as compared to a normal healthy intervertebral linkage with its constantly changing center of rotation and complex coupled motions, may impose abnormal forces on the facet joints and intervertebral ligaments.

With preservation of motion, the development of same level facet arthrosis may be reason for concern. A 14% increase in facet loads has been observed in a human osteo-ligamentous cadaver model of the CHARITÉ intervertebral disc replacement (DePuy Spine Inc., Raynham, MA).[57] A finite element analysis of a total disc replacement also showed high facet pressures (greater than 3MPa) and high ligament tensions (greater than 500 N).[58] Significant facet arthrosis was reported by Van Ooij in 41% of 27 patients at a mean of 53 months after undergoing CHARITÉ lumbar disc replacement.[59] Similarly, Lemaire reported the observation of progressive facet arthrosis in 11 of 107 patients after undergoing lumbar total disc replacement.[60] A more recent MRI investigation of 16 patients, each 2 years after total disc arthroplasty with the CHARITÉ device, also reported accelerated facet degeneration. Overall, 7 of 16 (44%) patients had progression of facet degeneration in the 2 years after arthroplasty. Those patients who had progression of facet degeneration had increased pain Visual Analog Scale (VAS) scores as compared to those without progression.[61] This potential effect of accelerated same segment disease may be related to limitations in implant motion characteristics, which transfer forces to the facet joints.[62] It may also be related to the ongoing natural history of lumbar facet arthrosis, which is a well-established age-related disease. It should be noted, however, that there have been no high-quality controlled studies specifically evaluating the risk of "same segment disease" after total disc arthroplasty or other motion-sparing technologies.

## SUMMARY

There is evidence to suggest that the risk for progression of adjacent segment degeneration and development of adjacent segment disease may be related to both the natural history of spondylosis and to the presence of a neighboring fusion. The relative risk of each of these factors is not well understood, however, and conflicting data exist in the literature. Additionally, evidence to support the hypothesis that arthroplasty can reduce the risk of adjacent segment disease is not yet well established. Each disc arthroplasty device has specific motion characteristics with its relative merits and limitations. None fully re-create the elegant motion characteristics of the native disc. It is not known how closely an arthroplasty implant must mimic normal motion mechanics to successfully achieve its goals of preserving overall spinal kinematics and preserving adjacent levels in a lasting fashion. A more complete understanding of the causal relationship between fusion and adjacent segment disease and additionally between arthroplasty and adjacent segment (or same segment) disease is critical to a successful development and implementation of this burgeoning arthroplasty technology.

## REFERENCES

1. Eck JC, Humphreys SC, Lim TH, et al: Biomechanical study on the effect of cervical spine fusion on adjacent-level intradiscal pressure and segmental motion. Spine 27:2431–2434, 2002.
2. Weinhoffer SL, Guyer RD, Herbert M, Griffith SL: Intradiscal pressure measurements above an instrumented fusion. Spine 20:526–531, 1995.
3. DiAngelo DJ, Roberston JT, Metcalf NH, et al: Biomechanical testing of an artificial cervical joint and an anterior cervical plate. J Spinal Disord Tech 16:314–323, 2003.

4. Lee CK, Langrana NA: Lumbosacral spinal fusion: a biomechanical study. Spine 9:574–581, 1984.
5. Boden SD, McCowin PR, Davis DO: Abnormal magnetic resonance scans of the cervical spine in asymptomatic subjects. J Bone Joint Surg Am 72:1178–1184, 1990.
6. Gore DR, Sepic SB: Anterior cervical fusion for degenerated or protruded discs: a review of 146 patients. Spine 9:667–671, 1984.
7. Boden SD, Davis DO, Dina TS, et al: Abnormal magnetic-resonance scans of the lumbar spine in asymptomatic subjects: a prospective investigation. J Bone Joint Surg Am 72:403–408, 1990.
8. Panjabi MM: Experimental determination of spinal motion segment behavior. Orthop Clin North Am 8:169–180, 1977.
9. Ishii T, Mukai Y, Hosono N, et al: Kinematics of the subaxial cervical spine in rotation: in vivo three-dimensional analysis. Spine 29:2826–2831, 2006.
10. Ishii T, Mukai Y, Hosono N, et al: Kinematics of the cervical spine in lateral bending: in vivo three-dimensional analysis. Spine 31:155–160, 2006.
11. Ochia RS, Inoue N, Renner SM, et al: Three-dimensional in vivo measurement of lumbar spine segmental motion. Spine 31:2073–2078, 2006.
12. Ogston NG, King GJ, Gertzbein SD, et al: Centrode patterns in the lumbar spine: baseline studies in normal subjects. Spine 11:591–595, 1986.
13. Pearcy MJ, Bogduk N: Instantaneous axes of rotation of the lumbar vertebral joints. Spine 13:1033–1041, 1988.
14. Dvorak J, Panjabi MM, Novotny JE, Antinnes JA: In vivo flexion/extension of the normal cervical spine. J Orthop Res 9:828–834, 1991.
15. White AA, Panjabi MM: The basic kinematics of the human spine. Spine 3:12–20, 1978.
16. Eck JC, Humphreys SC, Lim TH, et al: Biomechanical study on the effect of cervical spine fusion on adjacent-level intradiscal pressure and segmental motion. Spine 27:2431–2434, 2002.
17. Hilibrand AS, Carlson GD, Palumbo MA, et al: Radiculopathy and myelopathy at segments adjacent to the site of a previous anterior cervical arthrodesis. J Bone Joint Surg Am 81:519–528, 1999.
18. Park JB, Cho YS, Riew D: Development of adjacent-level ossification in patients with an anterior cervical plate. J Bone Joint Surg Am 87:558–563, 2005.
19. Katsura A, Hukada S, Saruhasji Y, Mari K: Kyphotic malalignment after anterior cervical fusion is one of the factors promoting the degenerative process in adjacent intervertebral levels. Eur Spine J 10:320–324, 2001.
20. Oda I, Cunningham BW, Buckley RA, et al: Does spinal kyphotic deformity influence the biomechanical characteristics of the adjacent motion segments? An in vivo animal model. Spine 24:2139–2146, 1999.
21. Weinhoffer SL, Guyer RD, Herbert M, Griffith SL: Intradiscal pressure measurements above an instrumented fusion. Spine 20:526–531, 1995.
22. Rao RD, David KS, Wang M: Biomechanical changes at adjacent segments following anterior lumbar interbody fusion using tapered cages. Spine 24:2772–2776, 2005.
23. Ghiselli G, Wang JC, Bhatia NN, et al: Adjacent segment degeneration in the lumbar spine. J Bone Joint Surg Am 86:1497–1503, 2004.
24. Emery SE, Bohlman HH, Bolesta MJ, Jones PK: Anterior cervical decompression and arthrodesis for the treatment of cervical spondylotic myelopathy: two to seventeen-year follow-up. J Bone Joint Surg Am 80:941–951, 1998.
25. Bohlman HH, Emery SE, Goodfellow DB, Jones PK: Robinson anterior cervical discectomy and arthrodesis for cervical radiculopathy. Long-term follow-up of one hundred and twenty-two patients. J Bone Joint Surg Am 75:1298–1307, 1993.
26. Davis HL: Increasing rates of cervical and lumbar spine surgery in the United States, 1979–1990. Spine 19:1117–1123, 1994.
27. Dohler JR, Kahn MR, Hughes SP: Instability of the cervical spine after anterior interbody fusion: a study on its incidence and clinical significance in 21 patients. Arch Orthop Trauma Surg 104: 247–250, 1985.
28. Wu W, Thomas KA, Hedlund R: Degenerative changes following anterior cervical discectomy and fusion evaluated by fast spine echo MR imaging. Acta Radiol 37:614–617, 1996.
29. McGrory BJ, Klassen RA: Arthrodesis of the cervical spine for fractures and dislocations in children and adolescents: a long term follow-up study. J Bone Joint Surg 76:1606–1616, 1994.
30. Shinomiya K, Okamoto A, Kamikozuru M: An analysis of failures in primary cervical anterior spinal cord decompression and fusion. J Spinal Disord 6:277–288, 1993.
31. Baba H, Furusawa N, Imura S, et al: Late radiographic findings after anterior cervical fusion for spondylotic myeloradiculopathy. Spine 18:2167–2173, 1993.
32. Goffin J, Geusens E, Vantomme N, et al: Long-term follow-up after interbody fusion of the cervical spine. J Spinal Disord Tech 17:79–85, 2004.
33. Kellgren JH, Lawrence JS: Osteoarthrosis and disc degeneration in an urban population. Ann Rheum Dis 17:388–397, 1958.
34. Gore DR, Sepic SB, Gardner G: Neck pain: a long-term follow-up of 205 patients. Spine 12:1–5, 1987.
35. Matsumoto M, Fujimura Y, Suzuki N, et al: MRI of cervical intervertebral discs in asymptomatic subjects. J Bone Joint Surg Br 80:19–24, 1998.
36. Gore DR, Sepic SB: Anterior cervical fusion for degenerated or protruded discs: a review of one hundred forty-six patients. Spine 9:667–671, 1984.
37. Gore DR, Sepic SB: Anterior discectomy and fusion for painful cervical disc disease: a report of 50 patients with an average follow-up of 21 years. Spine 23:2047–2051, 1998.
38. Baba H, Furusawa N, Imura S, et al: Late radiographic findings after anterior cervical fusion for spondylotic myeloradiculopathy. Spine 18:2167–2173, 1993.
39. White AP, Biswas D, Smart LR, et al: Utility of flexion–extension radiographs in evaluating the degenerative cervical spine. Spine 32(9): 975–979, 2007.
40. Brodke DS, Zdeblick TA: Modified Smith-Robinson procedure for anterior cervical discectomy and fusion. Spine 17:S427–S430, 1992.
41. Boden SD, McCowin PR, Davis DO: Abnormal magnetic resonance scans of the cervical spine in asymptomatic subjects. J Bone Joint Surg Am 72:1178–1184, 1990.
42. Robertson JT, Papadopoulos SM, Traynelis VC: Assessment of adjacent-segment disease in patients treated with cervical fusion or arthroplasty: a prospective 2-year study. J Neurosurg Spine 3:417–423, 2005.
43. West JL III, Bradford DS, Ogilvie JW: Results of spinal arthrodesis with pedicle screw-plate fixation. J Bone Joint Surg Am 73:1179–1184, 1991.
44. Frymoyer JW, Hanley EN Jr, Howe J, et al: A comparison of radiographic findings in fusion and nonfusion patients ten or more years following lumbar disc surgery. Spine 4:435–440, 1979.
45. Kanayama M, Hashimoto T, Shigenobu K, et al: Adjacent-segment morbidity after Graf ligamentoplasty compared with posterolateral lumbar fusion. J Neurosurg 95:5–10, 2001.
46. Kuslich SD, Danielson G, Dowdle JD, et al: Four-year follow-up results of lumbar spine arthrodesis using the Bagby and Kuslich lumbar fusion cage. Spine 25:2656–2662, 2000.
47. Kumar MN, Jacquot F, Hall H: Long-term follow-up of functional outcomes and radiographic changes at adjacent levels following lumbar spine fusion for degenerative disc disease. Eur Spine J 10:309–313, 2001.
48. Gillet P: The fate of the adjacent motion segments after lumbar fusion. J Spinal Disord Tech 16:338–345, 2003.
49. Lee CK: Accelerated degeneration of the segment adjacent to a lumbar fusion. Spine 13:375–377, 1988.
50. Rahm MD, Hall BB: Adjacent-segment degeneration after lumbar fusion with instrumentation: a retrospective study. J Spinal Dis 9:392–400, 1996.

51. Lehmann TR, Spratt KF, Tozzi JE, et al: Long-term follow-up of lower lumbar fusion patients. Spine 12:97–104, 1987.
52. Penta M, Sandhu A, Fraser RD: Magnetic resonance imaging assessment of disc degeneration 10 years after anterior lumbar interbody fusion. Spine 20:743–747, 1995.
53. Throckmorton TW, Hilibrand AS, Mencio GA, et al: The impact of adjacent level disc degeneration on health status outcomes following lumbar fusion. Spine 28:2546–2550, 2003.
54. Ghiselli G, Wang JC, Hsu WK, Dawson EG: L5-S1 segment survivorship and clinical outcome analysis after L4-L5 isolated fusion. Spine 28:1275–1280, 2003.
55. Huang RC, Tropiano P, Marnay T, et al: Range of motion and adjacent level degeneration after lumbar total disc replacement. Spine J 6:242–247, 2006.
56. Wai EK, Santos ERG, Morcom RA, Fraser RD: Magnetic resonance imaging 20 years after anterior lumbar interbody fusion. Spine 31:1952–1956, 2006.
57. Goel VK, Grauer JN, Patel TCh, et al: Effects of CHARITÉ Artificial Disc on the implanted and adjacent spinal segments mechanics using a hybrid testing protocol. Spine 30:2755–2764, 2005.
58. Denoziere G, Ku DN: Biomechanical comparison between fusion of two vertebrae and implantation of an artificial intervertebral disc. J Biomech 39:766–775, 2006.
59. Van Ooij A, Oner FC, Verbout AJ: Complications of artificial disc replacement: a report of 27 patients with the SB Charite disc. J Spinal Disord Tech 16:369–383, 2003.
60. Lemaire JP, Skalli W, Lavaste F, et al: Intervertebral disc prosthesis: Results and prospects for the year 2000. Clin Orthop 337:64–76, 1997.
61. Phillips FM, Diaz R, Pimenta L: The fate of the facet joints after lumbar total disc replacement: a clinical and MRI study. Spine J 5:75S, 2005.
62. Huang RC, Wright TM, Panjabi MM, Lipman JD: Biomechanics of nonfusion implants. Orthop Clin N Am 36:271–280, 2005.
63. Lunsford LD, Bissonette DJ, Jannetta PJ, et al: Anterior surgery for cervical disc disease. Part 1: Treatment of lateral cervical disc herniation in 253 cases. J Neurosurg 53(1):1–11, 1980.

CHAPTER 13

# Statistical Outcome Interpretation of Randomized Clinical Trials

**Fred H. Geisler**

## KEY POINTS

- Student's t-test is not the appropriate test to analyze non-normally distributed data because by definition the test assumes a normal distribution.
- A more appropriate statistical test for analysis of non-normally distributed data is a non-parametric test such as the Wilcoxon Rank Sum test, which is appropriate for a non-normal data distribution.
- Given the distribution of the ODI and VAS scores at two years in the US FDA IDE CHARITÉ randomized trial, it is clear that a non-parametric test is the appropriate statistical test to use when analyzing the ODI and VAS data from this clinical trial.
- The non-parametric analysis of ODI and VAS scores demonstrated that subjects enrolled in both the treatment and the control groups had highly significantly improved scores at all time points compared to baseline, including the two-year follow-up ($P < 0.001$). Significantly lower ODI and VAS scores occurred in the CHARITÉ Artificial Disc group compared to the central fusion group at all postoperative time points, including the two-year follow-up ($P < 0.05$). These results demonstrate superiority of arthroplasty over fusion in indicated patients, according to these key clinical measures.
- Multipoint, non-validated FDA a priori clinical success criteria are an inappropriate assessment of clinical outcomes that cannot be easily explained to patients. Validated measures such as scores from ODI and VAS questionnaires are appropriate in discussing clinical outcomes and more useful in explaining the risks and benefits of a given procedure to patients.

## INTRODUCTION

After the common cold, low back pain is the second most common reason for visits to primary care physicians.[1] Up to 80% of individuals in the United Sates experience low back pain at some point in their lives.[2] Approximately 5% of this group (much of which is due to degenerative disc disease (DDD) will progress to a condition of chronic back pain, the leading cause of pain and disability in the United States.[3,4] The exact incidence and prevalence of degenerative disc disease is unknown because many cases are asymptomatic and therefore do not trigger physician visits.[5]

Nonoperative care for chronic low back pain includes allowing time for a natural healing mechanism, physical therapy, exercise, stretching, epidural steroid injections, and chiropractic care. Approximately 870,000 cases[6,7] with degenerative disc disease and a posteriorly directed dislodged disc fragment occur with compression of the exiting or transversed nerve root at the disc level, thereby producing sciatic pain and mechanical traction clinical signs. In cases refractory to nonsurgical care, a discectomy or a microdiscectomy may be necessary for pain relief.

A spinal fusion is the most common surgical treatment for DDD of the lumbar spine. More than 200,000 lumbar fusion procedures are performed in the United States each year, although not all of them directly treat DDD (Merrill Lynch Orthopaedic Industry Model, 9/1/04). After surgery, it may take from 6 months to 6 years for mature healed fusion bone to develop, and rehabilitation of the patient to be completed, to achieve maximum successful clinical benefit of the procedure.

Lumbar artificial disc technology has been used in Europe for more than 21 years, and the first disc was implanted in the United States at Texas Back Institute by Dr. Scott Blumenthal in March 2000 at the start of the Food and Drug Administration (FDA) IDE trial. Therefore, lumbar arthroplasty is a relatively new procedure to treat lumbar DDD in the United States when compared with spinal fusion. The hypothesized benefits of arthroplasty over fusion with significant clinical benefit include (1) reduction or elimination of disc-derived (also known as discogenic) pain, (2) restoration and maintenance of normal segmental range of motion and sagittal balance, and (3) potential reduction or retardation of progressive adjacent-level DDD necessitating further surgical intervention[8] by not only reducing the forces and angulation of the adjacent level compared with a fusion but also normalizing the adjacent level biomechanics.

The FDA approved the world's first lumbar artificial disc, the CHARITÉ Artificial Disc (DePuy Spine, Raynham, MA) on October 26, 2004, for use in the United States.[9] In doing so, the FDA followed the recommendation of its expert Orthopaedic

Financial Disclosure: The author acknowledges consulting and research relationships with the manufacturer of the CHARITÉ artificial disc (DePuy Spine, Raynham, MA.)

and Rehabilitation Devices Panel, which on June 2, 2004, unanimously recommended approval.[10] The FDA decision was based on the results of a prospective, randomized, controlled clinical trial comparing lumbar artificial disc replacement with anterior lumbar interbody fusion, and 20 years of worldwide experience. The FDA approval meant that the manufacturer could market the device as safe and effective for the treatment of one-level lumbar DDD in indicated patients at either the L4-5 or L5-S1 level.

This clinical trial was the first in the history of spine surgery to compare two *different* surgical treatments for lumbar DDD using a multicenter, prospective, randomized, controlled study design. The results of the study were published in peer-reviewed journals including *Journal of Neurosurgery* in September 2004,[8] and *Spine* in July 2005.[11,12] Because of the prospectively specified noninferiority design of the study and the FDA required a complex success/failure criteria, the primary conclusion of the study for FDA labeling purposes was that clinically, treatment with artificial disc replacement was at least as good as a fusion procedure.

The author presents here new Level I Medical Evidence that surgical treatment with single level arthroplasty is not only at least as good as a fusion procedure (FDA label), but that reduction in pain and disability improvement are *highly statistically superior* in patients receiving treatment with lumbar arthroplasty compared with both baseline and an anterior fusion procedure. A more rapid decrease in pain and disability (postoperative healing/recovery) was also noted in the CHARITÉ group compared with the fusion group. It is notable that these scales are validated clinical scales. The complex criteria that the FDA used to analyze the CHARITÉ was a multipoint criteria agreed on before initiation of the study that statistically is a nonvalidated clinical scale.

## MATERIALS AND METHODS

A multicenter, prospective, randomized, controlled trial was performed under an FDA-approved protocol (IDE# G990303). Local IRB approval was obtained at all 14 study sites, and all subjects enrolled in the study signed the study informed consent form. The trial incorporated a noninferiority design with a 2:1 randomization, treatment with artificial disc replacement, versus the control, a fusion procedure. Enrollment in the study constituted 71 subjects in an initial nonrandomized treatment phase (approximately five cases per site) and then a total of 304 subjects in the randomized phase, 205 in the treatment group and 99 in the control group. Subjects in the control group underwent an anterior lumbar interbody fusion procedure with BAK threaded fusion cages (Zimmer Spine, Minneapolis, MN) and bone graft. Subjects were assessed clinically and radiographically preoperatively, and at 6 weeks, and then at 3, 6, 12, and 24 months postoperatively. Demographics, inclusion/exclusion criteria, subject accountability, clinical outcomes, and all other detailed study information conforming to the CONSORT checklist were previously described by Blumenthal et al in *Spine*, in July 2005.[11]

The Oswestry Disability Index (ODI) is a 10-question validated measure (score 0–100) of disability and pain in the low back pain population.[13] Subjects were required to complete an ODI questionnaire and a 0 to 100 Visual Analog Scale (VAS) pain questionnaire preoperatively and at each follow-up visit.

## STATISTICAL METHODS

The statistical analysis of the ODI and VAS scores performed for the FDA and reported in the paper by Blumenthal et al required the use of the prespecified Student's t-test. This methodology was prespecified in the statistical plan of the protocol prior to (1) FDA approval of the protocol, (2) subsequent subject enrollment, and (3) before the results/distributions of the data were known. In the FDA-approved protocol, the methodology could not be altered post hoc for FDA labeling claims. Using Student's t-test, mean ODI and VAS scores were significantly better in the treatment group compared to the control group at all follow-up time points except for the 2-year follow-up.[11] These results, combined with the non-inferiority study design of the pre–agreed-on multipoint scale, resulted in the primary conclusion of the study, that treatment with artificial disc replacement is at least as good as a fusion procedure in properly indicated patients.

However, the Student's t-test assumes a normal distribution of data. The ODI and VAS scores reasonably approximate a normal distribution at baseline. At the 2-year follow-up, the endpoint of the study, the distributions are heavily non-symmetric and skewed, and are clearly not normally distributed (Fig. 13–1). Student's t-test, very simply, is not the appropriate test to analyze non-normally distributed data because, by definition, the test assumes a normal distribution.

A more appropriate statistical test for analysis of non-normally distributed data would be a nonparametric test such as the Wilcoxon Rank Sum test, which is appropriate for a non-normal data distribution. The author performed a separate analysis of the ODI and VAS scores using the Wilcoxon Rank Sum test. All subjects enrolled in both the nonrandomized and randomized phases of the treatment group ($n$ = 276) were compared to the study control group (the complete FDA IDE dataset). The data used for this analysis was the exact same data submitted to the FDA as part of the post-marketing application submission. This was *not* a subset analysis.

## RESULTS

Both the ODI and VAS scores had almost identical initial mean values for each of the two groups (treatment and control). Thus, the initial randomization worked by balancing the groups in this study and no baseline corrections were necessary or used in the analysis of this data.

The nonparametric analysis of ODI and VAS scores demonstrated that subjects enrolled in both the treatment and the control groups had highly significantly lower scores at all time points compared with baseline, including the 2-year follow-up ($P < 0.001$). The improved scores in both groups are (1) sustained over the 2-year period, (2) monotonically decreasing, and (3) more than twice the difference considered to be of minimum clinical significance.[14] This triad makes a placebo effect of surgery for the observed improvement unlikely. Furthermore, inspection of the recovery curves demonstrates significant improvement at 6 weeks with maintenance to 2 years (Figs. 13–2 and 13–3).

Patients in the treatment group obtained a greater proportion of the total 2-year recovery in this early phase of the postoperative

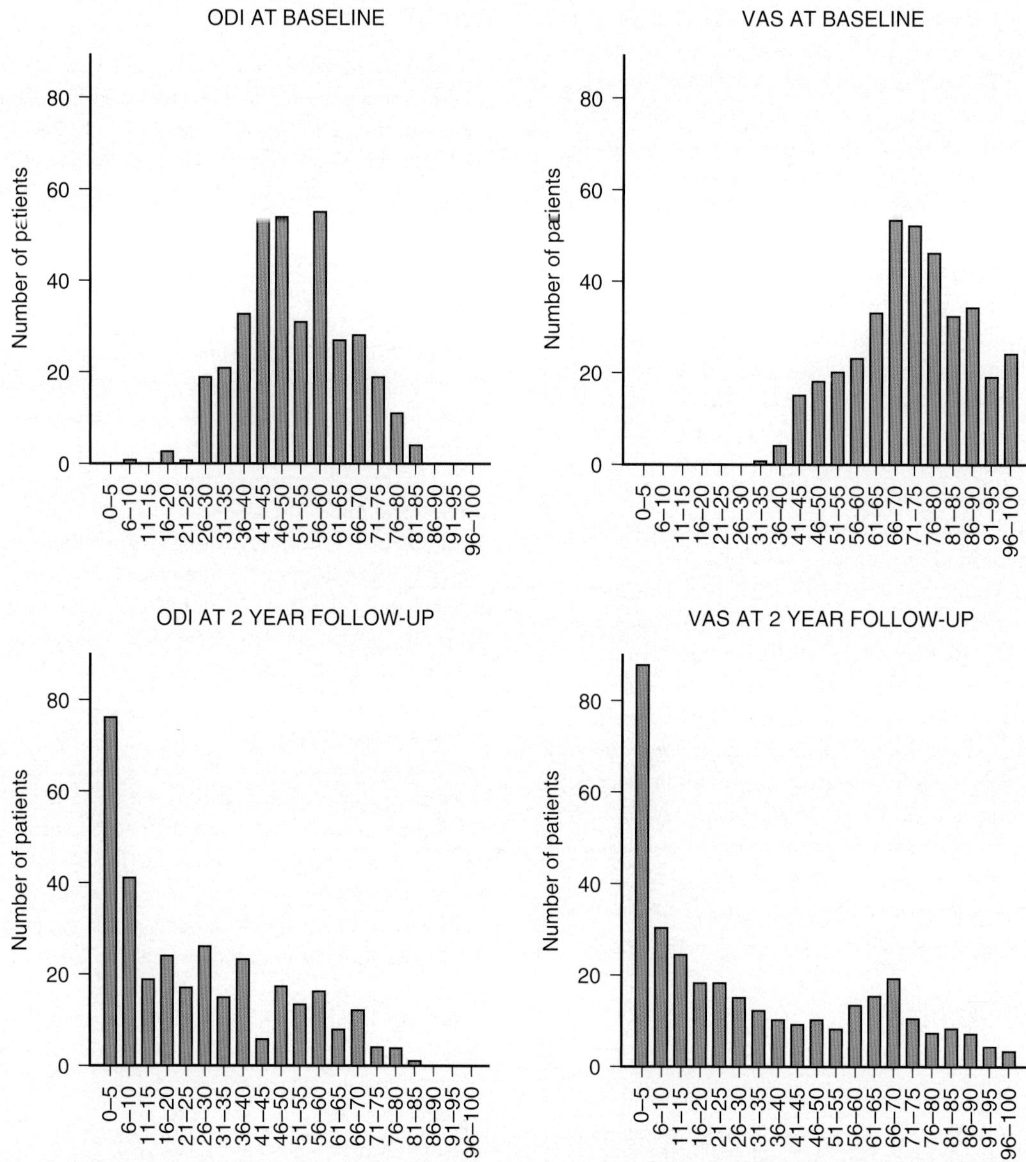


■ **FIGURE 13–1.** Distribution of visual analog scale pain scores and Oswestry Disability Index scores for all subjects in both the treatment and the control groups. A reasonable approximation of a normal distribution of scores is evident at baseline. However, at 2-year follow-up, the distributions are not normally distributed but have a large skew toward the low cut-off end of both scales (favorable clinical response).

period in both clinical indexes. Additionally, statistically significant lower scores occurred in the CHARITÉ Artificial Disc (DePuy Spine, Inc., Raynham, MA) group compared with the control fusion group at all postoperative time points, including the 2-year follow-up ($P<0.05$). These results demonstrate superiority of arthroplasty over fusion in indicated patients *using these two key clinical measures* and a major improvement (highly significant) from baseline in both treatment groups. The control group scores closely followed the results of the BAK cage IDE study described by Kuslich et al in 1998.[15]

## DISCUSSION

Given the distribution of the ODI and VAS scores at 2 years shown in Figure 13–1, it is clear that a nonparametric test is the appropriate statistical test to use when analyzing the ODI and VAS data from the CHARITÉ Artificial Disc clinical trial. This new analysis does not and cannot change the primary FDA study conclusion, that arthroplasty is "at least as good as" a fusion procedure. This limitation of labeling claims occurred because the FDA study was conducted with a non-inferiority design, with prespecified criteria for clinical success. Furthermore, FDA claims of clinical superiority cannot emanate from noninferiority studies that are not a priori powered sufficiently to demonstrate superiority of one treatment over another.

However, an improvement in the ODI score was a primary clinical endpoint of this study, and improvement in the VAS score was a secondary clinical endpoint. These two clinical outcome measures are the most relied on measures of clinical outcome following low back surgery. There is no doubt following this analysis that subjects receiving arthroplasty attained superiority in

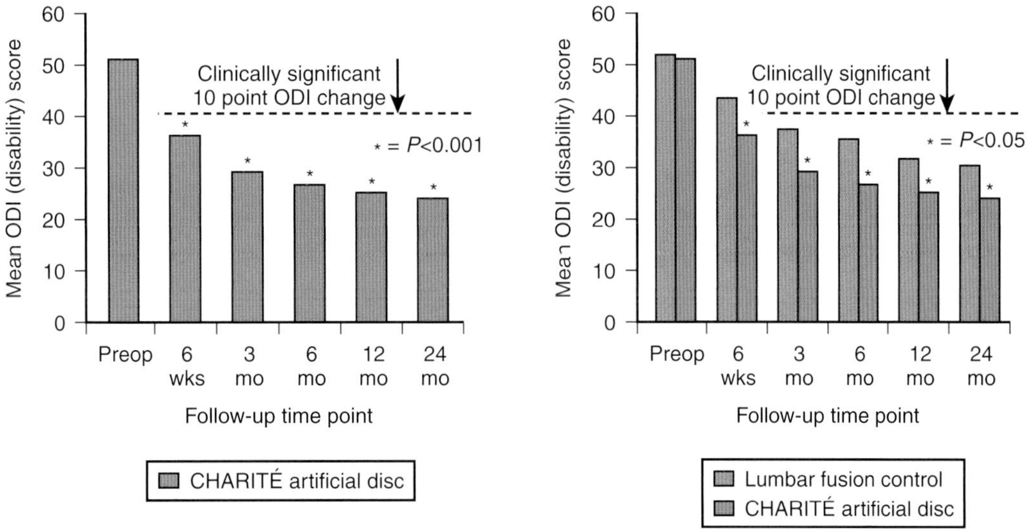


■ **FIGURE 13–2.** Mean Oswestry Disability Index (ODI) scores at baseline and at each protocol-specified follow-up time point through 2 years. The dotted line indicates the ODI score necessary for minimum clinical improvement (10 points).[14] **A,** Mean scores for 276 subjects in the CHARITÉ Artificial Disc treatment group. There was a significant difference in level of disability at all time points compared with baseline ($P<0.001$), Wilcoxon Rank Sum test. **B,** Means scores for subjects in the treatment group compared to 99 enrolled subjects in the control group. There was a significant difference in the treatment group with respect to disability, compared to the control group at all postoperative time points ($P<0.05$), Wilcoxon Rank Sum test.

improved pain and disability level compared with their baseline levels at all follow-up time points, and superiority in pain and disability level compared with fusion, the historical standard of care when the study began.

Deyo et al have pointed out in a number of publications that in their view, many treatments for low back pain are ineffective, including osteopathic manipulation,[16] chiropractic care,[17] physical therapy,[17] transcutaneous electrical nerve stimulation therapy,[18] and fusion.[19,20] Critics of lumbar arthroplasty cite mixed short-term[21–24] and long-term[25] results, with the CHARITÉ Artificial Disc and review articles[26,27] written before publication of the U.S. trial, as the primary reason why arthroplasty is not a

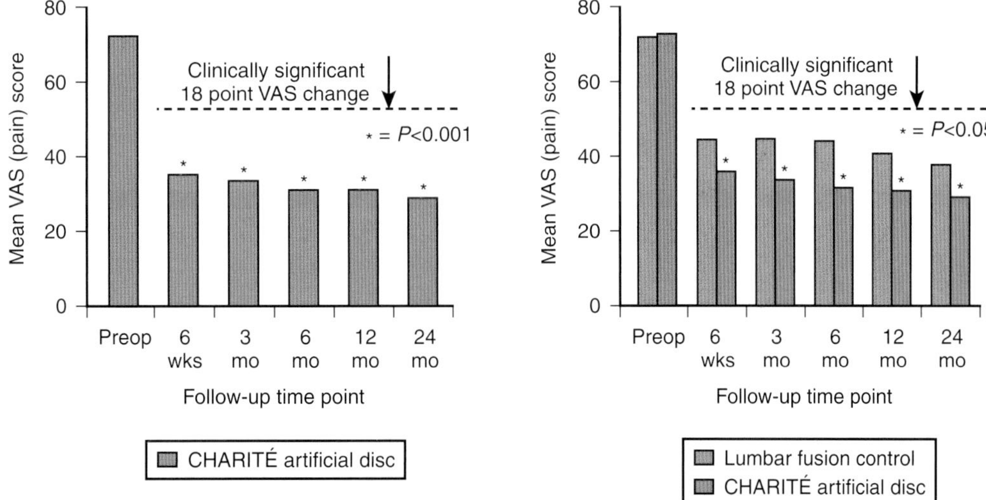


■ **FIGURE 13–3.** Mean visual analog (VAS) pain scores at baseline and at each protocol-specified follow-up time point through 2 years. The dotted line indicates the VAS score necessary for minimum clinical improvement (19 points).[14] **A,** Mean scores for 276 subjects in the CHARITÉ Artificial Disc treatment group. There was a significant difference in pain at all time points compared with baseline ($P<0.001$), Wilcoxon Rank Sum test. **B,** Means scores for subjects in the treatment group compared with the 99 enrolled subjects in the control group. There was a significant difference in the treatment group with respect to pain, compared to the control group at all postoperative points ($P<0.05$), Wilcoxon Rank Sum test.

reasonable treatment for discogenic low back pain (Level IV Medical Evidence). Yet other more favorable long-term results in large patient cohorts are often only offhandedly considered[28–31] (Level IV Medical Evidence).

Lumbar arthroplasty with the CHARITÉ Artificial Disc has been performed outside the United States for more than 20 years, and as McAfee[32] eloquently pointed out, the overwhelming majority of the early disc arthroplasty cases were performed with widely variable indications; basic, rudimentary instrumentation; different sizing options; nonexistent diagnostic testing; and a lack of fundamental understanding of lumbar spine biomechanics. These early issues and failures were well known to the clinical trial investigators at the time the FDA IDE study protocol was developed. In fact, it was with this knowledge of the prior successes and failures that led to the inclusion and exclusion criteria, and surgical technique used in the FDA IDE study. Thus, the FDA IDE study was designed to provide Level I Medical Evidence on the efficacy and safety of treatment with lumbar arthroplasty that was learned from the earlier experience; to better define the appropriate patient selection, surgical technique, and implant sizing. The prior lumbar artificial disc clinical information has been analyzed, and clinical and surgical techniques have been refined through the 20-year history of the device. If this historical review of the prior series had not occurred, then the clinically superior results presented here would not have been possible. Using the historical data and clinical experience to criticize the FDA IDE results in a vacuum, without considering the advancements described above, seems particularly unfair and unscientific.

As for safety, which is also a continuing criticism of arthroplasty, the same historical literature is often cited, almost always without proper context and without any relevance to today's indications, implants, instrumentation, and knowledge. And again, contemporary information about complications in today's arthroplasty patients has been presented at dozens of medical meetings over the past 3 years, and that information is published in the literature.[11, 33–35] Revision rates for fusion are just as high or higher than those for disc replacement.[35,36] There is no evidence that the incidence of complications with or without necessitating revision is higher in patients who have undergone arthroplasty compared with patients who have undergone fusion. There are, however, differences in the type of potential problems.

Decades ago, fusion was the standard of care for surgical treatment of degenerative conditions of the hip and knee. This fusion standard was replaced in the ensuing years with artificial joint arthroplasty, which today is the standard of care for surgical treatment of these conditions in indicated patients. Often cited as the grandfather of modern hip arthroplasty, John Charnley's early ideas for avoiding fusion of the hip[37–39] were not readily accepted.[40,41] Though Charnley's work began in the late 1950s, the first hip replacement in the United States was not performed until 1969, with the first appearance in the U.S. literature in 1970.[42] Modern disc replacement has taken a similar track, with the third-generation CHARITÉ Artificial Disc developed and used in Europe as early as 1987[43] and the first procedure performed in the United States in March 2000.

As previously discussed, Deyo et al have denounced every nonoperative and operative treatment for low back pain, including fusion and now disc replacement. Despite this criticism, there are, in fact, multiple prospective, multicenter low back fusion studies describing good results published in the peer-reviewed literature.[15,44–46] All of these studies were performed under FDA-approved protocols with narrow indications, as was the CHARITÉ clinical trial.

Highly significant improved pain and level of disability versus baseline in indicated disc replacement patients is not in question. Superior pain reduction and disability level compared with the current standard of care is not in question. Detractors of surgical intervention for low back pain patients decry the lack of Level I data, and then when Level I data demonstrating superior outcomes are produced, the surgical intervention is still criticized as "too new," "ineffective," or "unsafe," despite extraordinary evidence to the contrary. Level II, III, IV, and V data do not trump Level I data. Lower levels of published data exist for every single treatment in medicine. If lower levels of data are allowed to trump Level I data, then nothing in medicine would be proven safe and effective, and if that is the case, why perform Level I studies at all?

## REFERENCES


1. White AA 3rd, Gordon SL: Synopsis: Workshop on idiopathic low-back pain. Spine 7:141–149, 1982.
2. Bertagnoli R, Kumar S: Indications for full prosthetic disc arthroplasty: a correlation of clinical outcome against a variety of indications. Eur Spine J 11(2):S131–S136, 2002.
3. Errico TJ: Lumbar disc arthroplasty. Clin Orthop Relat Res 435:106–117, 2005.
4. Davis TT, Delamarter RB, Sra P, et al: The IDET procedure for chronic discogenic low back pain. Spine 29:752–756, 2004.
5. Healy JF, Healy BB, Wong WH, et al: Cervical and lumbar MRI in asymptomatic older male lifelong athletes: Frequency of degenerative findings. J Comput Assist Tomogr 20:107–112, 1996.
6. Frymoyer JW: Back pain and sciatica. N Engl J Med 318:291–300, 1988.
7. Zitting P, Rantakallio P, Vanharanta H: Cumulative incidence of lumbar disc diseases leading to hospitalization up to the age of 28 years. Spine 23:2337–2343; discussion 43–44, 1998.
8. Geisler FH, Blumenthal SL, Guyer RD, et al: Neurological complications of lumbar artificial disc replacement and comparison of clinical results with those related to lumbar arthrodesis in the literature: Results of a multicenter, prospective, randomized investigational device exemption study of Charite intervertebral disc. Invited submission from the Joint Section Meeting on Disorders of the Spine and Peripheral Nerves, March 2004. J Neurosurg Spine 1:143–154, 2004.
9. Food and Drug Administration: CHARITÉ Artificial Disc summary of safety and effectiveness. PMA number P040006. October 26, 2004.
10. Federal Register: Panel Transcript: Orthopedic and Rehabilitation Devices Panel of the Medical Devices Advisory Committee, 2004.
11. Blumenthal SL, McAfee PC, Guyer RD, et al: A Prospective, Randomized, Multicenter Food and Drug Administration Investigational Device Exemption Study of Lumbar Total Disc Replacement with the CHARITÉ™ Artificial Disc Versus Lumbar Fusion, Part I: Evaluation of Clinical Outcomes. Spine 30:1565–1575, 2005.
12. McAfee PC, Cunningham B, Holsapple GA, et al: A Prospective, Randomized, Multicenter Food and Drug Administration Investigational Device Exemptions Study of Lumbar Total Disc Replacement with the CHARITÉ™ Artificial Disc Versus Lumbar Fusion, Part II: Evaluation of Radiographic Outcomes and Correlation of Surgical Technique Accuracy With Clinical Outcomes. Spine 30:1576–1583, 2005.

13. Fairbank JC, Couper J, Davies JB, et al: The Oswestry low back pain disability questionnaire. Physiotherapy 66:271–273, 1980.
14. Hagg O, Fritzell P, Ekselius L, et al: Predictors of outcome in fusion surgery for chronic low back pain: A report from the Swedish Lumbar Spine Study. Eur Spine J 12:22–33, 2003.
15. Kuslich SD, Ulstrom CL, Griffith SL, et al: The Bagby and Kuslich method of lumbar interbody fusion: History, techniques, and 2-year follow-up results of a United States prospective, multicenter trial. Spine 23:1267–1278; discussion 79, 1998.
16. Andersson GB, Lucente T, Davis AM, et al: A comparison of osteopathic spinal manipulation with standard care for patients with low back pain. N Engl J Med 341:1426–1431, 1999.
17. Cherkin DC, Deyo RA, Battie M, et al: A comparison of physical therapy, chiropractic manipulation, and provision of an educational booklet for the treatment of patients with low back pain. N Engl J Med 339:1021–1029, 1998.
18. Deyo RA, Walsh NE, Martin DC, et al: A controlled trial of transcutaneous electrical nerve stimulation (TENS) and exercise for chronic low back pain. N Engl J Med 322:1627–1634, 1990.
19. Deyo RA, Nachemson A, Mirza SK: Spinal-fusion surgery—the case for restraint. N Engl J Med 350:722–726, 2004.
20. Deyo RA, Weinstein JN: Low back pain. N Engl J Med 344:363–370, 2001.
21. Cinotti G, David T, Postacchini F: Results of disc prosthesis after a minimum follow-up period of 2 years. Spine 21:995–1000, 1996.
22. Zeegers WS, Bohnen LM, Laaper M, et al: Artificial disc replacement with the modular type SB Charite III: 2-year results in 50 prospectively studied patients. Eur Spine J 8:210–217, 1999.
23. van Ooij A, Oner FC, Verbout AJ: Complications of artificial disc replacement: a report of 27 patients with the SB Charite disc. J Spinal Disord Tech 16:369–383, 2003.
24. Griffith SL, Shelokov AP, Buttner-Janz K, et al: A multicenter retrospective study of the clinical results of the LINK SB Charite intervertebral prosthesis: The initial European experience. Spine 19:1842–1849, 1994.
25. Putzier M, Funk JF, Schneider SV, et al: Charité total disc replacement—clinical and radiographical results after an average follow-up of 17 years. Eur Spine J 2005, published online October 28, 2005.
26. Gamradt SC, Wang JC: Lumbar disc arthroplasty. Spine J 5:95–103, 2005.
27. de Kleuver M, Oner FC, Jacobs WC: Total disc replacement for chronic low back pain: background and a systematic review of the literature. Eur Spine J 12:108–116, 2003.
28. Lemaire JP, Skalli W, Lavaste F, et al: Intervertebral disc prosthesis: Results and prospects for the year 2000. Clin Orthop 337:64–76, 1997.
29. Lemaire JP, Carrier H, Sari Ali E, et al: Clinical and radiological outcomes with the CHARITÉ™ artificial disc: A 10-year minimum follow-up. J Spinal Disord 18:353–359, 2005.
30. David T: Lumbar Disc Prosthesis: Five Years Follow-up Study on 96 Patients. Presented at the 15th Annual Meeting of the North American Spine Society (NASS). New Orleans, Louisiana, 2000.
31. David T: Lumbar disc prosthesis: an analysis of long-term complications for 272 CHARITÉ Artificial Disc Prostheses with minimum 10 year follow-up. Spine J 4:S50–S51, 2004.
32. McAfee PC: Comments on the van Ooij article. J Spinal Disord Tech 18:116–117, 2005.
33. David T: Revision of a Charite artificial disc 9.5 years in vivo to a new Charite artificial disc: Case report and explant analysis. Eur Spine J 14:507–511, 2005.
34. Regan JJ, McAfee PC, Blumenthal SL, et al: Evaluation of surgical volume and the early experience with lumbar total disc replacement as part of the investigational device exemption study of the Charite Artificial Disc. Spine 31:2270–2276, 2006.
35. McAfee PC, Geisler FH, Saiedy S, et al: Revisability of the CHARITÉ Artificial Disc Replacement—analysis of 688 patients enrolled in the U.S. IDE Study of the CHARITÉ Artificial Disc. Spine 31:1217–1226, 2006.
36. Blumenthal SL, McAfee PC, Geisler FH, et al: Response to the editorial and points of view regarding the IDE Study of the CHARITÉ™ Artificial Disc. Spine 30, 2005. Linked via *Article Plus* to Zindrick et al E388–390.
37. Charnley J, Wright JK: A spring exerciser for arthroplasty of the hip joint. J Bone Joint Surg Br 33B:634–635, 1951.
38. Charnley J: Surgery of the hip-joint: present and future developments. Br Med J 5176:821–826, 1960.
39. Charnley J: Arthroplasty of the hip: A new operation. Lancet 1:1129–1132, 1961.
40. Chapchal G: [Critique of arthroplasty of the hip joint with special reference to further therapy following defective results.] Ann Univ Sarav [Med] 6:280–281, 1958.
41. Chapchal G: [Critical remarks on arthroplasty of the hip with reference to further treatment in poor results.] Medizinische 12:560–564, 1958.
42. Nelson JP, Talbott RD, Glassburn AR Jr: Charnley total hip arthroplasty—a preliminary report. Rocky Mt Med J 67:25–26, 1970.
43. Link HD: History, design and biomechanics of the LINK SB Charite artificial disc. Eur Spine J 11(2):S98–S105, 2002.
44. Brantigan JW, Steffee AD, Lewis ML, et al: Lumbar interbody fusion using the Brantigan I/F cage for posterior lumbar interbody fusion and the variable pedicle screw placement system: two-year results from a Food and Drug Administration investigational device exemption clinical trial. Spine 25:1437–1446, 2000.
45. Burkus JK, Gornet MF, Dickman CA, et al: Anterior lumbar interbody fusion using rhBMP-2 with tapered interbody cages. J Spinal Disord Tech 15:337–349, 2002.
46. Ray CD: Threaded titanium cages for lumbar interbody fusions. Spine 22:667–679; discussion 679–680, 1997.

CHAPTER 14

# Socioeconomic Impact of Motion Preservation Technology

**Richard D. Guyer** and **Donna D. Ohnmeiss**

## KEY POINTS

- Expanding number of new technologies makes this an exciting time in spine care.
- Traditionally, FDA approval led to reimbursement for new technologies from insurers; however, currently rising costs and financial motives of both the medical and insurance industries have led to denial for reimbursement in many instances, even after FDA approval.
- Cost effectiveness studies are essential in this age of new technologies and rising healthcare costs.
- Perhaps the technologies that can be most readily accepted on a large-scale basis will be those that can decrease costs compared to the current standard of care for the same condition.
- Demands for demonstrated care improvement and cost effectiveness will change the development and evaluation process of new implants.

## INTRODUCTION

At no time in the history of back pain have there been as many advancements as are currently being seen. There is great excitement generated by the potential of motion-preserving technologies. Intuitively, these new implants are appealing to physicians and patients alike in that the concept of allowing motion rather than eliminating it is so simple and clearly desirable. The new devices may allow not only for motion but may allow for an earlier rehabilitation and return to activities because no time is required for the bone graft to incorporate as is the case with fusion. Also, the potential problem of accelerated deterioration of the segment or segments adjacent to the operated segment may be reduced. However, this enthusiasm must be tempered with several aspects of reality. First, the new implants must prove themselves clinically to provide benefit to patients. Traditionally, this was addressed in the Food and Drug Administration (FDA)–regulated trials required to get approval for marketing in which the safety and effectiveness of new treatments had to be found to be at least as good as the current standard of care for the same condition. However, in an age of ever-increasing healthcare costs, there is a new variable in the spine care arena that has not previously had to be addressed. That is cost effectiveness.

The costs related to back pain are enormous. Katz reported that in 2005 dollars, the total costs related to low back pain ranged between $100 and $200 billion a year.[1] In the work arena, 5% of workers consume 75% of the costs for work-related low back pain. Certainly with these staggering figures in mind, there is a potential for cost-effective treatment. There is big money in the spine. In 2003, the total revenue of U.S. spinal device manufacturers was $2.5 billion dollars.[2] Although this figure is attractive to investors and manufacturers, it may be alarming to those paying the bills for the devices.

With the development of total disc replacements, nucleus replacements, dynamic posterior stabilization devices, and the promise of tissue regeneration, there is no doubt that there will be a shifting of how dollars are spent in the spine care arena. In a review by Singh et al,[3] a report was cited that projected that by the year 2010, more than 47% of the fusion market may be transferred to dynamic devices. They projected that the revenue generated in the spine arthroplasty market in the United States 5 years after approval for use will be more than $2 billion.

Another important factor that is changing the environment of the spine is the increasing role of surgeons in device design and development. Physicians are seeking to enhance or replace income deteriorating by reduced reimbursements. Also, as any other group of inventors, they desire to receive benefit for their intellectual property that goes on to be developed into viable clinical products. The concept of dynamic spinal implants has created a venue for surgeons to be highly active in the device development process. Weiner and Levi[4] provided an overview of the potential impact, positive and negative, of the profit motive on spine surgery. They state that surgeons driven by a desire to enhance income by becoming involved with the development and evaluation of new technologies may perform unnecessary surgery and push the market on unproven technologies. However, the authors also realized that without the allure of profit, there may not be sufficient funding available to support the development and evaluation of new technologies. This could result in a cessation or at least significant slowdown of advances in patient care. Considering the high socioeconomic costs of back pain, advances in effective care are greatly needed.

In traditional economic models, when new technologies are initially introduced and only one company holds the patent or possesses another form of exclusivity for marketing, the price is initially high, and the item is considered somewhat of a luxury. As more companies enter the market with similar products to create market competition, the price of the item tends to decrease and the use increases. After this process, then the prices increase to keep pace with the cost of living and economics of the time. Lieberman[5] provided an overview of the economics of spinal implants and discussed how some traditional economic models are not seen in the spine market. He noted that traditionally, there are relationships of supply and demand. He noted that although there have been few truly innovative changes in pedicle screws from 1990 to 2000, the price range rose from $135 to $160 to $225 to $700. Although the increase was not attributed to development costs or increases in manufacturing costs, it was attributed to what the market would bear. In discussing this same information, Hochschuler[6] noted that with many new items on the market, such as computer-related technology, the costs are initially high, but with time and competition, the costs decrease in the absence of dramatic changes in the technology. As with pedicle screws, the number of companies offering pedicle screws on the market increased, and the cost did not decrease but rather increased during the 10-year period.

Perhaps one of the problems with trying to apply traditional economic models to the spine market is that the roles are not so clear cut. Traditionally, the consumer is primarily the one who selects the item to purchase, pays for it, and is the end user. In the spine implant arena, the picture is not so clear. The patient is the end user of the device, insurers typically bear the majority of the burden for paying for the item with the patient also paying part of the costs, and often the surgeon is the one who decides on the specific item that will be purchased, although he or she is not the primary user or pays nothing for the item. Manufacturers typically target the surgeons with marketing and to a lesser extent in recent years, primarily due to expansion to the Internet, to patients, with the patients then discussing with their physicians which device they want. We have experienced this recently with total disc replacement. With the availability of information on the Internet, both reliable and not reliable, patients are now asking more questions about the specific implant that may be used. In some cases, they have already decided which particular brand of total disc replacement is best for them and will then try to find a surgeon who will use it. The picture becomes grayer when considering the increasing ethical concerns caused by the relationships between physicians and industry, with the concern being that the choice of implant to use will be influenced by these financial relationships.

In the United States, the economics may also be more difficult to analyze and address than in other countries owing to the system of healthcare delivery. In many countries, all aspects of healthcare are addressed by the government. In the United States, there are numerous insurance companies involved. This may become important in the cost analysis. For example, in foreign countries, the government is responsible for all costs, including surgery, postoperative care, disability, and so on. In this scenario, the societal costs, that is, the total cost of care, including lost work time is all absorbed by the same entity. In the United States, one insurer may have the policy for covering the healthcare cost such as surgery, but another insurer may be responsible for the disability policy. Therefore, there may not be as much willingness to pay more for a surgery even if over the long term there is benefit owing to a rapid return to work. One company is bearing a higher cost than the alternative treatment for someone else to gain benefit later on.

True cost-effectiveness studies are needed to evaluate new spine technologies. This includes the obvious items such as implant cost, hospital costs, and so on. However, what are typically missing are the extended costs of care, or the lack thereof. Such costs include rehabilitation, medication, time off work, future medical care for the same problem or treatment of complications arising from it. In the United States, it is very difficult to retrieve comprehensive costs data for medical treatment. The problem is complicated by patients being treated by multiple doctors and no central depository for data concerning the care or its cost. In other countries, the data collection may be much more easily accomplished through centralized registries; however, the generalizability of the data across international economies and cultures is highly questionable. Until comprehensive data can be captured in relation to costs for various treatments, we will be forced to reply on only a partial or short-term data set to evaluate. At best, cost models can be constructed to compare treatments. But models are only as good as the assumptions on which they are constructed, and unfortunately, they are easily criticized by those who do not like the outcomes of the projections from the models. Also, in the United States, there are a myriad of problems related to cost modeling in the arena of costs versus charges. This is mainly in the eyes of the beholder. That is, models may be built on hospital costs, but the costs to individuals or insurers may be greater and vary depending on contract or region of the country. Also, these models do not address the costs of a person being out of work. This is perhaps one of the greatest dollar costs encountered in back pain patients. Not only is there the cost related to disability payment to the individual but also the societal cost of the individual not being in the workforce. To further complicate the issues surrounding new technologies, they are being introduced in an age of rapidly increasing medical care premiums, scrutiny of the ethics of financial relationships between physicians and manufacturers, as well as potential concerns about the role of venture capitalists investing in spine implants.

One recent cost-effectiveness study of the spine involved a review of 11 spinal fusion studies (nine of which were IDE trials) in which the physical component score (PCS) of the SF-36 was compared with three other well-accepted procedures: total hip replacement, total knee replacement, and coronary artery bypass graft (CABG) surgeries.[7] The data used came from the Centers for Medicare and Medicaid Services (CMS) and All Payer Data, and the study analyzed cost of the procedures per clinically relevant unit change in the PCS. They found that fusion was more cost effective than CABG, about the same as total knee replacement, and less than total hip replacement. The authors concluded that although results of cost-effective analyses may vary with populations and cost estimates used, the cost effectiveness of fusion was comparable to commonly accepted procedures. In that study, of note is that all but two of the studies included in the analysis were IDE trials. In such studies, the investigators must adhere rigorously to the selection criteria. Also, the protocols do not allow for "add on" items such as graft extenders, image guidance, anterior plates, and so on. These two factors taken together may have helped to improve effectiveness through more stringent selection criteria and reduce cost by rigorous adherence to treatment protocol. Another study found that spinal decompression was 1.5 times as cost effective as total hip replacement.[8] With the promise that bone morphogenetic protein (BMP) holds for increasing the fusion rate, there is concern about the cost. This has been analyzed by Ackerman et al,[9] and it was found that although the initial treatment costs are greater with BMP, these costs are offset with time owing to the decrease rate of failed fusion and future care-related costs.

A recent study performed an economic comparison of total disc replacement (TDR) to anterior lumbar interbody fusion (ALIF) with autograft, ALIF with BMP and tapered cages, and posterior lumbar interbody fusion PLIF with pedicle screws using autograft.[10] The analysis included costs related to the surgery itself and also an analysis of the costs during the following 24 months to include costs related to complications and re-operations. Both the hospital and long-term costs were significantly less in the TDR group than in any of the three fusion groups. The hospital costs were 12% to 36.5% greater in the fusion groups. In the 24-month follow-up model, the costs were 84% to 100% greater in the fusion groups compared to the TDR group. This study is likely the first of many addressing the cost-effectiveness of motion preservation technology.

Any economic model can be criticized, since the results projected from such models can only be as good as the assumptions upon which the models are based. However, as more cost models emerge for the spine and more data become available, it is likely that there will be some basic models that gain large-scale acceptance against which new technologies will be compared. In some ways, the evolution of such cost models may not be so different from what we saw evolve years ago to produce generally accepted models and protocols for biomechanical testing and, more recently, computerized biomechanical models. No doubt as the models are increasingly used, healthcare providers will become familiar with the terminology related to cost-effectiveness analyses as well as the basic concepts of the models used.

One of the areas with possibly the greatest potential for demonstrating cost effectiveness is motion-preserving implants that also are minimally invasive, such as the interspinous spacers. One such implant is the X STOP, which is designed for implantation under local anesthesia during outpatient surgery and has great potential for cost effectiveness. Less invasive technology may expand the current market by making operative treatment feasible in patients who would otherwise not be surgical candidates. This may be seen with technologies with a high safety profile and are viable treatment replacements for much more invasive procedures. Examples of such treatments are osteoplasty procedures and interspinous implants. Both of these technologies can be used in patients who may otherwise be considered poor candidates for much more invasive, and risky, surgery to treat the same problems. The interspinous devices, such as the X STOP, may expand the market by including patients who may otherwise not be considered surgical candidates. It is designed to treat stenosis, primarily found in older patients. The traditional treatment for the same problem is open decompression with or without fusion. The risk associated with such surgery, particularly in older patients, may make it a less appealing treatment option. However, the fact that the interspinous device is designed for outpatient surgery requiring local anesthesia may make it a safe treatment option in patients who may be considered poor candidates for more extensive spine surgery. If the effectiveness of such implants can be demonstrated, the costs are certainly reduced compared to the alternatives owing to the reduced operative time, reduced length of hospital stay, and reduced complications associated with more extensive surgery. However, there should be concern that owing to the decreased risks associated with this type of implant compared with traditional open decompressive surgery, it does have the potential deficit of being used in patients who are poorly indicated for the procedure and thus likely to compromise the results. In order for such treatments to be cost effective, surgeons must adhere to the appropriate indications and not be tempted to use new devices because they feel compelled to "do something" for the patient and traditional surgery is not indicated.

Although the lumbar spine has been the focus of most studies related to surgery and dynamic implants, the cervical spine should not be overlooked. It was reported that between the years of 1990 and 2000, the rate of surgery for degenerative cervical spinal conditions rose from 29 to 55 per 100,000 adults.[11] The proportion of anterior fusion procedures rose sharply from 17.8% to 69.5% during this time. Conversely, the rate of decompressive surgeries not involving fusion declined from 70.5% to 24.6%. Other data in that report found that although the percentages of older patients and patients with comorbidities increased, the perioperative complication rate did not. The mean length of hospital stay was reduced by more than 50%; however, the inflation-adjusted hospital charges increased by 48%, exceeding the $2 billion mark. No doubt this rapidly increasing arena of surgery and charges will attract much attention from those wanting to sell, as well as those who must bear the burden of paying the expenses. The data that was not reported was how these changes in treatment practice and charges affected outcome for patients, and also if these perioperative costs were later offset with reduced treatment costs. However, in the current era of wanting to control costs and focus on current cash flow and profits, absorbing higher costs earlier and waiting several years for total treatment costs to balance out may not be particularly attractive to payers.

## HOW CAN COST EFFECTIVENESS BE IMPROVED?

It seems reasonable that the key to widespread acceptance of motion-preserving technology is cost effectiveness. The concept of cost effectiveness is simple; however, definitively calculating it is difficult. The two primary factors are, of course, the cost and the effectiveness. The cost of the treatment takes into account many factors. The most obvious factors are the actual costs related to the surgery. These include the implants, surgeon fees, anesthesiologist fees, assistant or access surgeon if used, operating room time, intraoperative imaging, supplies, and the cost associated with each day spent in the hospital following the procedure. However, other costs must be considered as well. These include any diagnostic tests required (may be particularly relevant if use of image guidance is planned). Perhaps the most difficult costs to capture are the postoperative costs. These include medications, rehabilitation, orthotics, physician office visits, diagnostic studies, costs related to evaluating and treating complications, and the costs related to the patient being out of the workforce.

By reducing any of these costs, the cost effectiveness can be improved. One example of the potential for motion-retaining technology to reduce total care costs is in the postoperative period. Traditionally, patients who underwent fusion surgery have been limited to minimal activities during the time allowed for boney incorporation of the bone graft to occur. However with TDR, patients can participate in rehabilitation as soon as the incision has healed and can engage in all exercise activities except for those requiring extreme extension. This quicker participation in rehabilitation should accelerate the patient's overall recovery time and produce a more rapid return to work after surgery.

The other route to improve cost effectiveness of new technology is to improve the outcomes. Not only do some of the implants make more rapid return to work possible, they may also reduce the damage to musculature, as is the case with minimally invasive procedures, which may facilitate rehabilitation and physical functioning. In a recent article by Soegaard et al,[12] they suggested that cost effectiveness in patients who underwent fusion may be favorably affected by reducing or eliminating factors related to less desirable outcomes. They found that smoking and psychological factors negatively affected cost effectiveness because these factors reduce the benefit of the surgical intervention. They suggested that addressing such factors with individual patients may lead to improved cost effectiveness of the procedures investigated. This same strategy may be beneficial to employ for motion-retaining technologies to maximize the benefits of the new treatments. Careful patient selection has always been a key to good outcomes. Poor patient selection can lead to greatly reduced cost effectiveness because such patients generally represent those who have less than desirable results and who consume financial resources after surgery related to continued time off work, medication use, additional diagnostic evaluations, and, possibly, reoperation.

One good example of poor selection criteria is presented in the following case report. A 24-year-old man presented to our clinic complaining of persistent severe low back pain following TDR performed at another facility. Those who elect to criticize new technology may be quick to use this case as an example of failure of the implant. In reviewing the patient's information, we found that he had undergone TDR 10 months earlier. The patient's body mass index was more than 40. The patient's size would present a challenge for surgeons very experienced with anterior spine surgery. Unfortunately, the surgeon did not yet have a lot of experience with TDR implantation. The TDR surgery required several hours to perform. On the surface, this patient may be seen as a failure of the new technology. However, he more likely represents one surgeon's failure to employ rigorous patient selection criteria.

Data must be continuously collected for new implants. Although the 510(k) process is attractive to manufacturers because it allows rapid access for devices deemed to be similar to existing technology, it does not require the collection of data for assessment of the technology, nor is the cost of the implant considered. In theory, an expensive ineffective item could be approved for marketing that adds costs to a surgical procedure, without adding any benefit. Although the 510(k) process allows earlier marketing, it is likely that manufacturers will need to pursue studies to prove their products' effectiveness before insurance reimbursement or large-scale acceptance among physician users and hospitals is achieved.

## WHAT MIGHT THE FINANCIAL FUTURE OF MOTION PRESERVATION TECHNOLOGY BE?

In the near future, it seems inevitable that there will have to be much work performed in the area of cost effectiveness of spinal surgery. This fits well with the ongoing evolution of pay-for-performance and quality assurance initiatives. All of these changes will require careful data collection for outcomes and delineation of the indications, as well as openness on the part of surgeons to report their results, good and bad, in patients who were ideal and less than ideal candidates for the procedures they elected to perform. Payers need to be willing to delineate what evidence they will be comfortable with in order to reimburse for new treatment, even after FDA-regulated trials have demonstrated the implants to be as safe and effective as existing technologies. In the planning of new devices, engineers and manufacturers must take into account the cost of the implants they want to take to market. New technologies that are most likely to be readily successful will need to be designed to incorporate minimally invasive techniques, to decrease hospital costs (operating room time, outpatient surgery versus multiday stays, and so on), to allow rapid return to activities and to cost less than existing alternatives. Although these may be lofty goals, they are not likely unattainable. However, one question remains, who will pay for the series of studies needed to optimize the cost effectiveness of new treatments? Although manufacturers may be able to combine some of the cost-effectiveness assessment in with the IDE trials, this puts more burden on the sponsors who are already investing heavily in the development of the implants. Also, there is already growing criticism and skepticism of industry-sponsored research. Insurers have an interest in optimizing cost effectiveness; however, it is unlikely that they will be willing to sponsor large-scale clinical studies. Individual clinics may be able to take on part of the burden, but with the reduced reimbursements, there is little motivation to invest in clinical trials. There may be a tendency to look to governmental agencies for funding. However, the available resources are decreasing, and competition for such funding is increasing. Also, would there be bias toward funding only a few academic centers that may, or may not, represent the back pain population across the country?

Much of the cost of back pain is the indirect costs related to time away from work. Ekman et al[13] reported that indirect costs constitute about 84% of the total societal costs of back pain. With this figure in mind, one avenue for cost effectiveness may be the treatments that can return workers back to the workplace more quickly. This may come through the technology of tissue regeneration. If such a treatment can be designed so that it has a high safety profile, the socioeconomic potential is tremendous. Ideally, such a treatment would be safe enough so that it could be administered early after injury or significant pain onset. If the patient fails to respond to exercise and medication, then go to the tissue regeneration injection. No more waiting 6 months or longer for more invasive surgery. This would allow treatment before patients potentially become chronic pain patients and adjust to living without working.

We have already seen payers denying new technology such as TDR even after FDA approval. The argument is that there is not enough evidence and not enough follow-up to justify the implants. However, the evidence available from the multicenter trial[14] satisfied the FDA criteria for approval based on safety and effectiveness. Also, long-term data from Europe, in the more than 10-year follow-up range, provided support that the devices remain safe and effective during the long term. There are several issues related to demanding long-term follow-up (defined to be 10 years or more) in the United States before granting reimbursement and widespread acceptance of new implants. By the time the device is accepted, it may well be obsolete compared with the technology developed during this time. Of greater importance, if the technology is promising in IDE trials and approved for marketing by the FDA but denied by insurers, how should patients be treated during this time period? Should the standard of care be employed and no new technology covered by insurance until the first patients reach 10-year follow-up? This scenario is not one that is likely acceptable to patients. Also, considering the cost of conducting the trial and gaining approval from the FDA, manufacturers cannot afford to continue a 10-year study with no devices being sold during that interim. It is more likely that there should be a compromise and continued data collection to monitor the long-term safety and effectiveness of new technology; however, once initial safety and effectiveness have been demonstrated to the FDA's satisfaction, insurers should be willing to pay for the implants, provided that the cost effectiveness is comparable with the current standard of care and proper selection criteria is employed.

## DISCUSSION

Perhaps the most relevant question is can we identify who is most likely to be helped by which technology. This is particularly important when considering technologies that add costs to existing procedures such as image guidance systems. Although such technology may be helpful in difficult cases, it is likely not cost effective if applied to more routine cases performed by highly experienced surgeons. One problem is who will pay for the studies needed to differentiate which patients need more expensive surgery to maximize their outcome and which patients do not need it. Also, how can physicians communicate to insurers that a particular patient needs a more expensive procedure to enhance safety or effectiveness of a surgical treatment when the patient is assigned the same diagnostic code as one in whom a less expensive procedure is acceptable?

Some other questions to consider include:

- Will the lack of reimbursement and acceptance of new technologies be such a great disincentive to industry and investors that the funding to support developing promising new technologies will slowly shift to other areas of investment that may offer a greater return on investment?
- At the same time, can a society support uncontrolled increasing costs of an item as crucial as optimal healthcare?
- Can a reasonable compromise be reached before either of these undesirable events become the new reality in spine care?
- We may be approaching an age of combining total disc replacement with dynamic posterior stabilization and use of image guidance to implant the devices. This may lead to the cost of elective spine surgery soaring into the range of $100,000. Can a correlative benefit of such a great cost be demonstrated?

What needs to happen to maximize the economics of motion-retaining devices? Treatment costs must be considered in the development of new technologies. Although there are some wonderfully intriguing advancements possible, they must be proven to be cost effective, not just an exciting additional cost, or a more expensive means to achieve outcomes similar to what are already being achieved. One key may be focusing on the development of minimally invasive procedures using simple implant designs. This may already be evolving with the interspinous implants. However, one of the most important areas to address may be differentiating which specific technology is most appropriate for which specific subgroup of patients. Can the subgroup of patients in which image-guided surgery provides benefit proportional to its cost be identified so that the cost effectiveness is realized, by reducing the costs related to complications associated with poor device placement while not unnecessarily increasing the costs in patient subgroups in which there is likely no benefit associated with the added cost of using the technology? However, one difficult question looms—who will pay for the research needed to identify subgroups of patients and the most cost-effective treatments for each? The most obvious answer is that there should be motivation for whoever is most likely to realize financial benefit from the findings. However, this is difficult to determine. Manufacturers and investors may view the refined indications as limiting the scope of their product and thus decreasing revenue from sales. This may be true in the short term, but over the long term, they may gain from being able to enjoy demonstrated cost effectiveness in that subgroup rather than deal with across-the-board denials due to the expense and lack of data to support the use of their technology. Insurers also have much to gain in the optimal matching of treatment with specific subgroups of patients. Although slow acceptance of new treatments may initially appear cost effective, it may be detrimental long-term due to complications resulting from not using new technology (such as preventing adjacent segment deterioration) or losing the potential savings of reduced recovery time.

All spine care providers must take responsibility for the appropriate adoption of technology. Otherwise, the opportunity to advance care for patients with back pain is likely to come to a standstill, or worse, existing care options diminish for lack of cost-effectiveness data. Surgeons must be properly trained to use new devices and techniques. This comes through attending educational training courses, observing those with experience, and having proctors present for their initial cases. Perhaps the most important factor is using appropriate patient selection. If one desires to go outside the strictly defined indications, one must do so cautiously. Some of the selection criteria are in place to assist with patient safety and to increase the likelihood of a favorable outcome. For implants such as TDR, these include lack of osteoporosis, pars fractures, significant facet degeneration, and so on. Other selection criteria may be optional for the surgeons who are well experienced with a device, but should not be undertaken by those who do not have experience with that device. For example, for the first TDR patients, surgeons should select single-level degeneration, preferably at the L5–S1 level, in a thin patient with no previous abdominal surgery in the region of the affected disc. After many cases, one may want to expand to two-level TDR in well-selected patients. In addition to adherence to selection criteria, all surgeons should maintain at least a registry of their cases, and notes on any complications and variances from selection criteria. Only through the recording and public reporting of this information can the potential cost effectiveness of new technology be addressed. The physicians and professional organizations such as the North American Spine Society (NASS), American Association of Neurological Surgeons (AANS), Congress of Neurological Surgeons (CNS), and Spine Arthroplasty Society (SAS) must take the lead in this or they will be led by outside forces such as insurers, who already have much data.

This is an exciting time in spine surgery. It is also a time for surgeons to take on an increasing level of responsibility. The temptation of new technology is great. Better care for patients is desired by all, and most patients want the latest treatment. However, new technology can only be accepted once it is proven to be safe and effective. In the past, this was primarily addressed through noninferiority studies regulated by the FDA. The bar for acceptance is being raised. Not only must the new treatment be as effective and safe as the current standard, it must also be cost effective. Cost effectiveness requires several entities coming together to maximize patient care. First, manufacturers must make the implants available for use at a cost low enough to justify their use but high enough to realize a fair profit. Surgeons have a great responsibility in employing rigorous patient selection criteria. Without this, the effectiveness of the device will be compromised, thus reducing the overall cost effectiveness of the implant. Also, payers need to be willing to pay for new implants that have been approved for marketing when surgeons are employing the appropriate patient selection criteria, and the cost of such implants is no greater than the current standard of care, or if a greater cost-effectiveness benefit can be established. Although spine surgeons are not used to investing in maintaining a registry of their cases and outcomes assessment, this is becoming more feasible with current technology and is more needed now than ever before. If surgeons cannot demonstrate the effectiveness of the treatments they think are best for their patients, such treatments may no longer be paid for by insurers, and there are very few patients who can afford cash payment for such treatments.

Promising new technology is emerging rapidly. However, for the promise to be realized, all of those involved, including physicians, investors, payers, and manufacturers, must be willing to work together to optimize patient care. Only through ongoing evaluation of new technologies can the indications be refined to the point providing each patient with the best care available for his/her particular problem. However, patients meeting the rigorous selection criteria should be able to receive the optimal treatment without being limited by their insurers. Manufacturers must balance the demands of their investors for revenue with the long-term gains of not losing out entirely due to overaggressive use of their products. Physicians must not become too aggressive in using new technology so as to compromise results by not adhering to basic principles of appropriate patient selection and take on the responsibility to track their own results and share the information with their peers. Only with progressive cycles of assessment, redefining indications, and evaluating outcomes can real progress be made to optimizing patient care by maximizing cost effectiveness of motion-preserving technologies.

## REFERENCES


1. Katz JN: Lumbar disc disorders and low-back pain: socioeconomic factors and consequences. J Bone Joint Surg [Am] 88:21–24, 2006.
2. The Burton Report: The cost of lumbar "fusion." www.burtonreport.com/InfSpine/SurgStabilCost.htm.
3. Singh K, Vaccaro AR, Albert TJ: Assessing the potential impact of total disc arthroplasty on surgeon practice patterns in North America. Spine J 4:195S–201S, 2004.
4. Weiner BK, Levi BH: The profit motive and spine surgery. Spine 29:2588–2591, 2004.
5. Lieberman IH: Disc bulge bubble: spine economics 101. Spine J 4:609–613, 2004.
6. Hochschuler SH: Presidential address. Spine Arthroplasty Society. May 2006, Montreal, Canada.
7. Polly D Jr, Branch C Jr, Burkus K, et al: SF-36 PCS benefit/cost ratio of lumbar fusion comparison to other surgical interventions. Bergen, Norway, International Society for the Study of the Lumbar Spine, June 2006.
8. Fleischer GD, Lam J, Shah R, et al: A comparison of the cost effectiveness of lumbar decompression surgery and total hip arthroplasty in a matched cohort using quality adjusted life years as a determinant of utility. Bergen, Norway, International Society for the Study of the Lumbar Spine, June 2006.
9. Ackerman SJ, Mafilios MS, Polly DW Jr: Economic evaluation of bone morphogenetic protein versus autogenous iliac crest bone graft in single-level anterior lumbar fusion. Spine 16S:S94–S99, 2002.
10. Guyer RD, Tromanhauser SG, Regan JJ: An economic model of one-level lumbar arthroplasty vs. fusion. Spine J 7:558–562, 2007.
11. Patil PG, Turner DA, Pietrobon R: National trends in surgical procedures for degenerative cervical spine disease: 1990–2000. Neurosurgery 57:753–758, 2005.
12. Soegaard R, Christensen FB, Christiansen T, Bunger C: Costs and effects in lumbar spinal fusion: A follow-up study in 136 consecutive patients with chronic low back pain. Eur Spine J, e-pub, 2006.
13. Ekman M, Johnell O, Lidgren L: The economic cost of low back pain in Sweden in 2001. Acta Orthop 76:275–284, 2005.
14. Blumenthal SL, McAfee PC, Guyer RD, et al: A Prospective, Randomized, Multi-Center FDA IDE Study of Lumbar Total Disc Replacement with the CHARITÉ™ Artificial Disc vs. Lumbar Fusion: Part I—Evaluation of Clinical Outcomes. Spine 30:1565–1575, 2005.

PART

# II

# Surgical Considerations of Motion Preservation Surgery of the Spine

CHAPTER 15

# Technique of Anterior Exposure of the Lumbar Spine

Bauer E. Sumpio

**KEY POINTS**

- Retroperitoneal approach to the anterior spine is a safe and expeditious technique that provides excellent anterior exposure of L3-S1 vertebrae.
- Advantages of the paramedian retroperitoneal approach include the avoidance of entry into the peritoneal cavity and need for abdominal wall muscle transaction.
- Appropriate instrumentation with visualization afforded by good lighting and retraction is key to obtaining safe and adequate exposure of the lumbar discs.
- Precise knowledge of the relationship of the lumbar bodies with the vascular, genitourinary, and nerve structures is critical to providing safe exposure of the anterior surface.
- Early ligation of the ascending lumbar (ileolumbar) vein is recommended when exposing the L4-L5 bodies.

## INTRODUCTION

Anterior lumbar interbody fusion (ALIF) and disc replacement are increasingly common procedures for the management of a number of spinal problems such as pseudoarthrosis, degenerative joint disease, and internal disc disruption from malignancy, infection, or trauma. Exposure of the anterior portion of the lumbar discs can be obtained through either a transperitoneal or extraperitoneal approach using a variety of skin incisions.[1–3] The retroperitoneal approach is the preferred procedure because it can be performed through small skin incisions and obviates the need for bowel retraction. Because mobilization of vascular structures and the ureters is generally necessary, it is common for vascular, urologic, or general surgeons to assist the spine surgeon with the exposure of the lumbar discs.

## TECHNIQUE

### Patient Preparation

Although a standard fluoroscopic operating room table is adequate, we have found that it is easier for the operator to perform the procedure when standing between the legs of the patient. We, therefore, utilize a radiolucent cystoscopy OSI bed that allows attachment of two leg boards that can be split apart. Once the patient has undergone induction of anesthesia, we place a Foley bladder catheter and secure pneumatic compression stockings to both legs.

### Skin Incision

Although the positions of the lumbar discs are fairly constant, we routinely use lateral and anteroposterior fluoroscopy to mark the skin over the disc spaces of interest (Fig. 15–1). This maneuver is helpful in minimizing the length of the skin incision. For a retroperitoneal approach to the lumbar spine, we usually employ a left paramedian incision for exposing L4-L5 and more cephalad disc spaces and a right paramedian incision for L5-S1 disc centered on the skin marking. Although the L5-S1 disc can be approached from either side, the rationale for selecting a right-sided incision initially is to spare the left retroperitoneum for recurrent disease of the L5-S1 disc or subsequent disc involvement at higher lumbar levels. A transverse skin incision is also acceptable for most single-level cases and some 2-level cases. In thin females, a Pfannensteil incision is commonly utilized and with adequate retraction can provide excellent visualization of not only the L5-S1 disc but also the L4-L5 disc. If a transperitoneal approach is contemplated, the standard midline incision is utilized.

### Entry into Retroperitoneal Space

For the retroperitoneal approach, the external oblique fascia is identified and incised close to the midline (Fig. 15–2A). The rectus muscle is mobilized posteriorly to its lateral extent past the inferior epigastric vessels (Fig. 15–2B). Care should be taken in handling these vessels since rectus sheath hematomas have been reported as a result of a ruptured inferior epigastric artery.[4] Visualization of the semilunar line of Douglas (Fig. 15–2C) is important since it marks the transition of the separation of the aponeurosis of the transversus oblique and posterior internal oblique layer from

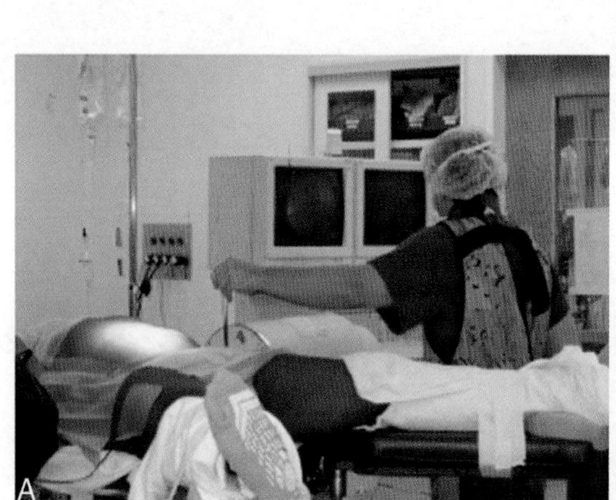

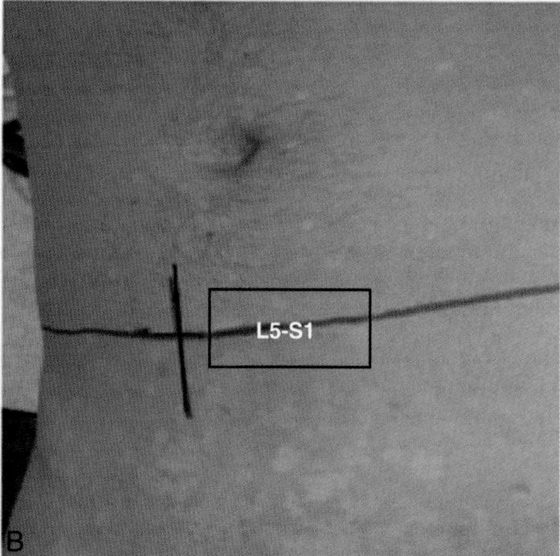


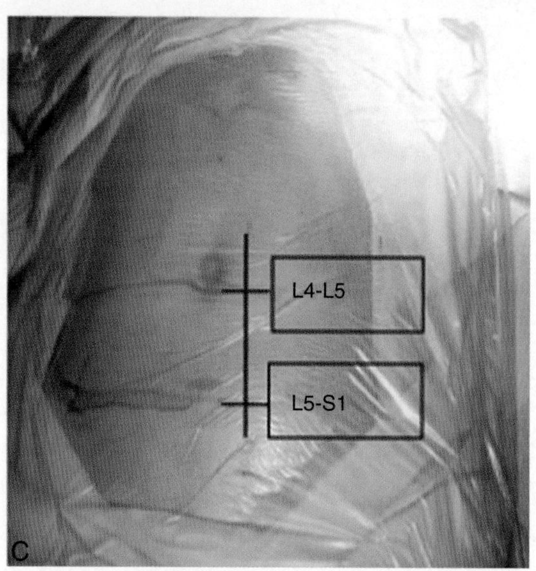


■ **FIGURE 15–1.** **(A)** Use of lateral and anteroposterior fluoroscopy to identify the disc spaces of interest. **(B)** Skin marks indicating proposed right paramedian incision for an L5-S1 disc procedure. **(C)** Skin marks for a left paramedian incision for combined L4-L5 and L5-S1 procedure.

the anterior internal oblique muscle fibers. Caudad to this anatomic line, the retroperitoneal space can be easily developed by sweeping the peritoneum in a lateral to medial direction and off the overlying posterior rectus sheath superiorly (Fig. 15–3A). The posterior sheath can then be safely incised in a vertical orientation, preserving the integrity of the peritoneum, allowing easy retraction of the peritoneal contents. The peritoneum and ipsilateral ureter are easily mobilized off the psoas muscle and the ipsilateral iliac artery and vein are identified (Fig. 15–3B). Violations into the peritoneal cavity should be promptly repaired with an appropriate absorbable suture to prevent further enlargement of the rent and to avoid spillage of bowel into the retroperitoneal space being developed. Injury to the ipsilateral ureter is uncommon, unless there is fibrous scarring from previous procedures.[5]

Exposure in the retroperitoneum and anterior lumbar spine is aided by the use of a self-retaining retractor, the SynFrame, (Synthes, West Chester, PA), which has multiple blades of varying length that are attached to a swivel clamp that can be anchored on a retractor ring (Fig. 15–4). The swivel clamp allows for multiple axes of articulation of the blades which enable easy and safe visualization of the deep structures.[6]

## Mobilization of Blood Vessels

The aorta and the inferior vena cava and their respective branches and tributaries lie anterior to the vertebral column. To safely dissect the anterior surface of the lumbar bodies, knowledge of their spatial relationship to these blood vessels is important[7,8] (Fig. 15–5A). The abdominal aorta usually divides on the left side of the L5 body into the common iliac arteries. The middle sacral artery arises from the back of the aorta at this bifurcation and descends in the middle of the L4-S1 vertebrae. The right common iliac artery is somewhat longer than the left, and passes more obliquely across the body of L5 (Fig. 15–5B). The arteries are separated from the bodies L4

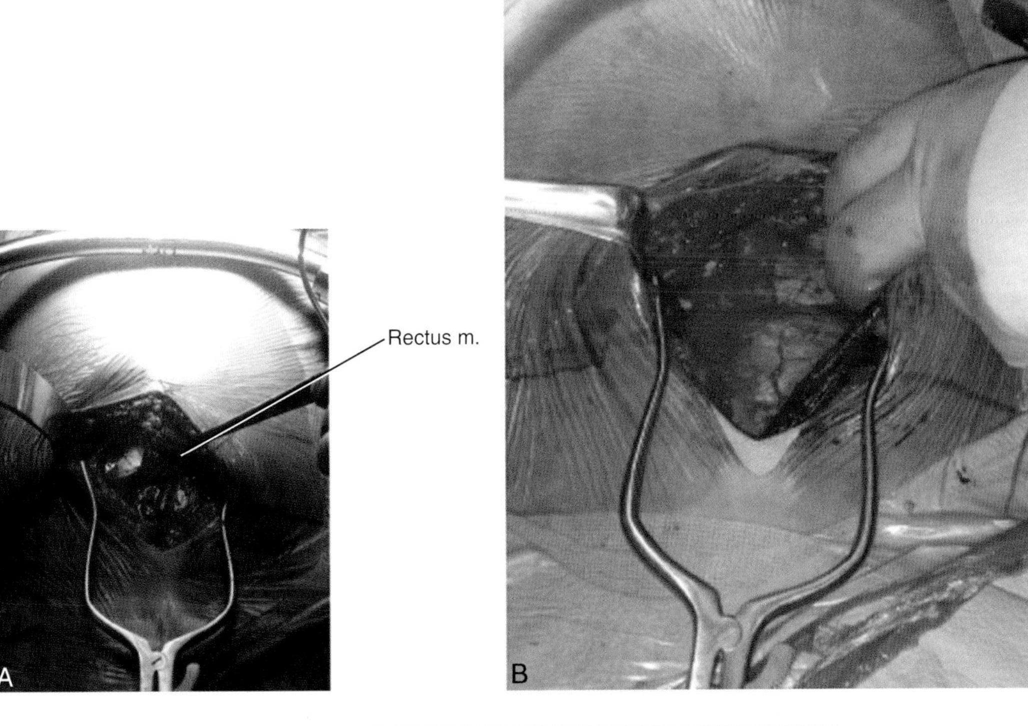


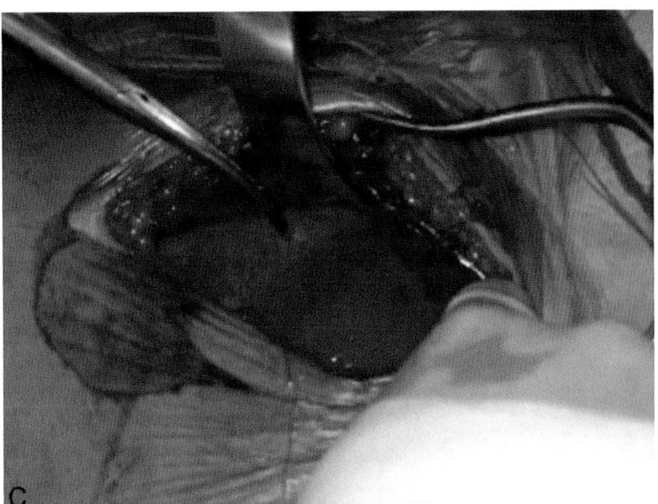


■ **FIGURE 15–2.** **(A)** After the skin incision is made and deepened through the subcutaneous tissue, the external oblique fascia is identified and incised close to the midline. **(B)** Mobilization of rectus muscle posteriorly to its lateral extent past the inferior epigastric vessels. **(C)** Clamp pointing to the semilunar line of Douglas.

and L5 by fibrocartilage and the common iliac veins and inferior vena cava. The right iliac arteries are just medial to the inferior vena cava and the right common iliac vein.

The left common iliac vein lies partly medial to, and partly behind, the left iliac arteries. The common iliac veins join each other at an acute angle at the L5 body to form the inferior vena cava. The left common iliac vein courses initially on the medial aspect of the left iliac artery, but then runs behind the right common iliac artery. Each common iliac vein receives the ileolumbar, and sometimes a lateral sacral vein. The left common iliac vein also drains the middle sacral vein. It should be emphasized that venous anomalies are not infrequent,[8] and therefore it is important to exercise caution when anatomic variants are encountered (Fig. 15–6).

For exposure of the L5-S1 disc, it is usually easy to dissect between the iliac vessels to expose the sacral promontory (see Fig. 15–5B). This is because in three-fourths of cases the bifurcation of the aorta occurs below the L4 vertebra with only less than 10% occurring below L5.[7] The common iliac vessels are mobilized laterally, and the middle sacral vessels are divided to provide complete exposure. Generally, blunt dissection is all that is then required to expose the fibrocartilage overlying the disc.

For exposure of discs higher than L5-S1, it is necessary to mobilize the overlying aorta and inferior vena cava medially. Because the bifurcation of the aorta and the inferior vena cava is usually below the L4 body, it is almost impossible to approach the L4-L5 disc between the iliac vessels. The risk of thrombosis

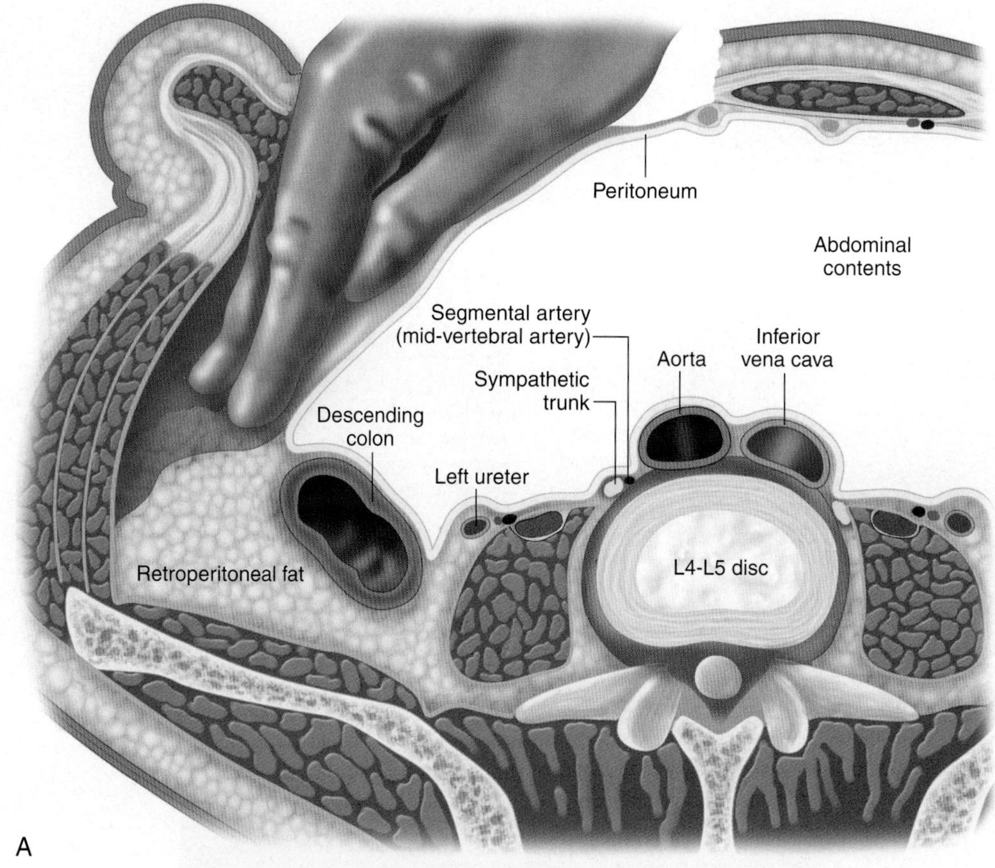


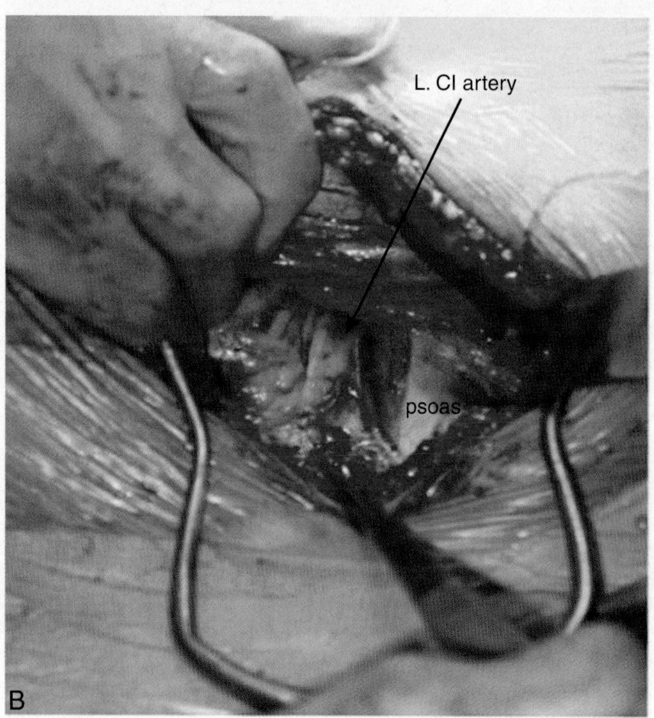


■ **FIGURE 15–3.** **(A)** Schematic depicting mobilization of the peritoneal cavity during a retroperitoneal approach **(B)** Intraoperative photograph showing the retroperitoneal space and the underlying psoas muscle and adjacent common iliac vessels.

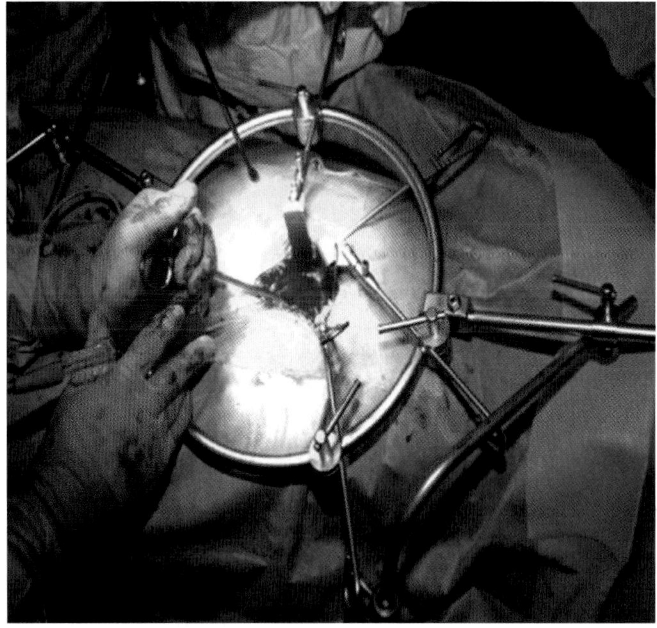

■ **FIGURE 15–4.** Self-retaining retractor (SynFrame, Synthes, West Chester, PA), which has multiple blades of varying length that are attached to a swivel clamp that can be anchored on a retractor ring.

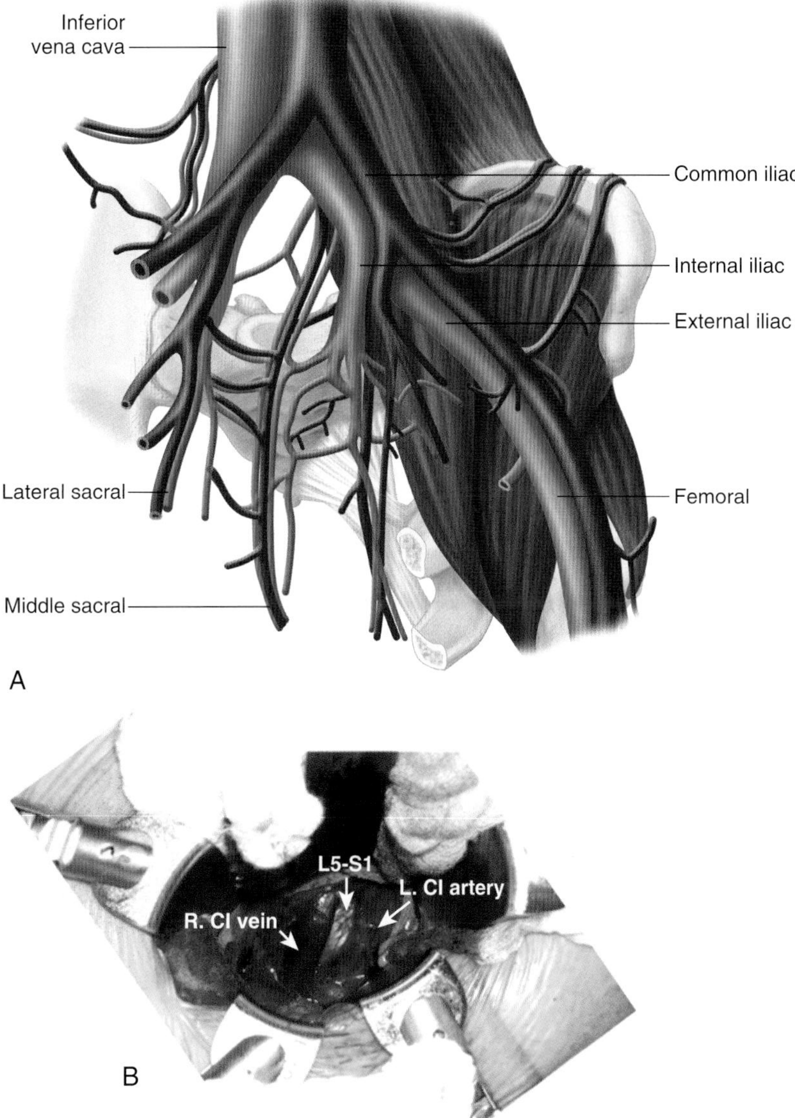


■ **FIGURE 15–5.** **(A)** Anatomic relationship of the common iliac vessels (from reference 7). **(B)** L5-S1 exposure approached from a right paramedian incision. The head of the patient is at the top and the feet toward the bottom. Note that the dissection for the L5-S1 disc space (L5-S1) is between the right common iliac vein (R. CI Vein) and the left common iliac artery (L. CI Artery).

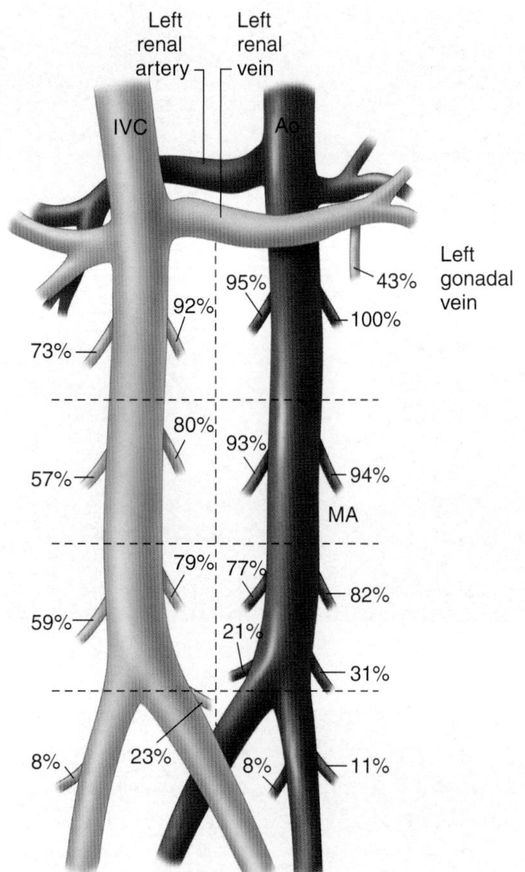


■ **FIGURE 15–6.** Frequency of venous anomalies encountered during the dissection of the anterior lumbar spine. *(Adapted from Baniel J, Foster RS, Donohue JP. (1995) Surgical anatomy of the lumbar vessels: implications for retroperitoneal surgery.* J Urol. *153: 1422–1424.)*

of the iliac arteries or veins, if not actual tearing of the vessels, because of excessive retraction is extremely high and may be limb or life threatening. The safest approach for the lumbar discs is to divide the segmental vessels that emanate from the aorta and vena cava to facilitate the medial retraction of these vessels. When the L4-L5 disc is being exposed, special attention should be paid to the ileolumbar or ascending vein, a large venous branch overlying the L5 body and draining into the lateral left common iliac vein (Fig. 15-7). We generally dissect this vessel completely, early in the procedure, and divide it. The L5 root often runs in close proximity to this branch and should be identified and avoided. In the rare cases where the ascending branch is left intact, one must be cognizant to avoid undue traction on the left iliac vein, as major hemorrhage can result from minor injuries.

## Other Technical Considerations

Meticulous attention to detail is essential when obtaining anterior exposure of the lumbar spine to the vascular, neurological, and urological structures which could be potentially injured. Excessive retraction on arteries or veins may lead to thrombosis, if not frank laceration. Use of the bipolar electrocautery may reduce the chance of inadvertent damage to nerve fibers. Retroperitoneal lymphatics must be ligated if crossed to prevent lymph leak that may be a nidus for infection or prolonged ileus.

## COMMENT

Anterior exposure of lumbar discs has become an increasingly popular approach to the treatment of disc disease. This strategy has several advantages over the posterior approach, including the

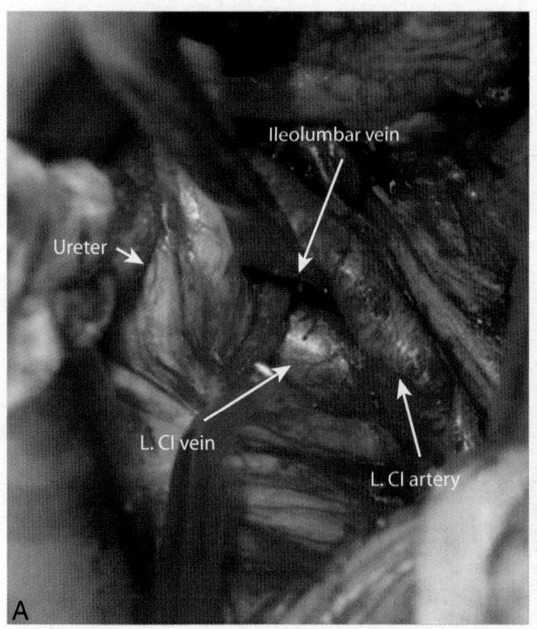


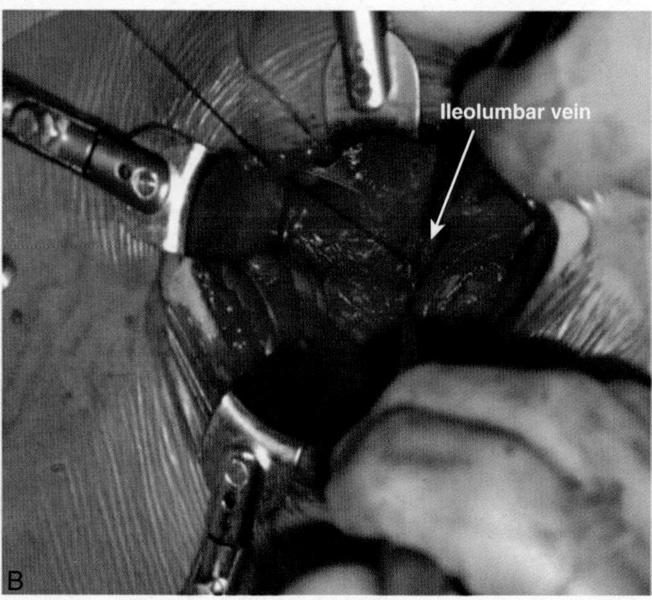


■ **FIGURE 15–7.** L4-L5 exposure approached from a left paramedian incision. **(A)** The head of the patient is toward the upper left corner and the feet toward the lower right corner. The left common iliac vein (L. CI vein), left common iliac artery (L. CI artery), ureter, and ileolumbar vein are depicted. The left common iliac artery is retracted laterally to expose the ileolumbar vein off of the left common iliac vein. Note the L5 nerve root running lateral to the left iliac artery. **(B)** Silk ligature around the ileolumbar vein.

reduced incidence of nerve damage and avoidance of paraspinal muscle trauma, the ability to get a more complete disc excision, and therefore placement of a larger interbody fusion device, and decreased hospital stay.[1,2,3,5]

Potential complications of the anterior approach are numerous because of the anatomic structures and the technical demands; the avoidance and management of these complications will be discussed in detail in the following chapter. Nevertheless, the open retroperitoneal exposure for anterior spine surgery is a safe and rewarding technique. Because of the distinct advantages of accessing the entire disc as opposed to the posterior approach, as well as the emerging technique of spinal disc arthroplasty, demand for anterior lumbar procedures will only increase. Other techniques, such as laparoscopy has not shown any advantage to the open technique; however, larger prospective randomized trials are still necessary.[9] The lumboscopic aproach is a promising new technique to gain access to the retroperitoneal space with similar complication rates to the open technique, and it has the theoretical advantage of decreased hospital stay and convalescent time, but experience is limited.

Open retroperitoneal exposure to the lumbar and lumbosacral vertebral bodies can be performed safely and should be in the repertoire of the general and vascular surgeon. Although a few centers have experienced orthopaedic spine surgeons with comparable complication rates, we believe that a combined multidisciplinary approach maximizes the various surgical skills of the orthopaedic and vascular or general surgeon, reducing complication rates in anterior spinal surgery.

## REFERENCES

1. Gumbs A, Shah R, Yue J, Sumpio BE: The open anterior paramedian retroperitoneal approach for spine procedures. Arch Surg 140:339–343, 2005.
2. Brau S, Delamarter RB, Schiffman ML, et al: Vascular injury during anterior lumbar surgery. Spine J 4:409–412, 2004.
3. Bianchi C, Ballard JL, Abou-Zamzam AM, et al: Anterior retroperitoneal lumbosacral spine exposure: Operative technique and results. Ann Vasc Surg 17:137–142, 2003.
4. Graham J, Reardon M: Rectus sheath hematoma after anterior lumbar fusion. Spine J 12:1377, 1991.
5. Sumpio B, Gumbs A: Revision open anterior approaches for spine procedures. Spine J 7(3):280–285. E pub Jan. 30, 2007.
6. *http://products.synthes.com/prod_support/Product%20Support%20Materials/Technique%20Guides/SPINE/SPTGSynFrameJ2887L.pdf#search=%22synframe%22*
7. Gray H: Anatomy of the Human Body. Philadelphia, Lea & Febiger, 1918.
8. Baniel J, Foster RS, Donohue JP: Surgical anatomy of the lumbar vessels: Implications for retroperitoneal surgery. J Urol 153:1422–1424, 1995.
9. Zdeblick TA, David SM: A prospective comparison of surgical approach for anterior L4-L5 fusion: Laparoscopic versus minianterior lumbar interbody fusion. Spine 25:2682–2687, 2000.

CHAPTER 16

# Management of Complications of the Anterior Exposure of the Lumbar Spine

**Kristina Spate** and **Bauer E. Sumpio**

**KEY POINTS**

- Major complications of anterior exposures are rare but include vascular injury, vascular thrombosis, genitourinary injury, and retrograde ejaculation.
- A careful preoperative history and physical examination are essential in identifying patients at higher risk for complications.
- Understanding anatomic relationships of vital structures involved in the procedure is important in the prevention of an injury.
- Early recognition of a complication is essential for a positive outcome.
- Prompt management of complications can improve clinical outcomes.

## INTRODUCTION

With the growing number of lumbar spine procedures being performed, the need for efficient and adequate exposure to the anterior lumbar spine has increased. Unlike the traditional posterior approach to the spine, use of an anterior exposure involves either a transperitoneal approach or a retroperitoneal approach.[1] Owing to the nature of the procedure, the complications may involve, but are not limited to, vascular, neurologic, and urologic structures (Tables 16–1 and 16–2). There are many different strategies to manage these complications, but the most important factor in obtaining a positive clinical outcome is early recognition. This can be provided by the surgeon only if he is cognizant of the potential complications for a specific patient while obtaining a thorough preoperative history and physical examination, while performing the procedure, and when he also has a high index of suspicion during the postoperative period.

## VASCULAR COMPLICATIONS

The occurrence of blood vessel injury during an anterior lumbar procedure can be potentially life threatening for the patient if the problem is not recognized and rectified promptly during or immediately following the procedure. Recent reports have demonstrated an overall incidence of vessel injury to be relatively low at 1.9%.[2] The mobilization of the iliac vessels during the dissection places the patient at potential risk for arterial or venous disruption or thrombosis (Fig. 16–1).

Preoperative work-up should include a careful history and physical examination. The history should document whether the patient suffers from symptoms such as claudication or rest pain, or if he has undergone any revascularization procedures in the past. The patient's physical examination should note the presence of pedal pulses, chronic leg edema, or any long-term ulcers suggestive of peripheral arterial or venous disease. If there are any positive findings on history or physical examination, further laboratory evaluation of the patient's preoperative vascular status will need to be obtained.[3] An ankle brachial index is helpful in evaluating a patient during the initial physical. If the suspicion for symptomatic peripheral arterial disease is high, the need for further diagnostic tests may be necessary and include the use of complete duplex ultrasonography, pulse volume recordings, and plethysmographic tracings. Depending on the results of these diagnostic tests, the patient may be deemed a high risk for vascular complications before the elective lumbar procedure. All patients should have a physical examination that contains documentation of pedal pulses before the procedure. This will serve as a useful reference when monitoring a patient through the procedure and postoperative course. A lateral lumbar radiograph is useful for evaluating the presence of calcifications in the aorta or iliac vessels. In a prior study, this was not considered a contraindication to performing an anterior lumbar exposure.[2] The radiograph might demonstrate the presence of osteophytes, which have been noted to make the dissection of vessels more difficult. Preoperative ultrasound or imaging studies are not routinely used if the patient does not have symptoms suggestive of peripheral arterial disease; however, an arteriogram or venogram may need to be obtained if the patient is undergoing a revision of an anterior lumbar exposure.[4] The presence of scar tissue could potentially alter the anatomy, placing the vessels at higher risk of injury when the operation is approached without the knowledge of aberrant anatomy.

In patients at risk for arterial compromise, an oxygen saturation monitor can be placed on the patient's lower extremities in order

**TABLE 16–1. Table of Potential Complications**

**Vascular Complications**
Arterial injury
Arterial thrombosis
Venous injury
Venous thrombosis

**Urological Complications**
Ureter transection
Retrograde ejaculation

**Neurologic Complications**
Iliohypogastric nerve injury
Ilioinguinal nerve injury
Genitofemoral nerve injury
Femoral nerve injury
Sympathetic chain injury

**Miscellaneous**
Prolonged ileus
Psoas abcess
Wound infection
Hernia
Pseudomeningocele
Rectus muscle hematoma

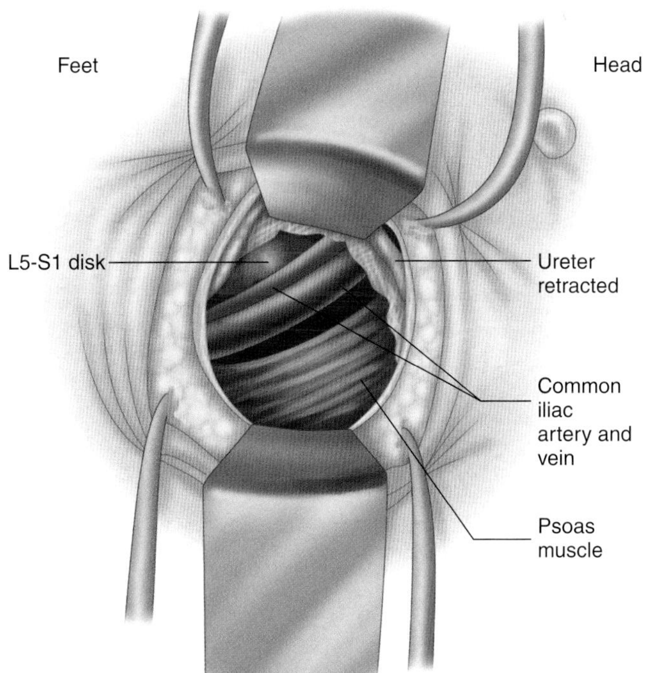


■ **FIGURE 16–1.** The view of the L5-S1 disc in relation to the left common iliac artery and vein. Retraction of the vessels is required to obtain adequate exposure of the disc space.

to provide continuous monitoring of the arterial flow to the lower extremities. This method has been found effective in monitoring iliac artery compression.[5] A desaturation below 90% is considered to be an indication of early signs of ischemia. The placement of retractors on the lumbar spine during the procedure often correlates with desaturation of the lower extremities with full recovery after the removal of the retractors. It is important to evaluate the patient for left iliac arterial thrombosis if the desaturation does not improve on the removal of the retractors. It should be noted that most of the patients who had signs of desaturation were able to withstand a temporary duration of iliac artery compression of up to one hour.[5]

The incidence of vessel injury was found to be the highest during the anterior approach of L4-L5, where care must be taken to identify the ileolumbar vein. The ileolumbar vein, also called the ascending lumbar vein, often drains into the lateral left common iliac vein and should be carefully identified, ligated, and divided (Fig. 16–2). Failure to identify and divide this branch may result in excessive traction on the left iliac vein, resulting in tearing of the vessels. It has been suggested that adequate distal mobilization of the left iliac artery down to the femoral canal also reduces overstretching of the artery, subsequently decreasing the occurrence of small intimal tears. If small arteriotomies are encountered, they are frequently primarily repaired without any further sequelae.

Arterial thrombosis is another complication that is encountered during the procedure. A prior study noted the incidence of left iliac artery thrombosis to be 0.45%.[2] The diagnosis is made clinically by the presence of a cool, mottled lower extremity; loss of palpable pulses; and decreased oxygen saturation on the affected extremity. Before the closure of the abdomen, it is necessary to note the presence of a palpable common iliac pulse. If the situation is encountered where there is a loss of the common iliac pulse, a common iliac thrombus should be suspected, and a thrombectomy can be performed using a Fogarty balloon catheter. Following the thrombectomy, return of good blood flow accompanied by the

**TABLE 16–2. Table of Complication Rates**

| | Brau[2] | Brau[2] | Sumpio[4] | Rajaraman[11] | Sasso[8] | Tiusanen[7] |
|---|---|---|---|---|---|---|
| Arterial thrombosis | 6/1315 (0.45%) | — | — | — | — | — |
| Venous injuries | 19/1315 (1.4%) | — | — | 4/60 (6.6%) | — | — |
| Compartment syndrome | 2/1315 (0.15%) | — | — | — | — | — |
| DVT | — | 7/684 (1.02%) | 1/9 (11%) | 1/60 (1.6%) | — | — |
| Somatic neural injury | — | — | 1/9 (11%) | 3/60 (5%) | — | — |
| Retrograde ejaculation | — | 1/684 (0.14%) | 1/9 (11%) | — | 6/146 (4.1%) | 9/40 (22.5%) |
| Ureteral disruption | — | — | 1/9 (11%) | — | — | — |
| Wound infection | — | 3/684 (0.43%) | — | 2/60 (3.3%) | — | — |
| Postoperative ileus | — | 4/684 (0.58%) | 1/9 (11%) | 3/60 (5%) | — | — |
| Hernias | — | 2/684 (0.29%) | — | — | — | — |

DVT, deep vein thrombosis.

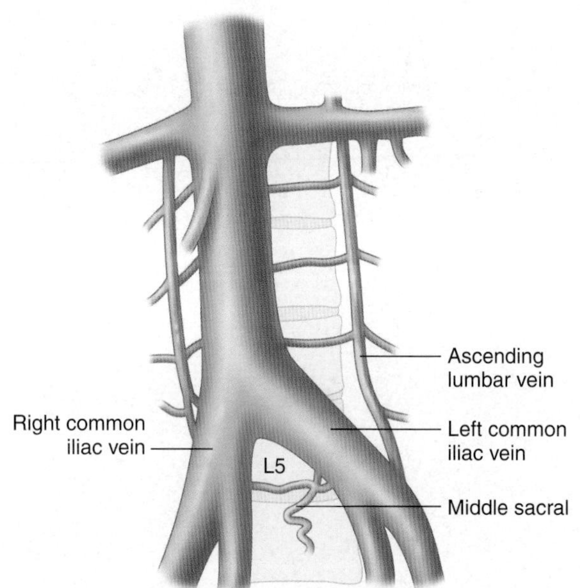


■ **FIGURE 16–2.** The relationship of the ascending lumbar vein (also known as ileolumbar) to the left common iliac vein. This venous tributary should be identified, ligated, and divided during the anterior exposure to prevent excessive traction.

return of a palpable pulse must be demonstrated. On-table angiography may be used post-thrombectomy for further evaluation if needed. In patients who have had ischemia for more than 2 hours, prophylactic calf fasciotomies may be required. The most significant long-term sequelae in these patients are the presence of residual sensory and muscular deficits in the affected extremity. The delay in diagnosis and treatment of patients with this condition had a significant impact on the patients' recovery following these complications.

Major vein lacerations had a reported incidence of 1.4% to 3% in prior studies.[4,5] The majority of injuries are found to occur to the left common iliac vein, but injuries to the inferior vena cava and lumbar veins have also been reported while performing the procedure. Primary repair of venous lacerations, when possible, is the preferred management of this complication. In the case of an injury to the inferior vena cava, venorraphy is usually successful in controlling the bleeding, but in extreme cases, ligation of the inferior vena cava and common iliac veins may be performed. The latter may have the resultant long-term sequelae of chronic leg edema but provides a prompt and effective way to aid in minimizing blood loss.

Postoperative deep venous thrombosis can occur following the anterior exposure to the lumbar spine. However, studies have not been performed to evaluate if the occurrence is higher following this operation compared with other procedures. When this complication is encountered, the treatment regimen includes anticoagulation, and an inferior vena cava (IVC) filter if indicated. Many surgeons routinely use pneumatic compression stockings to prevent the occurrence of deep venous thrombosis.

## UROLOGIC COMPLICATIONS

Given the nature of extensive dissection necessary during anterior lumbar spine exposures, the performing surgeon must be aware of the possibility of urologic complications. Genitourinary complications range from transection of the ureter to postoperative retrograde ejaculation. As with the vascular evaluation, a careful preoperative history is critical in identifying patients who may be at greater risk for urologic complications. For example, a preoperative history from the patient may reveal a history of prior retroperitoneal surgery such as colonic resection or certain gynecologic procedures. This may suggest the presence of extensive scar tissue in the retroperitoneal space, placing this subset of patients at higher risk for genitourinary injuries. It is also imperative that a preoperative history determine whether the patient suffers from symptoms of erectile dysfunction before the operation.

The use of preoperative ureteral stents in revisions involving prior anterior lumbar procedures has been advocated to prevent ureteral injuries due to the extensive scar tissue that may pose a challenge during these procedures.[4] If the ureter is partially transected during the procedure, a primary closure over the ureteral stent is generally recommended. For uncomplicated upper and middle third ureteral injuries, ureteroureterostomy is the procedure of choice. For injuries below the pelvic brim, ureteroneocystostomy may be needed. On rare occasions, the ureteral injury may not be identified until the postoperative period. Patients with a ureteral injury may present with fever and abdominal or flank pain. Ultrasound may be a useful diagnostic tool with potential therapeutic effects if a urinoma is identified and requires drainage. Many reports advocate for the placement of a percutaneous nephrostomy tube following initial drainage to allow for urinary diversion followed by a definitive repair.[6]

Retrograde ejaculation is a complication that derives from an iatrogenic injury to the superior hypogastric plexus during the procedure and is an underestimated complication following these procedures. The incidence of this complication had been reported to range from 0.42% to 5.9%.[7,8] The ejaculatory response is composed of synchronous events involving the contraction of the bladder neck musculature innervated by the superior hypogastric plexus.[8] This nerve plexus resides in the retroperitoneal space in close proximity to the lumbosacral junction and overlies the origin of the common iliac artery, making it vulnerable to injury during dissection and mobilization (Fig. 16–3). Injury to the superior hypogastric plexus results in bladder neck incompetence during ejaculation, resulting in the flow of semen into the bladder. A study evaluating retrograde ejaculation occurrence during anterior lumbar exposures found the transperitoneal approach to have a much higher incidence of this complication compared with the retroperitoneal approach.[8] The transperitoneal approach almost necessitates dissection on top of the superior hypogastric plexus, accounting for the increased damage to this nerve plexus. In contrast, dissection in the retroperitoneal approach mobilizes the plexus within the peritoneum; sweeping it from left to right offers greater protection to this delicate structure (Fig. 16–4). It should also be mentioned that most of the patients who suffered from this complication had a significantly greater blood loss during their operation than patients who did not develop this condition, potentially suggesting that these patients had a more difficult dissection making them more prone to this complication. Many surgeons advocate for preoperative storage of patient semen before the operation in younger male patients.

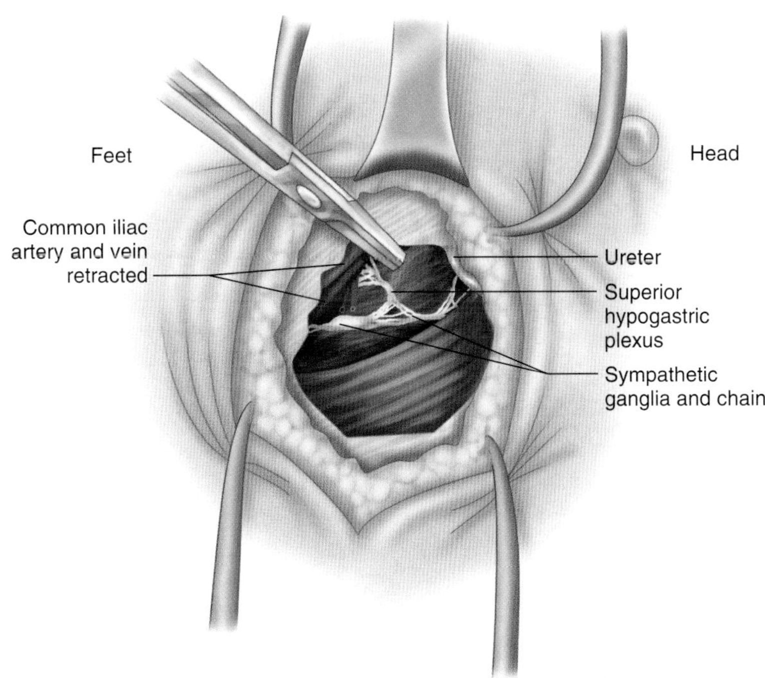


■ **FIGURE 16–3.** The superior hypogastric plexus and sympatheic chain. Preservation of the superior hypogastric plexus prevents retrograde ejaculation. The sympathetic chain, when inured, will cause temperature variation in the lower extremity on the ipsilateral side of the injured nerve.

## NEUROLOGIC COMPLICATIONS

Neurologic complications may occur during the exposure of the anterior spine and can leave a patient with chronic motor or sensory deficits depending on the involved nerve. The neurologic complications that have been described following this procedure are injuries to the iliohypogastric nerve, ilioinguinal nerve, genitofemoral nerve, femoral nerve, the sympathetic chain, and superior hypogastric plexus (Fig. 16–5). The iliohypogastric nerve, ilioinguinal nerve, genitofemoral nerve, and the sympathetic chain are primarily sensory nerves and are present in the postoperative period with dysthesias. In contrast, injury to the femoral nerve results in motor deficits to the affected limb. Injury to the superior hypogastric plexus results in retrograde ejaculation. Postoperative radiculopathies may also develop following the procedure but are usually not a result of the exposure but rather lumbar nerve root impingement from instrumentation and therefore are not discussed in this chapter.

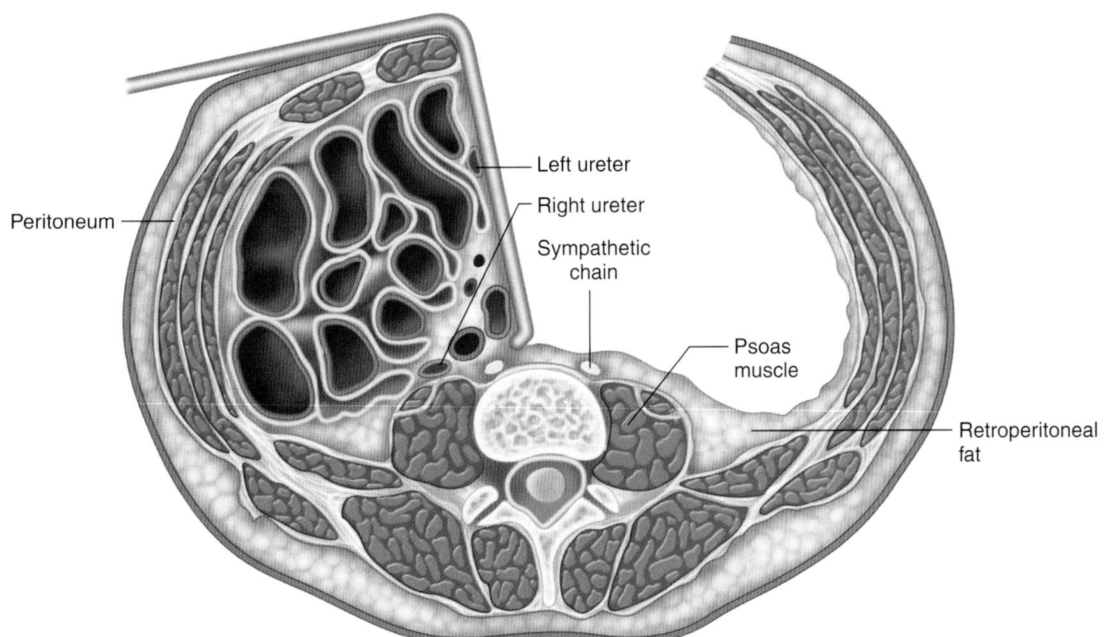


■ **FIGURE 16–4.** A cross-sectional view of the retroperitoneal space through an anterior retroperitoneal approach. Note that the bowel contents are mobilized and retracted to one side within the peritoneum, providing protection of the peritoneal contents and the ureters.

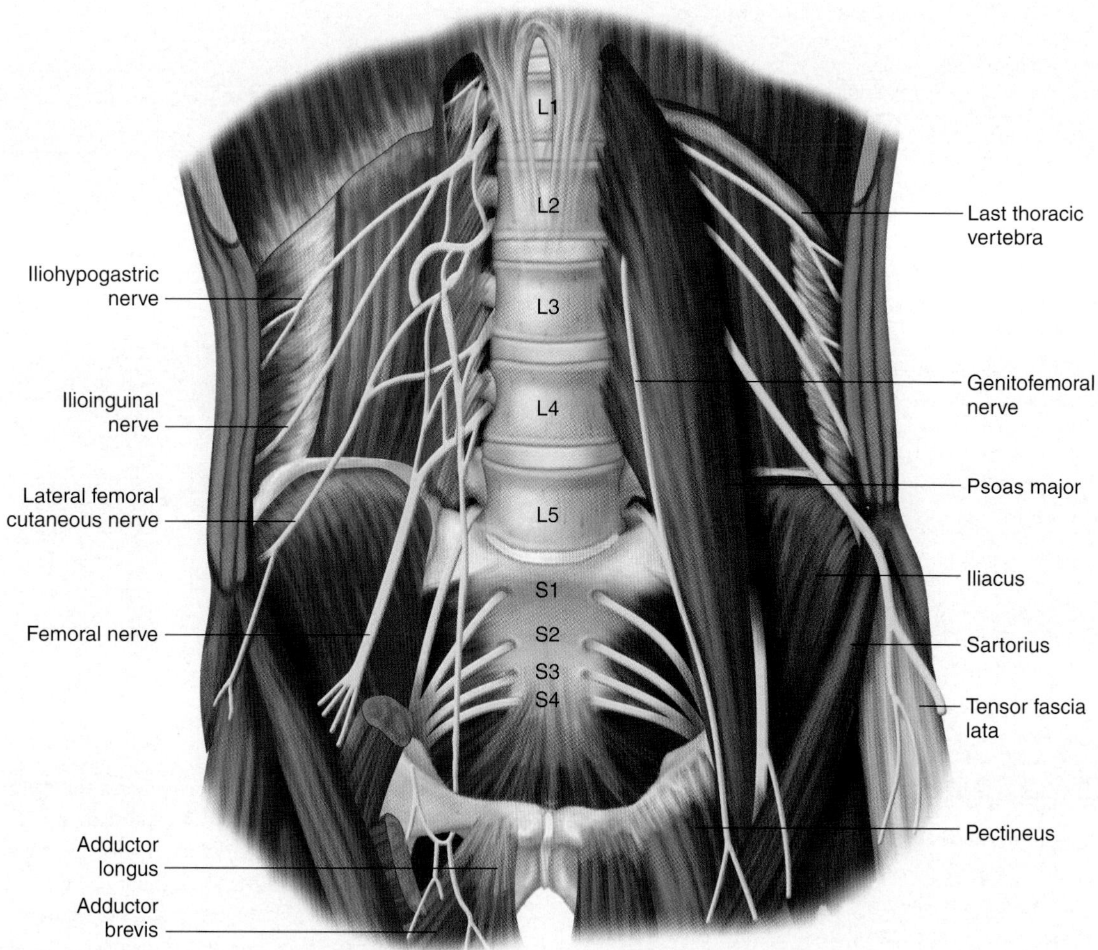


■ **FIGURE 16–5.** Iliohypogastric nerve, ilioinguinal nerve, gentiofemoral nerve, femoral nerve, and lumbar plexus. These nerves are vulnerable to injury during anterior exposure of the lumbar spine.

Injuries to nerves can occur from several mechanisms such as overstreching, blunt trauma, compression, hypoxia, and entrapment. Pain with a burning quality is usually the presenting symptom when a sensory nerve in this region is injured. The diagnosis is usually established with the clinical presentation, but differential nerve blocks may be used if there is any difficulty with the diagnosis. The general principles in treatment include alleviation of nerve compression, rehabilitation, and the use of analgesics. If necessary, therapeutic nerve blocks or nerve transection may be used if prior attempts at conservative management have been attempted and failed.

Injury to the iliohypogastric nerve is rare but could be potentially injured during the exposure of the higher lumbar regions. The location provides itself for injury as it passes through the psoas muscle, extending diagonally along the anterior surface of the quadratus lumborum (see Fig. 16–5). This nerve serves as motor innervation to the transversus abdominis and the internal oblique muscles. Its sensory distribution is the groin and the symphysis pubis region. When injury to this nerve occurs, patients may describe a pulling or throbbing sensation, which can occur many years after the surgery. Their physical activity may be limited owing to the aggravation of the nerve. As mentioned earlier, conservative therapy should first be initiated. If conservative therapy fails, nerve blocks and transection of the nerve in the retroperitoneal space may be attempted in order to improve the patient's symptoms.

The occurrence of ilioinguinal nerve injury is also rare in anterior exposures but should be discussed to aid in obtaining a differential diagnosis. The ilioinguinal nerve courses along a similar route just inferior to the iliohypogastric nerve until it enters the inguinal canal about 2 cm medial to the anterior superior iliac spine and then courses just beneath the anterior leaf of the inguinal canal as it exits out the superficial inguinal ring to become a sensory nerve to the overlying skin (see Fig. 16–4). The nerve supplies sensory innervation to the groin and inner thigh. The diagnosis is confirmed by blocking the nerve with local anesthetic injected 2.5 to 3 cm medial and inferior to the anterior superior iliac crest. Desensitization of this nerve can be achieved by multiple nerve blocks to achieve long-term pain relief for these patients.[9]

The genitofemoral nerve can sustain an injury during this procedure as the nerve runs through the psoas muscle and emerges near its medial border opposite the third and fourth lumbar vertebrae (see Fig. 16–5). It descends retroperitoneally and crosses behind the ureter. The genital branch supplies the skin of the genital region, whereas the femoral branch supplies the skin of the femoral triangle. When this nerve is injured, these patients will complain of burning paresthesias and pain in the groin and medial thigh.[9] Transection of the nerve can be accomplished if conservative treatment is unsuccessful.

Injury to the sympathetic chain during the exposure is also a neurological complication that may occur during the procedure. The lumbar sympathetic chain is located on the lateral aspect of the vertebral bodies (see Fig. 16–3). The patient will present with a warmer extremity on the affected side owing to the loss of sympathetic vasoconstriction. Patients may also note a slight swelling or discoloration on the affected side as well. The majority of patients improve with conservative management.

Femoral nerve injury has been described during an anterior exposure as it lies in close proximity to the psoas muscle prior to traversing beneath the inguinal ligament. Injury to the femoral nerve will present with a weakness or absence of the patellar reflex and a notable weakness or paralysis of the quadriceps muscle. A case report of two patients who suffered from femoral nerve palsy following the operation has been described.[10] Previous reports have described the mechanism of this condition to be an iliacus muscle hematoma causing nerve compression. The surgeons describing their complications following anterior lumbar interbody fusions proposed this injury was attributed to a tight constriction of the nerve by a portion of the psoas while the muscle was in maximum stretch during the operation.

## MISCELLANEOUS COMPLICATIONS

There are several other complications that have been associated with the procedure that are worthy of discussion but do not fit in a particular category. Postoperative ileus, defined as an ileus lasting more than 4 days, has been described with an incidence of 0.6%.[12] Prolonged ileus may be related to prior abdominal surgeries, extensive dissection, retroperitoneal hematoma formation, major interoperative fluid shifts, or excessive narcotic use. It is intuitive that a retroperitoneal approach may have a lower occurrence of postoperative ileus than a transperitoneal approach due to less manipulation of peritoneal contents (see Fig. 16–4). Regardless of the approach performed, these patients may be successfully managed conservatively with nasogastric decompression, intravenous fluids, and minimal use of narcotic medications. The diet may be slowly advanced as bowel function returns.

Wound infections are an additional reported complication. The incidence of wound infection has been cited as being as low as 0.4–3.3%.[11,12] These were mostly uncomplicated infections that resolved with drainage and antibiotics. The incidence of postoperative hernias was reported to occur at a rate less than 0.3%.[12] These primarily occurred in larger patients and were primarily asymptomatic.

Rectus sheath hematomas have been described following an anterior approach to the lumbar spine. A case report described a patient who became tachycardic, pale, and diffusely tender at the postoperative site after a paroxysm of severe coughing 3 days following the operation.[13] Surgical exploration found the hemorrhage to be a result of a ruptured inferior epigastric artery. To prevent this complication, careful attention should be made to preserve the epigastric vessels if they are encountered during the surgical approach through the rectus sheath. If these vessels are severely injured, it may be necessary to ligate them.

The development of a psoas abcess was not reported in the large studies; however, one case report described a patient who developerd a psoas abcess after an anterior spinal fusion in the late postoperative period.[14] The classic symptoms of a psoas abcess are fever, leukocytosis, and pain with extension and internal rotation of the hip described as a "psoas sign." Drainage of the abcess, antibiotics, and the removal of hardware is the treatment for this condition.

Development of an anterior pseudomeningocele following an anterior lumbar fusion was described in a 35-year-old woman following anterior lumbar interbody fusion. The pseudomeningocele presented as a large abdominal mass.[15] The mass appeared large and cystic in nature, and upon further analysis of cystic fluid revealed to be cerebrospinal fluid suggestive of a pseudomeningocele. A cystoperitoneal shunt was placed and allowed for gradual drainage of the cerebrospinal fluid (CSF) into the abdominal cavity, allowing the cyst to gradually decrease in size.

## CONCLUSION

With the increasing demand for safe and efficient exposure of the anterior lumbar spine, knowledge of potential complications is critical for the surgeons performing the procedure. The management of the complications depends on the nature of the complication. Prudent attention to detail is essential when obtaining exposure of the vascular, neurologic, and urologic structures that could be potentially injured. Clinical reports demonstrate that with the judicious use of caution, the anterior exposure of the lumbar spine can be performed with low complication rates.

## REFERENCES

1. Gumbs A, Shah R, Yue J, Sumpio BE: The open anterior paramedian retroperitoneal approach for spine procedures. Arch Surg 140:339–343, 2005.
2. Brau S, Delamarter RB, Schiffman ML, et al: Vascular injury during anterior lumbar surgery. Spine J 4:409–412, 2004.
3. Collins K, Sumpio B: Vascular Assessment. Clin Podiatr Med Surg 17:171–191, 2000.
4. Sumpio B, Gumbs A: Revision open anterior approaches for spine procedures. Spine J 7(3):280–285, 2006.
5. Brau S, Spoonamore MJ, Snyder L, et al: Nerve monitoring changes related to iliac artery compression during anterior lumbar surgery. Spine J 3:351–355, 2003.
6. Fry D, Milholen L, Harbrecht PJ: Iatrogenic ureteral injury: Options in management. Arch Surg 4:454–457, 1983.
7. Tiusanen H, Seitsalo D, Osterman K, Soini J: Retrograde Ejaculation after anterior interbody fusion. Eur Spine J 4:339–342, 1995.
8. Sasso R, Kenneth Burkus J, LeHuec J-C: Retrograde ejaculation after anterior lumbar interbody fusion: Transperitoneal versus retroperitoneal exposure. Spine J 28:1023–1026, 2003.
9. Perry CP: Peripheral neuropathies presenting as chronic pelvic pain. J Am Assoc Gynecol Laparosc 7(2):281–287, 2000.
10. Papastefanou S, Stevens K, Mulholland R: Femoral nerve palsy: An unusual complication of anterior lumbar interbody fusion. Spine J 19:2842–2844, 1994.

11. Rajaraman V, Vingan R, Roth P, et al: Visceral and vascular complications resulting from anterior lumbar interbody fusion. J Neurosurg 91:60–64, 1999.
12. Brau SM: Mini-open approach to the spine for anterior lumbar interbody fusion: Description of the procedure, results and complications. Spine J 2:216–223, 2002.
13. Graham J, Kozak J, Reardon M: Rectus sheath hematoma after anterior lumbar fusion. Spine J 12:1377, 1991.
14. Hresko M, Hall J: Latent psoas abcess after anterior spinal fusion. Spine J 17:590–593, 1992.
15. Kolawole T, Patel P, Ur-Rahaman N: Post surgical anterior pseudomeningocele presenting as an abdominal mass. Comp Radiol 11: 237–240, 1987.

CHAPTER 17

# Lateral Approaches to the Lumbar Spine: Anterolateral Transpsoatic Approach

Rudolf Bertagnoli

## KEY POINTS

- The anterolateral transpsoatic approach (ALPA) has been developed to bypass risks of a posterior approach to the lumbar spine disc space. These risks are weakening and removal of ligament and bone material, as well as affection of nerve tissue.
- Compared with traditional anterior and posterior approaches, it is more secure in total or partial disc arthroplasty because it saves anterior longitudinal ligaments (ALL) and posterior longitudinal ligaments (PLL), and therefore, segment stability is maintained. It is also useful for fusion procedures. It can be used from the left and right side.
- A limitation, however, is in the L5-S1 region where lateral access is possible only by means of osteotomy through the iliac crest, and here, the vascular topography around the disc is different and bears more risks.

## INTRODUCTION

A treatment strategy for disc degeneration is either partial or total disc arthroplasty. Numerous devices are currently in use. Historically, the surgical strategy used to implant these nucleus replacement devices was an open posterior approach. But this approach bears some risks associated with the procedure, such as mechanical weakening through removal of ligament and bone material. A damage to the facet joints induces painful perifacetogen reactions and nerve tissue damage due to the necessary exposure of the dura, the traversing and exiting nerve roots and epidural scarring and bleeding should be kept in view. Implant expulsions as a consequence of the defect in the posterior longitudinal ligament (PLL) and posterior annulus have been observed as well. The anterolateral transpsoatic approach (ALPA) was developed to bypass the risks associated with the posterior approach[1,2] and to access the largest possible area of the disc without important anatomic structures. With the ALPA the access to the disc is made laterally through the psoas muscle, which minimizes the chance of damage to the osseoligamentous tension band structures. Specially the PLL and ALL, the strongest tension bands that are mainly controlling segment, are not disturbed at all, and therefore flexion/extension, the most important movement pattern in the lumbar spine, will not lead to dislocation in this direction. The evacuation of the nucleus as well as the implantation of the prosthetic device is also eased owing to the greater exposure of the disc from a lateral approach. Other authors have introduced the term XLIF90° (eXtreme Lateral Interbody Fusion), but the method is the same as the precursor ALPA approach.[3]

## INDICATIONS

Although the ALPA approach was initially developed for nucleus replacement arthroplasty, total disc replacements as well as fusion procedures are possible through this approach. This atraumatic, muscle-sparing access bypasses the risks of the posterior approach and at the same time eases the implantation process by providing a greater exposure of the disc. It allows an easy introduction of the artificial disc and the closure of the annulus after implantation.

## LIMITATIONS

Although ALPA is suitable for disc surgeries at levels L2 to L5, access to L5-S1 is possible by means of an osteotomy through the iliac crest.[4] The advantages of approaching the disc without having interference with important anatomic structures unfortunately is not possible in L5-S1 owing to the specific vascular anatomic topography, with the iliac vessels being located on the anterolateral and lateral aspect of the disc.

## OPERATIVE TECHNIQUE

### Positioning

To perform the ALPA approach, the surgeon should ideally stand behind the patient (Fig. 17–1). The patient is positioned in a strict 90-degree lateral decubitus position on an adjustable surgical table (Fig. 17–2). This is in contrast to the anterior lumbar interbody fusion (Mini-ALIF)[5], where the patient is positioned at a 60- to 70-degree angle (Fig. 17–3) and the surgeon is recommended to stand in front of the patient. Stable fixation is necessary to prevent shifting during the surgical procedure. If necessary, the patient's arms and legs can be supported also. It is recommended to flex

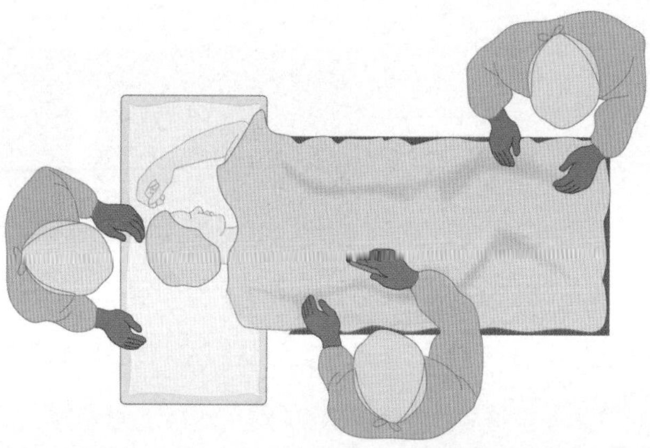

■ **FIGURE 17–1.** Surgeon stands behind the patient *(right)*.

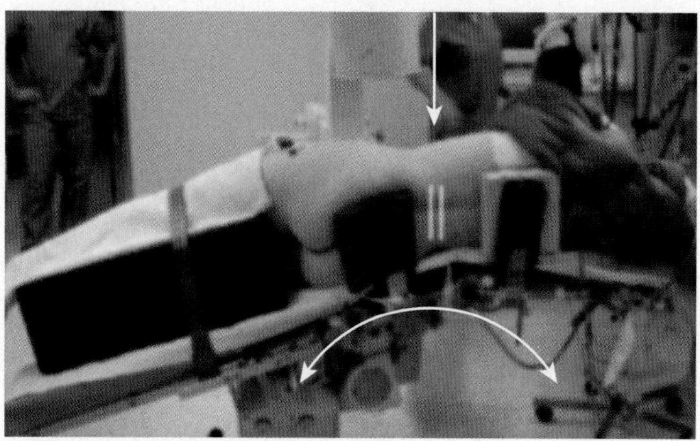

■ **FIGURE 17–2.** Patient positioning: 90 degrees lateral decubitus position, perpendicular adjustment of the segment by tilting the surgical table.

the table slightly to arch the patient to increase the distance between the iliac crest and the rib cage. To guarantee precise and easy working in the disc space, the table is tilted as long as the affected vertebra(e) is in a perpendicular position to the floor (see Fig. 17–2). This allows an optimal instrument orientation and reduces the risk of end plate damage. This exact position can be achieved only by using fluoroscopic imaging. The perpendicular projection of the disc space to the skin is marked by using a K-wire for identification (Fig. 17–4).

## Incision, Disc Exposure

To maximize the working angle away from the spinal canal, the surgeon stands behind the patient (see Fig. 17–1). Parallel to the fibers of the external oblique muscle, a 3- to 4-cm incision is made obliquely over the target area. Then the three layers of the abdominal muscles (external oblique, internal oblique, and traversus muscles) are bluntly dissected in the direction of the fibers. Self-retaining retractors are used and placed in the wound to keep the surgical field open. The psoas muscle is then approached retroperitoneally.

The anatomic safe zone with a width of approximately 2 to 3 cm through the psoas muscle corresponds with the lateral middle third of the disc (see Figs. 17–3, 17–5). A deviation too far toward the anterior margin of the lumbar spine must be avoided to keep the risk of injury of the sympathetic nerve and major blood vessels as small as possible. A deviation too far to the posterior region is also unfavorable because the exiting nerve roots of the spine as well as the lumbar plexus can be damaged (Fig 17–6). To minimize the risk of a damage of the exiting nerve roots or the lumbar plexus, an additional nerve root detection device can be used (NeuroVision, NuVasive, Inc.). The fibers of the psoas muscle will protect the sympathetic nerve chain in its anterior portion and the exiting nerve roots in their posterior portion if the access is carried out correctly in a strict lateral path through the muscle in the middle of the lateral aspect of the disc (Fig. 17–7). In a blunt dissection, the fibers of the psoas muscle are separated in a longitudinal direction. The surgical field is kept open with long self-retaining systems (e.g., Synframe, Synthes Inc., West Chester, PA; MaXess, NuVasive Inc., San Diego, CA) (Fig. 17–8). The use of retractor blades facing directly posterior should be avoided to reduce the risk of neuropraxy. Isolated blades in conjunction with the NeuroVision system are very helpful in this regard.

## Annulus Incision, Annulotomy

In preparation of the implantation procedure of the device, an annular flap is created in the outer annulus layers. This flap can later be securely closed after the implantation of the device. To access the nuclear cavity, a single midannular incision is performed through the remaining annulus layers.[6]

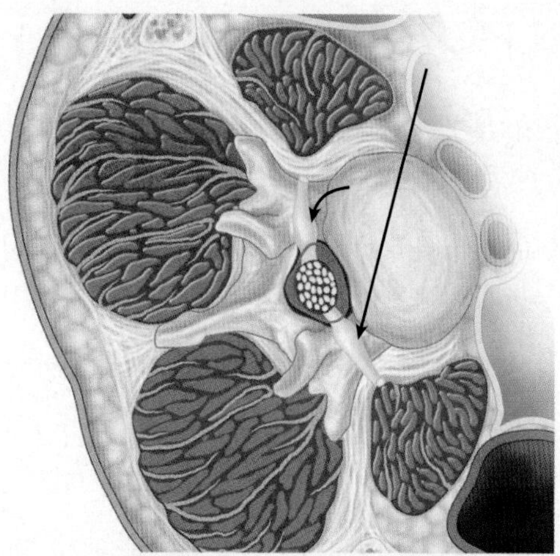

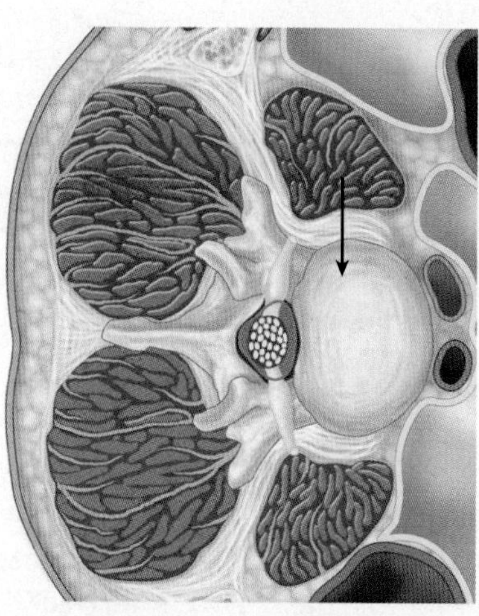

■ **FIGURE 17–3.** Access direction with conventional mini-ALIF *(left)* and with ALPA approach *(right)*.

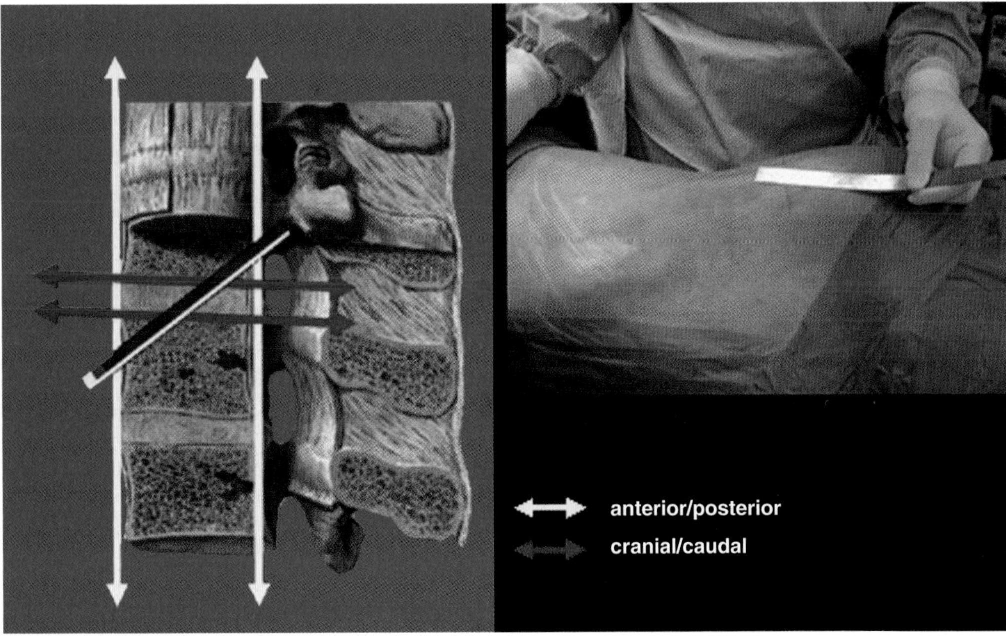


■ **FIGURE 17–4.** Anterior and posterior segment borders in projection to the skin level are marked with yellow lines; superior and inferior border of the disc space is marked with red lines; Oblique skin incision centered over the disc space is marked with a black line.

## Nucleus Excision, Wound Closure

The nucleus material is removed by means of pituitary rongeurs, suction devices, or automatic shaver systems after dilating the incised lateral annulus layers. In using nucleus arthroplasty devices, damage of the cartilagineous end plate or fractures of the bony portion of the end plates should be strictly avoided. Subsequently, all nucleus pulposus material is removed to create a big enough cavity for the finally expanded device.

The complete evacuation of the disc cavity is of utmost importance for a successful implantation of a prosthetic nucleus device. To achieve this, fluoroscopic imaging should be applied to determine whether additional nucleus material must be removed. Water-soluble contrast agents should be used alternatively; endoscopes can be used as well for checking the adequate preparation of the disc. Finally, the nucleus arthroplasty device can be implanted with specific instruments. The procedure is finalized by refixation of the annulus flap and removal of the retractors that allow the psoas muscles to readapt to each other (Fig. 17–9). Wound closure is attained with adaptation sutures of the three abdominal muscle layers.

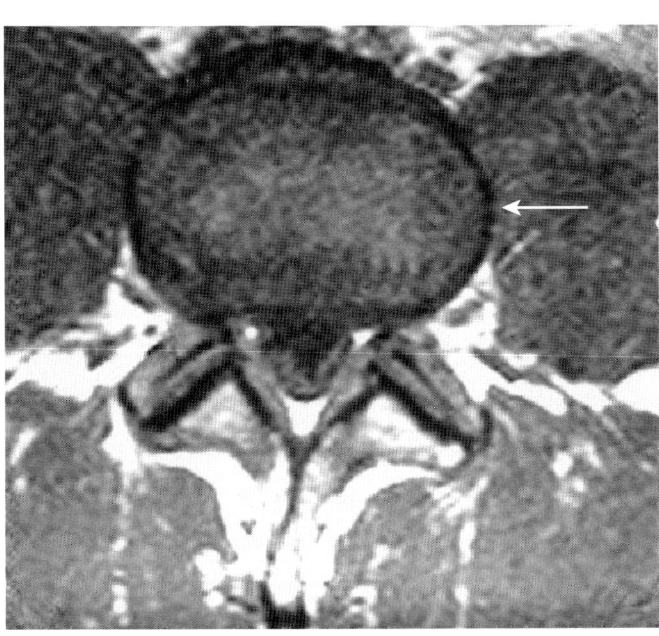

■ **FIGURE 17–5.** ALPA access route compared to mini-ALIF.

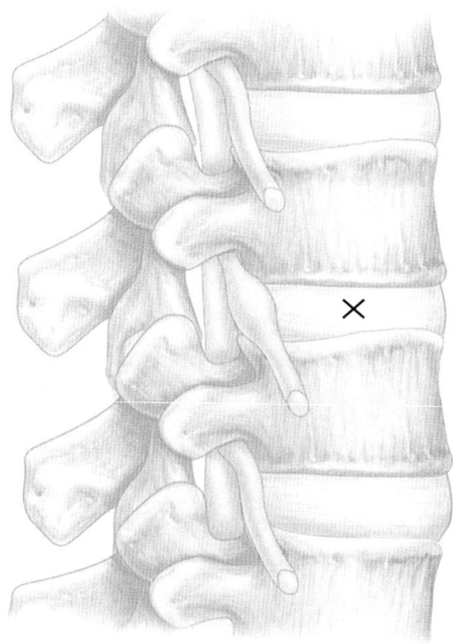

■ **FIGURE 17–6.** Disc space is accessed in an orthograde lateral way.

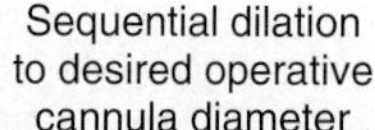
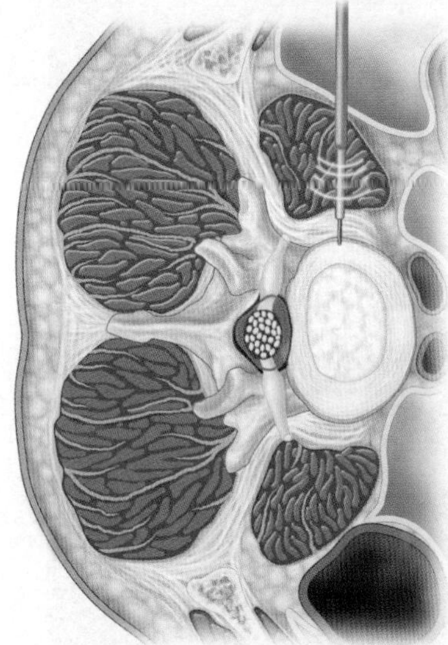


■ FIGURE 17–7. Sequential dilatation.

## COMPLICATIONS AND AVOIDANCE

A possible complication of the ALPA technique is induction of neuropraxia of the exiting nerve roots or the plexus. This injury may happen when pressure is applied with a posterior retraction blade and the nerves in between the retractor blade and the spinal process are compressed. Therefore, special attention should be given to this detail to minimize the occurrence of this side effect.

## CONCLUSION

The ALPA surgical technique can be used for nucleus replacement as well as for interbody fusion (XLIF90°). It has several advantages over traditional posterior and anterior approaches: First, there is no disturbance to important posterior and anterior structures while accessing the intervertebral disc. ALPA also makes the implantation of the device much simpler because it allows lateral

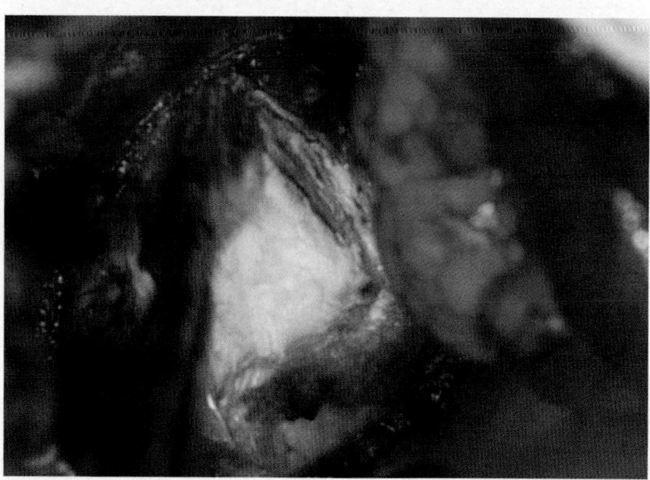

■ FIGURE 17–8. Annulus flap.

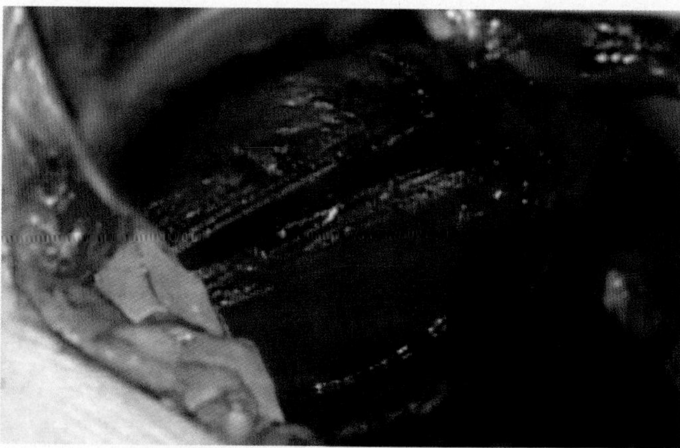

■ FIGURE 17–9. Closure of splitted psoas muscle.

access to the disc space. The implants can be inserted parallel to the canal, which requires much less manipulation for achieving optimal alignment of the device and reduces the risk of penetrating the spinal canal. Owing to the lateral access, the strong anterior/posterior tension band structures (ALL, PLL) can be kept intact. The classic risk factors of anterior approaches such as vascular complications or retrograde ejaculation can be almost completely avoided. Another advantage of ALPA is the possibility of carrying out the approach from the left as well as from the right side of the patient in the same quality. Therefore, reexposure problems of anterior approaches through the same side with an significantly increased risk of complication no longer exist.

Owing to a lot of advantages, the ALPA approach is a promising alternative to the posterior and anterior approach for intradiscal surgeries. Continuing studies will provide better understanding of its risk/reward ratio.

## REFERENCES

1. Bertagnoli R: Anterior mini-open approach for nucleus prosthesis: A new application technique for PDN. Lecture at the 13th annual meeting of the International Intradiscal Therapy Society (IITS), June 8–10, 2000, Williamsburg, Virginia.
2. Bertagnoli R, Vazquez RJ: The AnteroLateral TransPsoatic approach (ALPA): A new technique for implanting prosthetic disc nucleus devices. J Spinal Disord Tech 16(4):398–404, 2003.
3. Ozgur BM, Aryan HE, Pimenta L, Taylor WR: XLIF (eXtreme Lateral Interbody Fusion): A novel surgical technique for anterior lumbar interbody fusion. Spine J 6:435–443, 2006.
4. Pimenta L, Filipe F, Schaffa T: The transiliac endoscopic approach for implantation of prosthetic disc-nucleus devices. Presented at the 10th International Conference on Lumbar Fusion and Stabilization, Cancun, Mexico, 2001.
5. Mayer HM: The ALIF concept. Eur Spine J 9(1):S35–S43, 2000.
6. Ahlgren BD, Vasvada A, Brower RS, et al: Annular incision technique on the strength and multidirectional flexibility of the healing intervertebral disk. Spine 19:948–954, 1994.

CHAPTER 18

# Minimally Invasive Posterior Approaches to the Lumbar Spine

**Jean-Charles Le Huec, Richard Blondet Meyrat,** and **Stephane Aunoble**

## KEY POINTS

- Minimally invasive posterior lumbar approaches have been developed to provide the widest exposure through the smallest opening. A smaller opening reduces iatrogenic injury to the surrounding tissue, resulting in decreased postoperative pain, shortened hospital stay, and greater patient satisfaction.
- Minimal access techniques are safely performed using the operating microscope, the endoscope, or both.
- The muscle-splitting tubular retractor system has created new possibilities in accessing the posterior spine, allowing virtually every open posterior lumbar procedure to be performed minimally invasively.
- There are three basic posterior lumbar approaches: midline, paramedian, and far lateral. Each of these approaches offers a different view of the posterior elements, conferring advantages and disadvantages in treating specific pathologic conditions.
- Minimally invasive posterior lumbar surgery is technically demanding and involves a steep learning curve. A thorough understanding of the anatomy is imperative.

## INTRODUCTION

Minimally invasive procedures have become the standard for the management of a multitude of pathologic conditions in various surgical disciplines. Recent advances in microsurgical techniques and endoscopy have made minimally invasive approaches to the lumbar spine a safe alternative to traditional open approaches. A smaller incision and direct access to the area of pathology decrease iatrogenic injury to the surrounding structures. Minimally invasive surgery to the posterior spine has been shown to reduce postoperative pain and shorten postoperative recovery, leading to reduced hospital cost and greater patient satisfaction.

Minimally invasive surgery differs from open surgery in that the access to the area is "minimal." Once the target is identified, the techniques and instruments for the crucial portion of the procedure do not differ. The goal of minimally invasive surgery is to provide the greatest exposure through the smallest opening. Minimally invasive approaches to the posterior lumbar spine have been developed to provide direct access to areas of interest with minimal injury to the surrounding structures. Minimal access reduces soft tissue injury by minimizing muscle retraction and eliminating the removal of important soft tissue attachments. In addition, resection of bone is minimal or absent, preserving spine stability.

Several studies have shown that open lumbar surgeries can cause ischemia and denervation of the paraspinal musculature, which may lead to muscle atrophy and pain.[1,2] The multifidus muscle is particularly susceptible to injury during posterior spinal surgery because its nerve supply, the medial branch of the posterior rami, is often injured during retraction. Dysfunction of this muscle has been proposed as a mechanism in "failed back" syndrome. This appears to be especially true in open fusions through a midline approach, which often require long incisions above and below the spinal levels to be fused, detachment of the paraspinal muscles from the spinous process, and prolonged muscle retraction. Minimally invasive approaches provide direct access to the area of pathology, resulting in smaller incisions and reducing trauma to the surrounding musculature.

The posterior approaches for minimally invasive lumbar surgery are based on classic approaches originally described to treat specific lumbar conditions. Three of these approaches will be described: midline, paramedian, and far lateral. Advances in microsurgery and endoscopy have helped evolve less traumatic retraction systems, providing narrower corridors for these approaches. The operating microscope and the microsurgical techniques pioneered by Caspar, Williams, and Yasargil have helped create the first generation of minimally invasive retracting systems in the late 70s.[3] Refinement in endoscopic techniques during the late 80s and early 90s[4–7] has led to the development of the tubular retractor system for microendoscopic discectomy in 1997. This retractor system has revolutionized minimally invasive spinal surgery. Its use has expanded to almost all surgeries of the posterior lumbar spine, including canal decompression, removal of far lateral disc herniation, posterior lumbar interbody fusion (PLIF), and transverse lumbar interbody fusion (TLIF).

## MIDLINE APPROACH

The cause-and-effect relationship between disc herniation and sciatica was established by Mixter and Barr in 1934.[3] This important discovery sparked the evolution of posterior approaches to the disc space. A midline approach to the disc space was developed by Love in 1942. This well-known approach takes advantage of the familiar midline anatomy to help guide the surgeon to the area of pathology. For this reason, it has been the standard approach used to gain access to the spine.

Love's classic approach requires extensive muscle dissection and significant resection of the posterior elements to access the disc space. In response, a minimally invasive midline approach to the disc space was introduced by Yasargil and Caspar in 1977. Their "microdiscecomy" was made possible through the advances brought forth by the inception of the operating microscope in the 1950s. The improved illumination and magnification rendered by the microscope allowed easy identification of deep-seated structures. In addition, microsurgical techniques and refined instruments allowed access to the disc space with minimal manipulation of the neural structures. The smaller incision, decreased blood loss, and reduced soft tissue disruption have helped turn discectomies into an outpatient procedure.

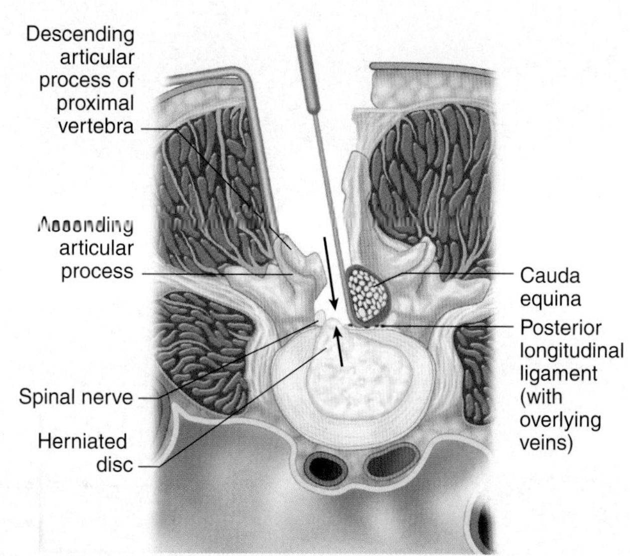


■ **FIGURE 18–2.** Axial view of the minimally invasive midline approach used for microdiscectomies.

### Technique (Microdiscectomy)

A midline incision of 15 to 20 mm is made over the correct interspace.[3] The lumbodorsal fascia is divided 2 mm lateral to its insertion on the spinous process. A subperiosteal dissection is performed, exposing the inferior one third of the superior lamina, the ligamentum flavum, the medial facet, and the upper portion of the inferior lamina. A Williams retractor is positioned, and the microscope is brought into the field (Fig. 18–1). The inferior lamina, medial facet, and superior lamina surrounding the interspace are removed using a combination of a drill and Kerrison rongeur (Fig. 18–2). The remainder of this procedure is described elsewhere in this book.

## PARASPINAL APPROACHES

Paraspinal approaches provide a direct corridor to the facet-transverse process complex leaving the supraspinalis and interspinalis ligaments intact. Watkins first described a paraspinal approach in 1959.[8] It involved the splitting of the lateral border of the sacrospinalis muscles and the ileocostal muscle. It was introduced to facilitate posterolateral fusions. This approach is now referred to as the far lateral approach and is used to treat far lateral disc herniations. In 1968, Wiltse described a more medial paraspinal approach involving the division of the sacrospinalis muscle between its multifidus and longissimus components.[9] This approach is also called the paramedian approach. It provides a direct corridor to the posterolateral elements of the spine. Originally described for the treatment of spondylolisthesis, this approach has been used for the removal of far lateral disc herniations, decompression of far out syndrome, spinal canal decompression, insertion of pedicle screws, posterolateral lumbar arthrodesis, and lumbar interbody fusions. A novel muscle-splitting paraspinal approach using a tubular retractor system was introduced by Foley and Smith in 1997.[10] This gave surgeons great flexibility in choosing an approach irrespective of anatomic planes.

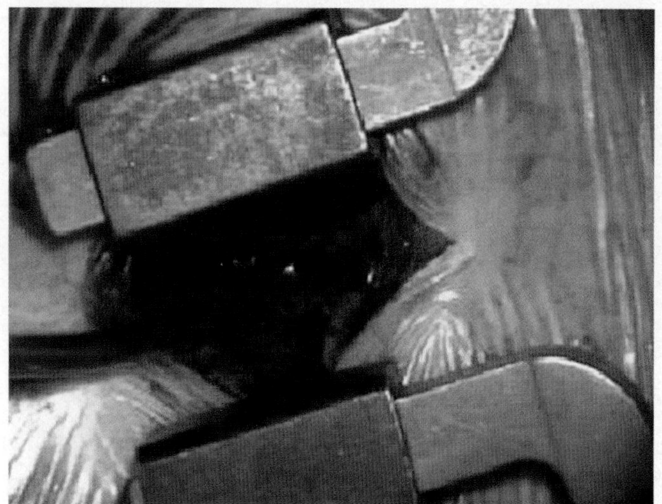

■ **FIGURE 18–1.** Microdiscectomy incision made possible by the development of less traumatic retracting system.

### Paramedian Approach (Wiltse Technique)

The Wiltse technique[11] involves the separation of the sacrospinalis muscle along an avascular plane between the multifidus and longissimus components (Fig. 18–3). A fibrous cleft between these two muscles can usually be identified using perforating vessels arising from the cleavage plane as a landmark (Fig. 18–4).

#### Technique

An incision is made about 4 cm lateral to the midline on the side of pathology. Next, the superficial muscular fascia is divided exposing the underlying sacrospinalis muscle. The intermuscular space between the multifidus and longissimus muscles can be found by identifying a set of perforating vessels exiting from within the cleft and draping over the sacrospinalis muscles (see Fig. 18–4). These vessels are often the only anatomic landmark leading to the cleavage plane. Once these vessels are coagulated, the intermuscular space is

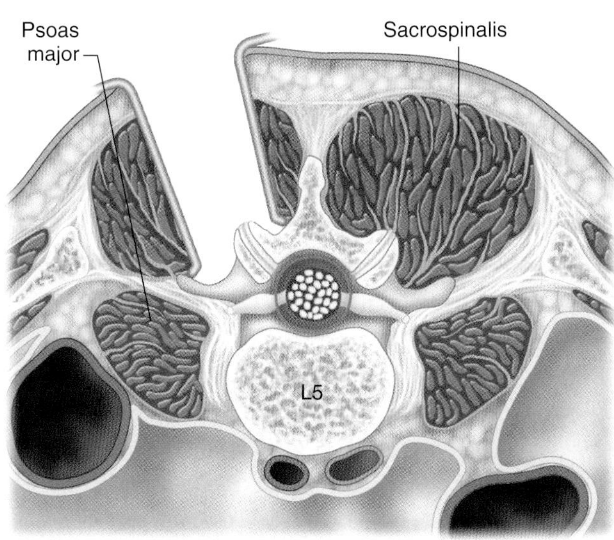


■ **FIGURE 18–3.** Axial view illustrating the division of the multifidus and longissimus muscles, leading directly to the facet-transverse process complex.

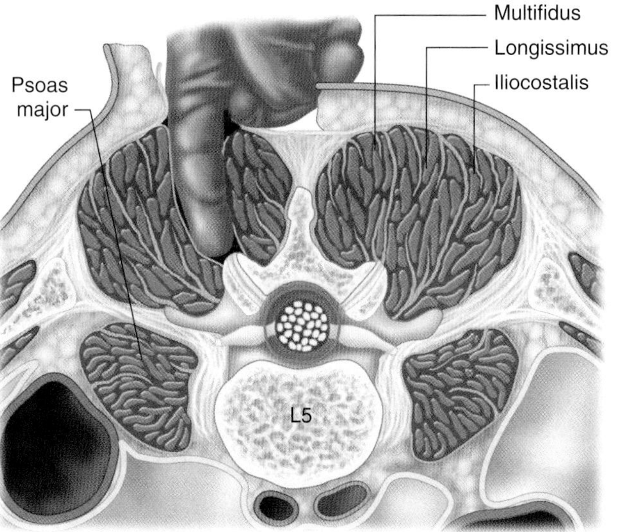


■ **FIGURE 18–5.** Once the perforating vessels are coagulated, the intermuscular space between the multifidus and longissimus muscles can be easily divided by digital manipulation.

divided manually with a finger (Fig. 18–5). The fibrous cleft is more easily identified caudal to the transverse process of L4 because it gradually disappears above this level. The posterior ramus of the L3 nerve can sometimes be encountered using this approach at more cranial levels. It must be carefully identified to prevent injury (Fig. 18–6).

This technique easily exposes the transverse and articular processes from L3 to the sacrum with minimal injury to the surrounding muscles. In addition, preservation of the interspinous ligaments and the muscle attachment to the posterior elements reduces iatrogenic instability.

## Far Lateral Approach (Watkins' Technique)

The far lateral approach allows the surgeon to access the lateral spinal structures without the need to remove any bone.[12] Compared with the classic midline approach and Wiltse's paramedian

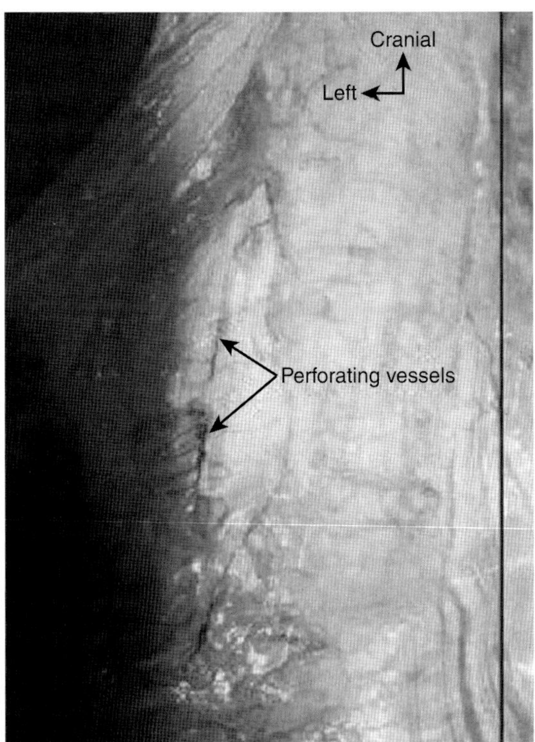


■ **FIGURE 18–4.** Perforating vessels seen exiting from within the intermuscular space between the multifidus and longissimus and draping over the sacrospinalis muscles.

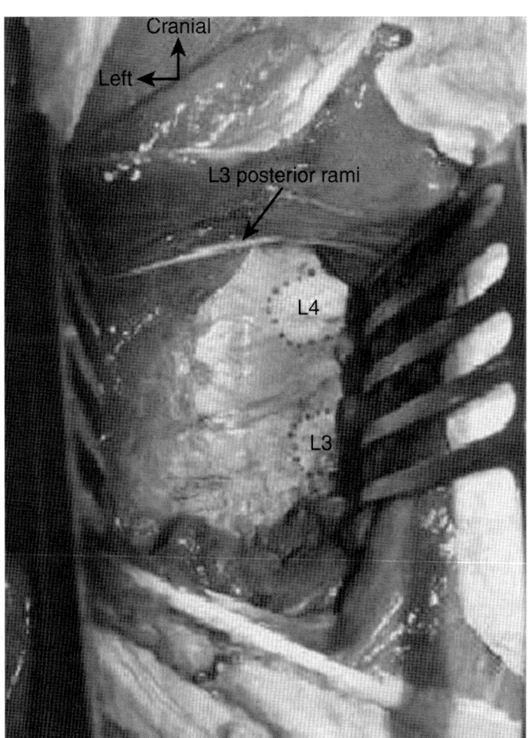


■ **FIGURE 18–6.** An illustration depicting the L3 posterior ramus as it courses laterally just cranial and dorsal to the L4 transverse process. This nerve is vulnerable to injury if it is not dissected carefully.

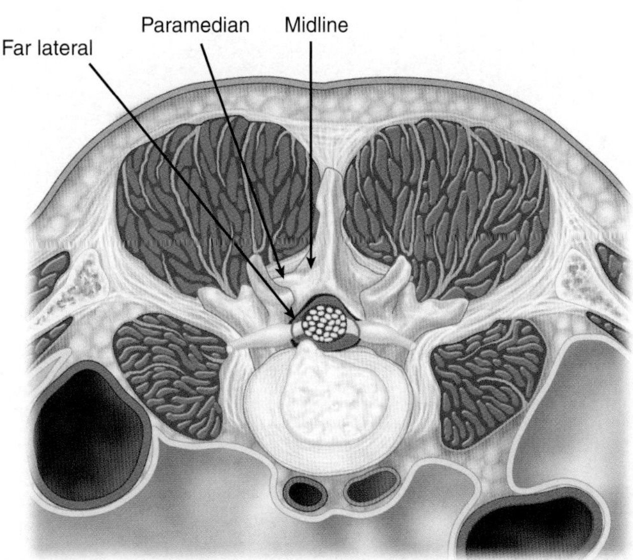


■ **FIGURE 18–7.** Illustration showing the different angles of approach through the midline, paramedian, and far lateral route.

approach, this approach produces a more oblique corridor, enabling the surgeon to directly visualize the intervertebral foramen and the lateral aspect of the vertebral bodies (Fig. 18–7). Consequently, it has become a preferred approach for the treatment of far lateral herniated discs.

The midline interlaminar approach has been the classic approach for far lateral disc pathologies. The anatomy is familiar to most surgeons, and the exposure allows clear visualization along the length of the nerve root inside and outside the foramen. This approach requires extensive resection of the facet joint. It is particularly useful in cases in which decompression of the canal and the foramen is warranted.[13] However, in cases for which a far lateral disc herniation is the sole pathology, this approach has fallen out of favor for the less invasive and more direct intertransverse approach.

The intertransverse approach can be accomplished by either the paramedian route or the far lateral route. The paramedian route provides direct access to the posterior osseous elements adjacent to the facet joints with less soft tissue retraction laterally. Its less oblique course to the intervertebral foramen provides a similar orientation as the midline approach[14] (see Fig. 18–7). Owing to its relative posterior access, the paramedian approach may still require significant bone resection to visualize far lateral pathology. The far lateral route is, on the contrary, more oblique and provides excellent visualization of the lateral spinal structures without the need to remove any bone. Good knowledge of the anatomic features of the intervertebral foramen and intertransverse space is mandatory.

The far lateral approach spares the attachment of the paraspinal muscles to the posterior elements, preserves the facet joints, and provides direct access to lateral spinal pathology. In addition, the ligamentum flavum and epidural fat are left untouched, minimizing epidural scarring. This approach has been shown to reduce postoperative discomfort and promote a speedy recovery.[15] Furthermore, the stability of the spine is preserved, minimizing iatrogenic spondylosis.

### Technique

Understanding the anatomy is essential.[14] The key to the far lateral approach is early identification of the lateral branch of the posterior primary ramus.[14] This leads to the ventral nerve root and to rapid localization of the intervertebral foramen. Care to not injure the segmental artery located just cranial and dorsal to the exiting nerve root is important as well (Fig. 18–8).

A vertical incision is made about 10 cm from the midline. Once the fascia is divided, the iliocostalis muscle is split in a 30-degree line to the horizontal (Fig. 18–9).

The bases of the transverse processes are identified with the finger, and the corresponding level is checked using fluoroscopy. The lateral branch of the posterior ramus can be felt with the finger as it crosses obliquely through the muscle fibers. It is followed ventromedially where it crosses the caudal transverse process and penetrates the medial aspect of the intertransverse fascia. This nerve is followed down to its origin ventral to the intertransverse fascia, where the ganglion and the ventral nerve root can be found exiting the intravertebral foramen (see Fig. 18–8). A plug of fat at the intravertebral foramen must be removed to visualize these structures. The transverse process and the facet joint are exposed by reflecting soft tissue, and the isthmus is defined by reflecting muscle from the pars interarticularis. The intertransverse fascia is removed in a superomedial-to-inferolateral direction beginning at the junction between the isthmus and the superior transverse process. Far lateral disc herniations can displace the nerve root dorsally and laterally, often above the intertransverse fascia. Care must be taken to not injure the nerve when removing the intertransverse fascia. Once the content of the extraforaminal space is exposed, discectomy proceeds in the standard fashion.

## Paraspinal Muscle-Splitting Approach Through the Tubular Retractor System

Foley and Smith described the microendoscopic discectomy (MED) system in 1997 to perform minimally invasive, endoscopic-guided discectomies.[10] MED was previously reported as an oral presentation and abstract by Destandau.[16–18] In contrast to percutaneous approaches, it combined standard lumbar microsurgical techniques with endoscopy, enabling surgeons to successfully address free-fragment disc and lateral recess stenosis.[19]

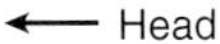


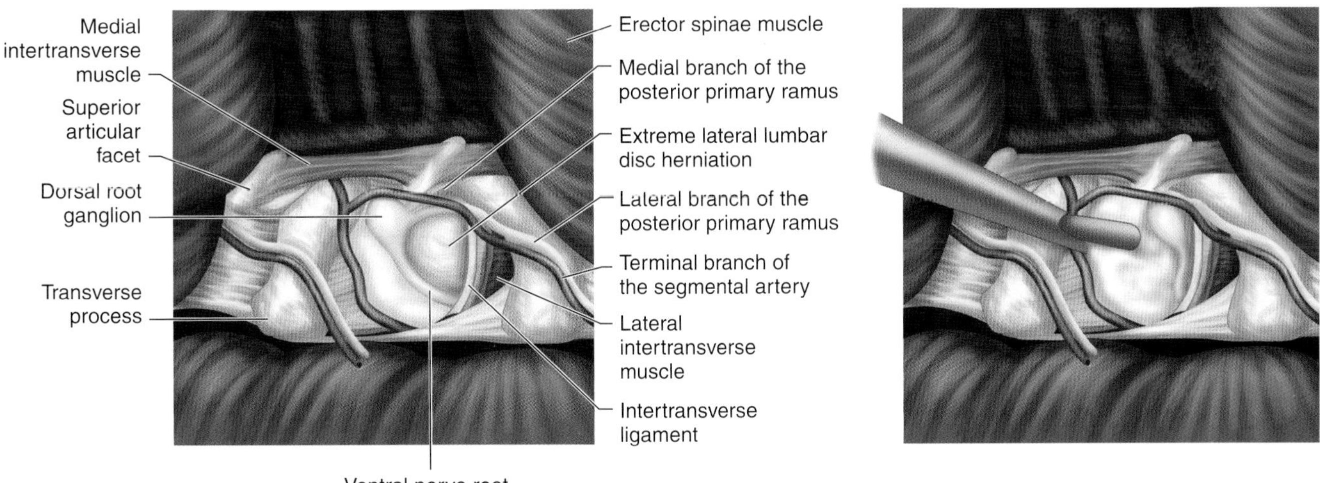


■ **FIGURE 18–8.** **A,** Drawing depicting the the extraforaminal space after the removal of the intertransverse ligament. Note the root ganglion pushed dorsally and cranially. Special care must be exercised when removing the soft tissue away from the intertransverse space. Note the proximity of the segmental artery to the root. **B,** Illustration showing the removal of a far lateral disc with a pituitary rongeur.

The concept of MED is not new. The use of endoscopy in the lumbar spine can be traced back as early as 1938 by Poole.[20] The introduction of the percutaneous nucleotomy by Hijikata in 1975[21] served as a catalyst for the evolution of posterior lumbar endoscopy. This procedure completely relied on fluoroscopy because the 7-mm working portal did not allow the operator to visualize the disc space. In 1986, Schreiber took Hijikata's technique a step further by using an endoscope on the contralateral side to allow direct observation of the insertion of the instruments into the disc space (biportal access).[6] Percutanous endoscopic techniques were further refined by Mayer and Brock in the early 1990s.[5] Kambin described the arthroscopic microdiscectomy in 1991, facilitating the removal of intra-annular, subligamentous, and extraligamentous herniations.[4] This was accomplished using biportal access through triangulation into the intervertebral disc using a 2.7-mm glass arthroscope combined with a videodiscoscope. The introduction of the tubular retractor in 1997 made endoscopic discectomy feasible through a single working channel. Combining both endoscopic and microscopic techniques, this procedure allowed the removal of all types of disc herniations, including those that had migrated in caudal and cephalad directions.

The MED system consists of four components: a tubular retractor system, a light source (endoscope providing a light source), image guidance (i.e., fluoroscopy), and modified instruments (Fig. 18–10). The tubular retractor introduces a novel muscle-splitting approach to the posterior lumbar spine involving a series of sequential soft tissue dilators that establishes a corridor through the paraspinous muscles to the area of interest.[22] The tubular retractor system can be used for any of the posterior lumbar approaches provided the corridor does not exceed the length of the retractor (20 cm). A video-assisted endoscope allows direct visualization of the nerve root and the surrounding structures. For this reason, MED is frequently called video-assisted discectomy. Fluoroscopy helps define the correct level and confirms the location of the tubular retractor. Long bayoneted instruments have been devised to allow smooth passage through the retractor without obstructing direct view (Fig. 18–11).

The initial MED system had several limitations and has been replaced by the METRx system (Medtronic Sofamor Danek, Memphis, TN). The METRx offers improved image quality, decreased endoscopic diameter, variable tubular retractor size, increased available working room within the tubular retractor, and decreased per-case cost. The tubular retractor has been

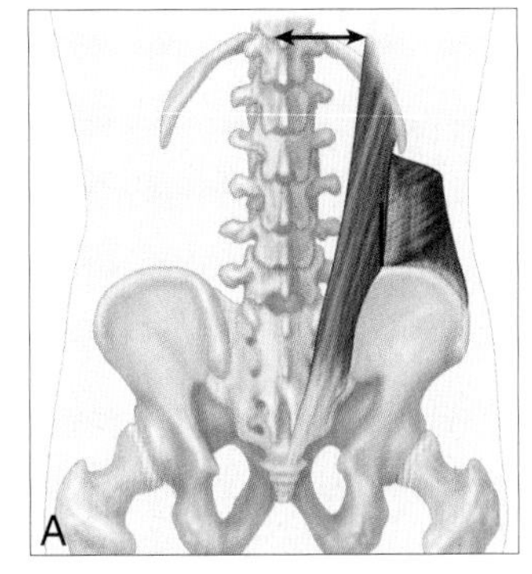


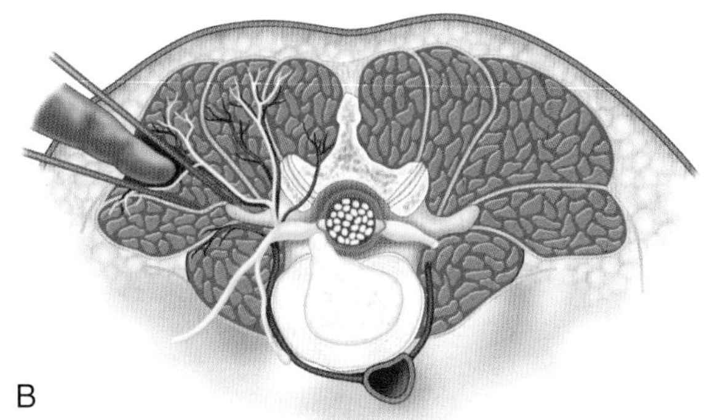


■ **FIGURE 18–9.** **A,** The far lateral approach. The iliocostalis muscle is split at 30 degrees from horizontal toward the transverse process. The lateral neurovascular branch can be palpated, which when followed, will direct to the root canal. Note the dorsally displaced nerve root by the far lateral disc. **B,** Far lateral skin incision 10 cm lateral to the midline.

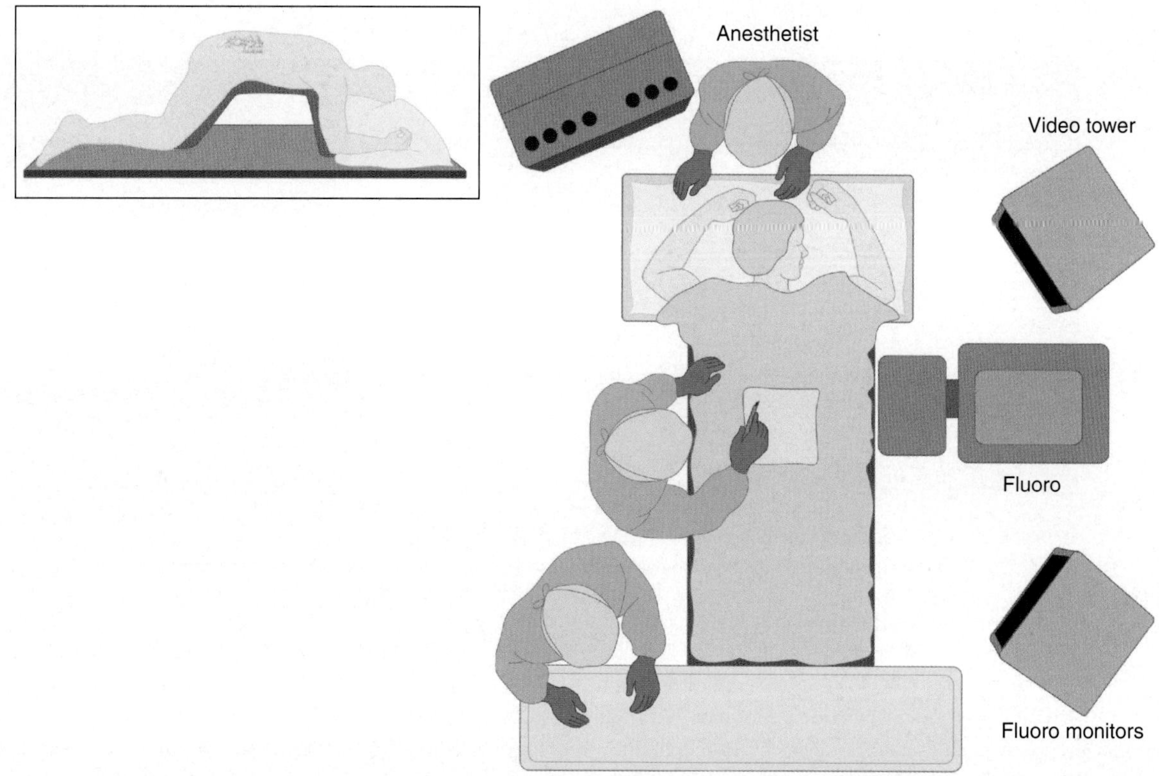


■ **FIGURE 18–10.** Operating room setup for MED procedure.

modified to accommodate the use of a microscope, allowing for three-dimensional visualization and improved image quality. Because the microscope is familiar to many surgeons, the METRx system is more user friendly than its predecessor. Nevertheless, the endoscope remains a vital component of this system because it allows the surgeon to visualize beyond the confines of the tubular retractor, for example, during a contralateral decompression from an ipsilateral approach. In addition, video-assisted endoscopy allows unobstructed use of long bayoneted instruments in and out of the retractor tube, whereas the microscope forces the surgeon to look straight down the tube, often obstructing the flow of instruments through the tube. The muscle-splitting technique by tubular dilation reduces tissue trauma, decreases postoperative pain and discomfort, shortens hospital stays, and allows a quicker return to activities of daily living. By maintaining the integrity of normal anatomic tissue structures, iatrogenic spinal instability is minimized.

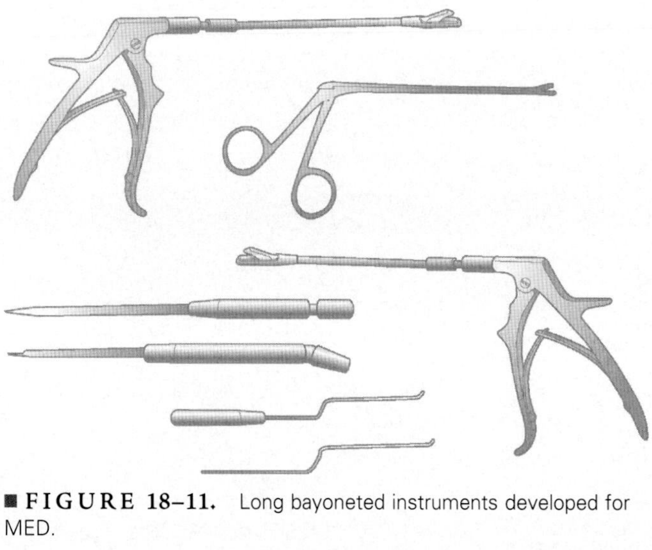

■ **FIGURE 18–11.** Long bayoneted instruments developed for MED.

Microendoscopic lumbar surgery involves a steep learning curve. One study concluded approximately 30 cases are required to gain a full command of this technique.[23] Endoscopy takes surgery from a direct line of sight to one in which visualization of the operative field is projected on a two-dimensional video monitor placed in front of the surgeon. This requires significant hand-eye coordination made especially difficult when working through a narrow working space.[24] The lack of depth perception and the scope limitations (e.g., color, restricted view) can make visiospatial orientation challenging. Perhaps the most difficult tasks to master are the angle of approach and the extent of movement of the tip of the tube during wanding. Therefore, a thorough knowledge of anatomy is critical to navigate safely.

### Technique (Modified for Microendoscopic Discectomy)[15]

Figure 18–10 illustrates a typical operating room setup for MED.[22] Using lateral fluoroscopy, a 20-gauge spinal needle is inserted into the paraspinal musculature approximately 1.5 cm lateral to the midline on the symptomatic side of the patient at the appropriate level. The tip of the needle should be positioned directly over the disc space. Next, a 16-mm vertical incision, the length of the diameter of the tubular retractor, is made at the puncture site. Under fluoroscopic guidance, a guidewire (K-wire) is inserted through the incision and directed over the junction between the inferior edge of the superior lamina and the medial facet. It is firmly anchored to the bone, taking precautions not to enter the interlaminar space and risk neural injury.

The first of four dilators is inserted over the K-wire using a twisting motion toward the lamina and docked on bone. The K-wire is removed, and lateral fluoroscopy is performed to confirm the first dilator's location over the disc space. Next, the paraspinal musculature is swept off the laminar edge using the tip of the dilator (Fig. 18–12). This facilitates the removal of soft tissue from the lamina, allowing placement of the tubular retractor and the endoscope. The dilator tip should be kept in the subperiosteal plane to minimize blood loss. Once again care must be taken not to enter the spinal canal.

The second, third, and fourth dilators are sequentially placed over the initial dilator down to the lamina, followed by placement of the tubular retractor over the final dilator (Fig. 18–13). A flexible arm, secured to the table, is connected to the tubular retractor to keep it in a locked position. The endoscope is inserted into the tubular retractor and secured (Fig. 18–14). The endoscope can be rotated anywhere along the circumference of the tubular retractor. Magnification can be adjusted by moving the endoscope toward or away from the field.

The remaining soft tissue over the lamina and interlaminar space is removed by a combination of a long-tip insulated Bovie and a pituitary rongeur. Soft tissue is removed from the lateral edge of the tube toward the center of the tube. Using a technique called wanding, the tubular retractor can be angled in different directions expanding surgical access from pedicle to pedicle through the original incision. Wanding also allows the area of interest to be at the center of the operative corridor, maximizing visualization. In order to prevent soft tissue from entering the field during wanding, a downward pressure is applied during movement of the retractor. The microdiscectomy proceeds in much the same way as in an open procedure described in other parts of this book.

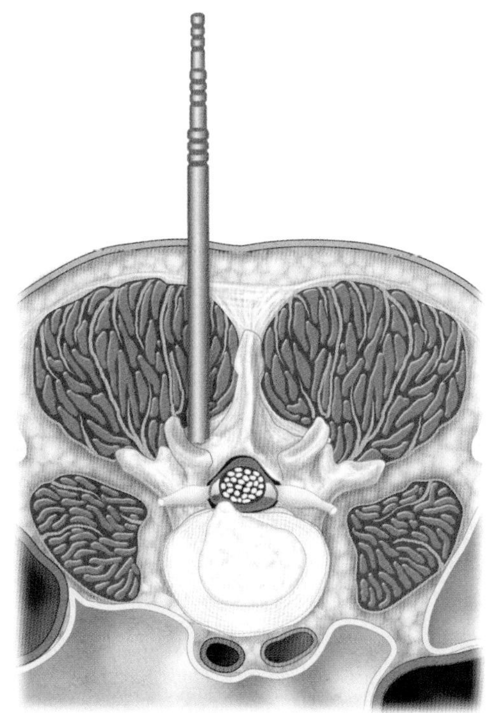

■ **FIGURE 18–13.** The sequential dilators used to split the muscle and create a corridor for the placement of the tubular retractor.

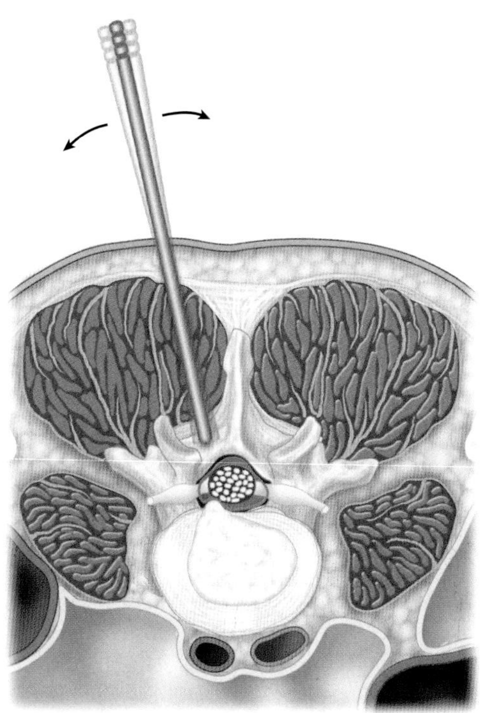

■ **FIGURE 18–12.** The sweeping motion used when removing soft tissue away from the lamina with the initial dilator.

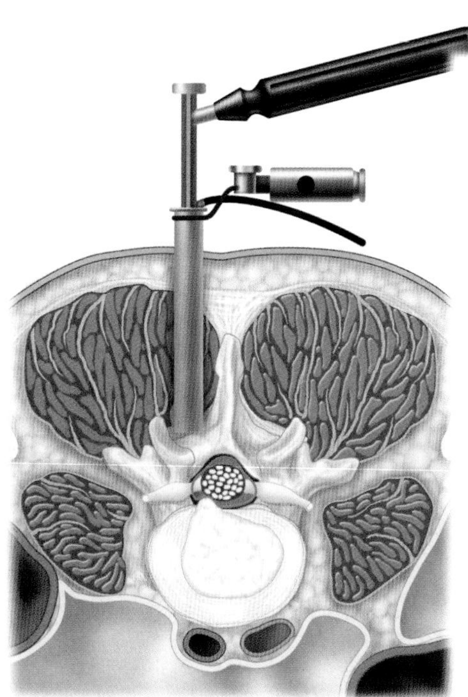

■ **FIGURE 18–14.** The tubular retractor in place with the endoscope inserted through it.

## REFERENCES


1. Kim KT, Lee SH, Suk KS, Bae SC: The quantitative analysis of tissue injury markers after mini-open lumbar fusion. Spine 31:712–716, 2006.
2. Stevens K, Spenciner DB, Griffths KL, et al: Comparison of minimally invasive and conventional open posterolateral lumbar fusion using magnetic resonance imaging and retraction pressure studies. J Spinal Disord Tech 19:77–86, 2006.
3. Maroon JC: Current concepts in minimally invasive discectomy. Neurosurgery 51(2):137–145, 2002.
4. Kambin P, Savitz MH: Arthroscopic microdiscectomy: An alternative to open disc surgery. Mt Sinai J Med 67:283–287, 2000.
5. Mayer HM, Brock M: Percutaneous endoscopic discectomy: Surgical technique and preliminary results compared to microsurgical discectomy. J Neurosurg 78:216–225, 1993.
6. Schreiber A, Suezawa Y: Transdiscoscopic percutaneous nucleotomy in disc herniation. Orthop Rev 15:35–38, 1986.
7. Ditsworth DA: Endoscopic transforaminal lumbar discectomy and reconfiguration: A postero-lateral approach into the spinal canal. Surg Neurol 49:588–598, 1998.
8. Watkins MB: Posterolateral bone grafting for fusion of the lumbar and lumbosacral spine. J Bone Joint Surg 41:388–396, 1959.
9. Wiltse LL, Bateman JG, Hutchinson RH, Nelson WE: The paraspinal sacrospinalis-splitting approach to the lumbar spine. J Bone Joint Surg Am 50:919–926, 1968.
10. Foley KT, Smith MM: Microendoscopic discectomy. Tech Neurosurg 3:301–307, 1997.
11. Vialle R, Wicart P, Drain O, et al: The Wiltse paraspinal approach to the lumbar spine revisited. Clin Orthop Relat Res 445:175–180, 2006.
12. O'Hara LJ, Marshall RW: Far lateral lumbar disc herniation: The key to the intertransverse approach. J Bone Joint Surg Br 79:943–947, 1997.
13. Ozveren MF, Bilge T, Barut S, Mustafa E: Combined approach for far lateral lumbar disc herniation. Neurol Med Chir (Tokyo) 44:118–123, 2004.
14. O'Brien MF, Peterson D, Crockard A: A posterolateral microsurgical approach to extreme-lateral lumbar disc herniation. J Neurosurg 83:636–640, 1995.
15. Tessitore E, De Tribolet N: Far-lateral lumbar disc herniation: The microsurgical transmuscular approach. Neurosurgery 54:939–942, 2004.
16. Destandau J: A special device for endoscopic surgery of lumbar disc herniation. Neurol Res 21:39–42, 1999.
17. Destandau J: Aspects techniques de la chirurgie endoscopique des hernies discales foraminales lombaires. Neurochirurgie 50:6–10, 2004.
18. Destandau J: Traitement des hernies discales lombaires par endoscopies. Proceedings Société Française Arthroscopie pp 21–22, 1997.
19. Sivakumar J, Kim D, Kam A: History of minimally invasive spine surgery. Neurosurgery 51(2):1–14, 2002.
20. Pool JL: Direct visualization of dorsal nerve roots of the cauda equina by means of a myeloscope. Arch Neurol Psychiattr 39:1308–1312, 1938.
21. Hijikata S, Yamgishi M, Nakayama T, Oomori K: Percutaneous discectomy: New treatment method for lumbar disc herniation. J Toden Hosp 5:5–13, 1975.
22. Perez-Cruet MJ, Foley KT, Isaacs RE, et al: Microendoscopic lumbar discectomy: Technical note. Neurosurgery 51(5):S129–S136, 2002.
23. Nowitzke A: Assessment of the learning curve for lumbar microendoscopic discectomy. Neurosurgery 56:755–762, 2005.
24. Perez-Cruet MJ, Fessler RG, Perin NI: Review: Complications of minimally invasive spinal surgery. Neurosurgery 51(5): S26–S36, 2002.

CHAPTER 19

# Lumbar Endoscopic Posterolateral (Transforaminal) Approach

Christopher A. Yeung, Victor M. Hayes, Farhan N. Siddiqi, and Anthony T. Yeung

## KEY POINTS

- The patient is positioned to obtain true anteroposterior (AP) and lateral views before needle placement; this will avoid radiographic parallax error and malpositioning of the needle, cannula, and endoscope.
- *Initial needle trajectory and placement is essential* because it will ultimately determine the endoscopic field of view. Optimum needle position is determined based on the pathology or region being addressed (see Figs. 19–5 through 19–7). The bony constraints of the iliac crest and foramen (facets and lateral vertebral body) restrict needle and scope trajectory, especially at L5-S1; therefore, perfect trajectory and placement are crucial.
- Fluoroscopy should be used to confirm location if there is *ANY uncertainty* about anatomy or location during endoscopy.
- Start the endoscopy using the "Inside-out" Yeung Endoscopic Spine Surgery (YESS)[1] technique (see Box 19–1), accessing the intervertebral disc first, which is always safe! This technique is especially important during the initial learning curve. Beginning the endoscopy before reaching the disc annulus can make recognition of foraminal anatomy more difficult and can increase the likelihood of nerve root injury except in special situations in which the patient's anatomy or the pathoanatomy justifies an alternate technique. Examples of specific situations that require an "outside-in" technique are removal of the lateral facet to get into the L5-S1 disc or a large far lateral disc sitting on the exiting nerve root and pushing it into the foramen.
- It is recommended that the patient be *awake and alert* until the endoscope is within the disc space to avoid nerve injury. Avoiding excessive sedation before this point in the procedure is crucial, especially during needle insertion, and dilator and cannula passage. We recommend against the use of a general anesthetic such as propofol.

## INTRODUCTION

Open posterior approaches to the lumbar spine are used to access the intervertebral disc when performing fusion procedures. Presently, this approach is the gold standard for accessing and removing herniated discs and decompressing the spinal canal. The posterior (transcanal) approach has inherent morbidity and approach-related limitations with regard to accessing the disc space and delivery of an interbody device. These approaches require a midline incision, muscle and ligament stripping, prolonged muscle retraction, partial facet and lamina resection, and both nerve root and dural retraction, which promote epidural scarring.

Although minimally invasive techniques use smaller incisions using dilators and tubular retractors that reduce muscle retraction, they still require the same amount of bone resection and dural retraction to expose the disc or pathology safely. Hence, even minimally invasive posterior approaches do not remove the morbidity associated with bony resection (i.e., instability) nor do they avoid epidural scarring, which can make revision surgery difficult. Delivery of an interbody device (cage or total disc replacement [TDR]) using an open posterior approach is also limited by the constraints of excessive bony resection, the distance between the exiting and traversing nerve roots, and the degree of "safe" retraction required to expose the disc. The morbidity and limitations associated with open posterior approaches have motivated surgeons to develop alternative approaches to access the spinal canal and intervertebral discs.

A fluoroscopically guided endoscopic method for accessing and removing herniated lumbar discs was introduced by Yeung and reported by Tsou.[2] This technique uses a transforaminal approach to the intervertebral disc combined with a unique endoscope (with a working channel), specially designed instruments, and use of the YESS technique to address the pathology. This transforaminal endoscopic approach was founded on principles of accessing the disc space through Kambin's triangle[3] (Fig. 19–1) in the hidden "safe zone" between the exiting and traversing nerve roots. The YESS technique expands on this approach using an "Inside-out" technique to safely gain access to the disc, remove any herniated material, and explore the epidural space, lateral facets, foramen, and the traversing and exiting nerve root.

For most spine surgeons, the transforaminal approach is unfamiliar. Access to this region through an open posterior approach requires significant dissection, bony resection, and soft tissue retraction (usually through a transforaminal lumbar interbody fusion [TLIF] approach) while still limiting visualization of lateral foraminal anatomy (the lateral superior articular process [SAP]) frequently implicated in failed back surgery syndrome. Technologic advances and new instruments have now expanded the scope

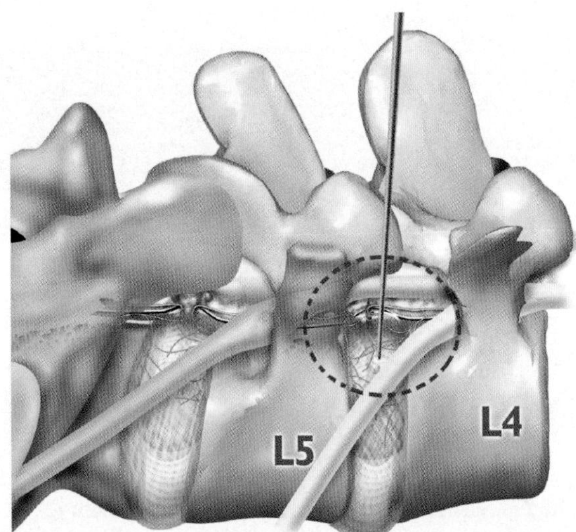


■ **FIGURE 19–1.** The transforaminal endoscopic approach was founded on principles of accessing the disc space through Kambin's triangle in the hidden "safe zone" between the exiting and traversing nerve roots.

of pathology that can be addressed using a transforaminal endoscopic approach in the lumbar spine. This chapter describes the YESS technique and its use to safely access the lumbar spine through an endoscopic transforaminal approach. We also discuss the indications, benefits, and pitfalls of using this approach to access the disc, foramen, and spinal canal.

## INDICATIONS/CONTRAINDICATIONS

Current indications for the use of an endoscopic posterolateral approach to the lumbar spine include contained central and paracentral disc herniations,[4] foraminal and far lateral disc herniations, recurrent herniations, small nonsequestered extruded disc herniations, symptomatic annular tears, synovial cysts, biopsy and débridement of discitis, decompression of foraminal stenosis, visualized total nuclectomy (before nucleus replacement), visualized discectomy, and end plate preparation before interbody fusion or total disc replacement (TDR) implantation. Because the technique uses local anesthesia with mild sedation, patients with the forestated pathology who are considered "too high risk" for general anesthesia can receive treatment safely through this approach and are excellent candidates.

Contraindications include any pathology not accessible from the posterolateral endoscopic approach. This may include some extruded sequestered disc herniations, extruded migrated disc herniations (migrated >20% of vertebral body superiorly or inferiorly), recurrent or virgin disc herniations with associated epidural scarring, moderate to severe central canal stenosis, and hard calcified herniations. These contraindications are considered relative contraindications dependent on the surgeon's technical experience and comfort level. More experienced endoscopic surgeons can gain greater access to pathology by using advanced techniques for bone removal of ostoephytes, stenosis, and the posterolateral corner of the vertebral body before addressing the pathology. Other relative contraindications include inadequate support staff or equipment to successfully perform procedure and uncooperative patients.

## DESCRIPTION OF THE DEVICE

Approaching the spine through an endoscopic posterolateral (transforaminal) approach is best accomplished by the use of a specially designed endoscope and instruments. There are a couple of competing endoscopic systems available, but the most widely used and the authors' preferred system is the endoscopic spine surgery system from Richard Wolfe Medical Instruments, (Vernon Hills, IL) (Fig. 19–2). The current outer diameter of the cannula is 7 mm, which is well within the dimensional constraints of foraminal anatomy (Fig. 19–3). The rigid endoscope houses a 3.1-mm working channel (which is capable of accepting specialized instruments), an irrigation channel, a light source, and a video camera. Specialized instruments include straight and hinged pituitary rongeurs, straight and flexible suction-irrigation shavers for mechanical tissue removal, a flexible bipolar radiofrequency probe (Ellman International Oceanside, NY; trigger-flex bipolar probe) for hemostasis, tissue modulation and manual probing, and a side-firing Holmium-YAG laser (Trimedyne, Inc., Lake Forest, CA) for precise tissue and bony ablation. A standard arthroscopic tower and monitor are also required to visualize the endoscopy. Recording equipment for capturing video and still pictures is optional.

## BACKGROUND OF SCIENTIFIC TESTING/CLINICAL OUTCOMES

Current peer-reviewed literature on outcomes of endoscopic transforaminal spinal procedures is described for discogenic pain from annular tears, discitis, lumbar disc herniations, recurrent lumbar disc herniations, central and lateral spinal stenosis, and failed back surgery syndrome.[2,5–8] Surgical outcomes of posterolateral endoscopic discectomy for contained lumbar disc herniations are comparable with that for traditional open trans-canal microdiscectomy[7,8] but with lower surgical morbidity and faster recovery time.

## CLINICAL PRESENTATION AND EVALUATION

A careful preoperative history, physical examination, and meticulous review of the plain radiographs and magnetic resonance imaging scan (MRI) are essential before attempting an endoscopic transformaminal approach regardless of the pathology being addressed. Attention to specific anatomic relationships is important to determine whether the approach is safe and feasible, and to ensure that there are no contraindications. Note the level of the iliac crest in relation to the disc space being accessed to determine the optimum needle trajectory. We also recommend checking the axial MRI images to evaluate the relationship of the lateral facets to the disc space, making sure the needle can pass into the disc space without significant bony obstruction. Access to the disc may or may not require partial resection of the lateral facet (especially and L5-S1) before entering the disc, but this can be anticipated by a detailed preoperative review of the patient's MRI and radiographs.

**PARTIAL INSTRUMENT SET FOR SELECTIVE ENDOSCOPIC DISCECTOMY (not to scale)**

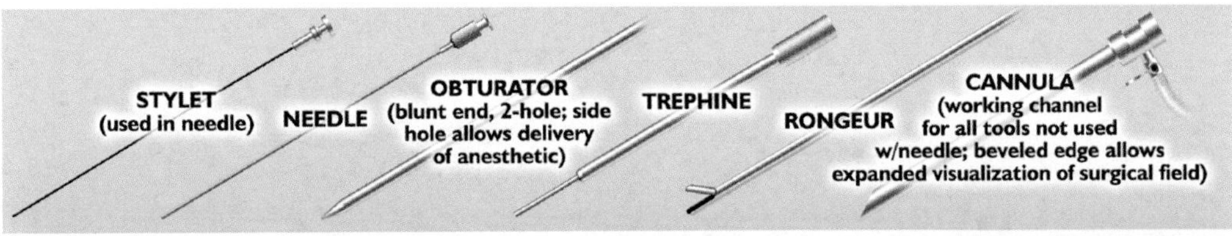


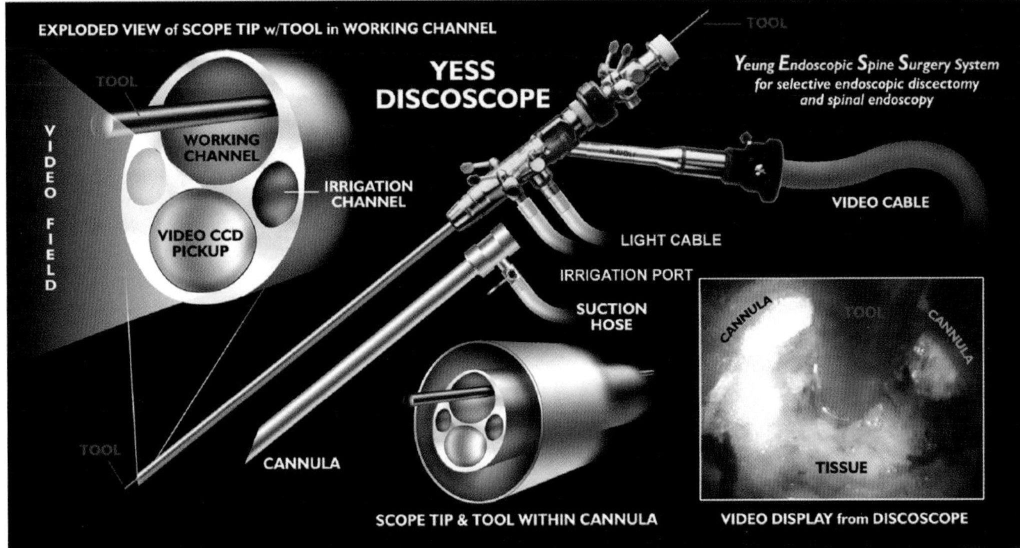


■ **FIGURE 19–2.** Endoscopic spine surgery system from Richard Wolfe Medical Instruments, Vernon Hills, IL.

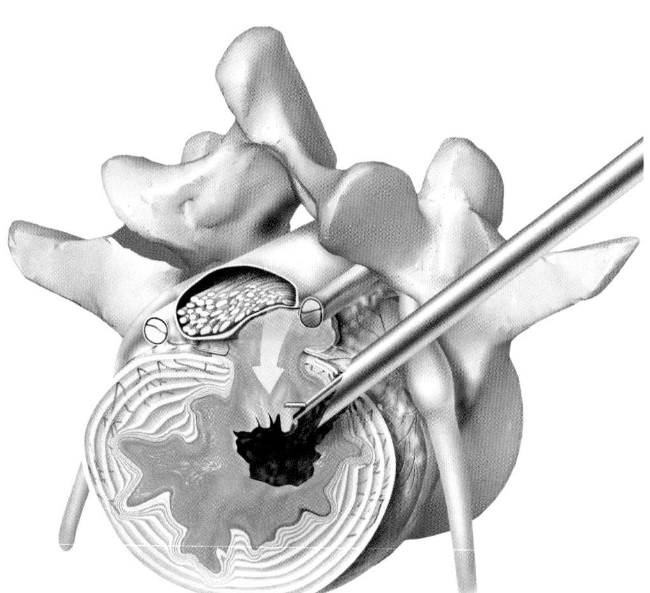

■ **FIGURE 19–3.** For a paracentral herniated nucleus pulposus, the beveled cannula is ideally positioned at the base of the herniation. This allows the surgeon to grasp the base of the herniation and pull it into the disc and out the cannula. Cutting any intact annular fibers between the cannula and the base of the herniation prior to pulling the herniation, prevents the annular fibers from pinching off the apex of the herniated nucleus pulposus.The current outer diameter of the cannula is 7mm, which is well within the dimensional constraints of foraminal anatomy.

## OPERATIVE TECHNIQUE

### Anesthesia

Although some experienced international endoscopic surgeons prefer general anesthesia, the authors recommend mild sedation and local anesthesia so that the patient is awake and responsive throughout the procedure. The patient can then provide real-time feedback in case of nerve irritation from instrument pressure or retraction, adding a layer of safety and allowing the surgeon to adjust the instruments accordingly. The skin, needle tract, and annulus are anesthetized with half percent lidocaine. This allows anesthesia without motor block of the nerve roots. Throughout the procedure, the patient can receive mild sedation and analgesia with midazolam (Versed) and fentanyl. We recommend against using general anesthetics like propofol, which can produce temporary total analgesia and may cause airway concerns if the patient becomes overly sedated.

### Position

The patient is prone on a hyperkyphotic frame with a radiolucent table. The endoscope is on one side, and the fluoroscopic unit is on the opposite side of the patient (Fig. 19–4).

### Procedure

The instructions below are a step-by-step surgical technique and protocol for accessing the disc space using an endoscopic transforaminal approach. **Optimal needle placement is the most crucial**

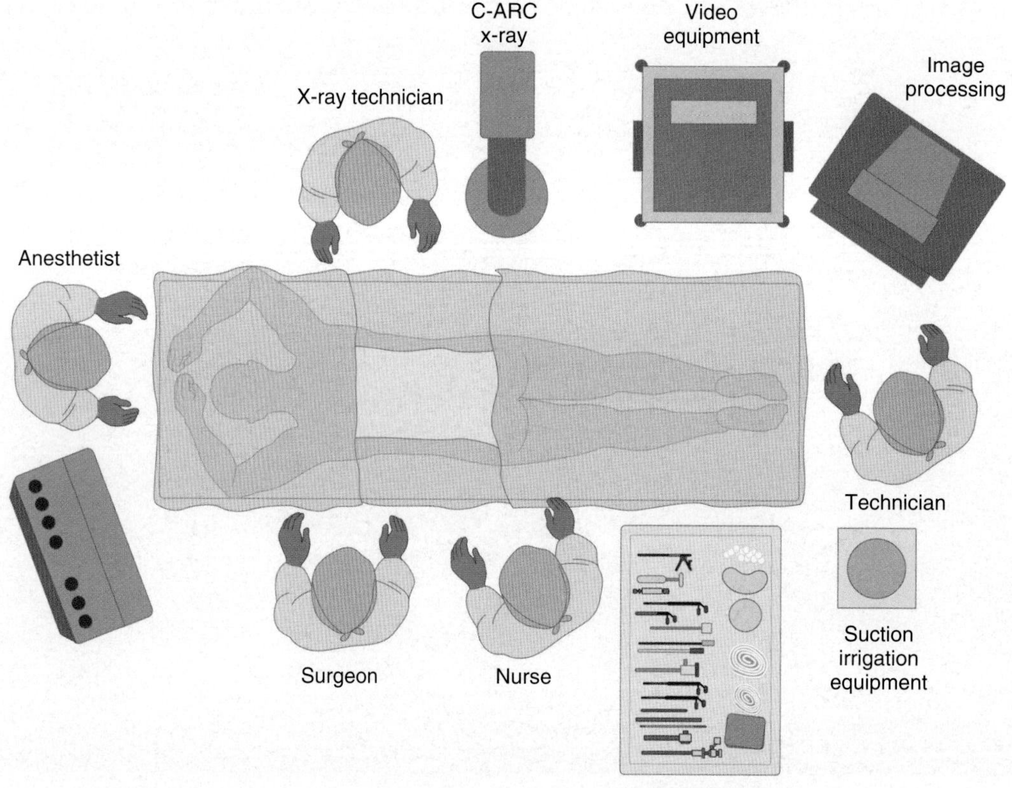


■ **FIGURE 19–4.** The patient is prone on a hyperkyphotic frame with a radiolucent table. The endoscope is on one side, and the fluoroscopic unit is on the opposite side of the patient.

**step of the procedure and is based on the type of pathology being addressed (see Box 19–1).**

Using a thin metal rod as a radio-opaque marker and ruler, lines are drawn on the skin to mark surface topography for guidance using biplane C-arm needle placement. These surface markings help identify three key landmarks for needle placement: the anatomic disc center, the annular foraminal window (centered within the medial and lateral borders of the pedicles), and the skin window (needle entry point).

- Using a metal rod as radio-opaque marker and ruler, draw a longitudinal line over the spinous processes to mark the midline on the posteroanterior (PA) view.
- Draw a transverse line bisecting the targeted disc space to mark the transverse disc plane on the PA view. The intersection of these two lines marks the anatomic disc center (Fig. 19–6).
- On the lateral view, draw the disc inclination plane from the lateral disc center to the posterior skin. This line should bisect the disc and be parallel to the end plates. This line determines the cephalad/caudal position of the needle entry point. When drawing this disc inclination line, the tip of the metal rod should be at the lateral anatomic disc center. The distance from the rod tip to the plane of the posterior skin is measured by grasping the rod at the point where the posterior skin plane intersects it (Fig. 19–7).
- This distance is then measured on the posterior skin from the midline along the transverse plane line.

**BOX 19–1. TECHNICAL "PEARLS" AND BASIC PRINCIPLES OF THE YESS TECHNIQUE: AVOIDANCE OF POTENTIAL COMPLICATIONS**

1. Use the "Inside-out" technique: Start the endoscopy by first entering the disc and then address the pathology accordingly.
2. Sometimes (especially at L5-S1) partial lateral facetectomy may be required prior to entry into the disc. Dock the long or short beveled cannula on the facet, resect the SAP undersurface from 3 o'clock to 12 o'clock (right sided approach) or 12 o'clock to 9 o'clock (left sided approach) until you can gain safe entry into the disc space. Protect the exiting nerve with the cannula, then use the standard "Inside-out" technique.
3. The disc is the safest and best starting point. Both the disc and bone and safe harbors, you can dock on these structures initially.
4. It is of extreme importance to use the specially designed cannulas with a penfield-like extension (Figure 19-5) to protect the exiting nerve when working in the foramen.
5. The patient is awake so use this to your advantage!! If significant leg pain is experienced, stop and reevaluate the patient; ask them about the distribution of the pain and re-assess position using fluoroscopy to prevent complications.
6. When bleeding is encountered, advance the scope back into the disc and slowly pull back the scope, cauterizing the bleeders from inside to out.
7. Use the "Inside-out" technique to your advantage: Once you are within the disc, the herniation is between you and the affected nerve, which is advantageous because it protects the nerve from iatrogenic injury. When possible remove the herniation by pulling the herniation into the disc space and then out the cannula.

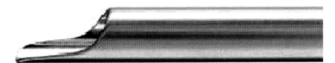

■ **FIGURE 19–5.** Cannula with a penfield-like extension specifically designed to protect the exiting nerve when working in the foramen.

- At the lateral extent of this measurement, a line parallel to the midline is drawn to intersect the disc inclination plane line. This intersection marks the skin entry point, or "skin window," for the needle (Fig. 19–8).
- The skin window's lateral location from the midline determines the trajectory angle into the foraminal annular window. A 45-degree needle trajectory to the disc should place the needle tip in the true anatomic disc center. If you are attempting to access the posterior one third of the disc, then the optimum skin window is more lateral (1–2 cm) and the needle trajectory angle is less acute (25–30 degrees in the coronal place).
- Alternatively one can place the rod tip at the anterior portion of the disc when measuring the disc inclination plane. This produces a longer measurement to the posterior skin plane, thus placing the skin window more lateral. This is actually the preferred method. This coordinate system of finding the optimal anatomical landmarks for instrument placement will help decrease the steep learning curve for needle placement and eliminate the less accurate "down the tunnel" method favored by radiologists and pain management physicians.
- The positive disc inclination plane of the L5-S1 disc is noteworthy. A steep positive inclination line (lordosis) positions the optimal skin window more cephalad from the transverse plane line, avoiding the "high iliac crest." A flatly inclined L5-S1 disc will position the optimal skin window with the iliac crest obstructing the trajectory of the needle. The skin window will have to start more medial to avoid the iliac crest, and sometimes the lateral and ventral portion of the superior articular facet (SAP) must be resected to allow for posterior needle placement in the disc.
- The first neutrally aligned disc inclination plane is usually at L4-L5 or L3-L4. A neutrally aligned disc inclination plane is in the same plane as the transverse plane line; thus, the skin window is in line with the transverse plane line. A negatively inclined disc, often at L1-L2 and L2-L3, places the skin window caudal to the transverse plane line.

### Needle Placement

Once the starting point and needle trajectory are determined, the skin window and subcutaneous tissue are infiltrated with one-half percent lidocaine. A 6-inch-long, 18-gauge needle is then inserted from the skin window at the desired trajectory (coronal plane) and passed anteromedially toward the anatomic disc center. Infiltrating the needle tract with one-half percent lidocaine as you are advancing the needle will anesthetize the tissue tract, avoiding pain when the dilator is passed later in the procedure. Tilt the C-arm beam parallel to the disc inclination plane (the Ferguson view) while advancing the needle toward the disc to avoid parallax error. At the first bony resistance or before the needle tip is advanced medial to the pedicle, turn the C-arm to the lateral projection. Avoid advancing the needle tip medial to the pedicle during the initial approach because doing so risks inadvertent traversing nerve root and dural puncture.

Most frequently (and ideally) the first bony resistance encountered is the lateral facet. Increase the trajectory angle to aim ventral to the facet and continue the approach toward the foraminal annular window. Turning the needle bevel to face dorsal helps the

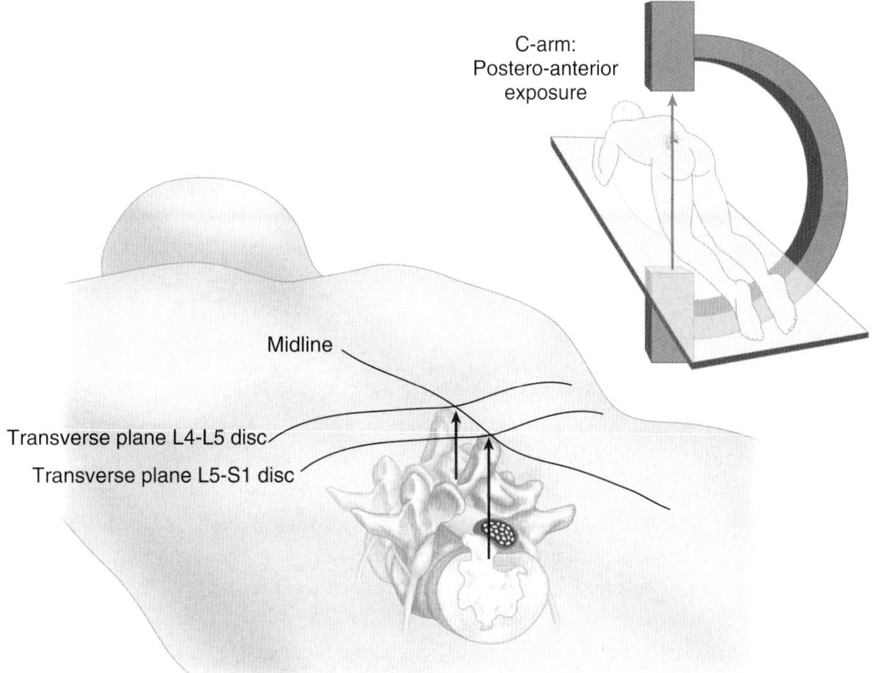


■ **FIGURE 19–6.** Postero anterior fluoroscopic exposure enables topographic location of spinal column midline and transverse planes of target discs. Intersections of drawn lines mark PA disc centers.

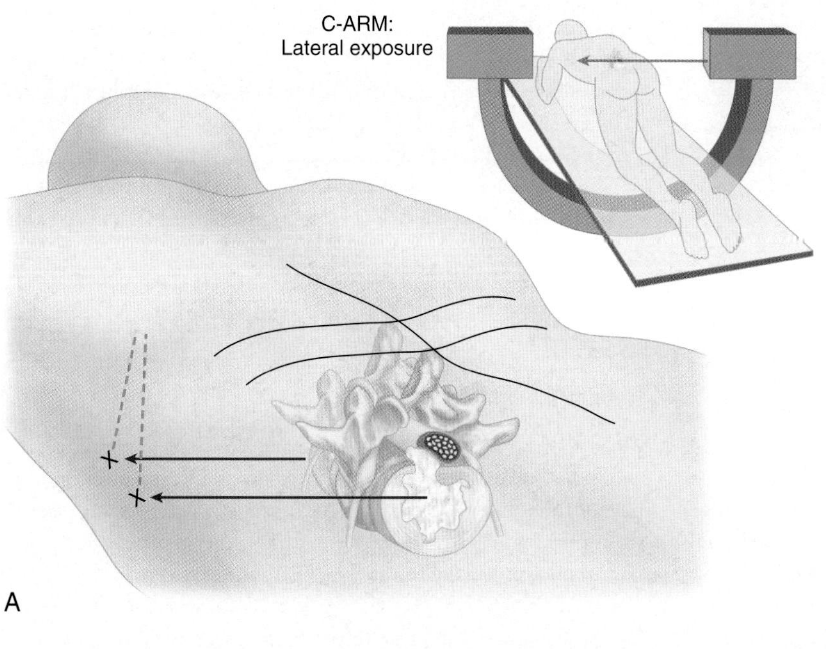


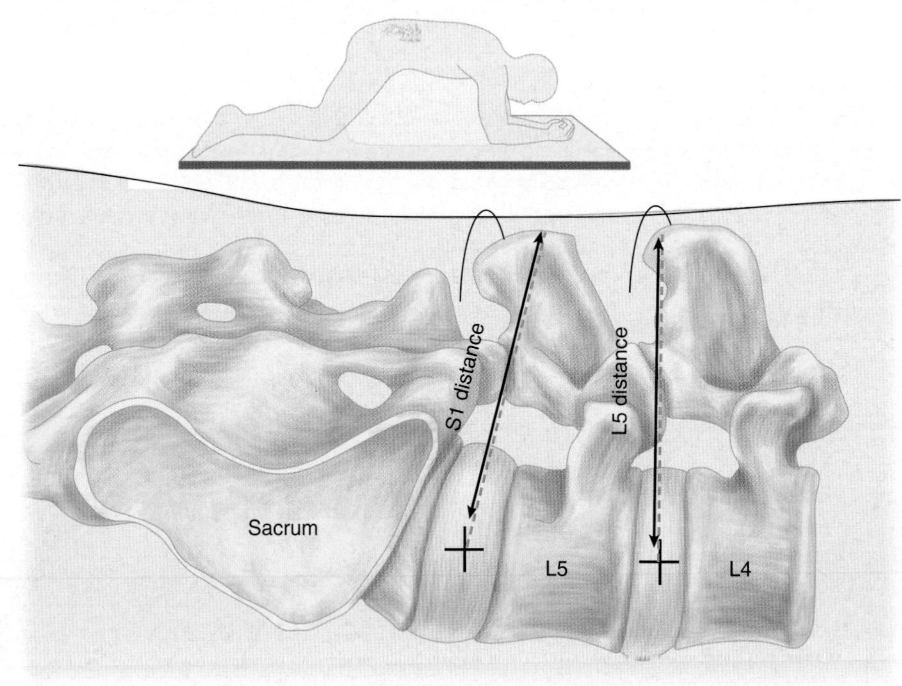


■ **FIGURE 19–7.** **A,** Lateral fluoroscopic exposure enables topographic location of the lateral disc center and allows visualization of the *plane of inclination* for each disc. **B,** The distance between lateral disc center and posterior skin surface plane is measured along each *disc inclination line.*

needle tip skive off the undersurface of the facet, but if the needle then deflects too much, reversing the bevel may allow the needle to fenestrate the ventral facet capsule and hug the bony facet when the exiting spinal nerve is irritated in the course of needle placement. If the trajectory is less than ideal by visualizing the trajectory angle, the skin window can be adjusted to approximate the ideal trajectory angle. The C-arm lateral projection should confirm the needle tip's correct annular location. In the lateral view, the correct needle tip position should be just touching the posterior annulus surface. In the posteroanterior view, the needle tip should be centered in the foraminal annular window. The two above-mentioned views of the C-arm confirm that the needle tip has engaged the safe zone, the center of the foraminal annular widow.

While monitoring the posteroanterior view, advance the needle tip through the annulus to the midline (anatomic disc center). Then check the lateral view. If the needle tip is in the center of the disc on the lateral view, you have a central needle placement, which is good for a central nucleotomy. Ideally, the needle tip will be in the posterior one third of the disc, indicating posterior needle placement if you are attempting to access herniations.

A mixture of 9cc Isouue 300 with 1cc indigo carmine dye is then injected to perform evocative chromadiscography. This mixture allows good radio-opacity on fluoroscopy and intraoperative light-blue chromatization of the pathologic nucleus and annular fissures, which helps guide the targeted fragmentectomy.

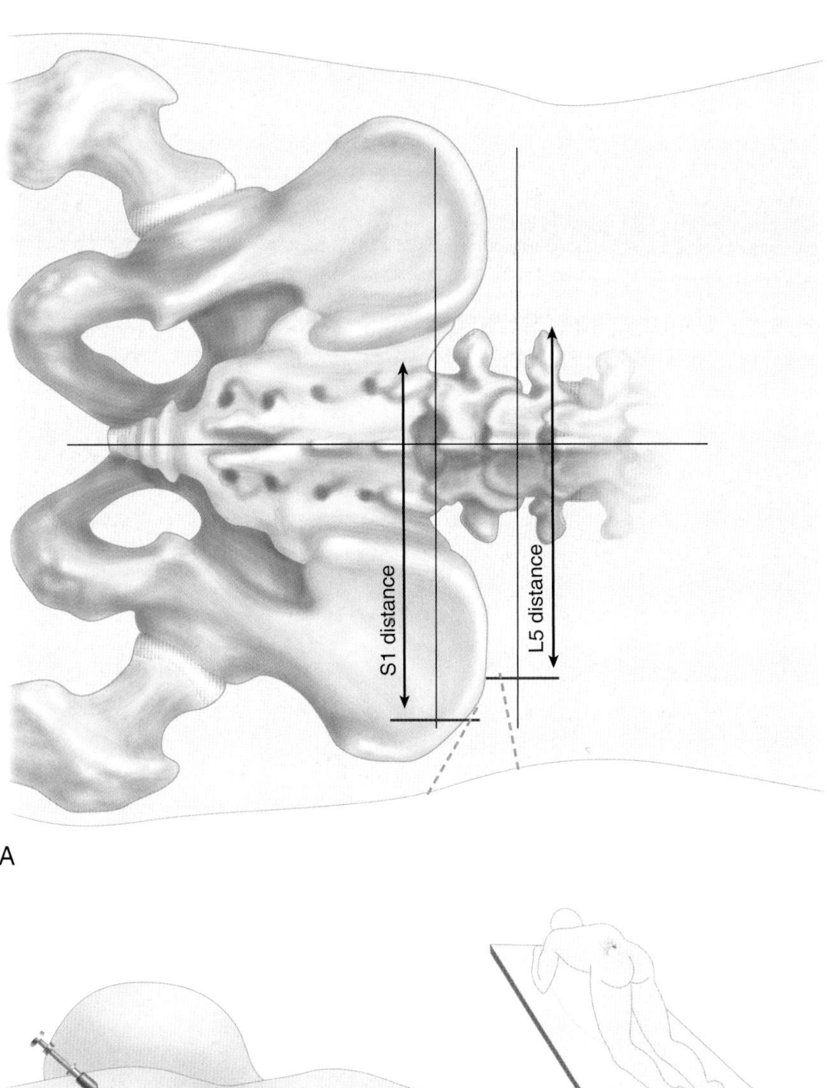


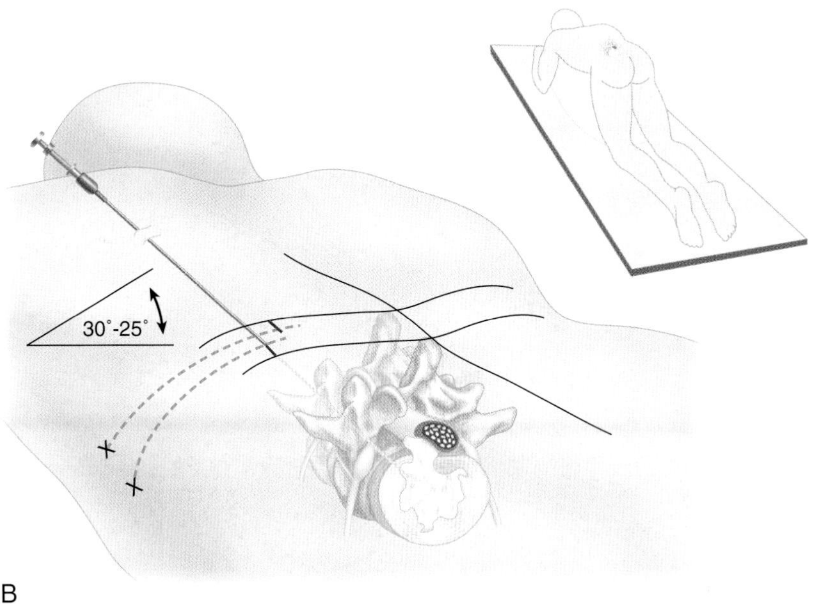


■ **FIGURE 19–8.** **A,** The distance is then measured from the midline along the respective transverse plane line for each disc. At the end of this measure, a *line parallel to midline* is drawn to intersect each *disc inclination line*. This intersection marks the skin entry point or "skin window" for each target disc. **B,** Needle is inserted at entry point toward the target disc at an angle 30 to 25 degrees to the surface skin plane. This trajectory will determine the path of all subsequent instrumentation.

## Instrument Placement

Insert a long thin guide wire through the 18-gauge needle channel. Advance the guide wire tip 1 to 2 cm deep into the annulus, and then remove the needle. Slide the bluntly tapered tissue-dilating obturator over the guide wire until the tip of the obturator is firmly engaged in the annular window. An eccentric parallel channel in the obturator allows for four-quadrant annular infiltration using small incremental volumes of one-half percent lidocaine in each quadrant, enough to anesthetize the annulus but not the nerves. Hold the obturator firmly against the annular window surface and remove the guide wire. Infiltrate the full thickness of the annulus through the obturator's center channel using lidocaine.

The next step is the through-and-through fenestration of the annular window by advancing the bluntly tapered obturator with a mallet. Annular fenestration is the most painful step of the entire procedure. Advise the anesthesiologist to heighten the sedation level just prior to annular fenestration. Advance the obturator tip deep into the annulus and confirm on the C-arm views. Now slide the beveled access cannula over the obturator toward the disc. Advance the cannula until the beveled tip is deep in the annular window. Remove the obturator and insert the endoscope to get a view of the disc nucleus and annulus. The subsequent steps depend on the goal of the procedure and pathology being addressed. The basic endoscopic method to excise a noncontained paramedian extruded lumbar herniated disc through a uniportal technique is described here. Different steps are used for other pathology and are beyond the scope of this chapter.

### Performing the Discectomy

First enlarge the annulotomy medially to the base of the herniation with a cutting forcep. The side-firing Holmium-YAG laser can also be used to enlarge and widen the annulotomy. This is performed to release the annular fibers at the herniation site that may pinch off or prevent the extruded portion of the herniation from being extracted. Directly under the herniation apex, a large amount of blue-stained nucleus is usually present, similar to the submerged portion of an iceberg (Figs. 19–9 and 19–10). The nucleus here represents migrated and unstable nucleus. The endoscopic rongeurs are used to extract the blue-stained nucleus pulposus under direct visualization (Fig. 19–11; also see Fig. 19–3). The larger straight and hinged rongeurs are used directly through the cannula after the endoscope is removed. Fluoroscopy and surgeon feel guide this step. By grabbing the base of the herniated fragment, one can usually extract the extruded portion of the herniation. Initial medialization and widening of the annulotomy reduce the prospect of breaking off the apex of the herniation. The traversing nerve root is readily visualized after removal of the extruded herniation (Figs. 19–12 and 19–13).

Next perform a bulk decompression by using a straight and flexible suction-irrigation shaver (Endius Inc., Plainville, MA). This step requires shaver head c-arm localization before power is activated to avoid nerve/dura injury and anterior annular penetration. The cavity thus created is called the working cavity. The debulking process serves two functions. First, it decompresses the disc, reducing the risk for further acute herniation. Second, it removes the unstable nucleus material to prevent future reherniation.

Inspect the working cavity. If a noncontained extruded disc fragment is still present by finding blue-stained nucleus material posteriorly, then these fragments are teased into the working cavity with the endoscopic rongeurs and the flexible radiofrequency trigger-flex bipolar probe (Ellman International, Oceanside, NY) and removed. Creation of the working cavity allows the herniated disc tissue to follow the path of least resistance into the cavity. The flexible radiofrequency bipolar probe is used to contract and thicken the annular collagen at the herniation site. It is also used for hemostasis throughout the case.

The vast majority of herniations can be treated via the uniportal technique. Sometimes for large central herniations, the disc needs to be approached from both sides, which is called the biportal technique.

### Postoperative Care

Because it is recommended that this technique be performed under local anesthesia, most procedures that use the approach can be performed as an outpatient procedure with same-day patient discharge. Most patients require only brief postoperative monitoring depending on the amount of sedation given. The postoperative restrictions are dependent on the pathology being addressed. Small annulotomies are made during the scope insertion into the disc; therefore, postoperative activity restrictions should be similar to that of an open lumbar discectomy. This activity modification will allow adequate time for scar formation over the annulotomy defect and to prevent herniation/reherniation.

### Complications and Avoidance

There is peer-reviewed literature on the complication rates associated with spinal surgery performed through an endoscopic

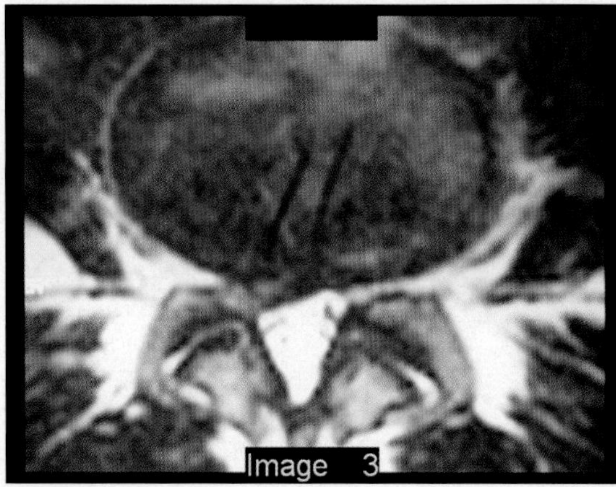


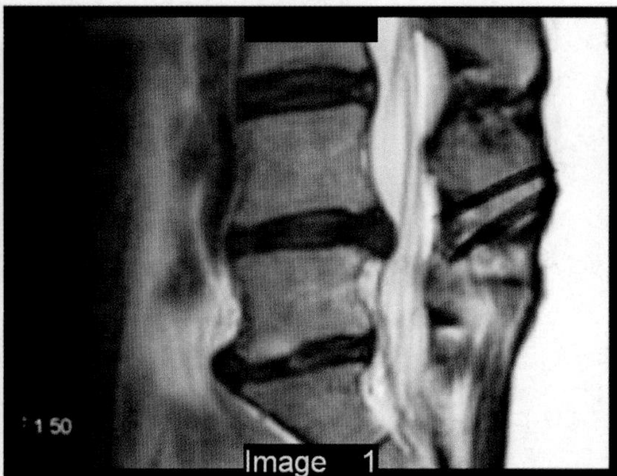


■ **FIGURE 19–9.** Preoperative axial and saggital MRI showing a right paracentral herniated nucleus pulposus. This is the same patient shown in the DVD clip.

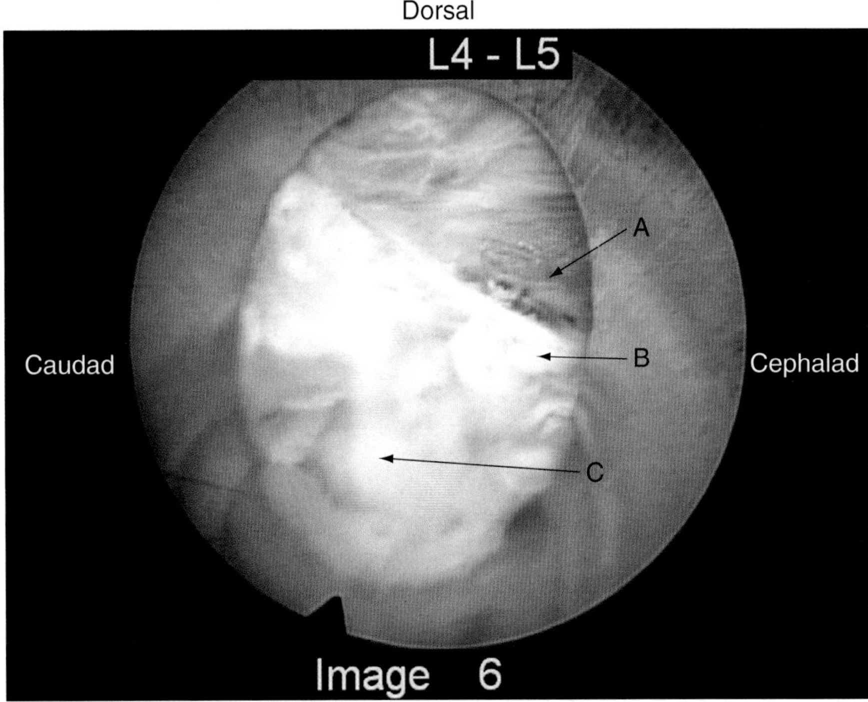


■ **FIGURE 19–10.** The initial endoscopic view shows the epidural space with epidural fat in the upper third of the picture **(A)**, the thinned out white posterior annular fibres in the middle third **(B)**, and the blue-stained (from indigo carmine) base of the herniated nucleus pulposus (HNP) **(C)**.

transforaminal approach.[2,5–7] Potential complications of the endoscopic transforaminal approach include nerve dysesthesias (5%–15% transient) (1.9%), persistent sensory deficit (1%), deep infection (0.65%), discitis (0.05%), dural tear (0.3%), thrombophlebitis (0.65), bowel injury (0.004%), vascular injury (0%), and respiratory distress requiring intubation (0%).[7]

Complications can be avoided by strictly adhering to the details in the Key Points section earlier and principles of the YESS technique listed in Box 19–1. Avoidance of complications is enhanced by the ability to clearly visualize normal and pathoanatomy, the use of local anesthesia and conscious sedation rather than general or spinal anesthesia, and the use of a standardized needle placement protocol.

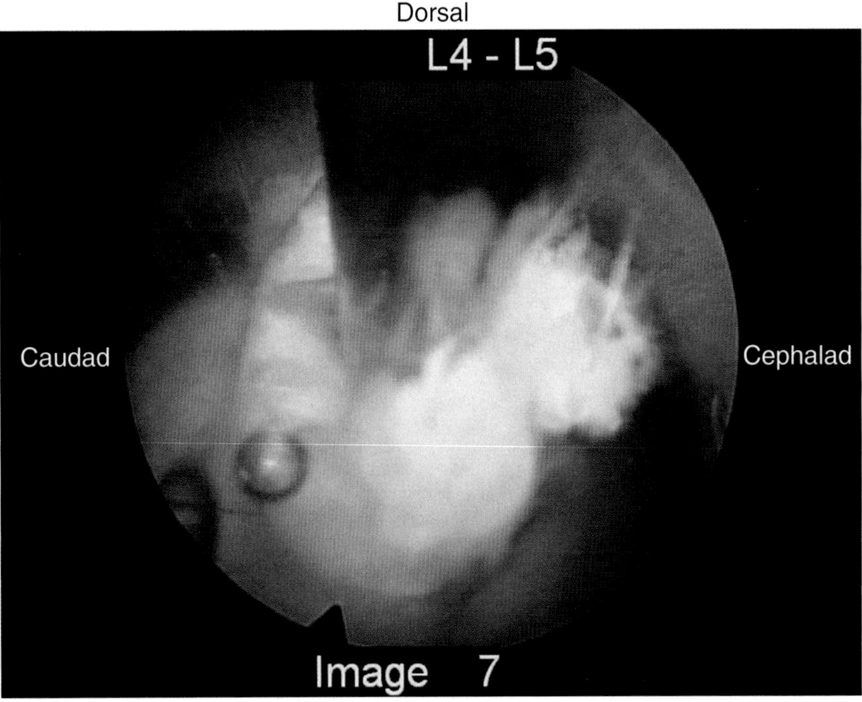


■ **FIGURE 19–11.** After cutting the annular fibers to enlarge the annulotomy medially, pituitary rongeurs grasp the base of the HNP to remove it.

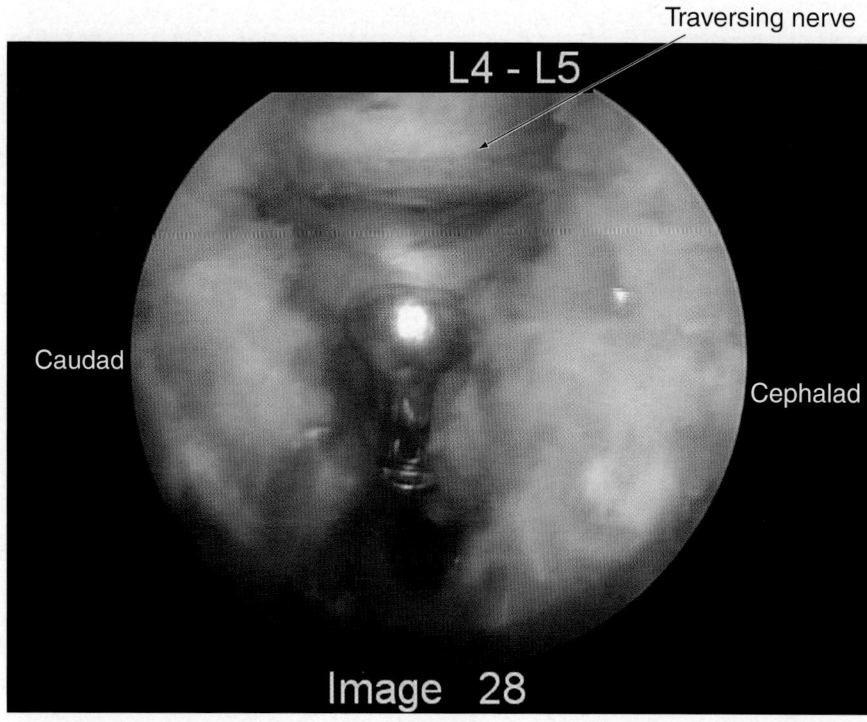


■ **FIGURE 19–12.** An accessory portal (Biportal technique) is utilized from the contra lateral left side to allow insertion of larger articulating instruments to reach more dorsally. The Endius flexible pituitary is shown here grasping the posterior annulus and posterior longitudinal ligament. The traversing nerve root is clearly decompressed.

The entire procedure is usually accomplished with the patient remaining comfortable during the entire procedure and should be done without the patient feeling severe pain except when expected, such as during evocative discography, annular fenestration, or when instruments are manipulated past the exiting nerve. Local anesthesia using half-percent xylocaine allows generous use of this dilute anesthetic for pain control and still allows the patient to feel pain when the nerve root is manipulated. Thus, the awake and aware patient serves as the best indicator to avoid any nerve irritation/damage. Dural tears can be treated with a visualized blood patch and observation because there is no "dead space" for cerebral spinal fluid collection or drainage.

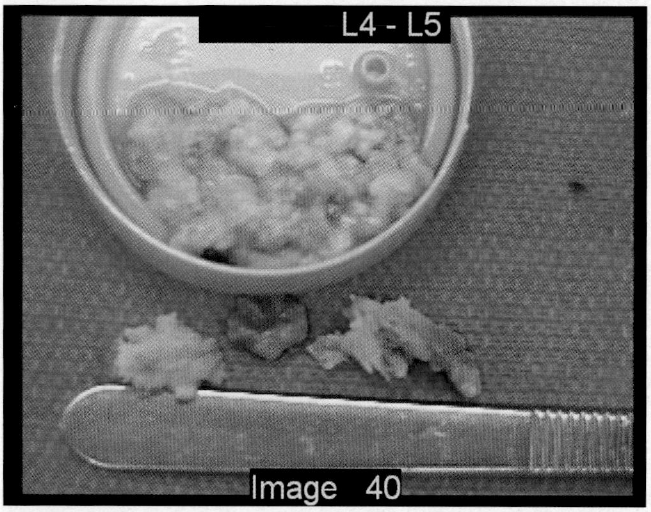

## CONCLUSIONS/DISCUSSION

The endoscopic transforaminal approach is safe and efficacious but does require a unique combination of skills not typically used by spine surgeons. Prior experience with discography, epidural injections, and arthroscopic experience is helpful in reducing the learning curve. Most spine surgeons are unfamiliar and uncomfortable with the endoscopic transforaminal approach; therefore, the learning curve is a major obstacle to more widespread use of this technique. Some surgeons believe that the potential for inferior outcomes that is associated with the learning curve of this approach may not be justified when open posterior approaches dictate high success rates and outcomes. Perhaps this is why this transforaminal approach is seldom used by spinal surgeons despite the fact that the technique was first described by Kambin in 1991.[9,10] However, new implants and instruments and technologic advances have made this approach safer, easier to learn, and a versatile option for effective delivery of implants to the disc space. The benefits of using muscle-spreading techniques under local anesthesia (avoiding general anesthesia) to access the foraminal anatomy and disc space cannot be denied.

## FUTURE CONSIDERATIONS

Perhaps the best new indication for the use of this technique and approach is in the realm of motion preservation (nucleus replacement) or minimally invasive anterior stabilization. One advantage of this approach stems from its ability to approach the disc through the

■ **FIGURE 19–13.** The removed disc fragments are shown here. Note the differential coloring of the fragments. The red part is the inflamed extruded portion and the blue/white part is the nucleus that was still within the disc.

foramen, avoiding the morbidity associated with dural scarring encountered in revision lumbar surgery. The presence of scar tissue makes traditional posterior lumbar interbody fusion techniques difficult or impossible, but an interbody fusion through an endoscopic transforaminal approach would avoid this issue. A biportal endoscopic fusion technique can be used to perform a radical discectomy with burring of the end plates under direct visualization and subsequent delivery of a cage and bone graft. Transforaminal anatomy will limit size of implant that can be delivered; however, this problem can be overcome by using expandable interbody or graft containment devices.

This approach is also applicable as a vehicle for visualized total nuclectomy with end plate preservation and delivery of a nucleus replacement prosthesis. Endoscopic nuclectomy can be performed under direct visualization before implanting an expandable nucleus replacement or possibly a disc replacement. Expandable nucleus replacement devices such as the DASCOR nucleus replacement prosthesis (Disc Dynamics Inc., Eden Prairie, MN) and the Neudisc (Replication Medical Inc., New Brunswick, NJ) are well suited for this route of delivery (see Chapter 53).

## REFERENCES

1. Yeung AT: Minimally invasive disc surgery with the Yeung Endoscopic Spine System (YESS). Surg Tech Int 8:1–11, 1999.
2. Tsou PM, Yeung AT: Transforaminal endoscopic decompression for radiculopathy secondary to intra-canal non-contained lumbar disc herniations: outcome and technique. Spine J 2:41–48, 2002.
3. Kambin P: Percutaneous lumbar discectomy: Review of 100 patients and current practice. Clin Orthop 238:24–34, 1989.
4. Lee SH, Uk Kang B: Operative failure of percutaneous endoscopic lumbar discectomy: a radiologic analysis of 55 cases. Spine 31: E285–E290, 2006.
5. Jang JS, An SH, Lee SH: Transforaminal percutaneous endoscopic discectomy in the treatment of foraminal and extraforaminal lumbar disc herniations. J Spinal Disord Tech 19:338–343, 2006.
6. Ahn Y, Lee SH, Park WM, Lee HY: Posterolateral percutaneous endoscopic lumbar foraminotomy for L5-S1 foraminal or lateral exit zone stenosis: Technical note. J Neurosurg 99(3 suppl):320–323, 2003.
7. Yeung AT, Tsou PM: Posterolateral endoscopic excision for lumbar disc herniation: Surgical techniques, outcome, and complications in 307 consecutive cases. Spine 27:722–773, 2002.
8. Mayer HM, Brock M: Percutaneous endoscopic discectomy: surgical technique and preliminary results compared to microsurgical discectomy. J Neurosurg 78:216–225, 1993.
9. Schaffeer JL, Kambin P: Percutaneous posterolateral lumbar discectomy and decompression with a 6.9-millimeter cannula: Analysis of operative failures and complications. J Bone Joint Surg (Am) 73:822–831, 1991.
10. Kambin P: Posterolateral percutaneous lumbar discetomy and decompression. *In* Kambin P (ed): Arthroscopic Microdiscectomy: Minimally Intervention in Spinal Surgery. Baltimore, Williams & Wilkins, 1991, pp 67–100.

CHAPTER 20

# Cervical Approaches: Anterior and Posterior

**Domagoj Coric** and **Daniel M. Oberer**

## KEY POINTS

- Cervical disc arthroplasty offers several theoretical advantages over anterior cervical discectomy and fusion (ACDF) in the treatment of cervical spondylosis.
- Anterior and posterior approaches to the cervical spine for arthroplasty mimic standard exposure for cervical degenerative disc disease, trauma, and other common pathologic entities.
- Special considerations relating to anterior cervical arthroplasty include emphasis on true midline orientation as well as meticulous carpentry relating to end plate preparation and resection of the uncovertebral joints.

## INTRODUCTION

Cervical disc arthroplasty offers several theoretical advantages over anterior cervical discectomy and fusion (ACDF) in the treatment of cervical spondylosis.[1–3] ACDF results in loss of mobility at the operated level or levels and places increased stress on adjacent levels above and below the fusion.[1,4–9] These stresses may lead to a higher incidence of segmental degeneration and, possibly, instability.[10–12] Disc space arthroplasty achieves identical decompression of the neural elements, but preserves motion and elasticity at the operated level, and may potentially decrease the occurrence of adjacent segment degeneration.[13–19]

Anterior and posterior approaches to the cervical spine for arthroplasty mimic standard exposure for cervical degenerative disc disease, trauma, and other common pathologic entities. But, several important differences need to be taken into account. Special considerations relating to anterior cervical arthroplasty include emphasis on true midline orientation as well as meticulous carpentry relating to end plate preparation and resection of the uncovertebral joints (Table 20–1).

## ANATOMY

The standard anterior approach to the cervical spine is made in the avascular plane medial to the carotid sheath and sternocleidomastoid muscle and lateral to the esophagus and trachea. The two layers of the cervical fascia, superficial and deep, are sequentially encountered. The superficial fascia contains the platysma muscle. The deep fascia has three layers: superficial, middle, and deep, which overlie the prevertebral space.[20–23]

The carotid sheath (carotid artery, internal jugular vein, and vagus nerve) lies deep to the sternocleidomastoid muscle and is retracted laterally with the muscle. The recurrent laryngeal nerve arises from the vagus nerve. The recurrent laryngeal innervates the larynx above the vocal cords. Most subaxial cervical levels can be accessed above the omohyoid muscle, which can be mobilized as needed. The longus colli muscles symmetrically border the ventrolateral aspect of the vertebral bodies. The cervical sympathetic trunk lies laterally on the anterior aspect of the longus colli muscle. The vertebral artery, the first branch of the subclavian artery, usually enters the foramen transversarium at C6, and exits at C1. The artery lies immediately lateral to the uncovertebral joint, which marks the lateral aspect of the disc space. The distance between the medial aspects of the uncovertebral joints in the subaxial spine is ~15 mm.[21,23]

## ANTERIOR APPROACH

The patient is positioned supine on the operating room table. Care is taken to insure neutral positioning, and to avoid extension, which is generally employed with standard ACDF. The head is secured in the midline position. The shoulders are taped down to facilitate optimal fluoroscopic visualization. Elbows should be padded, and care must be taken to avoid excessive traction to the upper trunk of the brachial plexus (Fig. 20–1). A standard transverse skin incision is made in a natural skin crease, and routine sharp dissection is performed through the superficial cervical fascia. The platysma is entered longitudinally along the axis of its fibers, perpendicular to the incision. Sharp dissection is carried down to the anterior border of the sternocleidomastoid muscle, which is also mobilized laterally. The middle layer of the deep cervical fascia is sharply incised, and blunt finger dissection is performed medial to the carotid sheath and down to the deep cervical fascia in the prevertebral space. The prevertebral deep fascia is then dissected rostrally and caudally off the anterior longitudinal ligament using a Kittner dissector. Proper localization is confirmed with lateral fluoroscopy. Care is taken to preserve the normal anatomy before electrocautery and placement of retractors.

**TABLE 20–1. Key Points for Anterior Cervical Arthroplasty**

| |
|---|
| Neutral positioning |
| Identify midline anatomically early and confirm with true AP flouroscopy |
| Drill end plates parallel—avoid cancellous bone |
| Drill uncovertebral joints to accomplish bilateral proximal foraminotomies |
| Do not oversize implants |

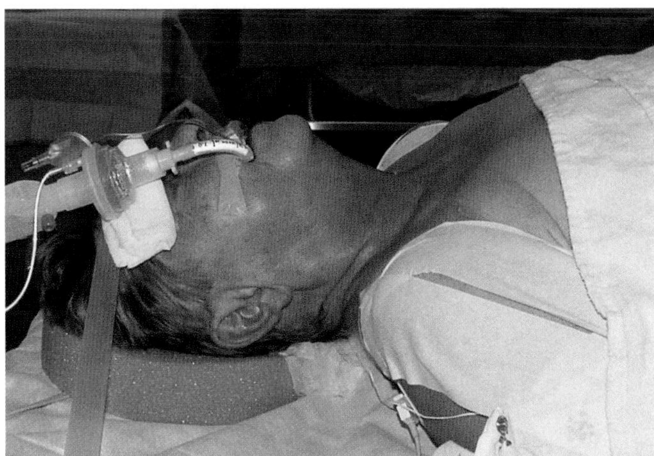

■ **FIGURE 20–1.** Neutral positioning.

In order to tentatively identify the midline, use the colli muscles and the natural slope of the anterior vertebral bodies as landmarks. The vertebral body is preliminarily marked in the midline using Bovie electrocautery. The longus colli muscles are then mobilized using bipolar electrocautery along the venous plexus that runs on their medial border, taking care to avoid the cervical sympathetic trunk in the anterolateral portion of the muscles. A self-retaining retractor system of choice is employed. Anterior osteophytes should be removed to allow for an accurate assessment of the true anterior vertebral body, which is found using direct visualization and lateral fluoroscopy. If the arthroplasty system utilized allows for placement of distraction pins, they should be placed in the midline (Fig. 20–2).

Complete discectomy is performed in the standard fashion with curettes and pituitary rongeurs.

Following discectomy, attention is turned to decompression. A thorough decompression is essential to the success of cervical arthroplasty. This is an important differentiating factor from ACDF. With ACDF, several factors contribute to clinical success: (1) direct decompression of the symptomatic side, (2) indirect decompression due to restoration of foraminal height, and (3) loss of motion. Conversely, cervical arthroplasty is largely dependent on direct decompression, owing to the fact that indirect decompression is limited by the size of the arthroplasty device (generally only 5 or 6 mm) and maintenance of motion. Additionally, proper fit of the arthroplasty device is dependent on meticulous preparation of the disc space. A high-speed drill is used to remove the cartilaginous end plates, taking care to preserve the bony end plates. Exposure of the cancellous bone can predispose to heterotopic ossification and subsidence.[24–26] The inferior and superior end plates are drilled down until they are parallel. The uncovertebral joints are resected bilaterally and equally until proximal foraminotomies are completed. Bilateral decompression and parallel end plates are crucial to allow for proper sizing, fit, and midline placement of the artificial disc (Fig. 20–3). Generally, cervical arthroplasty devices are anchored to the vertebral bodies with keel or tooth fixation or by milling or screw fixation of the vertebral body end plate.[14,17,28] Long-term stability is dependent on proper sizing and fit in the interbody space. The decompression includes resection of the posterior longitudinal ligament to expose the dura and proximal nerve roots bilaterally. Posterior osteophytes and hypertrophied uncal spurs are removed using Kerrison rongeurs and currettes.

The specifics of cervical artificial disc placement are dependent on each unique arthroplasty device. But, generally, after decompression, attention is turned to artificial disc placement which consists of (1) midline verification, (2) sizing, and (3) disc placement. Midline verification is accomplished by placing distraction posts or a localizing device in line with the spinous processes using anteroposterior (AP) fluoroscopy (Fig. 20–4). Trials are used to determine proper AP and lateral sizing and fit. Lateral flouroscopy is used to confirm good fit by demonstrating excellent apposition of the end plates to the trial without intervening radiolucency (Fig. 20–5). The goal is to maximize vertebral end plate coverage

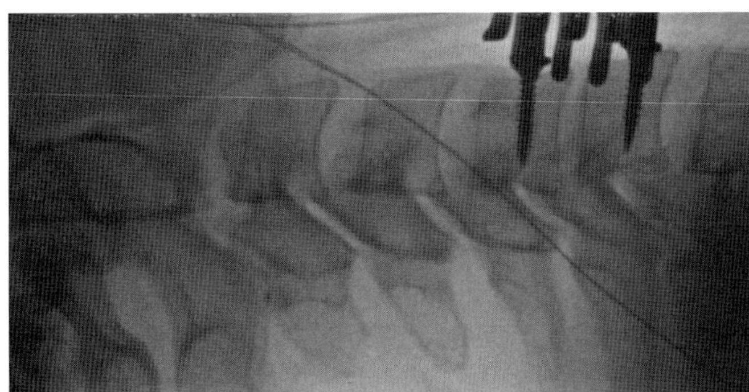

■ **FIGURE 20–2.** Parallel distractor pin placement.

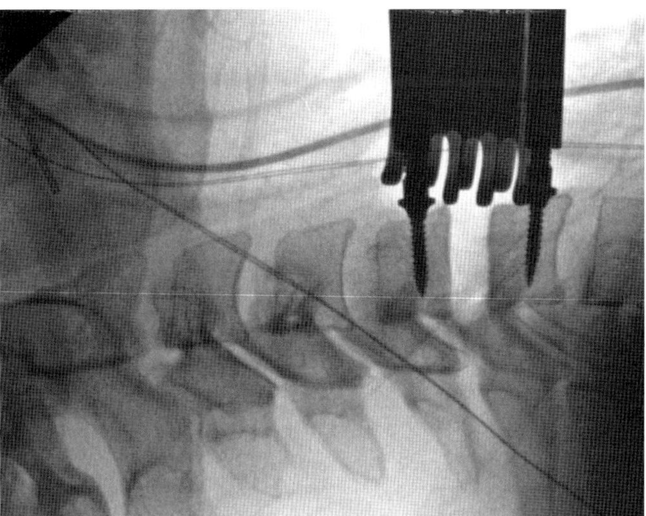

■ **FIGURE 20–3.** Disc space preparation with parallel end plates and resection of uncovertebral joints.

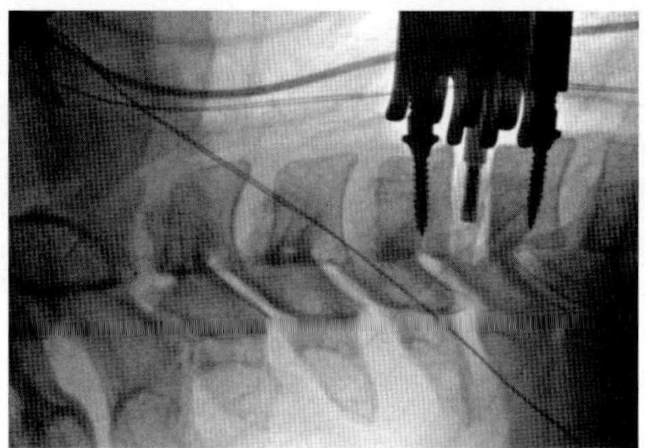

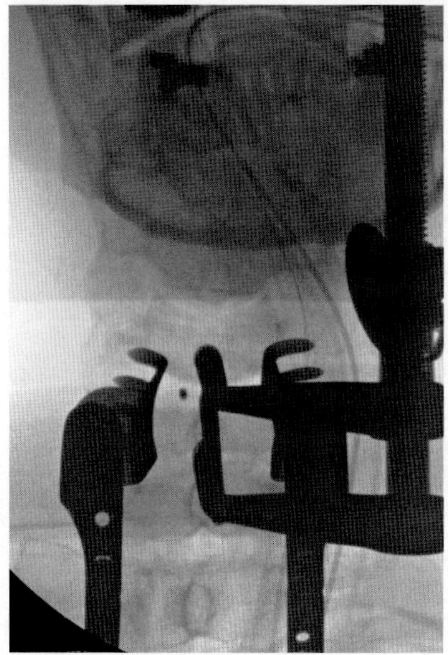

■ **FIGURE 20–4.** Midline verification. Note alignment of distractor pins and midline finder with spinous processes on true anteroposterior flouro image.

in order to minimize subsidence and risk of malpositioning. With keel-based devices, keel cutting precedes final disc placement (Fig. 20–6). The arthroplasty device is then placed in the disc space using lateral fluoroscopic guidance (Fig. 20–7). Appropriate fit of the artificial disc is important, because oversizing or malposition (off-midline in the AP plane or too anterior or posterior in the lateral plane) can lead to limitation of motion and subsidence (Fig. 20–8). Oversizing can lead to limitation of motion or segmental kyphosis. For two-level artificial disc placement, proper sizing and midline placement are especially critical for technical and clinical success (Fig. 20–9).

Closure involves reapproximating the platysma and subcutaneous layer of the skin with Vicryl suture followed by skin closure with Dermabond (Fig 20–10). Patients are mobilized out of bed without bracing on the day of surgery and are usually discharged home within 24 hours.

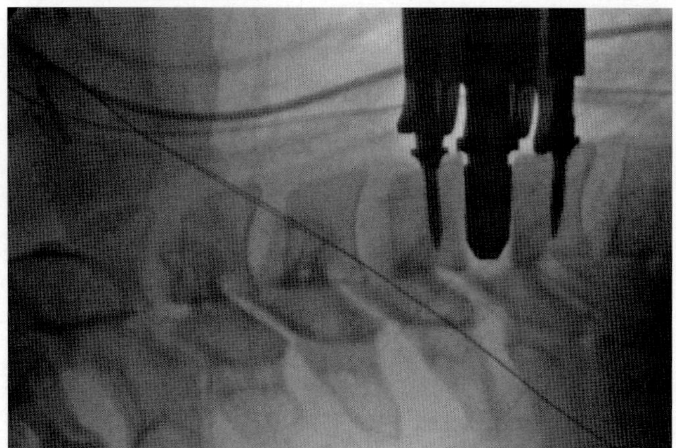

■ **FIGURE 20–5.** Sizing. Note lack of lucency between trialer and end plates.

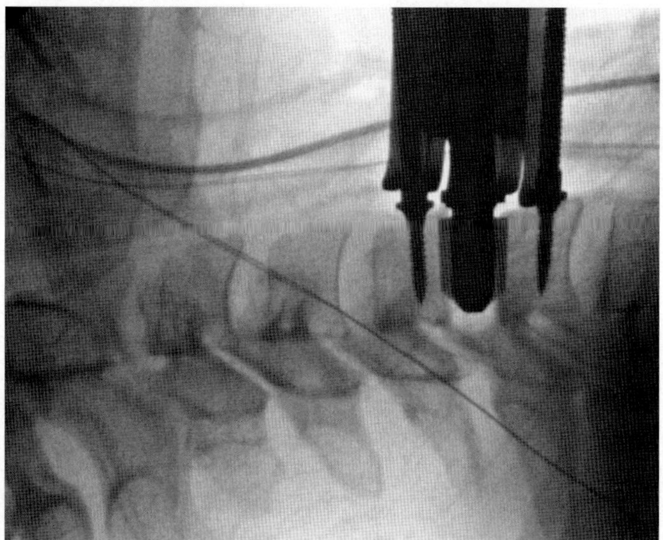

■ **FIGURE 20–6.** Keel cutting.

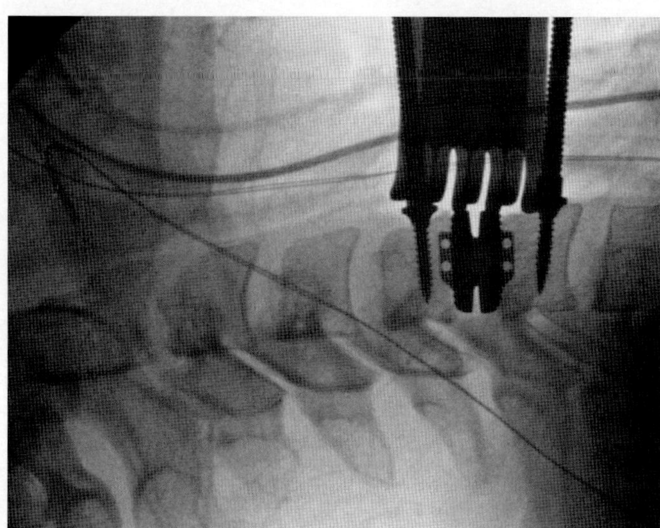

■ **FIGURE 20–7.** Kineflex|C (Spinal Motion, Inc., Mountainview, CA) artificial disc placement.

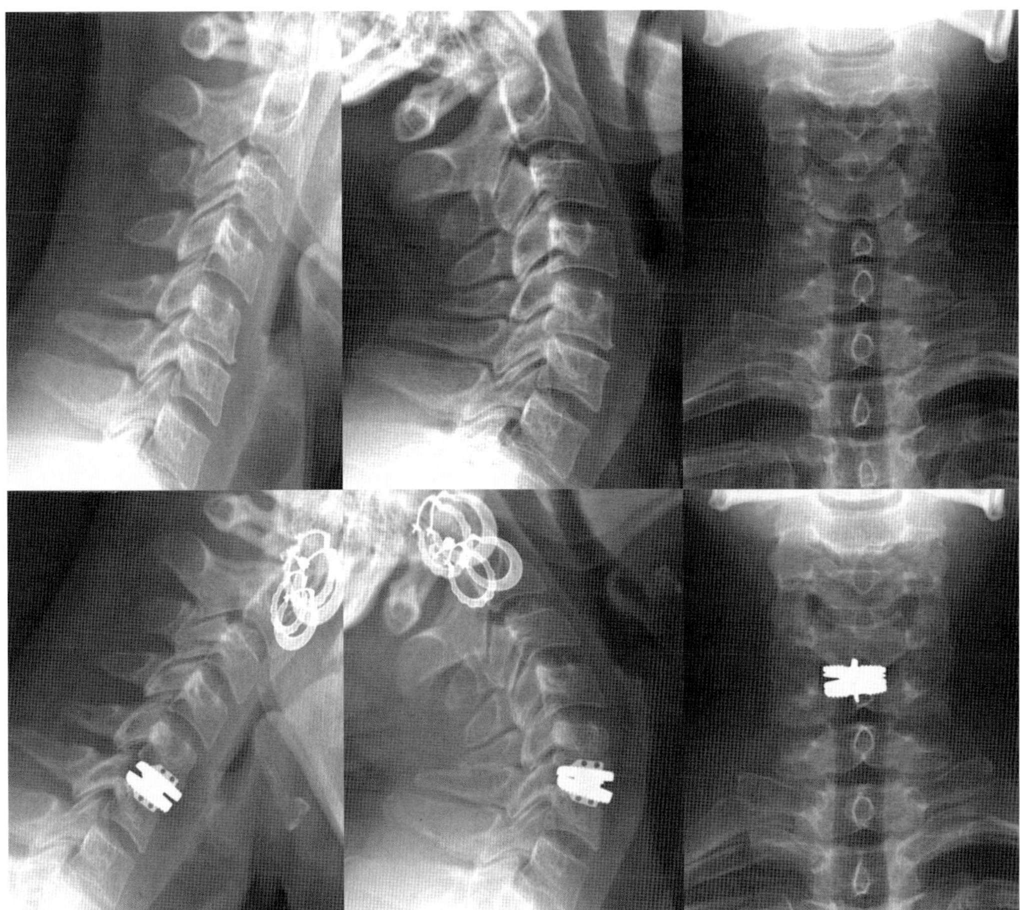

■ **FIGURE 20–8.** *Top*, Preoperative anteroposterior and lateral flexion/extension radiographs. *Bottom*, Postoperative anteroposterior and lateral flexion-extension radiographs. Note restoration of disc space height with maintenance of motion and midline disc placement.

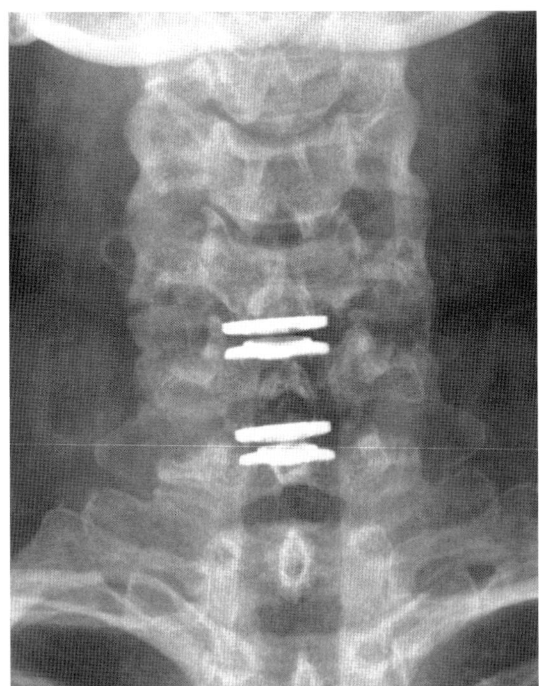

■ **FIGURE 20–9.** Two-level DISCOVER (DePuy Spine, Inc., Raynham, MA) artificial disc placement.

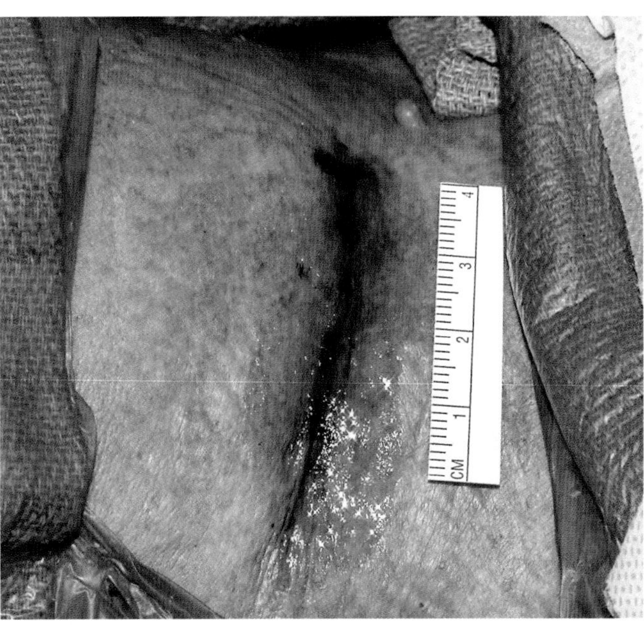

■ **FIGURE 20–10.** Standard skin closure following a two-level artificial disc placement.

## POSTERIOR APPROACH

The posterior approach is not appropriate for access to the disc space, because the spinal cord cannot be manipulated, and the facet joints and vertebral arteries impede access. For surgery on the posterior elements, the patient is placed prone on chest and hip rolls, and all pressure points are padded. The head is secured in Mayfield headframe and pins are used to ensure maximum stability and to control proper alignment. Spinal alignment and localization are established with radiograph or flouroscopy. A standard midline incision is made in the avascular plane, the ligamentum nuchae. Muscle dissection and blood loss are minimized with proper retraction of the soft tissues using Cobb elevators and cerebellar retractors, and dissection is performed subperiostially. It is helpful to use the sharpened end of a Penfield 1 to dissect the soft tissue off the lateral masses and the facet joints. This can prevent venous injury and damage to the joint capsules caused by electrocautery. The wound is closed in layers, with special attention paid to approximating the muscle layers, and closing the fascia tightly.

## REFERENCES

1. Aronson N, Filtzer D, Bagan M: Anterior cervical fusion by the Smith-Robinson approach. J Neurosurg 29:396–404, 1968.
2. Coric D, Finger F, Boltes P: The Bryan Cervical Disc prospective, randomized, controlled study: Early clinical results from a single investigational site. J Neurosurg 1:31–35, 2006.
3. Mummaneni P, Haid R: The future in the care of the cervical spine: Interbody fusion and arthroplasty. J Neurosurg 2:155–159, 2004.
4. Bailey RW, Badgley CE: Stabilization of the cervical spine by anterior fusion. J Bone Joint Surg Am 42:565–594, 1960.
5. DiAngelo D, Roberston J, Metcalf, N, et al: Biomechanical testing of an artificial cervical joint and an anterior cervical plate. J Spinal Disord Tech 16:314–323, 2003.
6. Hunter L, Braunstein E, Bailey R: Radiographic changes following anterior cervical fusion. Spine 5:399–401, 1980.
7. Matsunaga S, Kabayama S, Yamamoto, T, et al: Strain on intervertebral discs after anterior cervical decompression and fusion. Spine 24:670–675, 1999.
8. Pospiech J, Stolke D, Wilke H, Claes L: Intradiscal pressure recordings in the cervical spine. Neurosurgery 44:379–385, 1999.
9. Wang J, McDonough P, Endow K, et al: The effect of cervical plating on single-level anterior cervical discectomy and fusion. J Spinal Disord 112:467–471, 1999.
10. Bohlman HH, Emery SE, Goodfellow DB, Jones PK: Robinson anterior cervical discectomy and arthrodesis for cervical radiculopathy: Long-term follow-up of one hundred and twenty-two patients. J Bone Joint Surg Am 75:1298–1307, 1993.
11. Emery S, Bohlman H, Bolesta M, Jones P: Anterior cervical decompression and arthrodesis for the treatment of cervical spondylotic myelopathy: Two- to seventeen-year follow-up. J Bone Joint Surg Am 80:941–951, 1998.
12. Hilibrand A, Carlson G, Palumbo M, et al: Radiculopathy and myelopathy at segments adjacent to the site of a previous anterior cervical arthrodesis. J Bone Joint Surg Am 81:519–528, 1999.
13. Bertagnoli R, Yue J, Pfeiffer F, et al: Early results after ProDisc-C cervical disc replacement. J Neurosurg 4:403–410, 2005.
14. Cummins B, Robertson J, Gill S: Surgical experience with an implanted artificial cervical joint. J Neurosurg 88:943–948, 1998.
15. Goffin J, Van Calenbergh F, van Loon J, et al: Intermediate follow-up after treatment of degenerative disc disease with the Bryan cervical disc prosthesis: single-level and bi-level. Spine 23:2673–2678, 2003.
16. Mummaneni P, Burkus J, Haid R, et al: Clinical and radiographic analysis of cervical disc arthroplasty compared with allograft fusion: A randomized controlled clinical trial. J Neurosurg 6:198–200, 2007.
17. Sekhon LHS: Cervical arthroplasty in the management of spondylotic myelopathy. J Spinal Disord Tech 16:307–313, 2003.
18. Sekhon LHS, Sears W, Duggal N: Cervical arthroplasty after previous surgery: results of treating 24 discs in 15 patients. J Neurosurg 3:335–341, 2005.
19. Wigfield C, Gill S, Nelson R, et al: Influence of an artificial cervical joint compared with fusion on adjacent-level motion in the treatment of degenerative cervical disc disease. J Neurosurg 96:17–21, 2002.
20. Cloward RB: The anterior approach for removal of ruptured cervical discs. J Neurosurg 15:602–617, 1958.
21. Farey ID: Anterior approach to the cervical spine. *In* Zdeblick TA, (ed): Anterior Approaches to the Spine. St. Louis, Quality Medical Publishing, 1999, pp 47–74.
22. Robinson RA, Smith GW: Anterolateral cervical disc removal and interbody fusion of cervical disc. Bull Johns Hopkins Hosp 96:223–224, 1955.
23. Saunders RL: Ventral subaxial cervical spine anatomy. *In* Benzel E (ed): Surgical Exposure of the Spine: An Extensile Approach. Park Ridge, IL, American Association of Neurological Surgeons, 1995, pp 21–26.
24. Bartels R, Donk R: Fusion around cervical disc prosthesis: case report. Neurosurgery 57:194, 2005.
25. Parkinson JF, Sekhon L: Cervical arthroplasty complicated by delayed spontaneous fusion: case report. J Neurosurg 2:377–380, 2005.
26. Pickett GE, Sekhon LHS, Sears WR, Duggal N: Complications with cervical arthroplasty. J Neurosurg 4:98–105, 2006.
27. Goffin J, Casey A, Kehr P, et al: Preliminary clinical experience with the Bryan cervical disc prosthesis. Neurosurgery 51:840–847, 2002.
28. Wigfield C, Gill S, Nelson R, et al: The new Frenchay artificial cervical joint: Results from a two-year pilot study. Spine 27:2446–2452, 2002.

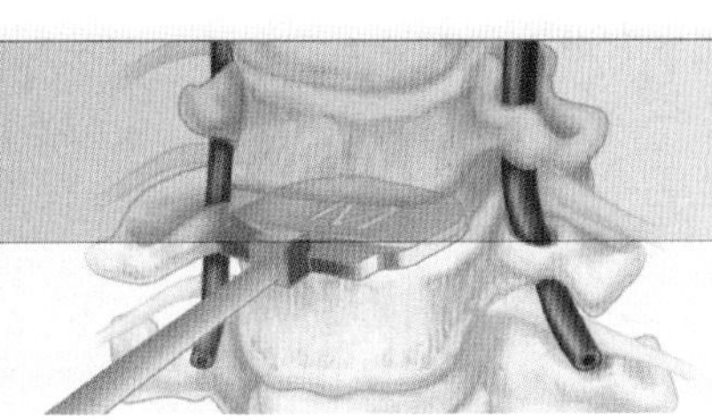

PART

# III

# Cervical Total Disc Arthroplasty

CHAPTER 21

# Primary Indications and Disc Space Preparation for Cervical Disc Arthroplasty

Jacob M. Buchowski and K. Daniel Riew

## KEY POINTS

- The indications for cervical disc arthroplasty are nearly the same as for anterior cervical discectomy and fusion: namely radiculopathy and myelopathy due to retrodiscal compression.
- Arthroplasty should not be performed for myelopathy caused by congenital stenosis, ossification of posterior longitudinal ligament (OPLL), or any other etiology that causes retrovertebral compression; in addition, arthroplasty should not be performed in patients with ankylosing spondylitis, diffuse idiopathic skeletal hyperostosis (DISH), facet arthropathy, ongoing or chronic cervical spine infection, severe osteoporosis, patients who are likely to become unstable with the procedure, and patients with axial neck pain as the solitary symptom.
- Neutral positioning of the neck is critical for end plate preparation and arthroplasty placement to avoid placing the arthroplasty device in a too kyphotic or lordotic position.
- Successful disc space preparation requires light decortication of both the inferior and superior end plates, removal of all posterior vertebral osteophytes, and a thorough foraminal decompression.
- When performing cervical disc arthroplasty in patients with spondylotic radiculopathy or myelopathy, a more thorough and wider uncinate and osteophyte resection is required than in patients in whom a fusion is performed, because continued motion across the segment may lead to recurrence of spondylosis when compared with cervical fusion procedures in which it would be unusual for spurs to recur once a solid fusion is obtained.

## INTRODUCTION

Anterior cervical discectomy and fusion (ACDF) for spondylotic myelopathy and radiculopathy affecting one or two cervical levels has proved to be one of the most effective and successful procedures in spine surgery both clinically and radiographically.[1–5] Despite the overall success of the procedure, however, there are significant disadvantages of fusing motion segments. The primary disadvantage is the potential risk of inducing accelerated adjacent segment degeneration, which has been estimated to occur with an incidence of 2.9% per year following ACDF, with 25.6% of patients having symptomatic adjacent segment degeneration 10 years following surgery.[6] Treatment of degenerated segments adjacent to a prior fusion can be problematic, usually requiring plate fixation, which can increase the risk of dysphagia and potential for instrumentation failure.[5,7–9] Therefore, although single- and two-level ACDF remains an effective treatment of myelopathy or radiculopathy, the drawbacks of the procedure have sparked a great interest in cervical disc arthroplasty, which although it is an infant technology compared with ACDF, has the potential to eliminate the disadvantages of ACDF while allowing similar (or even improved) clinical outcomes. The goals of the cervical disc arthroplasty are to maintain or restore intervertebral height, spinal balance, and mobility, and to avoid adjacent segment degeneration.[8,9]

## INDICATIONS FOR CERVICAL DISC ARTHROPLASTY

The indications for cervical disc arthroplasty are nearly the same as for anterior cervical discectomy and fusion: namely radiculopathy and myelopathy due to retrodiscal compression.[5,8,10–15] More specifically, cervical disc arthroplasty is indicated in patients with cervical degenerative disc disease and symptoms or signs of cervical myelopathy and radiculopathy (with or without neck pain) requiring surgical treatment at one to two and, occasionally, three levels. Patients should have evidence of disc herniation or cervical spondylosis resulting in myelopathy or radiculopathy. Because most patients with new-onset neck and arm pain and findings secondary to disc herniation improve within 6 weeks with nonoperative treatment measures, patients undergoing cervical disc arthroplasty should have failed an extensive nonoperative treatment program lasting at least 6 weeks and consisting of anti-inflammatory pain medications, physical therapy, and other modalities such as injections, neck bracing, and so on. Obviously, patients with neurologic deficits or signs of acute or progressive myelopathy and weakness with confirmed spinal cord compression should undergo a decompression without delay. Patients should have signs of the underlying pathology on physical examination consisting of an abnormal reflex, sensation, or motor strength in the appropriate dermatome/myotome. Radiographic work-up should consist of plain radiographs (including anteroposterior, lateral, flexion, extension, and oblique views), and advanced imaging (usually a magnetic

**TABLE 21–1. Clinical Indications for Cervical Disc Arthroplasty**

1. Radiculopathy attributable to cervical disc degeneration at one to three levels
2. Myelopathy attributable to cervical disc degeneration at one to three levels with retrodiscal disease
3. Radiographic evidence of cervical disc herniation or spondylosis at one to three levels
4. Symptoms and findings present between C3 and T1
5. Failure of nonoperative treatment (minimum of 6 weeks)

resonance imaging [MRI] scan or a computed tomographic myelogram, especially in patients with contraindications to MRI).[5,8,10–16] The focal compressive lesion or lesions (whether due to a disc herniation or spondylotic changes) should be easily identified on these studies. The indications for cervical disc arthroplasty are summarized in Table 21–1.

## CONTRAINDICATIONS FOR CERVICAL DISC ARTHROPLASTY

Arthroplasty should not be performed for myelopathy caused by congenital stenosis, ossification of posterior longitudinal ligament (OPLL), or any other etiology that causes retrovertebral compression. Arthroplasty is a disc-based procedure that allows for only decompression of retrodiscal pathology. Hence, it cannot address retrovertebral compression.

Arthroplasty should not be performed in patients with ankylosing spondylitis, OPLL, or diffuse idiopathic skeletal hyperostosis (DISH). The contraindication for patients with ankylosing spondylitis and DISH is not that the procedure will cause significant problems but that the arthroplasty will result in an eventual fusion. Whether this is really the case or not remains to be determined, but arthroplasty devices have been known to spontaneously fuse, and these patients are already predisposed to autofusion. In patients with OPLL, motion preservation may result in new bone formation behind the device, resulting in cord compression. Therefore, we believe that OPLL is an absolute contraindication to arthroplasty.

Another contraindication for cervical disc arthroplasty includes patients who are likely to become unstable with the procedure. These include patients who have had prior cervical laminectomy.[5,8,10–15] For the same reason, patients with posterior column instability or those with an acute fracture or subluxation should not undergo the procedure. If a patient has a traumatic disc herniation without ligamentous or bony instability, then an arthroplasty procedure is likely to be successful. Whether arthroplasty is contraindicated owing to instability following laminaplasty remains to be determined. It is possible that this might be dependent on the type of laminaplasty that has been performed, because different laminaplasties will produce different degrees of instability.

Patients with an ongoing or chronic cervical spine infection should also not undergo the procedure. Although a stable fusion is often the best treatment for an acute or chronic infection, motion preservation surgery with a foreign body is likely only to aggravate the existing infection.

Facet arthrosis is often mentioned as a contraindication to arthroplasty. However, in our opinion, this should be revised to state that facet arthrosis causing neck pain should be a

**TABLE 21–2. Clinical Contraindications for Cervical Disc Arthroplasty**

1. Prior cervical laminectomy
2. Structural instability of the cervical spine
3. Acute fracture
4. Presence of facet arthropathy causing neck pain
5. History of recent cervical spine infection
6. Ankylosing spondylitis
7. Rheumatoid arthritis with instability
8. Ossification of posterior longitudinal ligament (OPLL)
9. Diffuse idiopathic skeletal hyperostosis (DISH)
10. Osteoporosis and related metabolic bone diseases
11. Myelopathy due to retrovertebral compression
12. Morbid obesity that precludes anterior approach

contraindication to arthroplasty. It is clear that there are some patients who have facet arthrosis and have little to no neck pain. If such a person develops a disc herniation causing radiculopathy or myelopathy, we believe that it is not unreasonable to perform an arthroplasty. The problem lies in the fact that most patients with a herniated disc will also complain of neck pain, and it is unclear how much of this pain is arising out of the disc herniation versus facet arthrosis.

Other contraindications include severe osteoporosis. In such cases, the device may subside or extrude and a fusion is likely to be a safer alternative. Finally, in contrast to patients with isolated mechanical low back pain and no lower extremity symptoms or neurologic signs who are ideal candidates for lumbar disc arthroplasty, patients with axial neck pain as the solitary symptom are not considered ideal candidates for cervical disc arthroplasty. Although they, too, may benefit from cervical disc arthroplasty, there is no evidence for this at the present time. The contraindications for cervical disc arthroplasty are summarized in Table 21–2.

## SURGICAL APPROACH

Different arthroplasty systems use different methods for preparing the disc space. Some require the use of proprietary distraction systems, whereas others require preparation of the end plate before decompressing the disc space. In this chapter, we will address only the generic method of decompressing the disc space that is applicable to nearly all arthroplasty systems.

### Patient Positioning

To perform the procedure, the physician positions the patient in a supine position on a radiolucent table to allow imaging in both the anteroposterior (AP) and lateral planes to localize and identify the affected levels and to provide imaging assistance throughout the case. A closed Jackson frame/table (OSI, Orthopaedic Systems, Inc., Union City, CA) works well for this purpose, although obviously any radiolucent table that can be used in conjunction with fluoroscopy can be used.

Neutral positioning of the neck is critical for end plate preparation and arthroplasty placement. If the neck is hyperextended, then during end plate preparation, an excessive amount of the posterior end plate needs to be removed to produce parallel surfaces (Fig. 21–1). This can result in a malpositioned (kyphotic)

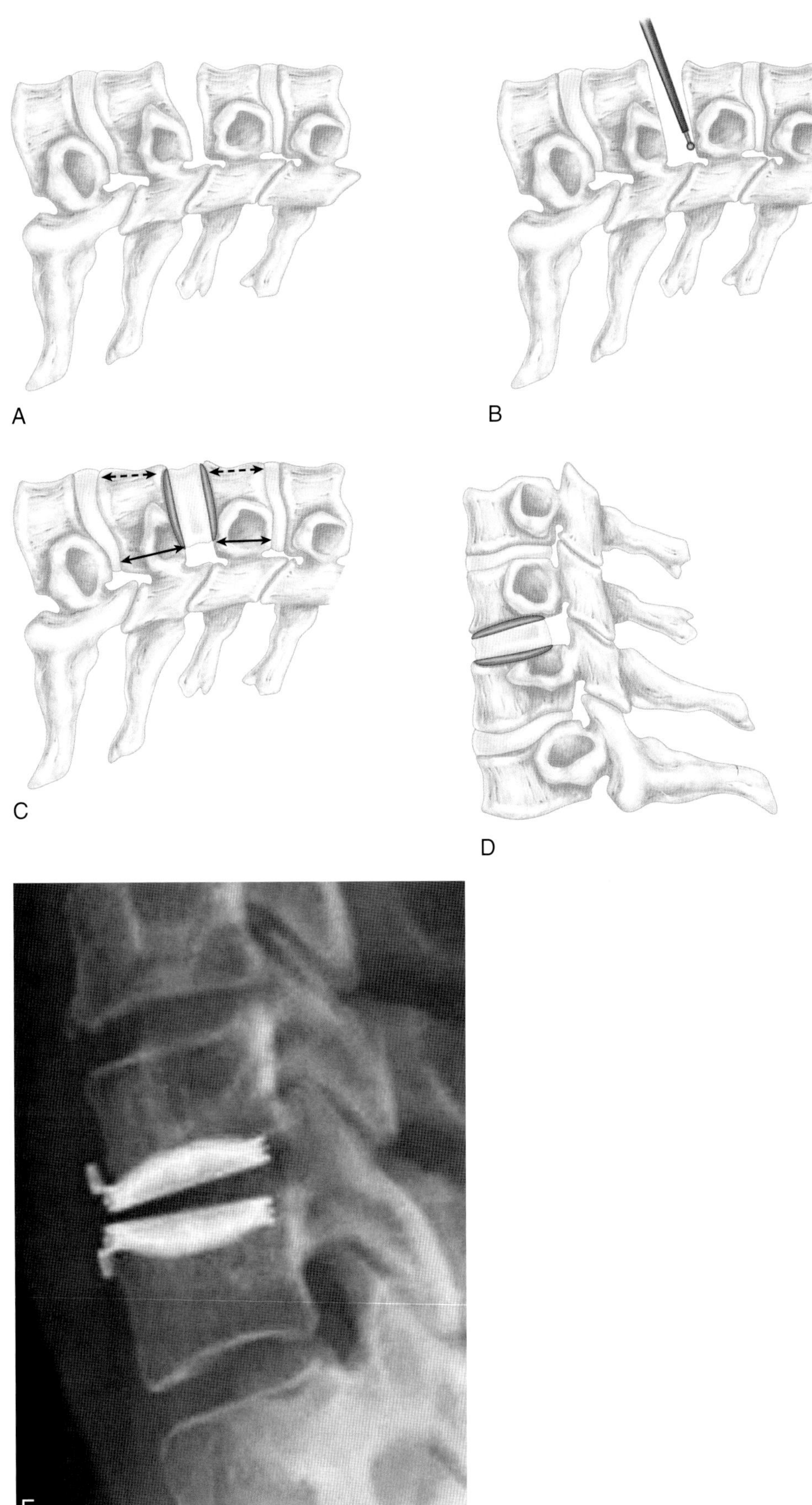


■ **FIGURE 21–1.** **A,** The figure depicts a neck that has been positioned in hyperextension. Note that the posterior aspect of the disc space is narrowed, compared with the anterior. **B,** If the end plates are milled to have parallel surfaces, then more of the posterior end plate needs to be removed. **C,** With the artificial disc in place, the anterior aspect of the vertebral body *(dashed arrows)* is longer than the posterior body *(solid arrows)*. The consequence of this is not evident until the patient stands and the disc is loaded. **D,** Once the patient stands, it is evident that the prosthesis is placed in a kyphotic position. This is true, even if the patient's overall cervical alignment may be in a neutral or lordotic position. **E,** Note that this prosthesis is minimally kyphotic, because more of the posterior than anterior end plate has been removed. Nevertheless, the overall cervical alignment is neutral. If the prosthesis is in kyphosis, then it may limit how much flexion this motion segment can achieve.

prosthesis, especially when placing unconstrained devices such as the Bryan disc (Medtronic Sofamor Danek, Memphis, TN). Conversely, if the neck is placed in a kyphotic position, too much of the anterior end plate is removed and the prosthesis is placed in too lordotic a position.

## Exposure

The anterior cervical spine is exposed using a standard Smith-Robinson approach. A standard or specialized retractor system is used to retract the soft tissues and allow visualization of the spine. After the spine is exposed and the level which is to be addressed is identified, we elevate the longus colli. We use an electrocautery to separate the muscle from its attachment to the bone and disc. We then switch to using a Penfield 2 dissector to elevate the longus farther laterally, because this prevents inadvertent injury to an aberrant vertebral artery. We elevate the muscle past the uncinate and over the foramen transversarium. This allows for thorough decompression of the uncinate region, as well as accurate determination of the midline.

## Disc Space Preparation

We then remove all anterior osteophytes with a burr or a Laksell rongeur, such that the anterior margin of the disc space is smooth with the rest of the body. Any remaining osteophytic lipping at the disc space is likely to cause errors in placement of the disc. We often find that palpating the space is the best way to determine if the osteophyte removal is adequate.

We next incise and remove much of the disc material. Typically, a #15 scalpel is used to cut the width of the anterior annulus, and a pituitary rongeur is used to remove the initial disc fragments. Attention should be paid to the location of the lateral border of the vertebral body so as to avoid damaging the vertebral artery. Once the initial discectomy is performed, we carefully identify the lateral borders of the uncinate. A small curette (typically a 2 mm) is used to identify and denude the uncovertebral joint of cartilaginous material. When performing this maneuver, care should be taken to prevent accidental injury to the vertebral artery with the curette. Scraping the uncinate in a lateral direction can injure the vertebral artery.

Once the uncinates are cleaned out bilaterally, it is easy to determine where the midline of the disc space is (Fig. 21–2). This allows for accurate placement of the distraction pins. Furthermore, it is easier to make sure that the artificial disc is placed in the center of the disc space. Another technique to determine the midline is to mark the midpoint with an electrocautery, before elevating the longus colli.

At this point, some arthroplasty devices require end plate preparation before the decompression, whereas others permit the decompression first. For the latter type, pins are fixed into the vertebral

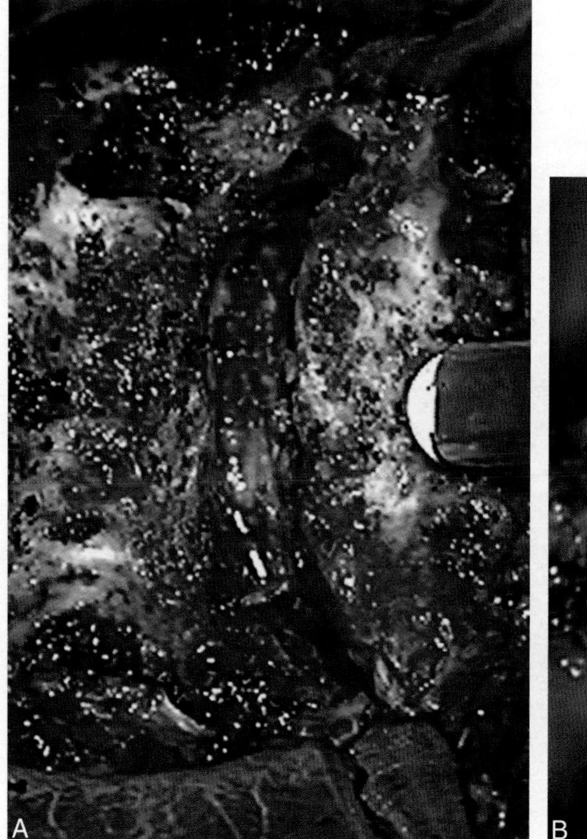


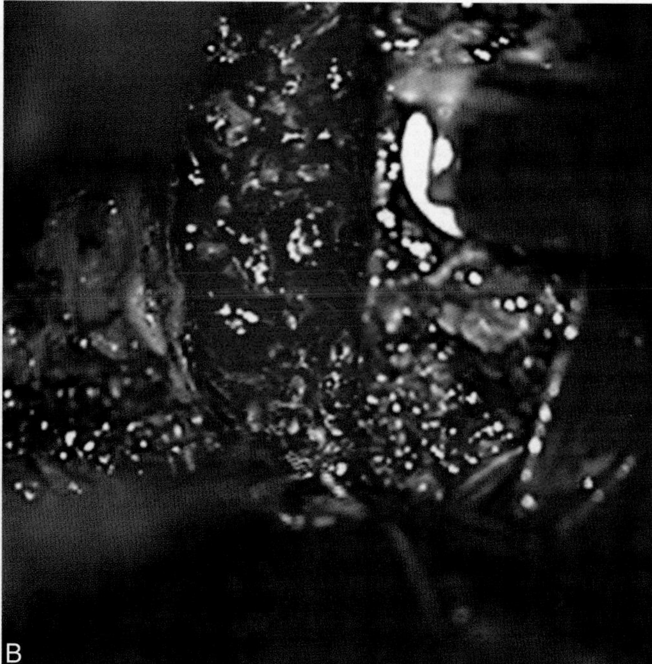


■ **FIGURE 21–2.** **A,** Penfield #2 dissectors are placed lateral to the uncinate bilaterally to demonstrate the lateral extent of the exposure. **B,** A clinical intraoperative photograph demonstrating the use of a small curette to identify and decorticate the uncovertebral joint.

bodies to allow distraction across the disc space. It is important to place the pins in the midline so as to avoid asymmetric distraction across the disc space, which could lead to uneven loads across the total disc arthroplasty device or creation of a scoliotic deformity.

The burr is then used to remove any remaining cartilage and lightly decorticate the inferior end plate of the cephalad vertebra initially anteriorly and then deeper down to the posterior longitudinal ligament, removing any remnants of the posterior annulus during the process. Removing the anterior portion of this end plate also allows for better visualization of the disc space. Care must be taken to minimize the removal of this end plate as different arthroplasty systems have different requirements for end plate removal. A similar maneuver is then used to remove any remaining cartilage and minimally decorticate the superior end plate of the caudal vertebra. The goal is to fashion the end plates so that they are parallel to each other and "squared off" to allow placement of the arthroplasty device, while maintaining the majority of the natural end plates to support the stresses associated with motion across the disc space and to prevent end plate collapse.

## Decompression

All posterior vertebral osteophytes must be removed, preferably with a burr (Fig. 21–3). When performing a fusion, it is not absolutely necessary to remove these osteophytes, because they often remodel with time. However, when performing a cervical disc arthroplasty, osteophytes must be removed, because they may cause continued or worsening symptoms with motion preservation and may even increase in size with time. After these osteophytes are removed, we apply bone wax to the bleeding cancellous bone not only to stop the blood loss, but more important, to help prevent recurrence of the osteophytes. If there is a large disc herniation, we routinely explore behind the posterior longitudinal ligament for any invaginated fragments.

Once the central decompression is completed, attention is turned to decompressing stenotic foraminae (Fig. 21–4). A currette is used to remove any remaining cartilage within the uncovertebral joint and to determine the lateral margin of the uncinate. We then use a matchstick burr to decompress the stenotic foramen. With a high-speed matchstick burr, most of the cutting is done on the side of the burr. Therefore, the tip of the burr can lightly rest on the posterior longitudinal ligament, and even briefly on the dura, without perforating the soft tissues. Great care must be taken to avoid injury to the vertebral artery during the foraminal decompression. To help identify the lateral border of the vertebral body (beyond which is the vertebral artery), a Penfield 4 or 2 can be placed just lateral to the uncinate to help retract the soft tissues and to orient the surgeon (see Fig. 21–2A). Occasionally, a partial or subtotal uncinate resection is necessary to achieve a thorough decompression. We try to avoid performing bilateral complete uncinatectomies, because the uncinates contribute to overall spinal stability and kinematics. This has been carefully documented in at least two biomechanical studies: McAfee et al[17] has recently shown that resection of one uncinate allows preservation of rotational stability with an unconstrained prosthesis, whereas resection of bilateral uncinates may lead to instability. In another study, Snyder et al[18] showed that cervical range of motion increases significantly with progressive resection of the uncovertebral joints, with maximum range of motion in all planes seen in specimens with complete bilateral uncinatectomies.

Although we prefer to use a burr to perform the decompression, a small (1-mm) Kerrison rongeur can be used instead to perform the foraminal decompression. The danger with the Kerrison rongeur is that the tip of the device is placed blindly into the foramen and it can inadvertently injure the root or the vertebral artery. In addition, if the foramen is already severely stenosed, inserting even a 1-mm rongeur can further compress and injure the root. The risk of root injury with a Kerrison rongeur is further increased if the patient's neck has been placed in extension, a position which further narrows the foramen.

To summarize, it is important to realize that when performing cervical disc replacement in patients with spondylotic radiculopathy or myelopathy, a more thorough and wider uncinate and osteophyte resection will need to be performed than in patients in whom a fusion is performed, because continued motion across the segment may lead to recurrence of spondylosis when compared with cervical fusion procedures in which it would be unusual for spurs to recur once a solid fusion is obtained.

Once the central and lateral decompression is completed and the end plates are prepared, in most systems, sizing trials are used to determine the appropriate size of the prosthesis.[13–16] In general, the trial device should fit snugly within the disc space. If the device is too tight, the ligaments that surround the segment may be too taut and cause posterior neck pain and limit motion; on the other hand, if the trial is too loose, the intervertebral height may be too small, leading to foraminal stenosis and poor function of the device. Once the proper size is determined, the final device matching the size of the trial is inserted into the interspace, usually under fluoroscopic guidance. Final placement of the device is then confirmed in both the AP and lateral planes. The wound is then irrigated and closed in the usual fashion. Postoperative immobilization is not necessary. A clinical example of cervical disc arthroplasty is shown in Figure 21–5.

## CONCLUSIONS

In summary, cervical disc arthroplasty is a novel and exciting technology, which holds a lot of promise and provides an alternative to fusion. Although many questions remain, the most important potential advantages include motion preservation and prevention or postponement of adjacent segment degeneration. Despite these potential advantages, it is important to realize that careful surgical technique will be necessary to achieve both short- and long-term clinical success. More specifically, careful end plate preparation and a thorough decompression (both central and foraminal) need to be performed in order to maximize the chance of success.

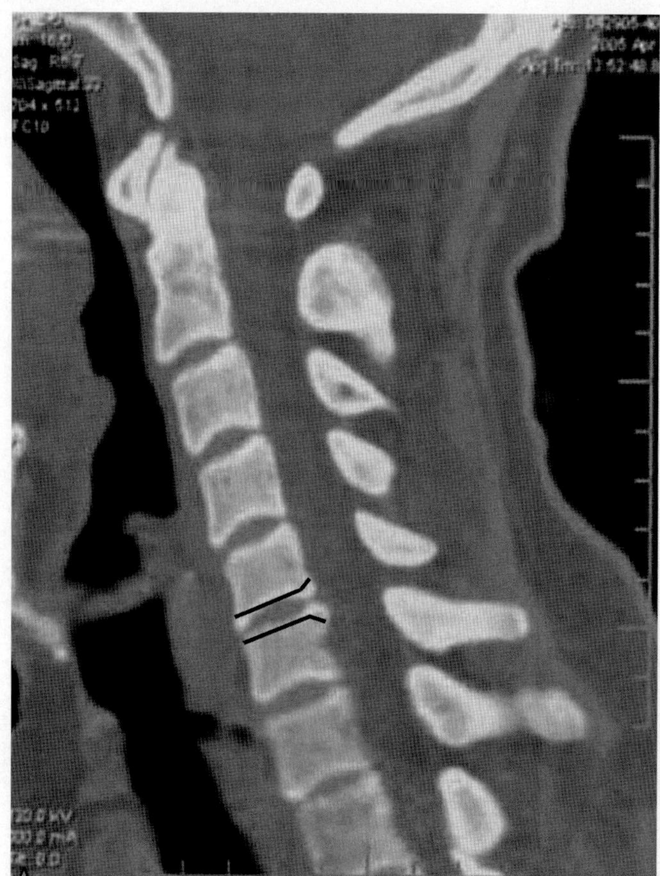

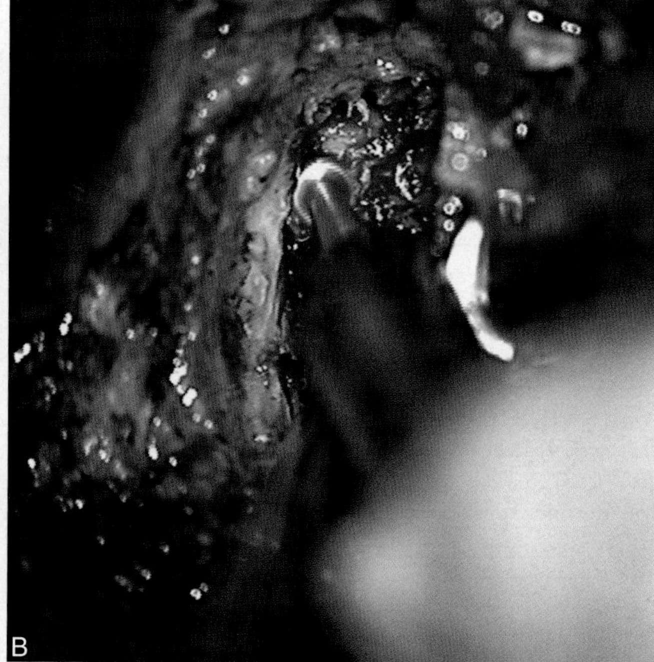

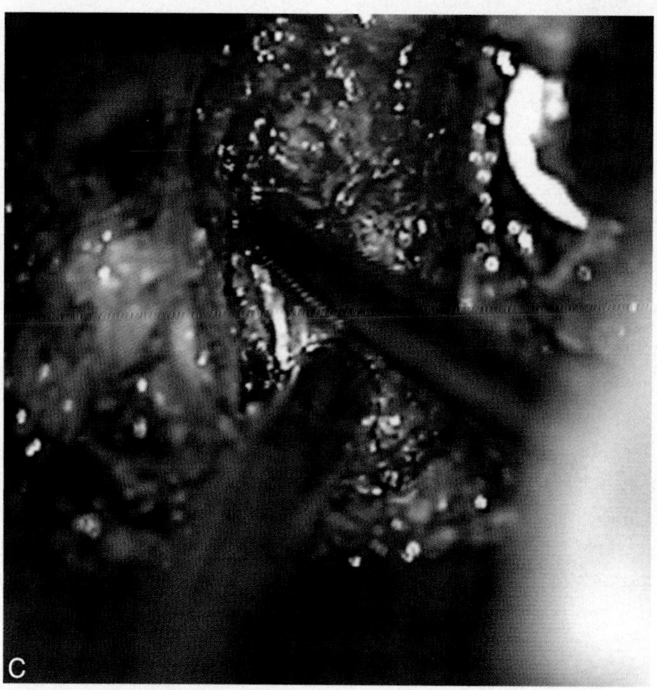

■ **FIGURE 21–3.** **A,** A sagittal computed tomography reconstruction demonstrating the amount of end plate and posterior vertebral osteophyte resection necessary to achieve a thorough central decompression. **B,** A clinical intraoperative photograph demonstrating the use of a matchstick carbide burr to decorticate the end plates and posterior vertebral body osteophytes. **C,** A clinical intraoperative photograph demonstrating a thorough central decompression. Note that following the decompression, the posterior vertebral body osteophytes have been resected and an angled curette can be safely positioned behind the vertebral body.

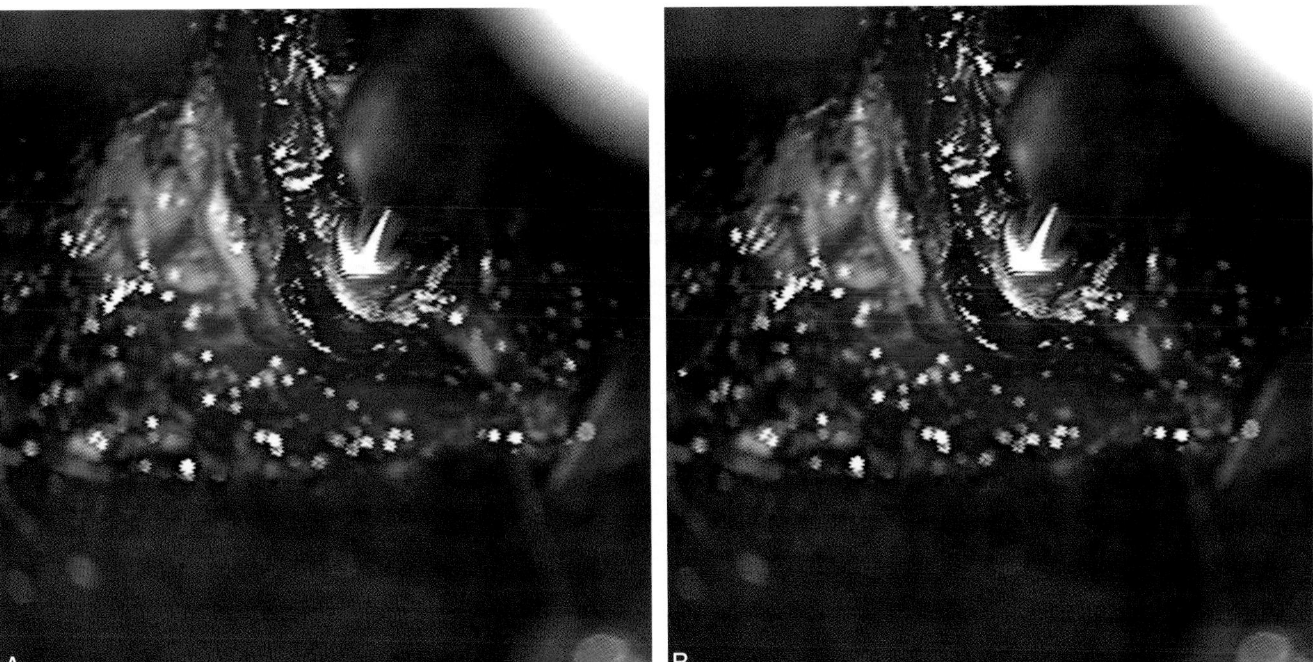

■ **FIGURE 21–4.** **A,** A clinical intraoperative photograph showing the use of a bur to thin out the uncinate and decompress the foramen. **B,** A clinical intraoperative photograph demonstrating a partial uncinate resection and foraminal decompression. Note the curette showing the location of the foramen.

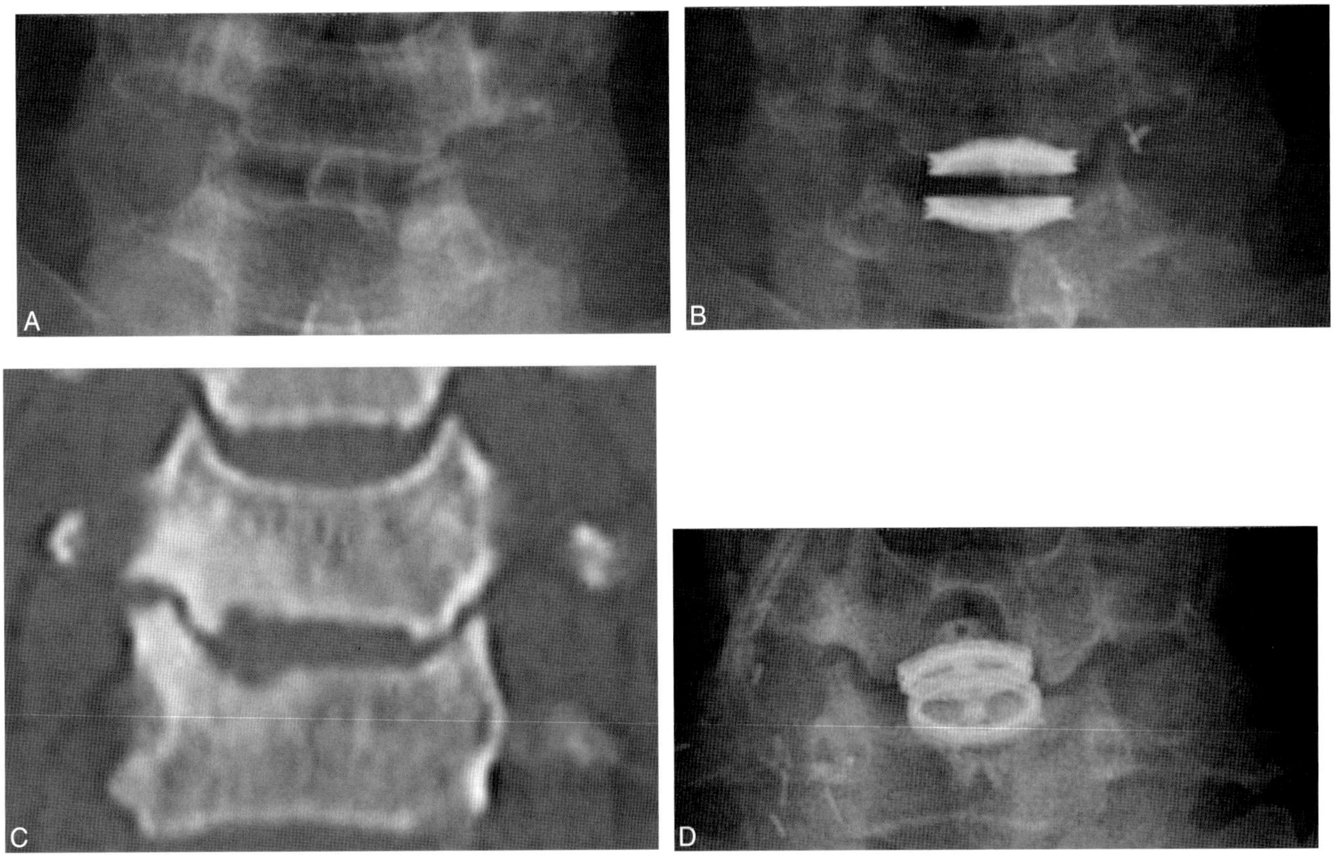

■ **FIGURE 21–5.** **A,** An anteroposterior (AP) plain radiograph of a 43-year-old man with C6-C7 spondylosis and radicular symptoms. Note the presence of large uncovertebral joint spurs at C6-C7. **B,** A postoperative AP plain radiograph showing the cervical disc arthroplasty at C6-C7. Note that the uncovertebral spurs present on the preoperative radiographs have been resected. **C** and **D,** A preoperative CT and postoperative AP plain radiograph demonstrating uncinate decompression and cervical disc arthroplasty at C6-C7. Note that the C7 uncinate has been squared off bilaterally to thin it down. Then a posterior foraminotomy was completed bilaterally, without completely resecting the uncinate. The disc appears overlapped, because the radiograph is not a true AP of the prosthesis. The posterior vertebral body osteophytes have been resected.

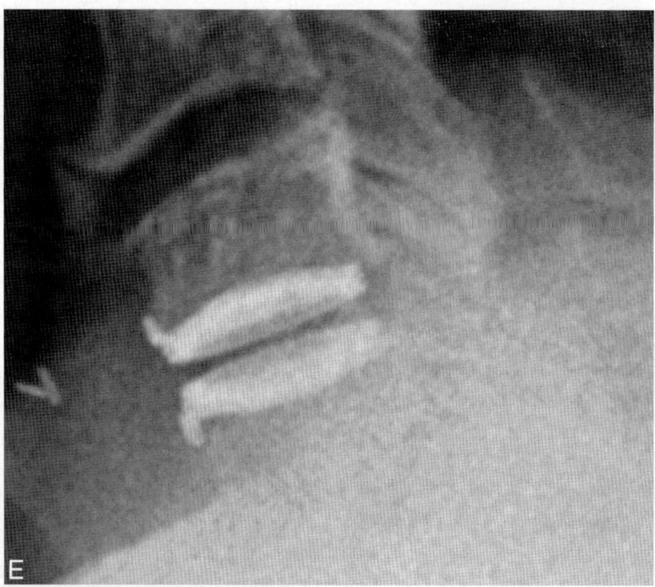


■ **FIGURE 21–5. Cont'd.** **E,** The lateral radiograph demonstrates the resection of posterior osteophytes.

## REFERENCES


1. Emery SE, Bolesta MJ, Banks MA, et al: Robinson anterior cervical fusion: comparison of the standard and modified techniques. Spine 19:660–663, 1994.
2. Bohlman HH, Emery SE, Goodfellow DB, et al: Robinson anterior cervical discectomy and arthrodesis for cervical radiculopathy. Long-term follow-up of one hundred and twenty-two patients. J Bone Joint Surg Am 75:1298–1307, 1993.
3. Brodke DS, Zdeblick TA: Modified Smith-Robinson procedure for anterior cervical discectomy and fusion. Spine 17:S427–S430, 1992.
4. Williams JL, Allen MB, Harnkess JW: Late results of cervical discectomy and interbody fusion: some factors influencing the results. J Bone Joint Surg Am 50:277–286, 1968.
5. Acosta FL, Ames CP: Cervical disc arthroplasty: general introduction. Neurosurg Clin N Am 16:603–607, 2005.
6. Hilibrand AS, Carlson GD, Palumbo MA, et al: Radiculopathy and myelopathy at segments adjacent to the site of a pervious anterior cervical arthrodesis. J Bone Joint Surg Am 81:519–528, 1999.
7. Hilibrand AS, Yoo JU, Carlson GD, et al: The success of anterior cervical arthrodesis adjacent to a previous fusion. Spine 22:1574–1579, 1997.
8. McAfee PC: The indications for lumbar and cervical disc replacement. Spine J 4:177S–181S, 2004.
9. Albert TJ, Eichenbaum MD: Cervical disc replacement: goals of cervical disc replacement. Spine J 4:292S–293S, 2004.
10. Durbhakula MM, Ghiselli G: Cervical total disc replacement, part I: rationale, biomechanics, and implant types. Orthop Clin N Am 36:349–354, 2005.
11. Bertagnoli R, Duggal N, Pickett GE, et al: Cervical total disc replacement, part II: clinical results. Orthop Clin N Am 36:355–362, 2005.
12. Phillips FM, Garfin SR: Cervical disc replacement. Spine 30: S27–S33, 2005.
13. Traynelis VC: The Prestige cervical disc. Neurosurg Clin N Am 16:621–628, 2005.
14. Papadopoulos S: The Bryan cervical disc system. Neurosurg Clin N Am 16:629–636, 2005.
15. Chi JH, Ames CP, Tay B: General considerations for cervical arthroplasty with technique for Prodisc-C. Neurosurg Clin N Am 16:609–619, 2005.
16. Pimenta L, McAfee PC, Cappuccino A, et al: Clinical experience with the new artificial cervical PCM (Cervitech) disc. Spine J 4:315S–321S, 2004.
17. McAfee PC, Cunningham BW, Hayes V, et al: Biomechanical analysis of rotational motion after disc arthroplasty: implications for patients with adult deformities. Spine 31:S152–S160, 2006.
18. Snyder J, Ghanayem A, Rinella A, et al: Effect of partial versus total uncovertebral joint excision in cervical total disc replacement. Presented at the 34th Annual Meeting of the Cervical Spine Research Society, Palm Beach, Florida, November 30–December 2, 2006.

CHAPTER 22

# The Bryan Artificial Disc

**Rick Sasso** and **Larry Martin, Jr.**

## KEY POINTS

- In a prospective, randomized trial, the Bryan disc group demonstrated statistically significant better functional outcomes compared with the cervical fusion cohort.
- At 2 years' follow-up, there are statistically significant improvements in the neck disability index, the neck pain and arm pain visual analog pain scores (VASs), and the SF-36 physical component score.
- In a prospective trial, there were no intraoperative complications, vascular or neurologic complications, spontaneous fusions, device failures, or explantations in the Bryan cohort.
- More motion was retained in the disc replacement group than the plated group at the index level ($P < 0.006$ at 3, 6, 12, and 24 months); the disc replacement group retained an average of 7.9 degrees at 24 months. In contrast, the average range of motion in the fusion group was 0.6 degrees at 24 months.

## INTRODUCTION

The cervical spine is a linkage of specialized joints and, like other joints, may be the source of significant pain and functional incapacity with age, trauma, and subsequent degeneration. However unlike other major joints, the traditional perception is that motion in the cervical spine is not a necessity and has been routinely sacrificed for pain relief and functional recovery. For more than 50 years, anterior cervical discectomy and fusion (ACDF) has been the treatment of choice for cervical disc disease. Numerous studies have demonstrated the kinematic and biomechanical limitations inherent in this procedure in addition to the potential to accelerate adjacent segment degeneration. Thus, intervertebral disc replacement has been designed to remedy these shortcomings. Duggal et al[1] confirmed preservation of motion in Bryan disc replacement–treated spinal segments with a mean range of motion of 7.8 degrees at 24 months. Sasso[2] described normal flexion-extension motion (6.7 degrees) in comparison to ACDF of 0.6 degrees at 24 months postoperatively. In addition, abnormal motion at the adjacent segment of a fusion was demonstrated. An increase in anterior or posterior translation at the cephalad adjacent level in patients with arthrodesis occurred while the Bryan arthroplasty retained normal translation for the same amount of flexion/extension at the adjacent level.

## INDICATIONS/CONTRAINDICATIONS

Indications for cervical arthroplasty include patients with radiculopathy or myleopathy at a single level owing to a focal herniated nucleus pulposus or uncovertebral osteophyte from C3 to C7 (Fig. 22–1). The intent is to use an arthroplasty as an alternative to arthrodesis after neural decompression. Contraindications include severe myelopathy secondary to retrovertebral osteophytes, multilevel disease, chronic infection, osteopenia, and posterior facet arthropathy.

## DESCRIPTION OF THE DEVICE

The Bryan disc (Medtronic Sofamor Danek, Memphis, TN) is a one-piece, biarticulating, metal on polymer, semiconstrained device with a variable instantaneous axis of rotation[3,4] (Fig. 22–2). The component is composed of two titanium alloy shells that have a porus coating at the bone-implant interface, which promotes ingrowth of bone providing long-term stability (Fig. 22–3). Jensen reported adequate and reproducible bone ingrowth into the Bryan Cervical Disc end plates.[5] Each shell has an anterior flange to articulate with the inserting device and also prevent posterior migration. The polyurethane nucleus between the shells is surrounded by a sheath creating a pseudocapsule over time. Saline is used as a lubricant inside the sheath. This also provides a hydraulic dampening effect under axial loads that allows shock-absorbing characteristics to the Bryan artificial disc (Fig. 22–4).

## BACKGROUND OF SCIENTIFIC TESTING AND CLINICAL OUTCOMES

Goffin et al[6] published results from a multicenter European study and found success rates in single-level Bryan Cervical Disc replacements at 6 months, 12 months, and 24 months of 90%, 86%, and 90%, respectively. In a bilevel study, success rates at 6 months and 1 year were 82% and 96%, respectively. At 1 year, flexion-extension range of motion per level averaged 7.9 degrees in the single-level arm and 7.4 degrees in the bilevel arm (Fig. 22–5). Complications included three hematomas, three subsequent decompressions, and one repair of pharyngeal and esophageal injury. One patient had migration of the

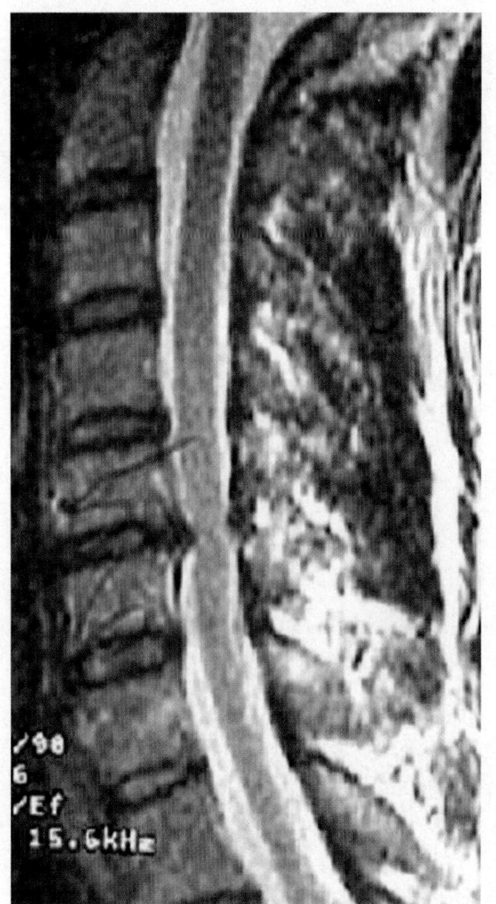

■ **FIGURE 22–1.** Preoperative magnetic resonance imaging scan with a focal disc herniation at C5–C6 causing a C6 radiculopathy.

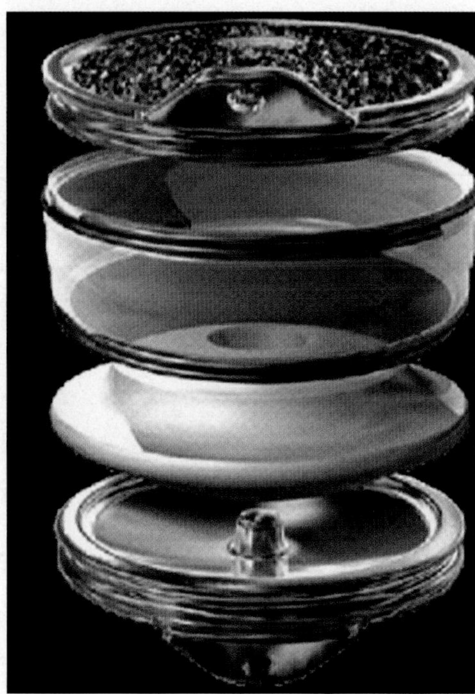

■ **FIGURE 22–2.** The Bryan Cervical Disc Replacement: titanium shells with an intervening polyurethane nucleus wrapped by a polyurethane sheath.

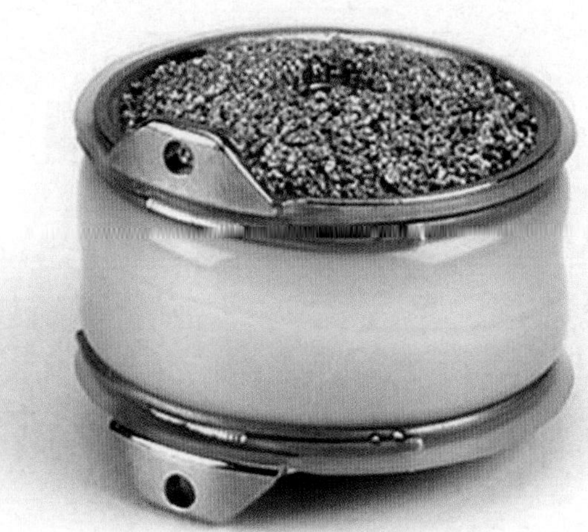

■ **FIGURE 22–3.** The titanium porous end plates of the Bryan cervical disc arthroplasty.

implant, but it was not greater than the 3.5-mm radiographic threshold. Sekhon[7] performed arthroplasty on 22 patients with myelopathy and 24 controls. Their study found both groups had significant arm and neck pain relief. The SF-36 and neck disability index scores reflected improvement, with numerically better results in the Bryan disc group but the results not statistically significant. The only complications were one hematoma and one required a fusion.

Anderson et al[8] reported on 73 patients with greater than 2-year follow-up. Forty-five patients rated excellent, seven rated good, 13 rated fair, and eight rated poor. SF-36 functional data demonstrated significant improvement from preoperative to 3-month postoperative time points and remained stable at 2 years after surgery. They reported no evidence of subsidence, and 89% of all patients had at least two degrees of motion. There was one early anterior device migration associated with a partially milled cavity.

Sasso et al[9] published data on 99 patients from a multicenter randomized trial. At 2-year follow-up, neck disability index for the Bryan group was statistically better than that for the controls

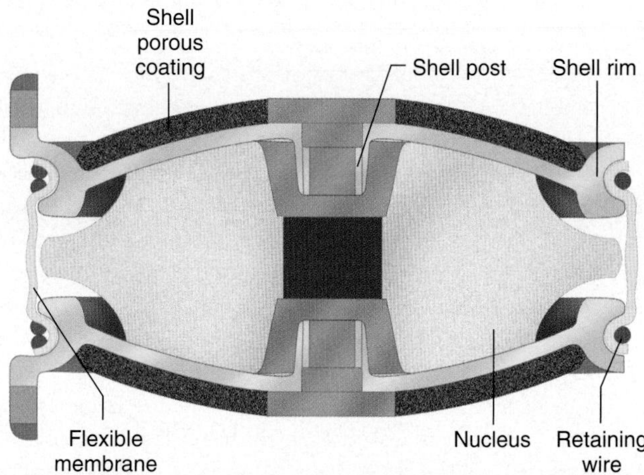


■ **FIGURE 22–4.** Cross-section of the Bryan artificial disc with the titanium shells surrounding a polyurethane nucleus in a saline fluid bath.

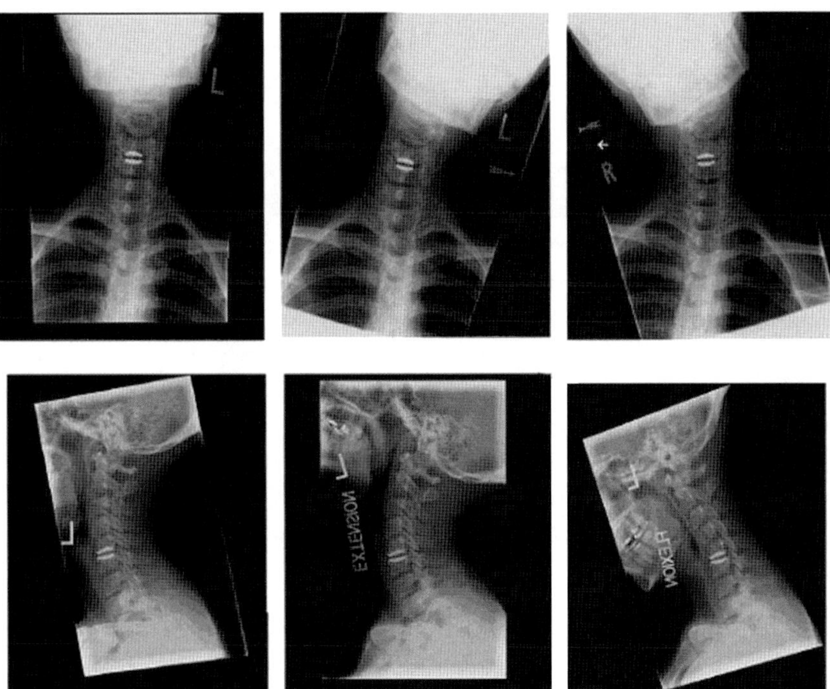

■ **FIGURE 22–5.** Anteroposterior side-bending and lateral flexion-extension radiographs after Bryan artificial cervical disc replacement.

(Fig. 22–6). Arm pain VAS score was statistically better in the Bryan group compared with that of the the control group. Neck pain VAS in the Bryan group was also statistically better than in the control group (Fig. 22–7). Flexion-extension motion in the Bryan disc group at 24 months was 6.7 degrees compared with 0.6 degrees in the control group.

## OPERATIVE TECHNIQUE

Preoperative clinical and radiographic assessment is essential as in all operative procedures. Preoperative computed tomography (CT) scan allows determination of the exact dimensions of the disc space and use of a template to identify the appropriate size of the Bryan disc. Patient positioning is in a neutral orientation. Hyperextension should be avoided. This technique is a variation to the standard anterior fusion in which the neck is often intraoperatively in hyperextension by inserting a roll under the shoulders. Cervical artificial discs should be inserted in a neutral standing position. This is best facilitated by putting the rolled towel under the neck rather than the shoulders and raising the head by placing it on a folded towel. The position should approximate standing with the back against a wall and the head also against the same wall.

The cervical spine is accessed via a standard Smith-Robinson approach. Decompression is then performed at the affected level.

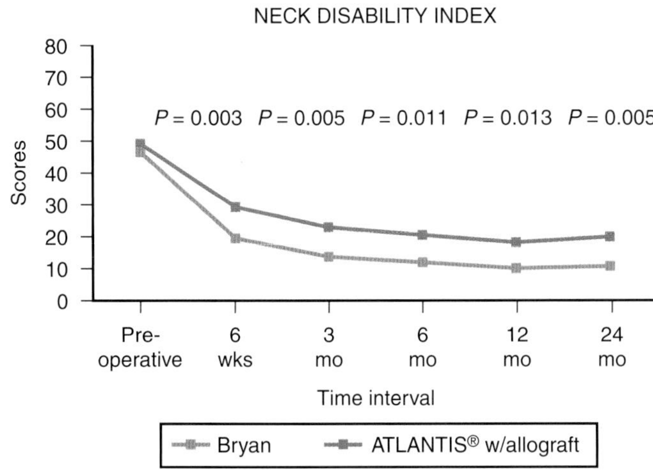


■ **FIGURE 22–6.** Neck Disability Index with statistically significant improvement of the Bryan disc replacement over the control fusion group at all time points postoperatively.

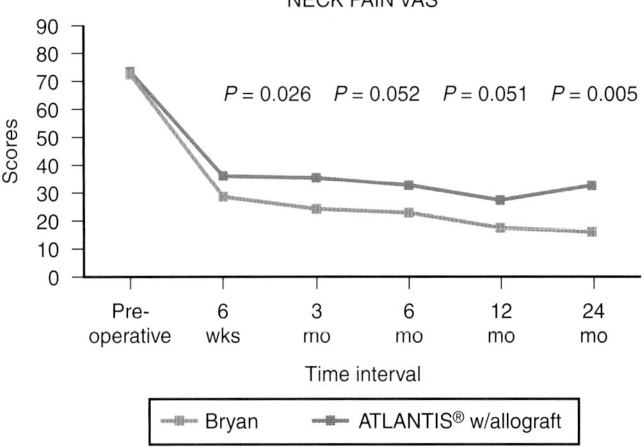


■ **FIGURE 22–7.** Neck Pain Visual Analog Scale with statistically significant improvement of the Bryan disc replacement over the control fusion group at 12 and 24 months postoperatively.

A milling technique using a jig creates concave surfaces on each vertebral end plate to match the convex porous-coated titanium end plates of the Bryan disc. The correct size of Bryan disc is determined using a combination of intraoperative techniques and preoperative radiographic studies. The center of the disc space is determined intraoperatively using a jig, which defines the uncovertebral joints and finds the center between these structures. A gravitational referencing system determines the sagittal angle of the disc space. With knowledge of the center of the disc space, a milling fixture is anchored to the vertebral bodies (Fig. 22–8). This fixture controls the cutting tools that mill the end plates to the exact geometry of the device end plates, providing immediate stability. Lateral fluoroscopy assists in determining the diameter of the implant. Final decompression of the foramen and spinal canal can be performed after preparation of the end plates. When motion-sparing devices are implemented, it is extremely important to completely decompress the neural structures, including the contralateral asymptomatic foramen. This is a significant variation to the standard fusion procedure in which the neural structures are protected by the lack of motion. The uncovertebral joints should not be sacrificed bilaterally in artificial disc replacement; however, aggressive decompression unilaterally is acceptable.

The Bryan disc is filled with sterile saline (Fig. 22–9) and positioned on an inserter that attaches to the flanges on the anterior titanium shells (Fig. 22–10). An intervertebral distracter allows atraumatic insertion of the prepared Bryan disc (Fig. 22–11). Appropriate placement is confirmed with anteroposterior (AP) and lateral fluoroscopy before skin closure (Fig. 22–12).

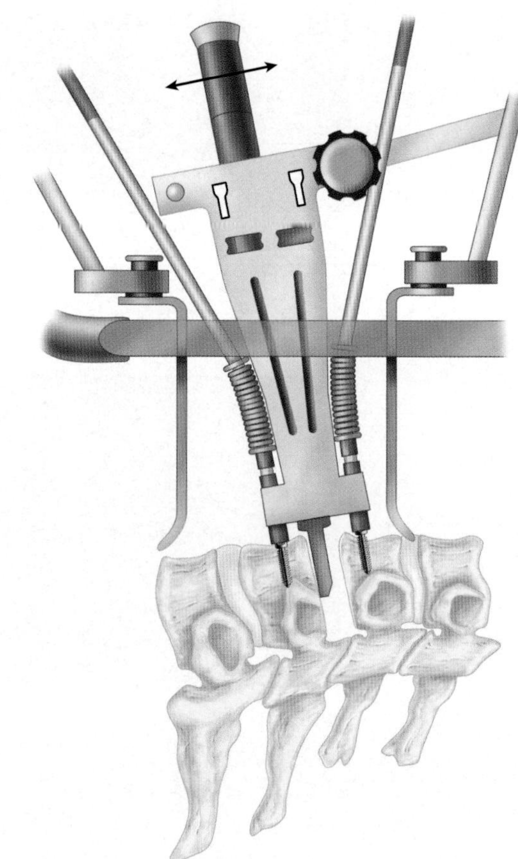

■ **FIGURE 22–8.** Milling jig preparing the end plates for the Bryan disc.

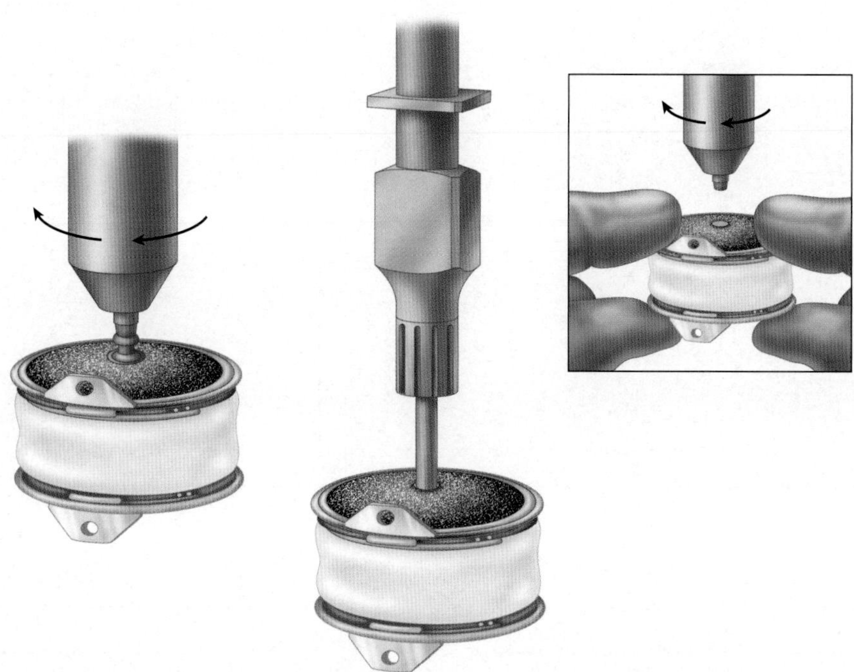

■ **FIGURE 22–9.** Before implanting the Bryan disc, it is filled with saline and set screws seal the infusion port.

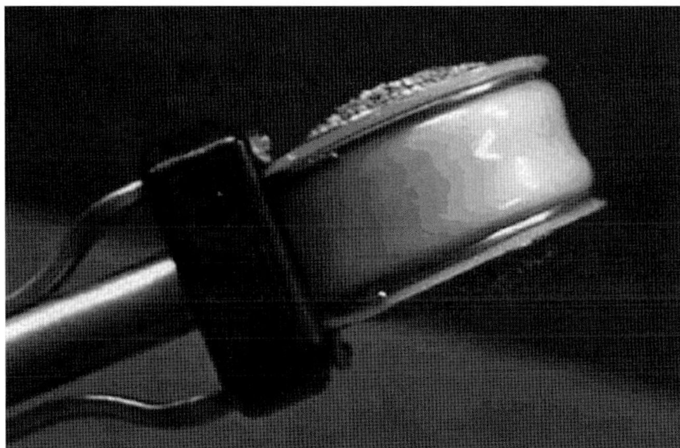

■ **FIGURE 22–10.** Bryan disc attached to inserter.

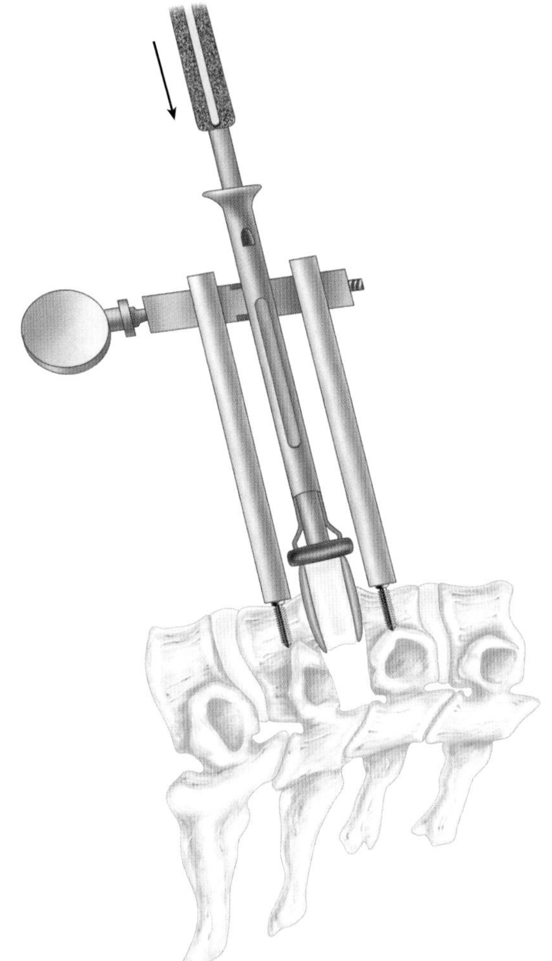

■ **FIGURE 22–11.** The Bryan disc placed into the prepared interspace.

## POSTOPERATIVE CARE

After implantation of the Bryan artificial disc, no cervical collar is needed. Patients are routinely discharged the same day of surgery. Patients are allowed to mobilize their neck immediately and return to work when comfortable. Traynelis et al[10] found in a prospective, randomized trial that patients undergoing Bryan cervical disc replacements returned to work statistically earlier than those having a fusion after cervical decompression.

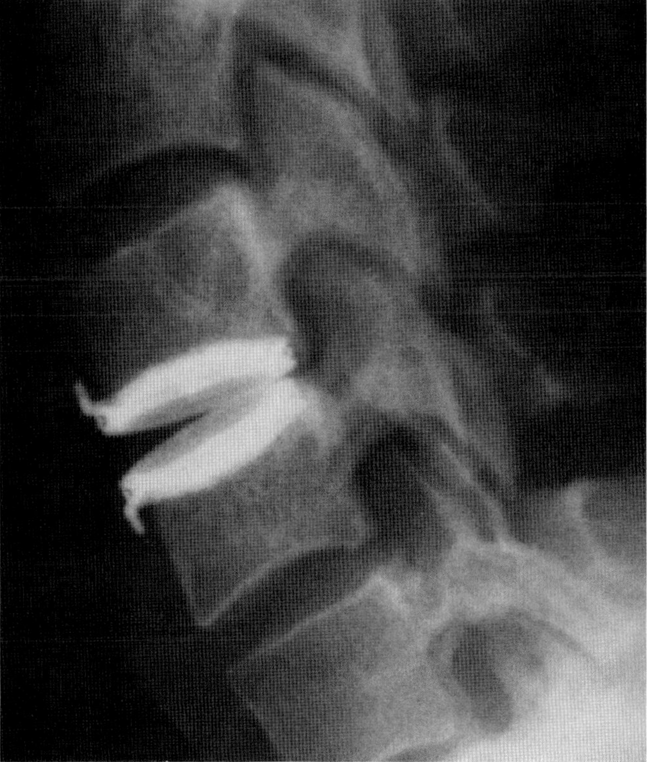

■ **FIGURE 22–12.** Postoperative lateral radiograph after Bryan cervical disc replacement.

## CONCLUSIONS/DISCUSSION

Disc arthroplasty was developed to maintain motion to hypothetically reduce the risk of future adjacent segment degeneration. Other advantages are thought to be earlier return to activity and reduced surgical morbidity. Six devices are undergoing investigation by the U.S. Food and Drug Administration. The differences in materials, design, and implantation techniques on their performance are unknown. Preclinical testing for durability, stability, bony ingrowth, and inflammatory reactions show that current designs are meeting established criteria for success.

Early follow-up of human studies are encouraging, demonstrating at least as good outcomes with the advantage of motion preservation. Complications are few and manageable, and have not resulted in catastrophic neural injury. The rate of revision has been low. Longer follow-up is needed to determine if these devices can function over time and whether there will be an implant-to-host or host-to-implant reaction.

Although far from being an accepted standard, the concept of artificial disc replacement is gradually becoming a reality. The possibility of being able to minimize adjacent segment degeneration is exciting; however, much more intermediate and long-term outcome-based data are going to be necessary to prove that this technology supersedes the current gold standard of anterior fusion. Biomechanical studies demonstrate that disc replacement creates less adjacent level strain than fusion. With time, it is hoped that long-term studies will prove that this correlates to a lower incidence of adjacent level degeneration.

Wear studies suggest that there may be less potential for aseptic loosening than in large joint arthroplasty, although the reality of this will be borne out only with more follow-up time. Although early reports of success in the United States with the total disc replacement suggest that the intended effects are being achieved, the final results of arthroplasty with these devices and of cervical arthroplasty are pending the outcomes of long-term studies.

Prospective, randomized studies demonstrate the favorable outcomes of cervical disc arthroplasty using the Bryan disc in comparison to the gold standard (ACDF) at 24 months for the treatment of patients with cervical myelopathy and radiculopathy. At 2 years' follow-up, the Bryan artificial disc replacement demonstrated statistically significant improvements in the neck disability index, the neck pain and arm pain VASs, and the SF-36 physical component score compared with the control fusion population. The future looks bright for cervical arthroplasty, but further long-term studies are necessary.

## REFERENCES


1. Duggal N, Pickett E, Mitsis DK, et al: Early clinical and biomechanical results following cervical arthroplasty. Neurosurg Focus 17:E9, 2004.
2. Sasso RC, Best NM: Cervical kinematics after fusion and Bryan disc arthroplasty. J Spinal Disord Tech 2007 (in press).
3. Anderson PA, Sasso RC, Rouleau JP, et al: The Bryan Disc: Wear properties and early clinical results. Spine J 4:303S–309S, 2004.
4. Goffin J, Casey A, Kehr P, et al: Preliminary clinical experience with the Bryan Cervical Disc Prosthesis. Neurosurgery 51:840–845; discussion 845–847, 2002.
5. Jensen WK, Anderson PA, Rouleau JP: Bone ingrowth into the Bryan Cervical Disc. Spine 30:2497–2502, 2005.
6. Goffin J, Casey A, Kehr P, et al: Preliminary clinical experience with the Bryan Cervical Disc Prosthesis. Neurosurgery 51:840–845; discussion 845–847, 2002.
7. Sekhon LH: Cervical arthroplasty in the management of spondylotic myelopathy: 18 month results. Neurosurg Focus 17:E8, 2004.
8. Anderson PA, Sasso RC, Rouleau JP, et al: The Bryan Disc: wear properties and early clinical results. Spine J 4:303S–309S, 2004.
9. Sasso RC, Hacker R, Heller JG: Artificial disc versus fusion for the treatment of cervical radiculopathy: A prospective, randomized study. J Spinal Disord Tech 2007 (in press).
10. Traynelis V, Sasso RC, Anderson P: Return to Work Analysis of patients treated with an Artificial Cervical Disc or an Arthrodesis. North American Spine Society 21st annual meeting, September 26–30, 2006, Seattle, Washington.

CHAPTER 23

# The Prestige Cervical Disc

**Vincent C. Traynelis**

**KEY POINTS**

- The Prestige ST and LP are metal-on-metal total cervical disc replacements that provide anterior column support and replicate normal physiologic segmental motion.
- Immediate fixation is achieved with screws for the Prestige ST device and with rails for the Prestige LP device.
- A complete bilateral decompression must be achieved in all patients, and a precise fit between the vertebral bodies and the implants should be achieved.
- Patients receiving the Prestige ST have significantly improved early neck disability index scores and return to work sooner than patients treated with an arthrodesis.
- Cervical arthroplasty is contraindicated in patients with advanced spondylosis, instability, and significant deformity.

## INTRODUCTION

The Prestige device was developed by Mr. Brian Cummins, who attempted to address the shortcomings of cervical arthrodesis about 20 years ago by developing an artificial cervical disc in collaboration with the Department of Medical Engineering at Frenchay Hospital, Bristol, U.K. in 1989.[1] His pioneering efforts to create a metal-on-metal artificial cervical disc laid the foundation for the development of the Prestige ST and LP Cervical Disc Replacements (Medtronic Sofamor Danek, Memphis, TN).[2,3]

## INDICATIONS/CONTRAINDICATIONS

Arthroplasty is an option in patients with normal cervical spinal alignment and mobility and radiculopathy due to root compression resulting from a disc herniation or anterior osteophyte or myelopathy secondary to spinal cord compression from a soft disc herniation.[4] At present, there is controversy concerning whether arthroplasty is appropriate in patients with myelopathy due to hard disc herniations or central anterior osteophytes.

Arthroplasty is contraindicated in the setting of instability and significant segmental or global deformity. Patients without preexisting motion cannot be expected to regain mobility by implanting a total prosthetic disc replacement. A recent history of infection or osteomyelitis would preclude the use of a prosthetic disc device. Other potential contraindications include rheumatoid arthritis, renal failure, osteoporosis, cancer, and preoperative corticosteroid medication.

## DESCRIPTION OF THE DEVICE

The Prestige ST is constructed of stainless steel and consists of two articulating components attached to the cervical vertebrae with locking screws (Fig. 23–1).[5,6] The ball-and-trough design of the Prestige ST allows relatively unconstrained motion, which is comparable to that of a normal cervical spinal segment, including anteroposterior (AP) translation, which is physiologically coupled with sagittal plane rotation. The 2.5-mm anterior face is comparable to the thickness of the majority of anterior cervical plates. The surfaces that contact the vertebral end plates are grit-blasted to promote osteointegration.

The Prestige LP (Fig. 23–2) has a ball-and-trough articulation that is identical to that of the Prestige ST.[6] The Prestige LP is manufactured from a unique titanium ceramic composite material which is highly durable and image-friendly on computed tomography and magnetic resonance imaging scans. Initial fixation is achieved by means of a series of four rails, two on each component, which engage the vertebral bodies. A porous titanium plasma spray coating on the end plate contacting surfaces facilitates bone ingrowth and long-term fixation.

Both the Prestige ST and LP are available in a number of sizes, and specialized instrumentation for implantation has been developed for each.

## BACKGROUND OF SCIENTIFIC TESTING/CLINICAL OUTCOMES

The Prestige ST and LP each have been extensively tested for safety and durability. The materials from which they are constructed are nontoxic and have excellent wear characteristics, and the wear debris generated does not elicit an inflammatory response. Cadaveric and clinical studies have demonstrated that the Prestige articulation maintains normal physiologic motion of the cervical spine.[7,8] Prospectively collected data indicate that adjacent segment

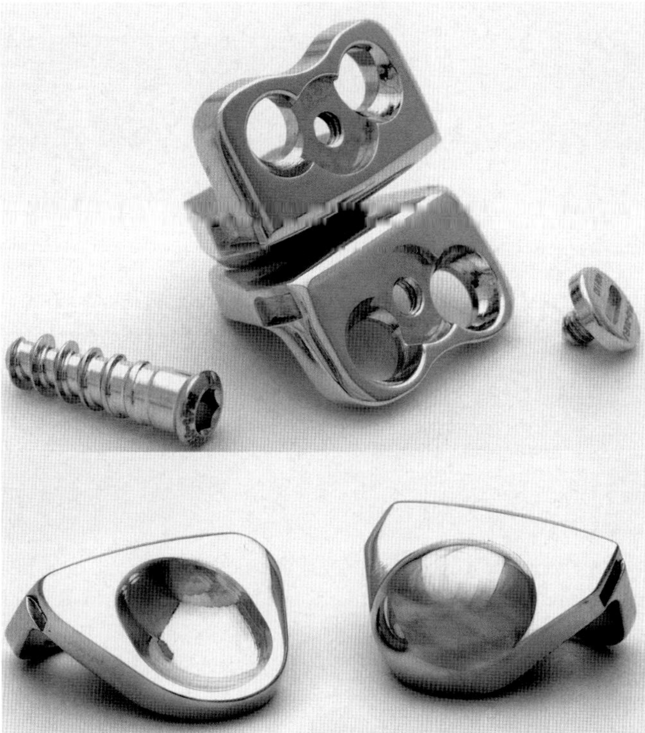

■ **FIGURE 23–1.** Prestige ST.

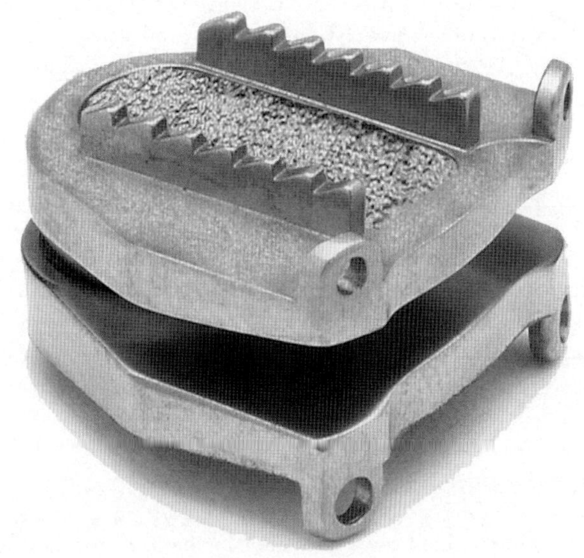

■ **FIGURE 23–2.** Prestige LP.

degeneration is less in patients treated with an arthroplasty as compared with an arthrodesis.[9] Patients treated with the Prestige ST have lower early neck disability index scores and return to work significantly earlier than patients treated with an arthrodesis.[10]

## CLINICAL PRESENTATION AND EVALUATION

Surgical candidates include those with significant neurologic symptoms owing to either nerve root or spinal cord compression secondary to subaxial cervical spondylosis. These patients should have failed nonoperative treatments such as activity modification, physical therapy, and medication. The evaluation should include imaging studies to visualize neural compression and dynamic lateral cervical radiographs.

## OPERATIVE TECHNIQUES

Cervical arthroplasty is performed under general anesthesia. The patient is positioned supine on the operating table, and the cervical spinal level to be addressed must be in the neutral position. It is preferable to perform these procedures with fluoroscopic guidance to ensure proper sizing and placement of the implant. The anterior cervical spine is exposed through a standard approach, and the disc is removed and all osteophytes resected. Particular attention should be directed toward removing osteophytes arising from the uncinate processes. The neural foraminal decompression should be bilateral and complete.

Anterior osteophytes are resected, and the vertebral end plates are denuded of cartilage and thinned until there are two parallel surfaces of subchondral bone. This is usually accomplished with a high-speed bur. A rasp may be used to help with this step. Care should be taken to avoid excessive thinning or violation of the end plates. Prestige sizing trials are placed into the interspace to determine the appropriate size of the prosthesis. Ideally, the trial device should fit snugly and cover the maximal amount of end plate surface that is safely possible. If it is too tight, the ligaments which surround the segment may become overly taut, thereby restricting motion. The trial device should be inserted in the proper orientation and in the midline. If it does not fit precisely, more end plate preparation is necessary.

## PRESTIGE ST

A final check of the interspace and anterior vertebral surfaces is performed by sweeping the anterior face profile trial medially and laterally. Any bony irregularities detected during this maneuver should be addressed.

A Prestige ST disc matching the interspace trial device is attached to the implant holder and inserted into the interspace. Holes are drilled and tapped using the guide in the implant holder and the bone screws placed. The implant holder is then detached from the Prestige ST implant. Two locking cap screws are engaged and tightened.

## PRESTIGE LP

The initial fixation of the Prestige LP is achieved through a series of four rails: two on each component, which engage the vertebral bodies. A rail cutting guide is inserted into the interspace, and two small holes are drilled into each vertebral body. A rail punch is used to connect these holes with the interspace. The Prestige LP is then loaded into the implant holder and gently tamped into place.

## POSTOPERATIVE CARE

Patients receiving Prestige artificial disc replacements are treated with nonsteroidal anti-inflammatory medications for 2 weeks following surgery. No bracing is necessary, and they may resume all activities when they desire except those that produce high-impact loading such as jogging, horseback riding, and so forth.

## COMPLICATIONS AND AVOIDANCE

Patients with instability and deformity should be treated with a fusion. Individuals with significant osteoporosis may be better served with a 360-degree fusion following decompression. Care should be taken to prevent the development of a postoperative kyphotic deformity. Maintenance of proper alignment requires that the patient be positioned such that the segment being treated is in neutral alignment. This will ensure a proper match of the spine with the implant because the device holder maintains the artificial disc in the neutral position during insertion.

Although heterotopic ossification has not been reported to occur in conjunction with the Prestige devices, it is probably optimal that patients receive nonsteroidal anti-inflammatory medications for 2 weeks following surgery, which may further reduce the risk of developing this entity.

## ADVANTAGES/DISADVANTAGES

The primary advantage of cervical arthroplasty is preservation of segmental motion. Single-segment reconstruction with the Prestige device appears to result in more rapid improvement following surgery and a decreased risk of developing adjacent segment disease as compared with arthrodesis. The ST device has a very secure initial fixation but is poorly imaged with magnetic resonance. The Prestige LP is imaging friendly.

## CONCLUSIONS/DISCUSSION

The Prestige ST and LP total cervical disc arthroplasty devices are an excellent means of preserving physiologic motion following anterior cervical decompression. Long-term results are helpful in determining the degree of benefit this technology provides in terms of limiting adjacent segment degeneration.

## REFERENCES


1. Cummins BH, Robertson JT, Gill SS: Surgical experience with an implanted artificial cervical joint. J Neurosurg 88(suppl 6):943–948, 1998.
2. Robertson JT, Metcalf NH: Long-term outcome after implantation of the Prestige I disc in an end-stage indication: 4-year results from a pilot study. Neurosurg Focus 17(suppl 3):E10, 69–71, 2004.
3. Wigfield CC, Gill SS, Nelson RJ, et al: The new Frenchay artificial cervical joint: Results from a two-year pilot study. Spine 27 (suppl 22):2446–2452, 2002.
4. Pracyk JB, Traynelis VC: Treatment of the painful motion segment: Cervical arthroplasty. Spine 30(suppl 16):S23–S32, 2005.
5. Traynelis VC: The Prestige cervical disc replacement. Spine J 4 (suppl 6):310S–314S, 2004.
6. Traynelis VC: The Prestige cervical disc. Neurosurg Clin N Am 16 (suppl 4):621–628, 2005.
7. DiAngelo DJ, Robertson JT, Metcalf NH, et al: Biomechanical testing of an artificial cervical joint and an anterior cervical plate. J Spinal Disord Tech 16(suppl 4):314–323, 2003.
8. Wigfield C, Gill S, Nelson R, et al: Influence of an artificial cervical joint compared with fusion on adjacent-level motion in the treatment of degenerative cervical disc disease. J Neurosurg 96(suppl 1):17–21, 2002.
9. Robertson JT, Papadopoulos SM, Traynelis VC: Assessment of adjacent-segment disease in patients treated with cervical fusion or arthroplasty: A prospective 2-year study. J Neurosurg Spine 3(suppl 6): 417–423, 2005.
10. Traynelis V, Anderson P, Hacker R, et al: Return to work analysis of patients treated with an artificial cervical disc or an arthrodesis. Spine J 6(5, suppl 1):63S–64S, 2006.

CHAPTER 24

# Porous Coated Motion (PCM) Cervical Arthroplasty

**Paul C. McAfee**

## KEY POINTS

- Porous Coated Motion (PCM) is a surface-replacement, no-anterior-profile, cervical arthroplasty with a large enough radius of curvature to allow physiologic translation in flexion-extension and side bending without a true "ball-and-socket" constraint.
- PCM is actually an array of implants designed to address a variety of indications, depending on the degree of instability and the amount of bone resected during the neurological decompression.
- The pilot study of 229 cases in Brazil is the first disc replacement study showing significantly greater improvement in clinical outcomes, Neck Disability Index (NDI), in multiple level cervical arthroplasty compared to single level disc replacement.
- The U.S. Investigational Device Exemption (IDE) study for the PCM is unique in that it includes cervical arthroplasty adjacent to a prior cervical fused vertebral level or arthroplasty in the treatment of adjacent segment disease.
- The modularity of the ancillary components (Fig. 24–1), such as the Modular Flange plate, Corpomotion device, and mobile-bearing inserts of the constrained PCM (PCM-C), allow increased stability even in cases of posterior facet joint capsular laxity.

## INTRODUCTION

Porous Coated Motion (PCM) (Cervitech, Inc., Rockaway, NJ) arthroplasty is one of five cervical disc replacement prostheses undergoing a prospective IDE trial. All five prostheses are currently under investigation with no final approval; however, the experience outside the United States and the preclinical basic scientific data has begun to show promising advantages of arthroplasty versus arthrodesis in four areas.

First, there is less soft tissue dissection and less retraction of the esophagus with disc replacement. The current-generation cervical disc replacements have no anterior profile, whereas all cervical plate systems project anteriorly, with the incidence of postoperative dysphagia and dysarthria correlating with the thickness of the cervical plate.

Second, there is less transmission of additional load and strain to the adjacent cervical vertebral levels with anthroplasty. The adjacent intradiscal pressure is similar between nonoperated conditions and those undergoing disc replacements, which are both significantly less than levels adjacent to anterior cervical fusions.

Third, there has been a large series of prospectively enrolled cervical disc replacement demonstrating a significantly higher reoperation rate and adjacent level disease with cervical arthrodesis compared with a lower reoperation incidence with cervical disc replacement.

Fourth, with fusion, the outcomes deteriorate as the number of vertebral levels of treatment increase, whereas with cervical disc replacement, the outcomes remain consistent, even with increasing levels of implantation.

## INDICATIONS/CONTRAINDICATIONS

### Description of the Device

The name "Porous Coated" highlights the ingrowth capabilities of the TiCaP-coated CHARITÉ (DePuy Spine Inc., Raynham, MA) device used worldwide since 1998. McAfee et al[1] measured the amount of bony ingrowth and calculated, through a computerized microscopic imaging system called the Bioquant-histomorphometric analysis, at the metal-bone interface (bone contact area/total end plate area) that the mean ingrowth was 47.9%, with a standard deviation of ± 8.12%. The total range of ingrowth was 35.5% to 58.8%.

The term motion in "Porous Coated Motion" highlights the principles in Charnley's low-friction arthroplasty in which the bio materials ultra-high-molecular-weight polyethylene (UHMWPE) and cobalt chrome alloy allow motion with a minimum of frictional wear particulate.[2,3]

Conceptually, the PCM cervical disc replacement is more of a surface replacement in that it does not require a lot of bone resection or reaming. In addition, there are no fins or sharp projections from the prosthesis that would get embedded, requiring either hemicorpectomy or extensive bone grafting in a salvage situation. There are no external steriotactic frames that need to be bolted to the table, and there is no "blind reaming" under fluoroscopy at any time during the procedure. If the prosthesis can be placed in a "press-fit" fashion, then the low-profile standard version can be implanted. However, if the bony preparation is suboptimal or the anatomy is abnormal, such as in Klippel-Feil syndrome, then there is an augmented backup version of the prosthesis called the augmented PCM-C, which is fixed with screws to

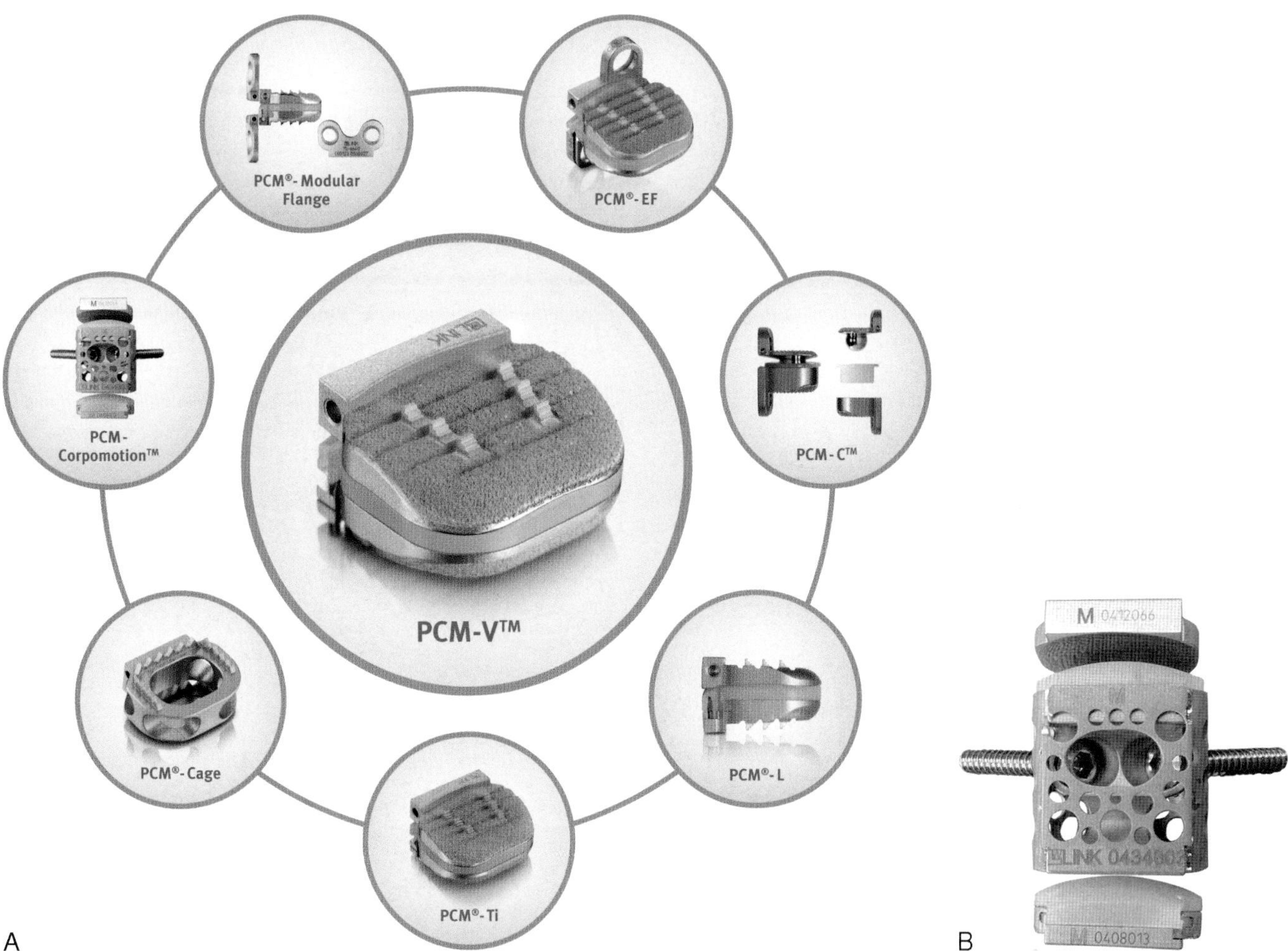


■ **FIGURE 24–1.** **A,** Modularity. Most modern total joint prostheses have a modular design to address a number of different indications of varying degrees of instability. Shown here are the PCM-V (center), the PCM Modular Flange for additional stability (top left), PCM-EF with excentric flange, the constrained version of the PCM-C, the lordotic version PCM-L, for sensitive patients the PCM-Ti, the Titanium fusion PCM cage, and the Corpomotion PCM for corpectomies. **B,** The PCM Corpomotion, which replaces a vertebral body and two adjacent intervertebral discs.

the anterior surface of the vertebral body. This armamentarium is analogous to performing a press-fit total hip replacement and having a long-stem femoral component available.

With the major design parameters of the cervical PCM prosthesis, the more conservative, traditional option was used: (1) the biomaterial, UHMWPE (7) (ISO 5834/2; ASTM 648) - wrought CoCrMo alloy (ISO 5832/12; ASTM F1537), articular bearing surface (rather than metal-on-metal or untreated titanium-on-UHMWPE interface);[3] (2) an optional unconstrained design rather than a ball-and-socket design; (3) the metal-bone porous ingrowth surface; (4) compression-molded sheet polyethylene, standard gamma irradiation sterilized, versus high cross-linked polyethylene; and (5) the maximum preservation of vertebral body bone stock as opposed to cutting a groove into the middle of the vertebral body, insertion of a fin possibly requiring a corpectomy for revision. Basically, the same amount of bone resection required for anterior spinal cord decompression is sufficient for preparation of the PCM disc, and excessive reaming or cumbersome table-mounted fixation jigs are not required.

### The Bearing Surface

The calculated wear rate of gamma-sterilized UHMWPE for hip joints is less than 0.152 mm per year. More favorable wear particulate and incidence of osteolysis have been described with UHMWPE-cross-linked either with radiation or peroxidase. The early wear rates in hip simulators of this newer configuration of UHMWPE are improved (0.015 mm/year); however, the highly cross-linked variety has a greater chance of plastic deformation owing to its reduced crystallinity and ultimate tensile strength, and, most important, reduction of tensile elongation at fracture.[4]

### Preclinical Background Work: Caprine Animal Model for Porous Coated Motion Cervical Arthroplasty

Animal model testing was completed. Twelve goats that underwent PCM cervical disc replacement at C3-C4 were followed for 6 months (Fig. 24–4).[5] There was no evidence of particulate debris, cytokines, cellular apoptosis, or membrane-bound tumor necrosis factor-α. The caprine model has been used to test a variety of brands and models of cervical disc replacements using the same criteria analogous to the baboon lumbar spine for testing a lumbar disc replacement: (1) similar anatomic dimensions between the caprine C3-C4 intervertebral disc and the human C5-C6 and C6-C7 discs; (2) similar ranges of motion in flexion-extension and axial compression; axial rotation is more restricted in the goat owing to larger uncovertebral joints, and the overall disc has more of a dome-like shape than that of the human; (3) human-sized cervical disc replacements can be used in the goat at C3-C4; and (4) it is absolutely a "worst-case" scenario with regard to evaluating the durability of the cervical prosthesis. The goats are ambulatory without a brace several hours after the surgery. They butt heads with each other, violently shaking and extending their cervical spines and occasionally leaping over 4-foot stockade fences, becoming completely airborne.

In more than 12 goats with the PCM device followed for 6 months, there were no significant perioperative complications in the animal model. There was no loosening, no osteolysis, and no translational instabilities associated with the device at 6 months postoperatively. The osteoconductive TiCaP coating provided some immediate advantages with friction during press-fit applications, and there was no significant anterior prosthesis subluxation for 6 months despite unrestricted cervical activity (see Fig. 24–4).

Figure 24–4 demonstrates the ability to image and assess the cervical spinal canal in the area of the prosthesis. This representative computed tomography (CT) scan axial image is through the maximum mass of the prosthesis, showing the preserved ability to rule out further compressive spinal cord lesions. At 6-month follow-up in the caprine model, there was an absence of cellular reaction and no granulation tissue response to any particulate wear debris.

## Background of Scientific Testing/Clinical Outcomes

### Clinical Food and Drug Administration Pilot Study

Preliminary clinical results of a cervical disc replacement using conventional conservative biomaterials (UHMWPE + CoCrMo) were analyzed. One hundred and forty patients underwent a total of 229 consecutive PCM cervical arthroplasties from C3–4 to C7-T1 (single level, 71 cases [Fig. 24–5]; double level, 53 cases; three levels, 12 cases; and four levels, 4 cases).[6] Indications were 102 patients with radiculopathy and 38 patients with cervical myelopathy. The neural decompression was a standard Smith-Robinson type anterior cervical decompression, followed by cervical arthroplasty. The procedure allows reconstruction of more unstable indications than previously reported with disc replacement. Twenty PCM cases had been performed as complex revision procedures in patients with prior instrumentation, including previous failed disc replacements, one cage plate, three patients with failed lordotic cages, three patients with fragmented polymethyl methacrylate, and 21 patients had presented with adjacent segment disease following anterior cervical discectomy and fusion (ACDF). One additional patient had presented with a fracture-dislocation at C4-C5 and a pseudoarthrosis at C3-C4 and C5-C6.

At mean follow-up of 26.7 months (range 12 to 42 months), all patients were neurologically intact. Mean EBL = 113 mL (range <50 to 850 mL). Mean length of surgery was 80.7 minutes (range 35 to 150 min). The length of hospital stay ranged from outpatient to 3 days, with 80% of patients discharged in less than 23 hours. Oswestry, visual analog scale (VAS), and Odoms outcome measures were improved as compared with published reports of ACDF with plates and cervical cages. The mean improvement in the Neck Disability Index (NDI) for the single cases was 37.6% versus the multilevel cases mean improvement in NDI, 52.6% ($P = 0.021$). The difference between the two was statistically significant. The mean improvement in the VAS showed the same relationship—single-level mean improvement was 58.4% versus the multilevel cases, in which the mean VAS improvement was 65.9%. The Odoms were also more improved for the multilevel versus the single-level group—93.9% versus 90.5% in the excellent, good, and fair categories. No external steriotactic frames or excessive reaming was required, and 87% of working patients were able to return to their baseline level of employment.

### Clinical Presentation and Evaluation

The indications for anterior cervical disc replacement are the same as those for anterior cervical decompression: radiculopathy or myelopathy caused by either one or two levels of anterior cervical compression (Table 24–1). Most surgeons would agree that a patient presenting with a compressive lesion causing arm weakness, paresthesia, and unremitting radicular pain with or without lower extremity hyperactive reflexes requires anterior cervical decompression. The only difference of opinion is what to do following anterior surgical spinal cord or nerve root decompression. The goals are to restore the intervertebral disc height and neuroforaminal height to prevent recurrence of neurologic compression.

## OPERATIVE TECHNIQUES (10 STEPS)

**STEP 1:** Figure 24–6 illustrates the ideal setup for a PCM implantation. The surgeon needs to be able to work around the C-arm in order to facilitate fine adjustments during the instrumentation. The overall guiding principle of the PCM is to not compromise the surgeon's decision making and ability to perform whatever neurologic decompression the surgeon believes is indicated. With a wide array of implants available worldwide, the decompression can extend through four disc spaces, include a corpectomy, and even span a level with facet joint laxity. There is a model of the PCM that is indicated. The instruments are also designed to be used with a microscope if the surgeon desires. The patient has to be placed in neutral position.

**STEP 2:** A standard Smith-Robinson exposure is performed, the inventor of the PCM having worked with George Smith, Robbie Robinson, Wayne Southwick, Lee Riley, and Henry Bohlman. The PCM is the outgrowth of the Johns Hopkins legacy of anterior approaches to the extensile approach to the cervical spine. What allows the PCM to be minimally invasive is the careful placement of the fixation pins, which are placed in parallel to the intervertebral disc space. Four different lengths of drill guides allow maximum exposure of the disc without putting a pin into the next disc space.

**STEP 3:** The Caspar Type Distractor can be locked in place to prevent inadvertent backing out. The cervical vertebra are never extended—the system is designed to give parallel distraction of the interspinous ligaments.

**TABLE 24–1. Indications/Contraindications for Cervical Disk Arthroplasty**

| | |
|---|---|
| Clinical inclusion criteria | Patients 20 to 60 years old<br>Degenerative disc disease with radicular or spinal cord compression<br>HNP C3-4 to C7-T1<br>Cervical myelopathy without myelomalacia<br>MRI-documented evidence of mechanical pressure on neurologic elements<br>Adjacent to a spinal fusion in the cervical spine (adjacent segment disease) |
| Contraindications | Metabolic and bone disease<br>Patients in terminal phase of chronic disease<br>Patients with pyogenic infection or active granulomatosis<br>Patients with neoplastic or traumatic disease of the cervical spine<br>OPLL<br>Severe facet joint arthritis |
| Indications for PCM-V (**Fig. 24–2**) | Radicular compression<br>Herniation of the nucleus pulposus of C3-C4 to C7-T1<br>Anterior medullary compression<br>Cervical spondylosis<br>Nuclear MRI evidence of mechanical compression of neural elements<br>Nontraumatic segmental instability<br>Neurologic compression of one or multilevel from C3–C4 to C7–T1<br>Primary degenerative disc disease<br>Degenerative adjacent segment disease |
| Indications for the "Modular Flanged" version (with screw fixation), in addition to the above, include: | Suboptimal carpentry, understood as an irregular cut in the preparation of the vertebral end plate<br>Loss of anterior vertebral body bone stock<br>Anterior vertebral subluxation greater than or equal to 3.5 mm<br>Anatomical variation or previous surgery predisposing the segment to higher loads |
| Indications for the (Constrained PCM ball-and-stocket) PCM-C disc arthroplasty with mobile-bearing inserts (**Fig. 24–3**). | Greater than or equal to 3.5 mm anterior translation of segmental motion<br>Posterior laxity of the facet joint capsular ligaments<br>Revision cervical arthroplasty with loss of more than 8.0 mm of anterior cervical spinal column bone stock |
| Indications for the PCM Corpomotion | The need for two adjacent levels of cervical disc replacement with a corpectomy, i.e., anterior decompression of the entire vertebral body between the two disc levels |

MRI, magnetic resonance imaging; OPLL, ossification of the posterior longitudinal ligament.

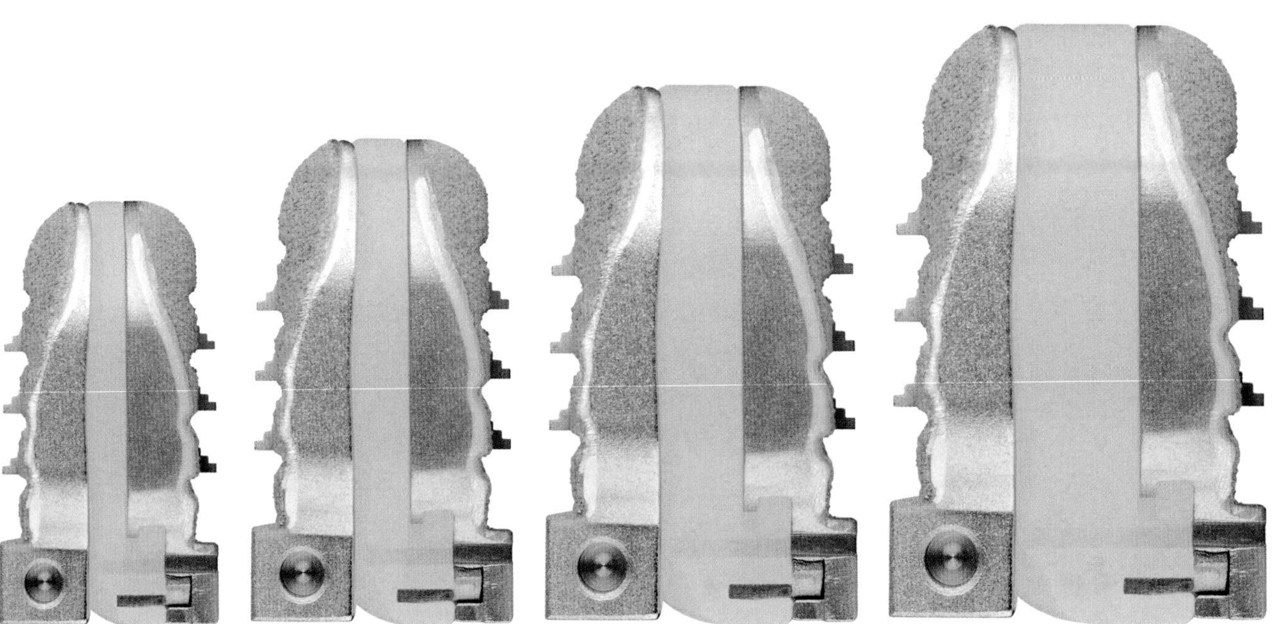

**FIGURE 24–2.** The PCM-V uses two rounded posterolateral corners that fit into the uncovertebral joints. Four different prosthetic heights are shown, 5.7 mm, 6.5 mm, 7.2 mm and 8 mm, depending on the desired ultra-high-molecular-weight polyethylene height.

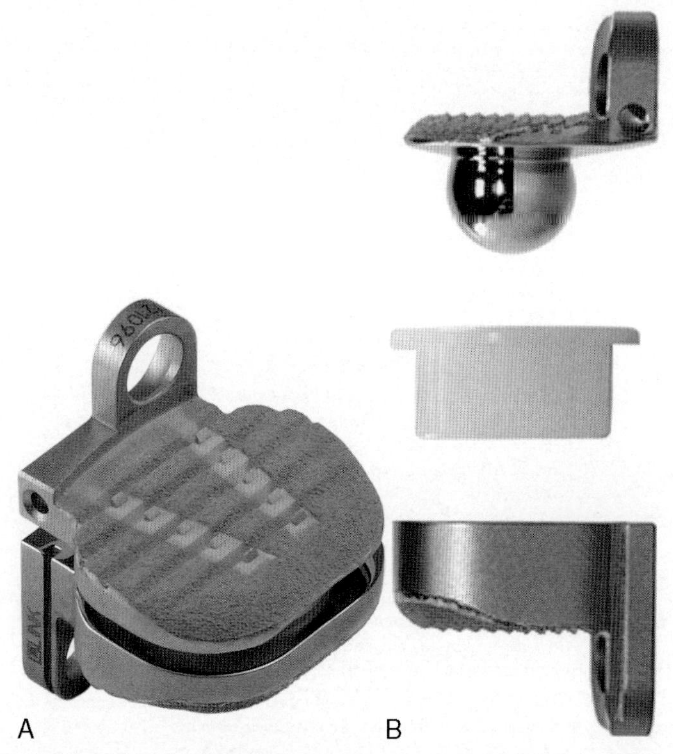


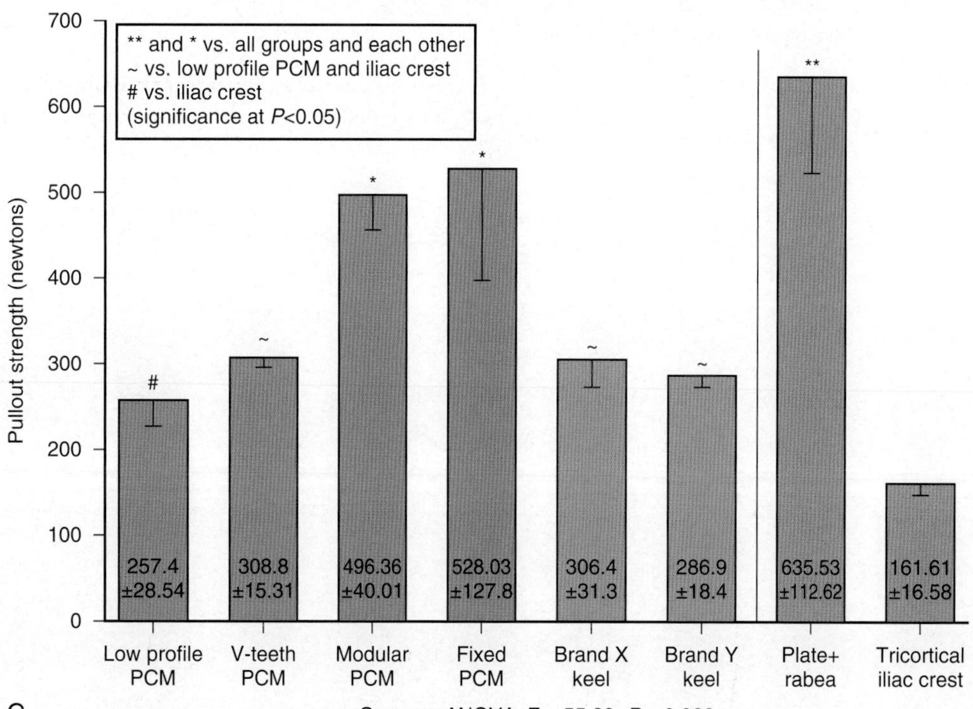


■ **FIGURE 24–3.** **A** and **B,** The constrained version of the Porous Coated Motion (PCM) prosthesis, the PCM-C with flanges and V-teeth fixation. **C,** The bar graph shows pull out tests of the metal-bone fixation of various prostheses. Notice that the anterior cervical discectomy and fusion plate and cage and the iliac bone graft alone comprise the two bars on the far right. The PCM with the V-teeth gives the same fixation as a keel without requiring specialized instruments for insertion. The V-teeth also made it possible to revise without having to perform a corpectomy, reported occasionally for the keeled prostheses.

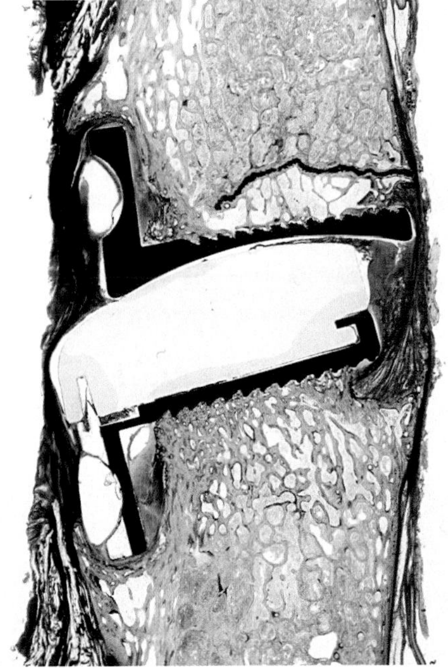


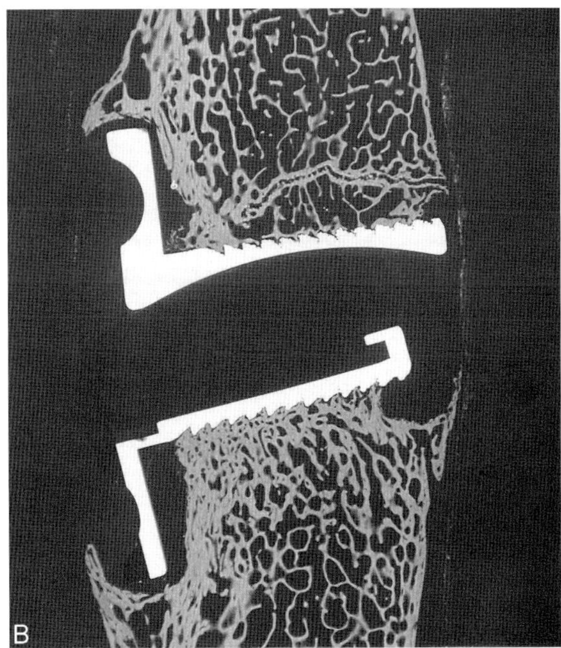


■ **FIGURE 24–4.** The Porous Coated Motion (PCM standard mode) prosthesis was inserted in a caprine model at C3-C4. Six goats were followed for 6 months, and 6 goats were followed for 1 year in order to evaluate the absence of wear particulate debris and lack of prosthetic loosening, and to calculate the percentage of bony ingrowth into the TiCaP porous surface. **A,** This is a sagittal histologic section 6 months after implantation, showing no fibrous tissue at the metal-bone interface. **B,** The corresponding microradiograph at 12 months shows superior ingrowth of the TiCaP bioactive material. There was no loosening of any of the 12 PCM prostheses in this caprine model.

**Step 4:** The posterior osteophytes and entire posterior longitudinal ligament are removed in their entirety. With motion preservation, it is not possible to predict whether a retained osteophyte will become symptomatic in the future, so they are all prophylactically removed during a thorough decompression. The end plates are prepared with Planer Rasps or barrel-shaped burrs.

**Step 5:** Five different sizers are used (alternatively called a "lollipop") to optimally cover the vertebral end plates with the correct footprint.

**Step 6:** Each end plate footprint size has two broaches, which are used in sequence (Broach A and Broach B). They are not used with force to move bone around, instead they are used to see where the vertebral bone "hangs up" and needs to be gently removed with either a high-speed burr or a curette.

**Step 7:** The most important PCM instrument is the prosthesis trial for each size and height. There needs to be good visualization of the metal-bone interface with the C-arm. The trial needs to reflect press-fit after removal of an anterior step-cut with a Terraced Reamer. The anterior edge of the prosthesis is recessed into the disc space, ensuring that the PCM sits flush with the anterior borders of the vertebrae. This minimizes the potential for esophageal irritation. If the PCM trial is correctly press-fit, then the Caspar distraction can be removed and the prosthesis trial will be stable in spite of its smooth surfaces due to the disc space ligamentotaxis. The trial is test run upward, downward, flexion, extension, side bending, and pull-out to evaluate stability. This is called the push-pull PCM press-fit trial test.

**Step 8:** Loading the PCM on the holding and insertion. The forceps is placed into the tracks located on the lateral margins of the rack. This method ensures accurate location of the holding pins and ridges of the holding and insertion forceps into the reciprocating holes on the superior pins and grooves on the inferior plate of the PCM prosthesis.

**Step 9:** The PCM is inserted into the disc space, top on the instrument showing to cranial, without impaction and under slight distraction. Special attention is paid to the posterior third of the disc space because it is important to get full coverage of the vertebral bodies.

**Step 10:** Final position of the PCM cervical disc. (See corresponding DVD for this step in particular). The final position of the PCM cervical disc is checked before final closure. It is important that the anterior edges of the implant seat flush with or just deeper that the bony surface. In addition, full coverage is required of the vertebral end plates, because it maximizes the implant's resistance to subsidence due to its unique scalloped and "V-teeth" design. This allows the implant to rest on the bony areas within the cervical body that has the most density. Under C-arm radiographic visualization the patient's neck is taken through a full range of motion to ensure that there is good ligamentous balance and good stability at the metal-bone interface. If there is any shifting of the prosthesis or any sizing issues, they can be corrected at this time. One would not think of doing a total hip or knee replacement without taking the knee through a range of motion intraoperatively. This is our analogous range-of-motion (ROM) check for optimal balance for the PCM intraoperatively. We actually ask the anesthesiologist to perform this function because (1) they are unscrubbed and (2) they will protect the patient's endotracheal tube during the range of motion testing for the PCM.

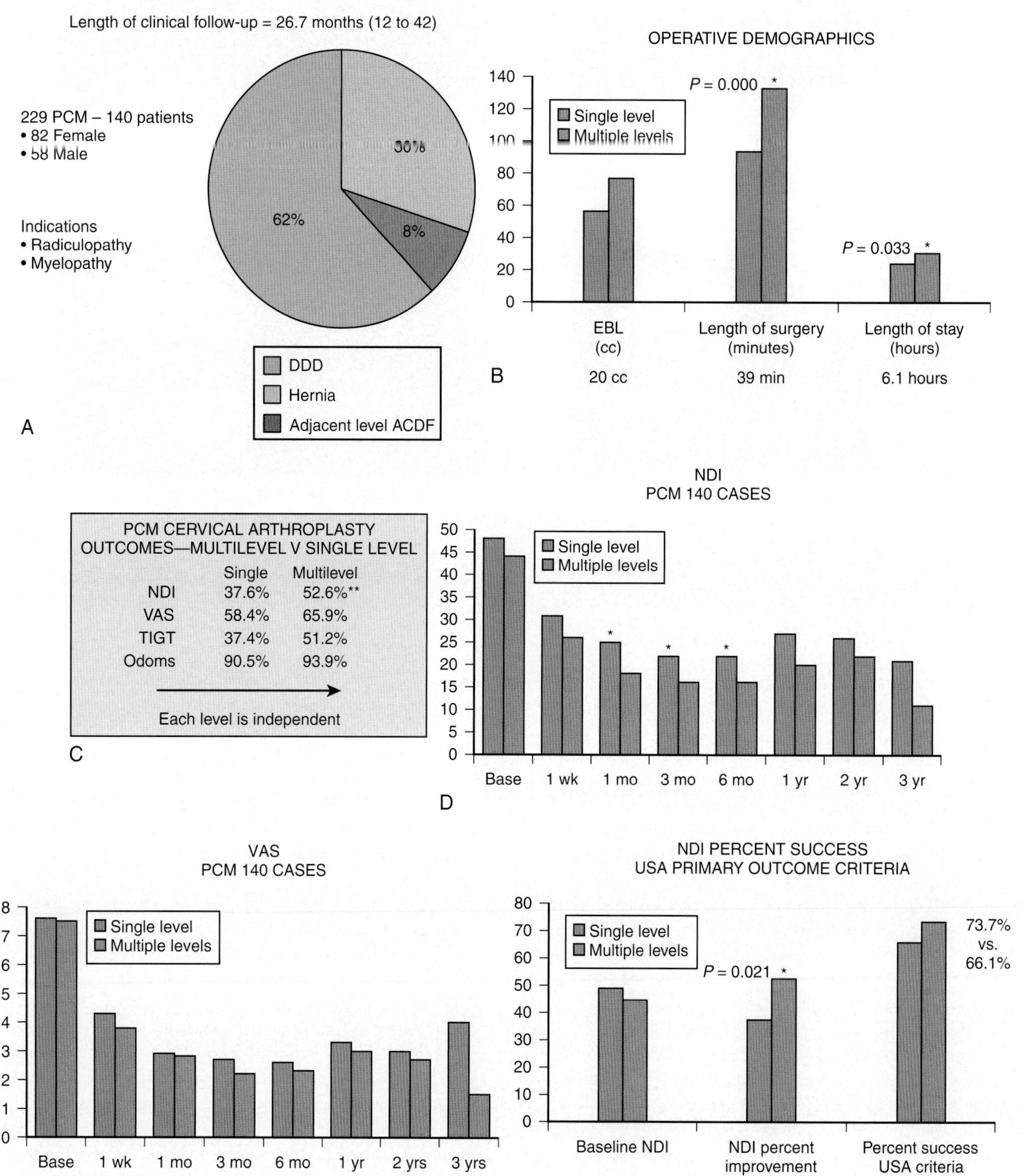


■ **FIGURE 24–5.** **A** to **F,** These figures summarize the clinical outcomes from the Porous-Coated Motion PCM Prosthesis Pilot Study in São Paulo, Brazil, under Luiz Pimenta. NDI, Neck Disability Index.

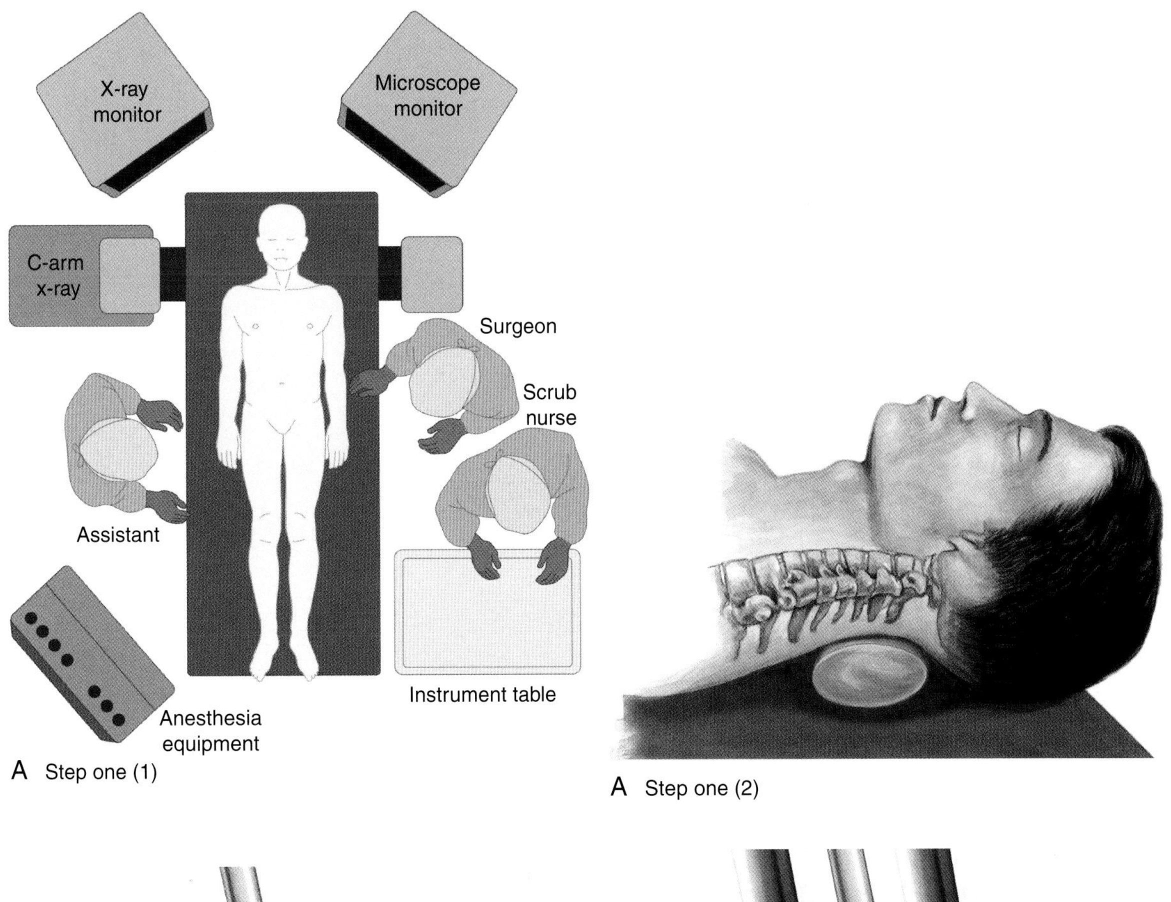


A Step one (1)

A Step one (2)

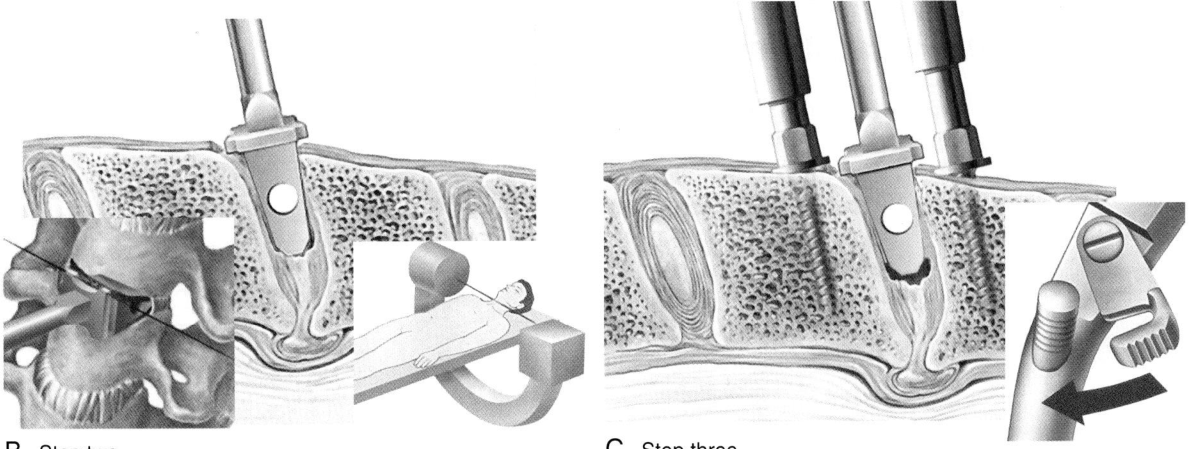

B Step two

C Step three

■ **FIGURE 24–6.** **A** to **J,** The 10 steps required for accurate porous-coated motion prosthesis implantation. A detailed explanation is in the text.

*(Continued)*

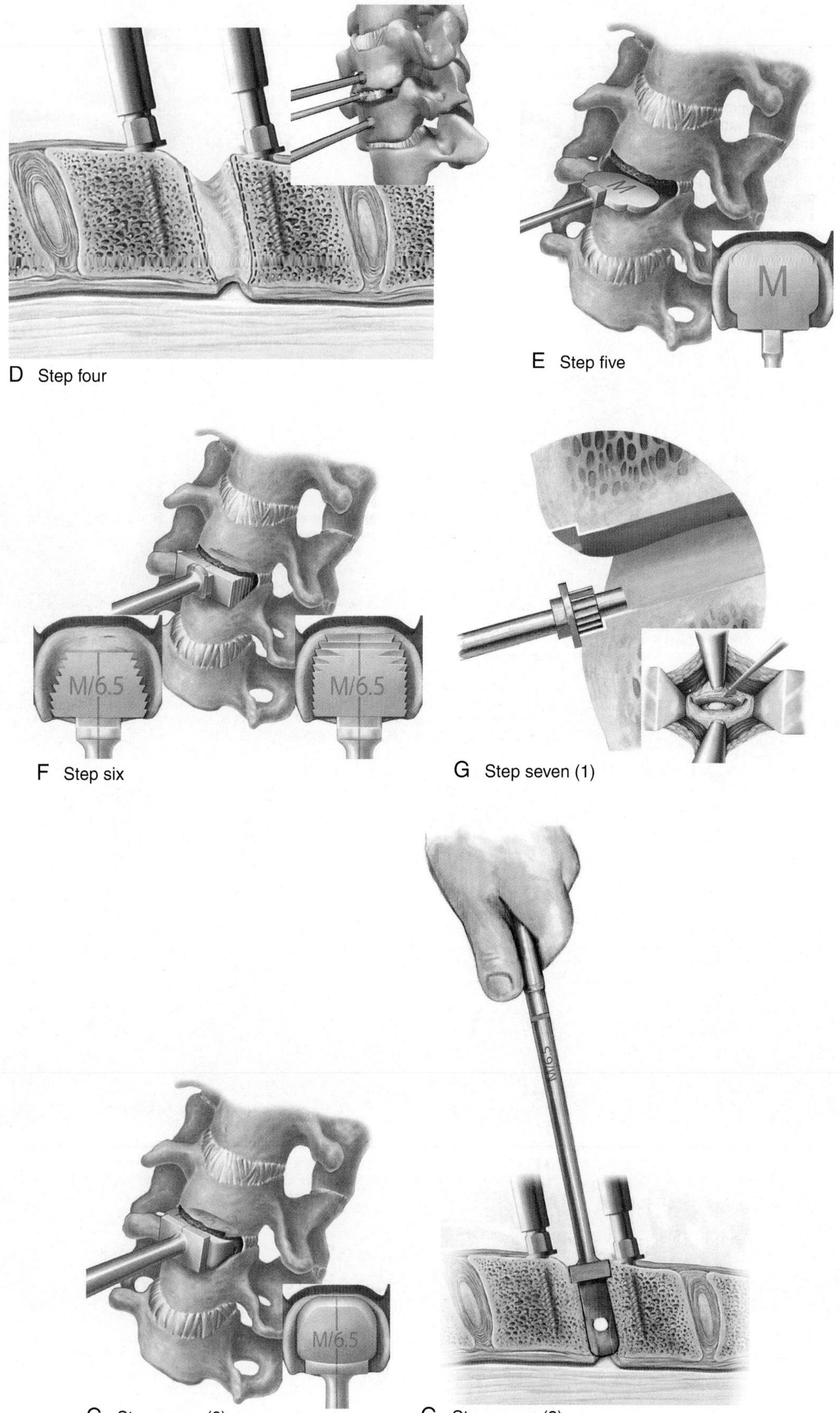


■ **FIGURE 24–6. Cont'd** **A** to **J,** The 10 steps required for accurate porous-coated motion prosthesis implantation. A detailed explanation is in the text.

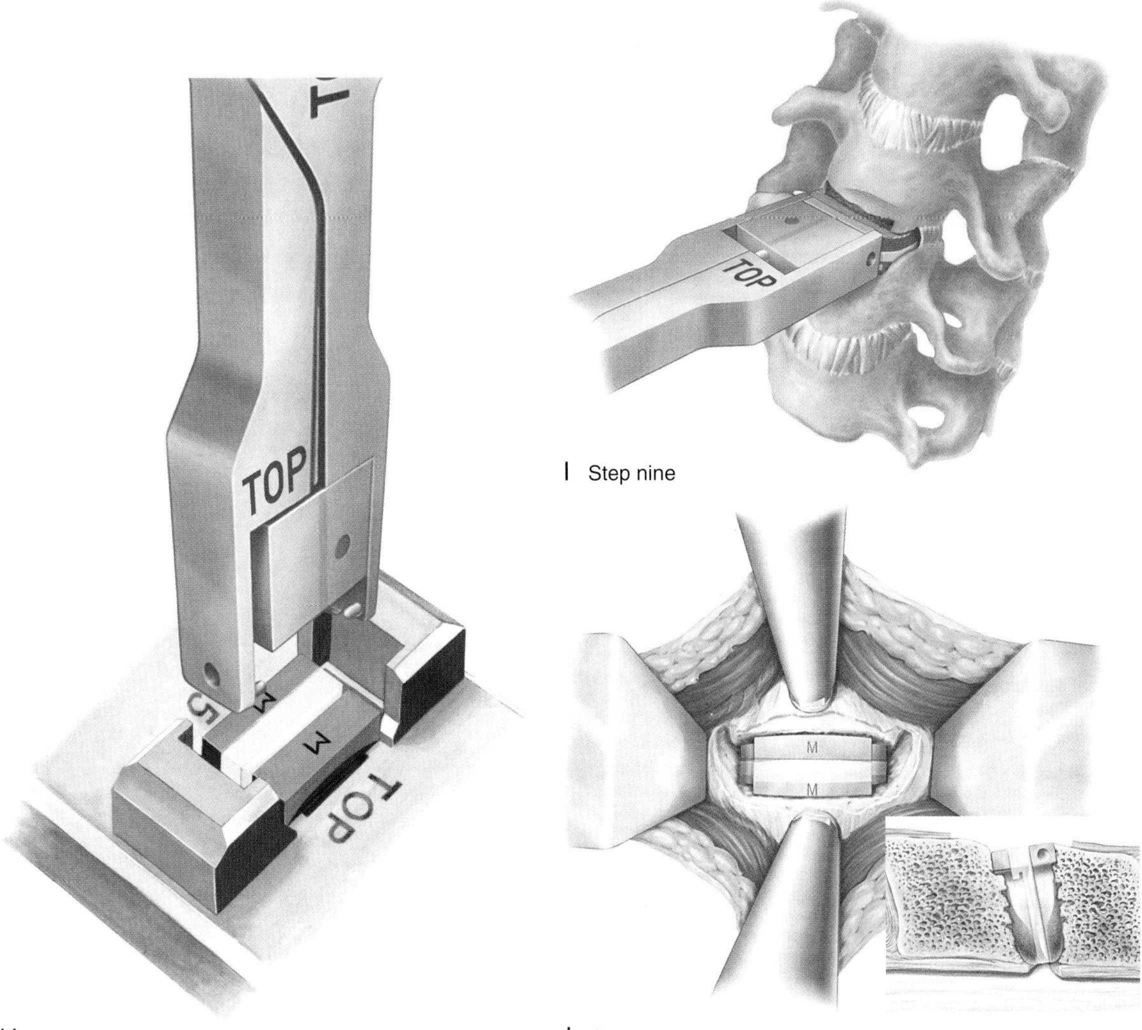


■ **FIGURE 24–6. Cont'd** **A** to **J**, The 10 steps required for accurate Porous Coated Motion prosthesis implantation. A detailed explanation is in the text.

## POSTOPERATIVE CARE

The patient is discharged usually within 24 hours for a one-level PCM implantation. A soft cervical collar can be used for 1 to 3 weeks. The important part of the rehabilitation is the active ROM of cervical spine mobilization, which can be started within 2 weeks. Weight training and high-impact loading is restricted for 8 weeks. Laboratory and animal test data reflected high CaP solubility of 18.3% in 7 days. That resulted in 73% direct bone/implant contact as opposed to only 49.8% at uncoated controls. It is important to limit impact loading and jarring to the neck for the first 2 months postoperatively. There are patients with a PCM prosthesis who have returned to professional sports. However, the restrictions are not due to the PCM prosthesis but rather due to the muscular conditioning that needs to occur over the first 6 postoperative weeks. The restriction of activity, therefore, is usually dependent on the speed of ligamentous and muscular recovery, not the PCM prosthesis characteristics.

## COMPLICATIONS

The best cohort of cases to study to determine the incidence of complications of the PCM is Luiz Pimenta's 229 consecutive prospective cases in São Paulo, Brazil (Fig. 24–7). There were no deaths, no infections, and no iatrogenic neurologic problems. Five reoperations were required—usually revised with low-profile devices with a PCM component augmented with screw fixation. Six patients had presented with translational instability and had undergone PCM-C, constrained prostheses augmented with screw fixation. One patient had 4 mm of anterior subluxation of the components in the first 3 months but was clinically asymptomatic with 10 degrees flexion-extension ROM 1 year postoperatively. There were two patients with intraoperative CSF leakage owing to the spinal decompression who had uneventful recoveries. A Kaplan-Meier implant survivorship analysis at 3 years for the cohort of 229 prostheses was 94.5% (confidence interval, 3.00 to .820) (Fig. 24–8).

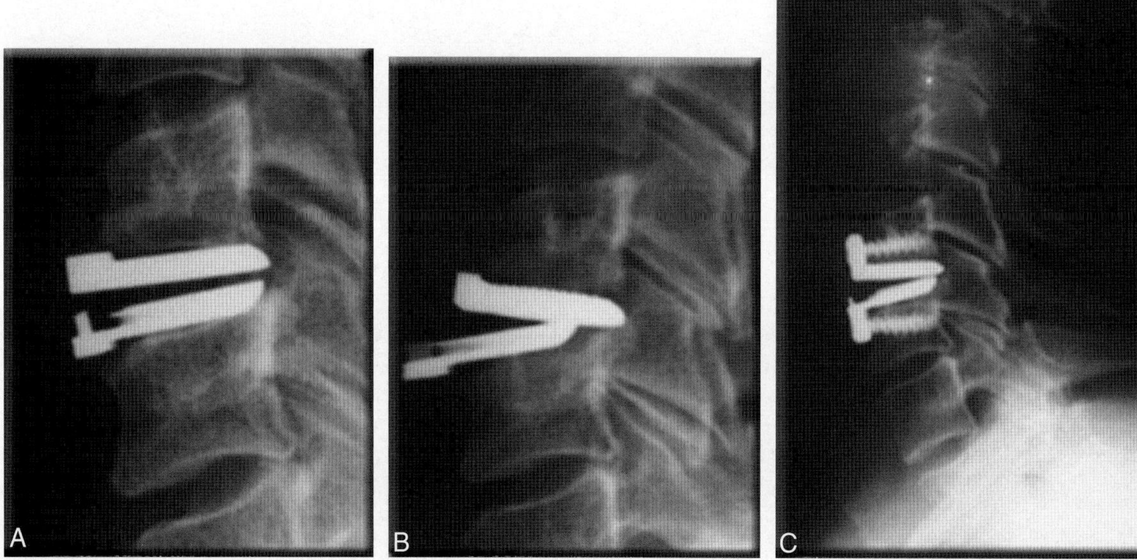


■ **FIGURE 24–7.** **A** to **C,** Complications. In more than 3 years with a consecutive series of 229 Porous Coated Motion prosthesis implantations, there was only one case that required conversion to a fusion. There were occasional cerebrospinal fluid leaks secondary to the difficulty of the decompression. There were four cases of heterotopic bone formation.

## Advantages/Disadvantages

### Differences in Rate of Instrumentation Failure: Fusions Versus Arthroplasty

Swank et al reported the pseudarthrosis rates after cervical corpectomy. The incidence increased as the length of the cervical plate got longer: one level, 10%; two levels, 44%; and three levels, 54%. In a similar fashion, Lowery and McDonough found that the incidence of hardware failures using Orozco plates increased as the number of cervical levels increased: one-level fusion, 20%; two-level fusion, 36%; three-level fusion, 71%; and four-level fusion, 80%. In the largest series yet discussed, Geisler et al[7] analyzed the reoperation rates in a total of 402 patients after cervical plate stabilization: one-level cases requiring reoperation (15/258), 5.8%; two levels requiring reoperation (7/107), 6.5%; three levels requiring reoperation (2/25), 8%; and four levels requiring reoperation (2/12), 16.8%.

This is not the trend or indicative of early reports of cervical arthroplasty in which each cervical vertebral level is biomechanically independent of the adjacent levels. With the PCM prosthesis (see Fig. 24–7) the incidence of reoperation does not increase

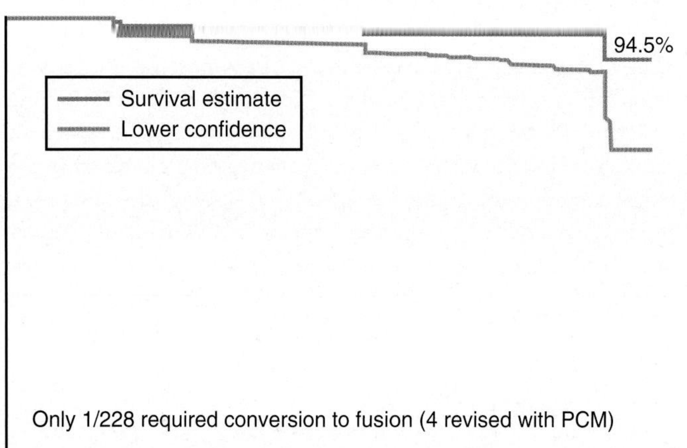


■ **FIGURE 24–8.** This is a survivorship analysis of the Pilot Study in Brazil focusing on the 229 PCM prosthesis. Notice that the calculated 5-year survivorship is 94.5%, which is encouraging for any orthopaedic total joint arthroplasty.

**ADVANTAGES/DISADVANTAGES: PCM**

**Advantages**

- Two components are composed of clinically familiar materials with a 50-year track record—UHMWPE and cobalt chrome.
- It is a nonconstrained, full motion implant.
- The sculpted form is designed to fit the cervical disc space, reducing the reaming and bone resection the patient undergoes.
- Primary fixation is achieved by forward facing ridges and "V-teeth" to provide initial security and allow for early patient mobilization.
- Secondary fixation and stability are pursued through an osteoconductive TiCaP coating on both the superior and inferior implant surfaces.
- Because the PCM implant is designed to "fit the void" rather than have the surgeon "ream a void to fit" the implant, bone preparation stages are significantly reduced, preserving maximum implant stability and shorter preparation times, with the associated benefits of reduced morbidity and shorter rehabilitation times.

**Disadvantages**

- With the current biomaterials in the U.S. IDE trial, an MRI can be performed to evaluate the adjacent cervical levels, but a CT-myelogram is required for optimal evaluation of the index cervical level. The PCM-Ti is available outside the United States but not in the United States at the current time.
- The PCM is currently only available inside the United States to participants in a prospective FDA clinical trial.

CT, computed tomography; FDA, U.S. Food and Drug Administration; IDE, Investigational Device Exemption; PCM, Porous Coated Motion; UHMWPE, ultra-high-molecular-weight polyethylene.

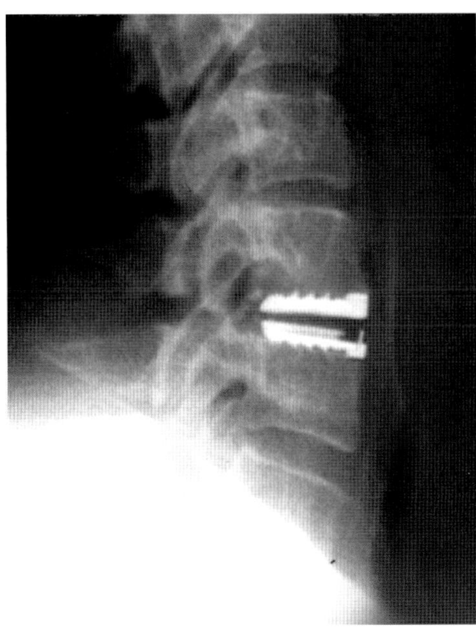

■ FIGURE 24-9. PCM-V in level 5-6.

proportionately higher as the number of cervical levels requiring instrumentation increases.

In short, the advantage of cervical arthroplasty is that the complications are not magnified by the number of vertebral levels treated in the same patient. Unlike cervical fusion, with cervical arthroplasty the outcomes at each level are independent. With cervical fusion, however, if the cervical plate fails at one level, it has failed to provide fixation at all levels.[8]

## CONCLUSIONS/DISCUSSION

The PCM investigators in the U.S. trial tend to be the most academic and accomplished cervical investigators.[9] By definition they are thoughtful, so they do not blindly "rack up the numbers" and thus the rate of enrollment might not be as fast as some of the competitors'.

Intermediate-length follow-up results outside the United States have shown that the PCM can be applied in cases of myelopathy and patients presenting with significant spinal cord compression. The PCM has been applied in more than 5,000 cases in 30 countries. The maintenance of neurologic integrity in patients with myelomalacia treated with the PCM needs to be born out throughout longer term follow-up of 10 years or more.

Thus far, nonsteroidal anti-inflammatory agents have not been required with the PCM in order to prevent heterotopic bone formation. These agents are apparently necessary as prophylactic treatment in other arthroplasty clinical trials.[10]

It will require a prospective randomized clinical trial of the PCM to show that a prosthesis intended as a surface replacement, with preservation of the vertebral end plates, can provide improved clinical outcomes and a lower reoperation rate.

It is hoped that a keeled prosthesis is not necessary as a primary implant because the revisions often require corpectomies and conversion to multilevel cervical fusion and instrumentation.

The PCM is not only the first cervical disc replacement, but it is the first motion preservation device to show significantly improved outcomes with multilevel versus single-level use with an outcome instrument validated by the Food and Drug Administration.

## CROSS-REFERENCES

Chapter 21: Primary Indications and Disc Space Preparation for Cervical Arthroplasty

Chapter 35: Cervical Disc Replacement Revisions: Clinical and Biomechanical Considerations

## REFERENCES


1. McAfee PC, Cunningham BW, Orbegoso CM, et al: Analysis of porous ingrowth in intervertebral disc prostheses: A non-human primate model. Spine 28:332–340, 2003.
2. McAfee PC, Cunningham BW, Dmitriev A, et al: Cervical disc replacement—porous coated motion prosthesis: A comparative biomechanical analysis showing the key role of the posterior longitudinal ligament. Spine 28:S167–S185, 2003.
3. McAfee PC: Artificial disc prosthesis: The Link SB Charité. *In* Kaech DL, Jinkins JR (eds): Spinal Restabilization Procedures. Philadelphia, Elsevier Science B.V., 2002, pp. 299–310.
4. Lewis GL: Properties of crosslinked ultra-high-molecular-weight polyethylene. Biomaterials 22:371–401, 2001.
5. Cunningham BW, Gordon JD, Dmietriev AE, et al: Biomechanical evaluation of total disk arthroplasty: and in-vitro human cadaveric model. Presented at the international meeting of advanced spinal technologies (IMAST), Montreaux, Switzerland, May 2002.
6. Pimenta L, McAfee PC, Cappuccino A, et al: Superiority of Multiple Cervical Arthroplasty Outcomes Versus Single Level Outcomes—229 Consecutive PCM Prostheses. Palm Beach, FL, CSRS, 2006.
7. Geisler FH, Caspar W, Pitzen T, Johnson TA: Reoperation in patients after anterior cervical plate stabilization in degenerative disease. Spine 23:911–920, 1998.
8. Goffin J, Calenbergh FV, Loon JV: Intermediate follow up after treatment of degenerative disc disease with the bryan cervical disc prosthesis: single-level and bi-level. Spine 28:2673–2678, 2003.
9. Hilibrand AS, Carlson GD, Palumbo MA, et al: Radiculopathy and myelopathy at segments adjacent to the site of a previous anterior cervical arthrodesis. J Bone Joint Surg 81-A:519–528, 1999.
10. McAfee PC, Cunningham BW, Devine JD, et al: Classification of Heterotopic Ossification (HO) in Artificial Disk Replacement. Proceedings of the 17th Annual Meeting of the North American Spine Society in Montreal, Canada. Spine J 94S–98S, 2002.

CHAPTER 25

# ProDisc-C Total Cervical Disc Replacement

**Rick B. Delamarter** and **Ben B. Pradhan**

**KEY POINTS**

- The ProDisc-C is a two-piece semiconstrained artificial cervical disc consisting of two metallic end plates and a polyethylene liner fixed to the bottom end plate.
- The semiconstrained mechanics of the device allow it to share shear (translational) forces with the posterior facet joints.
- The plasma sprayed finish and small keels on the end plates allow for immediate fixation as well as longer term bony ingrowth.
- The enrollment phase of a U.S. pivotal Food and Drug Adminstration (FDA) IDE study has been completed for this device, and the 2-year follow-up data for the entire multicenter cohort are being studied before likely full FDA approval for implantation.
- Multilevel disc replacements are possible with the ProDisc-C device and have been performed at two and three levels.

## INTRODUCTION

There have been limited published reports on the clinical results of cervical artificial disc replacement. Goffin et al[1] reported a 90% rate of good to excellent results at 1 to 2 years after cervical disc arthroplasty with the Bryan prosthesis. Wigfield et al[2] reported a 46% improvement in pain and a 31% improvement in disability 2 years after implantation of the Prestige cervical artificial disc. Our own institute[7] reported the early outcomes after ProDisc-C implantation, with significant reductions in visual analog pain and Oswestry disability scores. Longer term follow-up from the prospective, randomized, and controlled U.S. IDE trial at our center is reported in this chapter.

## INDICATIONS/CONTRAINDICATIONS

The inclusion and exclusion criteria for this device appear in Table 25–1, as listed for the pivotal U.S. Food and Drug Administration (FDA) clinical trials. The FDA has allowed some deviation from the strict requirements of the study on a carefully considered case-by-case basis, under the stipulation of "compassionate usage," such as for two- and three-level disc replacements for multilevel disease, disc replacement next to prior fusions to avoid fusion extension, and so on.

## DESCRIPTION OF THE DEVICE

The ProDisc-C prosthesis (Synthes, West Chester, PA) (Fig. 25–1) shares many of the physical characteristics of the ProDisc-L (Synthes, West Chester, PA) lumbar prosthesis. The device is essentially a ball-and-socket joint: The end plates are constructed of a cobalt-chrome alloy, and the articulating convex insert is made of ultra-high-molecular-weight polyethylene (UHMWPE). Both of these are proven materials with an extensive track record in hip and knee arthroplasty. Both upper and lower end plates have slotted keels and titanium plasma spray coating. These design characteristics allow for immediate fixation onto the vertebral end plates, as well as long-term fixation via bony ingrowth.

The UHMWPE insert is fixed onto the lower end plate. The kinematic philosophy of the ProDisc-C prosthesis again parallels that of the ProDisc-L. This is a semiconstrained device with a fixed axis of rotation. Rotation is allowed along all three axes. Translation is constrained. However, because the axis of rotation for the device actually lies inferior to the disc space, translation is not eliminated. Minute (~1 mm) anterior and posterior translational shift is allowed during flexion and extension (Fig. 25–2), as is seen physiologically. However, excessive translation is not allowed, protecting the facet joints from undue loading in the absence of the native disc. It is hoped that this method will prevent accelerated degeneration of the facet joints, which would otherwise bear the majority of the shear stabilization load in the presence of a nonconstrained artificial disc. However, the semiconstrained dynamics does shift shear load from the facets to the prosthesis-bone interface, highlighting the importance of the prosthesis fixation features mentioned earlier.

Based on human anatomic studies, four different prosthetic disc heights are available, ranging from 5 to 8 mm.[4,5] Disc height restoration is key in maintaining cervical lordosis and foraminal height. Similarly, six different footprint sizes are available. The largest allowable footprint size is necessary to optimize load distribution and to decrease risk of subsidence. Angular motion in the sagittal, coronal, and axial planes is also matched to physiologic intervertebral motion, which is important if abnormal loading or motion is to be avoided in the remaining unaffected segments. Again, based on human anatomic studies, the ProDisc-C device

TABLE 25-1. Inclusion and Exclusion Criteria for the U.S. IDE Clinical Trials for ProDisc-C

| Inclusion Criteria | Exclusion Criteria |
|---|---|
| 1. Symptomatic cervical disc disease in only one vertebral level between C3 and C7 defined as neck or arm (radicular) pain; and/or functional/neurologic deficit with at least one of the following conditions confirmed by imaging (CT, MRI, or x-ray studies):<br>a. Herniated nucleus pulposus;<br>b. Spondylosis (presence of osteophytes); and/or<br>c. Loss of disc height.<br>2. Age between 18 and 60 years.<br>3. Unresponsive to nonoperative treatment for 6 weeks or presence of progressive symptoms or signs of nerve root/spinal cord compression.<br>4. Neck Disability Index score greater than or equal to 15/50 (30%).<br>5. Psychosocially, mentally, and physically able to comply with the postoperative protocol.<br>6. Signed informed consent. | 1. More than one vertebral level requiring treatment.<br>2. Marked cervical instability on resting lateral or flexion-extension radiographs:<br>a. translation greater than 3 mm and/or<br>b. greater than 11 degrees of angular motion.<br>3. Has a fused level adjacent to the level to be treated.<br>4. Radiographic confirmation of severe facet joint disease or degeneration.<br>5. Known allergy to cobalt, chromium, molybdenum, titanium, or polyethylene.<br>6. Clinically compromised vertebral bodies at the affected level(s) due to current or past trauma, e.g., by the radiographic appearance of fracture callus, malunion, or nonunion.<br>7. Prior surgery at the level to be treated.<br>8. Severe spondylosis at the level to be treated as characterized by any of the following:<br>a. bridging osteophytes;<br>b. loss of disc height greater than 50%; or<br>c. absence of motion (<2 deg).<br>9. Neck or arm pain of unknown etiology.<br>10. Osteoporosis: If DEXA is required, exclusion defined as T score less than or equal to −2.5.<br>11. Paget's disease, osteomalacia, or any other metabolic bone disease.<br>12. Severe diabetes mellitus requiring insulin.<br>13. Pregnant or possible pregnancy in next 3 years.<br>14. Active infection—systemic or local.<br>15. Concurrent drugs that affect healing (e.g., steroids).<br>16. Rheumatoid arthritis or other autoimmune disease.<br>17. Systemic disease, including AIDS, HIV, hepatitis, and so on.<br>18. Active malignancy. |

AIDS, acquired immunodeficiency syndrome; CT, computed tomography; HIV, human immunodeficiency virus; IDE, Investigational Device Exemption; MRI, magnetic resonance imaging.

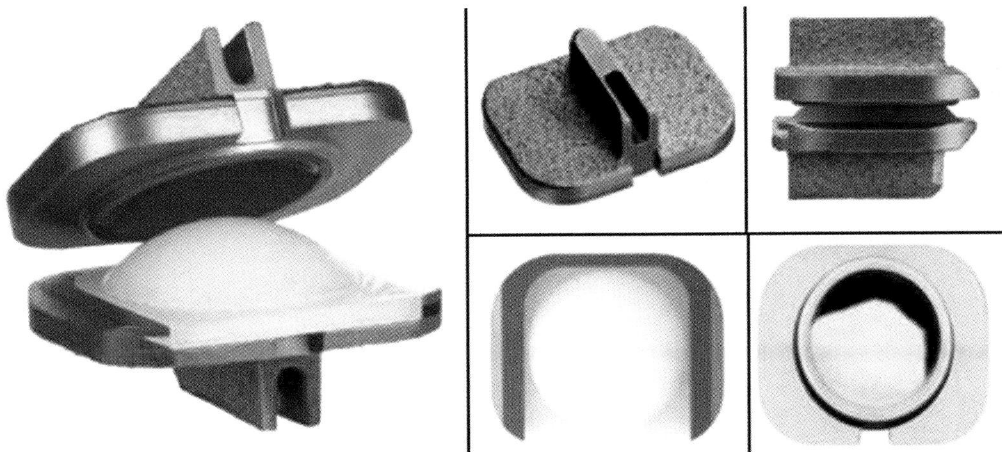

■ FIGURE 25-1. The ProDisc-C artificial cervical disc. *(Courtesy of Synthes, Paoli, PA).*

allows a maximum of 20 degrees of flexion-extension, 20 degrees of side-to-side bending, and 12 degrees of axial rotation.[6]

## BACKGROUND OF SCIENTIFIC TESTING/CLINICAL OUTCOMES

The first ProDisc-C implantation was performed in December of 2002. Since then, more than 6,000 prostheses have been implanted worldwide at the time of writing of this chapter. Multilevel disc replacements have also been performed. In the original European studies, there have been no device-related failures reported. The first implantation in the United States was performed at our center in August of 2003. Since then, more than 200 implantations have been performed in 15 centers across the country as part of the U.S. IDE study and many more as part of a "continued access" or "compassionate use" allowance by the FDA. The study enrollment phase is complete, with the FDA now analyzing the data for 2 years of follow-up.

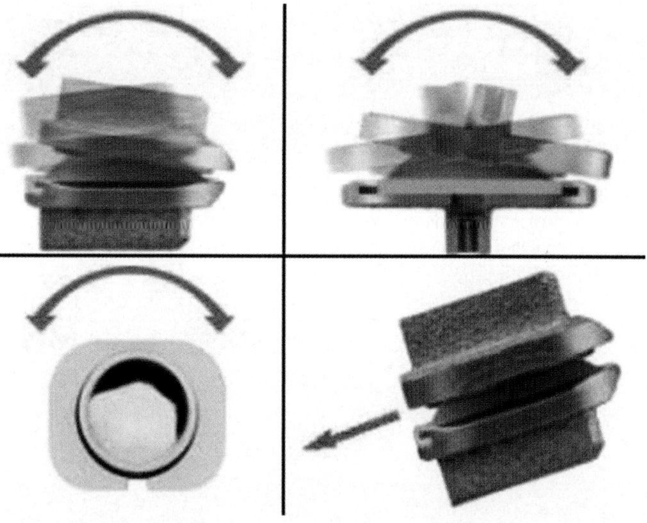

■ **FIGURE 25–2.** The ProDisc-C kinematics.

## The U.S. IDE Trial

Table 25–1 lists the eligibility criteria for the U.S. IDE study on spinal arthroplasty with the ProDisc-C device versus anterior cervical discectomy and fusion. In general, patients were selected for degenerative disc disease at one level between C3 to C7 causing intractable neck and or arm pain. Table 25–2 lists the demographic characteristics of the patients enrolled at our site for one-level disc replacements. Results for our first 48 patients were recently reported at the North American Spine Society annual meeting.[7] This included 14 disc replacement patients in the randomized trial, 19 disc replacement patients in the continued access one-level disc replacement group, and 15 patients who underwent fusion from the randomized trial. Randomization was performed at a 1:1 ratio to anterior cervical disc replacement (ACDR) versus anterior cervical discectomy and fusion (ACDF). Pain, disability, and range of motion were evaluated at preoperative, 6 weeks, 3-, 6-, 12-, and 24- to 36-month follow-up visits. Because not all patients had reached 36-month follow-up, they were included in with the 24-month follow-up group.

Clinical outcome scores revealed significant improvements in Visual Analog Scale (VAS) scores for both neck pain (Fig. 25–3) and arm pain (Fig. 25–4) and ODI scores (Fig. 25–5) for both ACDR and ACDF patients. By 3 months, VAS (neck) scores were down by more than half in both disc replacement and in fusion patients. VAS (arm) scores improved even more significantly in both groups by 3 months. Both of these improvements stayed significant at 24 months and later. ODI scores similarly decreased at more than 24 months in disc replacement and fusion patients respectively, reaching values one half or less of preoperative values at final follow-up. Although all of the outcome measures decreased significantly from preoperative status ($P < 0.05$), they were not seen to be significantly different between treatment modalities (disc replacement versus fusion, $P > 0.05$).

Average flexion-extension motion went from 9 degrees preoperatively to about 1 degree (essentially no motion) at more than 24 months postoperatively in the fusion group but was well preserved at about 12 degrees in the disc replacement group. Side bending went from 6 degrees to less than 2 degrees (essentially no motion) in the fusion group versus about 5 degrees in disc replacement patients. There were no major complications, technique or device-related, in any of the cases. Figure 25–6 represents the sagittal angular motion measured radiographically at the operated segment. As expected, motion is effectively eliminated at fusion levels, whereas angular motion is well preserved with the prosthetic discs.

So the conclusion of the U.S. IDE trial was essentially that ACDR preserves range of motion without compromising the results as compared with the current surgical standard of ACDF. It is hoped that in the long run, the preserved motion will decrease adjacent segment degeneration.

## OPERATIVE TECHNIQUE

A standard anterior approach to the cervical spine is performed. Any operating table that allows supine positioning and fluoroscopy of the neck can be used. No external traction of the spine is necessary. A transverse skin incision is made over the level being operated, after localizing either by anatomic landmarks or with a lateral radiographic image (a fluoroscopy machine is used for the duration of instrumentation with the ProDisc-C). After incising through the skin, subcutaneous fascia, platysma muscle, and superficial layer of the deep cervical fascia, blunt dissection is performed first between the strap muscles medially and the sternocleidomastoid laterally then the tracheoesophageal bundle medially and the carotid sheath laterally. The prevertebral fascia is then split to expose the disc space. Before the discectomy, another localizing radiograph is performed.

**TABLE 25–2. Patient Demographics**

| Patient Characteristic | ACDF (allograft + plate) ($n = 15$) | ACDR (ProDisc-C) ($n = 33$) | $P$-Value (NS is > 0.05) |
|---|---|---|---|
| Average age (years) | 42.5 | 40.1 | NS |
| Gender (% male: % female) | 33:67 | 20:80 | NS |
| Body mass index (BMI) | 24.9 | 23.7 | NS |
| Workman's compensation status | 27% | 20% | NS |
| Preoperative duration of neck pain (months) | 10.5 | 10.3 | NS |
| Active smokers | 1 (6.6%) | 4 (16.7%) | NS |

ACDF, anterior cervical discectomy and fusion; ACDR, anterior cervical discectomy replacement.

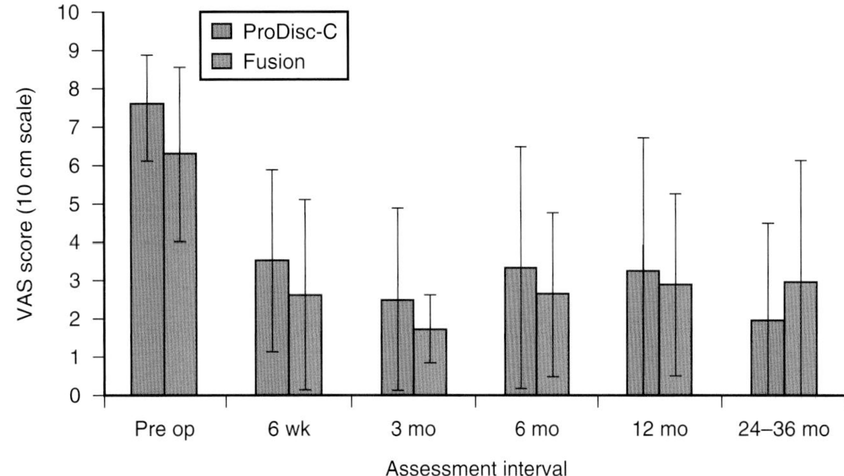


■ **FIGURE 25–3.** Visual Analog Scale (VAS) neck pain scores.

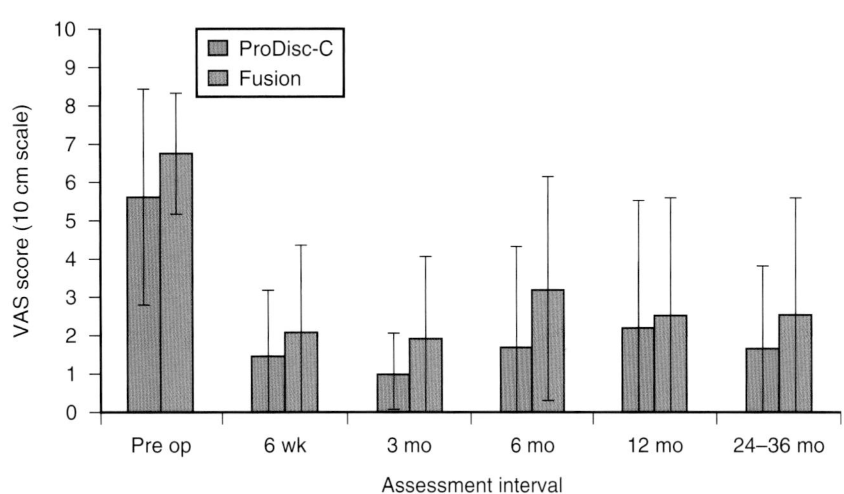


■ **FIGURE 25–4.** Visual Analog Scale (VAS) arm pain scores.

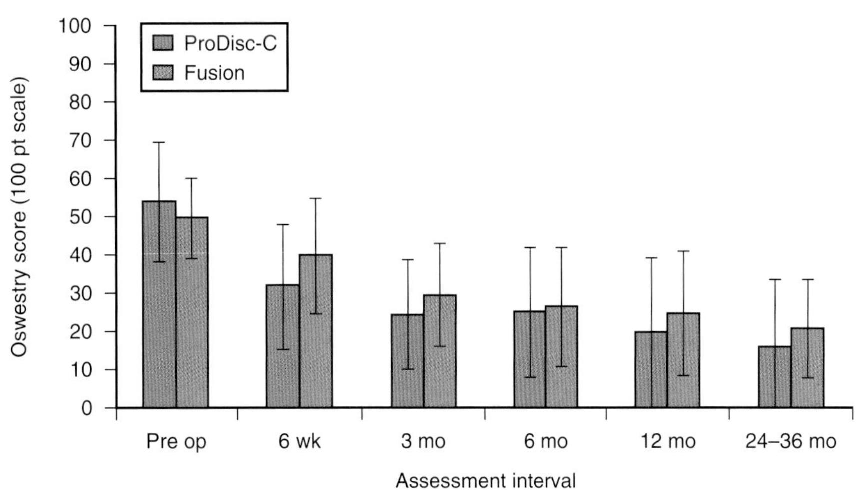


■ **FIGURE 25–5.** Oswestry Disability Index (ODI) scores.

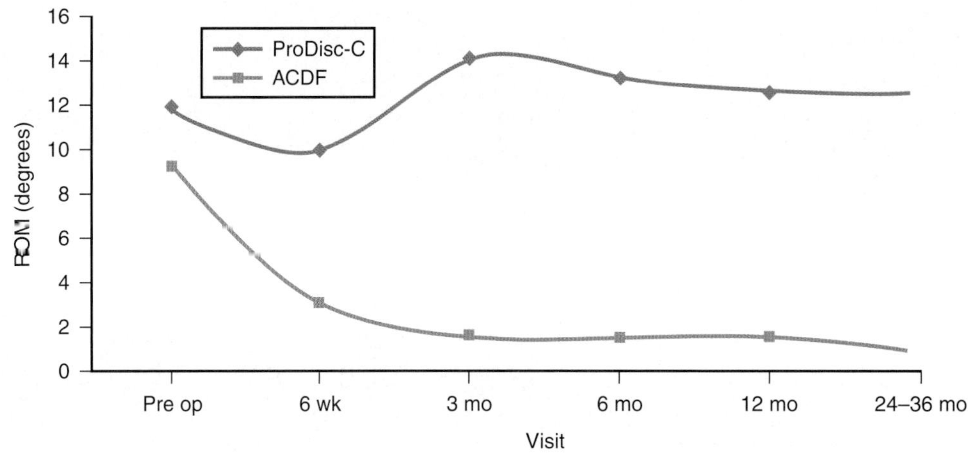


■ **FIGURE 25–6.** Sagittal angular motion in degrees.

Once the operative level is confirmed, self-retaining retractors are placed mediolaterally and superoinferiorly (Fig. 25–7). The fluoroscopy machine is positioned to allow anteroposterior and lateral imaging during the procedure. Midline in the anteroposterior plane is marked on the vertebral bodies spanning the operative disc, using the fluoroscopy machine. Manual discectomy is then performed.

Specialized pin distractors are then placed in the spanning vertebral bodies. These pins are actually fastened onto the distractor using nuts, making this device a rigid fixator (similar to an external fixator) rather than simply a distractor (Fig 25–7 and 25–8). Not only does this provide distraction for easier removal of disc tissue but it also provides rigid stabilization during instrumentation so that the relative alignment of the vertebral bodies is maintained. This prevents excessive jolting movements of the vertebral bodies and neural elements during impacting of the implant, and it also ensures precise and symmetric placement of the device keels within both vertebrae (avoiding any listhesis, see Fig. 25–8).

Disc resection is performed entirely manually, with minimal need for end plate preparation (e.g., burring, milling, and so on). The two keels and the porous-coated surfaces of the ProDisc-C provide enough initial fixation to obviate any end plate milling or preparation, which removes end plate bone and can risk loss of segmental lordosis and implant subsidence. Occasionally, osteophyte resection or end plate flattening with a bur or Kerrison rongeur may be necessary. The posterior longitudinal ligament may or may not be removed depending on the location of herniated disc or osteophyte.

Once the disc space is adequately cleared, trial sizing with the help of fluoroscopy is performed (see Fig. 25–8). The implant size that maximizes end plate coverage is chosen. Appropriate disc height is selected based upon the tightness of fit and the relative heights of the unaffected adjacent segments. Overstuffing or undersizing of the implant can both compromise stability and range of motion. Once the size of the implant is selected, an osteotome is slid over the trial (which acts as a stop) and malleted through the previously marked midline on the vertebrae to create a channel for the keels (see Fig. 25–8). A sharp chisel is followed by a box osteotome to widen the slot for the keels. This prevents excessive stress on the vertebrae during implant placement and also prevents posterior displacement of bony fragments. After the chiseling, the actual implant is then carefully malleted into place

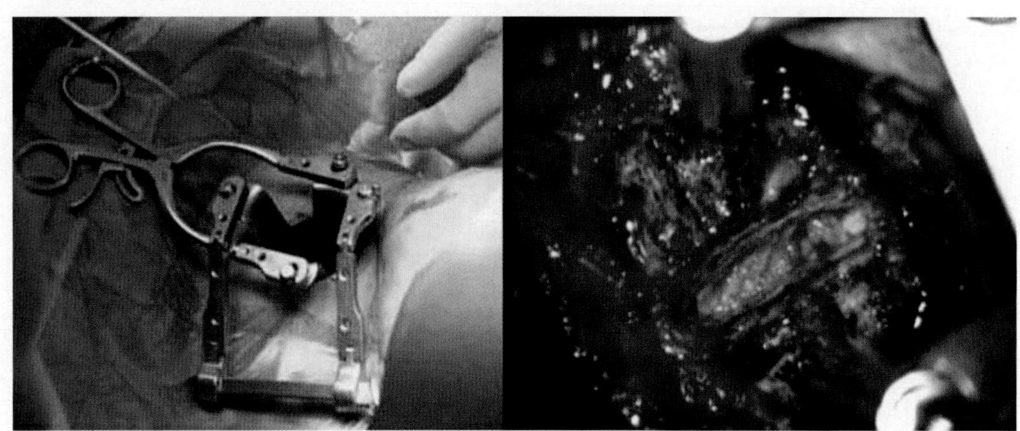

■ **FIGURE 25–7.** Anterior exposure and discectomy.

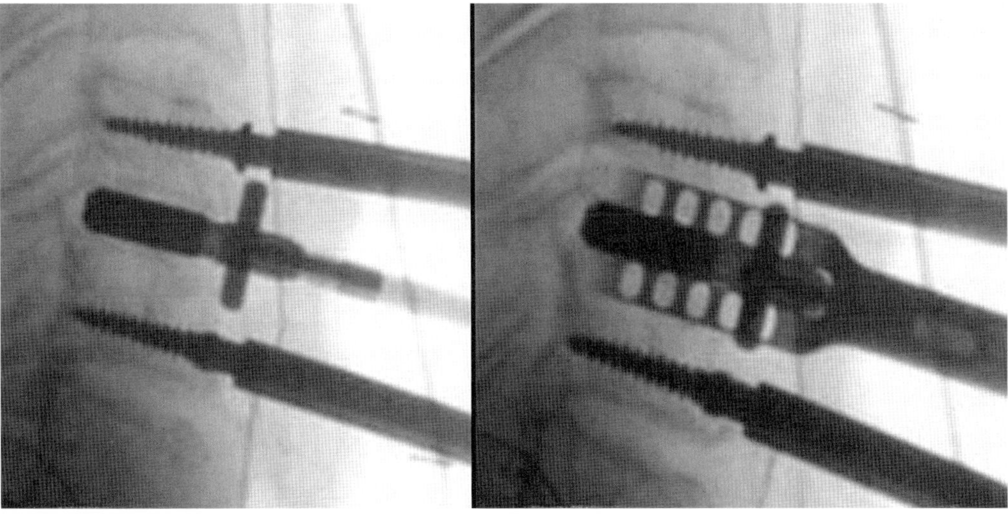

■ **FIGURE 25–8.** Trialing and chiseling under fluoroscopy.

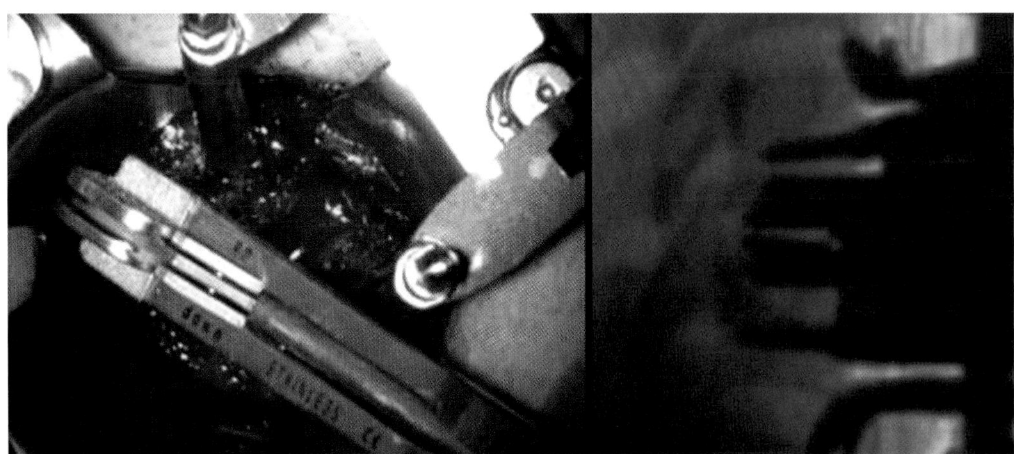

■ **FIGURE 25–9.** Insertion of prosthesis under fluoroscopy.

under fluoroscopic guidance (Fig. 25–9). The fixator, pins, and retractors are then removed, and closure is performed.

## POSTOPERATIVE CARE

A soft neck collar can be used for the first week or two to allow for wound protection. Otherwise there is no extensive postoperative protocol. Patients can return to work as soon as comfortable but should allow 6 weeks before returning to recreational sports or full duty (if the job is physically demanding).

## COMPLICATIONS AND AVOIDANCE

No major technique- or device-related complications were observed. Table 25–3 lists the complications for patients undergoing ACDR and ACDF. There was one revision surgery in each group. No device migration or subsidence requiring further treatment has been seen to date. This may be related to the screening out of osteoporotic patients, who would be high risk for such issues. The incidence of prolonged dysphagia, defined loosely as patient-subjective swallowing difficulty lasting more than 6 weeks, was

**TABLE 25–3. Complications From the U.S. IDE Study of ProDisc-C Versus ACDF**

| Complication | ProDisc-C (%) | ACDF (allograft + plate) (%) |
|---|---|---|
| Implant migration/subsidence | 0/33 (0) | 0/15 (0) |
| Nonunion | NA | 1/15 (6.7) |
| Revision surgery | 1/33 (3) | 1/15 (6.7) |
| Prolonged dysphagia | 2/33 (6) | 1/15 (6.7) |
| Postoperative swallow study, laryngoscopy, or other throat workup | 0/33 (0) | 0/15 (0) |
| Superficial infection | 1/33 (3) | 1/15 (6.7) |
| Deep infection | 0/33 (0) | 0/15 (0) |
| New transient symptoms* | 2/33 (6) | 2/15 (13.4) |

ACDF, anterior cervical discectomy and fusion; IDE, Investigational Device Exemption.
*Subsided by 6 weeks to 3 months after surgery.

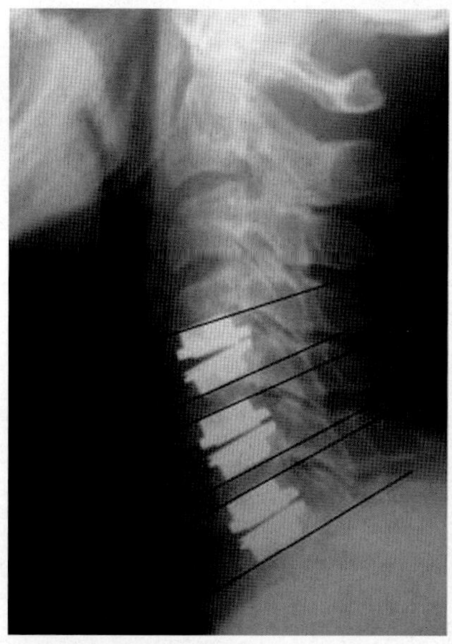
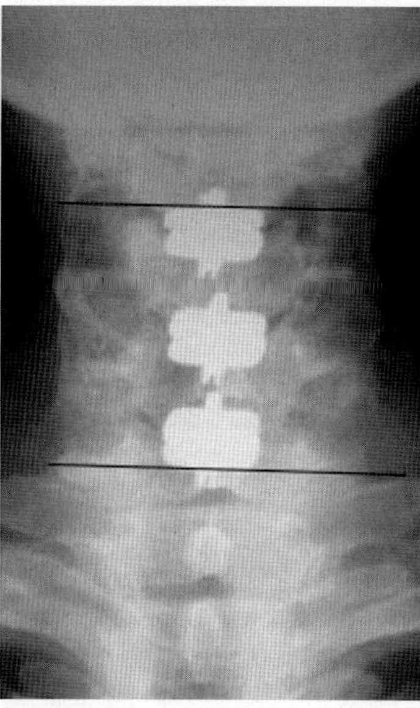

■ **FIGURE 25–10.** Example of multilevel cervical artificial disc replacement, 12 months after surgery.

minimal in either group. Patients claiming dysphagia were still eating a regular diet with solid foods. No swallow studies or any other post operative throat evaluations were needed for further persistent swallowing, breathing, or vocal difficulties in either study group. Transient new symptoms were observed in two patients each in the ACDF and ACDR groups. These were defined as spontaneous new-onset radiculopathy, numbness, or subjective weakness. All new symptoms subsided by 6 weeks to 3 months after surgery.

**ADVANTAGES/DISADVANTAGES: ProDisc-C TOTAL CERVICAL DISC REPLACEMENT**

| Advantages | Disadvantages |
|---|---|
| Semiconstrained motion is facet protective | Greater device-bone interface loading |
| Good fixation features (keels, coating) | Questionable risk of vertebral fractures (especially during multilevel use) |
| Familiar cobalt-chrome and polyethylene materials | Long-term data (5 to 10 years) from Class I data are still pending |
| No device protrusions beyond disc space | Questionable risk of polyethylene debris |
| Class I U.S. FDA clinical data available | |
| Multilevel disc replacements possible and clinical data also available (2 and 3 levels) | |
| Good experience: more than 6,000 implanted worldwide at time of writing (Aug 2006) | |
| Easily revisable (both approach and device extraction with designated instruments) | |

FDA, Food and Drug Administration.

## CONCLUSIONS/DISCUSSION

Our experience with the ProDisc-C artificial cervical disc suggests that cervical disc replacement is a viable surgical alternative to fusion for cervical disc degeneration and herniation, with preservation of motion and alignment at the treated vertebral levels and without compromising clinical outcomes. Although it is yet too early for the U.S. clinical trials to offer any definite proof of benefit against accelerated adjacent segment degeneration, the fact that normal intervertebral motion is preserved at the treated segment is encouraging. Longer term safety and efficacy studies are in progress.

This particular device has been used extensively for multilevel use, with as good or better clinical outcomes as compared with single-level surgeries and with good preservation of motion at each replaced level, good preservation of spinal alignment at each replaced level, and great patient satisfaction scores (Fig. 25–10). The technique and instrumentation are facile and streamlined, but the instruments continue to be refined still. One of the salient improvements has been in the way the keel cuts are made in the vertebrae: A drill with a protective guide has been built to seamlessly drill the keel grooves on the bone, thus minimizing the risk of vertebral splitting fractures, especially when performing multilevel disc replacement. The drill also minimizes malleting on the spine.

## REFERENCES


1. Goffin J, Van Calenbergh F, van Loon J, et al: Intermediate follow-up after treatment of degenerative disc disease with the Bryan Cervical Disc Prosthesis: single-level and bi-level. Spine 28:2673–2678, 2003.
2. Wigfield CC, Gill SS, Nelson RJ, et al: The new Frenchay artificial cervical joint: results from a two-year pilot study. Spine 27:2446–2452, 2002.
3. Delamarter RB, Pradhan BB: Indications for cervical spine prostheses, early experiences with ProDisc-C in the USA. Spine Art 1:7–9, 2004.
4. Panjabi M, Duranceau J, Goel V, et al: Cervical human vertebrae: quantitative three-dimensional anatomy of the middle and lower regions. Spine 16:861–869, 1991.
5. Yoganandan N, Lumaresan S, Printat F: Biomechanics of the cervical spine, Part 2: Cervical spine soft tissue responses and biomechanical modeling. Clin Biomech 16:1–27, 2001.
6. White A, Panjabi M: Clinical Biomechanics of the Spine. Philadelphia, J. B. Lippincott Co., 1990, pp 110–111.
7. Pradhan BB, Delamarter RB, Bae HW, et al: 2- to 3-Year Results with the ProDisc-C Cervical Disc Replacement from the US Clinical Trials. North American Spine Society annual meeting, Seattle, WA, September, 2006.

CHAPTER 26

# The NeoDisc Elastomeric Cervical Total Disc Replacement

Andre Jackowski, Alan McLeod, Christopher Reah, G. Bryan Cornwall, Lukas Eisermann, and Alexander W.L. Turner

## KEY POINTS

- The surgical technique for the NeoDisc device is less demanding than other cervical total disc replacement designs, in particular requiring less exactness in placing the device relative to the natural center of rotation.
- The materials used to construct the NeoDisc device are amenable to MRI investigation and do not obstruct x-rays.
- Biomechanically, the design of the NeoDisc device is closer to the natural cervical disc than a traditional articulating mechanical artificial disc. It will not impose a fixed center or arc of rotation on the disc level and offers an element of shock absorption.
- The NeoDisc device has very low wear rates in testing.
- Soft tissue ingrowth has been demonstrated in the NeoDisc device and has the potential to provide a secure long-term fixation.

## INTRODUCTION

The operation of anterior cervical decompression and interbody fusion has been a widely accepted surgical procedure in the treatment of radiculopathy or myelopathy since the original reports of Cloward in 1958[1] and Robinson and Smith in 1955.[2] Since that time, surgeons have employed these two operative techniques and their variations in the treatment of patients who present with persisting radicular pain and evidence of cervical compressive myelopathy.

Two considerations have led several researchers to investigate alternative forms of surgical treatment utilizing nonfusion technology. The first is that there is a small but significant number of patients who suffer complications in the form of either graft site donor pain or graft complications including collapse, expulsion, or nonintegration. The second consideration is the desire to maintain motion at the operated segment together with concern from a number of investigators that motion segment fusion can lead to accelerated adjacent-level degeneration and subsequent, adverse clinical sequelae.[3–6]

The rationale for developing and implanting a cervical disc prosthesis is that such a device may allow the following:

1. the maintenance of segmental mobility;
2. avoidance of altered adjacent segment mobility;
3. avoidance of or reduction in the incidence of adjacent motion segment disease;
4. the potential for more rapid functional recovery.

The design of an elastomeric artificial cervical disc prosthesis is influenced by the fact that the cervical disc is not a lubricated articulating synovial joint but is a deforming fibrocartilaginous joint. Elastomeric materials offer the potential to closely mimic the behavior of a natural intervertebral disc in a way that more traditional ball-and-socket devices cannot. Extensive initial testing was performed on a variety of elastomeric materials in conjunction with enveloping textile jackets and an artificial annulus or ligament in order to find the combination of materials that most closely mimics the natural joint. The design concepts for the NeoDisc are for the device to not only replace the disc but to also replicate the functions of the anterior and posterior longitudinal ligaments.

To reduce the learning curve associated with adopting a new technology, the surgeon should not have to radically alter his or her standard practice when doing an anterior cervical discectomy. That is, the ideally designed prosthesis fits a standard surgical defect following a microdiscectomy or Smith-Robinson decompression. There is no requirement for special jigs or templates and no need to mill the end plate or to alter the end plate to fit the device. By realizing these objectives, the operation time would be shortened rather than increased over current practice. Additionally, the ideal device is free of magnetic resonance imaging (MRI) and computed tomography (CT) scan artifact so as to allow for immediate and future patient investigations.

To achieve satisfactory integration with the implanted motion segment, the implanted device should achieve the following objectives:

1. allow for normal spinal biomechanics and not impose its own variable instantaneous access and rotation but adapt to the native axis of rotation;
2. not block motion within the patients normal range of motion;
3. allow coupled motions;
4. allow for a shock-absorption function.

To achieve immediate stability, the implant design incorporates fixation flanges that are anchored by traditional screws to the adjacent vertebral bodies. For long-term stability, the enveloping embroidered jacket has a naturally porous three-dimensional surface to allow adjacent end plate fibrous ingrowth. An elastomeric device can incorporate an artificial ligament to replicate the function of the anterior longitudinal ligament to avoid expulsion of the device either anteriorly or posteriorly during motion.

The biocompatibility of the materials used in the device is of great importance because any material that is to be implanted into the human body must have excellent biocompatibility to avoid failure of the device. The device, therefore, was manufactured using an elastomeric core and an enveloping jacket that are constructed of biomaterials that have an extensive clinical history within orthopaedic surgery, neurosurgery, and reconstructive surgery.

## INDICATIONS/CONTRAINDICATIONS

At the time of this writing, the NeoDisc (Nu Vasive, Inc., San Diego, CA) is under clinical use in studies that require regulatory approval to be conducted. Thus, at this stage, the inclusion-exclusion criteria have been tightly controlled in order to collect good quality data to support regulatory approval of the device. It is anticipated that in broader clinical usage, the indications will become broader in their scope. The indications and contraindications selected for the U.K. clinical trial are as follows:

### Indications

- Patients 18 years of age or older.
- Patients who, in the opinion of the clinical investigator, are suitable for the intended surgical procedure.
- Patients who have failed to adequately improve following at least an 8-week period of conservative management.
- Patients with evidence of spinal cord and/or nerve root compression causing myelopathy or radiculopathy that can be attributed to degenerative changes in a disc at a single cervical level corresponding with symptoms and confirmed using MRI, CT, or myelography within the last 6 months.
- Patients who are able to give voluntary, written informed consent to participate in this clinical investigation and from whom consent has been obtained.
- Patients who are, in the opinion of the clinical investigator, able to understand this clinical investigation, able to cooperate with the investigational procedures, and are willing to return to the hospital for all the required postoperative follow-up examinations.

### Contraindications

- Patients who, in the opinion of the clinical investigator, have an existing condition that would compromise their participation and follow-up in this clinical investigation.
- Patients who have compromised bone quality by osteoporosis, infection, inflammatory arthritis, or tumor.
- Patients who have had previous cervical spine surgery at the level being considered, including posterior surgery.
- Patients with evidence of instability, defined as greater than 3.5 mm sagittal-plane displacement (anterior translation of the anteroinferior corner of the moving vertebra) either on resting or on flexion-extension radiographic examination.
- Patients who require surgical intervention at more than one level of the spine.
- Patients with any active infection at time of surgery.
- Patients who have been clinically diagnosed with whiplash syndrome.
- Female patients who are pregnant or could be pregnant.
- Patients who are known drug or alcohol abusers or with psychological disorders that could affect follow-up care or treatment outcomes.
- Patients who have participated in a clinical investigation with an investigational product within 6 months before treatment.
- Patients who are currently involved in any injury litigation claims.

## DESCRIPTION OF THE DEVICE

The NeoDisc device is a multipart artificial disc intended to replace the function of the native intervertebral disc. The implanted device is composed of an elastomeric nucleus contained within an embroidered polyester fabric, secured by four bone screws. This device has two integral fixation flanges, each of which has a pair of fixation holes (Fig. 26–1). Fixation of the device occurs through three steps:

1. implantation with a secure interference fit;
2. supplementary mechanical fixation through anchoring of the flanges using bone screws;
3. additional biologic fixation through the process of soft tissue ingrowth in to the encapsulating polyester jacket of the device.

### Embroidered Jacket

The outer jacket of the NeoDisc device is a highly engineered textile, manufactured from polyester suture using a computer-controlled embroidery process. The use of embroidery allows for the individual placement of threads within the textile, where each thread size can also be chosen to optimize its strength/bulk characteristics. The complex design of the jacket includes an interdigitation of the fixation flanges. The jacket has two separate fixation flanges—the flange emanating from the superior surface passes through the flange that emanates from the inferior surface. The advantages of the NeoDisc textile design areas follow:

1. Conventional elastomeric artificial disc design concepts bond the elastomer to metallic end plates. In these designs, extension of the neck would subject the elastomeric core to a potentially damaging tensile load. However, for the NeoDisc with its textile encapsulation of the elastomeric core, as the flanges are pulled in opposite directions, it is a compression load that is passed to the core that the elastomer is ideally suited to withstand.
2. Secure fixation of the device combined with the ability to resist anterior device migration. It is during extension motions that grafts or implants are most likely to migrate anteriorly, but

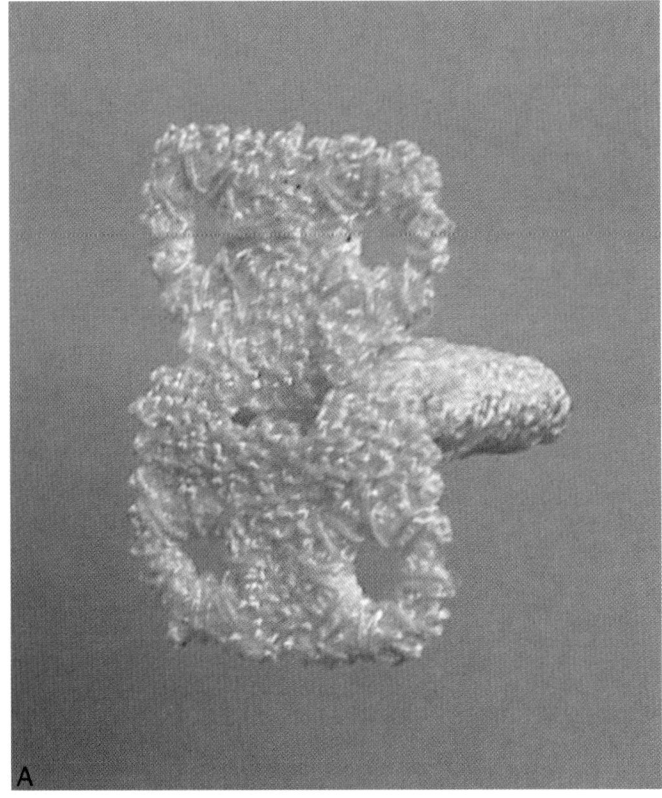


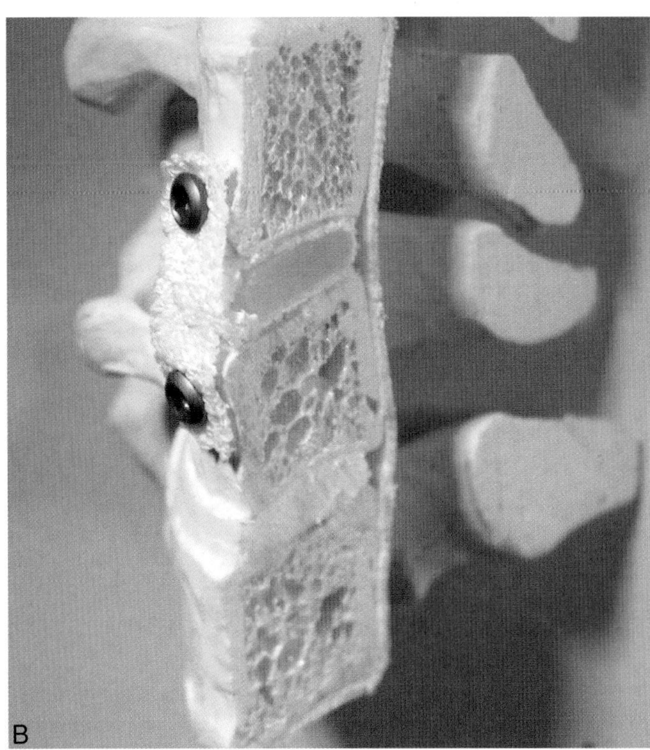


■ **FIGURE 26–1.** NeoDisc device. **A,** Photograph of the device illustrating the fixation flanges. **B,** Cross-sectional view of the device showing the construction.

for the NeoDisc, the more the neck is extended, the tighter the flanges are at the point where they interdigitate through each other. This has the effect of securely holding the main body of the device within the disc space.

3. Allow for a full range of motion. In extension, although a flat textile flange passing across or attached to the anterior surface of the device would help to prevent anterior migration, it would also act to limit extension. However, the interdigitated flanges not only prevent migration but they also still allow a natural extension motion. This is possible because in extension it is not only the flange that stretches but also the encapsulating fabric that is tensioned around the core.

Polyester was chosen as the material to construct the textile element of the NeoDisc because of its extensive history of successful clinical use in various devices where tissue ingrowth in to the device is desired; it has an extensive clinical history, particularly in vascular applications as a strong, stable, biocompatible material.

### Elastomeric Core

A medical implant-grade silicone is molded to form the compliant nucleus of the NeoDisc device. It is important to note that the silicone elastomer is solid and does not contain silicone gel. Solid silicone elastomers have been commonly used in a variety of biomedical devices for more than 40 years with a proven safety record.

## BACKGROUND OF SCIENTIFIC TESTING AND CLINICAL OUTCOMES

### Bench Top Mechanical Evaluation of the NeoDisc Device

#### Wear Testing

In order to test the size of implant most at risk of failure, the smallest available NeoDisc device was selected. Eight specimens of this size were tested.

Fluids used in medical device testing are typically either saline, bovine serum, or fetal calf serum. Using either bovine serum or fetal calf serum while testing a polyester textile implant will result in protein deposition on the textile, which would render all weight loss measurements meaningless because, even with soak controls, it will be impossible to allow for this variable. Thus, the test medium used for the NeoDisc device testing was saline. Each sample was tested in its own individual environment from which the fluid could be collected for particle analysis purposes.

The compressive load on the devices was maintained at an average of 100 N (± 5 N), as specified in ASTM standard F2423–05 as being a representative compressive load under which to conduct testing for cervical disc implants.

The three motions that occur within the cervical spine are flexion-extension, lateral bending, and axial rotation. For the ASTM test, the following motions are used: flexion-extension, ±7.5 degrees; lateral bending, ±6 degrees; and axial rotation, ±6 degrees. The requirement is for 10 million cycles of each load to be applied to the test sample. This can either be 10 million cycles of the motions combined together, or each motion can be applied individually.

In order to allow for the potential difference in results if the motion patterns were reversed, the following test procedure was used:

- Group A (devices 1, 2, 3, and 4) was tested for 10 million cycles of ± 7.5 degrees of flexion-extension motion, followed by a further 10 million cycles of ± 6 degrees of lateral bending, coupled with ± 6 degrees of axial rotation.
- Group B (devices 5, 6, 7, and 8) was tested for 10 million cycles of ± 6 degrees of lateral bending, coupled with ± 6 degrees of axial rotation, followed by a further 10 million cycles of ± 7.5 degrees of flexion-extension.
- Additional discs were set up as soak controls, with only a pure compressive load being applied throughout the testing.

The result was that all of the test specimens received a total of 20 million cycles of wear testing.

The test medium was collected from each station every 1 million cycles. The sample showing the greatest weight loss from each group in the test had its test medium analyzed at various timepoints. The analysis was performed in accordance with ASTM standard F1877–98.

Particle analysis of the wear-tested NeoDisc devices has demonstrated that throughout the test, the particulate stayed approximately consistent in terms of size and distribution. The Feret diameters based on both particle numbers and volume did not change significantly as the test progresseed, and the two samples were reasonably consistent with each other. Therefore, there does not appear to be a difference due to the order in which the motion pattern is applied to the specimens. The roundness, aspect ratio, and form factor also stayed similar throughout the tests. There is no evidence that the change in motion after the 10 million cycle changeover caused another running-in period in which the particles changed in their morphology. The polyester particles tend to be irregular and fibrous or flaky, whereas the silicone particles are mainly spherical or spheriodal.

At 20 million cycles, the average volumetric loss of material from the NeoDisc devices was 13.8 mg (approximately 11.2 mm$^3$). This corresponds to an average of 0.69 mg per million cycles of testing (0.56 mm$^3$ per million cycles). The 20 million cycle test can be considered to be a worst case test. It is unlikely that any device in clinical use will experience this quantity of large, exaggerated motions.

### Axial Compression Testing

To assess the safety of the implant under static and dynamic compression loading, a series of tests were conducted. Measurements of the loading required to create permanent height loss in the implant were performed. Also, the fatigue resistance of the implant design was evaluated in cyclic axial compression with dynamic loading. The discs were attached to the test frame by means of Delrin fixtures contoured to the geometry of the NeoDisc device as recommended by ASTM F2346.

The smallest specimen was selected as the worst case in order to test the implant with the highest applied stress. The smallest implant would be subjected to the highest stress because the same load applied to a smaller surface area leads to higher applied stresses.

Two dynamic test specimens were tested in saline at 37°C. A sinusoidal waveform with a maximum compressive load of 500 N was applied for 10 million cycles at a 5 Hz test speed. In this test, failure was defined as a loss of device height equivalent to 50% of the height of the elastomeric core.

Five static test specimens were tested in air at room temperature. Each sample had a 50 N preload applied. The device was compressed by half of the height of the elastomeric core and the corresponding force recorded. The load was then removed and the displacement at 50 N was determined.

The dynamic test specimens reached 10 million cycles without functional failure. The samples lost 0.13 and 0.18 mm of core height. For the static fatigue test samples, the load required to compress the discs by half the core height was between 4728 and 6975 N. The residual core heights were almost unaffected, with losses from 0 to 0.02 mm.

In conclusion, the endurance limit of the NeoDisc implant under dynamic axial compression testing was determined to be at least 500 N at 10 million cycles. Static axial compression to half of the core height did not cause damage or failure of the NeoDisc implant. The safety of the NeoDisc implant subjected to this loading mode was demonstrated by minimal height loss of the silicone core.

## Shear Compression

In order to assess the safety of the implant under shear loading, devices were tested in shear compression according to ASTM F2346.

The smallest specimen was selected as worst case in order to test the implant with the highest applied stress. The smallest implant would be subjected to the highest stress because the same load applied to a smaller surface area leads to higher applied stresses.

The discs were attached to the test frame by means of fixtures contoured to the geometry of the NeoDisc, as recommended by ASTM F2346. Delrin was used in the case of the dynamic testing and stainless steel for the static testing. Two dynamic test specimens were tested in saline at 37°C. A sinusoidal waveform with a maximum compressive load of 250 N was applied at an angle of 45 degrees to the test specimens for 10 million cycles. As with the pure compression test, failure was defined as a loss of device height equivalent to 50% of the height of the elastomeric core.

Five static test specimens were tested in air at room temperature. Each sample had a 50 N preload applied. The device was compressed by half of the height of the elastomeric core and the corresponding force recorded. The load was then removed and the displacement at 50 N was determined.

The dynamic shear test specimens reached 10 million cycles without functional failure. The samples lost 0.10 and 0.18 mm of core height. For the static shear test samples, the load required to compress the discs by half the core height was between 574 and 829 N. The residual core heights were almost unaffected with losses from 0 to 0.03mm.

In conclusion, the endurance limit of the NeoDisc implant under dynamic shear compression testing was determined to be at least 250 N at 10 million cycles. Static shear compression to half of the core height did not cause damage or failure of the NeoDisc implant. The safety of the NeoDisc implant subjected to this loading mode was demonstrated by minimal height loss of the silicone core.

## PUSHOUT (EXPULSION) TESTING

Soft tissue integration of the NeoDisc acts as long-term fixation. However, it is important to be sure that the fixation method is secure to prevent migration or expulsion of the implant. Thus, testing was conducted to determine the force required to expel the disc from a simulated disc space.

The discs were attached to the test jig by means of polyurethane foam blocks that formed a simulated disc space. As with clinical use, the devices were secured to the fixtures using four titanium alloy bone screws of the type used in the European clinical trial of the NeoDisc. The smallest specimen was selected as worst case in order to test the implant with the highest applied stress. The smallest implant would be subjected to the highest stress because the same load applied to a smaller surface area leads to higher applied stresses.

Five pushout test specimens were tested in air at room temperature. A compressive load of 100 N was applied to the discs through the foam blocks to simulate the compressive axial load in the cervical spine. Loading was applied on the posterior surface of the disc in order to force it out of the simulated disc space. In this test, failure was defined as pushing the NeoDisc fixation flange off the bone screws.

In the simulated pushout testing, an average of 238 N was required to dislodge the device and 293 N in order to expel it from the disc space. In each case, the failure mode was the polyester flange pulling over the head of the screw.

No failures of this type have been seen in clinical application at the time of this writing; there has also been no evidence of anterior or posterior movement displacement of any implanted NeoDisc.

The high load required to dislodge the NeoDisc and the stability of the device in clinical use have demonstrated that this potential failure mode is not a cause for concern.

### Biomechanical Testing

The NeoDisc device is intended to replicate as closely as possible the behavior of the natural disc. Biomechanical testing was initiated to examine the behavior of the implant under a variety of physiologic loading conditions. The results of biomechanical testing of the NeoDisc device have been presented at a number of international meetings and are the subject of preparation for publication in peer-reviewed journals (Yeh and Jackowski, 1996[7]; Jackowski and Yeh, 1997[8]; Jackowski and McLeod, 2002[9]).

To develop the cervical spine model, a total of 19 cadaveric cervical spines were harvested and fresh frozen (in an unembalmed state) at minus 18°C within 24 hours of the donor's death. Nine of the specimens were used to develop the in vitro cervical spine model that was the subject of a dotoral thesis entitled "The Preparation, Development and Analysis of an In Vitro Cadaveric Model of Cervical Spine Motion" (Yeh, 1997). The model monitored motion of vertebrae by the placement of small infrared reflectors mounted on the individual spinal vertebrae. MacReflex motion analysis equipment (Qualysis AB) monitored the output from an infrared camera that tracked the position of the markers.

To examine the behavior of the NeoDisc, the testing was conducted to monitor the spine in the following motions; flexion-extension, lateral bending, and axial rotation. The test monitored the behavior both for a multilevel spine and also on the individual motion segment. Four biomechanical representations were studied; the baseline was the behavior of the intact disc; the readings were then repeated after a microdiscectomy, and then after the implantation of the device, and finally after the motion segment had been mock "fused" with the aid of an anterior spinal plate.

The analysis demonstrated that the NeoDisc device retained natural motion to within 5% of the amount of movement that would be present with the natural disc. This compared with 58% more movement following a discectomy, in which the natural disc is removed and the disc space is left empty, and 68% less movement when a bone graft and plate were used. Analysis of the single motion segment demonstrated that the NeoDisc implant could preserve 93% of the mean proportional range of motion at the operated cervical levels and keep the increase in motion at adjacent cervical segments following surgery down to only 7%. Hysteresis loops for the single motion segment model were analyzed and demonstrated that the implanted NeoDisc device left a motion segment that was an extremely good match for the natural disc in terms of flexion-extension, lateral bending, and axial rotation motions.

The compliant nature of the NeoDisc device combined with mechanical function close to that of the natural disc offer the patient a very real possibility of avoiding long-term (specifically adjacent level) issues, if such issues can truly be attributed to mechanical alterations of the adjacent levels.

## ANIMAL DATA

### Implantation Data in an Ovine Model

It is widely accepted that there is no ideal animal model to evaluate the mechanical and kinematic performance of artificial discs. However, one of the key features of the NeoDisc device is the ability of the polyester to incite the ingrowth of soft tissue into the device. An ovine model was chosen as being the best animal model to use to demonstrate this effect

A total of 10 sheep received NeoDisc implants. The sheep were sacrificed at varying time points. In all cases, there were no signs of adverse reaction to the device and the sheep were both neurologically and physically normal during the length of the study. The following observations were noted:

In all cases of animal implantation, the polyester jacket was variably integrated by either fibrocartilage or by fibrous tissue, a result consistent with the historic use of polyester. The result is that the implant becomes a silicone core surrounded by a composite structure of polyester reinforced soft tissue. The tissue integration will serve to prevent the fibers of the textile jacket from being able to wear against each other. Fibrocartilaginous integration was seen at the anterior aspect of the intervertebral part of the implant. The fibrocartilage had undergone endochondral ossification on the external periphery of the implant to become continuous with the surrounding vertebral bone; in this sense, the tissue will serve to act as a biologic anchor to the device, rendering the fixation screws superfluous.

Examination of the tissues by a histopathologist demonstrated that there was no organized lymphoid tissue, indicating a lack of immune/allergic response to the device or any wear debris that may have been generated following implantation. In all of the sheep, there was no evidence of an immune or allergic response to the implanted materials. The fibrous tissue contained a far greater macrophage/macrophage polykaryon infiltrate than the fibrocartilage, and these cells showed their typical foreign body reaction to shed silicone and polyester fibers, as shown in Figure 26–2.

Bone resorption was noted in animals. At the 3-month time point, the definition of the end plates had been disrupted; by the 18-month time point, the end plates had clearly reconstituted and were in approximately the same position as preoperatively. The histopathologist hypothesized an initial fibroblastic activity with tissue penetration into the adjacent bone, followed by a process of maturation from fibroblastic to fibrocartilaginous tissue, which would be associated with a net gain in adjacent bone, thus explaining the difference in observations from the 3- to 18-month time points. The extent of the inflammation resulting from the presence of wear debris was consistent with the tissue reactions seen in other orthopaedic implants in the day-to-day practice of the histopathologist.

The observed tissue responses (to the debris from the NeoDisc device) are thought to be normal for a medical device and are not seen to be a cause for concern.

In summary, the animal trials provided macroscopic and histologic evidence of the tissue ingrowth. There were no unforeseen causes of wear debris, and the tissue response to the wear debris generated is seen to be in line with that in other medical devices.

## EPIDURAL APPLICATION OF PARTICULATE WEAR DEBRIS—AN IN VIVO RABBIT MODEL STUDY

To investigate the possible histopathologic effects on neurologic tissue caused by the release of wear debris from the NeoDisc device, an in vivo rabbit model was used.[10] It is unfeasible to collect significant volumes of particulate from the wear testing (and then subsequently clean and resterilize this particulate); thus, simulated wear debris was generated for use in the animal study.

The NeoDisc device is manufactured from silicone and polyester. Both of these materials produced wear debris during laboratory testing. Therefore, to provide pure sample particulate for each of these materials, samples of each type were processed separately. Particulate of a similar size and morphology to that collected during wear testing was generated by cryopulverization of each of the materials. For both materials, the particulate is mainly in the 1- to 50-μ size range. There were a significant number of submicron-sized polyester particles and some submicron-sized silicone particles. In line with particulate captured during wear testing, the polyester particles tended to be irregular flaky particles, and the silicone particles were mainly spherical or spheriodal.

For the epidural application study, a total of 30 New Zealand white rabbits were used. The animals were approximately 1 year old and 5 kg in weight. The animals were split into groups of 10 animals (five to be sacrificed at the 3-month interval and the remaining five to be sacrificed at 6 months). The first group of 10 animals was used as surgical controls. These animals had a sham operation in which the epidural area was exposed but no implantation took place. The second group of 10 animals was used to assess the silicone debris; for each of these, 3 mg of silicone particulate were applied to the epidural area of the lumbar spine. The third group of 10 animals was used to assess the polyester debris; for each of these, 3 mg of polyester particulate were applied to the epidural area of the lumbar spine.

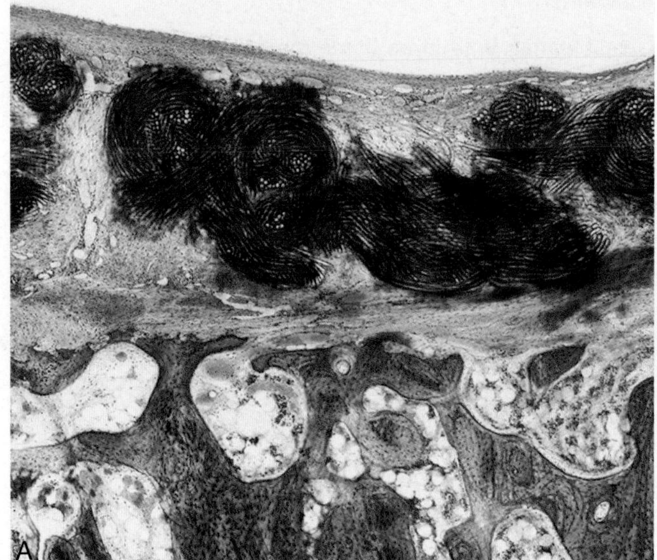


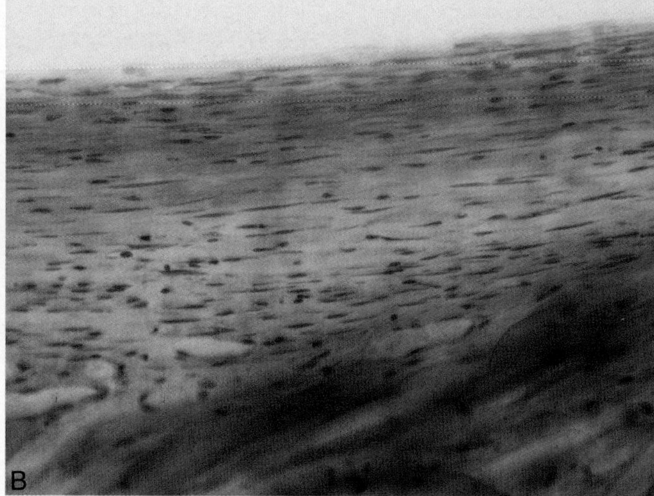


■ **FIGURE 26–2.** Histology showing fibrous tissue encapsulation of the polyester jacket at a survival time of 6 months in an ovine model. **A,** Overall view illustrating the elastomeric core and the fibrous tissue encapsulation around the polyester jacket. **B,** Higher magnification view showing the orientation of the fibroblasts adjacent to the elastomeric core at top and the relatively small number of macrophages.

The surgical technique for the implantation of the particulate was conducted with the animal positioned prone, aseptically prepared, and draped in sterile fashion. A midline skin incision of 4 to 5 cm in length was centered over the L5-L6 operative level. The L6 spinous process and L5-L6 supraspinous/interspinous ligament were then exposed using a periosteal elevator and electrocautery, as necessary. Most importantly the operative level bilateral facet capsules and joints were not exposed. The L6 spinous process and ligamentum flavum at L5-L6 were excised, permitting interlaminar exposure of the dural sac (5 mm diameter surface area). The membranous coverings and neural structures of the spinal canal were then accessible. The treatment materials were implanted in a sterile, dry format. To ensure that the spinal cord, nerve roots, and extramedullary vessels were not damaged, the surgical approach and material application techniques were performed using operating loupes. The control group consisted of epidural exposure alone.[10]

Following surgery, all of the animals in every group demonstrated a normal recovery, with no complications, and their behavior was unaffected.

The animals were sacrificed at 3 and 6 month intervals. At the time of necropsy, both experimental groups exhibited a greater amount of epidural fibrosis compared with controls. There were no signs of infection in any of the animals. Specimens taken from the epidural region were culture negative in every case.

The spinal cord and overlying fibrous tissues were examined using immunocytochemistry techniques. At the 3-month time interval, the number of macrophage-expressing cytokines present indicated no statistical differences between the control and study groups. In addition, there were no significant differences between the experimental and control groups with respect to activated macrophages. In general, macrophage activity was reported to be very low and was reported to be almost not observed in both of the experimental cases. At the 6-month time interval, the cytokine response from tumor necrosis factor-$\alpha$, tumor necrosis factor-$\beta$, interleukin-1$\beta$, and macrophages was essentially nonreactive. Interleukin-1$\alpha$ and interleukin-6 (IL-6) were reactive but not statistically different from the control groups.

Histopathologic analysis at both 3- and 6-month time intervals indicated there were no significant pathologic changes in the systematic tissues. All the systematic organs and organ systems demonstrated no issues of concern. It was postulated that lymphoreticular dissemination of both the silicone and polyester probably did occur. However, no evidence could be found in the tissues analyzed. In the control and study groups both at 3 and 6 months, there were increased concentrations of IL-6 cytokines. However, there were no statistical differences in cytokine activity between the study groups and the control. There were mild changes in cytokine and macrophage activity for the experimental groups, although the indication was that there was a normal distribution of myelin and the intracellular neurofibrilla network—characterizing the treatments as "without significant pathological changes at the three-month time interval." There was no evidence of cellular apoptosis, giant cell reaction, or other significant pathologic changes.

The study concluded that overall, based on the postoperative time period evaluated, there was no evidence of an acute neural or systematic histopathologic response to either the silicone or the polyester.

## CLINICAL PRESENTATION AND EVALUATION

The first two NeoDisc prostheses were implanted in two patients in July 2004 as part of a two-site European study regulated by the MHRA (the United Kingdom Regulatory Authority). The 1-year results on 14 patients treated were presented at the Spinal Arthroplasty Society meeting in Montreal in May, 2006. There were no adverse clinical or device-related events to report. Average blood loss during surgery was less than 15 mL, and the average operation time was less than 60 minutes. Neck pain assessed by Visual Analog Scale on a 100-point scale fell from an average of 38 preoperatively to 13 at 3 months and 8 at 12 months. The majority of patients presented with radiculopathy, and the visual analog arm pain score preoperatively was an average of 65, falling to 14 at 3 months, 9.5 at 6 months, and 11 at 12 months. Assessment of disability using the Neck Disability Index showed a reduction from an average of 24 on a 100-point scale preoperatively to 9 at 3 months, maintained at 10 by 12 months. Patients exhibited a range of flexion-extension segmental motion preopertively with an average of 8 degrees at the symptomatic level. Postoperatively, the average range of motion at the treated level was 6 degrees at the 3-month follow-up, 7 degrees at the 6-month follow-up, and 6 degrees of flexion-extension range of motion at the 12-month (1-year) follow-up. Postoperatively, all patients either maintained or recovered full neurologic function.

Clinical studies are ongoing. At the time of this writing, three patients have returned for 2-year clinical and radiologic follow-up examinations. The demonstrated flexion-extension ranges of motion for the three patients at the 2-year follow-up are 10, 6, and 9 degrees. The fourth patient was not able to attend his 2-year follow-up visit because he is on active military duty (with the U.K. armed forces) in Iraq at the time of this writing. All three patients continue to maintain excellent outcomes in terms of their clinical and functional outcomes with respect to the cervical spine. Repeat MRI imaging at 2 years has been performed and confirms that repeat imaging of the cervical spine and neural structures not only at adjacent levels but also at the operated levels is entirely possible in the presence of the NeoDisc device. Figures 26–3 and 26–4 demonstrate two patients from the European study. The first patient has radiculopathy, and the second patient has rapidly progressive myelopathy. The radiologic results for these two patients are shown in Figures 26–5 and 26–6.

At the time of this writing, a US IDE study is also under way.

## OPERATIVE TECHNIQUE

As described earlier, the design philosophy for the NeoDisc device is to minimize the necessity for the operating surgeon to alter his or her surgical technique; the implantation of the device does not involve the use of any specialized reamers, centering tools, or jigs. The procedure is performed with the patient under a general anesthetic, and the patient is positioned in a supine position with moderate head up tilt to reduce bleeding but with the neck being placed in a generally neutral position, avoiding excess flexion or extension. The surgeon performs the standard anterolateral approach and anterior cervical discectomy/decompression procedure. Because fusion is not the aim of the surgery, there is no requirement to prepare a bleeding end plate, but instead, only disc removal and decompressive techniques are needed. It is important to remove all disc material and

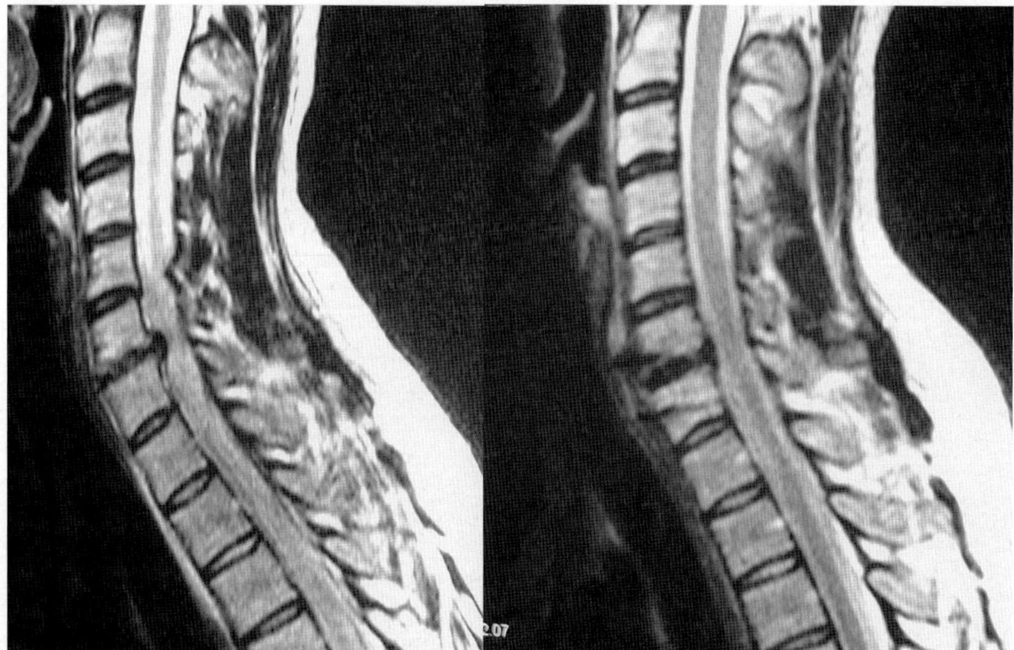

■ **FIGURE 26–3.** A C6-C7 NeoDisc arthroplasty performed for radiculopathy. This 37-year-old woman presented with severe right-sided radiculopathy affecting her C7 nerve root. A preoperative MRI scan demonstrated a C6-C7 predominantly right-sided compression due to a combination of osteophyte and soft disc prolapse. The one-year postoperative magnetic resonance imaging scan demonstrates removal of compressive pathology and restoration of disc height. The prosthesis is visible as a low-signal intensity within the C6-C7 disc space. There is minimal artifact present, attributable to the titanium anchor screws. The patient had complete relief of right arm radiculopathy.

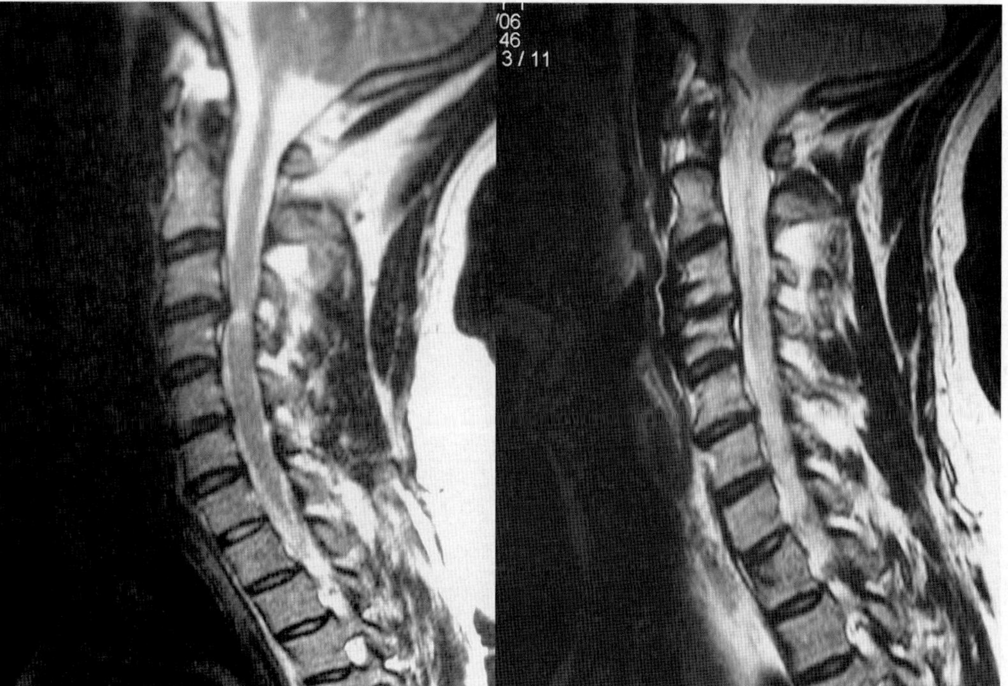


■ **FIGURE 26–4.** A C3-C4 NeoDisc arthroplasty performed for myelopathy. This 41-year-old man presented with myelopathy with bilateral arm and leg weakness and increased tone affecting all four limbs. The preoperative magnetic resonance imaging (MRI) scan demonstrates single-level cord compression at the C3-C4 level, predominantly due to a midline soft disc prolapse. Also apparent on the MRI scan is signal change within the spinal cord at this level. The two-year postoperative MRI scan demonstrates relief of spinal cord compression and return of normal signal within the cord. The NeoDisc prosthesis is visible as a low signal intensity within the disc space. There is minimal artifact due to the titanium anchor screws. The patient had complete relief of myelopathic symptoms and subsequently went on to become a personal fitness trainer and competed in half marathons.

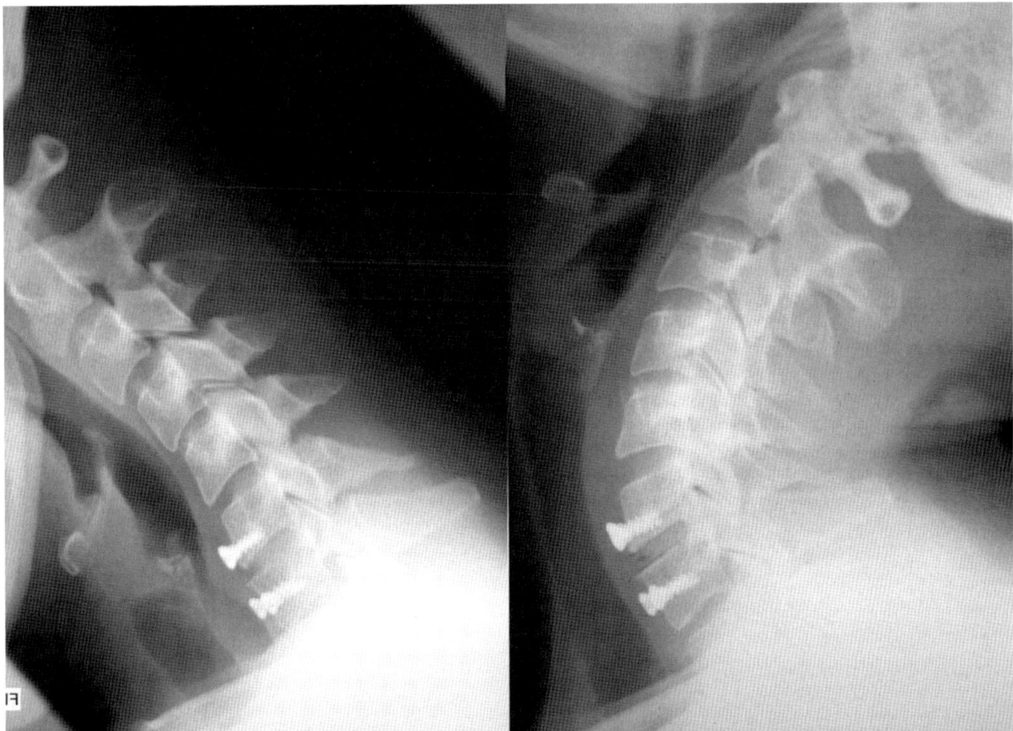

■ **FIGURE 26–5.** Flexion-extension radiograph of a C6-C7 NeoDisc arthroplasty for the patient shown in Figure 26–3.

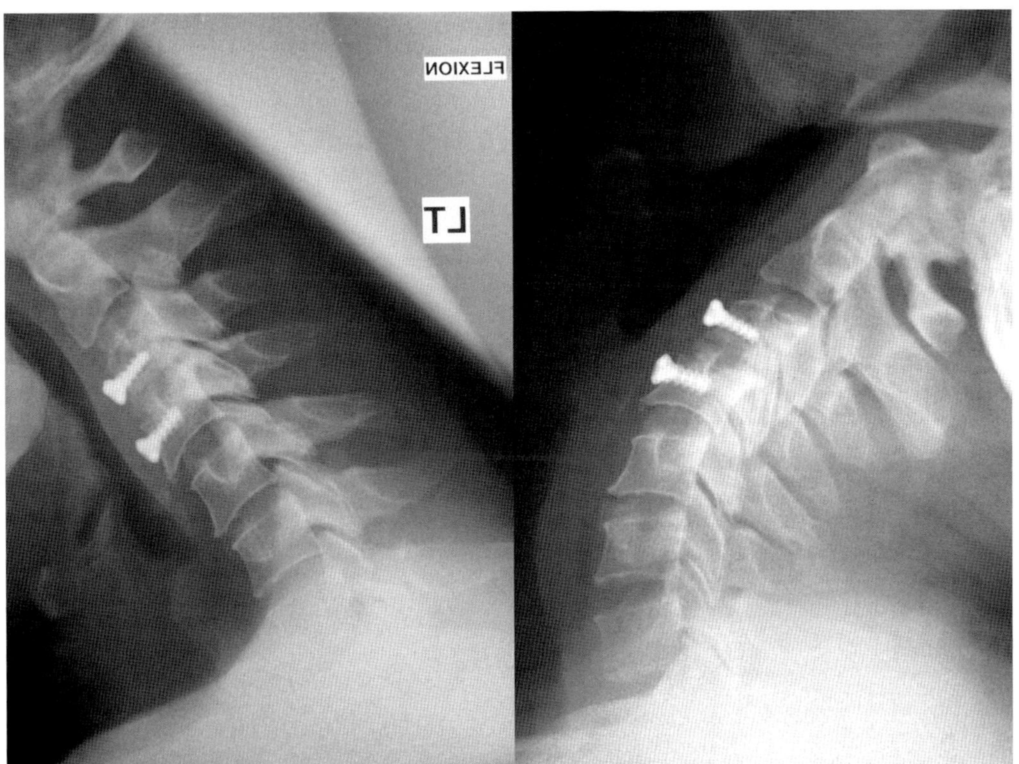

■ **FIGURE 26–6.** Flexion-extension radiograph of a C3-C4 NeoDisc arthroplasty for the patient shown in Figure 26–4.

compressive osteophytes or extruded disc to ensure relief of the patient's neurologic compression and symptoms. The posterior longitudinal ligament may be left or resected depending on the requirement to achieve satisfactory decompression of the compressed neural structures. When the surgeon is satisfied with the decompression, the NeoDisc trial sizers are inserted in a sequential fashion until a footprint and height of the trial are found that good fits as judged by visual examination, tactile feedback, and radiologic observation. Disc height should be restored to an appropriate level as judged by viewing adjacent disc spaces on an image intensifier. The sterile prosthesis is then selected to match the sizing trial and inserted into the disc space. This is achieved by the use of the insertion forceps, with recommended gentle traction under the chin while the device is inserted into the empty disc space. The device should fit fully within the disc space and be seated 1 to 2 mm deep to the anterior edge of the vertebral body. The securing textile flanges are positioned flat against the vertebral body, and a bone awl is passed through the flange hole to penetrate the anterior cortex of the vertebral body beneath. The bone screws are then placed through the flange holes, and the screws are secured in the normal manner until finger tight. This surgical technique is summarized in Video clip # 2. After securing the device, it may be useful to passively perform gentle flexion and extension of the patient's head and neck while observing the disc under direct vision and on the image intensifier (shown in Video clip # 3). This gives confirmation that the correct size of device has been selected and that it is seated securely within the disc space. The wound is closed in the usual manner, and a wound drain is recommended for the first 12 to 24 hours after surgery.

### Postoperative Care

Cervical collars are not required, and the patient is encouraged to move the head and neck as comfort allows and as normally as possible. It is recommended that a postoperative x-ray study is performed 24 to 48 hours after surgery to confirm correct position of the implant device. There are no unique recommendations or restrictions with regard to the NeoDisc device.

### Complications and Avoidance

In general terms, the risks of complications with the NeoDisc device are largely those of a standard anterior cervical decompression and interbody fusion. The patients in whom this device would be contraindicated are described under the earlier section on indications and contraindications and, broadly speaking, encompass patients who are at significant risk of infection or with poor-quality bone stock. Evidence of significant instability at the operative level is also a contraindication for use of this device.

**ADVANTAGES/DISADVANTAGES: THE NeoDisc ELASTOMERIC CERVICAL TOTAL DISC REPLACEMENT**

**Advantages**

The surgical technique is extremely simple, with no end plate milling or reaming. Detailed postoperative MRI and CT imaging of the spinal cord, nerves, and foraminae are easily obtainable. The device does not impose its own access of rotation but allows the axis of rotation determined by the patient's own anatomy. The device is available in a wide range of sizes. Surgical time is shorter than a standard ACDF with the possibility of less retraction on the soft tissue including the esophagus. The elastomeric core provides both mobility and axial compliance, acting as a more physiologic disc replacement. The polyester embroidered casing is designed to provide both immediate and long-term fixation. The interdigitated flanges provide immediate stability, preventing the anterior or posterior migration of the device. The embroidery also allows soft tissue ingrowth providing long-term fixation at the operative level.

**Disadvantages**

The currently employed titanium screws are associated with a small degree of MRI artifact. At present, there are only limited data with 2-year follow-up on a limited number of patients.

ACDF, anterior cervical discectomy and fusion; CT, computed tomography; MRI, magnetic resonance imaging.

## CONCLUSIONS/DISCUSSION

Cervical spine arthroplasty represents a developing and expanding area for designers and treating clinicians. Patient preference and pressures will increasingly lead to requests for artificial disc replacement in place of more traditional fusion procedures. Health economic pressures will require manufacturers and clinicians to demonstrate value for money invested and equal efficacy with the demonstration of preservation of segmental mobility. Long-term studies will be necessary before the full benefit of this technology can be determined.

The NeoDisc device represents the only currently available elastomeric textile prosthesis for cervical implantation. The operative procedure is simple and does not require the surgeon to learn new or demanding techniques or instrumentation. The device is highly compatible with all imaging modalities. Also, the potential to replace the titanium screws with nonmetallic anchoring devices will enable the device to become completely free of artifact on postimplantation MRI studies.

## REFERENCES

1. Cloward RB: The anterior approach for removal of ruptured cervical discs. Neurosurgery 15:62–67, 1958.
2. Robinson RA, Smith GW: Anterolateral cervical disc removal and interbody fusion for cervical disc syndrome. Bull Johns Hopkins Hosp 96:223–224, 1955.
3. Goffin J, Geusens E, Vantomme N, et al: Long term follow up after interbody fusion of the cervical spine. Presented at the annual meeting of the Cervical Spine Research Society, Charleston, SC, Nov–Dec 2000.
4. Goffin J, Van Loon J, V Calenberg F, et al: Long term results after anterior cervical fusion and osteosynthetic stabilisation for fractures and/or dislocations of the cervical spine. J Spinal Disord 8:500–508, 1995.
5. Hilibrand A, Carlson G, Palumbo M, et al: Radiculopathy and myelopathy at segments adjacent to the site of a previous anterior cervical arthrodesis. J Bone Joint Surg Am 81:519–528, 1999.
6. Pospiech J, Stolke D, Wilke H, et al: Intradiscal pressure recordings in the cervical spine. Neurosurgery 44:379–385, 1999.
7. Yeh J, Jackowski A: Proceedings of the British Cervical Spine Society, 1996.
8. Jackowski A, Yeh J: 13th Annual Meeting of the European Cervical Spine Research Society. 1997, pp 26–28.
9. Jackowski A, McLeod A: Spine Arthroplasty II Symposia Montpellier, VT, 2002.
10. Cunningham BW, Orbegoso CM, Dmitriev AE, et al: The effect of spinal instrumentation particulate wear debris: An in vivo rabbit model and applied clinical study of retrieved instrumentation cases. Spine J 3:19–32, 2003.

CHAPTER 27

# Mobi-C

**Jacques Beaurain, Pierre Bernard, Thierry Dufour, Jean-Marc Fuentes, Istvan Hovorka, Jean Huppert, Jean-Paul Steib,** and **Jean-Marc Vital**

## KEY POINTS

- Mobi-C is a second-generation, three-piece nonconstrained cervical disc prosthesis.
- The implantation technique is simple and accurate without invasive preparation of the end plates, allowing a multilevel arthroplasty.
- Intermediate clinical and radiologic results were satisfactory at both early and late control, without device-related complication.
- Physiologic cervical motion is often restored after Mobi-C implantation.
- Additional long-term follow-up results are mandatory to further evaluate the effects of the motion restoration at both the implanted and adjacent levels.

## INTRODUCTION

Duplicating the cervical intervertebral disc's form and function with an artificial disc is challenging. Cervical disc arthroplasty offers several theoretical advantages compared with anterior cervical discectomy and fusion (ACDF). The stresses on adjacent levels above and below the fusion site may lead to higher incidence of degeneration and segmental instability. On the other hand, preservation of motion at the surgically treated level may potentially decrease the occurrence of adjacent-level degeneration.[1,2]

Several prostheses with different components and kinematic designs are now available for clinical use.[3] Among them, Mobi-C (LDR Médical, Troyes, France) was designed by a French team of orthopaedic and neurosurgeons with two main objectives: (1) attempt to replicate the normal cervical intervertebral disc motion as much as possible and (2) develop a device with well-known materials that is easily placed with a simple and reliable technique.

Mobi-C has a three-piece nonconstrained articulation with a polyethylene mobile nucleus moving between two Cr-Co plates that are designed to be as anatomic as possible.[4]

## DESCRIPTION OF THE DEVICE

The Mobi-C represents a metal-on-polyethylene device. It is composed of two spinal plates consisting of cobalt, chromium, 29 molybdenum ISO 5832-12 alloy, and an ultra-high-molecular-weight polyethylene mobile insert (Fig. 27–1). The inner contact surfaces of the superior and inferior plates are spherical and flat, respectively. The mobile insert is self-centering on the inferior end plate. Each movement of the superior plate induces the mobile insert to reposition on the inferior spinal plate. The inner contact surface of the superior plate is spherical, allowing a fully congruent contact surface with the convex spherical dome of the mobile insert.

The inner contact surface of the inferior plate is flat and contains two lateral stops that limit the mobility of the mobile insert by contacting the lateral surface of the insert. The lateral stops reduce the potential for migration of the mobile insert. Both the superior and inferior spinal plates contain two teeth rows that are located laterally on each plate to ensure the primary fixation. A titanium and hydroxyapatite plasma spray coating is applied to the bony interface surfaces of the superior and inferior plates. Different plate sizes are available (13 × 15, 13 × 17, 15 × 17, and 15 × 20, depth by length in mm). Different insert heights are available (5 mm, 6 mm, 7 mm), to restore the physiologic height of the disc.

The device allows for various degrees of mobility that include five independent degrees of freedom, two translational and three rotational. The five independent degrees of freedom are illustrated below (Fig. 27–2).

## BACKGROUND OF SCIENTIFIC TESTING

Testing was conducted with success to determine the mechanical properties of the Mobi-C Cervical Disc Prosthesis in accordance with applicable American Society for Testing and Materials (ASTM) standardized test methods for the following:

Durability/wear testing: The results demonstrated a 0.08% mass loss or a total of 0.24 $mm^3$ volumetric loss after 10 million cycles (1 million cycles = 1 year of clinical use; rate of wear = 0.024 $mm^3$/year).

Static and dynamic axial compression fatigue testing: Specimens were loaded until failure in compression and exhibited a mean initial peak load of 4,752 ± 309 N (normal axial loads in the cervical spine range from 70 to 150 N). Axial fatigue failure of the device is thus unlikely.

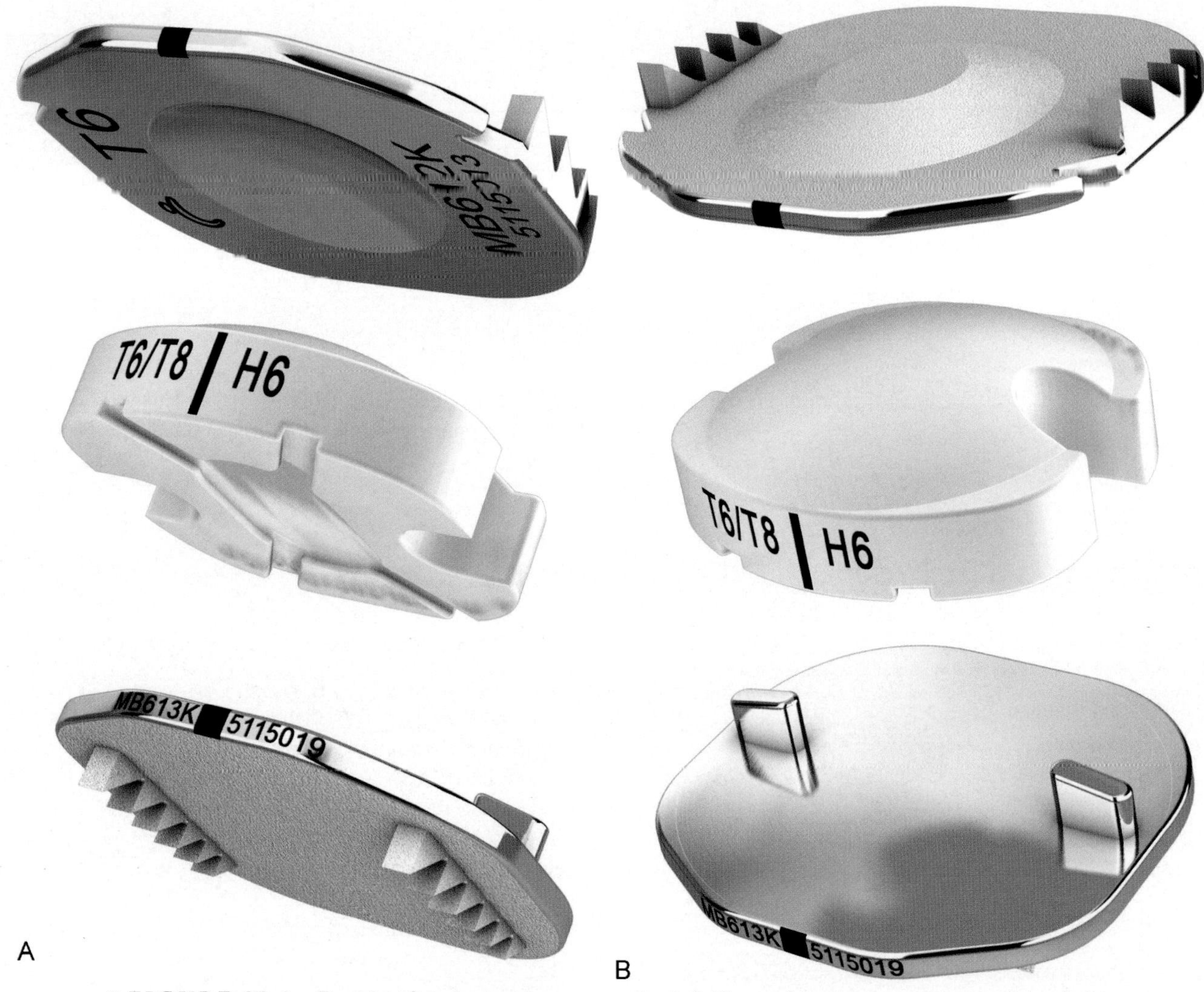


■ **FIGURE 27–1.** The Mobi-C device and its components. **A, B,** Views of the three components of the device.

Static and dynamic shear compression fatigue testing: Testing to 10 million cycles was completed at an applied load of 450 N with no observed failure (physiologic shear loads: less than 120 N).

Static subsidence testing: The devices exhibited a mean peak load of 1,090 ± 46 N without implant failure. Normal axial loads in the cervical spine range from 70 to 150 N.

Static expulsion testing for mobile insert and full device: An axial preload of 100 N was placed on the device, then the device and fixtures were rotated 90 degrees to test the expulsion resistance. The mobile insert was loaded with a posterior-to-anterior load. The inserts were loaded to failure (defined as movement of 3 mm) and exhibited a mean peak load of 143 ± 18 N without implant failure. The observed loads are comparable with the expulsion loads required to displace the entire device. Therefore, expulsion of the mobile inserts from the end plates is not anticipated under physiologic loading condition.

Mechanical testing demonstrated that the Mobi-C disc is adequate to provide an additional therapeutic option in maintaining motion segment position and spacing while preserving flexibility in the affected cervical vertebral level.

## CLINICAL AND RADIOLOGICAL EVALUATION

A multicenter clinical and radiologic prospective study is under way to assess the safety and efficacy of the Mobi-C implant in treating cervical degenerative disc disease (DDD). Ninety-two patients were enrolled across eight sites, between November 1, 2004 and January 31, 2006.

Indications were DDD at one or several levels between C3 and C7, leading to radiculopathy or myelopathy, or both. Surgery was performed only after failure of appropriate conservative medical treatment. DDD was confirmed through anterioposterior (AP) cervical x-ray studies, computed tomography, or magnetic resonance imaging. All patients signed the informed consent form.

Exclusion criteria are usual and include aging (>65 years old), noncompliance with the study protocol, osteoporosis, metabolic bone disease, congenital or post-traumatic deformity, infection, neoplasia, instability of the intersomatic space, or a narrow canal (<12 mm).

Autoevaluation was completed by the patient before and after the surgery, and included pain Visual Analog Scale (VAS 0 to 100), related to both neck and arm pain and Neck Disability Index functional score (NDI). After the surgery, the patient also completed a satisfaction index.

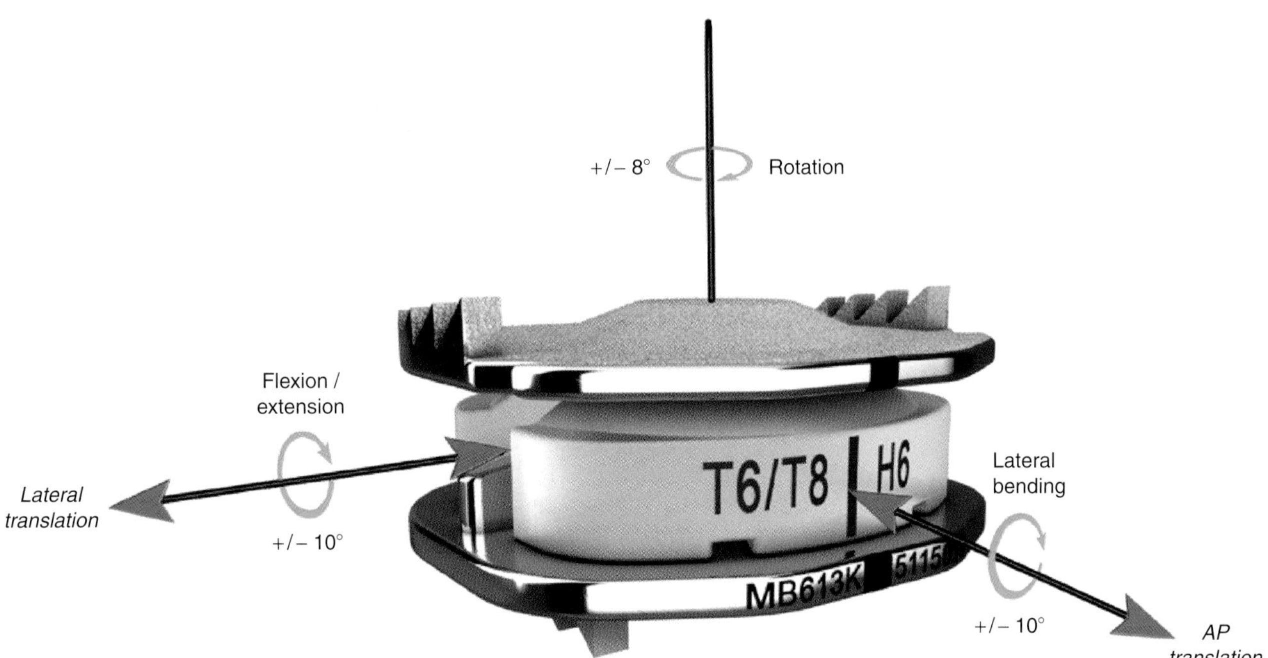


■ **FIGURE 27–2.** The five independent degrees of freedom of the Mobi-C device. Translation amplitude of the mobile insert is ± 1 mm in both lateral and anteroposterior directions.

Clinical evaluation included a detailed neurologic examination, and complications, analgesic requirements, and employment status were also documented.

Radiologic assessment included x-ray studies on AP cervical spine, and flexion-extension x-ray studies. Range of motion (ROM) and mean centers of rotation (MCRs) were measured segmentally, at the operative and adjacent levels, preoperatively and postoperatively at 1-year follow-up, with the Spine View software, using validated computerized techniques to ensure reproducibility.

Follow-up evaluation was performed at 6 weeks and 3, 6, and 12 months after the index surgery, considering that each patient will be followed-up for at least 2 years after surgery.

## Clinical Results

Mean age of the 92 enrolled patients is 43 years old (range 25 to 65 years); 46 patients are men, and 46 patients are women. The mean follow-up is 9 months (range 3 to 17 months), with 29 patients having a follow-up of 12 months or more. Eighty-three percent of the patients had no previous cervical surgery, and 15% of the patients had a previous fusion at an adjacent level. Eighty-two patients were operated on with Mobi-C at one level and 10 patients at two levels, distributed as follows: C3-C4 ($n$ = 1), C4-C5 ($n$ = 7), C5-C6 ($n$ = 42), C6-C7 ($n$ = 31), C7-D1 ($n$ = 1), C4-C5/C6-C7 ($n$ = 1), C4-C5/C5-C6 ($n$ = 2), and C5-C6/C6-C7 ($n$ = 7).

The mean operative duration was 84 minutes (range 40 to 190 minutes), which is quite similar to a standard ACDF procedure. The average hospital stay was 3 days (range 1 to 6 days), and the mean duration of sick leave following index surgery was 2.6 months.

As shown by VAS (Fig. 27–3) and NDI (Fig. 27–4) scores, the Mobi-C surgery had a strong impact on pain. The mean cervical pain VAS score is reduced by 75% after 1 year (see Fig. 27–3A), and the arm pain score (see Fig. 27–3B) by 74% (right arm) and

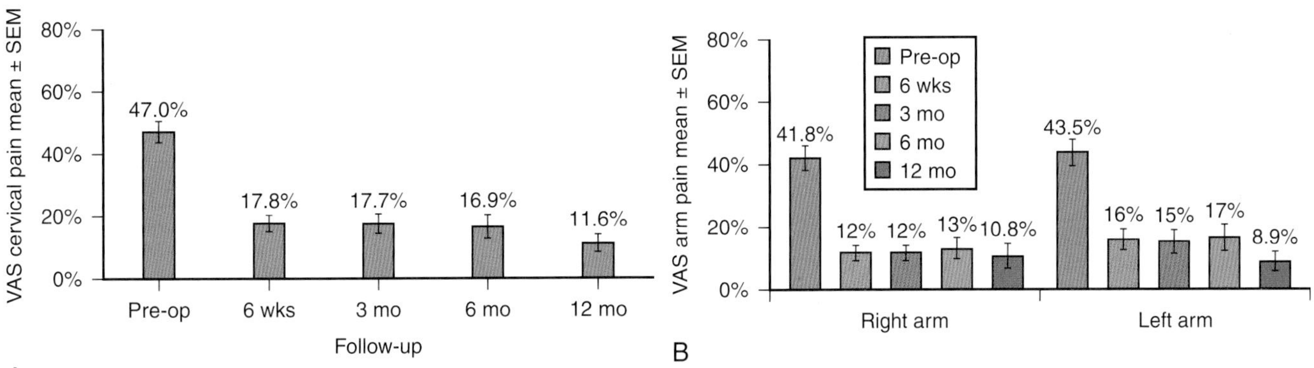


■ **FIGURE 27–3.** The Visual Analog Scale (VAS) scores for cervical **(A)** and arm **(B)** pain before and after the Mobi-C surgery. Evaluation was performed preoperatively, and at 6 weeks and 3, 6, and 12 months after the index surgery. Results are expressed as mean ± SEM.

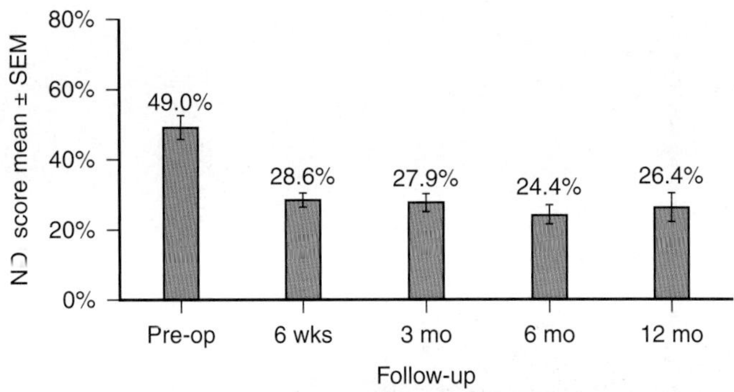


■ **FIGURE 27–4.** The Neck Disability Index (NDI) score before and after the Mobi-C surgery. Evaluation was performed preoperatively, and 6 weeks and 3, 6, and 12 months after the index surgery. Results are expressed as mean ± SEM.

80% (left arm). Seventy-four percent of the patients had an improvement of at least 50% of the VAS cervical pain score after 1 year compared with the preoperative score.

The mean NDI score was reduced by 46% after 1 year, with 52% of the patients having an improvement of their score of at least 50% after 1 year compared with the preoperative value. The Mobi-C surgery thus leads to an improvement of the pain symptoms within a few weeks, and most important, both pain decrease and functional improvement are maintained over the time.

One year after the surgery, 97% of the patients declared to be very satisfied or satisfied with the surgical procedure, whereas only 3% of the patients were not satisfied or dissatisfied (Table 27–1). Eighty-six and eighty-five percent of the patients were very satisfied or satisfied with cervical pain and arm pain, respectively.

### Radiographic Results

Radiologic evaluation has shown a restoration of the segmental mobility, because mean flexion/extension ROM of the treated level was 10.2 degrees (range 0 to 25 degrees) at the latest follow-up. Moreover, 93% of the prostheses were mobile (ROM > 2 degrees) at the last follow-up. Representative clinical cases are shown later (Fig. 27–5). There was no subluxation, no device migration, and no subsidence. Only one case of anterior ossification has been reported, which has been attributed to preoperative cervical kyphosis and to malposition of the device (too posterior) which led to a poor mobility after 1 year. No periprosthetic calcification was observed.

**TABLE 27–1. Satisfaction Index After the Mobi-C Surgery***

| | Very Satisfied (%) | Satisfied (%) | Not Satisfied (%) | Dissatisfied (%) |
|---|---|---|---|---|
| Intervention | 83 | 14 | 3 | 0 |
| Cervical pain | 38 | 48 | 14 | 0 |
| Arm pain | 37 | 48 | 11 | 4 |

*One year after the surgery, patients were asked to quote their satisfaction degree toward intervention benefit, cervical pain and arm pain.

In our MCR study, the Mobi-C device restored motion at the treated level without actual adjacent-segment compromise. The location of MCR varied between levels; it was generally located in the posterior half of the upper part of the inferior vertebral body (Fig. 27–6). Overall cervical motion (C2-C7) was moderately but significantly increased during late follow-up

## OPERATIVE TECHNIQUE

All of the surgical procedures are performed by senior surgeons. The patient is in supine position, under general anesthesia, with the neck in neutral position, and the head maintained in the straight position throughout the procedure. A standard right- or left-sided approach is taken to the anterior cervical spine. The midline is defined under AP fluoroscopic view. After a thorough discectomy, the intersomatic space is distracted by a vertebral distracter. Once the height restoration is obtained, the distraction is maintained by the Caspar retainer, providing access to the posterior disc space. After total disc material and osteophytes are removed and neuroforaminal decompression is completed, the end plates are prepared without any shaping or chiseling. Rather than recommending systematic and complete posterior longitudinal ligament (PLL) removal, we insist on performing a good release of the posterior part of the disc to ensure a parallel intervertebral space opening. To our opinion, a thin residual PLL layer has no mechanical influence on motion. Depth and width measurements allow the determination of the appropriate trial implant. The trials help to confirm the precise size of the implant, which is verified under fluoroscopic control. During this step, it is important not to exceed the height of the healthy adjacent discs and not to induce overdistraction of the facet joints. The prosthesis is gently impacted into the disc space using a specific inserter. An adjustable stop allows precise adjustments of the implant AP position. The primary anchoring optimization is obtained through compression with the Caspar. An x-ray control (AP and lateral view) must confirm the well positioning of the implant.

## POSTOPERATIVE CARE

The patient was out of the bed the day following the surgery without cervical collar and discharged from the hospital as soon as possible. There was no systematic postoperative medical treatment or physiotherapy.

## COMPLICATIONS

Postoperative complications were related to the cervical anterior approach: Two local hematomas and one cerebrospinal fluid leak have been reported without clinical consequence or reintervention, transient dysphagia ($n = 2$), bitonal voice ($n = 2$), and dysphonia ($n = 1$) have also been noted and were resolved within a few months. There was no device-related intraoperative complication.

One prosthesis had to be removed 4 months after the initial placement owing to persistent cervical pain and excessive mobility

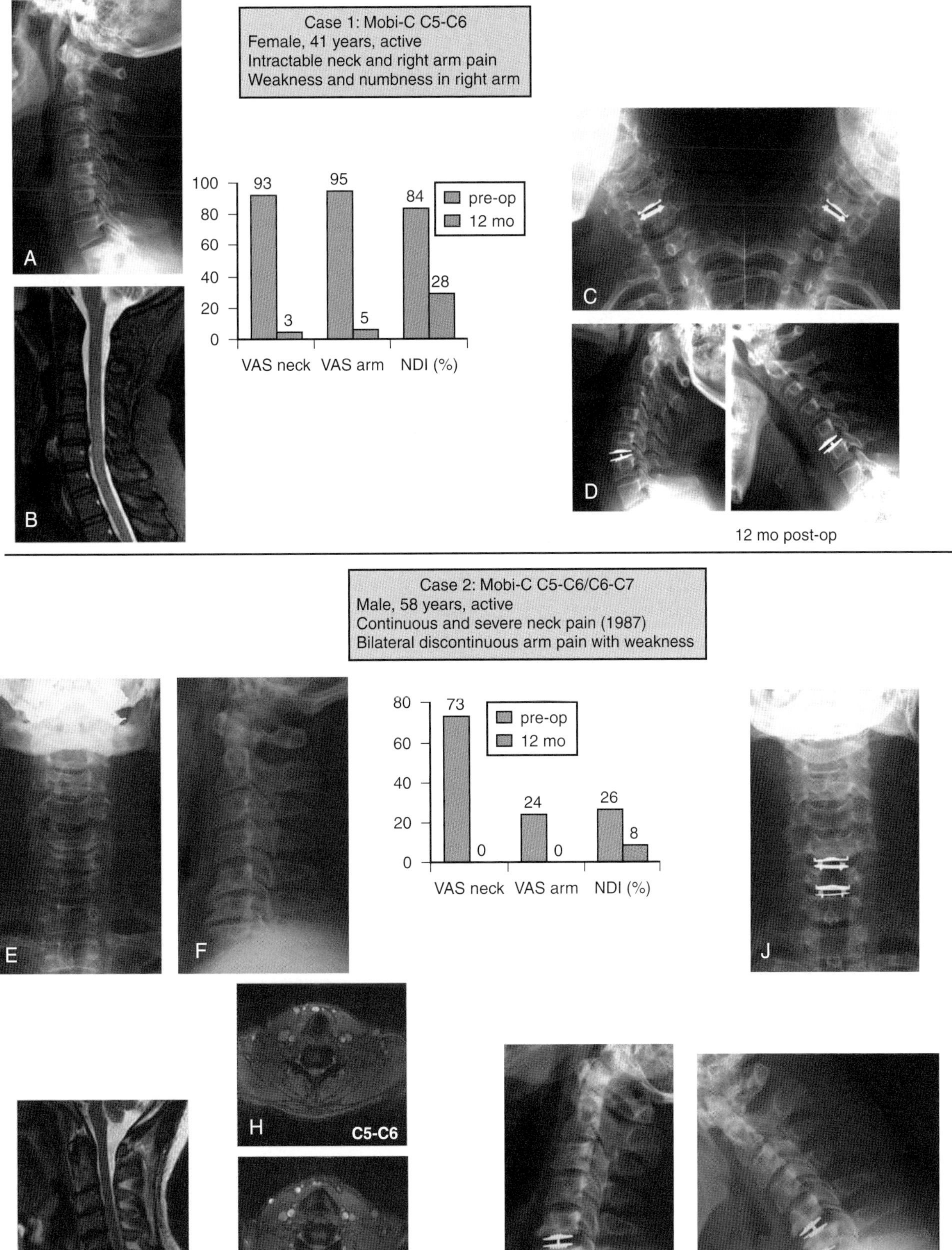


■ **FIGURE 27–5.** Clinical cases. VAS, Visual Analog Scale; NDI, Neck Disability Index.

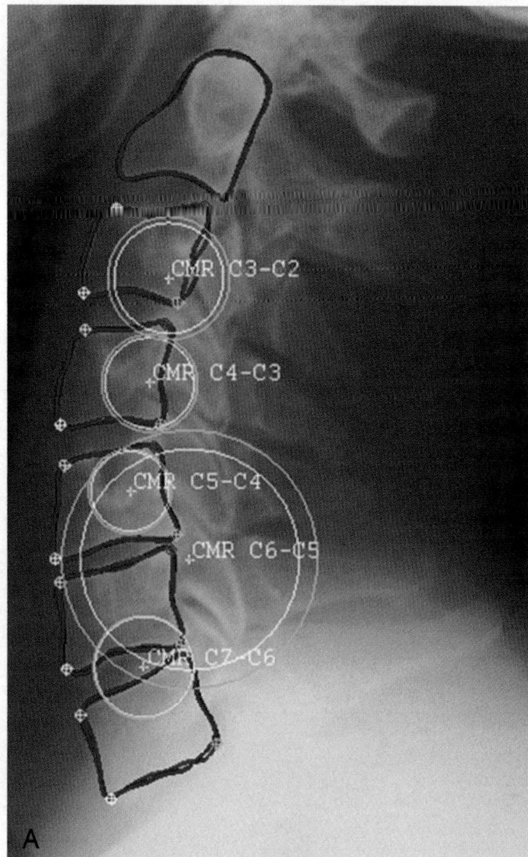


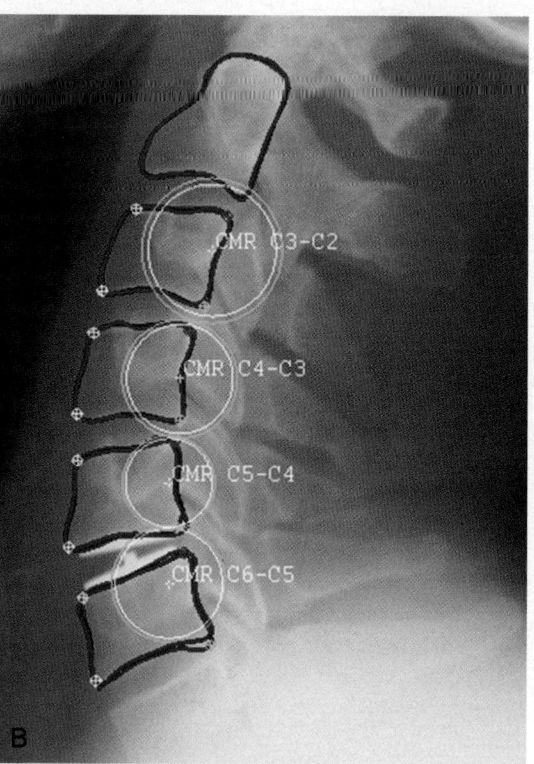


■ **FIGURE 27–6.** Physiologic restoration of the mean center of rotation (MCR) after Mobi-C surgery at the C5-C6 level. **A,** Calculation of MCR before surgery. **B,** MCR calculation 1 year after the surgery.

below a congenital cervical fusion block. The patient underwent fusion with an anterior cervical cage, resulting in a good clinical outcome.

## CONCLUSIONS/DISCUSSION

The Mobi-C prosthesis received approval to affix the CE Mark in 2004 and was first implanted in France in November 2004. The Mobi-C prosthesis is currently distributed in 20 countries in Europe, Asia, and Africa. As of September 2006, nearly 1000 Mobi-C devices have been implanted worldwide without any unanticipated adverse device effects.

In our study, more than 1-year follow-up demonstrates an excellent safety profile with no reported device-related complications, surgical re-interventions, or radiographic failures. Moreover, the data from the follow-up visits also demonstrate initial efficacy of Mobi-C with improvements in both pain and function as demonstrated by VAS and NDI scores, which confirms our preliminary results.[4]

The MCR study[5] shows that the Mobi-C device can restore the physiologic MCR position as defined by previous anatomic study, for each index level.[6] Calculation of the MCR at each follow-up timepoint indicates that sometimes this functional restoration may require a few weeks, even several months, depending probably on pain history duration.

This normal restoration of the index level segmental motion and the preservation of the adjacent level motion support the concept that arthroplasty may reduce adjacent degenerative disc disease compared to fusion.[5]

By comparison to constrained artificial discs, which require a definitive precise placement to reproduce a normal cervical kinematic, the nonconstrained Mobi-C device has a theoretical advantage: By this way, it should provide a better preservation of the MCR, and limit facets and ligament stresses. According to the MCR results of our study and the cumulated experience with Mobi-C implantation, we advise to center the device in the intersomatic space, rather than to push it to the posterior wall, as recommended for lumbar arthroplasty.

Whereas constrained devices require strong fixation systems such as keels or screws, the stability obtained with the four teeth rows and the coating of Mobi-C is proven to be sufficient. This design allows easy multilevel placement, without any risk of vertebral fracture or device conflict, even in small vertebral bodies.

Intermediate results on Mobi-C cervical disc prosthesis are very encouraging in this prospective ongoing study.

Of course, long-term follow-up will be needed to fully assess functionality of cervical disc replacement and its efficacy in preventing adjacent level early degeneration. We hope to answer these challenging questions in pursuit of our study, and with a prospective, multicentric, and randomized controlled clinical trial, which began in the United States in May 2006, in the context of an Investigational Device Exemption submission.

## REFERENCES

1. DiAngelo DJ, Robertson JT, Metcalf NH, et al: Biomechanical testing of an artificial cervical joint and an anterior cervical plate. J Spinal Disord Tech 16:314–323, 2003.
2. Goffin J, Geusens E, Vantomme N, et al: Long term follow-up after interbody fusion of the cervical spine. J Spinal Disord Tech 17:79–85, 2004.
3. Phillips FM, Garfin SR: Cervical disc replacement. Spine 30:S27–S33, 2005.
4. Bernard P, Vital JM, Dufour T, et al: A new mobile cervical prosthesis: Mobi-C. Preliminary results of a prospective study. Poster session, Global Symposium on Motion Preservation Technology, Spine Arthroplasty Society, 2005, New York.
5. Dufour T, Delecrin J, Beaurain J, et al: Calculation of centers of rotation in the cervical spine, before and after implantation of the Mobi-C cervical disc prosthesis. Global Symposium on Motion Preservation Technology, Spine Arthroplasty Society, 2006, Montréal, Canada.
6. Bogduk N, Mercer S: Biomechanics of the cervical spine, I: Normal kinematics. Clin Biomech 15:633–648, 2000.

CHAPTER 28

# The CerviCore Cervical Intervertebral Disc Replacement

**Jonathan R. Stieber, Jeffrey S. Fischgrund,** and **Jean-Jacques Abitbol**

**KEY POINTS**

- The CerviCore Intervertebral Disc is a cervical total disc replacement featuring metal-on-metal, saddle-shaped bearing surfaces.
- Indicated for the treatment of cervical radicular symptoms.
- Specialized insertion instrumentation facilitates accurate implantation.
- The CerviCore Intervertebral Disc is designed to replicate the motion of a native intact cervical disc.
- The procedure may be converted to a standard anterior cervical fusion if necessary at any stage of the procedure.

## INTRODUCTION

The CerviCore Intervertebral Disc (Stryker Spine, Allendale, NJ) prosthesis is an investigational device currently in a U.S. Food and Drug Administration (FDA)–approved Investigational Device Exemption (IDE) clinical trial. It is a semiconstrained cervical total disc replacement incorporating unique metal-on-metal, saddle-shaped bearing surfaces (Fig. 28–1). Following a standard anterior cervical decompression, the device is designed to preserve intervertebral motion by replicating the kinematics of the native cervical functional spinal unit. The CerviCore Intervertebral Disc is indicated for the treatment of cervical radicular symptoms associated with loss of disc height, disc/osteophyte complex, or herniated disc at a single level of the subaxial cervical spine from C3 to C7 resulting in upper extremity pain or neurologic deficit, or both. Specialized insertion instrumentation is designed to facilitate device implantation and minimize misalignment of the implant and other technical errors that may be associated with modular assembly and implantation.

## INDICATIONS

- Significant loss of disc height (>50% decrease), disc/osteophyte complex, or herniated disc at a single level between C3 and C7 on magnetic resonance imaging (MRI) or computed tomography, or both
- Clinical symptoms including radicular paresthesias in a dermatomal distribution or a progressive or acute onset functional neurologic deficit in a single nerve root distribution
- Failure of conservative treatment consisting of a minimum of 6 weeks of medical management, pain medication or injection therapy, physical therapy and/or physician-prescribed activity modification
- Clinically asymptomatic adjacent cervical levels
- Skeletally mature patients aged 18 to 65 who are nonsmokers

## CONTRAINDICATIONS

- Poor bone quality, osteopenia, osteoporosis, or a clinically compromised vertebral body structure at any cervical level due to acute or past trauma
- End plate incompetence at the level to be treated diagnosed on x-ray study or MRI such as a Schmorl's node, end plate fracture, or end plate herniation
- Metabolic bone disease or current medications that may interfere with normal bone metabolism
- Congenital or spontaneous fusion at the target or an adjacent level
- Cervical levels with less than 3 mm of preoperative disc height, evidence of ankylosis or localized kyphosis
- Pathology requiring concurrent posterior surgical treatment (Patients who have undergone prior laminectomy or laminotomy at a level other than the target level or adjacent levels may be indicated for treatment.)
- Significant radiographic instability at the target or an adjacent level, defined as >3.5 mm of translation, >11 degrees of angulation when compared with an adjacent level, and >3 mm spondylolisthesis, retrolisthesis, or spondylolysis
- Patients with severe facet joint arthritic changes at the target or an adjacent level
- Ossification of the posterior longitudinal ligament at any level
- Cervical spondolytic myelopathy (Myelopathy due to a recent [<12 months] soft disc herniation amenable to treatment with anterior discectomy may, however, be treated with the device.)
- Active systemic infection or infection at the operative site
- Allergy to components of the device, including cobalt, chromium, molybdenum, titanium, or nickel

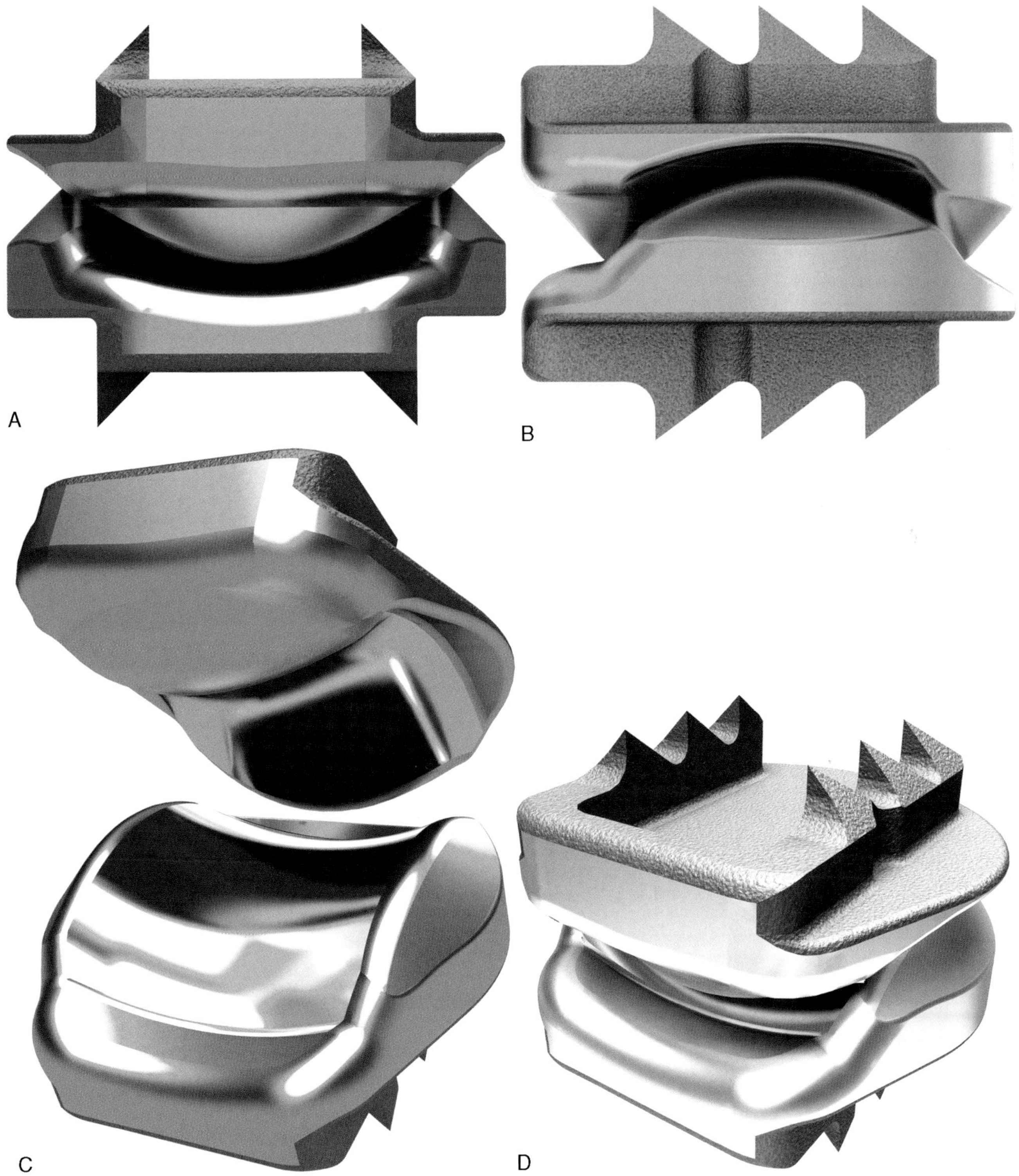


■ FIGURE 28–1. **A** to **D,** CerviCore Intervertebral Disc.

## DESCRIPTION OF THE DEVICE

The CerviCore Intervertebral Disc prosthesis is an all-metal device incorporating novel saddle-shaped bearing surfaces that are designed to replicate the kinematics of the native cervical functional spinal unit. The CerviCore device is composed of two opposing cobalt-chromium-molybdenum bearing surfaces backed with a titanium plasma spray coating to enhance osseous fixation. Two fins on each baseplate, each with three spikes, help achieve initial fixation. An anterior vertebral body stop decreases the chance of posterior placement or migration. The CerviCore Intervertebral Disc prosthesis is available in two footprint sizes (12 × 14 mm and 14 × 16 mm) and five intervertebral heights (5, 6, 7, 8, and 9 mm).

In the subaxial cervical spine from C3-C4 to C6-C7, the maximum physiologic range of motion is 10 degrees of flexion-extension, 11 degrees of lateral bending, and 7 degrees of axial rotation.[1] The saddle-shaped bearing surfaces of the CerviCore device are designed to allow lateral bending of ±7.5 degrees with a center of rotation located above the device and within the superior vertebral body, and flexion-extension of ±7.5 degrees with a center of rotation located below the device and within the inferior vertebral body. In contrast to designs that employ a ball-and-socket joint or single center of rotation, this unique design incorporating two separate centers of rotation is designed to more accurately reproduce physiologic motion.

The normal kinematics of the subaxial cervical spine couples limited distraction with axial rotation, and the innovative saddle-shaped bearing surface morphology of the CerviCore is designed to maintain this coupled motion. Different radii of curvature of the two saddle-shaped bearing surfaces allow approximately ±3 degrees of axial rotation before any axial distraction. Axial rotation beyond this threshold of approximately ±3 degrees initiates coupled axial rotation and distraction of the bearing surfaces. Cervical range of motion in situ is limited by soft tissue balance, the facet joints, and the uncovertebral joints. In biomechanical testing using an ovine model, the saddle-shape design was shown to be effective in establishing an incremental range of motion that is comparable to the native intact disc.[2]

## BACKGROUND OF SCIENTIFIC TESTING/CLINICAL OUTCOMES

The durability of a metal-on-metal bearing surface would be expected to exceed that of metal-on-polyethylene owing to material properties, including strength, hardness, and fatigue resistance. Cobalt, chromium, and molybdenum (CoCrMo) alloys are among the strongest, hardest, and most fatigue resistant of the metals used for joint replacement components. Given an average age of 35 years at the time of device implantation and a life expectancy of more than 85 years, the average patient would require a device with at least 50 years of longevity. It has been postulated that in 50 years, a device would be required to withstand 100 million cycles.[3] In bearing-surface validation, six samples were tested to 10 million cycles at both 70 N and 100 N. The total volume of cobalt debris was calculated to be 0.000002 $cm^3$ per million cycles, whereas chromium debris was 0.000216 $cm^3$ per million cycles. No evidence of cavitation or pitting was seen in photomicrographs. The bearing surfaces remained fully functional, with only minor burnishing and self-polishing marks. No component failed or demonstrated a loss of range of motion.[4]

## OPERATIVE TECHNIQUE

The principal purpose of the procedure is to address the primary disease, including spondylosis and the resultant neural compression. Implantation of the device requires adequate distraction, as well as contouring of the anterior vertebral body in order to permit proper and secure seating in the disc space. The end plates must also be adequately prepared for initial fixation and decorticated to facilitate ongrowth.

### Positioning and Surgical Approach/Exposure

General endotracheal anesthesia is used. The patient is positioned supine on a radiolucent table, with care taken to stabilize the head in a neutral position to prevent rotation during the procedure. The neck must be held in a neutral position for drilling of the reference pin holes and placement of the reference pins rather than in an extended position, as is common practice for an anterior cervical decompression and fusion. Placing a roll under the neck may aid in positioning; however, a bump or scapular roll placed underneath the shoulders may serve to undermine ideal positioning. After radiographically localizing the appropriate level, a transverse skin incision is completed. A standard ventral Smith-Robinson exposure is then performed to expose the disc space.

### Identification and Marking of the Midline

It is important for the CerviCore Intervertebral Disc to be positioned in the midline so that it may best replicate normal cervical motion, and this is accomplished with use of a template. The anterior surfaces of the adjacent vertebral bodies are made level using a cervical rongeur or motorized burr to remove anterior osteophytes. It is essential to complete this step before placing the template so that it may sit flush while identifying the midline. The lateral wings of the two template attachments serve to approximate the two width options of the CerviCore implant (Fig. 28–2). The selected template is then attached to the sizer/template handle. The vertical flanges of the template are then approximately aligned with the midline axis of the vertebral column, and the distal pin of the template is inserted into the center of the disc. Following satisfactory placement, the two tacks on the upper and lower flanges of the template are engaged by tapping lightly on the template handle (Fig. 28–3).

The template is then disengaged from the sizer/template handle, and fluoroscopy is used to confirm alignment of the template with the spinous processes, the uncovertebral joint, and the midline. In the event that the template is misaligned, the patient's head position should be examined as well as the alignment of the imaging equipment. If necessary, the template is repositioned and alignment is confirmed. Once the template has been properly

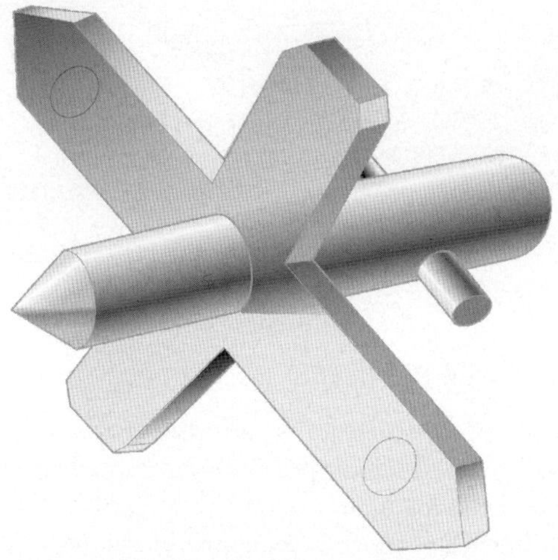

■ FIGURE 28–2. Template.

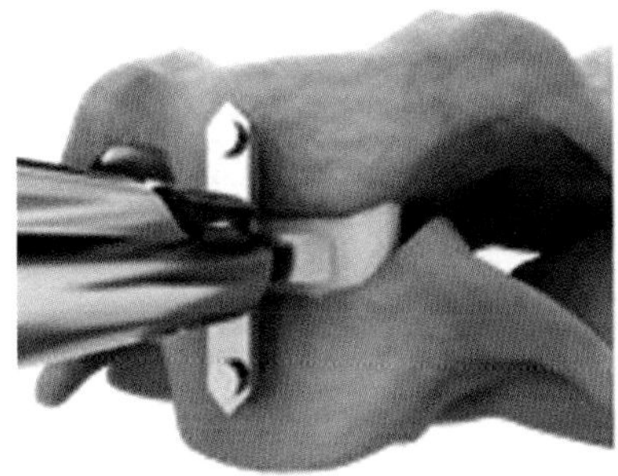

■ FIGURE 28–3. Template in position.

positioned and the midline of the adjacent vertebral bodies has been accurately identified, the midline of the adjacent vertebral bodies is marked. Care should be taken to ensure that the midline is well defined for subsequent steps of the procedure. After the midline has been marked, the template is removed.

## Insertion of Reference Pins

Two reference pins similar to Caspar pins are used to locate the subsequent steps of the procedure for disc space and end plate preparation, as well as insertion of the implant. Before insertion of the reference pins, a window is dissected in the anterior annulus that approximates the width of the CerviCore implant, and a provisional channel discectomy is performed in order to permit placement of the reference pin drill guide. For the procedure to proceed unhampered, sufficient disc material should be removed at this time to fit the actual implant. Before any further steps are taken, fluoroscopy is used to confirm resection of anterior osteophytes such that the anterior surfaces of the adjacent vertebral bodies are flush. Reference pins are employed during the procedure to maintain instrument alignment during end plate preparation and insertion of the implant. Because placement of the reference pins guides the subsequent steps of the procedure, care must be taken to ensure proper positioning. The reference pin drill guide is inserted into the disc space, aligned with the midline and with the guide head oriented in the sagittal plane. The alignment of the drill guide should be confirmed fluoroscopically so that it is parallel to the end plates on a lateral view. Once the reference pin drill guide is in place, a hole is drilled into each of the adjacent vertebral bodies with the drill bits provided (Fig. 28–4). The holes will be parallel and correctly distanced from the end plates.

After the reference pin holes have been drilled, the reference pin drill guide is removed and replaced with the reference pin insertion guide. Two sets of reference pins are provided in the instrument tray, standard (small threaded diameter) and rescue (large threaded diameter). The reference pin driver is used to insert the first standard reference pin (Fig. 28–5). Once inserted, the reference pin sleeve is placed over the first pin to stabilize the insertion guide. The second reference pin is inserted, and the driver sleeve and insertion guide are removed. At this point, the pins should be positioned in the midline, parallel to each other and the end plates. The reference pins are also used for distraction during the procedure in the manner of Caspar pins. Consequently, if a reference pin loosens during the procedure, it can be removed and replaced with the provided larger rescue pin.

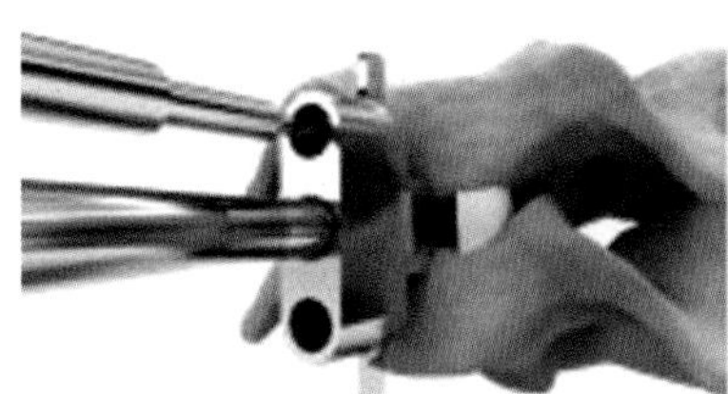

■ FIGURE 28–4. Drill holes using the reference pin drill guide.

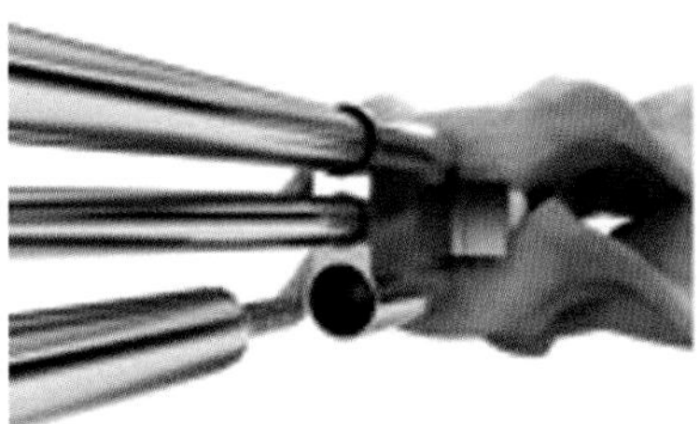

■ FIGURE 28–5. Reference pin driver with reference pin.

## Disc Space Distraction and Discectomy

The disc space must also be adequately distracted in order to permit implantation of the CerviCore Intervertebral Disc (Fig. 28–6). Distraction may also effect an indirect decompression of the neural foramina. Before distraction, the facet joints should be visualized fluoroscopically in order to monitor facet orientation.

The Caspar distractor is placed over the reference pins, and a distraction force is applied to the motion segment. Care should be taken to avoid overdistraction in excess of the height of the adjacent cranial disc space. Fluoroscopy should be employed to monitor disc height and facet separation and to confirm the appropriate distraction height while preventing overdistraction. Excessive distraction may lead to nerve or facet joint injury.

The initial discectomy and decompression should then be completed in the standard manner. The margins of the disc space should be cleared laterally to the uncinate processes and posteriorly to the spinal canal and neural foramina. An instrument such as a cylindrical burr with a 4- to 6-mm drill point, or curette, may be used to square off the bony end plates and remove the curvature of the superior end plate. In order to prevent undersizing of the implant, the end plates should be parallel to each other and relatively uniform. The decompression is then completed with attention to removal of any posterior osteophytes or soft tissue material that might inhibit full distraction of the posterior disc space. The posterolateral corners of the end plates and the posterolateral uncovertebral joints may be resected as needed for neural decompression. The lateral uncovertebral joints should be preserved

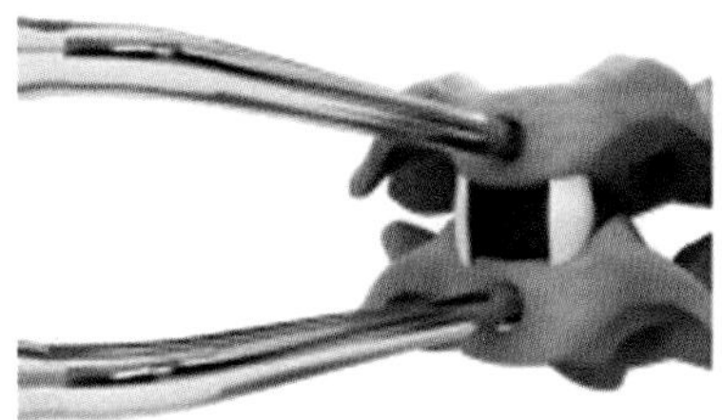

■ FIGURE 28–6. Caspar distractor applying distraction.

unless they are responsible for nerve root compression. Foraminotomies may be performed as indicated in order to address stenosis. It may be necessary to release the posterior longitudinal ligament in order to obtain optimal restoration of disc space height and postoperative range of motion. Ossification of the posterior longitudinal ligament is a contraindication for device placement.

After the Caspar distractor is removed, care should be taken to confirm that the reference pins are screwed in fully. It should also be noted that implantation of the CerviCore device requires a minimum of 5 mm of disc space distraction. If during any of the preliminary steps it is determined that the necessary distraction cannot be achieved without injury to the soft tissues or facet joints, the treatment should be converted to a standard anterior cervical fusion.

## Initial End Plate Preparation

Two fins on each baseplate provide initial fixation of the CerviCore Intervertebral Disc. Channels are cut for the fins before insertion of the device. In order to seat the device correctly, the appropriate channel depth must be achieved.

To create pilot holes for the end plate chisels, the fin drill guide is advanced along the reference pins and into the prepared disc space (Fig. 28–7). The position of the positive vertebral body stop should be visually confirmed so that it comes into full contact with both the superior and inferior vertebral bodies. The fin drill guide head should be parallel with the superior and inferior end plates and aligned in the sagittal plane. Four pilot holes are then drilled for the implant fins at precise locations in the end plates using the drill bits provided in the instrumentation set. A positive stop on the drill prevents overdrilling of the pilot grooves (greater than 10 mm in depth).

The fin drill guide is then removed and replaced with the chisel guide over the reference pins and into the disc space. Again, the positive stop on the chisel guide is checked to make sure that it comes into full contact with the adjacent vertebral bodies. The chisel guide must be fully seated to ensure that the channels are cut to the full depth. Failure to do so will prevent full and appropriate seating of the implant. The chisel guide handle should be parallel with the end plates and aligned in the sagittal plane. The first chisel is then advanced along the tracks of either the right or left side of the chisel guide and into the bone while applying positive pressure to the chisel guide to prevent it from backing out (Fig. 28–8). If necessary, gentle impaction may be added using the mallet included in the instrument set. Once the first chisel has been seated, the second chisel is inserted in the same manner in order to cut the second set of channels. Alternatively, both chisels may be advanced in tandem to cut both the right and left channels simultaneously. The chisels are then removed,

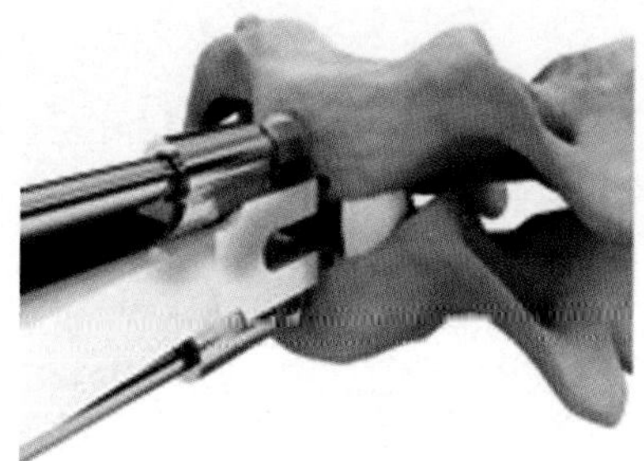

■ FIGURE 28–8. Chiseling of channels.

followed by the chisel guide. The slotted mallet may be used as a slap hammer with gentle force in order to remove the chisels from the disc space if required.

## Sizing

The disc space is then measured to determine the correct implant size. The smallest height implant that adequately restores the disc height should be selected. Because the sizers are chamfered at the leading end to facilitate insertion, care must be taken so that ease of insertion of the spacer does not mislead the surgeon to oversize the implant (Fig. 28–9). Sizers are provided in the same heights (5, 6, 7, 8, and 9 mm) and baseplate widths (14 and 16 mm) as the implants. The appropriate 5-mm (height) sizer with a width of either 14 or 16 mm is selected based on the size of the template used to identify the midline in the first step. The sizer is then attached to the sizer/template handle in the same manner that the template was secured to the handle and inserted into the disc space. Sequential sizers are used to gauge the desired implant height that will restore disc space height and tissue tension without overtensioning the annulus or causing injury to the soft tissue or neural structures. An implant should be chosen that covers at least two thirds of the anteroposterior depth of the end plates. Optimal sizing should result in a snug fit, with mild to moderate resistance to pull-out.

## Fin Track Preparation

The appropriately sized trial is then selected, corresponding to the final sizer (Fig. 28–10). The trial handle head is marked SUP (for superior) and INF (for inferior) to facilitate correct insertion of the trial. The trial is advanced over the reference pins and into the disc space with attention to align the fins of the trial with the prepared tracks in the end plates (Fig. 28–11). The mallet may be used for gentle impaction. Once the trial has been fully seated, it is removed from the disc space. Again, the slotted mallet

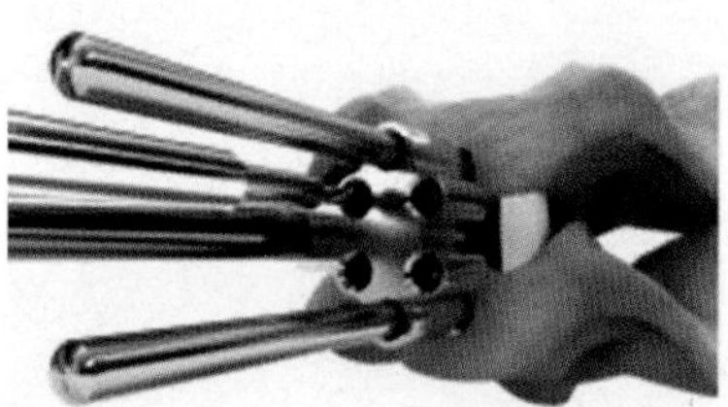

■ FIGURE 28–7. Fin drill guide in place over reference pins for drilling of the four pilot grooves.

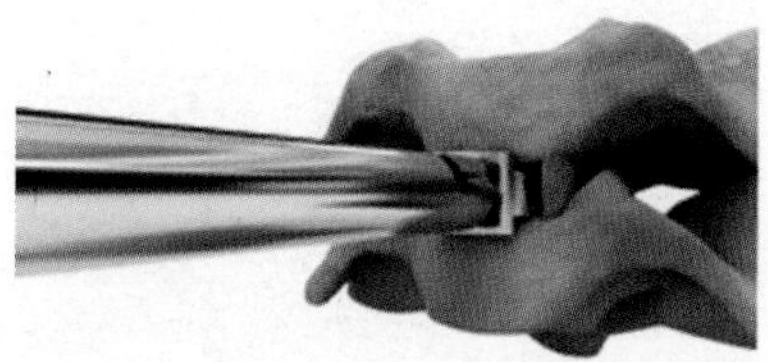

■ FIGURE 28–9. Insertion of sizer.

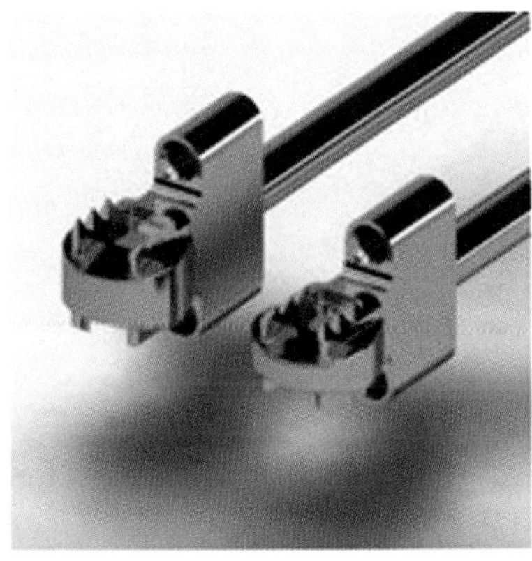

■ **FIGURE 28–10.** Trials (large and small).

may be used gently as a slap hammer to remove the trial from the disc space. Caution should be taken to both insert and remove the trial from the disc space with gentle force and at an angle parallel to the end plates in order to properly prepare the fin tracks, prevent damage to the end plates, and avoid the creation of bone fragments that could migrate into the canal or neural foramen.

### Device Insertion

The CerviCore Intervertebral Disc is provided as a single unit with the baseplates held together in parallel by a plastic implant dispenser. The appropriately sized implant is selected with height and baseplate dimensions that match the corresponding final sizer. The implant is attached to the head of the inserter using the implant dispenser, and the dispenser is then removed. The orientation of the implant is confirmed by checking that the exposed end of the implant is positioned with the bearing surface contour curving upward, i.e., "smiling" (Fig. 28–12). The head of the inserter, with the implant in place, is positioned so that the handle is oriented parallel to the end plates and slid over the reference pins. Before insertion of the implant, a final confirmation is performed both visually, to check that the implant fins are aligned with the fin tracks, and fluoroscopically, to verify that the angle of insertion of the implant is parallel to the end plates.

The implant is then advanced until the posterior margin of the device is in contact with the disc space and the four fins begin to enter the fin channels. The implant is further advanced into position by introducing the plunger through the inserter handle, thus providing gentle force to propel the plunger against the anterior surface of the CerviCore device. The device has been fully inserted and seated when the implant has completely disengaged from the inserter head and the anterior vertebral stops of the implant are in contact with the anterior vertebral margins of the adjacent vertebrae (Fig. 28–13).

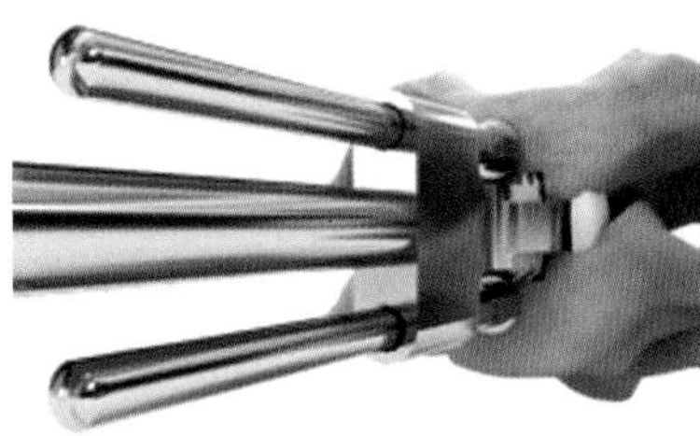

■ **FIGURE 28–11.** Insertion of trial over reference pins.

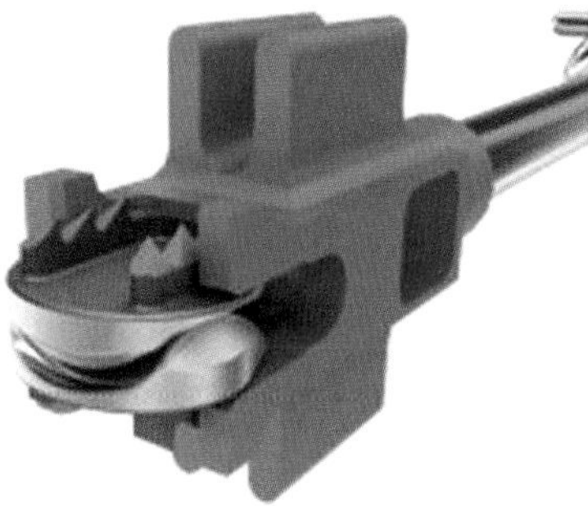

■ **FIGURE 28–12.** CerviCore Intervertebral Disc secured on inserter head/handle.

Final device sizing and positioning is confirmed fluoroscopically. The device can be positioned more posteriorly with a tamp, which is included in the instrumentation set. Gentle impaction may then be used to adjust the depth. Again, the device's anterior vertebral body stops will aid in preventing placement of the device too far posteriorly. These stops should ultimately be flush with the anterior face of the spine for proper positioning.

Once the implant has been fully inserted, the reference pins are removed (Fig. 28–14). A small amount of bone wax may be used to control bleeding from the vertebral body at these sites. Standard surgical closure is then performed for an anterior approach to the cervical spine.

## POSTOPERATIVE CARE AND REHABILITATION

A soft collar may be utilized for 1 to 2 weeks during initial wound healing, depending on patient comfort. Extension exercises are not recommended until at least 6 weeks postoperatively (Fig. 28–15).

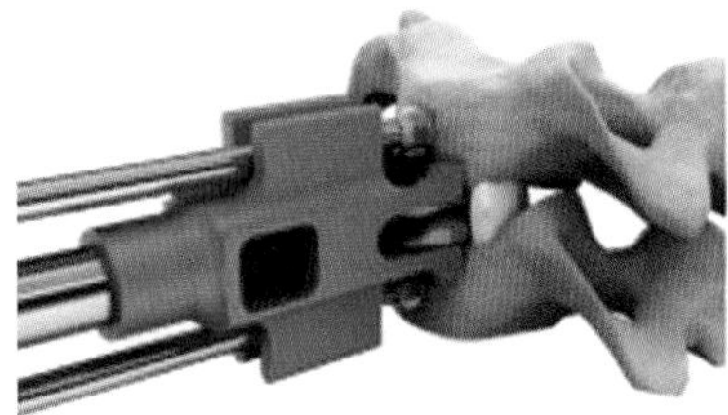

■ **FIGURE 28–13.** Advancement of the implant into the disc space.

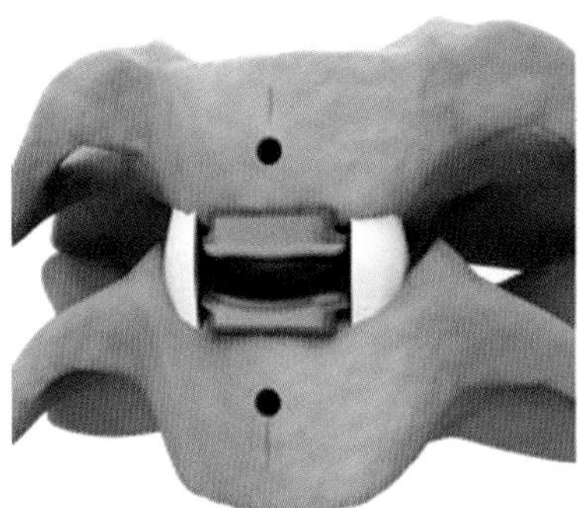

■ **FIGURE 28–14.** CerviCore Intervertebral Disc in situ.

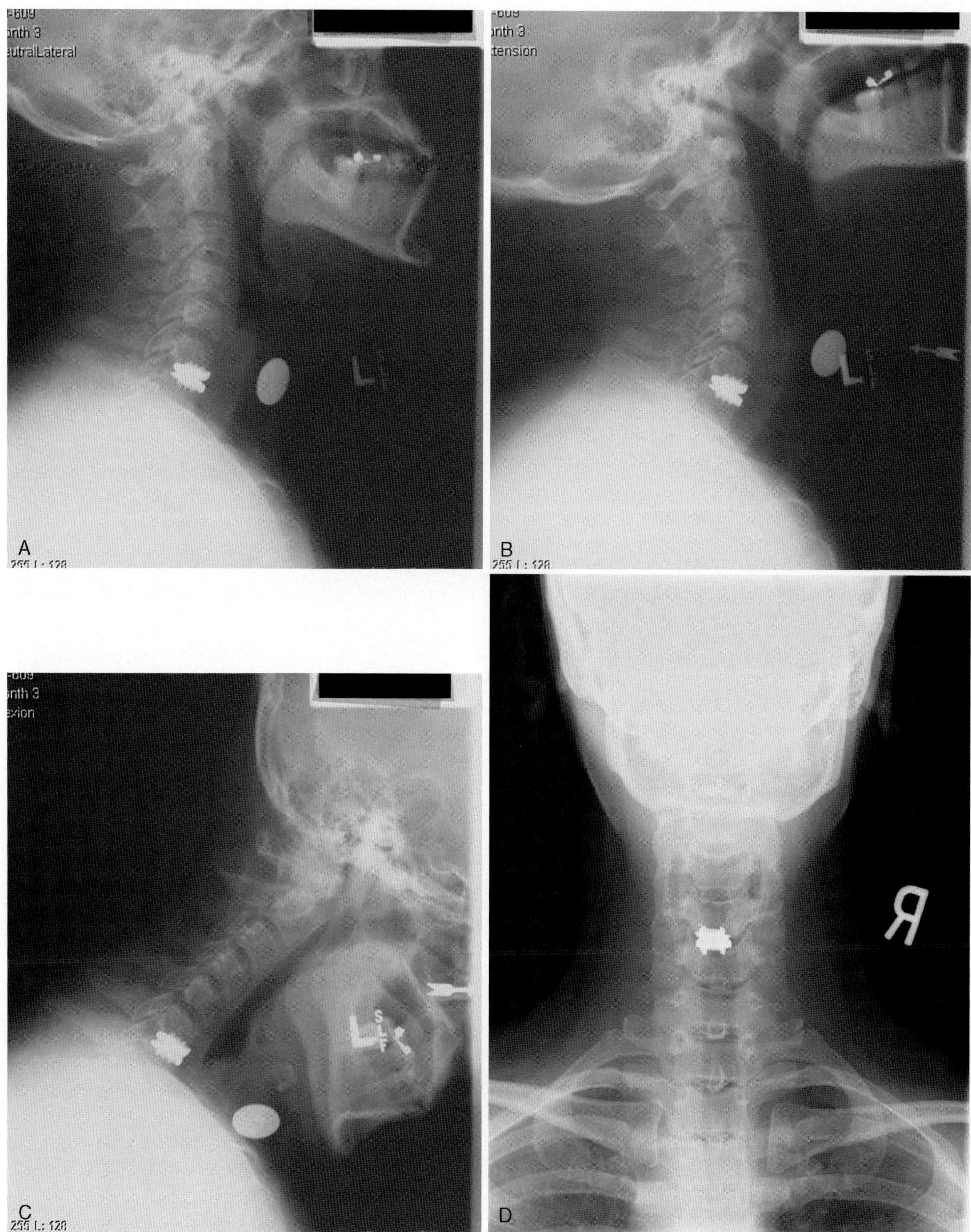

■ **FIGURE 28–15.** Three-month postoperative radiographs demonstrating flexion/extension and lateral bending. **A,** Neutral lateral radiograph of a patient following implantation of C6-C7 CerviCore Disc Replacement. **B,** Extension lateral radiograph. **C,** Flexion lateral radiograph. **D,** Anteroposterior (AP) radiograph.

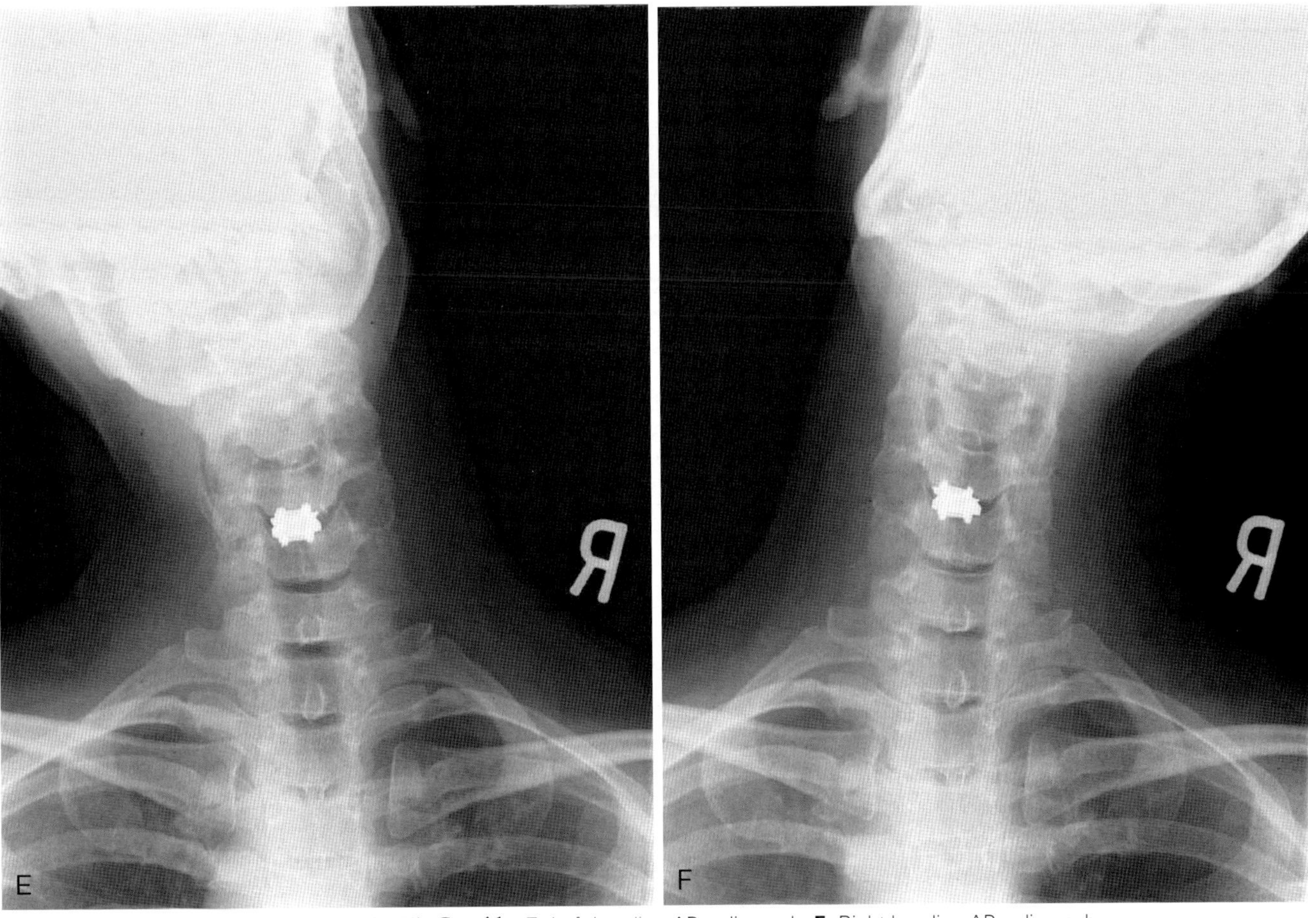


■ **FIGURE 28–15. Cont'd** **E,** Left-bending AP radiograph. **F,** Right-bending AP radiograph.

demonstrates postoperative range of motion at 3 months in both flexion-extension and lateral bending.

## REMOVAL OF THE DEVICE

Should it be necessary, the CerviCore Intervertebral Disc can be removed using the extractor tool included with the instrumentation. The curved distal tooth of the extractor is positioned under the anterior lip of the vertebral body stop in order to extract the device from the disc space. If required, gentle force may be applied to the extractor handle with the slotted mallet used as a slap hammer.

## COMPLICATIONS AND AVOIDANCE

The spectrum of complications associated with cervical disc replacement is similar to those encountered with anterior cervical decompression and interbody fusion. They include new neurologic deficits due to nerve root injury or edema, spinal cord contusion, or acute release of chronic neural compression. Moreover, acute neurologic deficits may result from mechanical problems such as migration of a fragment of residual disc or bone, compression from a residual osteophyte, acute epidural hematoma, or posterior migration of the device. Progressive neurologic deficit following the first week of recovery may be a sign of spinal instability or an epidural abscess. Dysphagia is common following anterior cervical surgery, usually from edema, but generally is self-limiting. Proper device positioning should be confirmed radiographically in cases that fail to resolve. Dysphonia may occur secondary to an injury of the recurrent laryngeal nerve. Limiting retraction and operative times as well as deflation and reinflation of the endotracheal tube balloon following placement of any self-retaining retractors may minimize injury to the recurrent laryngeal nerve. Infection, specifically vertebral osteomyelitis, should be ruled out in the event of delayed onset of cervical pain.

## CONCLUSIONS/DISCUSSION

At the writing of this chapter, the CerviCore Intervertebral Disc is under investigational status and is limited by U.S. law to investigational use. Anterior cervical decompression and fusion is a highly successful procedure with fusion rates exceeding 95% in well-selected patients and excellent clinical outcomes. Nevertheless, spinal fusion eliminates motion at the functional spinal unit and may contribute to a degenerative cascade in the cervical spine with adjacent segment degeneration leading to an average annual incidence of 3% of patients requiring further surgery for adjacent segment disease.[5]

When performed in appropriately indicated patients, cervical disc replacement may have a number of potential advantages over spinal fusion. By preserving or reestablishing motion at the functional spinal unit, the goals are twofold: Cervical motion may be preserved or improved, and the cascade of adjacent spinal segment degeneration may be impeded or prevented entirely. Following implantation, the cervical disc replacement is designed to articulate immediately, with recovery consisting of the anterior cervical wound and tissue healing alone. This period of recovery is expected to be substantially shorter than that required to achieve solid spinal fusion. Although a patient may wear a soft cervical orthosis for short-term postoperative comfort during wound healing, immediate stability can eliminate the need for the patient to wear a postoperative orthosis in order to enhance fusion.* Cervical disc replacement is a promising development in cervical spine surgery for the treatment of degenerative disc disease, and the CerviCore Intervertebral Disc incorporates a number of important potential advances in motion preservation technology.

*Nevertheless, time is required to establish long-term fixation of a cervical artificial disc, and so extension exercises should be avoided for a minimum of 6 weeks.

## REFERENCES


1. Dvorak J, Antinnes JA, Panjabi M, et al: Age and gender related normal motion of the cervical spine. Spine 17:S393–S398, 1992.
2. Valdevit A, Ryan T, Carannante F, et al: Incremental range of motion—A parameter to evaluate range of motion quality: Application to a saddle joint cervical disc replacement. Abstract presentation at the 53rd annual meeting of the Orthopaedic Research Society, San Diego, California, February 2007.
3. Hallab N, Link HD, McAfee PC: Biomaterial optimization in total disc arthroplasty. Spine 28:S139–S152, 2003.
4. Valdevit A, Kambic H, Errico JP, et al: Characteristics of a saddle joint—An alternative geometry for bearing surfaces. Abstract presentation at the 51st annual meeting of the Orthopaedic Research Society, Washington, DC, 2005.
5. Hilibrand AS, Robbins M: Adjacent segment degeneration and adjacent segment disease: The consequences of spinal fusion? Spine J 4:190S–194S, 2004.

CHAPTER 29

# SECURE-C Cervical Artificial Disc

**Scott A. Rushton, Joseph M. Marzluff,** and **Jeffrey McConnell**

## KEY POINTS

- The SECURE-C Cervical Artificial Disc is an articulating device intended to help alleviate pain and permit motion in the diseased cervical spine.
- The semiconstrained design features a sliding core that interfaces with a spherical surface on the superior end plate and a cylindrical surface on the inferior end plate.
- Serrated keels on the titanium plasma spray-coated end plates help to promote bone ingrowth and to secure fixation in the vertebrae.
- The device is composed of two cobalt-chrome alloy end plates and a central ultra-high-molecular-weight polyethylene core.
- Anteroposterior translation (1.25 mm) allows for a more physiologic moving instantaneous axis of rotation.

## INTRODUCTION

Neck and upper extremity radicular pain are common symptoms of cervical spine disease. Spinal cord compression, nerve root compression, herniated nucleus pulposus, degenerative spondylolisthesis, and other conditions are commonly treated by anterior cervical discectomy and fusion (ACDF) if surgery is necessary. Although treatment options including enhanced grafts, spacers, and plates have greatly improved over the past 20 years, the average clinical success rates for anterior cervical procedures are at approximately 75%.[1–4] Spinal fusion prohibits the normal motion in affected spinal segments and disrupts the normal biomechanical interactions between the vertebral bodies, disc, facets, and soft tissues, which may lead to secondary changes at adjacent levels.[5,6] There is a significant incidence of adjacent-level degeneration in the 5 to 10 years following fusion, with reports varying from 15% to 50%.[7–9] Over the past several decades, surgeons and researchers have investigated alternative motion-sparing nonfusion devices such as artificial discs. Several cervical disc replacement discs are currently under clinical investigation in the United States, including the ProDisc-C (Synthes, West Chester, PA), the Bryan Cervical Disc Prosthesis, Prestige Artificial Cervical Disc (both Medtronic Sofamor Danek, Memphis, TN), the PCM device (Cervitech, Inc., Rockaway, NJ), and the CerviCore (Stryker Spine, Allendale, NJ) devices. The U.S. Food and Drug Administration approved the initiation of a prospective randomized pivotal Investigational Device Exemption (IDE) clinical trial to evaluate the safety and effectiveness of the SECURE-C Cervical Artificial Disc (Globus Medical, Audubon, PA) compared with ACDF using the ASSURE (Globus Medical, Inc., Audubon, PA) cervical plate and allograft. Early results from three U.S. IDE centers are reported in this chapter.

## INDICATIONS/CONTRAINDICATIONS

Patients enrolled in the U.S. IDE clinical trial are 18 to 60 years old, have been diagnosed with single-level symptomatic cervical disc disease (C3-C7), have had no previous adjacent cervical fusion, have undergone 6 weeks of conservative therapy, and have met other inclusion/exclusion criteria as listed in Table 29–1. Patients agreed to undergo necessary preoperative and postoperative evaluations as specified in the follow-up schedule.

## DESCRIPTION OF THE DEVICE

The SECURE-C Cervical Artificial Disc is an articulating implant (Fig. 29–1) composed of two end plates and a central core, inserted using an anterior cervical approach. The superior and inferior cobalt-chrome alloy end plates feature serrated keels and a porous titanium plasma spray coating. The serrated keels are press-fit to provide immediate stabilization, whereas the end plate surface design features help promote long-term bony ongrowth and ingrowth.

The sliding core is composed of ultra-high-molecular-weight polyethylene (UHMWPE), with a spherical superior interface and a cylindrical inferior interface to fit with the metallic end plates. UHMWPE has been used extensively in hip and knee prostheses and has been shown to produce minimal wear. The device features allow anteroposterior (AP) sliding for more physiologic loading with a moving instantaneous axis of rotation (IAR). The design also eliminates dislodgement of the core, helping to protect facets from excessive loading.

SECURE-C is designed to permit motion in flexion-extension, lateral bending, and axial rotation. Motion is mediated by surrounding tissues, including the facets, interspinous ligament, posterior

**TABLE 29–1. Inclusion and Exclusion Criteria for the SECURE-C IDE Clinical Trial**

| Inclusion Criteria | Exclusion Criteria |
|---|---|
| 1. Symptomatic cervical disc disease (SCDD) in one vertebral level between C3-C7, defined as neck or arm (radicular) pain, or functional or neurological deficit, and radiographic confirmation (by CT, MRI, x-ray, etc.) of any of the following:<br>a) Herniated nucleus pulposus;<br>b) Radiculopathy or myelopathy;<br>c) Spondylosis (defined by the presence of osteophytes); or<br>d) Loss of disc height<br>2. Age between 18 and 60 years<br>3. Failed at least 6 weeks of conservative treatment<br>4. Neck Disability Index (NDI) Questionnaire score of at least 30 (as percentage of 50 point total)<br>5. Able to understand and sign informed consent form<br>6. Psychosocially, mentally, and physically able to fully comply with this protocol including adhering to follow-up schedule and filling out forms<br>7. Able to meet the proposed follow-up schedule at 6 weeks, and 3, 6, 12, and 24 months<br>8. Able to follow postoperative management program | 1. More than one vertebral level requiring treatment<br>2. Prior fusion surgery adjacent to the vertebral level being treated<br>3. Prior surgery at the level to be treated<br>4. Clinically compromised vertebral bodies at the affected levels due to current or past trauma<br>5. Radiographic confirmation of facet joint disease or degeneration, defined as apparent sclerosis or hypertrophy of the facets demonstrated on AP radiographs as a disruption of the normally smooth facet curve<br>6. Marked cervical instability on resting lateral or flexion-extension radiographs:<br>a) Translation greater than 3 mm and/or<br>b) More than 11 degrees of rotational difference from that of either adjacent level<br>7. Severe spondylosis at the level to be treated as characterized by any of the following:<br>a) Bridging osteophytes;<br>b) A loss of disc height greater than 50%; or<br>c) Absence of motion (<2 degrees)<br>8. Neck or arm pain of unknown etiology<br>9. Osteoporosis, osteopenia, Paget's disease, osteomalacia or any other metabolic bone disease<br>10. Pregnant or interested in becoming pregnant in the next 2 years<br>11. Active systemic or local infection<br>12. Known allergy to titanium, polyethylene, cobalt, chromium, or molybdenum<br>13. Taking medications or any drug known to potentially interfere with bone or soft tissue healing (e.g., steroids)<br>14. Rheumatoid arthritis or other autoimmune diseases<br>15. Systemic disease including AIDS, HIV, hepatitis<br>16. Active malignancy: A patient with a history of any invasive malignancy (except nonmelanoma skin cancer), unless he or she has been treated with curative intent and there has been no clinical signs or symptoms of the malignancy for at least 5 years<br>17. Neuromuscular disorders such as muscular dystrophy, spinal muscular atrophy, amyotrophic lateral sclerosis, etc.<br>18. Acute mental illness or substance abuse<br>19. Use of bone growth stimulator within past 30 days<br>20. Participation in other investigational device or drug clinical trials within 30 days of surgery<br>21. Prisoner |

AIDS, acquired immunodeficiency syndrome; CT, computed tomography; HIV, human immunodeficiency virus; IDE, Investigational Device Exemption; MRI, magnetic resonance imaging.

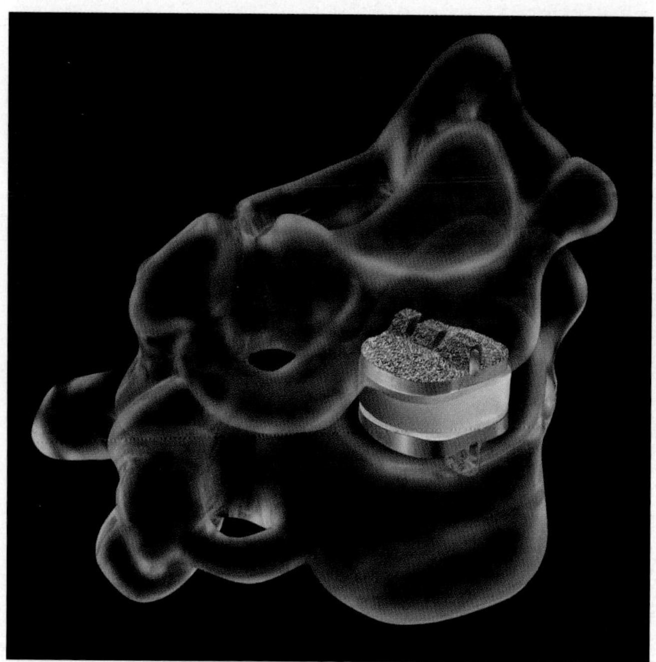

■ **FIGURE 29–1.** The SECURE-C Cervical Artificial Disc.

longitudinal ligament, and all surrounding musculature. The ranges of motion (ROMs) in the normal human spinal motion segment have been reviewed and reported[10] at up to 20 degrees in flexion-extension, up to 17 degrees in one side lateral bending, and up to 12 degrees in one side axial rotation. The SECURE-C Cervical Artificial Disc allows motion in flexion and extension up to 30 degrees (±15 degrees) and in lateral bending up to 20 degrees (±10 degrees). The design allows unlimited axial rotation, which is constrained by ligaments and posterior elements. The implant design is intended to provide 1.25 mm of AP translation during articulation, for a moving IAR in the sagittal plane, which is typically active in flexion and extension.[11]

Implants are offered in a variety of configurations to accommodate varied patient anatomy. Three implant footprints are available, with six core heights and lordotic (6 degrees) or parallel end plate configurations. The preferred size is large enough to fill most of the evacuated disc space anterior to posterior but not overstuff the disc space. The implant should rest within the apophyseal ring of the vertebral end plate, to minimize the potential for subsidence. Ideally, the device is centered just 1 to 2 mm posterior to vertebral midline to help approximate normal cervical spine biomechanics.

## OPERATIVE TECHNIQUE

Preoperative planners may be used with lateral and AP radiographs and magnetic resosnace imaging scans to estimate the SECURE-C disc size (lordosis, width, length, and height) to be implanted, using the levels adjacent to the operative level as guides. Standard anesthesia and preparation for an anterior cervical approach are used. The patient is positioned supine such that the neck is in neutral sagittal alignment, rather than in extension, which is typical for ACDF. A towel roll or intravenous bag may be used as support behind the neck. Lateral and AP fluoroscopy films are taken before draping to ensure proper positioning of the cervical spine. Fluoroscopy is used throughout the implantation procedure to visualize and confirm implant placement. Biplanar fluoroscopy is ideal if available.

A transverse skin incision is made over the desired operative level. The platysma muscle is sectioned, and blunt dissection is performed posteriorly and medially to the vertebral midline to visualize the disc space. The longus coli muscle is gently mobilized along both sides of the disc space. Self-retaining retractors are placed to visualize the disc space. A Caspar-type distractor is used in combination with grooved distraction pins that resist any sliding of the distractor. Distraction pins are placed superiorly in the vertebra above the operative level and inferiorly in the vertebra below, avoiding the locations for the small serrated keels on each device end plate. These pins may also be used as AP midline markers.

Partial discectomy is performed using standard disc preparation instruments, leaving the lateral annulus intact. Scrapers may be used to remove disc material and prepare the end plates for implantation. Burring and milling are not necessary and may damage vertebral end plates, increasing the risk of poor implantation or postoperative subsidence. Removal of osteophytes or mild end plate spondylosis may require the use of kerrison rongeurs or even a small burr. The posterior longitudinal ligament is usually resected when required to access the herniation or osteophyte.

Trials are used to determine the appropriate depth, length, and height of the SECURE-C implant for the disc space. Trials of various footprints, heights, and lordosis are used to determine the appropriate implant (Fig. 29–2A), with distraction released. The device is recommended to fit well within the disc space, with its midline 1 to 2 mm posterior from vertebral midline. Care should be taken in choosing a trial that does not overfill or underfill the disc space. Correct trial and implant placement must be confirmed with AP and lateral fluoroscopy.

A chisel matching the chosen trial's lordosis and height is selected. The chisel is slid over the trial and gently impacted until it is seated into the vertebral body, creating superior and inferior keel slots (see Fig 29–2B). Care must be taken to direct the chisel parallel with the vertebral end plates and the disc space, using fluoroscopy. Once the chisel is fully seated and both trial and chisel are confirmed to be in correct position, the chisel can be removed using a slap hammer, followed by the trial. Keel slots are cleared of bony debris using a nerve hook.

The SECURE-C end plates and polyethylene core are selected to match the chosen trial. The three implant components are assembled into the loading block, and an implant holder is then used to grasp the implant assembly as one unit for insertion. The SECURE-C device is inserted into the keel slots, using gentle impaction under fluoroscopic guidance. The implant holder is removed and may be further seated posteriorly using a single or double end plate positioner (see Fig. 29–2C) to reach its final position (see Fig. 29–2D). Distraction and retraction are removed, and the wound is closed using standard techniques.

## POSTOPERATIVE CARE

Standard procedures following spinal surgery are to be followed, with additional postoperative patient care for control and investigational patients recommended as follows: patients wear an external orthosis (i.e., soft cervical collar) until approximately 3 weeks following surgery; at 3 weeks after surgery, the collar is discontinued, and patients are referred to a physical therapy program for active range of motion exercises, postural exercises, and scapular stabilization. It is recommended that patients do not drive for 5 weeks, if possible. Patients are also requested to avoid repetitive bending or lifting and athletic activities for at least 6 months. Although not all patients fully comply with the protocol, the study is conservative in limiting excessive range of motion in the early postoperative period.

## CLINICAL PRESENTATION AND EVALUATION

SECURE-C has been implanted in more than 150 patients to date, with more than 245 patients enrolled, in the IDE clinical trial. Surgeries have been performed in 17 sites across the country. Clinical results from three centers and four operating surgeons have been pooled for this report. A total of 63 patients have been enrolled and had surgery at these three centers. Enrollment is under way, with completion anticipated within the next few months, and collection of patient follow-up evaluation data will be continued up to 2 years after surgery.

As described in Table 29–1, patients who met the eligibility criteria outlined in the IDE clinical trial were able to be enrolled in the study. The most common cause for enrollment was a degenerated or herniated disc. The first five patients at each site were not randomized and received the SECURE-C device. Thereafter, patients were randomized at a 1:1 ratio of SECURE-C cervical discs to ACDF. Pain and function outcomes (Neck Disability Index [NDI] and Visual Analog Scale [VAS] neck and arm pain) as well as disc height and range of motion were evaluated preoperatively, at 6 weeks, and at 3, 6, 12, and 24 months after surgery. Table 29–2 lists patient demographics, and Table 29–3 lists levels treated for the enrolled patients. The majority of surgeries were performed at C6-C7 and C5-C6. The number of patients reaching each follow-up evaluation is shown in Table 29–4.

Patient outcomes demonstrated significant improvements in NDI and VAS pain scores compared with the preoperative values (Figs. 29–3 to 29–6). NDI dropped significantly between preoperative and all postoperative follow-up evaluations for both SECURE-C and ACDF groups, with no significant difference between the two groups. Average NDI scores were reduced postoperatively by more than 75% in both groups, and average neck pain VAS was reduced by more than 65% in both groups. At the patients' most recent visits, 37/38 or 97.3% of SECURE-C patients and 23/25 or 91.7% of ACDF patients had more than 25% improvement from their preoperative NDI score. All outcomes

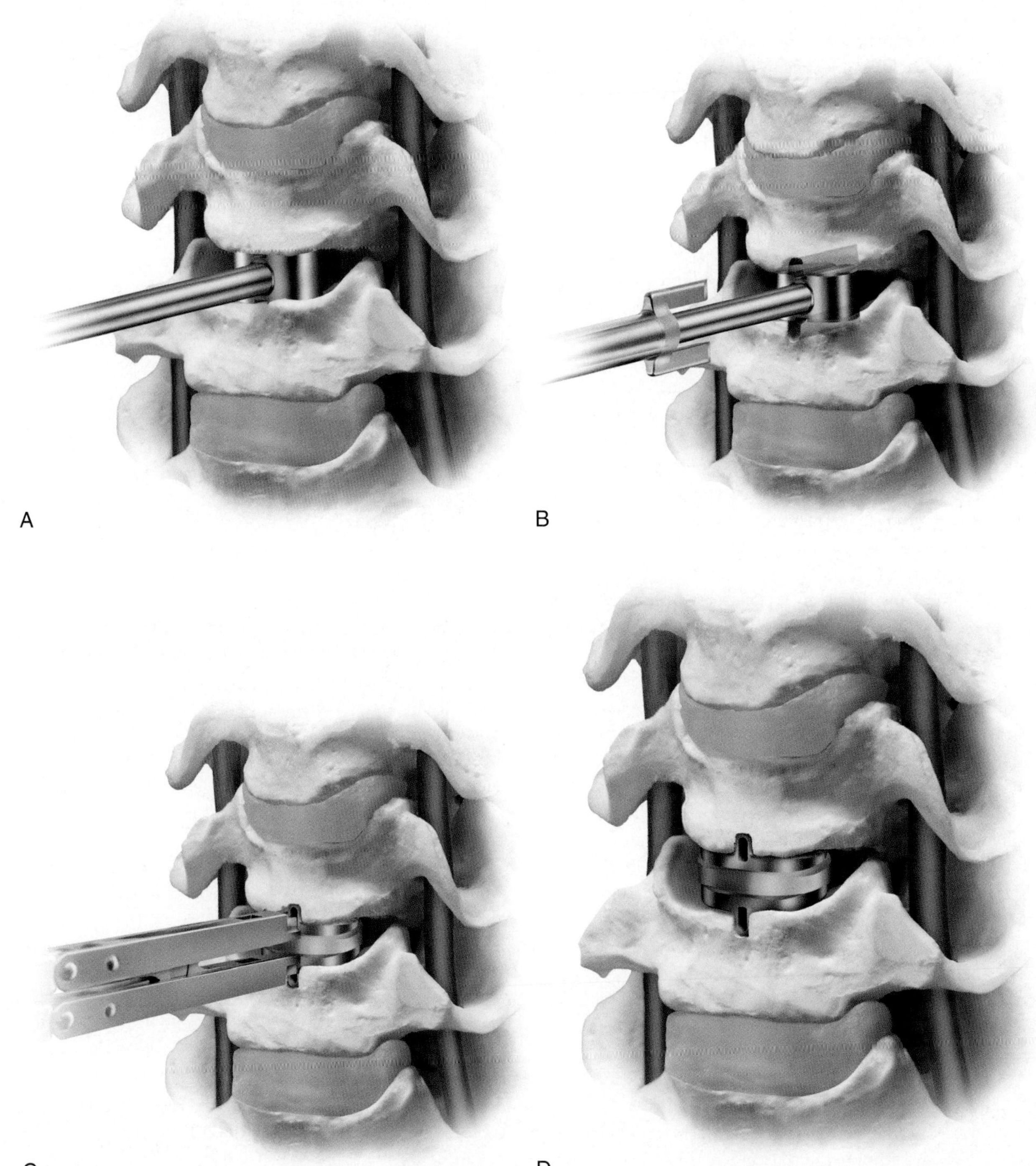


■ FIGURE 29–2. **A,** Trialing the disc space for the appropriate implant size (distractor and retractors removed for clarity for this and other technique images). **B,** Creating keel slots using guided chisels. **C,** Inserting and positioning the SECURE-C implant. **D,** Final position.

TABLE 29–2. Patient Demographic Variables

| Variable | First Five SECURE-C | Randomized SECURE-C | Randomized ACDF | Overall Total |
|---|---|---|---|---|
| Number of patients, *n* | 14 | 24 | 25 | 63 |
| Average age (yr) | 39.6 | 45.6 | 44.0 | 43.6 |
| Male (%):Female (%) | 57:43 | 58:42 | 44:56 | 52:48 |

ACDF, anterior cervical discectomy and fusion.

TABLE 29–3. Levels Treated

| Level | *n* (%) |
|---|---|
| C3-C4 | 0 (0) |
| C4-C5 | 4 (6) |
| C5-C6 | 27 (44) |
| C6-C7 | 31 (50) |

TABLE 29–4. Patients Reaching Each Postoperative Evaluation

| Group | Surgery | 6 Weeks | 3 Months | 6 Months | 12 Months | 24 Months |
|---|---|---|---|---|---|---|
| First 5 | 14 | 14 | 14 | 13 | 10 | 0 |
| SECURE-C randomized | 24 | 23 | 21 | 18 | 8 | 0 |
| ACDF randomized | 25 | 24 | 22 | 16 | 9 | 0 |
| **TOTAL** | **63** | **61** | **57** | **47** | **27** | **0** |

ACDF, anterior cervical discectomy and fusion.

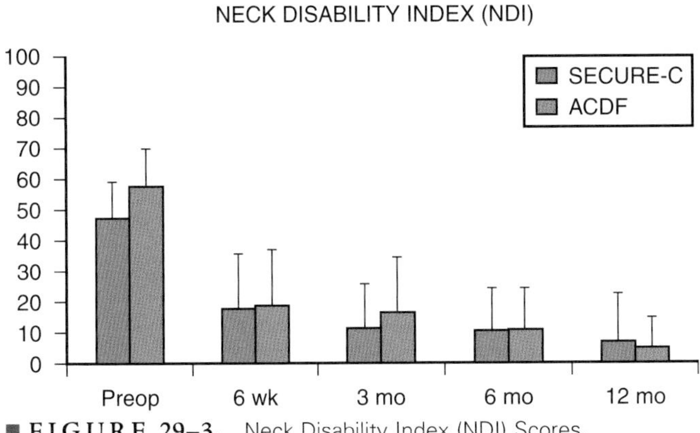


■ **FIGURE 29–3.** Neck Disability Index (NDI) Scores.

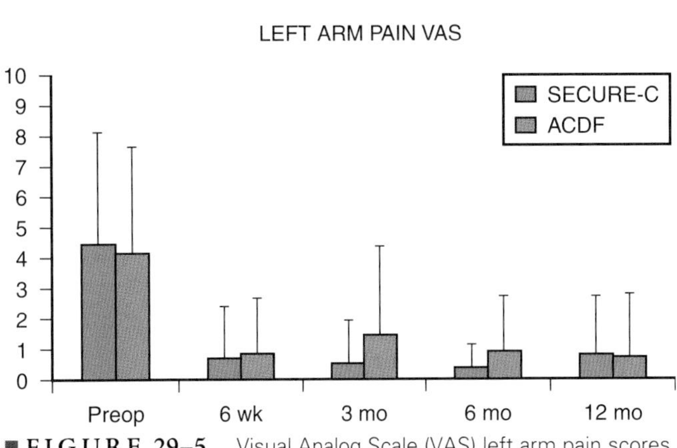


■ **FIGURE 29–5.** Visual Analog Scale (VAS) left arm pain scores.

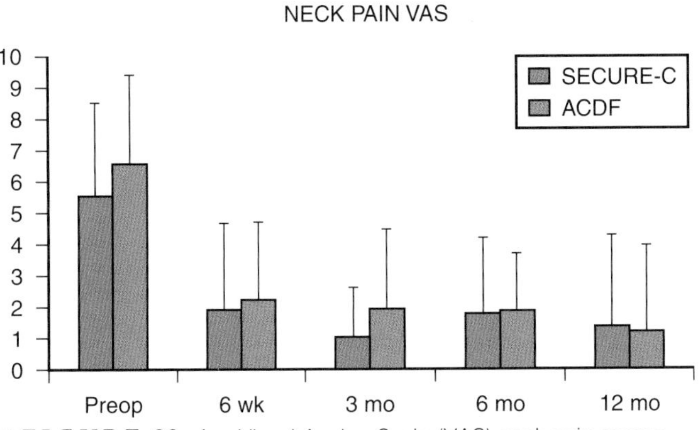


■ **FIGURE 29–4.** Visual Analog Scale (VAS) neck pain scores.

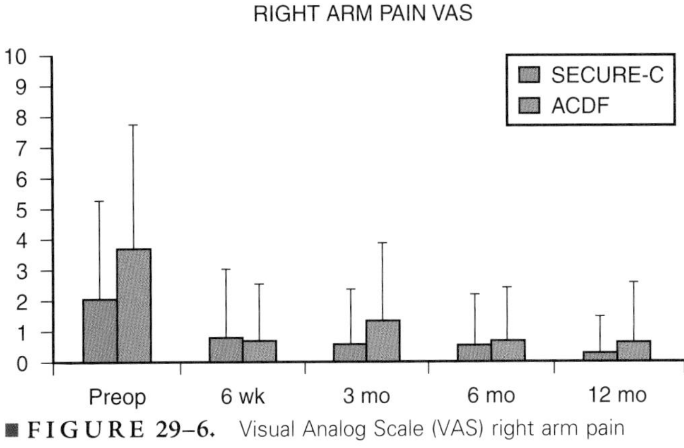


■ **FIGURE 29–6.** Visual Analog Scale (VAS) right arm pain scores.

exhibited reductions in pain and function from preoperative values ($P < 0.05$), but were not significantly different between treatment groups ($P > 0.05$).

Disc height and range of motion data are available for patients 6 months after surgery. Average disc height increased by 54.8% at 6 months and 52.6% at 12 months for the SECURE-C group and 16.0% at 6 months and 12.9% at 12 months for the ACDF group. For the SECURE-C group, the average range of motion was 9.0 degrees before surgery, 9.5 degrees at 6 months, and 8.0 degrees at 12 months, thereby maintaining preoperative motion. As expected in the ACDF group, the average range of motion was 7.2 degrees before surgery and was dramatically reduced to nominal levels of 1.5 degrees at 6 months and 0.7 degrees at 12 months. These data demonstrate the anticipated motion preservation for SECURE-C patients and motion elimination for fusion patients. Figure 29–7 shows 12-month postoperative films from a patient who received the SECURE-C device.

No patients had major complications or device-related adverse events. One adverse event was reported in a SECURE-C patient involved in a motor vehicle accident 24 days after surgery. There was no migration of the device, and the patient quickly recovered, reporting complete resolution of pain and no disability at all subsequent follow-up visits. Fusion evaluation will be based on 24-month postoperative films; however, no patients have reached this time point as yet.

## COMPLICATIONS AND AVOIDANCE

There were no major complications or device-related events in either the SECURE-C or ACDF groups. There have been no

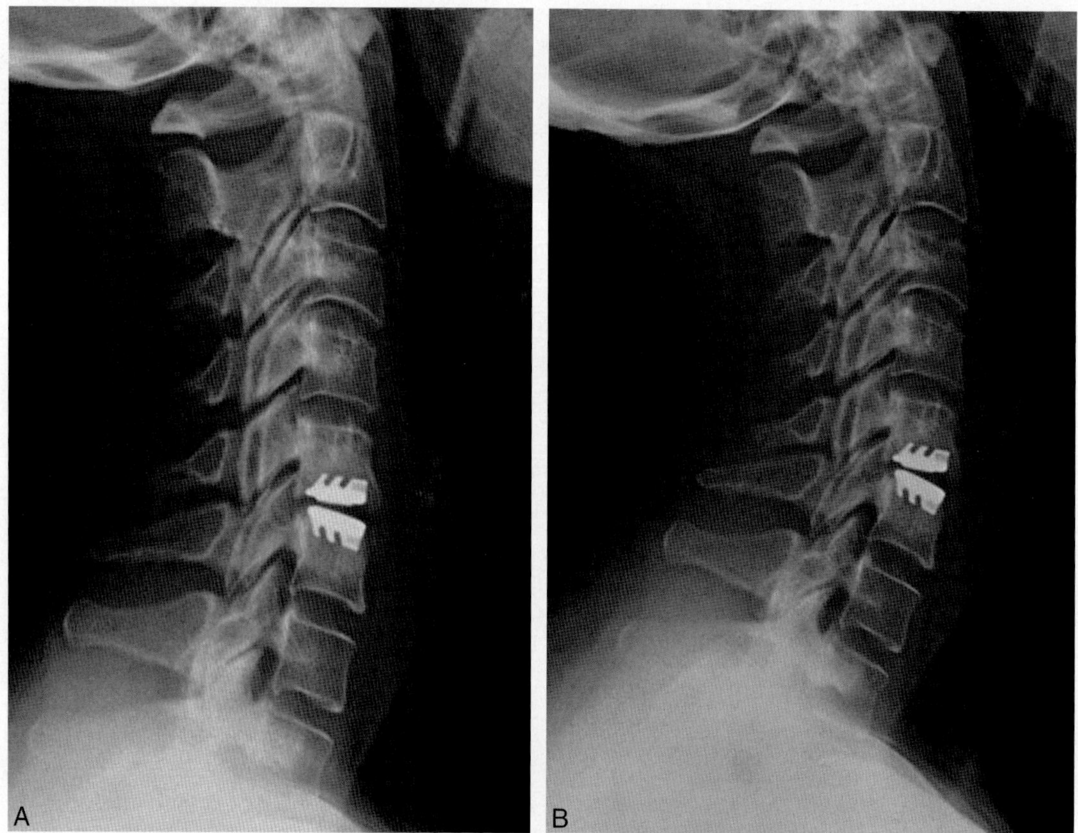


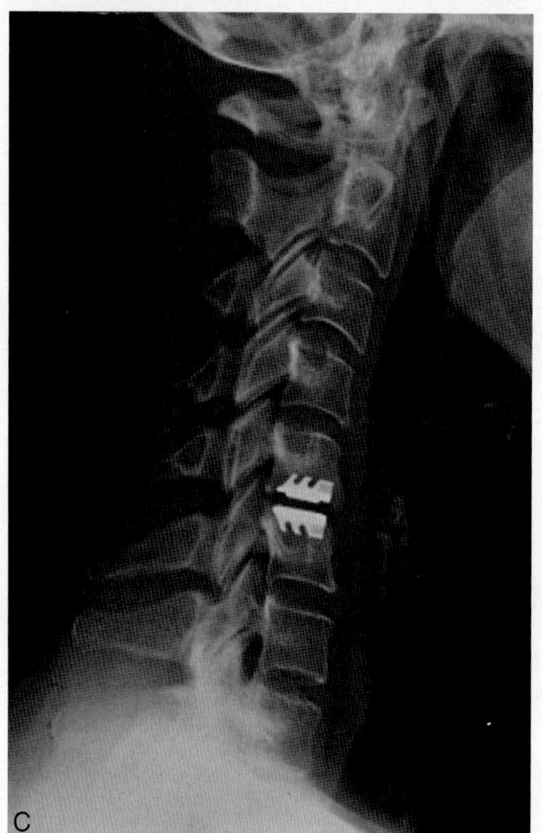


■ **FIGURE 29–7.** Postoperative films for SECURE-C patient at 12 months: **(A)** neutral lateral, **(B)** extension lateral, and **(C)** flexion lateral.

revision surgeries in either group. One patient required conversion to fusion due to the patient's small stature and corresponding small disc space; implanting the disc would have overstuffed the space and could have created additional complications.

### ADVANTAGES/DISADVANTAGES: SECURE-C DEVICE

| Advantages | Disadvantages |
|---|---|
| Familiar surgical approach | IDE study not yet completed |
| Known biomaterials (UHMWPE, CoCrMb) | Unknown multilevel outcomes |
| Device seated well within disc space | Long-term data >2 years not yet available |
| Dysphagia complications minimized | Long-term wear characteristics unknown |
| More physiologic motion | |
| Good clinical results in IDE study | |
| No technique-related complications | |
| No device-related complications | |

CoCrMb, cobalt, chromium, and molybdenum alloy; IDE, Investigational Device Exemption; UHMWPE, ultra-high-molecular-weight polyethylene.

## CONCLUSIONS/DISCUSSION

Our pooled multisite clinical experience demonstrates early favorable outcomes associated with the SECURE-C Cervical Artificial Disc. This new treatment for degenerative disorders of the cervical spine is a viable alternative to traditional fusion, which uses known methods of approach and discectomy. Early results suggest that motion is preserved and disc height is improved at the operative level. Long-term clinical safety and effectiveness of the device are yet to be determined and will be reported as enrollment concludes and patients reach their 2-year follow-up. Evaluation of adjacent level degeneration is of high interest and will be studied.

## REFERENCES

1. Goldberg EJ, Singh K, Van U, et al: Comparing outcomes of anterior cervical discectomy and fusion in workman's versus non-workman's compensation population. Spine J 2:408–414, 2002.
2. Bohlmann HH, Emery SE, Goodfellow DB, Jones PK: Robinson anterior cervical discectomy and arthrodesis for cervical radiculopathy: Long-term follow-up of one hundred and twenty-two patients. J Bone Joint Surg 75(A):1298–1307, 1993.
3. Bolesta MJ, Rechtine GR, Chrin AM: One- and two-level anterior cervical discectomy and fusion: The effect of plate fixation. Spine J 2:197–203, 2002.
4. Samartzis D, Shen FH, Lyon C, et al: Does rigid instrumentation increase the fusion rate in one-level anterior cerical discectomy and fusion? Spine J 4:636–643, 2004.
5. Hilibrand AS, Carlson GD, Palumbo MA, et al: Radiculopathy and myelopathy at segments adjacent to the site of a previous anterior cervical arthrodesis. J Bone Joint Surg 81A:519–528, 1999.
6. Robbins MM, Hilibrand AS: Post-arthrodesis adjacent segment degeneration. *In* Vaccaro A, Anderson DG, Crawford A, et al. (eds): Complications of Pediatric and Adult Spinal Surgery. New York, Marcel Dekker, 2004, pp 63–86.
7. Hilibrand AS, Carlson GD, Palumbo MA, et al: Radiculopathy and myelopathy at segments adjacent to the site of a previous anterior cervical arthrodesis. J Bone Joint Surg 81A:519–528, 1999.
8. Ishihara H, Kanamori M, Kawaguchi Y, et al: Adjacent segment disease after anterior cervical interbody fusion. Spine J 4:624–628, 2004.
9. Baba H, Furusawa N, Imura S, et al: Late radiographic findings after anterior cervical fusion for spondylotic myeloradiculopathy. Spine 18:2167–2173, 1993.
10. White AA, Panjabi MM: Clinical Biomechanics of the Spine, 2nd ed. Philadelphia, Lippincott Williams and Wilkins, 1990, pp 85–125.
11. Sengupta DK, Demetropoulos CK, Herkowitz HN, Serhan HA: Instantaneous axis rotation and its clinical importance in a healthy lumbar functional spinal unit. Roundtables in Spine Surgery 1:3–12, 2005.

CHAPTER 30

# Cerpass Cervical Total Disc Replacement

**Scott H. Kitchel, Lukas Eisermann, Alexander W.L. Turner, David Cutter,** and **G. Bryan Cornwall**

**KEY POINTS**

- Fixed-bearing total disc replacement
- Ceramic bearing
- All non-ferrous metal construction

## INTRODUCTION

To a typical patient, degenerative disc disease of the cervical spine manifests itself as a combination of neck and arm pain. It is well-accepted that the arm pain can be treated by decompression surgery. When the decompression is achieved through anterior discectomy, the surgeon is left with what may be a structurally unsound condition; thus following the decompression procedure, a stabilization procedure must be performed secondarily. The well-known solution is to place a structural graft or cage into the intervertebral space. Commonly, this construct is also associated with the placement of a titanium plate to enhance stability and thereby increase the chances for the level to successfully fuse.

The solution to the neck pain component has proved to be more elusive. Although the removal of the intervertebral disc does remove *a* potential pain generator, it does not remove *all* potential pain generators. The possibility that other nearby tissues are damaged—either as effects secondary to the degenerative condition (for example, arthritic facets due to excess loading secondary to disc collapse) or as separate primary conditions (for example, a ligament sprain) is not eliminated. Furthermore, the possibility that new neck pain is caused by the rigid stabilization should also be considered (for example, muscle atrophy at the fused level or increased stresses at adjacent levels). Finally, the possibility that all neck pain generators cannot be accurately diagnosed is an additional variable in the process.

It is thought that by replacing the rigid stabilization (the fusion construct) with a mobile stabilization device that allows bending motions while maintaining appropriate disc height, that some of the pain generators secondary to rigid fixation may not arise. For example, some authors have shown that the tissue pressure in adjacent intervertebral discs is lower after mobile stabilizations than after fusion stabilizations.[1,2] An added potential benefit may be that because the stresses and tissue pressures at the adjacent levels are decreased, there exists the potential that the rate of degeneration at the adjacent levels remains at a normal rate, as opposed to an accelerated rate adjacent to rigid stabilizations.[3]

Although all of these potential benefits make disc replacement procedures seem to be very appealing treatments in comparison to fusion procedures, they do not come without their own set of risks. The typical patient requiring a decompression treatment (and, thus, following stabilization treatment) is 35 to 45 years of age; thus, the chosen stabilization procedure must either last for several decades of life or must be designed in a manner that allows another treatment to be reasonably and safely performed.

When evaluating the potential risks associated with mobile stabilization versus the relatively known risks associated with rigid stabilization, the factor that stands out is the overall rate of re-operation of the cervical spine at any level. This is somewhat different than survivorship curves that have been commonly studied in the peripheral joints, because all levels must be taken into consideration, not only the operated level.

To that stated end, the key risk variable that the Cerpass design attempts to remove is complications related to wear of the bearing surfaces. Borrowing from the total hip experience, the Cerpass prosthesis (NuVasive, San Diego, CA) has been designed with toughened ceramic bearing surfaces to minimize the potential for wear debris generation. Alternative bearing surfaces for total hip replacement have been examined in many simulator studies and clinical retrieval studies. Although the specific details of individual designs may vary, the articulating surface is essentially a ball and socket joint. Thus, comparisons of the various articulating pairs or wear couples are more appropriate than in the disparate designs of spine arthoplasty. Greenwald and Garino[4] reviewed several different wear couples and found orders of magnitudes of difference in the amount of wear from these combinations of bearing surfaces. For purposes of comparison, the data are presented as volume of wear in cubic millimeters per year of loading:

- Metal on polyethylene had 55.7 $mm^3$/year
- Ceramic on polyethylene had 17.1 $mm^3$/year
- Metal on metal had 0.9 $mm^3$/year
- Ceramic on ceramic had 0.04 $mm^3$/year

Ceramic-on-ceramic wear surfaces thus represent significantly reduced amounts of wear than other comparable systems.

Another distinct advantage of ceramic articulating surfaces is the improved biocompatibility of ceramic wear debris compared with that of metal or polymer wear debris. Warashina et al.[5] performed a comparative study examining the biological effects of placing micron sized wear debris of two types of ceramics: alumina ($Al_2O_3$) and zirconia ($ZrO_2$), titanium alloy (Ti6Al4V), and high-density polyethylene (HDP) compared with a control in a murine calvarian defect. The study involved measuring the release of cytokines in response to the wear debris to examine the potential effects of osteolysis. The cytokines or bone resorbing mediators examined included tumor necrosis factor (TNF) and various interleukins including (interleukin-6 [IL-6], interleukin-α [IL-1α], and interleukin-1β [IL-1β]) from macrophages. Particles of HDP had the highest reactivity with a threefold increase in levels of IL-6, and the Ti6Al4V group had a twofold increase; both of these were significantly greater than the control. Although the $Al_2O_3$ and $ZrO_2$ had slightly elevated levels of IL-6, these were not significantly greater than the control. The biologic reactivity of ceramic wear particles is lower than that of metals and polymers, and because the amount of wear is lower as well, ceramic-on-ceramic bearing surfaces is an attractive solution for cervical spine arthroplasty.

## INDICATIONS/CONTRAINDICATIONS

Cervical total disc replacement is generally indicated for degenerative conditions in the absence of significant structural insufficiencies at the symptomatic level or levels. From a mechanical standpoint, the disc replacement will serve to maintain the intervertebral disc height, while allowing bending and rotational motions. Because the prosthesis restores only a portion of the function of the anterior column, structural deficiencies of the posterior elements at the affected levels should be carefully reviewed and generally be regarded as contraindications for disc replacement surgery.

Because the disc replacement allows bending motions to be maintained, adjacent level stresses are generally lower when compared with the stresses adjacent to fusion stabilizations. For the patient who presents with one clearly symptomatic degenerative level and one level that is degenerative and asymptomatic, disc replacement of the symptomatic level only may be an excellent treatment in comparison to either fusing the symptomatic level (which may hasten the degeneration of the adjacent level), fusing both levels, replacing both discs, or a hybrid construct having one level fused and one level replaced.

Patients who are thought to not benefit from disc replacement in the cervical spine include those having idiopathic deformities, iatrogenic deformities secondary to removal of portions of the bony elements of the posterior spine, and instabilities related to trauma.

Care should be taken to review the types of mechanical conditions that can be treated with different types of devices. Not every disc replacement will have the same indications and contraindications as every other device.

For example, one of the theoretical advantages of fixed bearings as opposed to mobile bearings is the relatively higher degree of joint stability that is achieved by the reconstruction. Hence, degenerative deformities may be corrected by a fixed bearing device but perhaps not by a mobile bearing device.

## DESCRIPTION OF THE DEVICE

The Cerpass device consists of titanium alloy end plates and ceramic bearing inserts (Fig. 30–1). In order to create a stable interface between the titanium and the ceramic, the ceramic component is swaged into the titanium end plate. This places the components into intimate mechanical contact with one another so that the ceramic bearing is fully supported by the metal end plate.

The device is provided in three footprints (denoted as small, medium, and large) and five heights per footprint (5, 6, 7, 8, and 9 mm) for a total of 15 devices in the basic kit. Owing to the fixed bearing articulation, the device has a superior and inferior orientation.

Titanium alloy and yttria-stabilized zirconia toughened alumina comprise the primary materials from which the device is constructed. A layer of plasma-sprayed hydroxyapatite is applied to the bone-contacting surface of each end plate in order to encourage bony ongrowth and thus appropriate device fixation.

A key advantage of the materials chosen in this construction is that there are no materials that can grossly interfere with MRI examinations postoperatively. While there is expected to be some image scattering related to the titanium in the device end plates, the effect compared to prostheses containing stainless steel or cobalt chrome in their construction is negligible.

## BACKGROUND OF SCIENTIFIC TESTING/CLINICAL OUTCOMES

Testing activities related to the Cerpass device are primarily centered on two areas of key interest. First, an evaluation of the ceramic construction and assembly process with the titanium end plates to ensure that the ceramic is of the highest quality and has not been damaged in-process; and second, bench-top mechanical evaluation of the prosthesis for fatigue and wear performance.

During the assembly process, the ceramic bearing components are inserted into a pocket in the titanium end plate, and then the pocket is deformed around the ceramic component to firmly capture and secure it by means of a swaging process. The swaging process works by applying several tons of pressure to the titanium in a controlled manner to produce a predictable deformation. This

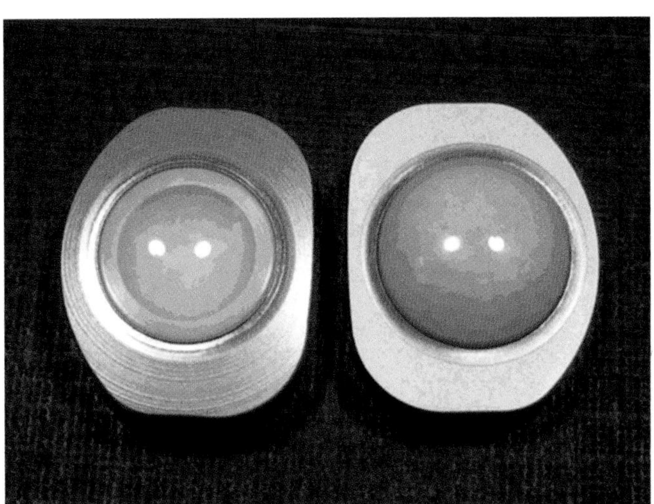

■ **FIGURE 30–1.** Photograph of the Cerpass device.

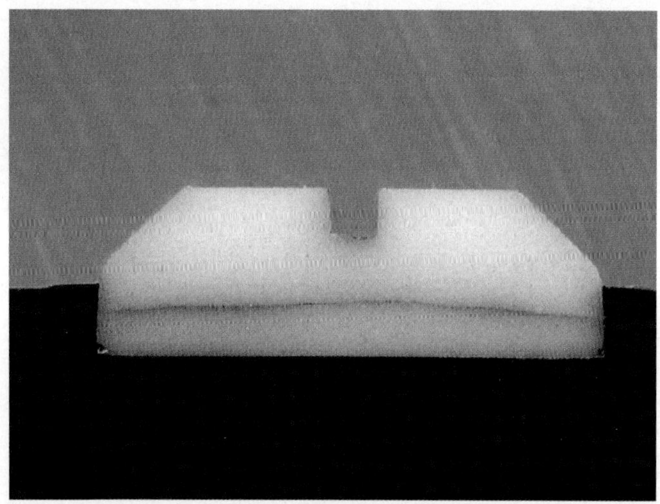

■ **FIGURE 30–2.** Cross-section of a test part intentionally cracked to determine manufacturing parameters. The swaging process essentially squeezes the ceramic bearing diametrically.

deformation in turn applies pressure to the ceramic. Some pressure is required in order to prevent the ceramic component from moving around in the pocket (e.g., micromotion), but too much pressure could crack the ceramic (Fig. 30–2).

To ensure that the process applies the correct amount of pressure, acoustic emissions are recorded from the devices during assembly. Cracks in the ceramic that are induced by the assembly process are readily identifiable in the acoustic spectra.

Properly assembled components have been tested in axial compression and for wear performance. Axial compression tests show that the prosthesis is expected to carry the in vivo load indefinitely without failure.

The most compelling property of the ceramic bearing becomes evident upon an examination of the wear data (Fig. 30–3). Devices were tested according to the American Society for Testing and Materials (ASTM) standard guide for evaluating spinal disc replacement wear (ASTM F2423) and showed on average 0.17 $mm^3$ wear debris generation at 5 million cycles, which is an extraordinarily low amount. To put this into perspective, in a very similar test format, the Bryan prosthesis (Medtronic Sofamor Danek, Memphis, TN) produced wear debris volume at a rate 28 times greater than the Cerpass prosthesis.[6,7] The testing reported by Anderson et al showed that in a 10 million cycle test, the Bryan prosthesis produced 9.6$mm^3$ of wear debris. The ASTM standard test is run with a constant load of 100 N to a total range of motion of 15 degrees.

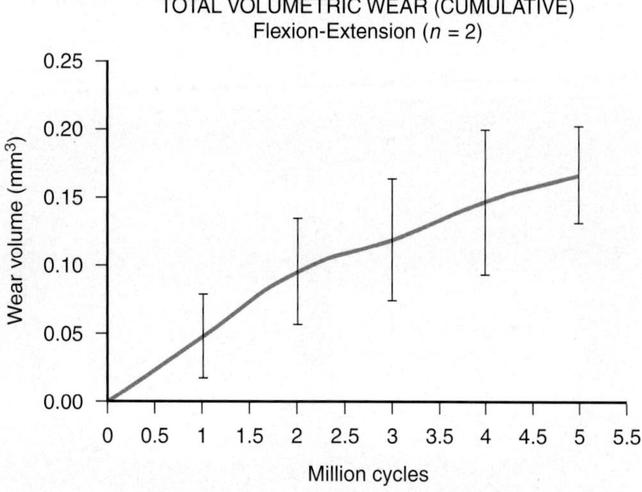


■ **FIGURE 30–3.** Wear data. Devices were tested according to the ASTM standard guide for evaluating spinal disc replacement wear (ASTM F2423) and showed on average 0.17 $mm^3$ wear debris generation at 5 million cycles.

## CLINICAL PRESENTATION AND EVALUATION

Like many articular bearing-based total disc replacements, the Cerpass prosthesis is designed for use in patients having degenerative disc disease of the middle and lower cervical spine. Radicular symptoms are generally treated by decompressive techniques, then the prosthesis maintains the disc height and allows continued motion of the joint.

## OPERATIVE TECHNIQUE

### Anesthesia

Standard anesthetic techniques for invasive cervical surgery should be used. There are no differences in anesthetic technique from traditional anterior cervical discectomy and fusion surgery.

### Position

The patient is positioned supine on the operating table, with the neck in a neutral position. The C-arm is positioned to allow lateral and anteroposterior views to be obtained during the procedure.

### Procedure

- A standard anterolateral approach is used to expose the operative level.
- Self-retaining retractor blades are used to retract the longus colli muscles and surrounding tissues.
- The centerline of the disc is determined and marked. It is helpful to use anteroposterior (AP) fluoroscopy to determine the midline.
- A pin-based spinal distractor is employed to apply distraction to the operative level.
- The discectomy is peformed. Kerrison rongeurs and curettes are used to remove bony spurs and excess osteophytes. There is no evidence to suggest that there exists a measurable or functional difference in clinical outcomes if the posterior longitudinal ligament is retained or resected.
- End plates are flattened for receiving the prosthesis by means of a rasp.
- Distraction is removed (it is not necessary to remove the pins, only to remove the tension from the distractor) and sizing trials are sequentially placed into the disc space from smallest to largest until a firm, snug fit is found. The largest footprint size possible should always be selected in order to minimize the chance for subsidence.

- The corresponding size prosthesis is opened and loaded onto the insertion tool.
- Distraction is reapplied to the operative level.
- The prosthesis is inserted into the disc space, taking care to align the device with the marked midline. AP fluoroscopy is used to check the midline position. Lateral fluoroscopy is used to verify the position of the posterior border of the prosthesis.

## POSTOPERATIVE CARE

The postoperative care should be considered routine for the Cerpass prosthesis. The surgeon may choose to prescribe a soft collar to be worn for several weeks postoperatively although this is not generally considered a requirement.

If magnetic resonance image (MRI) scanning is desired postoperatively, no special precautions need to be taken. The construction of the prosthesis is entirely titanium and ceramic materials, so there is no chance of dislodging the device with the magnetic field. Image scatter is limited to that typically seen adjacent to titanium implants.

## COMPLICATIONS AND AVOIDANCE

Patients having high degrees of instability or nondegenerative (e.g idiopathic) deformities are likely poor candidates for treatment with the Cerpass prosthesis. Additionally, patients having low bone density are at risk of subsidence if treated with an articulating total disc replacement.

Patients reporting high levels of neck pain in the absence of radicular pain rarely have good clinical outcomes from surgery. It is unlikely that the only (or indeed the primary) pain generator in these patients is the intervertebral disc, so treatment by removing and replacing the disc generally misses other potential pain generators.

### ADVANTAGES/DISADVANTAGES: CERPASS

**Advantages**

Extraordinarily low wear debris generation
Lower bioreactivity of ceramic wear debris than metallic or polymeric systems
Good MRI imaging properties
Standard, familiar surgical technique

**Disadvantages**

As with any ceramic implant, the potential for fractured bearing components exists.

Since the device-bone interface is limited to a roughened surface with spikes, patients with high degrees of instability should not be treated with the Cerpass prosthesis.

## CONCLUSIONS/DISCUSSION

Cervical disc replacement appears to be a promising treatment in the armamentarium of the spine surgeon. However, its key promise, the reduction of adjacent level degeneration, compared to fusion treatments remains yet to be proven.

The key measure for determining whether cervical disc replacement is truly an improvement over fusion procedures will be the long-term survivorship rate of both the device itself and of the intact intervertebral discs adjacent to it. We expect that the adjacent-level survivorship rates will be reasonably similar for the articulating disc replacements that are available or in development today. However, the survivorship rates of the devices themselves will vary. Devices will be removed for many reasons, some directly related to the device, and some not. One of the key reasons that we anticipate device removal to occur is the generation of wear debris leading to osteolytic reactions. By reducing the wear debris generation to an extremely low level, we believe the Cerpass device has the potential to have a very high survivorship rate.

## REFERENCES


1. Dimitriev AE, Cunningham BW, Hu N, et al: Adjacent level intradiscal pressure and segmental kinematics following a cervical disc arthroplasty: an in vitro human cadaveric model. Spine 30:1165–1172, 2005.
2. Wigfield CC, Skryzpiec D, Jackowski A, Adams MA: Internal stress distribution in cervical intervertebral discs: The influence of an artificial cervical joint and simulated anterior interbody fusion. J Spinal Disord Tech 16:441–449, 2003.
3. Cummins BH, Robertson JT, Gill SS: Surgical experience with an implanted artificial cervical joint. J Neurosurg 88:943–948, 1998.
4. Greenwald AS, Garino JP: Alternative bearing surfaces: The good, the bad, and the ugly. J Bone Joint Surg Am 83A:68–72, 2001.
5. Warashina H, Sakano S, Kitamura S, et al: Biological reaction to alumina, zirconia, titanium and polyethylene particles implanted onto murine calvaria. Biomaterials 24:3655–3661, 2003.
6. Anderson PA, Sasso RC, Rouleau JP, et al: The Bryan Cervical Disc: Wear properties and early clinical results. Spine J 4:303S–309S, 2004.
7. Anderson PA, Rouleau JP, Bryan VE, Carlson CS: Wear analysis of the Bryan cervical disc prosthesis. Spine 28:S186–S194, 2003.

CHAPTER 31

# Kineflex|C Cervical Artificial Disc

**James Robert Rappaport**

## KEY POINTS

- Kineflex|C is a total artificial disc designed to relieve symptoms and restore disc height while maintaining motion in the cervical spine.
- Kineflex|C is a metal-on-metal disc that has a semiconstrained core that allows for translation during flexion-extension, lateral bending, and axial rotation.
- Early clinical experience with the Kineflex|C artificial disc shows promising results for patients with degenerative disc disease (DDD).
- The implant technique for Kineflex|C is straightforward and similar to anterior cervical discectomy and fusion (ACDF) and to the Kineflex lumbar disc arthroplasty.
- Kineflex|C is a promising alternative to cervical disc fusion because it may minimize adjacent-level disc disease.

## INTRODUCTION

Cervical neck pain and neurologic symptoms associated with degenerative disc disease (DDD) are a significant cause of lost work time and account for very substantial costs to the healthcare system. Although the majority of simple disc herniation cases may resolve spontaneously or with conservative management, the progressive nature of cervical DDD is underscored by the research that finds 97% of patients with pre-existing DDD demonstrate progression 10 years later.[1]

Although a variety of therapeutic interventions are available for cases that do not respond to conservative therapy, including discectomy and various methods of interbody fusion, each presents limitations. Because of the potential for long-term complications associated with traditional surgical treatments, extensive research has been conducted to develop an intervertebral disc prosthesis.

## CURRENT TREATMENT MODALITIES

Traditionally, options for management of cervical DDD were principally limited to either conservative treatment (e.g., rest, therapy, analgesics) or removal of the disc through discectomy, with or without fusion at the affected level. A well-established, commonly performed cervical fusion procedure is anterior cervical discectomy and fusion (ACDF), which may be supplemented with anterior cervical plating or rigid internal fixation to further promote fusion.

In recent years, particularly due to increasing concern regarding the incidence of adjacent segment disease after fusion,[1] considerable research has been focused on the development of cervical arthroplasty. Each of these surgical treatment modalities is discussed in the following section.

### Discectomy

When conservative management does not yield adequate symptom relief, the first surgical measure that often may be attempted is a discectomy. Because damaged disc material may impinge on the spinal nerves, removal of this material frequently alleviates symptoms by eliminating the compression of spinal nerves. Satisfactory clinical results following cervical discectomy have been reported in the literature.[2] However, discectomy is not designed to resolve the patient's underlying pathology. As a result, discectomy is often combined with spinal fusion.

### Spinal Fusion

Spinal fusion effectively eliminates the motion segment between two vertebrae by use of a bone graft, thereby providing improved stability and decreased pain. A variety of graft materials may be used, including autograft bone, allograft bone, and others. Fusion may also involve use of instrumentation to stabilize the affected level and/or contain the graft, such as interbody cages and plating. Clinical success rates, using measures such as the Oswestry Disability Index (ODI) or the Neck Disability Index (NDI), are generally lower than fusion rates. One study, for example, found a 95% fusion rate at 6 months in patients treated with ACDF and a titanium fusion cage, but the success rate dropped to 70%, using an ODI score of 40 or less as the measure of success.[3]

A complication that has been the subject of increasing concern in the spinal literature is the possibility of the acceleration of adjacent-segment disease after cervical fusion, due to increased stress on adjacent unfused levels. Hilibrand et al[4] reported that 2.9% of patients per year required surgical intervention for symptomatic new onset adjacent-segment degeneration following ACDF; these researchers estimated a 25% cumulative rate of symptomatic adjacent-segment disease 10 years after ACDF.

Although the use of allograft material eliminates donor site complications, it carries a small risk of transmissible disease, as well as a risk of rejection reactions. Bone morphogenetic protein is another potential grafting option that became available in 2002 for use in the lumbar spine when U.S. Food and Drug Administration (FDA) approved Medtronic's InFUSE (Medtronic Sofamor Danek, Memphis, TN). Although the results of clinical trials are promising, this product is not yet approved in the United States for use in the cervical spine.

Rigid internal fixation devices have been used increasingly in addition to bone grafting in order to increase fusion rates. Anterior cervical plate fixation has been shown to improve successful arthrodesis rate after single-level ACDF. One study reported that fusion rates improved from 90% to 96% when cervical plate fixation was added to single-level fusions with allograft.[5] The same study also showed improvement from 72% to 91% in fusion rates for two-level cases with plating.

The implantation of metallic spinal cages into the disc space between two vertebrae is another method used to stabilize the spine and promote fusion. The cage also may be filled with graft material. Although fusion rates with the use of cages is generally greater than 90% in one-level procedures, complications do occur. Moreover, success rates with fusion cages decrease when the definition of success includes other factors in addition to fusion. The Investigation Device Exemption (IDE) clinical study of 202 patients who received the AFFINITY Anterior Cervical Cage System reported an overall success rate of only 68% at 24-month follow-up. Overall success was defined as fusion of the operative segment, successful pain and disability outcome, neurological success, and no revisions, removals, or supplemental fixation. Complications included 15 neurologic events, 29 spinal events, and 35 reports of neck or arm pain.

### Total Disc Replacement

The limitations of discectomy and spinal fusion procedures have resulted in significant interest in developing a total disc replacement. The goal is to develop an artificial disc that alleviates the pain associated with disc degeneration while preserving segmental range of motion and restoring stability.

Kineflex|C (Spinal Motion, Inc., Mountainview, CA) is a metal-on-metal, semiconstrained cervical artificial disc designed to relieve pain and maintain motion for the treatment of degenerative disc disease of the cervical spine. It has been used clinically since 2004, with more than 1,000 discs implanted worldwide. Kineflex|C is being investigated under an IDE clinical study in the United States that began in the summer of 2005, with completion of enrollment expected in the second quarter of 2007.

## INDICATIONS/CONTRAINDICATIONS

Appropriate patient selection is important for achieving optimal clinical outcomes. A summary of patient selection criteria from the IDE clinical study follows:

### Inclusion Criteria Overview

- Between 18 and 60 years of age
- Symptomatic disc at only one cervical level from C3-C7
- Have symptoms of radiculopathy in neck, one or both shoulders, and one or both arms
- Have at least 6 months of prior conservative treatment, the presence of progressive symptoms, or signs of nerve root compression
- Have a NDI demonstrating moderate disability (40 or higher)

### Exclusion Criteria Overview

- Marked cervical instability on lateral or flexion-extension X-ray study
    - Nondiscogenic neck pain or nondiscogenic source of symptoms
    - Radiographic confirmation of severe facet disease
    - Bridging osteophytes
    - Less than 2 degrees of motion at index level
- Severe myelopathy
- Metabolic bone disease

## DESCRIPTION OF THE DEVICE

The Kineflex|C Spinal System is designed to be used as a replacement for a degenerated or diseased cervical disc at one level from C3-C7 that is unresponsive to conservative management in subjects with single-level degenerative disc disease (DDD) with related pain. The spinal system is a three-piece modular design consisting of two cobalt chrome molybdenum (CCM) end plates and a fully articulating CCM core (Fig. 31–1). The system is available in two footprint sizes (size 1, 14 mm × 16 mm; and size 2, 16 mm × 18 mm).

The end plates are designated in three thicknesses relative to the disc (core) centerline and allow for assembled heights of 5.7 mm, 6.3 mm, and 7.1 mm (Fig. 31–2).

Each end plate exterior has a keel with two holes, a serrated edge surface, and a titanium plasma spray coating for bone ingrowth. The interior of each end plate has a polished concave bearing surface for evenly distributed contact with the convex-shaped core. The inferior end plate has a retaining ring to prevent extrusion of the core during movement (Fig. 31–3).

The Kineflex|C core is manufactured of CCM to which has been applied a highly polished finish. Only one size core is used with all the system combinations. The spinal system is implanted as one unit by means of the insertion instrument.

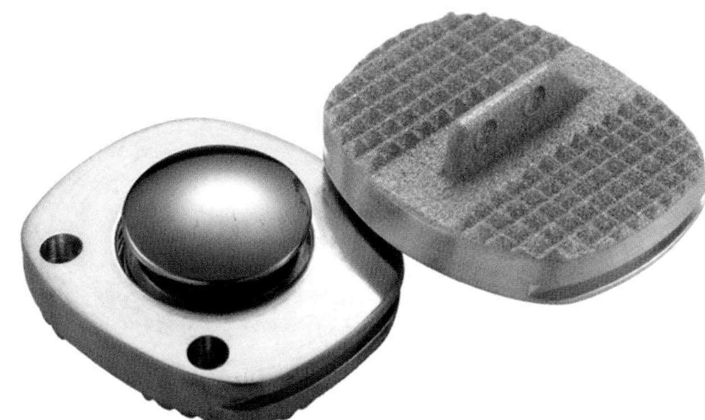

■ **FIGURE 31–1.** Kineflex|C cervical disc. The preassembled disc is shown, with core sitting in the inferior end plate. The disc is inserted assembled as one piece.

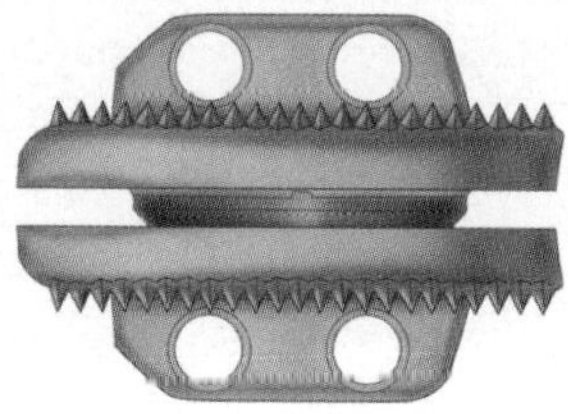
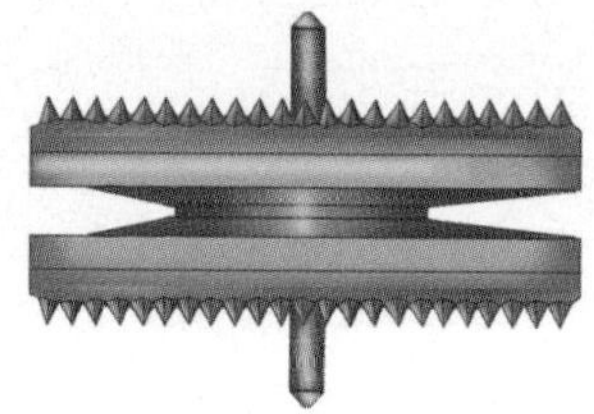

■ **FIGURE 31–2.** Kineflex|C cervical disc. Various viewpoints of the disc are shown as an assembled unit.

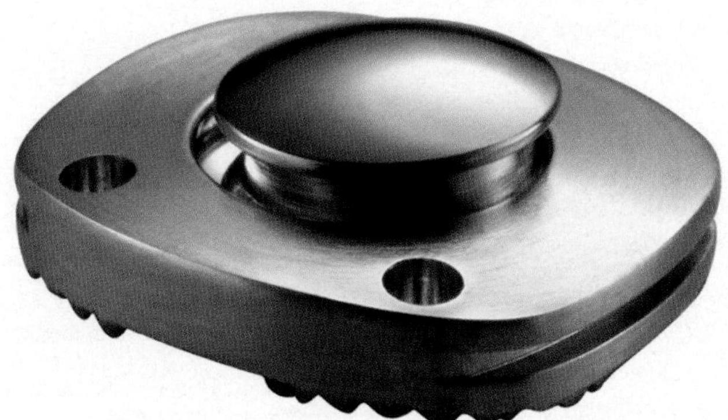

■ **FIGURE 31–3.** Cervical disc core in inferior end plate. The lower lip of the core sits in the inferior end plate, which has a matching interior surface designed to prevent the core from extruding out in situ.

## BACKGROUND OF SCIENTIFIC TESTING/CLINICAL OUTCOMES

A substantial body of preclinical mechanical testing has been performed on the Kineflex|C Spinal System, including static testing, monoaxial fatigue testing, and wear testing. These tests were performed in order to simulate the load and movement to which the discs would be exposed under in vivo conditions and to verify that the prosthesis could withstand static and fatigue load conditions, as well as to determine the wear characteristics of the prosthesis.

All of the tests were conducted in accordance with the protocols reviewed by FDA, and were based on the draft American Society for Testing and Materials (ASTM) standard for artificial disc testing.

### Static Testing

Static testing was performed in two loading conditions, axial compression and shear, in accordance with the ASTM Artificial Disc Testing Draft Standard.

#### Static Compression

The assembled disc was placed in an Instron machine with a 0- to 100- kN load capacity. The device was then loaded until either the maximum load permitted by the test fixture was reached, or mechanical failure of one of the device components occurred. Load and displacement data were recorded. The results demonstrated that there was no height reduction in any of the samples. The Kineflex|C substantially exceeded the strength of the vertebral bone and, therefore, was sufficient to withstand the worst case compressive forces anticipated in clinical use.

#### Static Shear

As in the compression test above, the test specimen was loaded until functional failure. Load and displacement data were recorded. No mechanical failures of the cores or end plates were observed.

### Dynamic Testing

#### Compression Fatigue Testing

Samples were tested under cyclic axial compressive loading to assess the suitability of the fatigue resistance of the device for in vivo use. Loads varied cyclically. The results demonstrated no measurable dimensional or mass changes in either the end plates or the core.

#### Shear Fatigue Testing

Samples were tested under cyclic shear compressive loading to assess the suitability of the fatigue resistance of the device for in vivo use. Loads varied cyclically. The results demonstrated no measurable dimensional changes or mass changes in either the end plates or the core.

#### Wear Testing

To evaluate the amount and size of wear particles generated by the Kineflex|C in vivo, test samples were cyclically loaded in a multiaxial motion simulator for 10 million cycles. A custom-loading fixture was constructed to test the prosthesis under a combination of cyclic flexion-extension, lateral bending, and rotation, corresponding to the types of in vivo movement that may be encountered.

To simulate in vivo cyclic loading conditions, ranges of motion were selected to conform to the ASTM Artificial Disc Testing Draft Standard.

Weighing and dimensional measurements of the prosthesis (end plates and core) performed after every million cycles showed an average volumetric loss for the prosthesis was approximately 3.84 $mm^3$ over the entire test, or 0.384 $mm^3$ per million cycles. Mass loss was approximately 32 mg, for an average of 3.2 mg per million cycles. This represents loss of only approximately 0.08% of the total prosthesis mass over 10 million cycles.

When the the observed wear rate for the Kineflex|C was compared with other results that have been reported in the literature, the wear rates are similar to other metal-metal discs, and significantly below volumetric wear rates reported for total hip arthroplasties (THAs). For example, Oskouian et al[6] reported a volumetric wear rate of 0.96 $mm^3$/million cycles in testing of an all-metal artificial disc. The authors note that this is approximately two orders of magnitude below the wear rates reported for metal THAs, which range from 50 to100 $mm^3$/million cycles. The Kineflex|C volumetric wear rate of 0.384 $mm^3$/M cycles is approximately one-third of the rate reported by Oskouian et al.[6]

Thus, both the materials used in the Kineflex|C and the amount of wear debris generated are consistent with previous prostheses that are currently undergoing clinical studies. In addition, there are in vivo animal data demonstrating that wear debris of this type and quantity are unlikely to generate an adverse biologic response.

Cunningham et al evaluated the neural and systemic tissue response to cobalt alloy particulate debris in an in vivo rabbit model up to 6 months. They placed 4 mg of cobalt alloy particles directly on the dura and compared the results with rabbits who had a sham procedure of dural exposure alone. At 3 months, the number of macrophage-expressing cytokines localized within the spinal cord and overlying tissues indicated no significant differences compared with the control group. Despite regions heavily laden with metallic particulate, histiocyctic reaction, and cytokine activity, the spinal cords indicated normal distribution of myelin and the intracellular neurofibrilla network. There was no evidence of cellular apoptosis, and all specimens were characterized as without significant histopathologic changes.

Finally, metal-on-metal THAs have been used clinically for more than 10 years with a strong safety record. Tipper indicated that histologic studies of periprosthetic tissues have not shown an inflammatory reaction to metal wear particles, and that MOM bearings show considerable potential as an osteolysis-free solution for younger patients.

In summary, the wear testing of the Kineflex|C demonstrates a wear rate that is similar to but generally lower than other all-metal disc prostheses that have been under clinical evaluation. Prior in vivo animal testing demonstrates that direct application of particles of the same material, and in extreme doses, to the dura does not trigger a significant adverse biologic response. Therefore, the observed wear characteristics of the Kineflex|C were determined to be appropriate for its intended use.

## CLINICAL PRESENTATION AND EVALUATION

Of the group of patients who are candidates for total disc replacement, there is a subset of those patients who would normally be considered candidates for ACDF. Just as when fusion is considered, there are multiple factors that can cause patients with similar pathology and physical findings to be categorized into radically different prognostic groups. Some of these factors are well known such as: workers' compensation issues, litigation, and socioeconomic factors. Other risk factors relate to physiology, such as a history of smoking. Unlike fusion, the total disc replacement does not stabilize the entire motion segment, so patients with preoperative instability may not be as effectively treated with a total disc replacement as with fusion. ACDF also effectively immobilizes the entire motion segment, including the facet joints. Therefore fusion has the potential to address both disc pathology and facet pathology. Cervical disc replacement addresses disc pathology and may improve facet pain to some degree, but it does have the potential to actually worsen any facet-mediated pain through increasing mobility at the motion segment.

The advent of the disc replacement has caused a shift in the consideration of the role of the facet joint in the pain mediation process. When evaluating a patient's candidacy for disc replacement, it is imperative that the surgeon first rule out facet-mediated pain and pathology. A total disc replacement will not immobilize or replace these joints. Plain x-ray studies, including flexion-extension views, may help rule out gross instability. The advent of total disc replacement has caused a greater scrutiny of the role of facet-mediated pain and has made clear the need for a grading system for degrees of facet pathology. It is hoped that such a grading system can distinguish between acceptable facet disease and facet disease that is too far advanced to be treated with total disc replacement. At present, a determination of clinically significant facet disease can be attempted by

1. Evaluation of the patients' symptoms, the nature of their pain, and aggravating factors. For example, pain with flexion usually indicates pain mediated by loading of the disc. Pain with extension may indicate pain mediated by facet joint loading.
2. Facet anesthetic injection or median branch blocks may also help determine if the facets are a significant part of the pain generator for an individual patient.

Preoperative evaluation of bone quality is just as important if not more so in the patient work-up for total disc replacement than it is for fusion. Bone quality must be adequate to support the disc end plates. All patients with risk factors for osteoporosis are checked preoperatively with a dual-energy x-ray absorptiometry scan.

Patients who have had previous anterior cervical surgery, whether related to the spine or unrelated, such as thyroidectomy, should undergo an ear, nose, and throat consultation to rule out an asymptomatic unilateral vocal cord paralysis. Doing so may help avoid the catastrophic complication of bilateral vocal cord paralysis. If a unilateral vocal cord paralysis is noted, then the surgical approach is planned from that side in order to avoid the unaffected recurrent laryngeal nerve on the opposite side. In the patient with bilateral normal functioning vocal cords, the side of approach is at the surgeon's discretion. Traditional teaching and older literature has stated that the left-sided approach was safer because the recurrent laryngeal nerve on the left side was anatomically somewhat less at risk. More recent studies have shown no difference between right- and left-sided approaches.[7]

Specific patient selection criteria from the Kineflex|C IDE clinical study were presented earlier in this chapter.

## OPERATIVE TECHNIQUE

The basic soft tissue dissection and exposure of the spine is the same for one-level ACDF and total disc replacement. The exposure required for total disc replacement may be somewhat less than that required for fusion. Therefore, a slightly smaller incision is generally made. There is less need for the extensive elevation of the longissimus coli muscles in a total disc replacement as compared with an anterior cervical discectomy and fusion in which exposure is required for an anterior plate. Although the third generation of cervical plates may be low profile, the artificial disc is a no-profile device. There is also no anterior footprint. There is no need for soft tissue dissection anterior to the vertebral body such as is required for cervical plating. Many of the techniques that ensure a safe ACDF are also used when performing a total disc arthroplasty.

## Anesthesia

Anesthesia is general endotracheal. Fiberoptic intubation is considered when a patient's range of motion while awake results in unacceptable neurologic symptoms. When self-retaining retractors are put into place, the endotracheal cuff pressure should be readjusted. This helps decrease the incidence of dysphonia.[7]

These procedures have very little blood loss. There is no need for the additional risk of hypotensive anesthesia.

## Position

The patient is positioned with the neck in a neutral position. The posterior aspect of the neck is supported with a firm contoured roll. The chin and neck are taped to secure their position. The shoulders are taped in a depressed position to allow intraoperative lateral x-ray study. The tape has been shown to be more secure than wrist band pulls and prevents over-distraction, which can result in nerve root or brachial plexus injury.

Casper distracter pins are used to apply distraction and control lordosis or kyphotic movement at the involved disc space.

Blunt self-retaining retractor blades are used against the esophagus. The small sharp-toothed blade is used towards the carotid artery but care is taken to place both blades underneath the elevated longissimus coli musculature.[8]

Accurate anteroposterior (AP) and lateral fluoroscopic views are crucial to technique even more so than with performing an anterior discectomy and fusion.

Points specific to the Kineflex|C surgical technique include an instrumentation set and implant design, which are very similar to the Kineflex lumbar disc design. This allows a surgeon to gain competency and confidence much quicker than would happen if he or she were required to learn two distinctly different techniques.

The modified mid-height keel allows for a more accurate initial intraoperative placement than a non-keeled device, yet avoids the potential complication of vertebral body fracture and compromise that has been associated with full-height keeled implants.

Because the disc goes in as one unit, there is no necessity for over-distraction to place the central core. This helps to reduce injury to soft tissues and ligaments, which otherwise could result in increased postoperative instability and pain.

## PROCEDURE

On completion of the disc space preparation, the implantation of the Kineflex|C artificial disc requires a straightforward six-step process:

**Step 1:** The first step is the determination of the vertebral body footprint using the end plate sizing instrument. Two footprint sizes are available (size 1, 14 mm × 16 mm; and size 2, 16 mm × 18 mm). This step is confirmed under fluoroscopy in a lateral view to confirm the posterior aspect of the end plate, and viewed visually from the anterior aspect to confirm boney coverage of the end plate (Fig. 31–4).

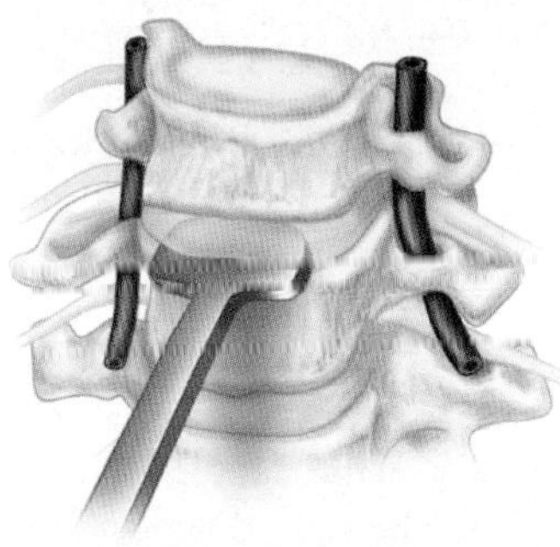

■ **FIGURE 31–4.** End plate sizing. Measurement of vertebral body for maximum and optimal coverage.

**Step 2:** The second step determines the disc height of the prosthesis using the distraction wedges. Three choices are available (5, 6, and 7). This step is performed under fluoroscopy in a lateral view, comparing the distraction wedge with the adjacent levels, with the intent of restoring the disc space back to a normal height (Fig. 31–5).

**Step 3:** The third step uses the midline verification instrument. This instrument is constructed from radiolucent material with metal markers on each side of the instrument shaft. Under fluoroscopic visualization in the AP view, the markers are used to locate the midline position by lining them up with the pedicles of the vertebrae above and below. The midline is then marked with a bovie (Fig. 31–6).

**Step 4:** The fourth step is the midline slot cut, performed under fluoroscopy in the lateral view, which is impacted until the required depth is achieved (Fig. 31–7).

**Step 5:** The fifth step is the initial insertion of the Kineflex|C prosthesis. The prosthesis is assembled and inserted as one piece. The initial insertion places the disc halfway into the disc space, ideally with one of the keel holes embedded in the vertebral body, with the other still exposed (Fig. 31–8).

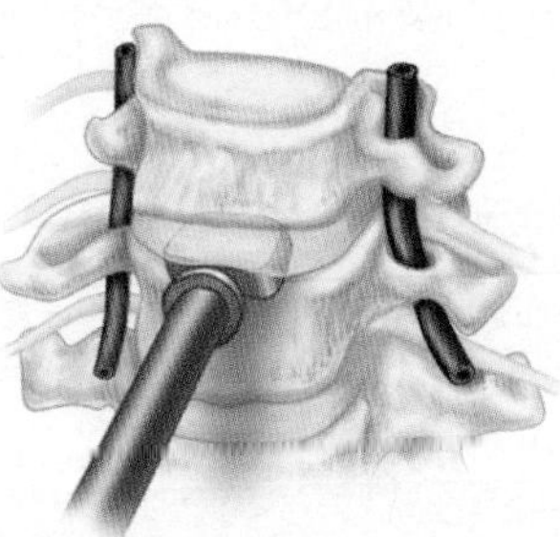

■ **FIGURE 31–5.** Distraction. Disc height is determined.

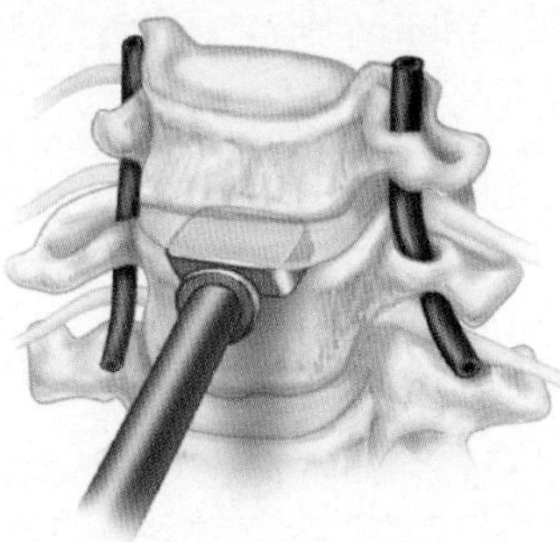

■ **FIGURE 31–6.** Midline verification. Specialized instrument determines midline location before cutting keel space.

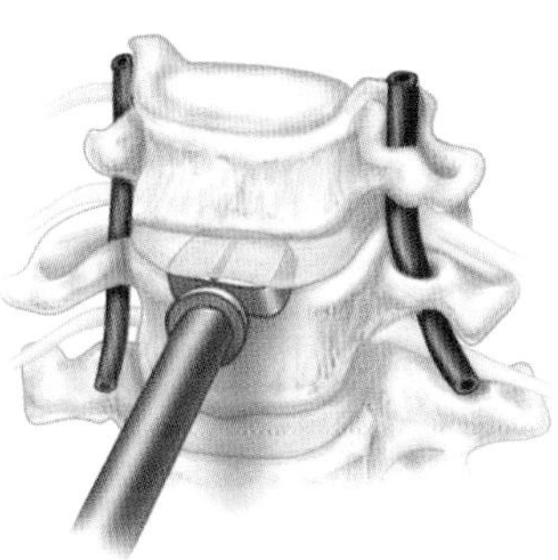

■ **FIGURE 31–7.** Midline slot cut. Keel space is cut using midline location.

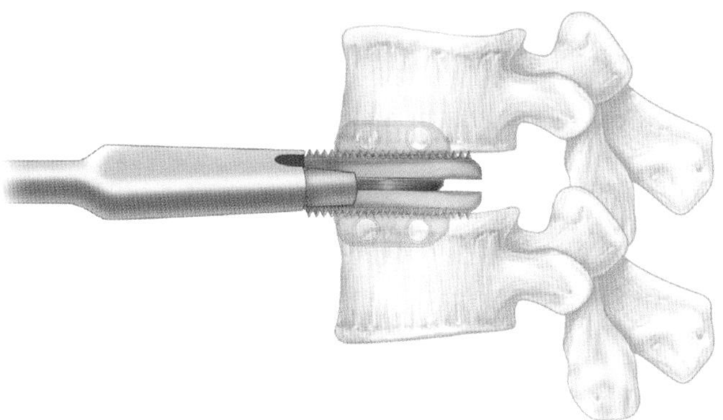

■ **FIGURE 31–8.** Initial insertion. Disc is partially inserted into disc space.

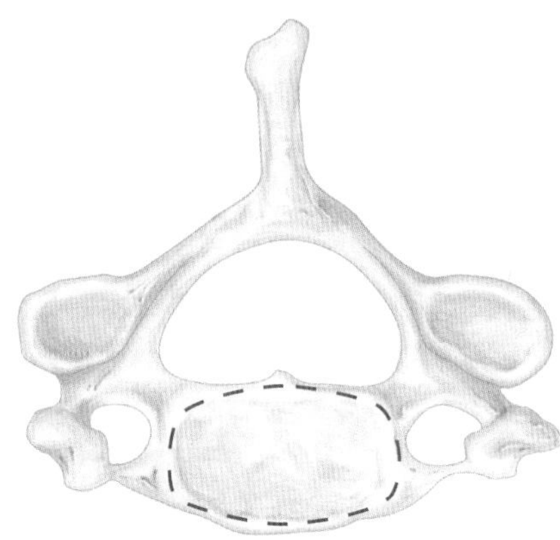

■ **FIGURE 31–10.** Final placement. Optimal final placement of disc over end plate.

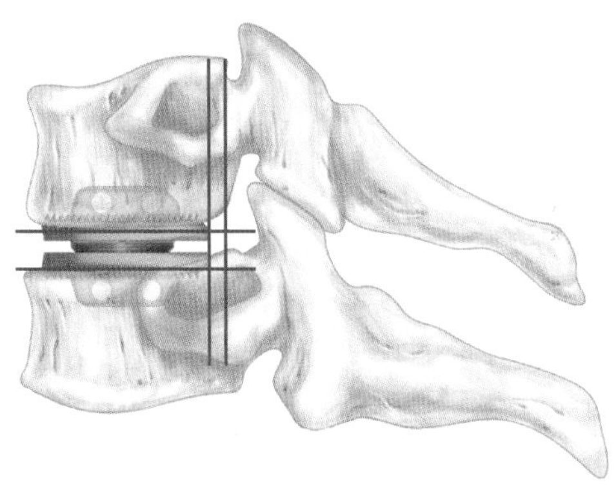

■ **FIGURE 31–11.** Final placement. Optimal orientation and location. End plates are parallel.

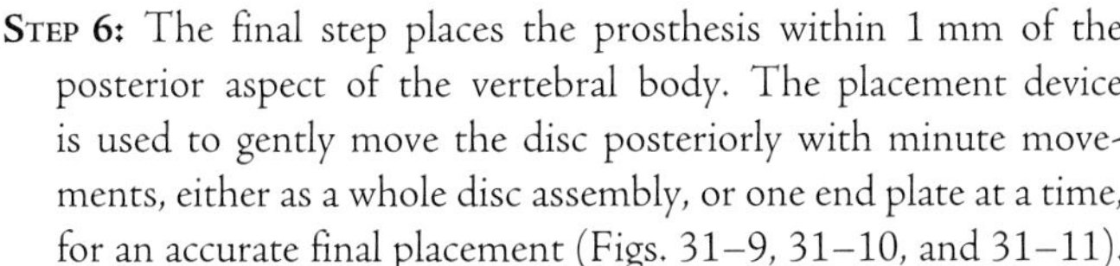

**Step 6:** The final step places the prosthesis within 1 mm of the posterior aspect of the vertebral body. The placement device is used to gently move the disc posteriorly with minute movements, either as a whole disc assembly, or one end plate at a time, for an accurate final placement (Figs. 31–9, 31–10, and 31–11).

The following MRI and x-ray images represent the treated disc space both before and after implantation. The disc herniation is seen at L6-L7 (Figs. 31–12 and 31–13). After implantation of the Kineflex|C disc, disc height and mobility are restored. X-ray images of the disc are shown in lateral bending and flexion-extension positions (Figs. 31–14 and 31–15).

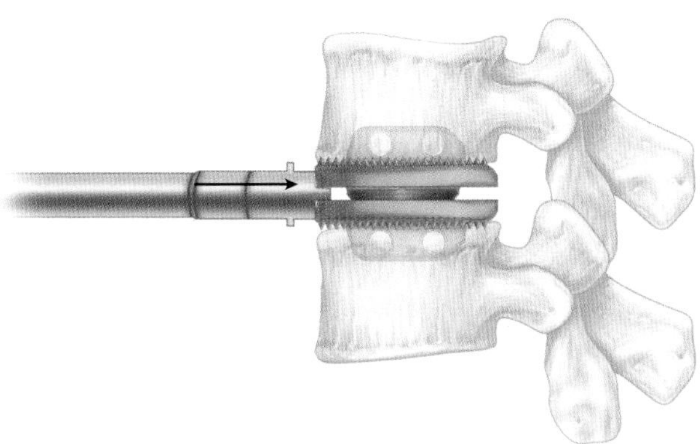

■ **FIGURE 31–9.** Final placement. Final advancement for optimal orientation and location of the disc.

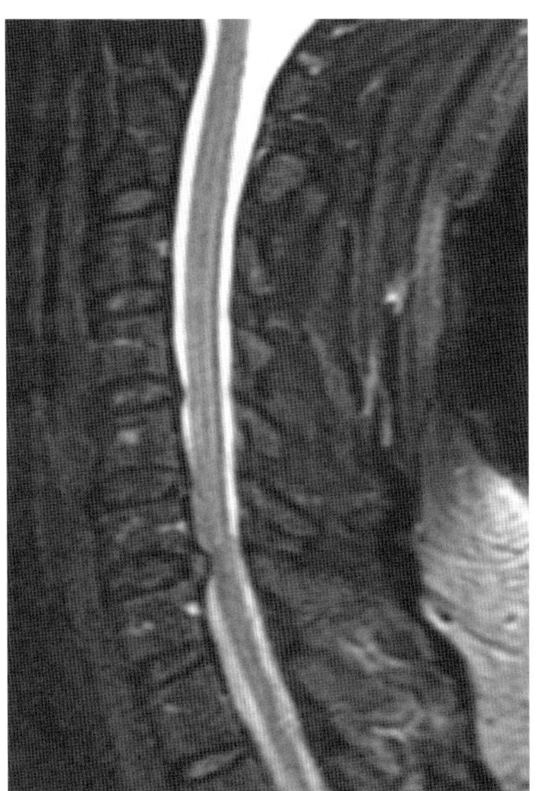

■ **FIGURE 31–12.** The disc herniation is seen at C6-C7.

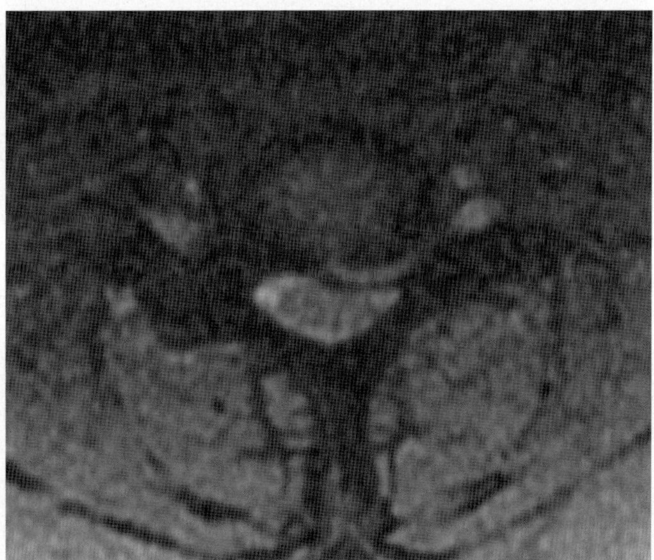

■ **FIGURE 31–13.** The disc herniation is seen at C6-C7.

## POSTOPERATIVE CARE

Patients use a soft collar for comfort, psychological support, and minimal physical support. Early active range of motion is encouraged. Passive range of motion through physical therapy is not required and is avoided. Patients are placed on a mechanical soft diet for 10 days or until swallowing becomes relatively normal.[9,10]

Postoperative physical therapy is prescribed on an individualized basis and is dependent upon the functional deficits that existed preoperatively. Follow up x-ray studies are done on a routine basis.

## COMPLICATIONS AND AVOIDANCE

A recent retrospective study using the Nationwide Inpatient Sample reported the incidence of complication with cervical surgery for spondylosis to be overall 3.93%. The incidence of complication with an anterior approach alone was lower than that with posterior fusion or combined anterior and posterior approaches.[11]

For anterior cervical discectomy in the State of California, complication rates include 1.8% infection, 0.3% cerebral spinal fluid leak, 0.09% recurrent nerve palsy. These complications can be avoided or reduced by surgically respecting the soft tissues. Infection can be decreased by use of prophylactic antibiotics and copious use of irrigation.

Dysphonia can be avoided by adjusting the endotracheal cuff tube pressure during the procedure. Potentially devastating bilateral recurrent laryngeal nerve injury can be avoided by  the vocal cords of any patient who has had previous anterior spine or neck surgery and choosing the side of approach appropriately.

Dysphagia and dysphonia can be reduced by placement of self-retaining retractors under the longissimus coli, and recalibration of the endotracheal tube cuff pressure after placement of the retractors.

Complications specific to disc replacement include subsidence of the implant through the bony end plate. Careful preservation of the end plate and placement of the implant can lower this complication.

Carefully balancing the soft tissue release around the disc space both anteriorly and posteriorly can help to avoid extrusion of the

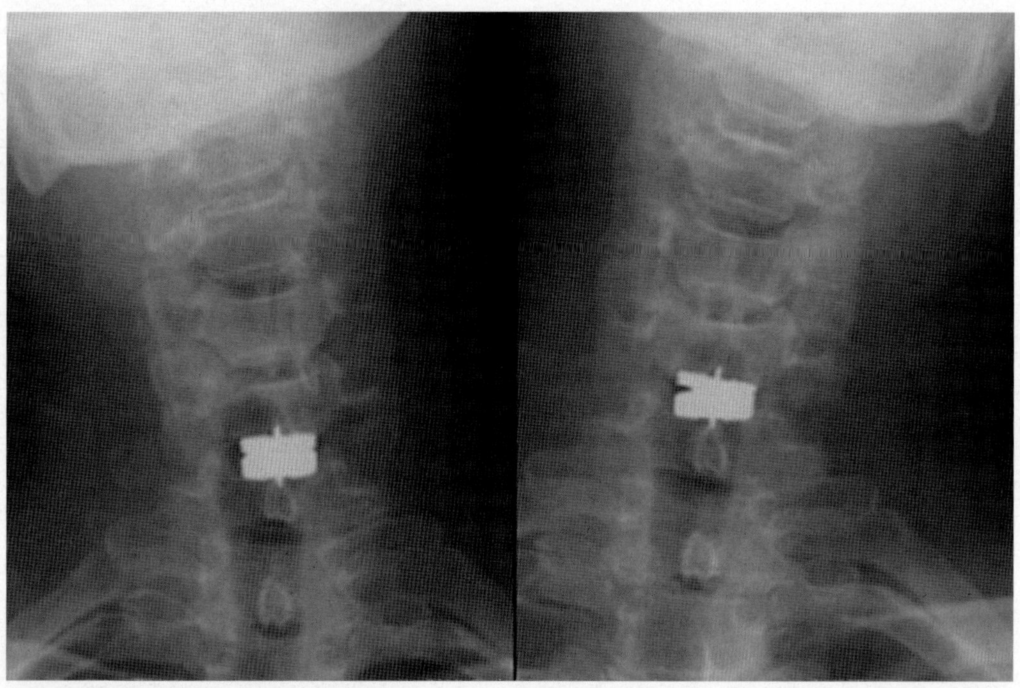

■ **FIGURE 31–14.** X-ray images of the disc are shown in lateral bending position. *(Courtesy of David B. Musante, MD, Triangle Orthopedic Associates, P.A., Durham, NC.)*

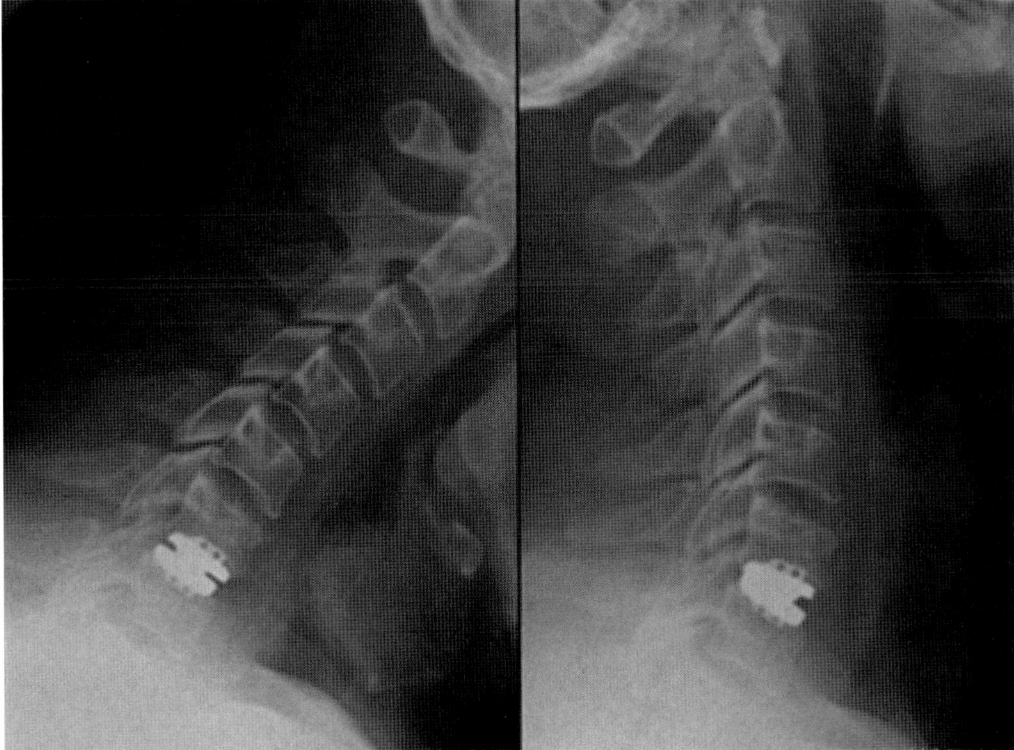

■ **FIGURE 31–15.** X-ray images of the disc are shown in flexion-extension positions. *(Courtesy of David B. Musante, MD, Triangle Orthopedic Associates, P.A., Durham, NC.)*

disc replacement implant anteriorly (i.e., the watermelon seed phenomenon).

Microscopic ACDF at one level is very safe and effective. But the risk of adjacent-segment disease after cervical fusion is an unacceptably high 2.9% per year in the first 10 years after treatment. The real advantage of total disc replacement may be seen in the long run if the incidence of adjacent-segment disease is decreased.[12–14]

Ironically some patients who highly value a return to normal cervical motion, such as an athlete in contact sports, may not benefit from the increased motion that a total disc replacement provides. A single-level ACDF has been documented to provide the stability needed to safely return to these types of activities.[15]

The edge of the indication envelope for total disc replacement remains to be defined. Additional challenges include increasing MRI compatibility. Challenges already met by the Kineflex|C include the following:

- Development of an easily reproducible safe and reliable implantation technique.
- Development of an implantation technique, which reliably restores disc space height and provides for a quick postoperative recovery.
- Development of a total disc implant that restores near-anatomic motion to the diseased spinal segment.

**ADVANTAGES/DISADVANTAGES: KINEFLEX|C.**

**Advantages**
Ease of implant
Restoration of disc height
Preserve motion
CCM is a durable material
Plasma titanium sprayed for bone in-growth fixation
Reproducible procedure
Eliminate need for bone graft/complications such as nonunions

**Disadvantages**
Imaging can be obstructed at the implant level
Lack of long-term clinical data

## REFERENCES


1. Hilibrand AS, Carlson GD, Palumbo, MA, et al: Radiculopathy and myelopathy at segments adjacent to the site of a previous anterior cervical arthrodesis. J Bone Joint Surg 81A:519–528, 1999.
2. Laing RJ, Ng I, Seeley HM, et al: Prospective study of clinical and radiological outcome after anterior cervical discectomy. Br J Neurosurg 15:319–323, 2001.
3. Moreland DB, Asch HL, Clabeaux RT, et al: Anterior cervical discectomy and fusion with implantable titanium cage: Initial impressions, patient outcomes and comparison to fusion with allograft. Spine J 4:184–191, 2004.
4. Hilibrand AS, Yoo JU, Carlson GC, et al: The success of anterior cervical arthrodesis adjacent to a previous fusion. Spine 22:1574–1579, 1997.
5. Kaiser MG, Haid RW, Subach BR, et al: Anterior cervical plating enhances arthrodesis after discectomy and fusion with cortical allograft. Neurosurgery 50:229–238, 2002.
6. Oskouian RJ, Whitehall R, Sami A, et al: The future of spinal arthroplasty: a biomaterials perspective. Neurosurg Focus 17:E2, 2004.

7. Apfelbaum RI, Kriskovich MD, Haller JR: On the incidence, cause and prevention of recurrent laryngeal nerve palsies during anterior cervical spine surgery. Spine 25:2906–2912, 2000.
8. Watkins R: Surgical Approaches to the Spine.
9. Riley LH, Skolasky RL, Alvert TJ, et al: Dysphagia after anterior cervical decompression and fusion: prevalence and risk factors from a longitudinal covert study. Spine 3022:2564–2569, 2005.
10. Rhyne AL, Siddiqi F, Darden DV, et al: Incidence of Postoperative Dysphagia Following Total Disc Replacement Versus Anterior Discectomy and Fusion with Instrumentation. Presented at the Cervical Spine Research Society, December 2005.
11. Marjorie C, Wang MD, Leighton Chan MPH: Complications and mortality associated with cervical spine surgery for degenerative disease in the United States. Spine 32:342–347, 2007.
12. Hillibrand AS, Robbins M: Adjacent segment degeneration and adjacent segment disease: The consequences of spinal fusion? Spine J 6:190S–194S, 2004.
13. D'Mitriev AE, Cunningham BW, Hu N, et al: Adjacent level intradiscal pressure and segmental kinematics following a cervical total disc arthroplasty: and in vitro human cataveric model. Spine 30: 1165–1172, 2005.
14. Eric JC, Humphries SC, Lynn PH, et al: Biomechanical study on the effect of cervical spine fusion on adjacent level intradiscal pressure and segmental motion. Spine 27:2431–2434, 2002.
15. Voccaro AR, Klein GR, Ciccoti M, et al: Return to play criteria for the athlete with cervical spine injuries resulting in stinger and transient quadriplegia/paresis. Spine J 2:351–356, 2002.

CHAPTER 32

# DISCOVER Artificial Cervical Disc*

Douglas G. Orndorff, Kornelis A. Poelstra, and Todd J. Albert

## KEY POINTS

- The DISCOVER Artificial Cervical Disc is a ball-and-socket design consisting of superior and inferior end plates manufactured from titanium alloy.
- The DISCOVER Artificial Cervical Disc features a spherical bearing surface between the titanium end plates and the ultra-high-molecular-weight polyethylene (UHMWPE) core. This bearing surface allows motion in all rotation directions—flexion, extension, lateral bending, and axial rotation.
- Each DISCOVER Artificial Cervical Disc assembly has been designed to provide 7 degrees of lordosis when implanted in the cervical spine and will be available in heights from 6 mm to 9 mm in 1-mm increments to accommodate varying patient anatomy.
- Previous neurotoxicity studies and reported clinical literature assessments for risk of osteolysis suggest that the wear rate and particle sizes in the DISCOVER Artificial Cervical Disc will be well tolerated by the body.

## INTRODUCTION

With the aging population, the development of cervical spondylosis is expected to increase. It has been shown that after age 40, up to 60% of the population has radiographic evidence of cervical spine degeneration and by age 65, 95% of men and 70% of women have at least one degenerative change radiographically.[1–3] Anterior cervical decompression and fusion (ACDF) has demonstrated successful treatment of symptomatic radiculopathy and myelopathy and has become the gold standard over the past 2 decades.[1]

## INDICATIONS AND CONTRAINDICATIONS

At this time, the definitive indications for cervical arthroplasty remain a matter of some debate. This investigational technique is typically reserved for individuals with symptomatic myeloradiculopathy secondary to a herniated nucleus pulposus or spondylosis who have failed conservative management and would otherwise undergo ACDF.[1] Although cervical disc replacements have already been used outside the United States to treat multilevel spondylotic disease, at this time, this technology is probably best suited for patients with degenerative changes limited to a single spinal segment.[1]

Contraindications to cervical disc replacement include any history of tumor or infection, significant osteoporosis, or any kyphotic deformity. In addition, arthroplasty is not recommended for patients with restricted preoperative range of motion (<3 degrees) or any radiographic evidence of pre-existing facet degeneration or adjacent segment disease.[1] Because the successful implantation of any prosthesis is dependent upon the ability to obtain clear intraoperative fluoroscopic images to ensure its proper positioning, cervical arthroplasty should be avoided in patients with morbid obesity or any other condition that might preclude the unobstructed visualization of the level of interest.

## DESCRIPTION OF THE DEVICE

### Design Considerations

With any prosthesis it is imperative to understand its specific design characteristics in order to formulate appropriate surgical techniques for its insertion, predict its long-term function, and anticipate potential complications related to its use. Principal design considerations for cervical disc replacement include kinematics, biomaterials of the articulating surfaces, implant dimensions, footprint geometry, and method of fixation.[1,4] According to Phillips and Garfin,[1] the ideal cervical disc replacement would be able to tolerate physiologic loads without premature fatigue or failure, exhibit superior wear properties, and be easily secured to the surrounding vertebral bodies. To protect the facet joints from abnormal biomechanical stresses, a cervical implant should also have an axis of rotation that is similar to that of the normal spine.[1]

There are primarily three classes of bearings that are used for cervical disc arthroplasty: constrained, semi-constrained, and unconstrained. A device is considered to be constrained if it includes a mechanical stop within the physiologic range of motion, whereas with a semi-constrained prosthesis, the mechanical stop is outside the normal range of motion. If an implant has no mechanical stop at all, it is classified as unconstrained. In addition, current cervical disc replacements may either employ a ball-and-socket

*Investigational Device (The DISCOVER Artificial Cervical Disc from DePuy Spine, Inc. [Raynham, MA] is an investigational device limited by federal law to only investigational use in the United States.)

articulation that generates rotational motion about a single point or a saddle type of joint that allows motion about multiple centers of rotation.

Constrained prostheses generally exhibit greater stability, and their fixed axis of rotation serves to minimize the shear forces on the facet joints. Unfortunately, these constrained devices place greater stresses on the implant-bone interfaces and are technically less forgiving, requiring more precise placement to effectively reproduce the natural axis of rotation of the cervical spine.[1] In contrast, because unconstrained implants allow some degree of translation, there is decreased stress concentration at specific points on the articulating surface, and they appear to be more forgiving in terms of their placement in the coronal and sagittal planes.[1] However, this lack of constraint provides less stability to the motion segment and can expose the adjacent facet joints to greater shear and torsional loads.[1,4] As a result, soft tissue tension is of the utmost importance in unconstrained devices.

As with total joint arthroplasty of the extremities, materials selection of cervical disc replacements is an important consideration. Stainless steel has not been widely implemented for cervical arthroplasty because of its tendency to produce artifacts in magnetic resonance imaging (MRI) scans and to corrode over long-term implantations. The end plates, as well as some of the articulating surfaces of most cervical prostheses currently in development, are composed of either cobalt-chromium or titanium, both of which have been used extensively for total joint arthroplasty because of their biocompatibility, resistance to corrosion, and superior biomechanical properties.[1,5]

Another factor that will be critical in determining the success of cervical disc replacement is implant stability. Long-term implant fixation is dependent upon solid bony ingrowth into the press-fit surfaces of the prosthesis.[1] For bone formation to occur, the implant must be stable, and the end plates must have adequate pore size and geometry. To facilitate this process, a number of surface coatings have been developed, including plasma-sprayed titanium, titanium wire mesh, aluminum oxide, porous cobalt-chromium, and materials such as hydroxyapatite and calcium phosphate. The stability of cervical disc replacements may also be augmented with keels or spikes, which can be located on the base plates, and some of these devices require supplementary screw fixation into the vertebral bodies.

## Device Design

The DISCOVER Artificial Cervical Disc is a ball-and-socket design consisting of superior and inferior end plates manufactured from titanium alloy. The inferior end plate is a two-piece design with a mechanically attached cross-linked ultra-high-molecular-weight polyethylene (UHMWPE). The DISCOVER Artificial Cervical Disc features a spherical bearing surface between the superior titanium end plate and the UHMWPE core. This bearing surface allows motion in all rotation directions—flexion, extension, lateral bending, and axial rotation. The UHMWPE was chosen as a bearing because it exhibits excellent wear properties (Fig. 32–1). Titanium was chosen as the end plate material because it exhibits excellent MRI compatibility.

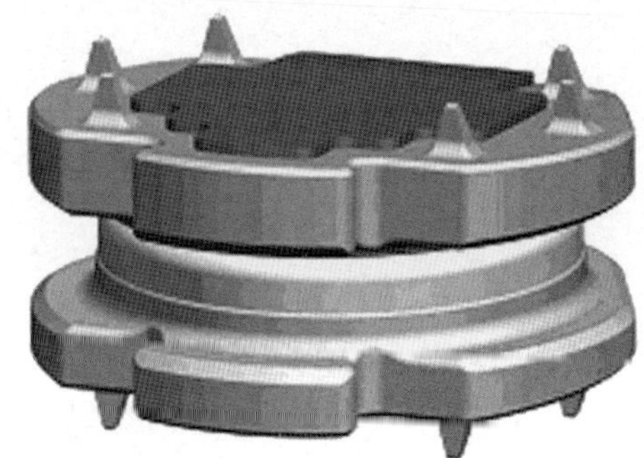

■ **FIGURE 32–1.** The DISCOVER Artificial Cervical Disc.

The trapezoidal implant footprint has been designed to reflect the natural bony geometry of the cervical vertebral end plates. The posterior edge of the superior implant component is rounded to provide ease of insertion as well as to accommodate the posterior rim on the inferior face of the upper vertebral body (Fig. 32–2). The implant's sizing scheme includes small, small extra-wide, medium, medium extra-wide, and large footprints. These options allow the surgeon to select a size that provides the greatest vertebral end plate coverage, with the goal of reducing the risk of subsidence. Each DISCOVER Artificial Cervical Disc assembly has been designed to provide seven degrees of lordosis when implanted in the cervical spine and will be available in heights from 6 mm to 9 mm in 1-mm increments to accommodate varying patient anatomy.

## Device Coating

The non-articulating (bone-contacting) surfaces of the DISCOVER Artificial Cervical Disc end plates are coated with a composite consisting of a first layer of titanium plasma spray and a second layer of hydroxyapatite. In order to maximize tooth penetration and therefore holding strength, the teeth are masked to prevent them from being coated with the titanium plasma spray.

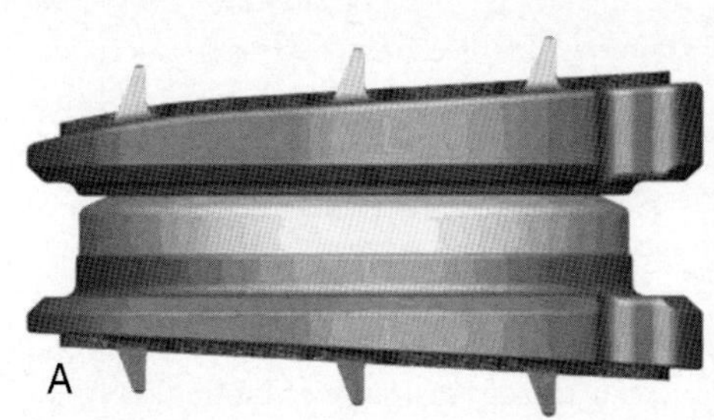


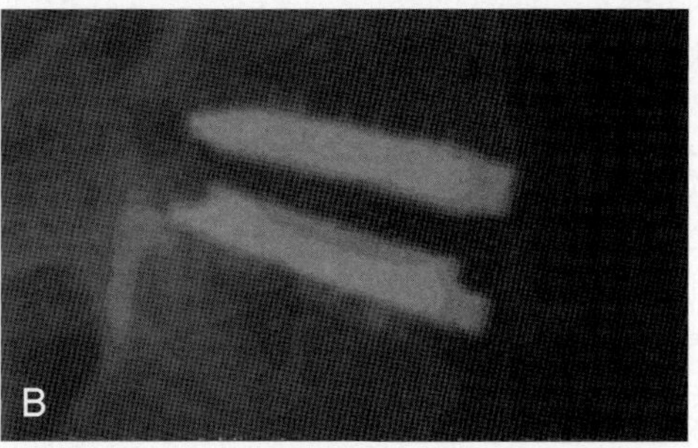


■ **FIGURE 32–2.** **A** and **B**, The posterior edge of the prosthesis is rounded to improve the insertion.

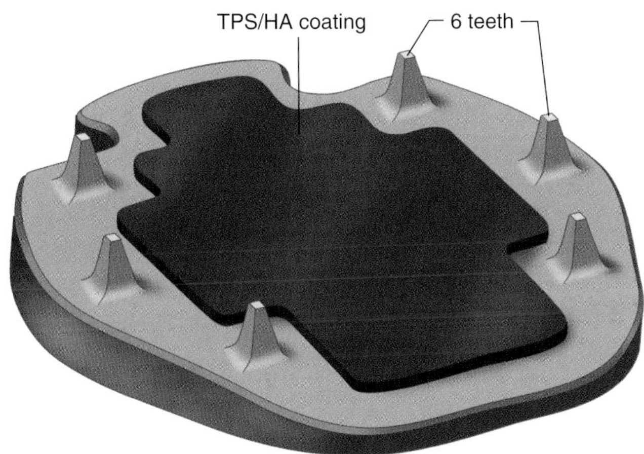


■ **FIGURE 32–3.** The end plates of the prosthesis have six teeth for immediate fixation as well as a sprayed coating to allow for bony ingrowth.

The six teeth that project from both the top and bottom end plates provide immediate fixation (Fig. 32–3). These teeth have a length of approximately 1 mm above the surface, sufficient to penetrate into the bony end plate and provide resistance to migration.

### Instruments

The instruments consisting of footprint sizing gauges, trials, and insertion instrumentation have been designed to aid the surgeon in optimal sizing and placement of the DISCOVER Artificial Cervical Disc, while mimicking the ACDF technique that surgeons are familiar with in anterior cervical spinal surgery. The principle of operation of the DISCOVER Artificial Cervical Disc is to replace key functions of the excised, degenerated intervertebral disc. The operating principles of the DISCOVER Artificial Cervical Disc are based on distribution and management of both static and dynamic loading forces exerted on the cervical spine (C3-C4 through C6-C7). Axial compression, compressive shear (both static and dynamic), and static creep testing were performed to ensure that the disc can withstand physiologic loads and is resistant to expulsion from the desired position.

### Wear Testing

Wear testing was conducted on test samples having identical bearing geometry and material composition to those of the DISCOVER implant assembly. Three of the smallest bearing radius implants and three of the largest bearing radius implants were tested simultaneously in combined flexion-extension, lateral bending, and axial rotation motions while subjected to a static axial compression load. Previous neurotoxicity studies and reported clinical literature assessments for risk of osteolysis suggest that the wear rate and particle sizes in the DISCOVER Artificial Cervical Disc will be well tolerated by the body. Further cadaveric testing has been performed to characterize the kinematics of the human cervical motion segments implanted with the DISCOVER disc. The results demonstrated that segmental motions in flexion-extension and axial rotation were restored to the intact levels at C5-C6 and C6-C7 motion segments.

## BACKGROUND OF SCIENTIFIC TESTING/CLINICAL OUTCOMES

ACDF has repeatedly demonstrated excellent results in the treatment of cervical decompression for myelopathy and radiculopathy; however, by limiting segmental motion, it may be responsible for adjacent level disease. Proponents of artificial disc replacement suggest that even though ACDF is clinically successful in the short term, fusion results in increased biomechanical stresses at adjacent segments that may hasten degeneration at those levels.[1–3] Eck et al[5] found a 73% increase in cranial and 45% in caudal disc pressures during flexion and increased intervertebral motion, especially rostrally. In essence, ACDF converts a functionally mobile triple joint complex into a fixed nonfunctional spinal unit that results in abnormal strain patterns at levels immediately adjacent to the fused segment.[1,5]

Baba et al[6] reported that an average of 8 years after ACDF, 25% of patients developed new onset spinal stenosis adjacent to the previously fused segments. Gore and Sepic[7] observed new spondylosis in 25% of 121 patients and progression of pre-existing spondylosis in another 25% of patients who had undergone prior ACDFs with a mean follow-up of 5 years. In addition they subsequently found that 14% of patients underwent additional surgery for adjacent level disease after ACDF.[6] Goffin et al[4] identified a 92% rate of adjacent segment disease after fusion over a mean of 8.6 years. Hilibrand et al[8] described the long-term follow-up of 409 patients who had previous ACDF procedures. They reported that 14% of patients had additional neck surgery over a 21-year period with an average annual incidence of development of adjacent level disease of 2.9%. The most common levels for adjacent segment disease were C5-C6 and C6-C7. Interestingly, they also demonstrated that ACDF performed at more than one level had a significantly lower rate of development of adjacent level disease than those fusions performed at a single level. One question that remains to be answered is whether ACDF actually does increase adjacent segment disease or whether it is just the natural progression in patients who are naturally predisposed to cervical spondylosis.

Considering cervical disc replacement, it is important to understand the specific kinematics, anatomy, and disease process of the cervical spine.[1] Biomechanical studies have demonstrated that cervical fusion alters adjacent level kinematics, and in cadaveric spines, it was demonstrated that a ball-and-socket design prosthesis can replicate physiologic motion at the affected and adjacent levels in flexion-extension and coupled motion.

## CLINICAL PRESENTATION AND EVALUATION

The typical patient who should be considered for the clinical study in the United States for cervical disc arthroplasty would be an individual with degenerative disc disease that is secondary to a herniated nucleus pulposus or spondylosis for whom conservative management has failed and would otherwise undergo ACDF.[1] A complete physical examination is imperative, assessing strength, evidence of pathologic reflexes, Spurling's or Hoffman's sign, and evidence of any specific level of compression. All patients should have plain radiographs with anteroposterior (AP), lateral, and flexion-extension views. MRI scan should be obtained to evaluate each specific level for spondylosis, disc herniation, status of the facets, and evidence of myelomalacia or intraspinal cord pathology. Conservative management should have consisted of physical therapy, nonsteroidal anti-inflammatory drugs (NSAIDs), followed by either epidural steroid injections or facet injections as deemed appropriate. After failure of conservative treatment or progression of symptoms, cervical disc arthroplasty should be considered as an alternative for ACDF.

## OPERATIVE TECHNIQUE

**STEP 1:** The patient should be placed under general anesthesia in supine position, with the neck in a physiologically neutral position. The skin should be prepped and draped in a sterile fashion, and the head should be in a neutral straight position. The head of the table should be elevated 30 degrees to decrease venous congestion, and the arms should be tucked to keep them out of the way. The incision is made to the left or right of the midline, depending on surgeon preference. The recurrent laryngeal nerve typically is found in a more predictable location between the trachea and esophagus on the left side. The right recurrent laryngeal nerve runs alongside the trachea in the neck after hooking around the right subclavian artery. In the lower part of the neck, it crosses from lateral to medial to reach the midline of the trachea and is more vulnerable during exposure.

**STEP 2:** A standard anterior approach to the cervical spine is performed. Once the desired cervical levels are visualized using fluorography before and during approach, it is important to mark the midline. The frontal midline can be identified by using the anatomic landmarks and fluoroscopy before placing a midline marker. All anterior osteophytes need to be removed. Once the midline has been identified and confirmed with an AP fluoroscopic image, a double-barrel guide is used for insertion of distraction pins into the vertebral bodies at the appropriate angle. Lateral fluoroscopy can be used to ensure that pins do not extend into the spinal canal and are parallel to the inferior end plates of the vertebral bodies; an AP fluoroscopic image is used to confirm frontal midline position of distraction pins (Figs. 32–4 and 32–5).

**STEP 3:** The next step is discectomy and end plate preparation as per surgeon preference, taking care to leave the lateral annulus intact. The posterior longitudinal ligament can be released in order to allow for parallel distraction, and rasps can be used to assist in end plate preparation. To achieve good bone-prosthesis contact, it is important to make the end plates as flat as possible within the footprint of the implant, while maintaining the integrity of the vertebral end plates. It is critical to pay particular attention to the supra-adjacent end plate, and care must be taken to avoid compromising end plate strength by removing too much cortical bone.

**STEP 4:** The final steps are trialing and implant insertion. Using a footprint sizing gauge to determine the appropriate size for the trial, a disc trial can be implanted to ascertain the appropriate height and fit of the final prosthesis. Disc trials are supplied in sizes corresponding to each prosthetic footprint and height. Using fluoroscopy, surface apposition at the bone-implant interface of the trial can be verified, and artificial implant height can be checked with adjacent discs to reduce the risk of overdistraction. During implant insertion, distraction across the disc space can be increased temporarily by using a vertebral distractor. The disc inserter that holds the implant is used to properly place the disc in the frontal midline, as indicated by the vertebral distractor pins. Fluoroscopy is needed to monitor the depth within the disc space. After the implant is disengaged from the disc inserter, the distraction can be released and final

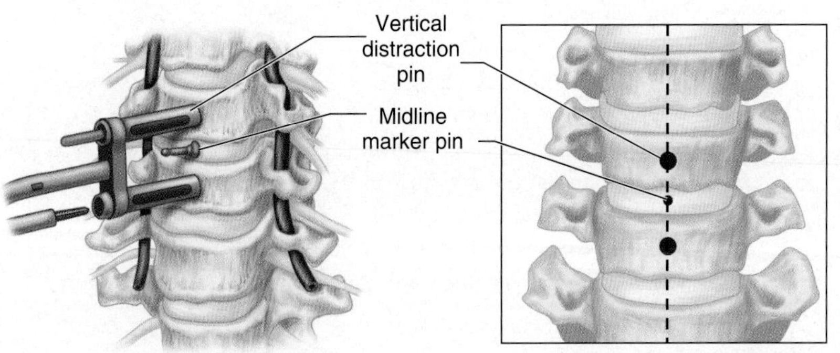


■ **FIGURE 32–4.** Placement of the midline marker and the double-barrel guide to determine the midline on anteroposterior fluoroscopy.

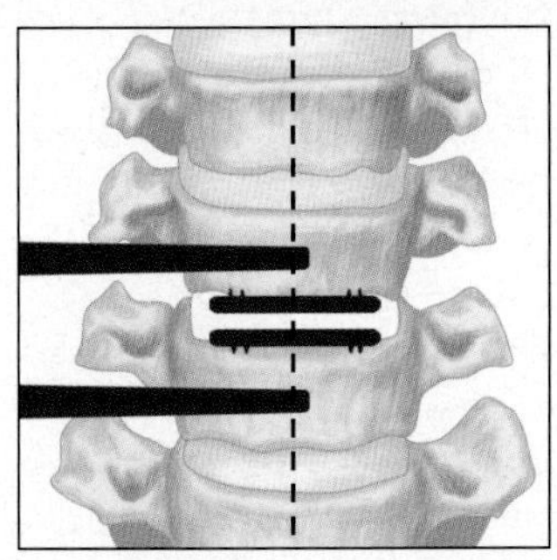

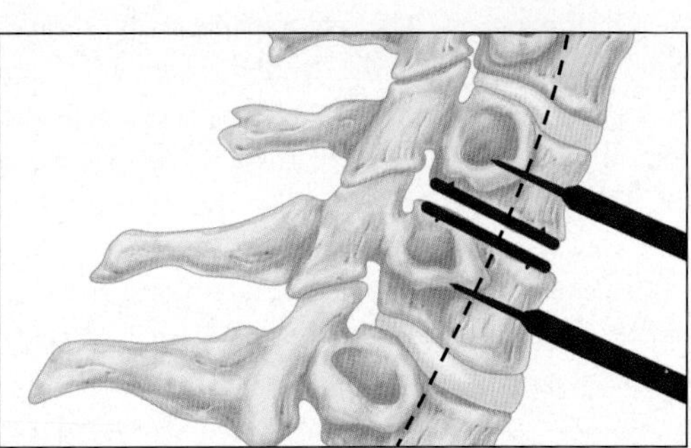

■ **FIGURE 32–5.** Final placement on anteroposterior and lateral fluoroscopy.

implant position can be checked. It must be emphasized that appropriate sizing is critical to enhance motion, and overstuffing must be vigorously avoided.

## POSTOPERATIVE CARE

External immobilization is not routinely required based on the nature of this operative intervention. Furthermore, some authors recommend a postoperative regimen of NSAIDs for all cervical arthroplasty patients in order to reduce the risk of developing heterotopic ossification,[1,7,10] although this can potentially reduce bony ingrowth on the titanium/hydroxyapatite coating.

## COMPLICATIONS AND AVOIDANCE

Cervical disc replacement is still investigational in the United States and still in its infancy outside the United States, and we have yet to experience some of the long-term complications that were seen with total hip and knee arthroplasty. These included aseptic loosing, osteolysis, infection, and complications during revision surgeries. To date, the follow-up from cervical disc arthroplasty is no longer than 3 years in U.S. clinical studies. Most of the reported complications involve perioperative complications that are maybe equivalent in incidence, but different in nature from those of ACDF. Intraoperative migration has been reported in two-level cases as well as delayed migration resulting in postoperative kyphosis.[9] HO and spontaneous fusion occurred in two patients and motion was preserved in 94 prostheses.[10] So far, approximately 25% of patients report neck pain in the late follow-up period, and there seems to be a trend toward increased kyphosis of the C2-C7 curve postoperatively. Goffin et al[4] reported on the European trial and documented seven complications (6.8%) in 103 one-level cases, and five complications (11.6%) in 43 two-level patients with an overall complication rate of 6.3% per year. The reported complication of the world literature for anterior cervical discectomy has an overall incidence of dysphagia (12.3%), hoarseness (4.9%), and unilateral vocal cord paralysis (1.4%) and recurrent laryngeal nerve injury are associated complications of the anterior approach.

### ADVANTAGES/DISADVANTAGES: DISCOVER ARTIFICIAL CERVICAL DISC

| Advantages | Disadvantages |
|---|---|
| Preserves motion | Novel technology |
| Decreased adjacent-segment disease | Possible osteolysis and bone loss |
| No need for allograft/autograft | Cost |
| No pseudarthrosis | Long-term effects on wear particles |

## CONCLUSIONS/DISCUSSION

Cervical arthroplasty represents a novel surgical procedure for degenerative cervical disc disease associated with symptoms of myelopathy, radiculopathy, or axial neck pain. The economic implications of motion-sparing technology must also be assessed to evaluate its cost-effectiveness, an important consideration in this era of limited health-care resources. Multiple prospective, randomized, controlled clinical trials with adequate follow-up will need to be performed before cervical arthroplasty may be regarded as an acceptable alternative to fusion for the treatment of cervical spondylosis.

## REFERENCES


1. Phillips FM, Garfin SR: Cervical disc replacement. Spine 30: S27–S33, 2005.
2. Boden SD, McCowin PR, Davis DO, et al: Abnormal magnetic-resonance scans of the cervical spine in asymptomatic subjects: A prospective investigation. J Bone Joint Surg Am 72:1178–1184, 1990.
3. Gore DR, Sepic SB, Gardner GM: Neck pain: a long-term follow-up of 205 patients. Spine 12:1–5, 1987.
4. Goffin J, Van Calenbergh F, van loon J, et al: Intermediate follow-up after treatment of degenerative disc disease with the Bryan Cervical Disc Prosthesis: single-level and bi-level. Spine 28:2673–2678, 2003.
5. Eck JC, Humphreys SC, Lim TH, et al: Biomechanical study on the effect of cervical spine fusion on adjacent-level intradiscal pressure and segmental motion. Spine 27:2431–2434, 2002.
6. Baba H, Furusawa N, Imura S, et al: Late radiographic findings after anterior cervical fusion for spondylotic myeloradiculopathy. Spine 18:2167–2173, 1993.
7. Gore DR, Sepic SB: Anterior discectomy and fusion for painful cervical disc disease: A report of 50 patients with an average follow-up of 21 years. Spine 23:3047–3051, 1998.
8. Hilibrand AS, Carlson GD, Palumbo MA, et al: Radiculopathy and myelopathy at segments adjacent to the site of a previous anterior cervical arthrodesis. J Bone Joint Surg Am 81:519–528, 1999.
9. Sekhon LH, Ball JR: Artificial cervical disc replacement: Principles, type and techniques. Neurol India 53:445–450, 2005.
10. Bertagnoli R, Yue JJ, Pfeiffer F, et al: Early results after ProDisc-C cervical disc replacement. J Neurosurg Spine 2:403–410, 2005.

CHAPTER 33

# The M6 Artificial Cervical Disc

**Alejandro A. Reyes-Sánchez, Avinash G. Patwardhan,** and **Jon E. Block**

## KEY POINTS

- The M6 Artificial Cervical Disc is designed to mimic the kinematics of the native disc, offering six degrees of freedom.
- A compressible polymer nucleus and woven fiber annulus allow axial compression, translation independent of rotation, and progressive resistance to motion.
- Simple operative technique using standard surgical instruments allowing one- or two-level application for the treatment of cervical radiculopathy.
- Durable design with optimized performance characteristics.
- Initial clinical experience suggests sustained clinical improvement through 12 months, with no device-related adverse events.

## INTRODUCTION

Restoring normal biomechanical function to a diseased cervical motion segment requires a total disc replacement device that mimics inherent disc kinematics. Almost all the first generation artificial cervical discs fail to replicate fully the normal viscoelastic disc structure, lacking internal elastic stiffness or restraint and axial compressibility.[1] Deprived of the full six degrees of freedom intrinsic to the native disc, these devices may function less than adequately and may not provide maximum clinical benefit to the patient.

The M6 Artificial Cervical Disc (Spinal Kinetics, Sunnyvale, CA) is a novel disc system designed to replicate the anatomic, physiologic, and biomechanical characteristics of the native disc by incorporating a compressible nucleus within a woven fiber annulus. These design features allow for natural kinematics, including axial compression, translation independent of rotation, and progressive resistance to motion resulting from a physiologically restrained construct. The resulting quality of motion closely mimics that of the native intervertebral cervical disc.

## DESCRIPTION OF THE DEVICE

The M6 Artificial Cervical Disc is an advanced-generation artificial disc intended to restore physiologic motion to a functional spinal unit when the native disc is diseased (Fig. 33–1). The core of the disc is composed of a polycarbonate urethane polymeric material that is surrounded by a polyethylene woven fiber construct. The compressible polymer core is designed to simulate the stiffness and function of the nucleus, and the fibers are designed to simulate the annulus. The fiber annulus is an assembly of high-tensile strength, ultra-high-molecular-weight polyethylene fibers wound in multiple redundant layers around the polymer nucleus, providing progressive resistance to motion. The core construct is attached to titanium alloy end plates to form the cervical disc prosthesis. This unique design enables the M6 disc to have all six degrees of freedom with independent angular motions in flexion-extension, lateral bending, and axial rotation, as well as independent translations along the three anatomic axes.

The prosthetic disc also has a polymer sheath encasing the core and fiber construct to inhibit any tissue ingrowth as well as capture any potential wear debris. The end plates are attached to the vertebral body through three low-profile keels on the superior and inferior surfaces. The keels provide acute fixation to the superior and inferior vertebral bodies within the intervertebral space. The end plates and keels are coated with porous titanium to promote bone-contact surface area and osseointegration.

## BACKGROUND OF SCIENTIFIC TESTING

A comprehensive battery of preclinical testing has been undertaken to evaluate the performance and safety of the device.

### Fatigue and Wear Testing

The functional and wear debris characteristics of the device, evaluated in flexion-extension, lateral bending, and rotational modes of motion, were tested through a minimum 10 million cycles in a physiologic solution under an axial compressive preload. The size, shape, quantity, and material composition of debris were determined after periodic evaluation of the testing solution. Functionality of the device was maintained throughout, with an acceptable level of wear debris.

### Static and Dynamic Characterization

Dynamic testing of the device was conducted at appropriate loads and torques through 10 million cycles. Fatigue-life characterization curves of load versus number of cycles in compression,

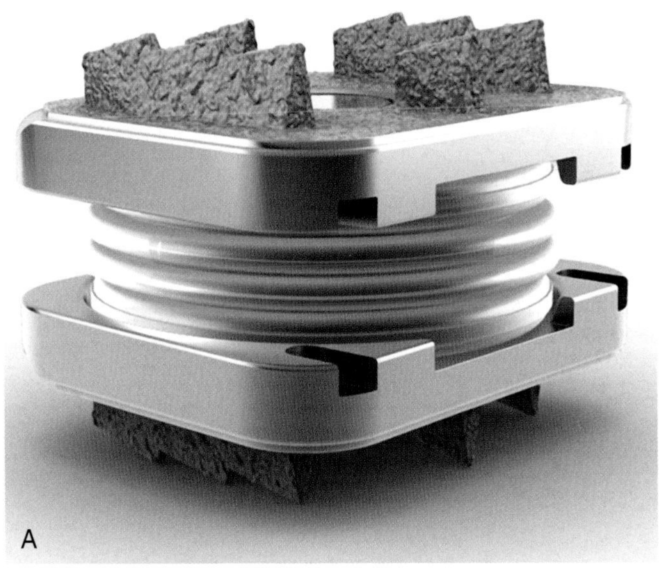


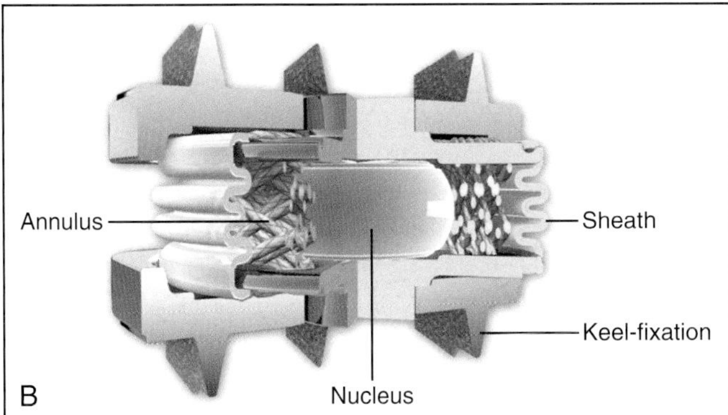


■ **FIGURE 33–1.** **A,** Graphic illustration of the M6 Artificial Cervical Disc (Spinal Kinetics, Sunnyvale, CA). **B,** Cut-away image of the disc illustrating a compressible polymer core to simulate the nucleus surrounded by woven fibers arranged circumferentially to simulate the annulus.

compression-shear, and torsional modes of motion were generated. Static testing was conducted to characterize maximum functional and mechanical failure limits. The results showed acceptable fatigue-life characterization curves with mechanical failure demonstrated well above normal physiologic loads.

### Creep and Stress Relaxation Testing

The device underwent creep testing, including an extended duration to simulate the sleep-wake cycle to evaluate stress relaxation. There was insignificant disc height loss predicted over the life of the device with nearly complete height recovery.

### Migration and Expulsion Testing

Following implantation of the device in cadaver cervical spine specimens, the artificial disc construct was subjected to natural range of motion (ROM) under normal and excessive loads. The device remained acutely fixed without notable migration in any direction.

### Biocompatibility

The device is composed of well-accepted and characterized biomaterials with a long history of use in medical device applications. Standard biocompatibility testing showed no evidence of tissue sensitization, irritation, or toxicity, either locally or systemically, and no indication of pyrogenicity or genotoxicity.

### Animal Implantation Studies

Two animal studies were undertaken to evaluate the in vivo characteristics of the device after long-term implantation. First, using a caprine model, the biological response of the implanted device after both one- and two-level spinal procedures was determined at 3, 6, and 12 months. Histopathologic assessment was conducted for the functional spinal units, including the spinal cord, periprosthetic tissues, and distant organs. There was no evidence of acute or systemic toxicity, no significant microscopic lesions, and minimal particulate material.

Second, using a rabbit model, the biologic response with respect to wear debris affecting the spinal cord was evaluated. Histopathologic assessment of the spinal cord and adjacent tissues 3 and 6 months after device implantation found acceptable cellular reaction with no evidence of systemic or neurotoxicity.

## BIOMECHANICAL EVALUATION

Three-dimensional kinematic assessment of cervical spines implanted with the M6 Artificial Cervical Disc was performed using fresh human cadaveric cervical spine specimens. In addition to quantifying the ROM, the ability of the implanted segments to replicate the kinematic signature of healthy cervical spine segments over the entire available ROM was also assessed.

Six human cervical spine specimens (C3-C7, 51.5 $\pm$ 5.5 yr) were tested in flexion-extension, lateral bending, and axial rotation. Flexion-extension was tested under a physiologic preload. Disc prostheses were implanted at C5-C6 with the prosthesis midline slightly posterior to the midpoint of the superior end plate of C6 vertebra.

The M6 Artificial Cervical Disc restored ROM in flexion-extension and axial rotation to previously reported physiologic norms. There was a loss of ROM in lateral bending; similar findings have been reported in the literature for other disc designs,[2] and this observation is likely related to the surgical implantation technique used in the in vitro study wherein the anterolateral annulus was retained to serve as an anterior tension band and the uncinate processes were left intact.

The kinematic signature of implanted segments approximated intact controls (Fig. 33–2), both qualitatively and in its quantitative measures. The center of rotation (COR) for flexion-extension motion of implanted segments was located posterior to the midpoint of C6 vertebra, similar to intact controls, and agreed well with the values reported in the literature for healthy subjects.[3]

Overall, the results of this kinematic assessment suggest that the M6 Artificial Cervical Disc allows restoration of physiologic quantity as well as quality of motion.

## OPERATIVE TECHNIQUE

As with cervical spinal fusion, surgical implantation of the M6 Artificial Cervical Disc uses a standard anterior approach. The target

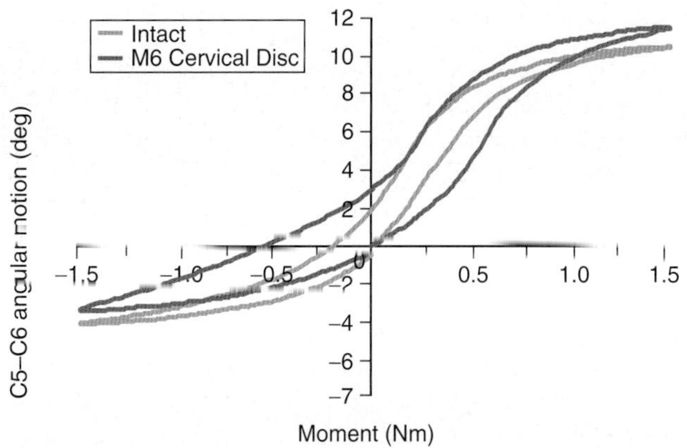


■ **FIGURE 33–2.** C5-C6 flexion-extension load-displacement curves. Biomechanical results showing the M6 Artificial Cervical Disc maintained total range of motion (ROM), with excellent quality of motion. The kinematic signatures of the intact disc and the M6 Artificial Cervical Disc are nearly identical.

disc space is identified and confirmed through fluoroscopy. Distractor pins and intervertebral distractors and spreaders are used, and a complete discectomy is performed with removal of all disc material to the posterior longitudinal ligament and uncovertebral junction. Anterior, lateral, and posterior osteophytes are removed, if present.

The surgical implantation of the disc requires M6 specific instruments to aid and ensure correct placement within the intervertebral space, including a trial implant to determine the appropriate size and position of the implant, a chisel to create keel tracks into the superior and inferior vertebral bodies, and an implant inserter to place the disc into the desired position (Fig. 33–3).

## CLINICAL EXPERIENCE

A single-arm prospective feasibility study was conducted in Mexico City to evaluate the preliminary safety and effectiveness of the M6 Artificial Cervical Disc in the treatment of patients with symptomatic cervical radiculopathy that was unresponsive to at least 6 weeks of conservative medical management.[4] A standardized battery of validated outcome measures, including the Neck Disability Index (NDI), an 11-point numeric pain severity scale, and the SF-36 Health Survey was administered pretreatment and at 6 weeks, 3, 6, and 12 months, postoperatively.

Entrance eligibility required a NDI score of 30% or higher at baseline and at least one positive neurologic sign. Thirty-two cases

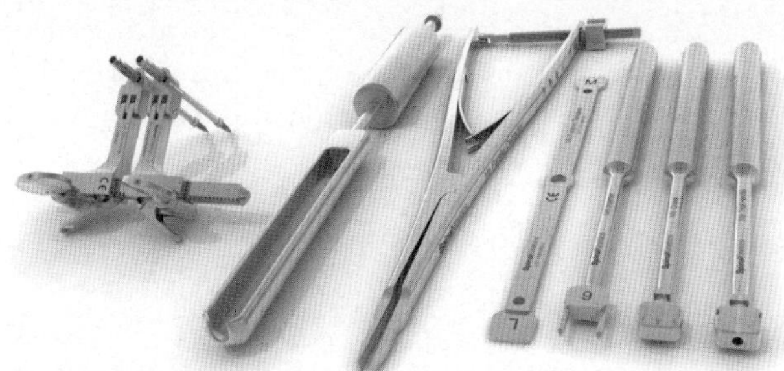

■ **FIGURE 33–3.** M6 surgical instrumentation.

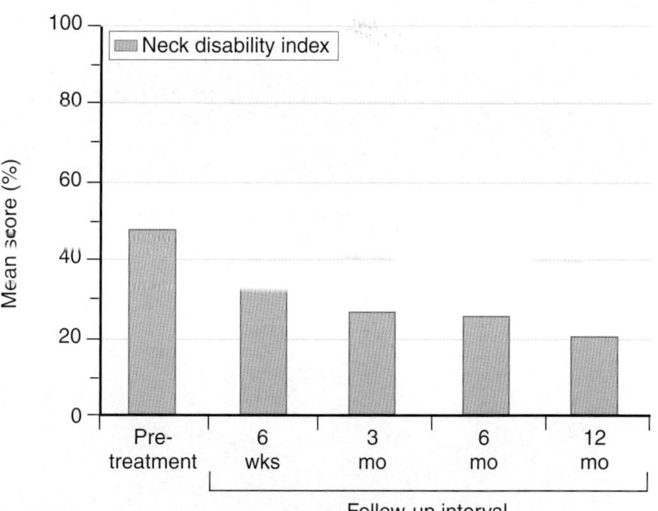


■ **FIGURE 33–4.** Mean Neck Disability Index (NDI) value pretreatment and at each follow-up interval. There was an average 59% improvement between baseline and 12 months ($P<0.0001$).

have been enrolled with 15 patients (mean age: 41.2 ± 10.6 y) reaching 12 months of postoperative follow-up. Ten patients underwent artificial disc implantation at one level, and five patients had two levels treated. The average duration of symptoms was approximately 24 months, and 6 patients (40%) were smokers.

The mean NDI score improved from 48.1% pretreatment to 20.4% at 12 months, representing an average 59% improvement ($P < 0.0001$) (Fig. 33–4). The mean arm pain score improved from 6.8 pretreatment to 3.2 at 12 months, representing an average 61% improvement ($P < 0.0001$) (see Fig. 33–5). The mean neck pain score improved from 7.2 pretreatment to 3.5 at 12 months, representing an average 50% improvement ($P = 0.0014$) (Fig. 33–5). The mean Physical Component Summary (PCS) and Mental Component Summary (MCS) scores of the SF-36 improved from

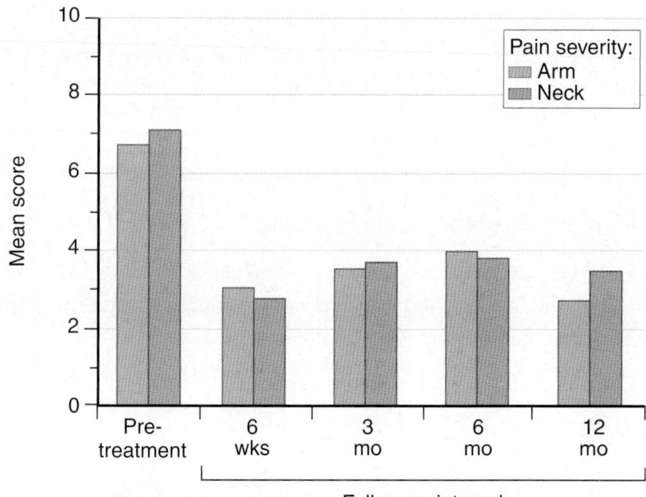


■ **FIGURE 33–5.** Mean arm and neck pain severity value pretreatment and at each follow-up interval. The average improvement over 12 months was 61% and 50% for arm and neck pain, respectively ($P<0.002$ for both comparisons).

34.7 and 43.6 pretreatment to 44.6 and 50.4 at 12 months, respectively ($P < 0.02$ for both comparisons).

Using dynamic flexion-extension radiographs, the mean ROM at the treated level was 12.3 degrees before surgery and 9.7 degrees by 12 months. Mean global ROM of the entire neck was approximately 47 degrees pretreatment and returned to this value by 12 months. Disc height at the treated level was 3.4 mm before surgery, improved to approximately 6 mm, and has remained constant through 12 months of follow-up (Fig. 33–6). There have been no cases of worsening neurologic status and no serious device-related adverse events, surgical reinterventions, or evidence of device migration, expulsion, or subsidence in this study group.

## DISCUSSION

Most patients with symptomatic and radiographically confirmed cervical radiculopathy who are unresponsive to at least 6 weeks of conservative medical care realize immediate and sustained clinical benefit from surgical treatment that includes en masse disc excision coupled with osteophyte removal to decompress the nerve roots at the affected level.[5–7] However, this procedure results in structural alterations that are less than optimal from an anatomic and biomechanical standpoint.[7] In fact, despite satisfactory clinical outcomes, cervical discectomy and neural decompression alone almost always result in disc space collapse.[5]

To maintain disc height and stability after discectomy, an interbody instrumented fusion procedure is commonly performed. Unfortunately, fusing the affected segment not only diminishes motion at the fused level[8] but has an untoward biomechanical effect on adjacent discs that, in essence, must compensate for the loss of natural motion in the fused segment.[9,10] The biomechanical modifications that occur after fusion have been shown radiographically to increase the risk of further disc degeneration and osteophyte formation at adjacent levels.[11,12] Although debate remains as to the short-term clinical importance of these radiographic changes,[13] it appears that there is a substantial possibility that new disease will develop at an adjacent level over the long term.[14]

In the case of degenerated large joints, fusion was abandoned long ago in preference of total joint replacement that provides motion preservation, returning nearly normal function to the patient. Similarly, artificial cervical disc replacement is emerging as a viable treatment alternative to fusion for the management of symptomatic compressive radiculopathies.[15,16] The designs of the first-generation artificial cervical discs evolved from large joint arthroplasty devices (e.g., ball and socket),[16–18] providing a certain degree of normal motion.[2] However, unlike large joints, the movement of the intervertebral disc joint involves complex coupled motions requiring all six degrees of freedom.[1,3] To date, these complex kinematic properties have been difficult to reproduce artificially.

## CONCLUSIONS

The M6 Artificial Cervical Disc represents more than an evolution of previous disc systems. It is intended to replicate the anatomic structure of the native disc with its artificial nucleus and annulus assembly, incorporating all six degrees of freedom in its kinematic

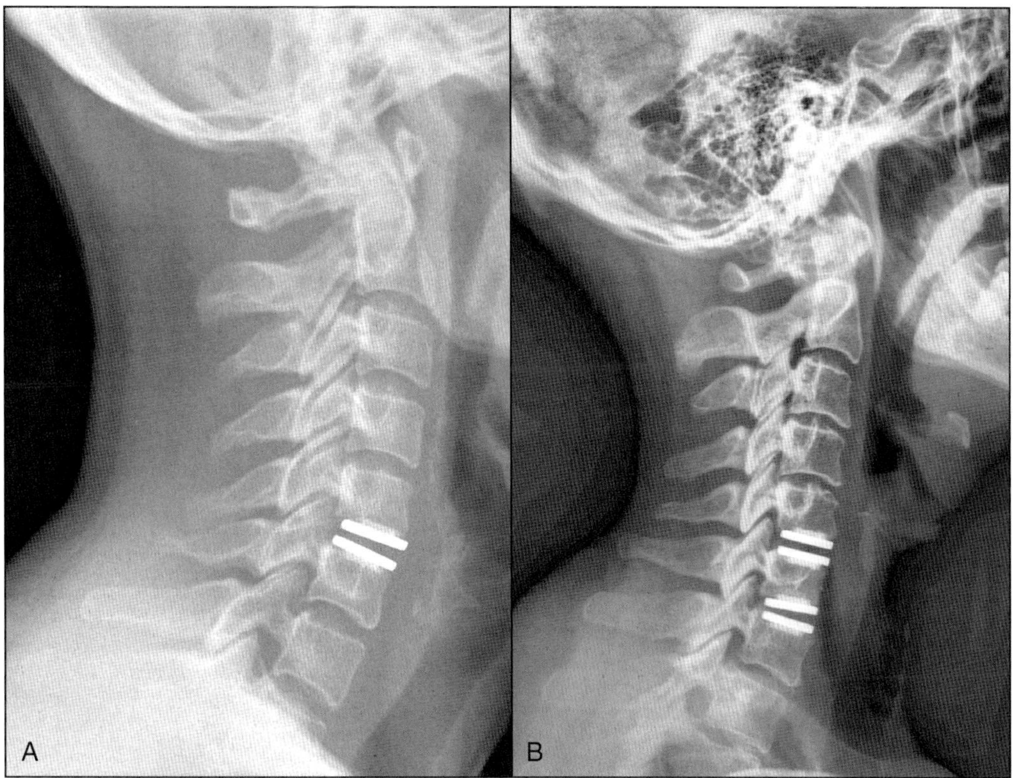


■ **FIGURE 33–6.** Neutral lateral view radiographs of M6 disc implantation at one level **(A)** and two levels **(B)** 12 months postoperatively. Movement of the facet joints at 12 months after surgery remains in physiologic parallel alignment, without notable angulation.

profile. Importantly, the novel design results in a physiologically restrained construct with progressive resistance to motion. Consequently, it can be considered a true next-generation advancement in artificial cervical disc replacement technology.

## REFERENCES


1. Sears WR, McCombe PF, Sasso RC: Kinematics of cervical and lumbar total disc replacement. Semin Spine Surg 18:117–129, 2006.
2. Puttlitz CM, Rousseau MA, Xu Z, et al: Intervertebral disc replacement maintains cervical spine kinetics. Spine 29:2809–2814, 2004.
3. Bogduk N, Mercer S: Biomechanics of the cervical spine, I: Normal kinematics. Clin Biomech 15:633–648, 2000.
4. Reyes-Sanchez A, Miramontes V, Olivrez LR, et al: Sustained clinical improvement following cervical disc replacement with a novel, next generation artificial disc: 12 month pilot results. Presented at the 7th Annual Meeting of the Spine Arthroplasty Society, Berlin, Germany. May 1–5, 2007.
5. Albert TJ, Murrell SE: Surgical management of cervical radiculopathy. J Am Acad Orthop Surg 7:368–376, 1999.
6. Carette S, Fehlings MG: Clinical practice: Cervical radiculopathy. N Engl J Med 353:392–399, 2005.
7. Chesnut RM, Abitbol JJ, Garfin SR: Surgical management of cervical radiculopathy: Indication, techniques, and results. Orthop Clin North Am 23:461–474, 1992.
8. Hilibrand AS, Balasubramanian K, Eichenbaum M, et al: The effect of anterior cervical fusion on neck motion. Spine 31:1688–1692, 2006.
9. Lopez-Espina CG, Amirouche F, Havalad V: Multilevel cervical fusion and its effect on disc degeneration and osteophyte formation. Spine 31:972–978, 2006.
10. Wigfield C, Gill S, Nelson R, et al: Influence of an artificial cervical joint compared with fusion on adjacent-level motion in the treatment of degenerative cervical disc disease. J Neurosurg 96:17–21, 2002.
11. Truumees E, Herkowitz HN: Adjacent segment degeneration in the cervical spine: Incidence and management. Semin Spine Surg 11:373–383, 1999.
12. Robertson JT, Papadopoulos SM, Traynelis VC: Assessment of adjacent segment disease in patients treated with cervical fusion or arthroplasty: A prospective 2-year study. J Neurosurg Spine 3:417–423, 2005.
13. Bartolomei JC, Theodore N, Sonntag VK: Adjacent level degeneration after anterior cervical fusion: A clinical review. Neurosurg Clin N Am 16:575–587, v, 2005.
14. Hilibrand AS, Carlson GD, Palumbo MA, et al: Radiculopathy and myelopathy at segments adjacent to the site of a previous anterior cervical arthrodesis. J Bone Joint Surg Am 81:519–528, 1999.
15. Acosta FL Jr, Ames CP: Cervical disc arthroplasty: General introduction. Neurosurg Clin N Am 16: 603–607, vi, 2005.
16. Phillips FM, Garfin SR: Cervical disc replacement. Spine 30: S27–S33, 2005.
17. Anderson PA, Rouleau JP: Intervertebral disc arthroplasty. Spine 29:2779–2786, 2004.
18. Guyer RD, Ohnmeiss DD: Intervertebral disc prostheses. Spine 28: S15–S23, 2003.

CHAPTER 34

# Complications of Anterior Cervical Approaches: Cervical Revision: Approach-Related Considerations

**Paul C. McAfee**

## KEY POINTS

- There is no comparison between the complexity of revision anterior approaches to the lumbar spine, which have a high incidence of vascular complications, compared to the relatively straightforward, low-complication incidence with revision anterior cervical approaches.
- The presence of prior anterior cervical fusion or prior anterior cervical surgery should not preclude a revision anterior cervical arthroplasty, even performed through the same incision or through the same side of the neck.
- The most common approach-related problems from revision anterior cervical approaches stem directly from adhesions to normal anatomic structures; therefore, the approach-related complications are predictable.
- The main considerations of revision anterior approaches are airway problems due to soft tissue edema, vocal cord paralysis, esophageal fistula, mechanical pressure on the esophagus creating dysphagia, and inadequate exposure to perform cervical disc replacement.
- The most common intraoperative consideration creating an obstacle to performance of a revision cervical arthroplasty is inadequate fluoroscopic visualization, usually due to the overlying radiodensity of the patient's shoulders.

## INTRODUCTION

The biggest difference or change in operative technique with cervical arthroplasty versus traditional anterior cervical fusion approaches as developed by Robbie Robinson and his co-workers at Johns Hopkins Hospital from 1953 to 2000[1–6] is that the procedure is done using fluoroscopy on a radiolucent table. Many of the operative illustrations and techniques and operative anatomic considerations outlined by Smith and Robinson in 1958[6] are still relevant—the main fascial layers, development of the interval between the carotid sheath laterally and the esophagus and tracheal in the midline, and avoidance of traction on the recurrent laryngeal nerve—favoring the incision on the left side of the patient's neck.

With cervical arthroplasty, there are simply too many adjustments to be made regarding prosthetic trials, rasps, intervertebral spacers, and distracting pins to depend on conventional one-shot radiographs. Because of the importance of surgeon orientation and disc space preparation, with cervical arthroplasty and especially with arthroplasty revision surgery, the patient needs to be placed on a radiolucent operating table. The procedure needs to be able to include anteroposterior (AP) and lateral fluoroscopy at any time during the procedure. The surgical team needs to wear protective lead aprons for radiographic shielding, and often the surgeon and the assistants need to be able to dissect and work around the sterile-draped image intensifier.

Operative positioning is important for anterior cervical primary and revision procedures because there should not be excessive cervical extension (Fig. 34–1). More extension can be tolerated for fusion procedures, but for cervical arthroplasty, the neck needs to be in a neutral position. Figure 34–1 shows too much extension and too much downward pressure on the shoulders which, in this case, created 24 hours of brachial plexopathy with bilateral lower brachial plexus weakness and arm pain. This resolved within 24 hours with observation only.

## OPERATIVE TECHNIQUE FOR ANTERIOR CERVICAL REVISION APPROACH

The patient should be in the supine position on a radiolucent operating table in 5 pounds of cervical traction with a roll under the thoracic spine to allow the shoulders to be gently taped inferiorly out of the surgical field. Ideally, before the surgical site is prepped and draped, a lateral C-arm fluoroscopic image should document good visualization of the vertebral disc in question.

A modified transverse or diagonal incision is made along the left side of the neck at the anterior border of the sternocleidomastoid muscle (Figs. 34–2 and 34–3). I advise using the left side of the neck for all revision approaches at C5-C6 or inferiorly because the recurrent laryngeal nerve is less susceptible to traction injury. At C5 or above, either the left or the right side is acceptable, usually opposite the previous procedure to facilitate a dissection through virgin anatomy.

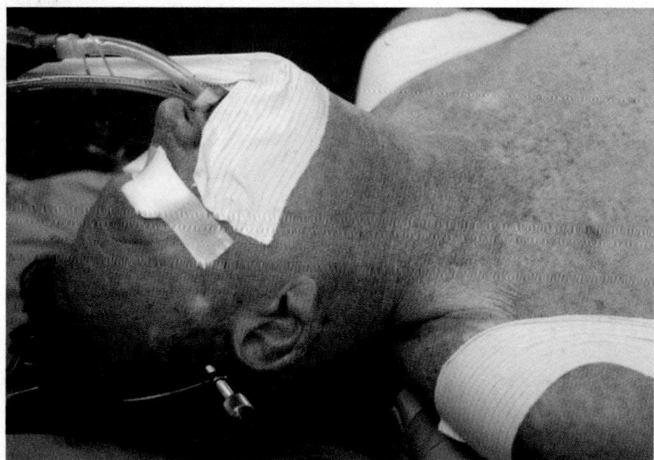

■ **FIGURE 34–1.** Correct operative positioning is important for revision anterior cervical approaches. This picture demonstrates excessive cervical extension, and the patient awoke with temporary brachial plexus lower trunk deficit, fortunately resolving within 24 hours.

The recurrent laryngeal nerves are branches of the vagus nerves.[7] The left recurrent nerve descends into the thorax in the carotid sheath and runs around the aortic arch. It ascends directly into the tracheoesophageal grove. It courses posterior to the inferior thyroid artery. In contrast, the right recurrent laryngeal nerve is variable in its location, so a revision procedure on the right side requires preservation of all nerves encountered. Occasionally, the right nerve is non-recurrent and does not course around the subclavian artery. Injury to the laryngeal nerve produces vocal cord paralysis, hoarseness, and a characteristic "bovine cough."

If the spine is not too heavily encased in soft tissue, the carotid tubercule or Chassaignac's tubercule on the sixth cervical vertebra can be palpated before the incision is made. This is the most consistent palpable skeletal landmark in the cervical spine. I usually check the position of the incision radiographically because the C-arm is already in place.

The surgeon must be thoroughly familiar with the four fascial planes of the neck. They consist of (1) the superficial fascia containing the platysma. Especially during revisions it is important to preserve and dissect the platysma because this is the important strength layer for the wound closure. (2) The next layer is the superficial layer of the deep cervical fascia surrounding the sternomastoid muscle; (3) the middle layer of the deep fascia that encloses the omohyoid, sternohyoid, sterothyroid, and thryohyoid muscles and the visceral fascia enclosing the trachea, esophagus, and recurrent nerve; and (4) the deep layer of the deep cervical fascia, which is divided into the alar fascia connecting the two carotid sheaths and fused midline to the visceral fascia and the prevertebral fascia covering the longus colli and scalene muscles.

The marginal mandibular branch of the facial nerve is found with the aid of a nerve stimulator by ligating and dissecting the retromandibular veins. If it is injured by traction or direct injury, the side of the patient's ipsilateral face and mouth will droop postoperatively (Fig. 34–4).

The anterior border of the sternocleidomastoid muscle is mobilized by longitudinally transecting the superficial layer of the deep cervical fascia. If the previous surgery has resulted in excessive fibrosis, then the omohyoid muscle can be transected—this serves at a gateway to the interval between the carotid sheath laterally and the esophagus medially. There are several vascular potential pitfalls that can be encountered during revisions—a cervical aortic arch

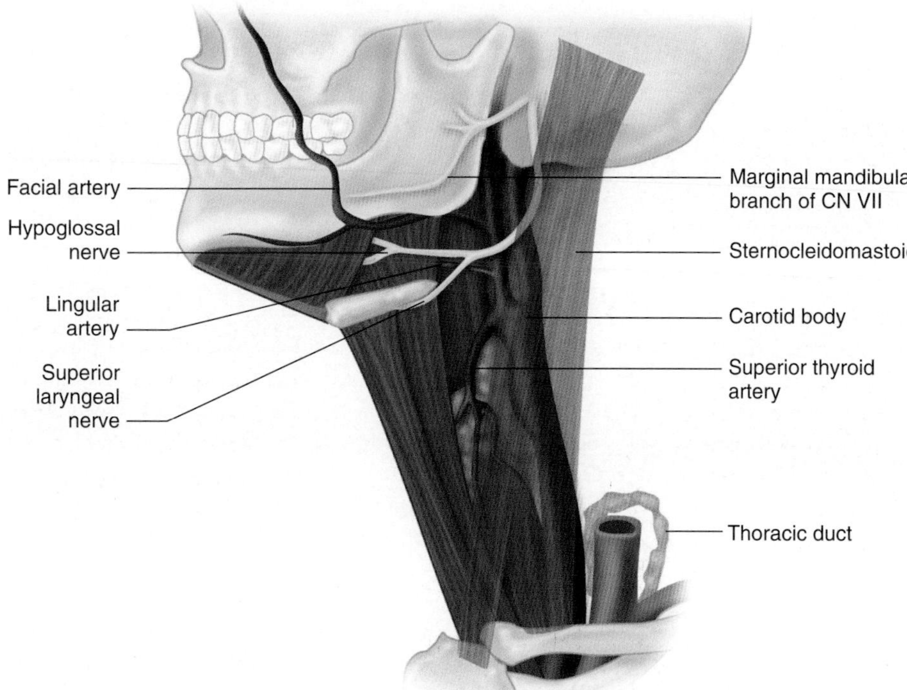


■ **FIGURE 34–2.** This illustration highlights the major structures of concern with a revision anterior cervical approach.

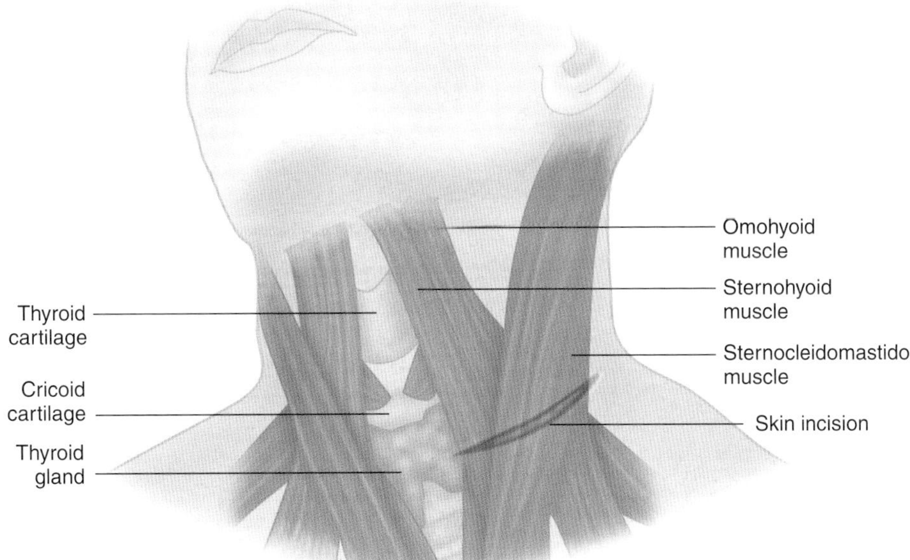


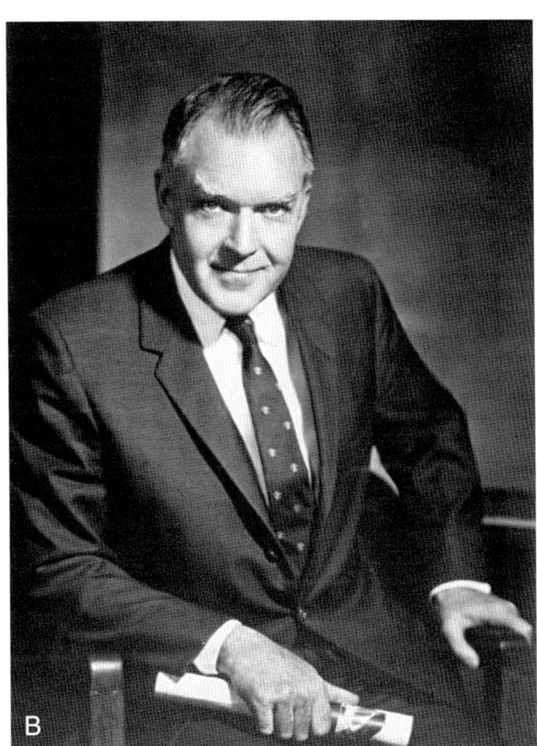


■ **FIGURE 34–3.** **A,** This is the location of the skin incision as originally described by Robbie Robinson in 1953. **B,** This is a picture of Robbie Robinson, Chairman of Johns Hopkins Orthopaedic Surgery, the original developer of the anterior approach to the cervical spine using the interval between the carotid sheath and the esophagus, originally used for surgical resection of esophageal diverticuli. Robinson trained a long legacy of spinal surgeons whose area of interest was the cervical spine including Southwick, Riley, Bohlman, Filtzer, Long, Dunn, Davis, and McAfee.

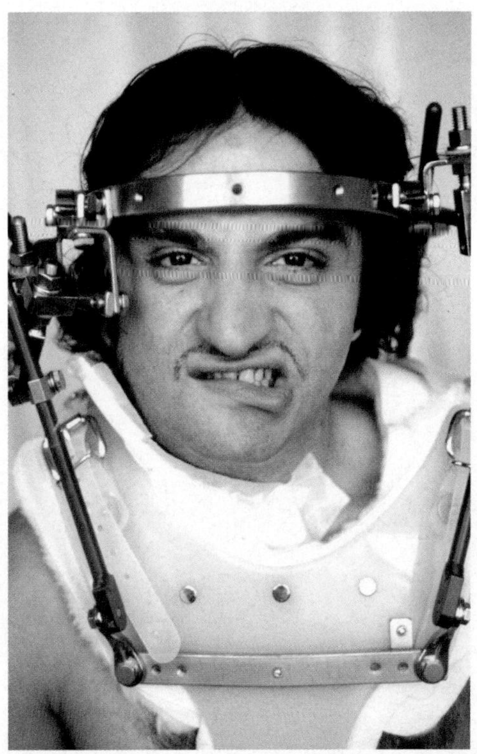

■ **FIGURE 34–4.** This patient with Klippel-Feil syndrome underwent a revision anterior approach and demonstrates injury to the marginal mandibular branch of the right facial nerve.

(Fig. 34–5), a carotid artery aneurism, or the thoracic duct entering the left subclavian or internal jugular vein. The cupola of the lung needs to be bluntly dissected free with lower approaches. I have been able to address the T2-T3 interspace through an anterior cervical approach, whereas occasionally it is difficult to visualize inferiorly even down to the C6-C7 disc space—the anatomic constraints are variable depending on a given patient's body habitus. The caudad extent of the anterior approach largely depends on the amount of kyphosis on the cervical spine and on the diameter of the patient's soft tissues of the neck (Fig. 34–6).

The hypoglossal nerve is the same diameter and close to the location of the superior thyroid artery so the two need to be separately identified. The hypoglossal nerve needs to be well protected and preserved in its transverse course behind the hypopharynx; a deficit of the hypoglossal nerve can cause severe symptoms of inadvertent tongue biting and trouble swallowing. The protruding tongue deviates towards the side of the damaged hypoglossal nerve (Fig. 34–7).

It is easier to enter the esophagus during a revision procedure and at the upper cervical levels as the hypopharngeal wall is thinner than the esophagus. The anesthesiologist can pass an esophageal stethoscope down the esophagus to assist the spinal surgeon's ability to palpate the esophagus or pass a strobe-lighted esophageal catheter, which will transilluminate the esophagus. If the esophagus is inadvertently entered, to prevent a life-threatening esophageal fistula (Fig. 34–8) from forming, the following sequence of steps needs to be taken:

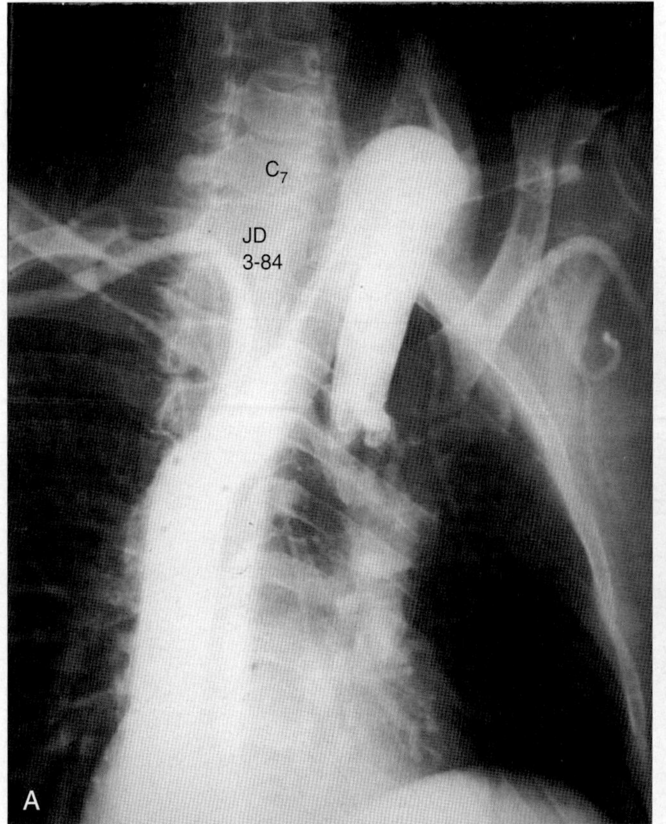


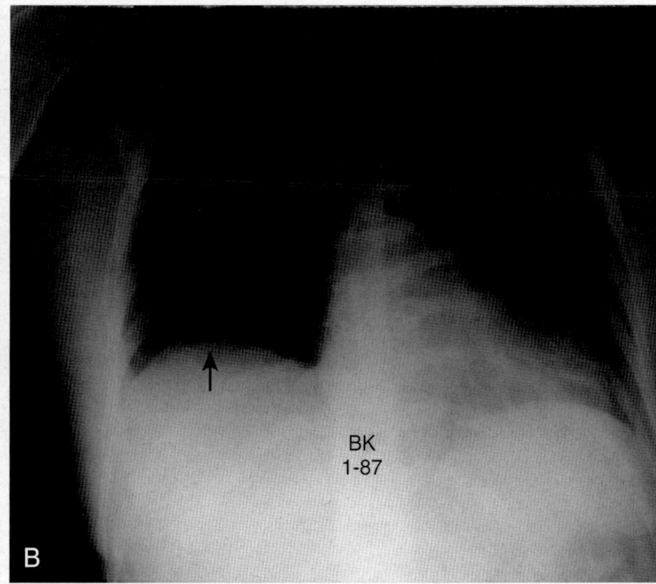


■ **FIGURE 34–5.** **A,** A high-riding cervical aortic arch would be nice to know about preoperatively. **B,** This patient demonstrates the importance of a preoperative chest radiograph, which demonstrated an elevated right hemidiaphragm due to phrenic nerve paralysis from a C3-C4 unilateral fracture-subluxation and nerve root injury.

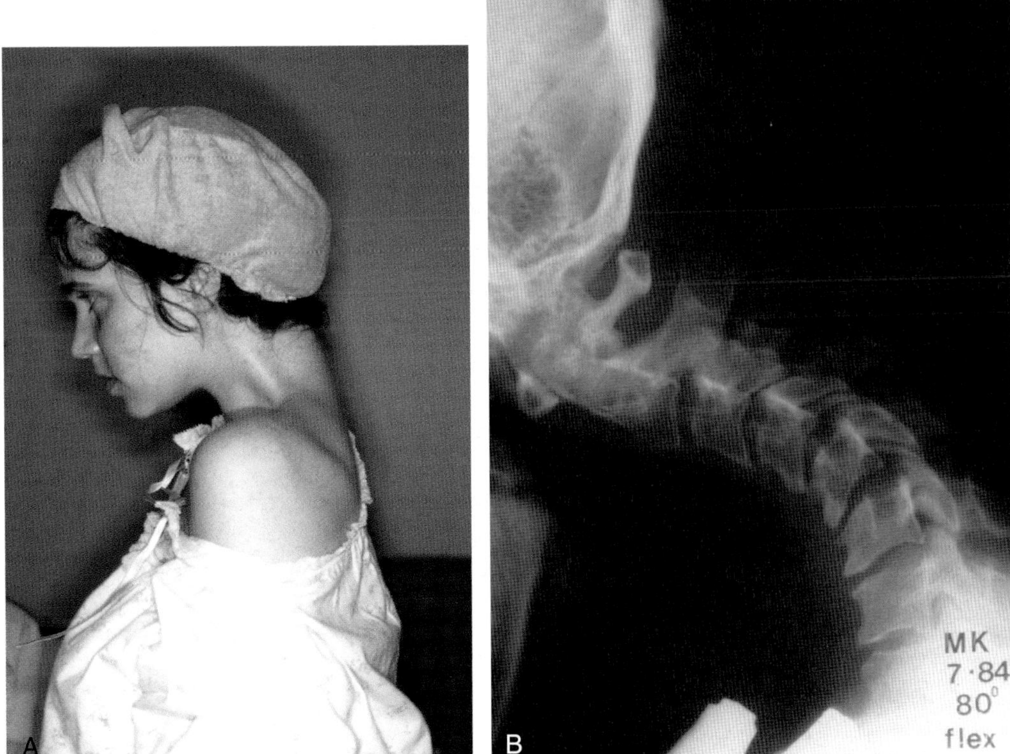


■ **FIGURE 34–6.** **A,** This clinical picture illustrates severe cervical kyphosis with hypertrophy of the trapezius muscle as the patient tries to counteract the muscular mechanical disadvantage of severe cervical kyphosis. **B,** The corresponding radiograph documents 80 degrees of kyphosis due to ligamentous instability at C4-C5, C5-C6, and C6-C7.

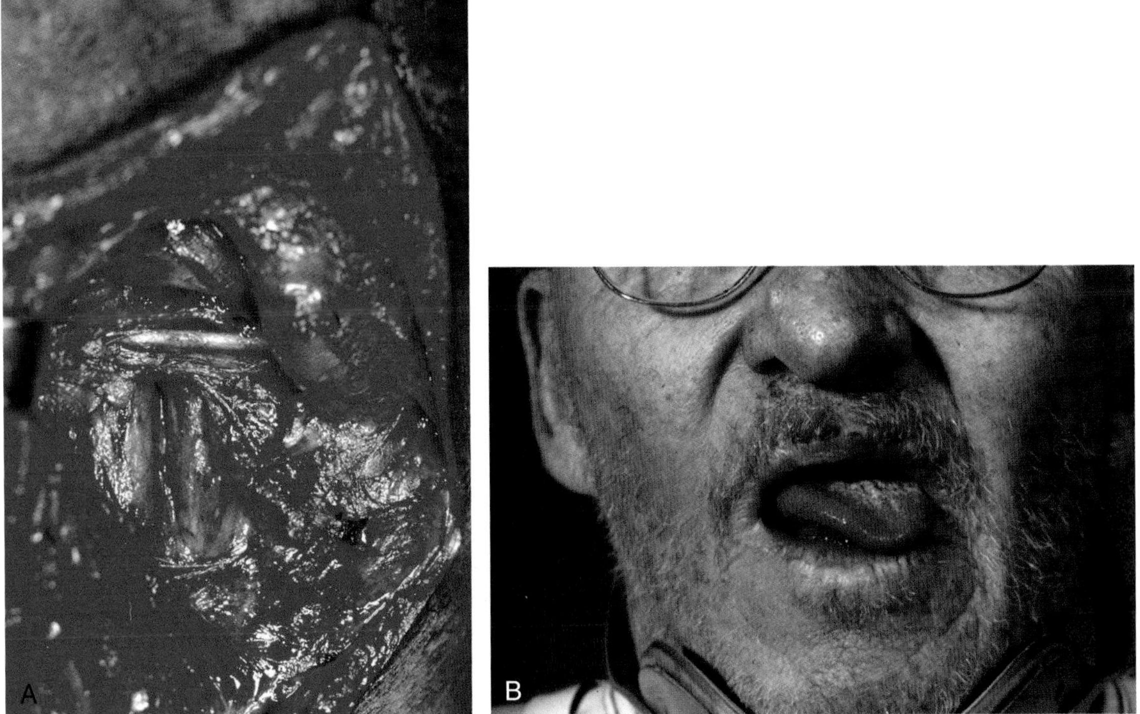


■ **FIGURE 34–7.** **A,** The course of the hypoglossal nerve is transverse anterior to the carotid sheath to the posterior aspect of the hypopharynx. **B,** Following a left-sided anterior cervical approach to C3-C4 and C4-C5, this patient demonstrated paralysis of the left hypoglossal nerve due to retraction. This spontaneously resolved in the first postoperative week.

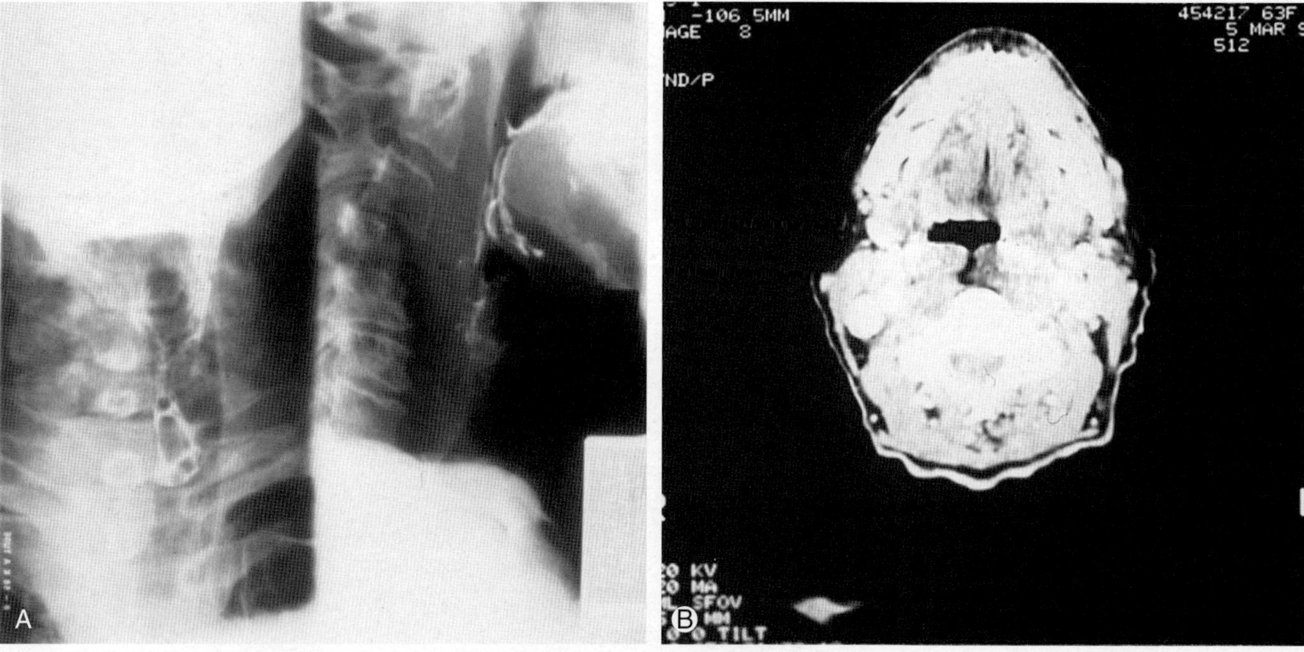

■ **FIGURE 34–8.** **A,** This 73-year-old woman was transferred from another hospital with an esophageal laceration after an anterior approach to C4-C5. Notice the large amount of soft tissue swelling behind the Gastrograffin-coated esophagus. **B,** The axial computed tomography image demonstrates air in a fistula communicating between the esophagus and the C4-C5 intervertebral disc space.

1. A feeding tube from the nose to the stomach (nasogastric feeding tube) needs to be placed by the anesthesiologist before the repair is undertaken.
2. The esophagus is repaired with absorbable horizontal mattress sutures, burying the knot within the esophagus.
3. The nasogastric feeding tube is left in place for 7 to 10 days as a gastric feeding conduit in order to protect the repair and prevent it from reopening and extending.

The superior laryngeal nerve is mobilized from its origin to its entrance into the larynx. This nerve is responsible for high-pitched phonation. The alar and prevertebral fascia are transected in the midline to expose the longus colli muscles, which run longitudinally. Usually the thyroid gland can be palpated but is kept medially. The stellate ganglion and cervical sympathetic trunk is on the anterior surface of the longus colli, and injury here results in Horner's syndrome, which is associated with miosis, anhydrosis, and ptosis (Fig. 34–9).

If the approach is high in the cervical spine, that is, above C2, then dislocation of the temporomandibular joint can be performed by placing a Steinman pin through the mandible and pulling the jaw to the opposite side (Fig. 34–10). The surgeon's orientation of the skeletal midline is particularly important during revisions or with anterior osteophytes. The key to midline orientation is to visualize the uncovertebral joints on each side. The surgeon's orientation regarding the midline of the cervical spine is maintained as the longus colli muscles are detached from the anterior surface of the vertebral bodies. It is essential to maintain this orientation throughout the anterior decompression of the spinal cord so that the decompression may be carried far enough laterally to decompress the spinal cord but not so far laterally as to endanger the vertebral arteries (Fig. 34–11). The vertebral artery, which is the first branch of the subclavian artery, usually enters the foramen transversarium of C6 and courses through the successive foramenae to C1. As a rule, I do not recommend using a high-speed burr until the discectomy is performed. The discectomy is helpful for orientation, does not create blood loss, and too many surgeons get disoriented removing bone stock with the high-speed burr. Furthermore, excessive reaming contributes to postoperative heterotopic ossification. I perform most of the decompression and bone removal with curettes and 1-, 2-, and 3-mm Kerrison rongeurs in order to preserve bone stock. The loss of blood during removal of vertebral osteophytes and bone can be minimized by the generous use of thrombin-soaked Gelfoam, bone wax, and bipolar cauderization of feeding vessels.

Revision motion preservation in the cervical spine is more difficult than comparable fusion procedures because one does not have the luxury of supplementing the anterior procedure with a posterior spinal stabilization procedure (Fig. 34–12). In addition, once the vertebral bone is removed, then it is gone. It cannot be replaced with bone graft or a prosthetic wedge. The barbershop rule pertains to revision cervical disc replacement—preserve bone stock during the early parts of the discectomy; you can always remove more later.

As a rule, with revision fusion procedures, the neck is extended, which opens up the disc space and allows the surgeon to pack it. However, the most common mistake with revision disc replacements is to "overstuff" the disc space and to leave the implant too anterior, so it functions as an arthrodesis cage. The second most common mistake is to burr away too much bone, removing the end plate, as fusion surgeons are accustomed to placing 8- to 10-mm bone grafts or spacers. With revision cervical disc replacement, one needs to preserve the vertebral end plates, preventing prosthesis subsidence, which means the most common thickness of prosthetic spacers are only 5 to 6.5 mm in total thickness.

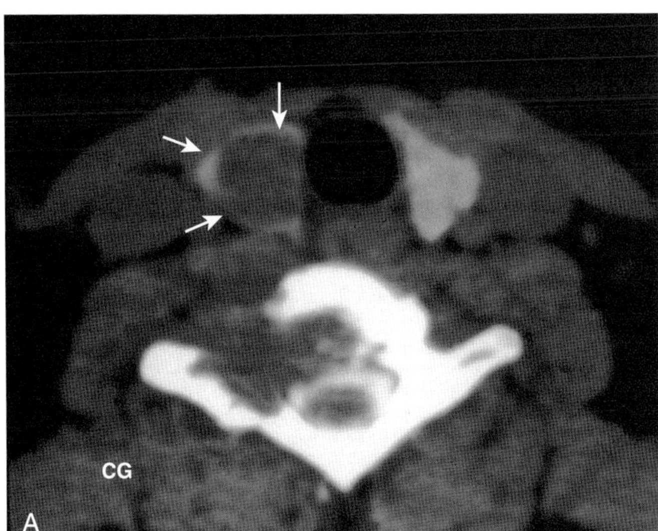


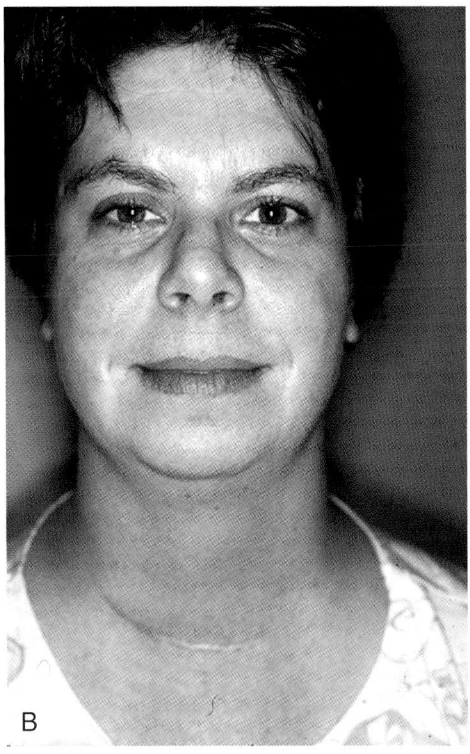


■ **FIGURE 34–9.** **A,** This computed tomography (CT) scan demonstrates a thyroid tumor that metastasized to the right aspect of the C7 vertebral body, causing this erosion on the CT myelogram. **B,** Following revision anterior resection of the right side of C7, the dissection had to extend more laterally than usual causing a Horner's syndrome. The pupillary constriction (miosis) and drooping right eyelid (ptosis) are evident, but the anhydrosis on the right side of the face had to be confirmed by history.

Once the prosthesis is inserted, remove the Caspar pins and check the prosthesis position and stability by having the anesthesiologist take the patient's head and neck through five complete flexion and extension ranges of motion. First of all, every total knee and total hip replacement surgeon understands the value of trial ranges of motion to check for ligamentous balance. Second, if there are "flexion gaps" or rocking of the prosthesis in extension or limitations of motion, one would rather find out on the operating table with the patient's neck open, where the prosthesis-bone interface can be directly examined, than find out there is a problem after the patient has been taken to the recovery room with the incision closed. Last, the anesthesiologist is the best person to take the patient's head and neck through a fluroscopically enhanced ROM because the anesthesiologist is the best person to protect the patient's airway during this maneuver. I have performed fluroscopically enhanced ROM intraoperatively in the cervical spine for over 20 years (more than 5,000 cervical spine procedures) and not had an airway complication due to this maneuver.

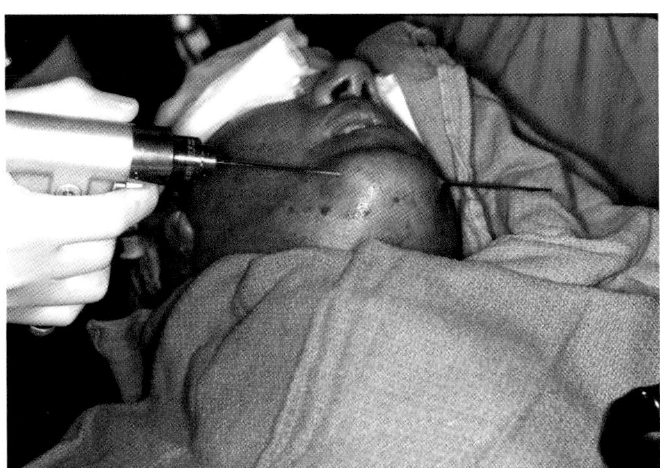

■ **FIGURE 34–10.** Steinman pin placed in the mandible to dislocate the jaw and allow improved access to the upper cervical spine.

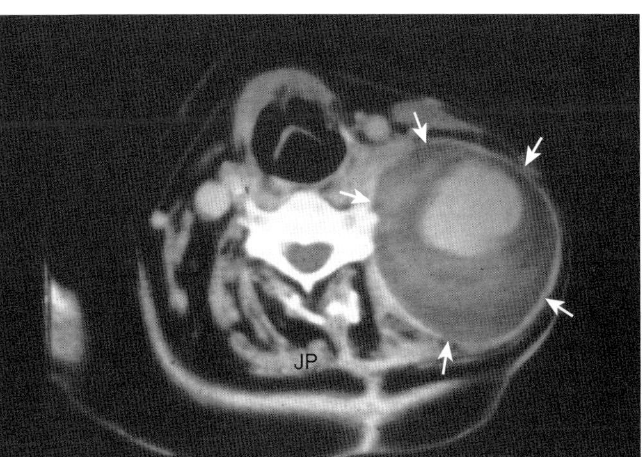


■ **FIGURE 34–11.** This is a revision anterior cervical approach gone wrong. The patient developed a 10-cm × 10-cm pulsatile mass postoperatively owing to penetration into the left vertebral artery. This is a contrast study documenting that active bleeding is still occurring as the arterial contrast leaks into the vertebral artery hematoma.

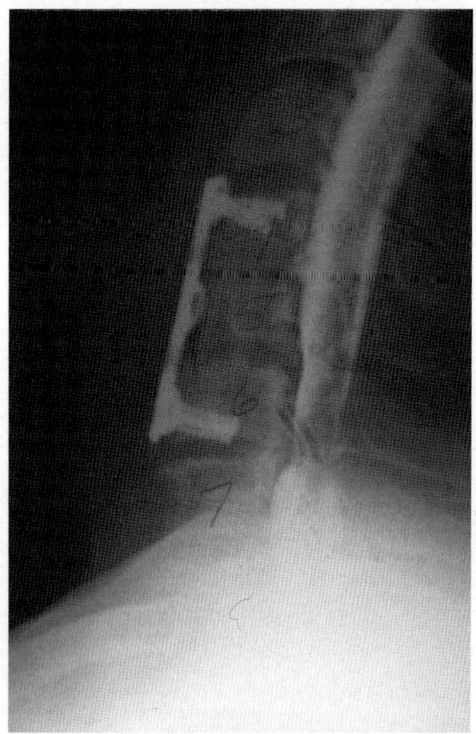

■ **FIGURE 34–12.** The C6–C7 disc space was damaged by misplaced screws so this compromises the bony end plate, which would anchor the cervical total disc replacement at C6-C7.

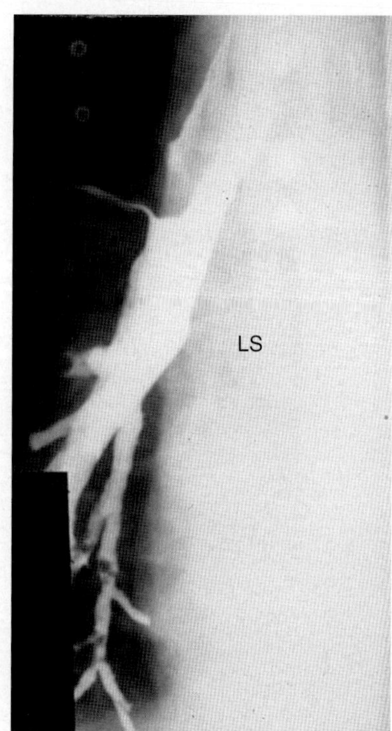


■ **FIGURE 34–13.** This patient underwent a Gastrograffin swallow for the work-up of dysphagia following an anterior cervical approach. The study was read by the radiology attending as a "Normal Bronchogram," which might indicate normal anatomy but indicates the severity of the patient's swallowing dysfunction, which required 3 weeks of clear liquid ingestion before the soft tissue muscular of the neck recovered enough for normal swallowing of regular food.

## DISCUSSION

Thus far, for the revision anterior approaches, usually in patients with prior anterior cervical discectomy and fusion who undergo a cervical total disc replacement, we have not altered the postoperative management. The patients have not required any orthoses, bracing, or physical therapy, which is different from primary cases. The postoperative instability or analgesic requirements have not been different. As a general rule, I would expect the complication rate to be higher, but I have not encountered this—I am simply more vigilant with regard to postoperative airway management. I keep the head of the patient's bed prophylactically elevated 30 degrees to reduce postoperative edema. I also have a low threshold for intensive care unit observation for the first 24 hours postoperatively following revision anterior cervical approaches. In revision approaches at the upper cervical spine, which is more of a factor with revision approaches at the C2 level and more cephalad, I also have a low threshold for keeping patients intubated overnight to avoid airway problems due to tracheal edema.

Common complications are sore throat, dysphagia, and hoarseness, and they can be minimized by gentle retraction. Hematoma formation causing respiratory obstruction can be minimized by meticulous inspection of all aspects of the wound before closure. Any persistent bleeding vessels are coagulated. If there is any doubt about adequate hemostasis or if there is any residual cancellous bone bleeding, then a soft tissue drain is used in the neck for 24 hours postoperatively.

A drain should also be used if there were any repairs of major branches of the carotid artery or internal jugular vein. The most common cause of vascular problems is not direct injuries but is due to misplaced teeth on self-retaining retractors, which is why I use hand-held retractors (Fig. 34–13). They can be radiolucent to permit better radiographic visualization. Self-retaining retractors causing sustained pressure on the esophagus are also responsible

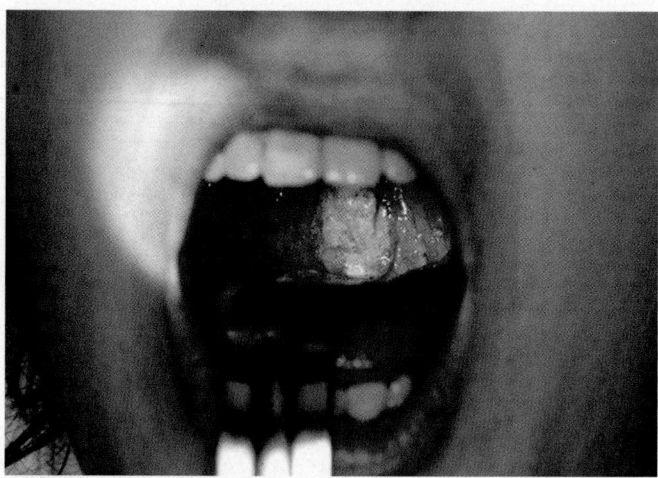

■ **FIGURE 34–14.** This is a 30-year-old woman who noted that a bone graft had eroded through the back of her mouth following anterior cervical fusion with an irregularly shaped bone graft. It required transoral removal.

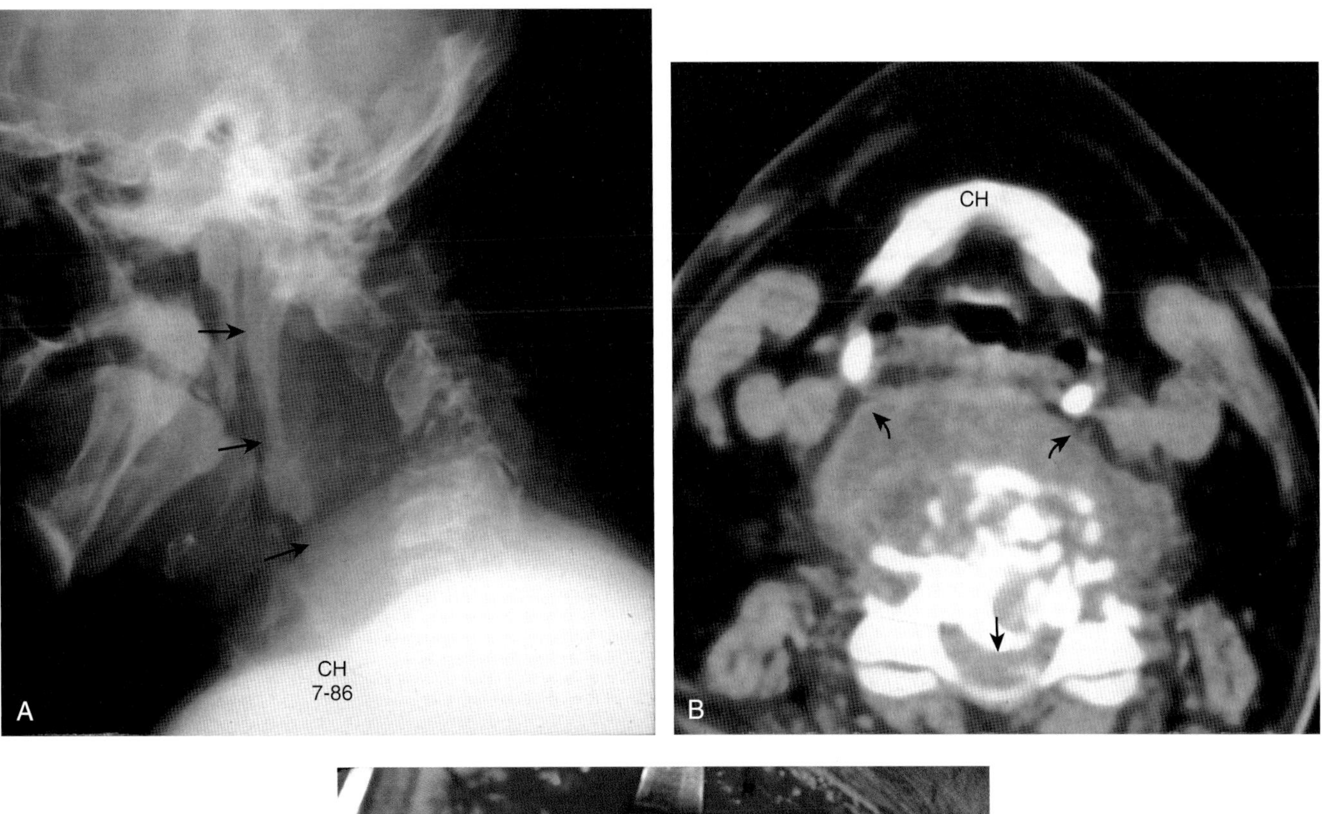


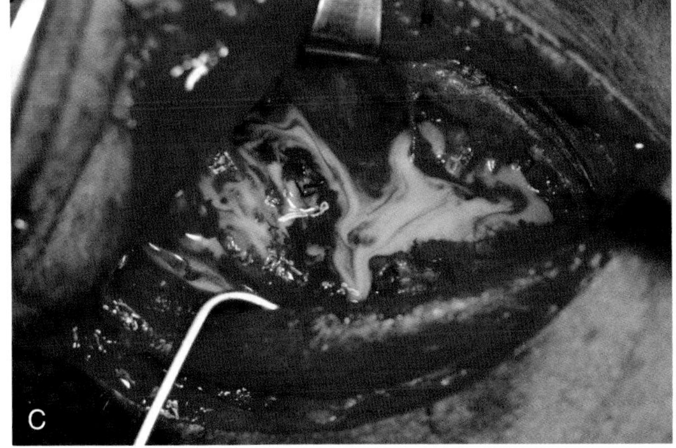


■ **FIGURE 34–15.** **A,** This is the soft tissue retropharyngeal swelling that occurred due to a *Staphlococcus aureus* anterior cervical infection. **B,** The computed tomography (CT) scan shows bony destruction and the extent of the soft tissue mass, which was erroneously interpreted by the admitting ENT attending as a neoplasm. **C,** With the anterior cervical approach, the purulence was obvious and the orthopaedic spinal team definitively treated the infection with a decompression and stabilization with iliac bone graft.

for late postoperative esophageal perforation. I have had patients referred from other hospitals who required gastric feeding tubes in treatment of esophageal perforations from sustained pressure from self-retaining neck retractors. I do not use them.

The last thing a surgeon should do before closing a revision anterior surgical exposure is to digitally palpate the anterior surface of the cervical reconstruction, whether it be bone graft, cervical plates, or a cervical disc replacement. The surgeon should not close if there are metal or bony protuberances that project anteriorly into the hypopharynx or the esophagus (Fig. 34–14). The surgeon should take a high-speed burr and smooth out any spikes of metal, bone, or tissue that project towards the mucosa of the alimentary tract.

Any anterior approach or surgery can be complicated by an infection. Figure 34–15 shows a pyogenic vertebral osteomyelitis that presented as an incomplete spinal cord deficit and a large anterior cervical soft tissue mass. A complete blood count, white blood cell count with differential, and an erythrocyte sedimentation rate with routine laboratory studies should be obtained on prospective revision anterior cervical approaches to ensure that the etiology is not an infection. This radiograph demonstrates that the process originated in the disc space, causing erosion, compared with a neoplastic process, which tends to originate in the vertebral bone initially.

The most serious complication of revision anterior cervical approaches would be neurologic spinal cord injuries. The exact incidence is not known for revisions, but there are two studies for all approaches. Flynn surveyed members of the American Association of Neurological Surgeons and reported a neurologic complication rate of 0.28% in 36,657 cases. Myelopathy occurred in 107 cases and radiculopathy in 138 cases. The Cervical Spine Research Society surveyed its members and found with 5356 cases the incidence was 0.64%. In summary, the exact incidence is not known for neurologic spinal cord injuries with revision approaches, but I always use continuous intraoperative spinal cord monitoring to provide every possible safety measure.

## REFERENCES


1. McAfee PC: The indications for lumbar and cervical disc replacement. Spine J 4:177S–181S, 2004.
2. McAfee PC: The advantages of cervical disc replacement for the treatment of degenerative disc disease. Curr Opin Orthop 17:233–239, 2006.
3. McAfee PC, Bohlman HH: Combined anterior decompression and posterior stabilization with circumferential spinal fusion: An analysis of twenty-four cases. J Bone Joint Surg 71A:78–88, 1989.
4. McAfee PC, Bohlman HH, Ducker TB, et al: One-stage anterior cervical decompression and posterior stabilization: A study of 100 patients with a minimum of two years of follow-up. J Bone Joint Surg [Am] 77A:1791–1800, 1995.
5. McAfee PC, Bohlman HH, Riley LH Jr, et al: Anterior retropharyngeal approach to the upper cervical spine (clivus to C-2). The evolution of the procedure at the Johns Hopkins Hospital representing a twenty five year experience. J Bone Joint Surg 69A:1371–1383, 1987.
6. Smith GW, Robinson RA: The treatment of certain cervical spine disorders by anterior removal of the intervertebral disc and interbody fusion. J Bone Joint Surg 40A:607–624, 1958.
7. Heller JG, Pedlow FX: Anatomy of the cervical spine. *In* Clark C (ed): The Cervical Spine. Philadelphia, Lippincott-Raven Publishers, 1998, pp 3–36.

CHAPTER 35

# Cervical Disc Replacement Revisions: Clinical and Biomechanical Considerations

**Luiz Pimenta, Roberto Díaz, Paul C. McAfee, Andrew G. Cappuccino, Bryan W. Cunningham, Hazem Nicola, Juliano Lhamby,** and **Ihab Gharzeddine**

## KEY POINTS

- Revision surgery–related approach complications are much easier to manage in the anterior cervical spine compared with those of the lumbar spine. This is primarily because the surgeon does not encounter the same complexity of problems with major vascular structures and adhesions.
- Primary surgical procedures and the revision procedures can be performed from the left or right side, provided care is taken to identify and protect the right recurrent laryngeal nerve.
- The same anatomic structures to use caution when retracting still come into play with revision approaches—the stellate ganglion laterally at C7 to avoid Horner's syndrome, the left side at T1 to avoid thoracic duct laceration, bilaterally at C3 to avoid injury to the superior laryngeal nerve, and all approaches need to delineate and protect the esophagus.
- The most common reason for cervical revision is inaccurate prosthesis sizing and subsequent prosthesis slippage.
- Provided the patient has good remaining bone stock without osteoporosis, a revision cervical total disc replacement (TDR) can be successfully performed using an augmented version of the cervical prosthesis, such as fixation with a modular plate, fixed flanges, screws, or a corpectomy replacement.

## INTRODUCTION

The indications for anterior cervical disc replacement are the same as for anterior cervical decompression and fusion (ACDF)—radiculopathy or myelopathy caused by either one or multiple levels of anterior cervical compression.[1–3] Most surgeons would agree that a patient presenting with a compressive lesion causing arm weakness, paresthesia, and unremitting radicular pain with or without lower extremity hyperactive reflexes requires anterior cervical decompression. The surgical objectives are to restore the intervertebral disc height and neuroforaminal height to prevent recurrence of neurologic compression. Although several surgical options are available to treat degenerative cervical spine disc disease, ACDF is currently the gold standard treatment, with satisfactory outcome in 90% to 95% of patients with single-level disease.[4] However, some problems have been identified, such as adjacent-segment disease,[5] perioperative immobilization, bone graft site morbidity, pseudoarthrosis, reoperation, and hardware failures.

Cervical disc arthroplasty has been introduced to enable restoration of postdecompression height and spinal alignment, with motion preservation and potential avoidance of adjacent level degeneration. White and Panjabi outlined the normal kinematics of the lower cervical spine, the restoration of which is the goal of cervical arthroplasty. Total disc replacement arthroplasty has been reported to restore motion in the cervical spine.[6]

One of the most beneficial aspects of ACDF is the exceptionally low rate of intraoperative and short-term postoperative complications. Decades of refinement in surgical and grafting techniques, combined with modern internal fixation technology, have rendered the procedure with relatively few complications. Cervical disc arthroplasty procedures, although undoubtedly benefiting similarly from these refinements represented in cervical spine surgery, will have to match the high standards set by the ACDF operation.

Complications in cervical disc arthroplasty procedures may be considered in the following categories: procedure related, implant related, fixation related, alignment related, stability related, and movement related (dynamic) varieties. A number of these complications, especially those in the procedure-related category, are familiar from traditional ACDF procedures.[7–10] However, the introduction of disc arthroplasty in the cervical spine does introduce new variations or new complications entirely, particularly in the latter category (Table 35–1).

In this study the Porous-Coated Motion (PCM) device (Cervitech Inc., Rockaway, NJ), a non-constrained cervical artificial disc prostheses,[5] was used. Conceptually, the PCM cervical disc replacement is a joint surface replacement providing an articulating surface in between two end plates that bond to the adjacent vertebrae. Bone resection typically required for ACDF is generally sufficient for preparation of the PCM prosthesis, and excessive reaming or table-mounted fixation jigs are not used. Excessive reaming probably contributes to the heterotopic ossification and "spontaneous" postoperative fusion across the vertebral levels bridged demonstrated

**TABLE 35–1. Categories of Cervical Disc Arthroplasty Complications**

| Complication | ACDF | Cervical Disk Arthroplasty |
|---|---|---|
| Procedure related | Esophageal injury<br>Laryngeal nerve injury<br>Vascular injury<br>Inadequate decompression<br>CSF leak | Esophageal injury<br>Laryngeal nerve injury<br>Vascular injury<br>Inadequate decompression<br>CSF leak |
| Implant related | Graft subsidence<br>Graft failure<br>Plate/screw breakage | Implant subsidence<br>Implant fracture<br>Implant wear<br>Translatory misalignment |
| Fixation related | Plate/screw loosening<br>Graft migration<br>Pseudoarthrosis | Implant loosening<br>Implant migration<br>Screw loosening |
| Alignment related | Loss of lordosis<br>Loss of disc height | Loss of lordosis<br>Loss of disk height |
| Stability related | Adjacent segment stress | Hypermobility<br>Traumatic instability |
| Movement related | None, if successful | Heterotopic ossification<br>Dynamic neural compression |

ACDF, anterior cervical discectomy and fusion; CSF, cerebrospinal fluid.

previously with cervical disc prostheses.[7] Therefore, the PCM was designed to avoid bone milling and reaming. In addition, vertebral end plate preservation is encouraged. Furthermore, there are no fins or sharp projections from the prosthesis to become embedded, facilitating revision, reducing the likelihood of either partial corpectomy or extensive bone grafting being required in a salvage situation. If the prosthesis can be placed in a press-fit fashion, then the low-profile standard version can be implanted. However, if the bony preparation is suboptimal or the anatomy is abnormal such as in Klippel-Feil syndrome, then there is a version of the prosthesis using screws to anchor to the anterior surface of the vertebral body. These design variations are similar to those described of other cervical disc prostheses. The biomaterials used in the manufacture of the PCM are the traditional ultra-high-molecular-weight polyethylene (UHMWPE) and cobalt chrome used in other conventional diarthrodial joint prostheses. The failure rate for cervical disc arthroplasty is unknown before this study. Although numerous studies show improvement in pain and function, details about the failures,[4] including approach and decompression complications, technical intraoperative complications, postoperative malposition, device displacement, arthrodesis, and infection, have not been presented. Also, different indications will likely require different revision strategies.

In the lumbar spine, the traditional options for failure of disc arthroplasty include (1) posterior fusion, (2) revision replacement, and (3) corpectomy and anterior fusion.[3] The goal of this prospective study is to determine if the situation is similar in the cervical spine.

## CLINICAL MATERIALS AND METHODS

Since December 2002, information on clinical and radiographic outcomes following cervical total disc replacement has been collected prospectively.

### Patient Population

Patients received implants at one level in 51% of the cases, two levels in 38% of the cases, three levels in 7% of cases, and four levels in 4% of cases. Indications were radiculopathy and cervical myelopathy. Approach and neural decompression were performed in a standard left-sided Smith-Robinson fashion, with complete decompression and posterior longitudinal ligament (PLL) removal followed by implantation of the PCM artificial cervical disc. The mean age of the patients was 45 years old (range: 28 to 63 years). Eighteen PCM cases were performed as complex revision procedures, including one previous Bryan disc replacement, one previous cage-plate fusion, three with failed lordotic fusion cages, and 12 patients presenting with adjacent-segment disease following previous anterior cervical disc fusion.

The 115 patients were selected according to the following criteria:

- Patients 20 to 65 years old.
- Degenerative disc disease with radicular or medullary compression.

The exclusion criteria were the following:

- Metabolic and bone disease.
- Patients in terminal phase of chronic disease.
- Patients with pyogenic infection or active granulomatosis.
- Patients with neoplastic or traumatic disease of the cervical spine.

Indications for the "press-fit" (no screws) model were as follows:

- Radicular compression.
- Herniation of the nucleus pulposus from C3-C4 to C7-T1.
- Anterior medullary compression.
- Cevical spondylosis.
- Nuclear magnetic resonance imaging evidence of mechanical compression of neural elements.
- Nontraumatic segmental instability.
- Neurologic compression of one, two, three, or four levels from C3-C4 to C7-T1.
- Primary degenerative disc disease.
- Degenerative adjacent-segment disease.

Indications for the "flanged" version (with screw fixation), in addition to those mentioned earlier, included:

- Suboptimal carpentry, understood as an irregular cut in the preparation of the vertebral end plate.
- Anterior vertebral subluxation greater than or equal to 3.5 mm (Fig. 35–1).

Contraindications to PCM disc arthroplasty were the following:

- Metabolic bone disease.
- Ossification of the posterior longitudinal ligament.
- Infection.
- Ankylosing spondylites.
- Spondylolisthesis with posterior element lesion.
- Narrow cervical canal, anteroposterior diameter less than 10 mm.
- Severe arthritis of the facet joints.

### Data Collection

For each eligible patient demographic group, employment status and return-to-work status were prospectively recorded. Operative details including the type of procedure (single, two, three, or four level), duration of the surgery, blood loss, complications, and the size of the device used were recorded. All patients enrolled underwent a complete neurologic examination before surgery and at each follow-up visit postoperatively. The Neck Disability Index (NDI), Visual Analog Scale (VAS), TIGT questionnaires, and Odom criteria were used to assess pain and functional outcomes preoperatively and on the 1-, 3-, 6-, 9-, 12-, 15-, 18-, 21-, 24-, and 27-month intervals after surgery. Static and dynamic cervical radiographs were obtained at 1 week, and then 1, 3, 6, 9, 12, 15, 18, 21, 24, and 27 months postoperatively. All adverse outcomes and complications related to the index procedure were noted.

## RESULTS

At the interval between 4 and 27 months follow-up, patients enrolled included 67 women and 48 men. The levels of disc implantation included the following: C3-4, 19 procedures; C4-5, 33 procedures; C5-6, 85 procedures; C6-7, 54 procedures; and C7-T1, 2 procedures. The mean length of surgery was 80.7 minutes. Blood loss ranged from 50 to 850 mL, with a mean of 113 mL. Almost all patients, (92%) were discharged within 24 hours of surgery. Patients did not require a cervical orthosis postoperatively. Procedures were performed at one level in 51% of patients, at two levels in 38%, at three levels in 7%, and at four levels in 4%. In six patients receiving two-level procedures, the implanted levels were not adjacent.

### Surgical Outcomes and Complications

#### Approach and Decompression Related

No approach-related complications with the standard Smith-Robinson technique occurred.[10] There were no permanent esophageal or tracheal injuries. No incorrect levels were operated. Two cases of cerebrospinal fluid leak occurred intraoperatively during the neurologic decompressive part of the surgical procedure. These were successfully resolved with fibrin glue and intraoperative tamponade, and there were no long-term sequelae. Two postoperative soft tissue hematomas occurred, but they were self-limited, did not require additional surgical drainage, and they both spontaneously reabsorbed.

#### Implantation Technique Related

No complications were presented during preparation of the end plates or device implantation procedures. No steriotactic frames were needed. Although implants were occasionally removed and reinserted intraoperatively following trial flexion-extension motion, short-term surgical re-exploration to replace or remove the prosthesis was necessary in two cases (Fig. 35–2).

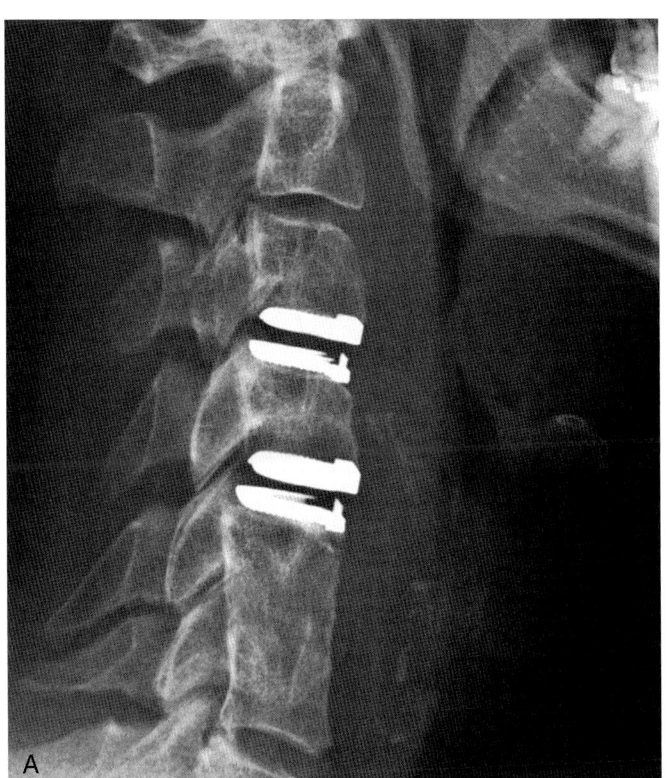


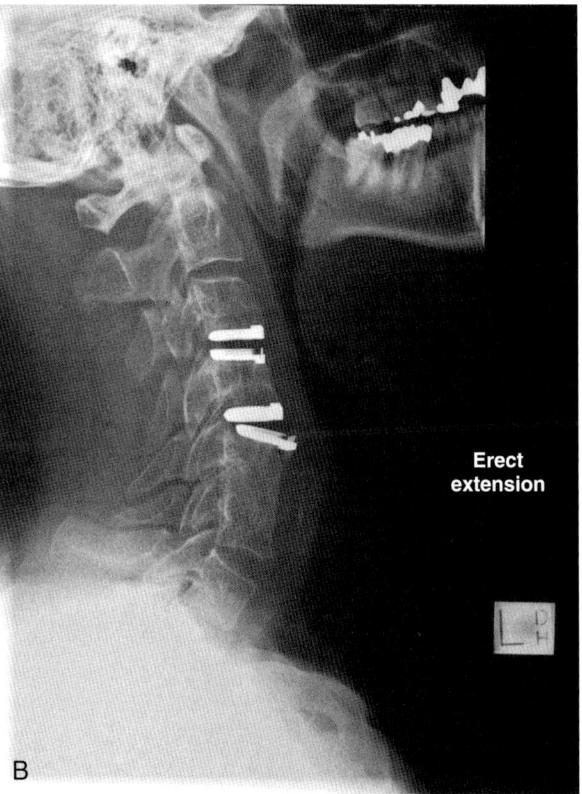


■ **FIGURE 35–1.** Head-on collision motor vehicle accident. **A,** This 42-year-old man underwent Porous-Coated Motion (PCM) cervical disc replacement at C3-4 and C4-5 above an adjacent-level fusion below at C5-6 without problems. The adjacent-level application is more exacting than virgin cases because the stresses are higher and often the spine has been fused in a kyphotic angulation. **B,** Unfortunately, she was involved in a head-on collision motor vehicular accident 3 months postoperatively and fractured the upper edge of the C5 vertebral body, dislodging the lower end plate of the prosthesis. The patient was neurologically intact.

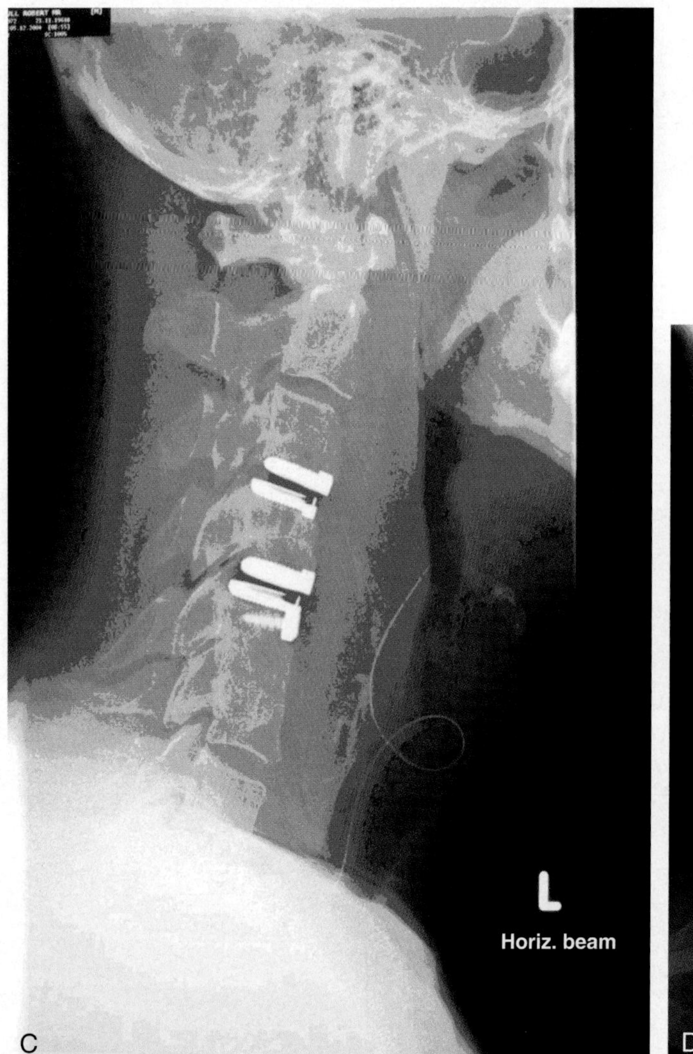


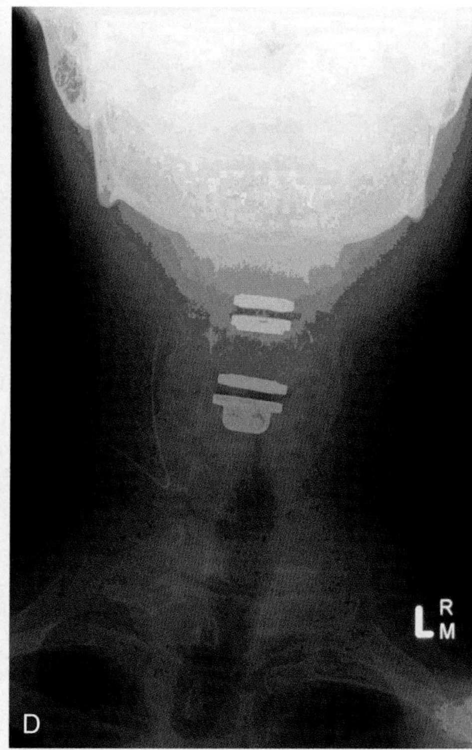


■ **FIGURE 35–1. Cont'd. C,** At surgery, the durability of the prosthesis was noted because the prosthesis itself had sustained no damage. It was able to be successfully anchored to the underlying fractured C5 vertebra with the use of the original version of the PCM prosthesis, the version with fixed flange with screws. The remaining three components of the PCM prosthesis were found to be secure by porous ingrowth at 3 months. **D,** This is the immediate anteroposterior view following revision illustrating good restoration of the artificial joint space despite the traumatic injury. This case demonstrates the advantages of a modular cervical spinal arthroplasty system.

Secondary to an excessive intraoperative extension position, two patients developed vertebral pseudosubluxation postoperatively. This abnormal translation alignment found in x-ray studies without clinical correlation never needed revision and preserved normal range of motion during further follow-up.

### Fixation Technique Related

No implant or screw loosening was seen (Fig. 35–3). The normal cervical spine motion is a synchronous harmonic fan. Four disc prostheses (2.05%) showed anterior device migration and needed revision with motion-preserving procedures. No iatrogenic motor or sensitive symptoms or signs were associated with this complication, and all cases were identified during incidental periodic radiographic review.

The first case was a 29-year-old woman with Klippel-Feil syndrome and myelopathy secondary to adjacent-level disease at C3-C4. She demonstrated rdiographically on the first postoperative day an anterior migration of the inferior component at C3-C4, without symptoms and signs. We revised the prosthesis simply by replacing the lower end plate with a taller UHMWPE core in the first 24 hours. Two years following this revision procedure, the patient remains asymptomatic (Fig. 35–4). The second case was a 53-year-old man, who presented with a C5-C6 disc herniation with radiculopathy. He underwent anterior cervical decompression and insertion of a PCM prosthesis, which in retrospect, was too large. Radiographs taken 3 months postoperatively showed an anterior migration of the inferior component, which was asymptomatic. This was revised with a more appropriately sized prosthesis with fixed flanges and screws to enhance stability (Fig. 35–5).

The last case was a 28-year-old man with C5-C6 radiculopathy, who developed avascular necrosis of the C5 vertebral body and refused an arthrodesis procedure. He developed cervical axial pain at 1-year follow-up. The patient's implant was successfully revised with a

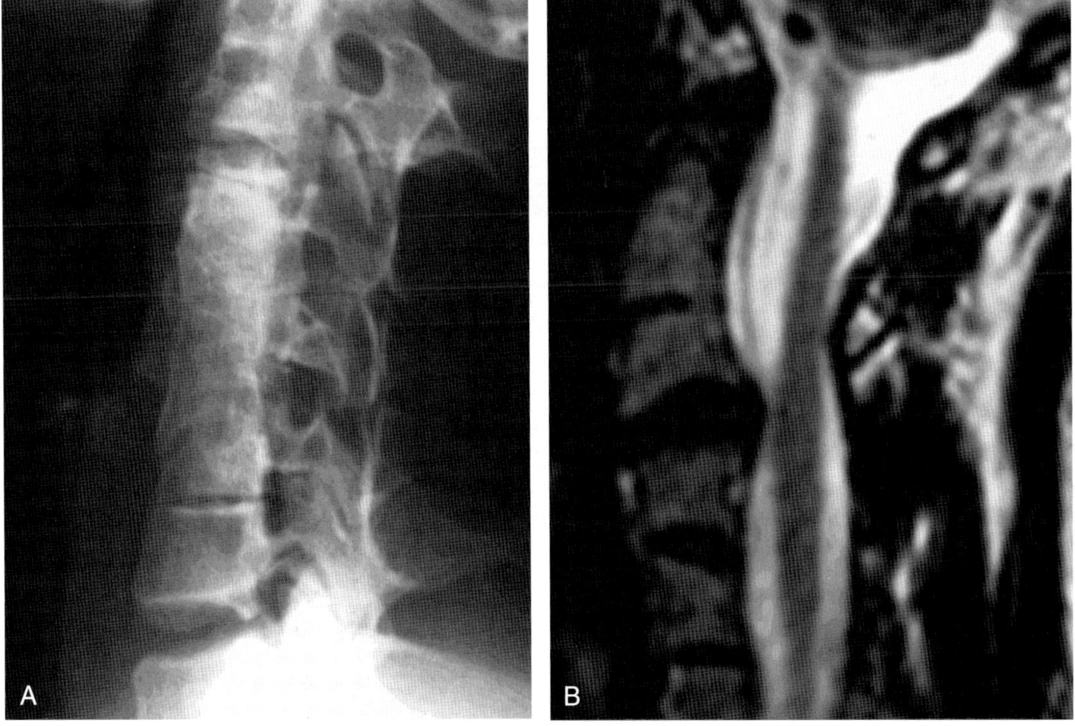


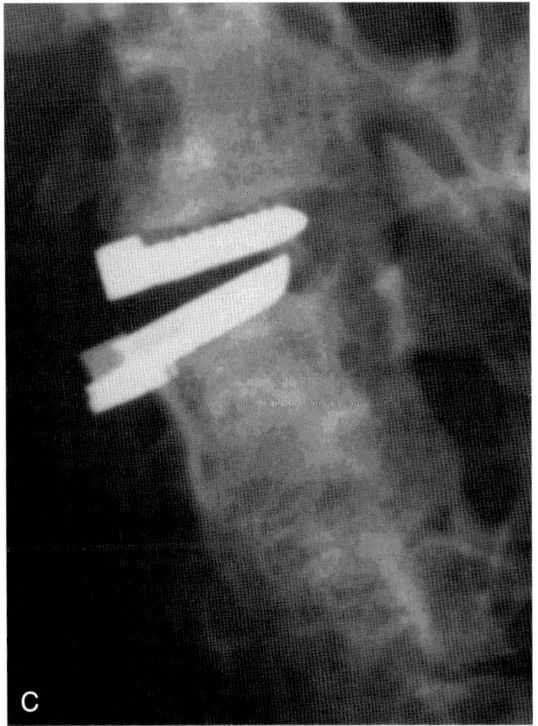


■ **FIGURE 35–2.** Klippel-Feil syndrome–redundant posterior longitudinal ligament (PLL). **A,** This 29-year-old woman had Klippel-Feil syndrome and adjacent-level disease at C3-C4 and at C7-T1 with myelopathy. She had previously undergone an anterior cervical cage arthrodesis at C6-C7 and could not afford to lose additional motion segments following neurologic decompression. **B,** The preoperative magnetic resonance imaging scan shows a redundant posterior longitudinal ligament at C3-C4. **C,** On the day after surgery, the prosthesis subluxed anteriorly owing to inadequate ligament tension across the annulus of the C3-C4 intervertebral disc space.

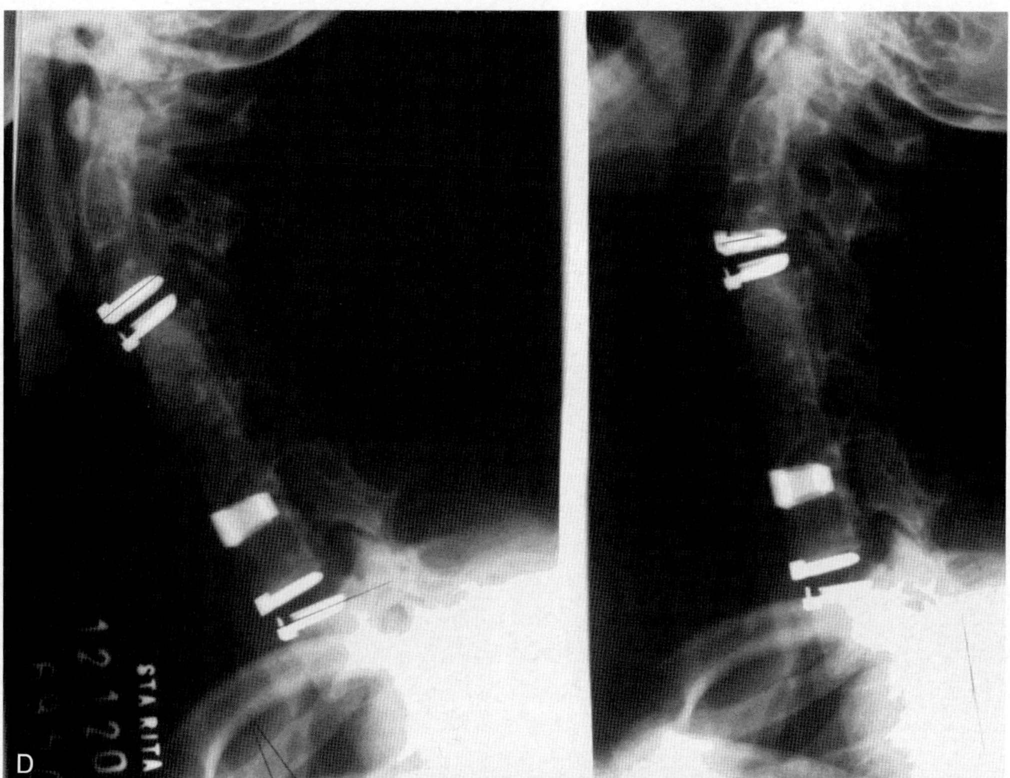

■ **FIGURE 35–2. Cont'd.** **D,** The prosthesis was easily revised 1 day after the original surgery simply by inserting a thicker, 8-mm, prosthesis with a taller ultra-high-molecular-weight polyethylene component. This is a flexion and extension lateral radiograph documenting 18 degrees of preserved motion 1 year postoperatively. The message in this case is that ligamentotaxis is important in contributing to the inherent stability of disc arthroplasty. At the time of the initial surgery, it should have been predicted that the redundant laxity of the PLL might have posed a problem. It is important, analogous to performing a total knee replacement, that the patient's neck is passively taken through a full range of motion intraoperatively under fluoroscopic control to evaluate the disc replacement stability—no component lift-off, no subluxation, and no restriction of motion. As documented on the next illustration, a smooth range of motion should be achieved.

dynamic PCM corpectomy device, which incorporates a disc replacement at C4-5 and a disc replacement at C5-6 (Fig. 35–6). The immediate means of fixation is provided by two reverse-direction cervical pedicle screws, oriented from an anterior to posterior direction. The long-term stability is provided by bony incorporation of autograft placed within the tubular mesh of the PCM prosthesis. Dr. Luiz Pimenta has had no complications thus far in an experience with three cases of the PCM corpectomy double-level replacement device.

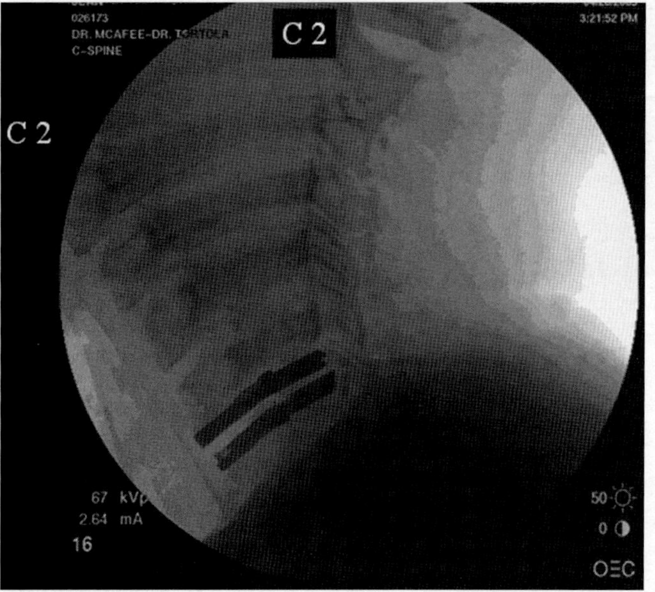


■ **FIGURE 35–3.** Physiologic fan-like motion pattern with the Porous-Coated Motion (PCM) device. This intraoperative fluoroscopic lateral image is a multiple exposure of a lateral cine picture following a PCM cervical disc replacement at C6-C7. It is important to note the fan-like pattern of motion of the vertebral bodies. Jan Goffin should be credited with this concept, which indicates synchronous motion of all seven cervical vertebra. If there is a fusion or restrictive motion, then a hinge-type motion pattern is observed instead of a fan-like motion pattern demonstrated above. If a patient has severe arthritis with restriction of motion at all vertebral levels, then a flagpole pattern of motion is observed. The image above is a reminder to check the flexion-extension and the side bending range of motion intraoperatively to ensure the prosthesis stability and confirm restoration of physiologic neck mobility.

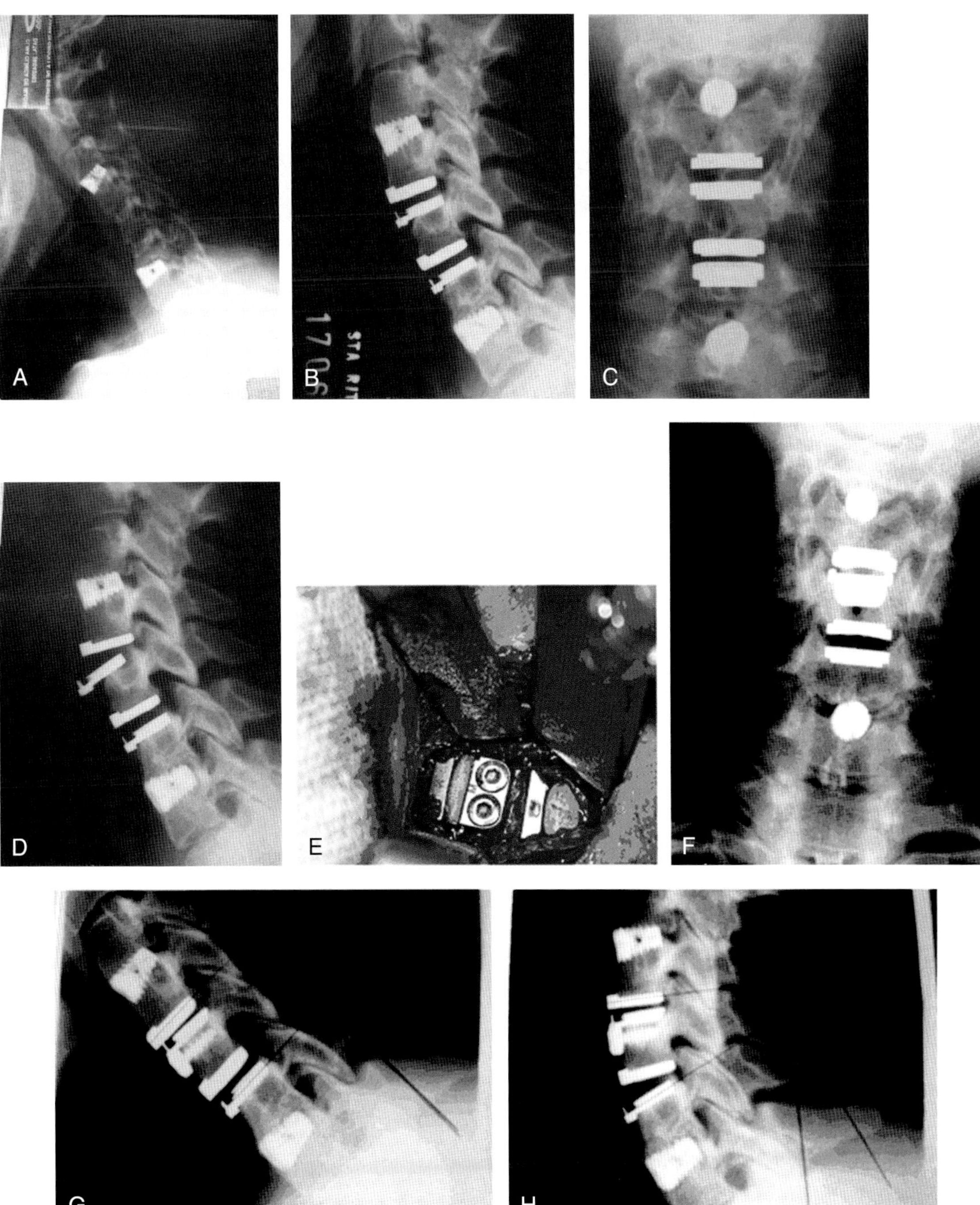

■ **FIGURE 35–4.** PCM requires good bone support for prosthetic end plates. This 39-year-old woman had previously undergone a cervical cage arthrodesis procedure at C3-C4 and C6-C7, highlighting the need for no additional restriction of motion. **A,** Unfortunately, she was locked in a kyphotic position with herniated discs at both intermediate levels. **B,** After PCM replacement and anterior releases at C5-C6 and C4-C5, her bilateral radicular pain resolved and her neck was in a more physiologic position with correction of kyphosis. **C,** The corresponding anteroposterior (AP) view. **D,** Five months postoperatively she had a severe fall that dislodged the caudal component in the C4-C5 interspace. In retrospect, there had not been sufficient bony support under the prosthesis at the superior corner of the C5 vertebral body (see Fig. 35–4B), and there had not been enough porous ingrowth at 5 months to compensate for this inadequate prosthetic anchorage. **E,** The intraoperative view after supplementing the inferior component of the C4-C5 level with two screws and an anterior prosthetic flange. **F,** The AP view after revision. **G,** The patient remains asymptomatic 9 months after reoperation, and she is neurologically intact. This flexion view documents that both prostheses are stable (C4-C5 and C5-C6). **H,** The extension view shows combined 26 degrees of flexion-extension mobility at both prosthetic levels, which was the identical range of motion following the primary disc replacement procedure.

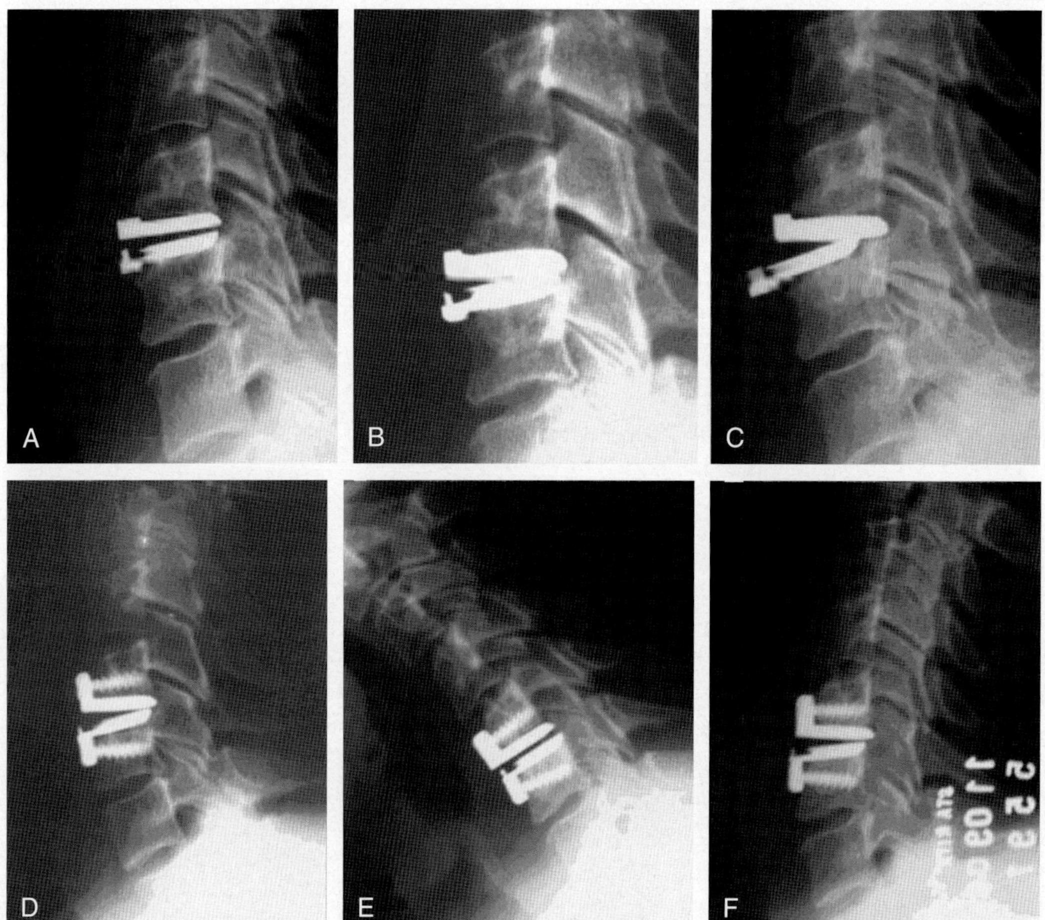


■ FIGURE 35–5. Intraoperative trial range of motion check is advised. This 53-year-old man presented with radiculopathy due to a herniated nucleus pulposis at C5-C6. **A,** A lateral radiograph in the early postoperative period shows a press-fit model Porous-Coated Motion (PCM) device in reasonable position, but the sizing is suboptimal. **B,** One month postoperatively the prosthesis looks too large and is overhanging anteriorly. Usually, the PCM prosthesis has no anterior profile and it can be countersunk entirely within the vertebral bodies. **C,** Three months postoperatively the radiographs disclose anterior device migration. At this point, a revision of the prosthesis is advised despite the fact that the patient was neurologically intact with no signs or symptoms of this complication. **D,** The patient was successfully revised with a more constrained version of the PCM prosthesis, a so-called fixed-flanged PCM anchored with screws. **E** and **F,** Flexion-extension x-rays at 6 months postoperatively documented good movement of the prosthesis following successful revision. All four out of 193 PCM prostheses that required reoperation in this series were successfully revised with motion-preserving procedures and none have required conversion to an arthrodesis.

### Alignment and Stability Related

No loss of disc height, hypermobility, or traumatic instability was encountered. The mean range of motion produced by the prosthesis was 8.3 degrees (range 4.1 to 16.5 degrees) in late follow-up. In two patients with preoperative kyphosis, the overall cervical alignment remained kyphotic postoperatively, although to a lesser degree. In the other patients, the kyphosis and sagittal balance were corrected after arthroplasty. There were no cases of prosthesis-induced kyphosis in this study (see Fig. 35–4).

### Movement Related

No iatrogenic neural deterioration occurred. One patient showed heterotopic ossification grade 3, without clinical symptoms. This study demonstrated that nonsteroidal anti-inflammatory agents are not necessary with the PCM prosthesis in order to prevent heterotopic ossification.

## CONCLUSIONS

In this prospective study, we treated patients with degenerative disc disease causing neurologic compression with single and multiple cervical disc replacement. In all the revisions, we were able to successfully implant another motion preservation device. Our preliminary results indicate that cervical arthroplasty with the PCM artificial disc provides favorable clinical and radiographic outcomes in a 2-year follow-up period. A reoperation rate of 2.05% appears to be an acceptable rate considering the investigative nature of this study. The levels of pathology treated in this pilot study are far more extreme than other reports of cervical arthroplasty—more multilevel implantations, more numerous adjacent-level cases, more patients with prior failed fusion procedures, Klippel-Feil syndrome—and the amount of preoperative cervical deformity was much more severe in this pilot study. It is hoped that by narrowing the indications that future PCM implantation series will have an even lower rate of reoperations. Other technical improvements

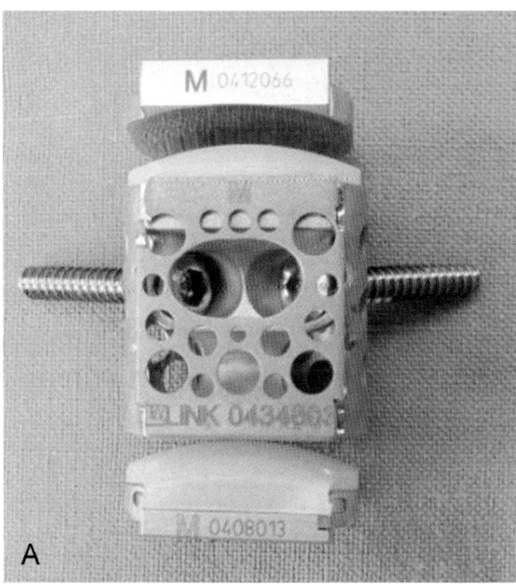


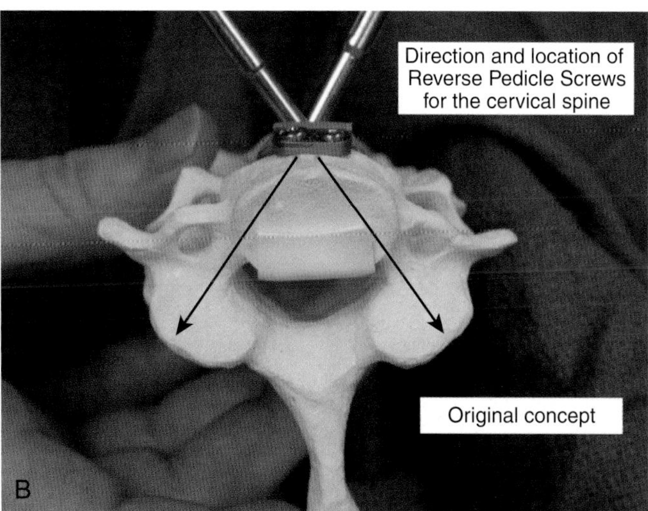


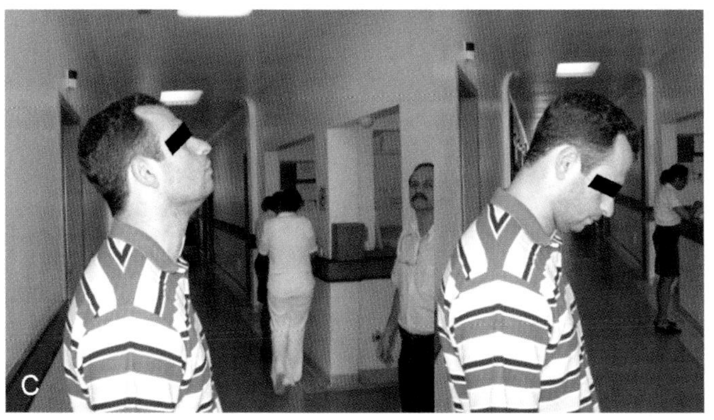


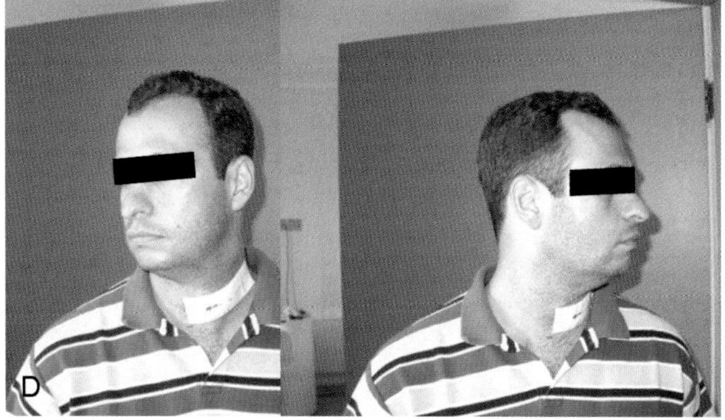


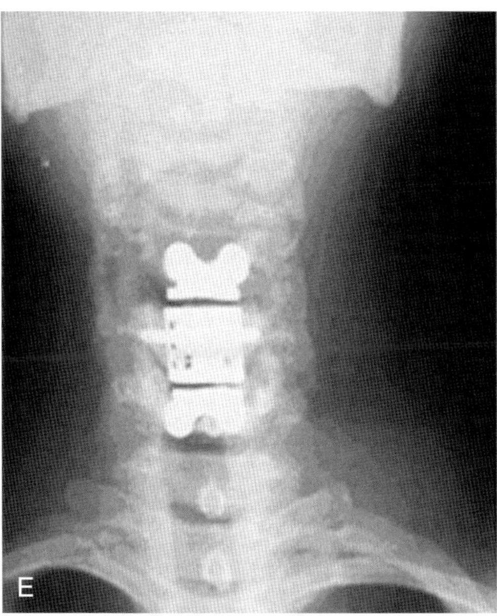


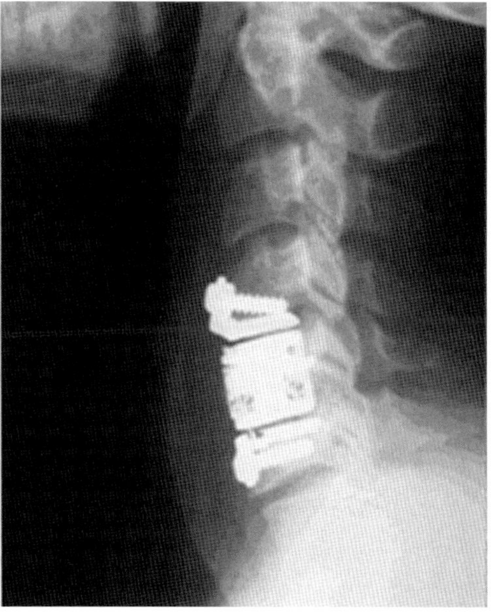

■ **FIGURE 35–6.** Porous-Coated Motion (PCM) corpectomy device with two adjoining cervical disc replacements. **A,** A 28-year-old man patient sustained a HNP at C5-6 and subsequently had avascular necrosis of the C5 vertebral body and required a formal C5 corpectomy with more extensive spinal canal decompression than could be obtained through a routine discectomy approach. The motion-preserving modular corpectomy PCM device was designed to replace the C5 and C6 motion segments. **B,** The immediate fixation of the revision PCM corpectomy device is provided by reverse pedicle screws, which are placed in an anterior-to-posterior direction down the cervical pedicles. Thus far, Luiz Pimenta has implanted three devices in this manner without complication. The screws are inserted under fluoroscopy in an oblique direction so the pedicles are visualized to prevent injury to the vertebral arteries. **C,** The immediate fixation is apparent 1 day postoperatively because the patient had the following flexion and extension clinically. He had already obtained full relief of his radiculopathy and was neurologically intact. **D,** One day following the PCM corpectomy instrumentation, the patient had 80% of normal cervical rotation and side bending. **E,** One year postoperatively, the patient has good restoration of C5 vertebral body height and preserved C4-5 and C5-6 motion. At this stage in follow-up, the bone graft within the vertebral body mesh has fused to the retained portions of the C5 vertebra.

we have adopted as a result of this landmark study are to routinely examine the prosthesis stability throughout the full lateral and side-bending range of motion intraoperatively with C-arm fluoroscopic visualization.

Assessment of the true short- and medium-term complication rates of cervical disc arthroplasty as compared with ACDF fusion will be determined by multi-institutional studies currently under way for U.S. Food and Drug Administration device approval. It is expected that the prospective randomized trials will also uncover a higher incidence of dysphagia, heterotopic bone formation, and a higher pseudathrosis rate occurring with the control groups. In the past, many clinical series have glossed over the problems occurring with translational-type plates, particularly in multilevel disease.

In conclusion, in this preliminary study, the PCM cervical disc replacement appeared to be a safe alternative for cervical reconstruction following spinal cord decompression, and it did not "burn any bridges." It is expected that any of these four revision cases could have been salvaged by a conventional fusion procedure. However, this was not necessary because all cases were successfully revised with a replacement prosthesis, that is, successful prosthesis revision. There is no question that this study proves that revision cervical procedures for failed disc replacement are far easier to perform than revision procedures for failed lumbar disc replacement procedures. The complication rate occurring with cervical disc arthroplasty appears to be acceptable, with a minimal incidence of both conventional and unique complications. Studies evaluating cervical disc arthroplasty must account for both varieties in their data collection efforts.

## REFERENCES


1. Pimenta L, McAfee PC, Capuccino A, et al: Clinical experience with new artificial cervical PCM (Cervitech) disc. Spine 4:315S–321S, 2004.
2. Bryan VE: Cervical motion segment replacement. Eur Spine J 11: S92–S97, 2002.
3. Cunningham BW, Gordon JD, Dmitriev AE, et al: Biomechanical evaluation of total disk arthroplasty: An in-vitro human cadaveric model. Presented at the International Meeting of Advanced Spinal Technologies (IMAST), May 2002, Montreaux, Switzerland.
4. Goffin J, Calenbergh FV, Loon JV, et al: Intermediate follow up after treatment of degenerative disc disease with the Bryan cervical disc prosthesis: Single-level and bi-level. Spine 28:2673–2678, 2003.
5. Hilibrand AS, Carlson GD, Palumbo MA, et al: Radiculopathy and myelopathy at segments adjacent to the site of a previous anterior cervical arthrodesis. J Bone Joint Surg 81A:519–528, 1999.
6. Pickett G, Mitsis D, Sekhon L, et al: Effects of a cervical disc prosthesis on segmental and cervical spine alignment. Neurosurg Focus 17:E5:30–35, 2004.
7. McAfee PC, Cunningham BW, Devine JD, et al: Classification of Heterotopic Ossification (HO) in Artificial Disk Replacement. Proceedings of the 17th Annual Meeting of the North American Spine Society in Montreal, Canada. Spine J 2:94S, 2002.
8. McAfee PC, Cunningham BW, Dmitriev A, et al: Cervical disc replacement-porous coated motion prosthesis: A comparative biomechanical analysis showing the key role of the posterior longitudinal ligament. Spine 28:S167–S185, 2003.
9. McAfee PC, Cunningham BW, Orbegoso CM, et al: Analysis of porous ingrowth in intervertebral disc prostheses: A non-human primate model. Spine 28:332–340, 2003.
10. Bohlman HH, Emery SE, Goodfellow DB, Jones PK: Anterior cervical disectomy and arthrodesis for cervical radiculopathy: Long-term follow-up of one hundred and twenty-two patients. J Bone Joint Surg Am 75:1298–1307, 1993.

CHAPTER 36

# Persistent Pain After Cervical Arthroplasty

Brian J. Sullivan, Gary A. Dix, and Thomas B. Ducker

## KEY POINTS

- A thorough neural decompression is essential for success in cervical arthroplasty. Residual neural compromise may cause symptoms that would not be seen in a successful anterior cervical discectomy and fusion (ACDF).
- The precise role of preoperative sagittal balance in cervical arthroplasty has yet to be elucidated. Producing or worsening kyphosis with cervical arthroplasty should be avoided.
- The function of the facet joints in persistent pain with cervical arthroplasty is incompletely understood. Avoiding arthroplasty in the face of significant facet arthropathy is advisable.
- Unlike a fusion, a functioning arthroplasty will never reach a steady state. Continued follow-up is desirable to monitor for device migration or failure and for heterotopic ossification.
- Candid long-term follow-up of cervical arthroplasty patients will be necessary to elucidate the causes and to reduce persistent pain following cervical arthroplasty.

## INTRODUCTION

Despite a relatively high rate of clinical success,[1] anterior cervical discectomy and fusion (ACDF) does have well-documented limitations and complications.[2] With promises of improved long-term clinical outcomes, cervical spine arthroplasty has seen a fairly recent surge in activity, because extensive research, a plethora of newly developed products, and multiple investigational trials have been devoted to this topic.[3,4] Proponents of cervical arthroplasty point to the biomechanical,[5,6] radiographic,[4,7] and clinical[8] data indicating that fusion may accelerate degeneration at immediately adjacent levels and beyond. The expectation is that cervical arthroplasty will provide enough mobility at the operated level to preserve and protect adjacent levels. Available data confirm encouraging clinical results; however, the fully realized protective effects of arthroplasty will require much longer term follow-up.

With the introduction of cervical arthroplasty, there will be unique causes for persistent pain following surgery. This chapter identifies some of these causes that have emerged in this relatively new field.

## CAUSES

### Inadequate Decompression

If an inadequate decompression of the neural elements is followed by a segmental fusion, the immobilization may provide a protective effect, with relief of symptoms. If foraminal osteophytes are incompletely resected, for example, immobilizing that disc space may produce relief of nerve root irritation, and possibly even resorption of the offending bone.

This is not the case for cervical arthroplasty. Many of the early pioneers stressed the importance of a very thorough, complete neural decompression (personal communication, Dr. Vincent Bryan, 1999). The mobility of the arthroplasty segment could, potentially, allow the nerve root to be drawn across incompletely resected disc or osteophyte material, resulting in symptoms.

Meticulous attention to detail of the decompression intraoperatively should be observed. In addition, a high index of suspicion should be maintained postoperatively for even relatively minor residual neural compression in the face of clinical symptoms.

### Kyphotic Deformity

Loss of preoperative cervical lordosis or worsening of preoperative kyphosis has been reported in up to 49% of patients treated with cervical arthroplasty.[9] The immediate and longer term clinical implications of this loss of sagittal balance have yet to be elucidated. There is concern that this phenomenon may affect the biomechanical function of not only the arthroplasty implant but the remaining levels of the cervical spine as well (Fig. 36–1).

Loss of sagittal balance could lead to abnormal stress on the facet joints, ligaments, and paraspinal musculature, resulting in axial cervical spine discomfort.[10] A more frank kyphotic deformity could result in post-arthroplasty radicular, even myelopathic, symptoms (Figs. 36–2 and 36–3).

Judicious preoperative planning with careful consideration of the sagittal balance needs to be conducted by the surgeon. Unlike ACDF procedures in which the use of a lordotic interbody graft can help restore more normal cervical lordosis, it is unclear whether

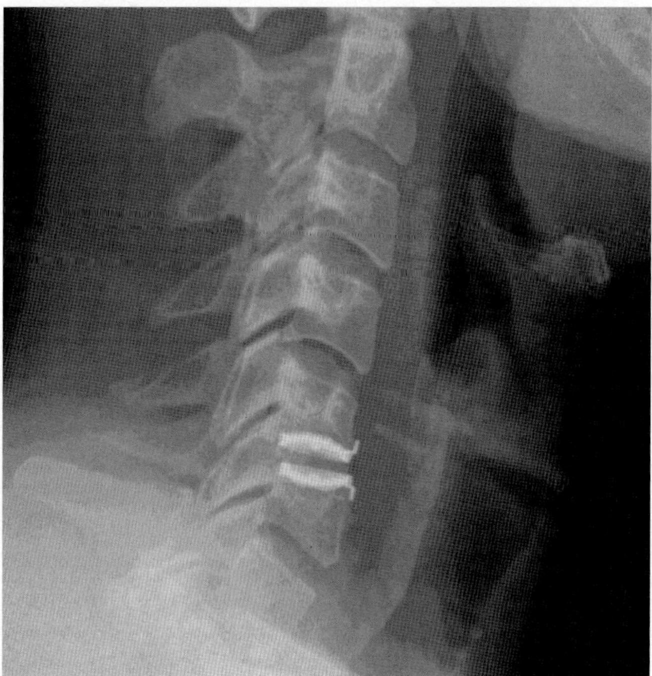

■ **FIGURE 36–1.** Immediate postoperative x-ray study of C5-C6 Bryan cervical disc arthroplasty. Note the early kyphosis.

the current generation of arthroplasty devices will improve, maintain, or worsen preoperative sagittal balance. Intraoperative sizing of the implant is believed to be a crucial step. In several early cases, undersizing of the implant was considered to be responsible for most of the postoperative kyphotic deformity.[9]

## Facet Disease

As is seen in ACDF,[1,2] persistent axial cervical spine discomfort has been reported following cervical arthroplasty. Pickett et al[9] reported that 25% of 74 patients treated with the Bryan cervical prosthesis complained of "varying degrees of neck pain." The Prestige ST cervical disc replacement ultimately showed improvement in the Neck Disability Index superior to that found with fusion at 12 and 24 months.[4] However, it should be noted that, in data submitted to the U.S. Food and Drug Administration (FDA) for the Prestige disc, 138 patients (50% of patients receiving the device) reported new or persisting neck, shoulder, or arm pain in various combinations at sometime during the follow-up period.[11] Notably, 47.9% of the fusion control patients reported similar complaints in this same study.[11]

Theoretically, a successful fusion will stop motion around painful facet joints at the treated level. A total disc replacement, on the other hand, will increase activity in these joints and potentially worsen pre-existing facet disease. Another concern is that "unbalancing" the facet joints intraoperatively with either overdistraction and insertion of an oversized prosthesis or undersizing and the introduction of kyphosis may lead to persistent axial pain.

The surgeon would do well to evaluate for facet disease from both a clinical and radiographic perspective preoperatively at the index level as well as adjacent levels. Intraoperatively, attempting to match the disc space height of the nearest healthy disc may be the best guideline until a better understanding of this issue evolves.

## Device Failure

Fortunately, the incidences of device failure and migration have been very low in the literature covering both cervical and lumbar arthroplasty.[9,12,13] No significant literature exists for device complications

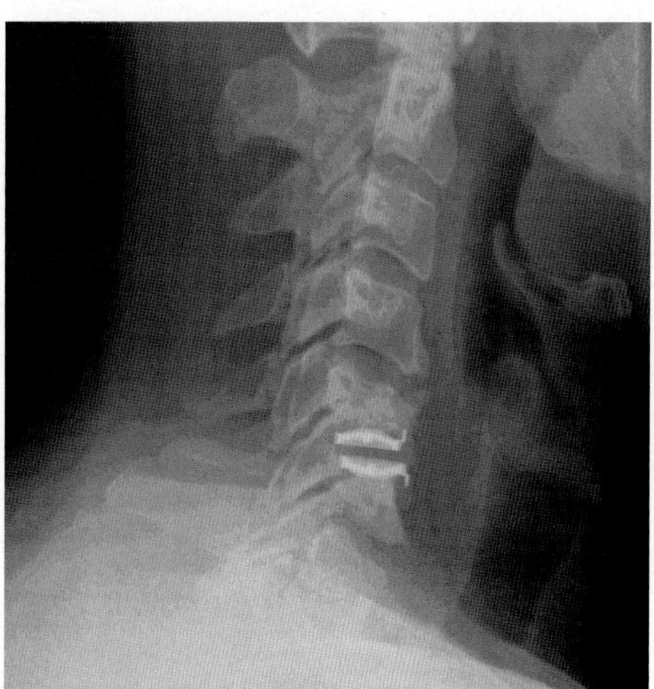

■ **FIGURE 36–2.** Two-year follow-up x-ray study same patient as Figure 36–1. Progression of kyphosis. Patient is asymptomatic and rates his clinical outcome as "excellent."

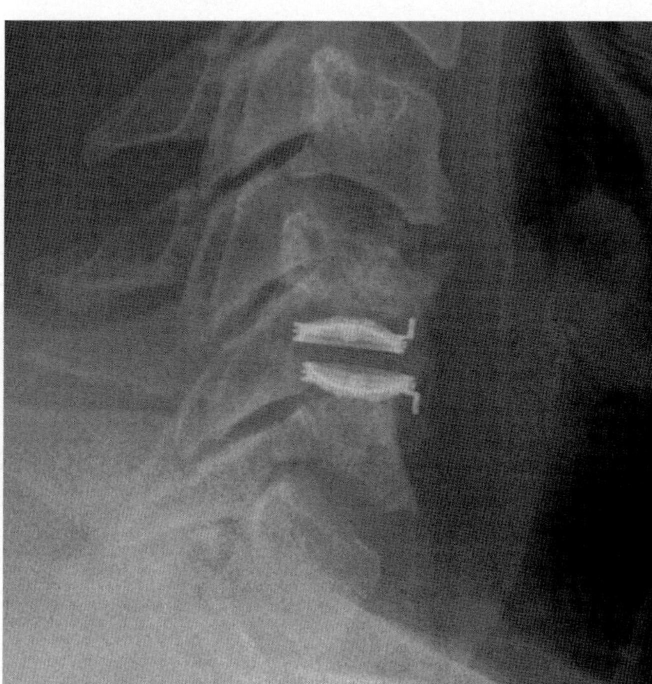

■ **FIGURE 36–3.** Close-up of C5-6 level reveals heterotopic ossification, pronounced adjacent-level disease, and sclerotic changes in C5 and C6 vertebral bodies.

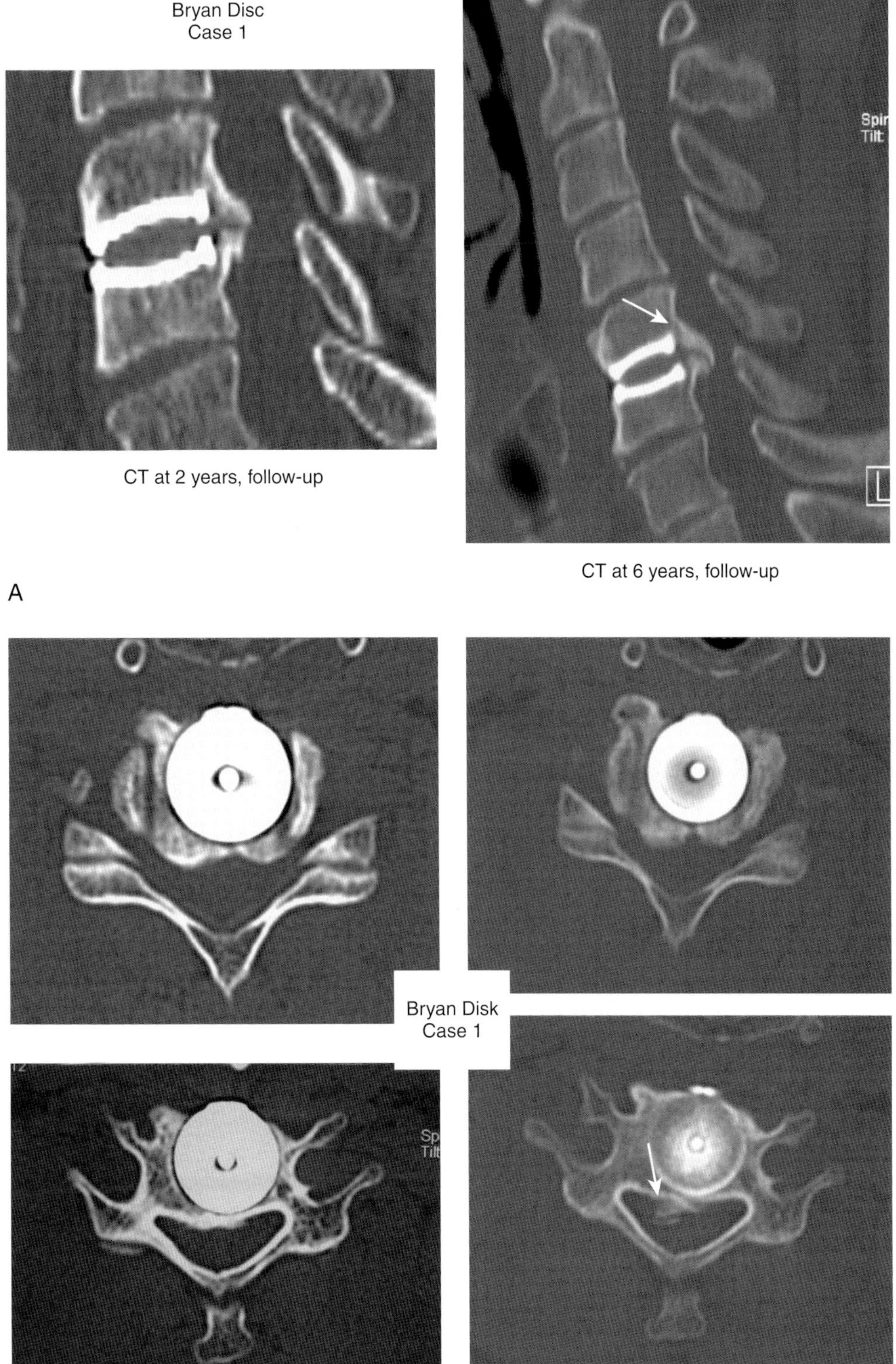


■ **FIGURE 36–4.** Shown are two cases of Bryan disc with 4 to 6 years' follow-up with recurrent pain and myelopathy due to extensive reformation of osteophytes within the spinal canal. The incidence of heterotopic bone formation associated with the Bryan arthroplasty is reported to be as high as 30%. Owing to the reaming and preparation of the vertebral end plates in order to retard the formation of heterotopic ossification, nonsteroidal anti-inflammatory agents are recommended with this prosthesis.

causing persistent pain. The reports of device migration[9,13] and a single report of device failure[9] have been apparently asymptomatic. The one group reporting a case of device failure noted excessive range of motion at the index level on preoperative studies.[9]

Device migration and device failure need to be carefully considered as causes of postoperative pain. Unlike a fusion, routine radiographic follow-up will need to be continued indefinitely, because a functioning prosthesis will never reach a steady state.

## Heterotopic Ossification

Heterotopic ossification (HO) is a well-documented phenomenon in total hip replacement; however, the incidence in vertebral arthroplasty is unclear. HO has been identified in 4% of cases implanted with a lumbar artificial disc, without significant effect on clinical outcomes.[13] In cervical disc arthroplasty, this may be more prevalent, with a recent study of 77 operated levels (in 54 patients) quoting an incidence of 66% for asymptomatic peridiscal HO (Figs. 36–3 and 36–4). In 10% of these cases, spontaneous fusion occurred by 1 year, without an increase in postoperative morbidity compared with published cervical disc arthroplasty data.[14] A recent case is described of persistent pain following artificial disc implantation, with subsequent radiographic HO proceeding to spontaneous fusion at the surgical level, which is thought to reproduce the symptoms for which the original operation was performed.[15] Therefore, it is possible that a higher incidence of persistent postoperative pain will result from the development of HO that may present following cervical arthroplasty.

## Other or Underappreciated Diagnoses

Classically described patterns of pain, weakness, and sensory change are used as guidelines for the diagnosis of cervical radiculopathy. The diagnostic picture may be complicated by overlapping distributions of nerve roots, anatomic variability, multilevel disease, and comorbid conditions. The latter may include amyotrophic lateral sclerosis, spinal cord pathology (such as syringomyelia and central cord syndrome), peripheral nerve entrapment syndromes

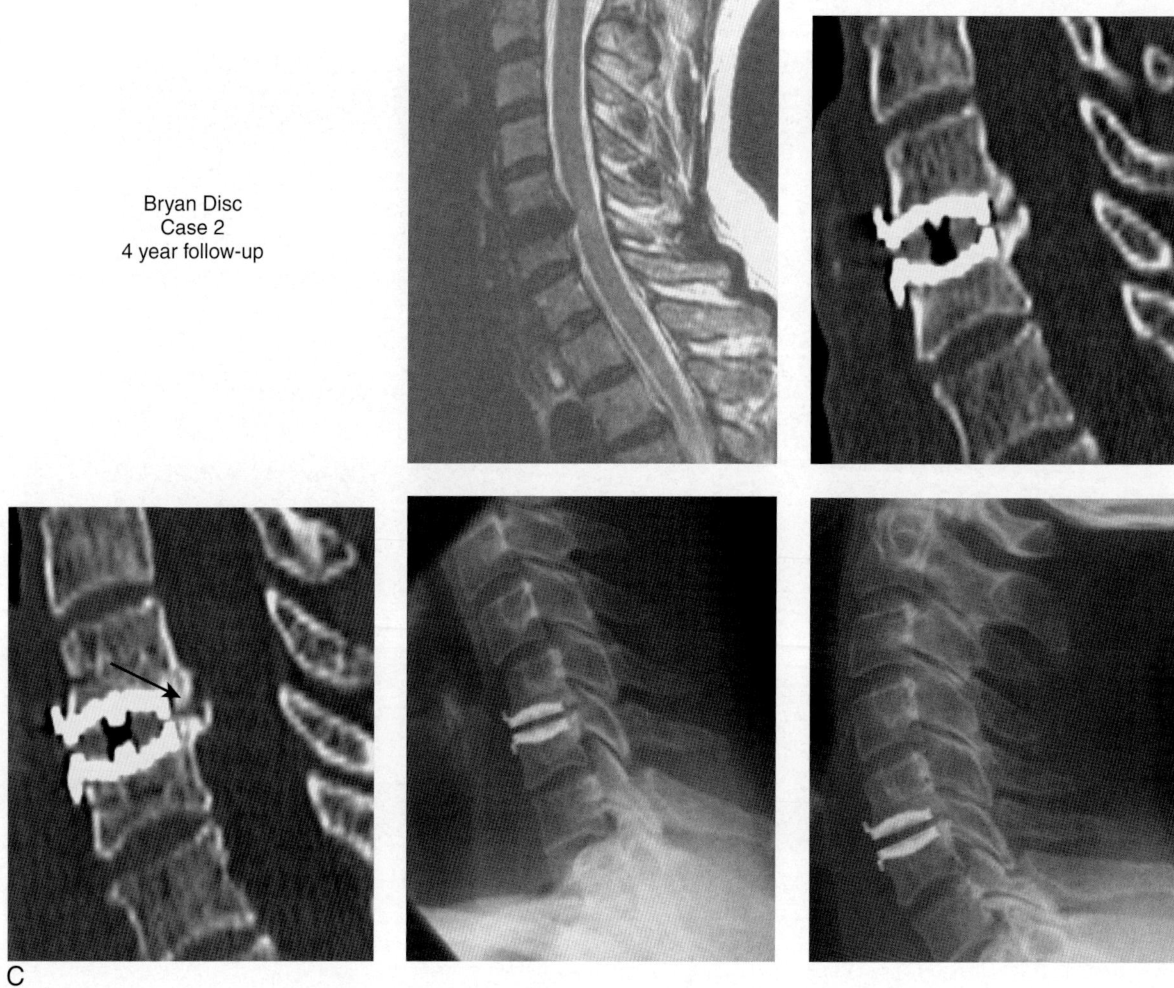


■ FIGURE 36–4. Cont'd.

(including carpal tunnel syndrome and ulnar neuropathy), brachial plexus injury or neuritis, thoracic outlet syndrome, Pancoast tumor, complex regional pain syndrome, and shoulder issues, such as rotator cuff tear and subacromial bursitis. Exclusion of these conditions is germane to the diagnosis of cervical radiculitis or radiculopathy, and further clinical evaluation with appropriate diagnostic tests should be considered, where applicable, for persistent pain following disc arthroplasty.

## CONCLUSION

This chapter lists six of the most likely causes for persistent pain following cervical disc arthroplasty. Of these, inadequate neural decompression and kyphotic deformity will likely account for a majority of the problems. However, a missed or inaccurate diagnosis along with device failure or migration is a major concern (Figs. 36–5 to 36–7).

Calcification around cervical arthroplasty devices may be a curse or a blessing. HO around a movable, functioning arthroplasty is undesirable. Once it is fused with no motion, however, one now has an ACDF with its associated benefits and difficulties.

Only candid, long-term follow-up will provide the data needed to make the necessary changes in patient selection, device design, and surgical technique that will reduce persistent pain following cervical arthroplasty.

DYSPHAGIA

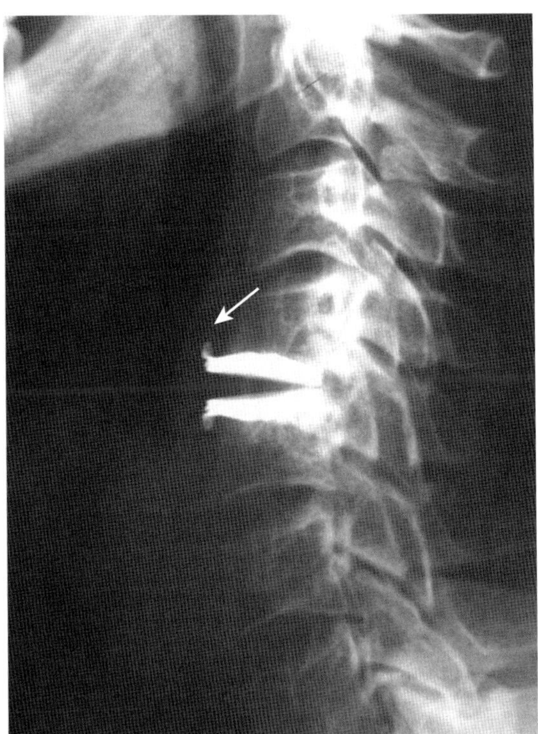

■ **FIGURE 36–5.** Care must be taken to recess the Bryan disc properly owing to the holding clips on the front of the prosthesis. This prosthesis had to be removed and converted to an arthrodesis owing to persistent postoperative dysphagia, reported as high as 20% at 2 years postoperatively.

PROSTHESIS MIGRATION

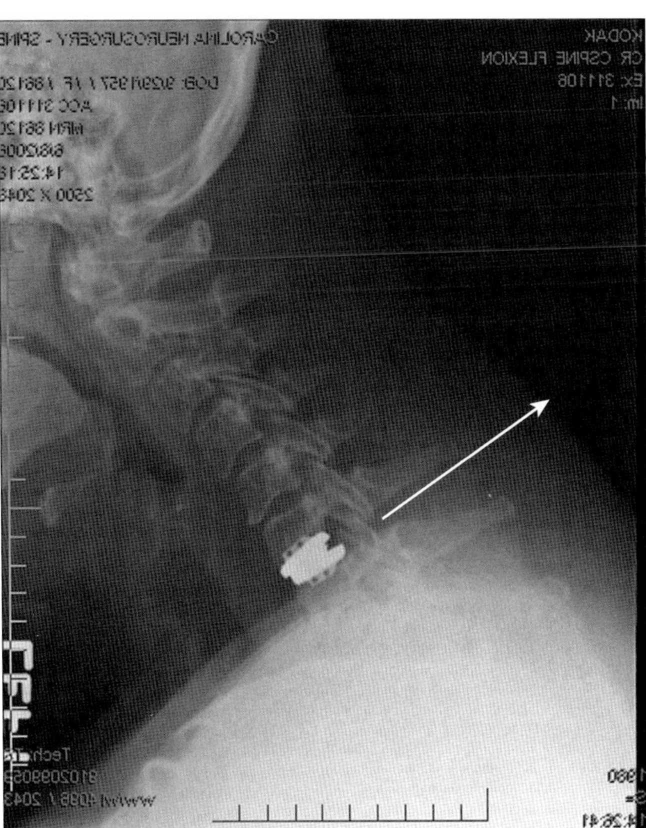

■ **FIGURE 36–6.** Implant posterior migration into the spinal canal can be not only a source of postoperative pain but postoperative neurologic deficit as well. Even a keeled prosthesis can migrate posteriorly if it is not ingrown in the first 8 postoperative weeks.

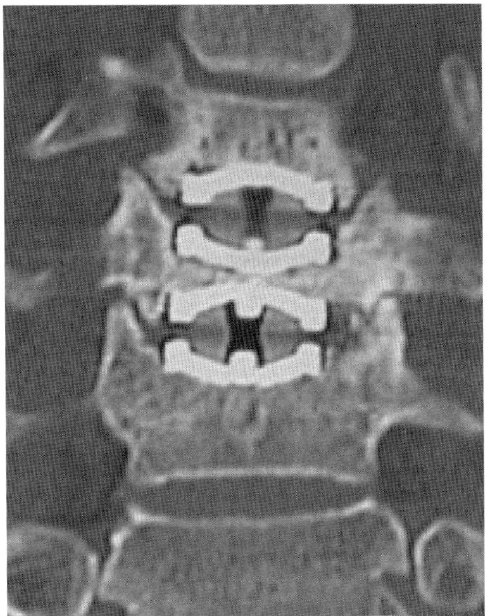

■ **FIGURE 36–7.** Overly vigorous reaming with the Bryan disc can cause an unstable pattern of loss of bone stock and avascular necrosis of the vertebral body in patients with small stature. The Bryan disc comes only in one height and requires removal of the bony end plates in order to achieve fixation. This can result in near-touching of two adjacent Bryan disc arthroplasties.

## REFERENCES


1. Goffin J, Geusens E, Vantomme N, et al: Long-term follow-up after interbody fusion of the cervical spine. J Spinal Disord Tech 17:79–85, 2004.
2. Taylor BA, Vaccaro AR, Albert TJ: Complications of anterior and posterior cervical approaches in the treatment of cervical degenerative disc disease. Semin Spine Surg 11:337–346, 1999.
3. Goffin J, Van Calenbergh F, van Loon J, et al: Intermediate follow up after treatment of degenerative disc disease with the Bryan Cervical Disc Prosthesis: Single-level and bi-level. Spine 28:2673–2678, 2003.
4. Mummaneni PV, Burkus JK, Haid RW, et al: Clinical and radiographic analysis of cervical disc arthroplasty compared with allograft fusion: A randomized controlled clinical trial. J Neurosurg Spine 6:198–209, 2007.
5. Eck JC, Humphreys SC, Lim TH, et al: Biomechanical study on the effect of cervical spine fusion on adjacent-level intradiscal pressure and segmental motion. Spine 27:2431–2434, 2002.
6. Galbusera MT, Raimondi M, Sassi M, et al: Biomechanics of the cervical spine after fusion and arthroplasty. J Biomech 39(3):418–425, 2006.
7. Kulkarni V, Rajshekhar V, Raghuram L: Accelerated spondylotic changes adjacent to the fused segment following central cervical corpectomy: magnetic resonance imaging study evidence. J Neurosurg 100(1 suppl):2–6, 2004.
8. Hilibrand AS, Carlson GD, Palumbo M, et al: Radiculopathy and myelopathy at segments adjacent to the site of a previous anterior cervical arthrodesis. J Bone Joint Surg Am 81:519–528, 1999.
9. Pickett GE, Sekhon LH, Sears WR, Duggal N: Complications with cervical arthroplasty. J Neurosurg Spine 4:98–105, 2006.
10. Katsuura A, Hukuda S, Saruhashi Y, Mori K: Kyphotic malalignment after anterior cervical fusion is one of the factors promoting the degenerative process in adjacent intervertebral levels. Eur Spine J 10:320–324, 2001.
11. Report of United States Clinical Study Results (G010188)—Prestige Cervical Disc System: www.fda.gov/ohrms/dockets/ac/06/briefing/2006-4243b1_02.pdf.htm. Accessed February 13, 2007.
12. Regan JJ, McAfee PC, Blumenthal SL, et al: Evaluation of surgical volume and the early experience with lumbar total disc replacement as part of the investigational device exemption study of the Charite Artificial Disc. Spine 31:2270–2276, 2006.
13. Tortolani PJ, Cunningham BW, Eng M, et al: Prevalence of heterotopic ossification following total disc replacement: A prospective, randomized study of two hundred and seventy-six patients. J Bone Joint Surg Am 89:82–84, 2007.
14. Parkinson JJ, Sekhon LH: Cervical arthroplasty complicated by delayed spontaneous fusion: Case report. J Neurosurg Spine 2:377–380, 2005.
15. Mehren C, Suchomel P, Grochula F, et al: Heterotopic ossification in total cervical disc replacement. Spine 31:2802–2806, 2006.

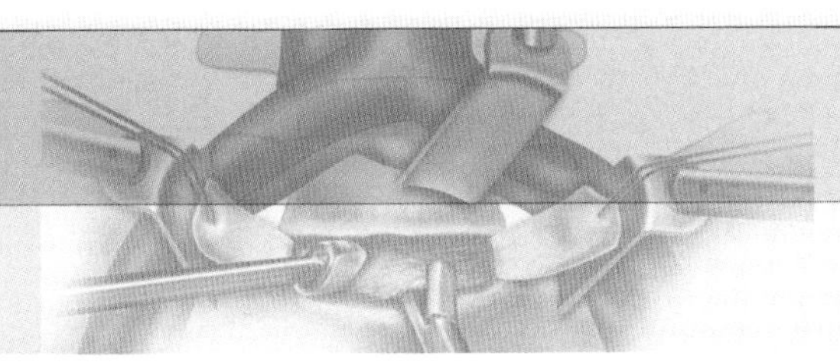

PART

# IV

# Lumbar Total Disc Arthroplasty

CHAPTER 37

# Disc Space Preparation Techniques for Lumbar Disc Arthroplasty

**Jorge Jaramillo** and **James J. Yue**

**KEY POINTS**

- Evaluate disc space before surgery in terms of degree of collapse, surgical level of surgery, and patient-related factors such as bone density and body mass index
- Surgeons unfamiliar with disc replacement surgery and advanced disc mobilization should begin with procedures with a preserved disc height of at least 50%.
- Mobilization of disc space may require careful release of posterior longitudinal ligament.
- Use of the David parallel distractor (Depuy Spine, Inc Raynham, MA USA) with slowly progressive and sequential assisted distraction is a relatively safe and time-efficient method for disc space mobilization.

## DISC SPACE PREPARATION TECHNIQUES FOR LUMBAR DISC ARTHROPLASTY

### Introduction: Preoperative Considerations

Proper disc space preparation and mobilization are essential for successful lumbar disc arthroplasty.[1–7] Whether the surgeon is implanting a total disc or nucleus device, distraction and mobilization are essential steps that must always be achieved to allow for proper functioning of a given device. If these critical steps cannot be achieved, other surgical options should be considered. The surgeon should appreciate that a given device does not produce motion in a given spinal segment. A device only maintains mobility that the surgeon has reintroduced.

Disc space preparation begins before the actual surgical procedure has been surgically initiated. The physical characteristics of the patient, such body mass index, history of prior abdominal surgeries or gynecological disease, and bone mineral density, should be carefully assessed. For example, a patient with a history of osteopenia and complete disc height collapse may not be an ideal candidate for an arthroplasty procedure. Anomalous segmentation should also be noted given the often varied vascular anatomy that can accompany these anomalies. Finally, the surgeon should assess end plate morphology for evidence of posterior end plate hooking (type II), central depressions (type III), anterior lipping (type IV), or combinations (type V) of these end plate types, which may influence the length of the surgical procedure and choice of implant type (keeled versus spiked) (Fig 37–1).

### Initial Perioperative Preparation

All patients should receive perioperative antibiotics, and a Foley catheter should be placed. Before prepping and draping, both an anteroposterior (AP) and a lateral fluoroscopic image should be obtained. The AP view should be obtained with the fluoroscopic C-arm at the zero-degree position such that the spinous process is midline and equidistant from each pedicle. If the pedicles are not equidistant, the patient's buttocks should be appropriately elevated to create a true AP view of the spine with the C-arm in a neutral position. Next, the C-arm is placed into the lateral position and appropriate skin markings are made anteriorly over the affected disc space. If appropriate imaging cannot be obtained, the surgeon is advised not to continue with the surgical procedure. Pulse oximetry may also be used to assess vascular status. In cases in which there is significant disc space narrowing, the surgeon may wish to place the affected level over the arch section of the surgical table to assist in gaining access to the intervertebral space. Anterior access can be assisted by flexing the table (lowering the foot of the bed) (Fig. 37–2). After anterior access to the intervertebral space and partial distraction have been achieved, the arch of the bed can be returned to a neutral position and the posterior disc space can be accessed.

### Disc Space Exposure

After an appropriate anterior retroperitoneal or transperitoneal approach to the lumbar spine has been achieved and once the disc space is exposed, the disc space should be reconfirmed on AP and lateral fluoroscopic images. It is crucial that the disc space be adequately exposed both medially and laterally as well as superiorly and inferiorly. Soft tissue structures should be protected with lap pads and self-retaining retractors preferably stabilized to a fixed

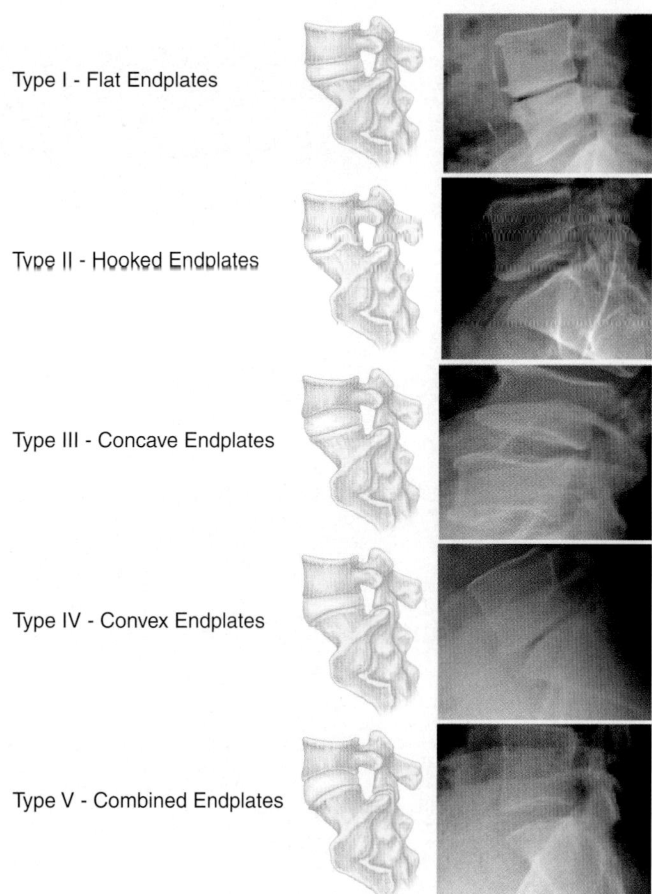


■ **FIGURE 37–1.** Vertebral End Plate Yue-Bertagnoli (VEYBR) Classification.

retractor ring. After disc space exposure, the midline of the vertebral body is identified on a true AP view. The midline is then marked in the adjacent vertebral bodies with the monopolar electrocautery, with a chisel, or with the placement of a cancellous self-drilling screw-pin in the superior vertebral body, about 5 mm above the anterior lip to avoid damage to the end plate (Fig. 37–3). This must be done immediately after the surgical approach, before the discectomy.

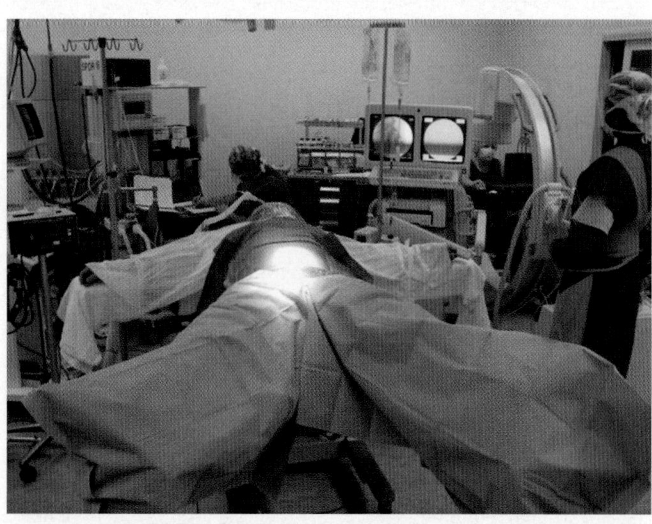

■ **FIGURE 37–2.** Patient positioning.

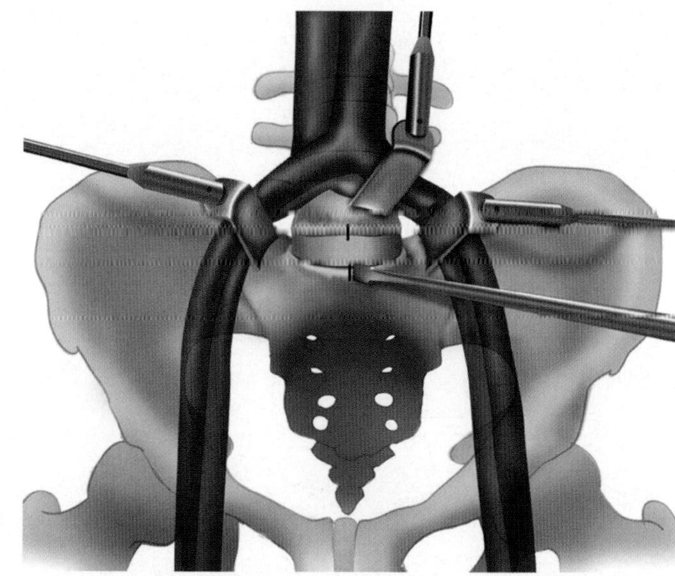

■ **FIGURE 37–3.** Midline marking.

## Discectomy

A complete discectomy is critical for adequate prosthesis implantation. This part of the procedure starts with an anterior annulectomy or anterior annulotomy if desired. The anterior annulectomy is performed with a 15-blade scalpel or with monopolar electrocautery at the junction of the annulus and end plate. In men, monopolar electrocautery should be avoided as much as possible to decrease the incidence of retrograde ejaculation. If an anterior annulotomy is preferred, an H-type incision is made using a midline incision to open the anterior annulus and then the blade is turned sideways to incise the superior and inferior annular attachments bilaterally as far as the width of the vertebral body. An annular open book flap is created on both sides (Fig. 37–4).

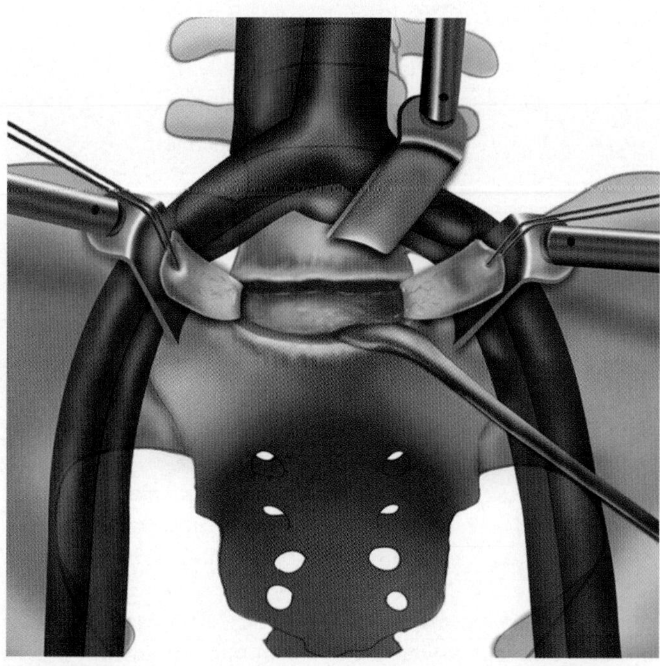

■ **FIGURE 37–4.** Retracted annulus and cartilaginous end plate elevation.

The flaps may be used to protect the eccentric vessels holding both ends of the flaps in position with a suture and taken outside the wound secured with hemostats. At the completion of the implantation, the anterior annular flaps may be closed using a number one absorbable suture, even though this has not shown any biomechanical advantage.

After annulotomy, the cartilaginous end plate is elevated away from the bony end plates using an end plate elevator. It is important not to disrupt the subchondral bone to prevent subsidence of the implant. Next, the remaining disc is removed using curettes (standard and ring), pituitaries, and Kerrison rongeurs. The disc is progressively removed from anterior to posterior. In addition, the discectomy is enlarged laterally to expose the vertebral body circumferential rim of cortical bone, leaving the lateral aspect of the annulus intact.

## Remobilization/Disc Space Distraction

As the disc is removed, sequential and progressive distraction is performed using an intervertebral distractor. To make visualization easier in the posterior compartment, it is possible to place a self-retaining bullet into the contralateral side of the interspace (Fig. 37–5). The last portion of the mobilization is removal of the posterior annulus and posterior longitudinal ligament (PLL). The posterior decompression is reserved for last owing to the possibility of epidural bleeding that can occur after removal of the posterior annulus and PLL. Although the posterior annulus should be opened to free the disc space and to allow good restoration of the disc height, it is not always necessary to excise the posterior longitudinal ligament. If additional mobilization is necessary or a nonmigrated extruded disc fragment must be excised, the PLL will need to be removed. Removal of the PLL can be performed in three steps. First, a small upward curved curette is placed behind the posterior border of the vertebral body first superiorly and then inferiorly (Fig. 37–6). This will isolate the PLL into a small ribbon. Next an appropriately sized Kerrison is placed behind the PLL and it is excised from one side to the other (Video #1). Note that epidural bleeding can occur during this phase. If bleeding does occur, a small amount of Floseal or Gelfoam usually adequately controls this bleeding. The goal of mobilization is to be able to distract the interspace with two-finger force using an intervertebral distractor (Fig. 37–7).

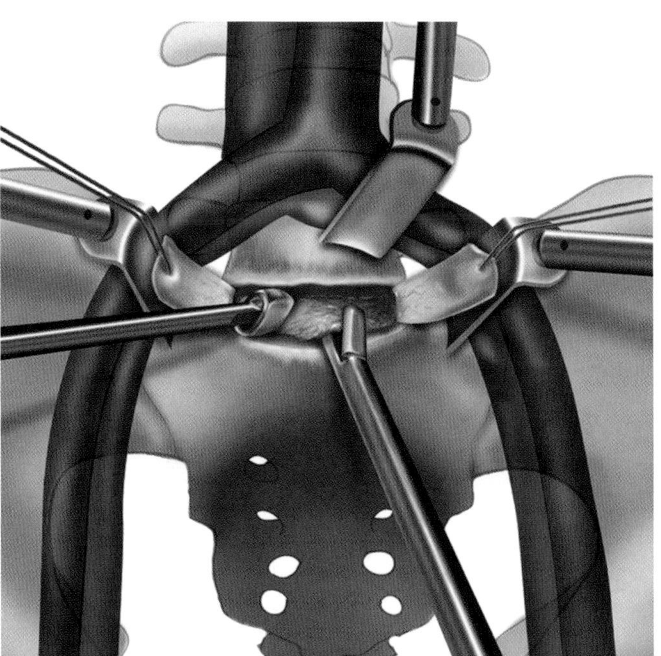

**FIGURE 37–5.** Bullet type distractor to hold open interspace with removable insertor handle during posterior decompression.

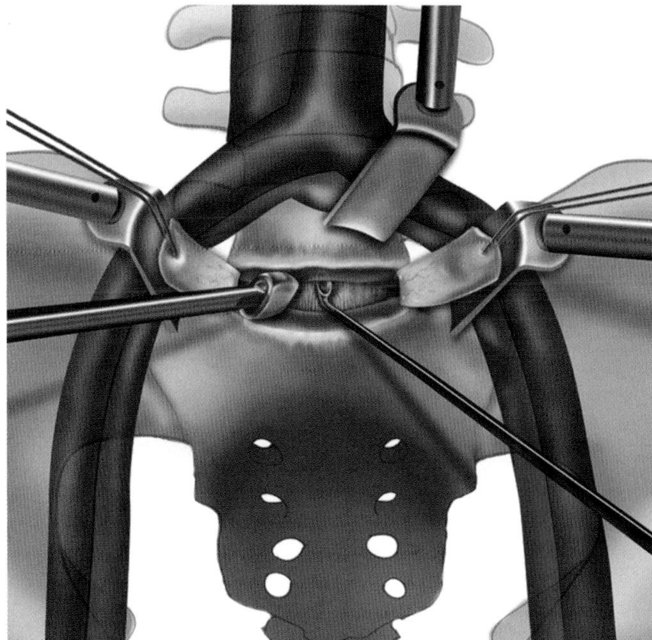

**FIGURE 37–6.** Releasing posterior longitudinal ligament with curved curette.

In certain cases, for instance, at a hyperlordotic L5/S1, failure to release the PLL when the posterior part of the disc space is vertically collapsed may result in a "fish-mouth" disc space with ample anterior distraction and inadequate posterior distraction. This makes posterior placement of the prosthesis difficult and increases the possibility of posterior end plate fracture during the insertion.

In cases of significant disc height loss in which routine mobilization does not produce a satisfactory degree of remobilization, the David parallel distractor (Depuy Spine, Inc, Raynham, MA, USA) (Fig. 37–8) can be a very useful additional tool. The device has two end plate sizes, #2 and #4. The largest end plate size that can fit into the interspace should be used. Next, concurrent sequential and progressive distraction is applied by inserting a bulled between the end plates and simultaneously squeezing the distractor. If remobilization does not occur after placing the 8- or 9-mm bullet, mobilization of the interspace will most likely not occur and distraction should be abandoned and a fusion should be performed. Posterior distraction should not exceed the normal posterior disc height of the levels above. Once the disc space has been distracted, the remaining disc material that may be contained within the buckled ligament is removed using a Kerrison or an intervertebral disc rongeur. The lateral annulus should be left intact in all cases.

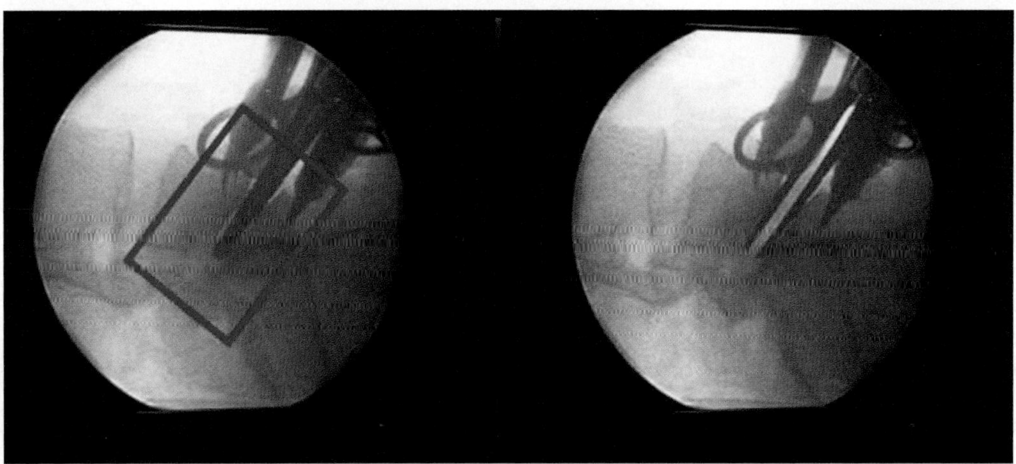

■ FIGURE 37–7. Disc space mobilization.

## End Plate Preparation

It is important to preserve the integrity of the subchondral osseous end plates, especially when the preoperative MRI shows Schmorl's nodes or other changes in the vertebral end plates. If the end plates are excessively concave, a burr or curettes may be used to flatten any irregularities of the end plates slightly, preserving as much of the osseous end plates as possible. Care must be taken not to damage the cortical end plate of the vertebral body to provide a firm base for mechanical stability after the implantation of the prosthesis and to reduce the potential for subsidence.

## CONCLUSION

Appropriate patient selection and meticulous surgical technique are paramount factors to enhance clinical and surgical outcomes.[8,9]

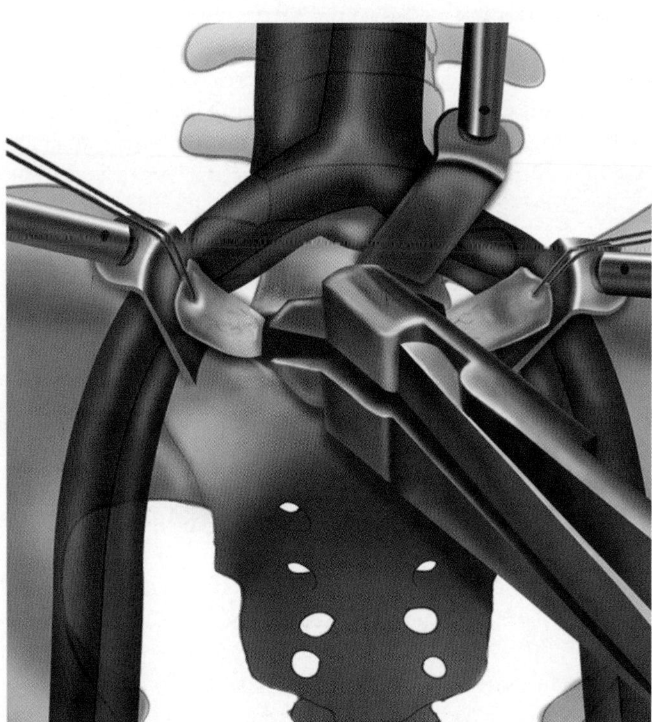

■ FIGURE 37–8. Distraction with a David distractor.

Disc preparation starts before beginning the surgical procedure. Preoperatively, the disc space should be assessed for degree of disc space collapse at the affected level and for the size of adjacent level normal discs to assess the likelihood of remobilization. Physical characteristics of the patient and surgical and gynecologic history should be obtained. Intraoperatively, the disc space must be cleared of all disc material and sequential progressive distraction should be performed. Attention to preserving subchondral bone is mandatory. Removal of the PLL should be performed if additional distraction is needed, if a disc fragment needs to be excised from the canal, or if there is a hyperlordotic or "fish-mouth" interspace. The lateral annulus should be preserved in all cases. In cases of difficult distraction, the surgeon may consider careful usage of the David distractor.

## REFERENCES


1. Aryan HE, Acosta FL Jr, Ames CP: The Charite Artificial Disc: insertion technique. Neurosurg Clin N Am 16:637–650, 2005.
2. Aryan HE, Acosta FL Jr, Ames CP: The ProDisc artificial disc: insertion technique. Neurosurg Clin N Am 16:651–656, 2005.
3. Bertagnoli R, Yue JJ, Shah RV, et al: The treatment of disabling multilevel lumbar discogenic low back pain with total disc arthroplasty utilizing the ProDisc prosthesis: a prospective study with 2-year minimum follow-up. Spine 30:2192–2199, 2005.
4. Bertagnoli R, Yue JJ, Shah RV, et al: The treatment of disabling single-level lumbar discogenic low back pain with total disc arthroplasty utilizing the Prodisc prosthesis: a prospective study with 2-year minimum follow-up. Spine 30:2230–2236, 2005.
5. Delamarter RB, Bae HW, Pradhan BB: Clinical results of ProDisc-II lumbar total disc replacement: report from the United States clinical trial. Orthop Clin North Am 36:301–313, 2005.
6. Delamarter RB, Fribourg DM, Kanim LE, et al: ProDisc artificial total lumbar disc replacement: introduction and early results from the United States clinical trial. Spine 28:S167–S175, 2003.
7. Geisler FH: Surgical technique of lumbar artificial disc replacement with the Charite Artificial Disc. Neurosurgery 56(Suppl 1):46–57, 2005.
8. Geisler FH, Blumenthal SL, Guyer RD, et al: Neurological complications of lumbar artificial disc replacement and comparison of clinical results with those related to lumbar arthrodesis in the literature: results of a multicenter, prospective, randomized investigational device exemption study of Charite intervertebral disc. J Neurosurg Spine 1:143–154, 2004.
9. Tropiano P, Huang RC, Girardi FP, et al: Lumbar total disc replacement. Surgical technique. J Bone Joint Surg Am 88(Suppl 1):50–64, 2006.

CHAPTER 38

# CHARITÉ Artificial Disc

**Scott L. Blumenthal** and **Donna D. Ohnmeiss**

## KEY POINTS

- The CHARITÉ Artificial Disc was the first total disc replacement used on a widespread basis, with the first disc implanted in 1984.
- There are favorable long-term follow-up data from Europe supporting the safety of the device as well as the clinical outcome.
- Results of the randomized study regulated by the U.S. Food and Drug Administration (FDA) demonstrated that the safety and effectiveness of the CHARITÉ was as good as, or better than, fusion in the treatment of disc-related pain.
- The implant preserves motion at the operated segment, even in long-term studies.
- Adherence to appropriate selection criteria is key for favorable results.

## INTRODUCTION

The concept for the CHARITÉ disc was developed by Karin Büttner-Janz and Kurt Schellnack working together in the Charité Hospital in Berlin, Germany, in the early to mid 1980s. They carefully analyzed the mechanics of the human disc and tried to design a device incorporating those properties. Motion was allowed through articulation between concave and convex surfaces. The core was also allowed to slide to mimic the anteroposterior (AP) movement of the disc nucleus during flexion and extension. The design incorporated two metallic plates with small anchoring teeth around the edges. There was a biconvex polyethylene core between the metal round plates. This device was subjected to extensive mechanical testing. The first of these total disc replacements was performed in 1984 and was implanted in 13 patients.[1] It was noted that the device sometimes subsided into the vertebral bodies. To address the potential problem of subsidence, the second generation of the implant incorporated "wings" on the plates to increase the load-bearing interface area with the vertebral bodies. This design was promising, and the device implanted into 36 patients. However, there were fractures on the endplates where the wings attached to the circular metal core. Helmut Link was involved with the design of the third and current disc. This design uses oval plates with a circular center. The only design modification since this 1987 model has been the inclusion of a bioactive coating on the surfaces of the endplates to encourage bony ingrowth and help prevent the potential for displacement. The recommended sterilization process for the polyethylene core was changed because the original may have been associated with increased wear of the device. There have been modifications to the insertion instrumentation and an increase in the number of options in the size of the prostheses and obliquity of the endplates. When reviewing the mechanics and clinical outcomes of total disc replacement (TDR) using the CHARITÉ (DePuy Spine Inc., Raynham, MA), it is very important to keep in mind the various designs. Results of the first two generations of the device have little bearing on evaluating the outcomes of the current design.

## INDICATIONS AND CONTRAINDICATIONS

The indications and contraindications for the CHARITÉ have been developed based on biomechanical principles, the design of the device, and clinical experience. The goal of patient selection is to avoid complications and maximize outcome. The primary indication for TDR is painful disc degeneration or disruption. The symptoms should have persisted for at least 6 months, and the patient should have participated in an active rehabilitation program. Diagnostic work-up should include thorough clinical examination, magnetic resonance imaging, and in most cases, discography.

Contraindications include items that may compromise the safety or integrity of the implant. The patient should not have vertebral factures at the implant levels. Patients with osteoporosis should not have TDR. The thinning bone may lead to fracture of the vertebrae or subsidence of the implant into the bone. Another contraindication is significant facet joint changes. This may compromise function of the motion segment, including the implant. Also, abnormal facets may be a source of symptoms not addressed by the artificial disc. This may lead to compromised results if the discogenic pain is addressed by the CHARITÉ, but the facet pain persists. If the facets are questionable but not to the point of possibly compromising device function, one may want to consider preoperative facet joint injections to rule out the facet as a pain generator. With respect to the facet joint, Büttner-Janz stated that the main item of interest is the presence of osteophytes.[2] The concern is that osteophytes may be maneuvered into the nerve roots due to the distraction of the disc space for the implant. In a study of the effect of facet condition on TDR outcome, Elders et al[3] found that there was no difference in the clinical outcomes with respect to the degree of facet arthrosis. However, the authors noted that in the moderate and severe arthrosis groups the number of patients was low and further investigation is needed with a larger number of patients to confirm their results.

As with any anterior spine surgery, there is added concern in patients with previous abdominal surgery. The exact location of the previous surgery should be considered with respect to the approach required for the disc level to be operated. As with any surgery, patients who have a strong psychological component to their ongoing pain complaints are likely to be poor TDR candidates. Screening by a psychologist familiar with chronic back pain patients should be undertaken.[4]

There may be some concern in performing TDR in patients with previous spinal surgery. However, if the structure of the spine has not been compromised by procedures such as a discectomy and the patient is otherwise a candidate for TDR, arthroplasty can be reasonably pursued. In a report by Leahy et al[5] on the ProDisc, results of TDR in patients with a previous discectomy were very similar to those in patients with no such previous surgery. The inventor of the CHARITÉ found that postdiscectomy patients are very good candidates for the device.[6] They found that leg pain was relieved in 83% of such patients and straight leg raising was negative in 93%.

## DESCRIPTION OF THE DEVICE

One of the fundamental issues with any implant is its biomechanical properties. The basic design concept for the CHARITÉ disc was to mimic the characteristics of the natural disc, combined with the concept of allowing motion through articulation of concave and convex surfaces (Fig. 38–1A and B) The implant has undergone extensive mechanical testing. The first of the tests were conducted on the early models designed in Germany to evaluate the ability of the disc to perform acceptably under the loads encountered in the human body.[2] Additional testing was performed on the subsequent modified designs of the disc to evaluate the safety of the implants under physiologic load.

The pattern of motion produced by the device was investigated compared with fusion cages and cages with pedicle screw constructs.[7] In flexion-extension, the CHARITÉ slightly increased movement compared with the intact spine (3%). The cages reduced motion by 57% and the addition of pedicle screws reduced it further by 93%. The center of rotation for the intact spine and the CHARITÉ was in the posterior one third of the operated segment with the implant mimicking the elliptical pattern of the center of rotation, as was seen with the intact spines. The implant was

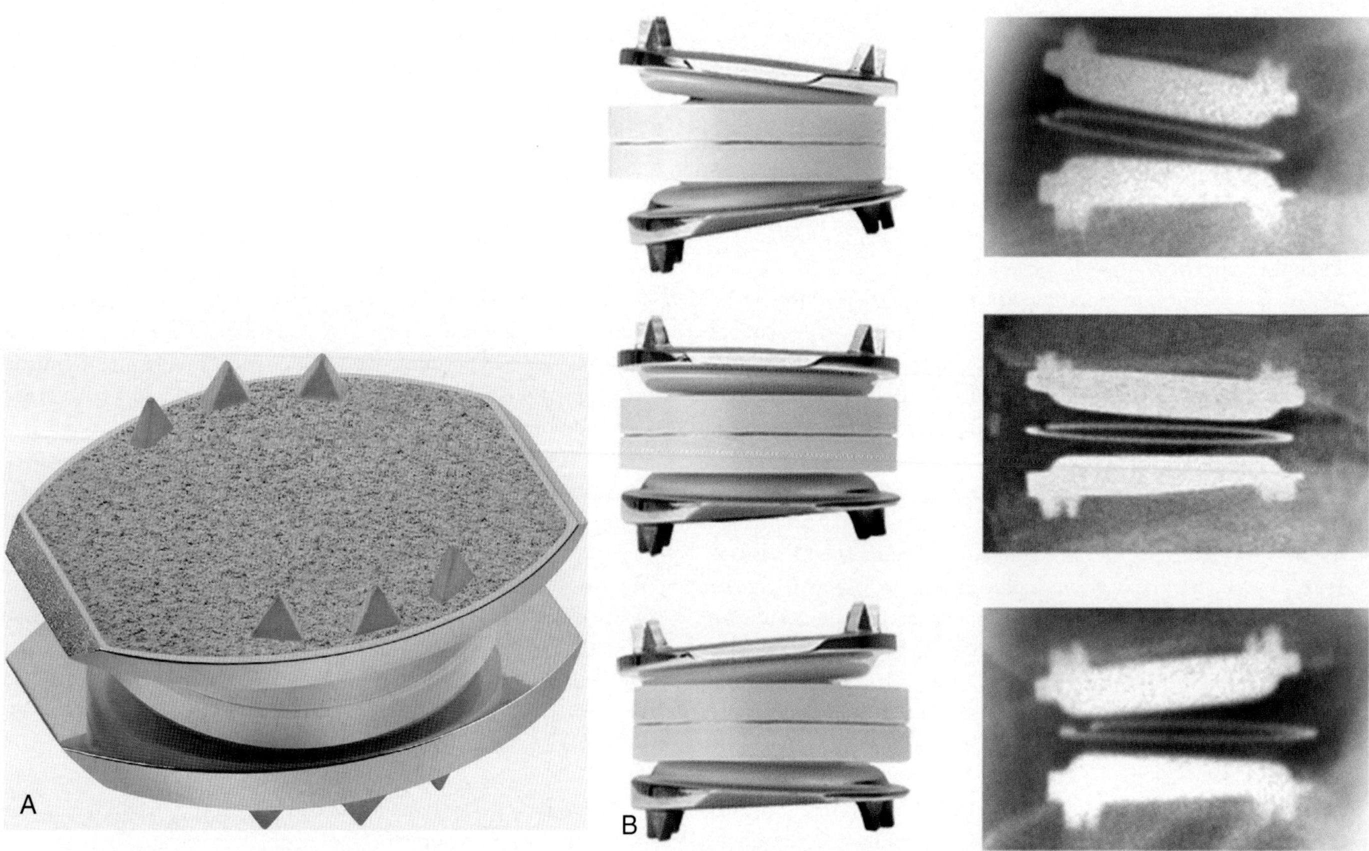

■ **FIGURE 38–1.** **A,** CHARITÉ Artificial Disc in an assembled form. **B,** Translation provided by the mobile core of the CHARITÉ Artifical Disc; also shown on plain flexion-extension radiographs. *(Reprinted with permission from DePuy Spine, Raynham, MA.)*

associated with a 44% increase in axial rotation. The cages reduced rotation by 29% and the addition of pedicle screws reduced rotation by 90%.

A biomechanical study investigated the function of two-level CHARITÉ implantation and possible surgical revisions.[8] One- and two-level CHARITÉ replacements preserved the motion of the operated and adjacent segments, and allowed more motion than TDR plus pedicle screws or screws plus femoral ring allograft simulating a 360-degree fusion. In terms of revision strategies for TDR, the TDR/pedicle screw construct was not significantly different from the femoral ring allograft with pedicle screws. Both of these constructs allows significantly less motion than the CHARITÉ alone. When analyzing the adjacent segment, L5-1, both the pedicle screw constructs increased segmental motion at this level, unlike the TDR.

Serhan et al[9] performed simulated testing with various combinations of one- and two-level CHARITÉ and fusions and investigated the motion patterns of the operated and adjacent segments. They found that single-level TDR preserved physiologic motion, and with two-level TDR, the motion was altered only at the L4-L5 level. With fusion, the motion was significantly altered with one- or two-level surgery. When testing combined TDR and fusion, they found that fusion at L5-1 combined with TDR at L4-L5 produced results similar to a single-level L5-1 fusion. This is supporting of the use of hybrid surgery, that is, combining fusion at the lower level with TDR at the upper level, in patients with two-level symptomatic disc degeneration.

One cadaveric study investigated the impact of increasing the disc space height on the facet joints.[10] They found that increased disc space height related to CHARITÉ implant caused a significant decrease in the overlap of the facets and increased facet joint space. It was stated by the authors that increasing the disc space height would result in facet joint subluxation.

The effect of device positioning on range of motion (ROM) has been investigated in a cadaveric study.[11] They found that placement posterior to midline increased the ROM level by approximately 3 degrees at the L5-1 and L4-L5 levels. Placement anterior to midline decreased ROM by about 3 degrees at L5-1 and almost 6 degrees at L4-L5.

## CLINICAL OUTCOMES

Since its introduction in the 1980s, there have been many clinical reports on the outcome of the CHARITÉ implant. These have dealt with the pain relief and function related to the device as well as the range of motion of the operated levels. The European literature offers long-term follow-up on results and complications related to the device. The Investigational Devise Exemption (IDE) trial regulated by the U.S. Food and Drug Adminstration (FDA) provides a prospective randomized study comparing the device to fusion.

Long-term follow-up results of the CHARITÉ Artificial Disc have been published by Lemaire.[12] He reported on a series of 100 patients with a follow-up of 10 to 13.4 years. An excellent outcome was reported for 62% of patients, with an additional 28% having a good result. David et al[13] recently reported the results of 10-year minimum follow-up (range 10 to 16 years) of 226 CHARITÉ patients, which is a total of 301 implants. Good or excellent outcome was noted in 78.8% of patients. Adjacent-level deterioration requiring reoperation occurred in 2.7% of patients. Immediate subluxation requiring reoperation was seen in 1.3% of cases. Posterior fusion and instrumentation for continued pain was undertaken in 8.4% of the study group. Facet arthrosis at the implanted level occurred in 10 patients (2.3%). In four patients, polyethylene core breakdown was noted that was attributed to the pre-1997 air sterilization process of the implant. Reoperation took place more than nine years after the initial surgery, and in two of the four patients, the patients received a new prosthesis. Putzier et al[14] reported 17-year follow-up on a series of 51 patients receiving 84 implants. They found that reoperation was undertaken in 11% of patients. However, the results of this study are not applicable to the current CHARITÉ because the study included patients receiving all three designs of the implant, which have not been available for use for the past 15 to 20 years. Also, the instrumentation for insertion of the implants was different from today's tools.

There have also been several studies offering shorter duration of follow-up. One of the earlier reports of clinical outcome of TDR was a 2-year follow-up of 46 patients by Cinotti et al.[15] They reported the overall success rate to be 63%. Factors related to a less favorable outcome were two-level replacements compared to single-level, previous spine surgery, and receiving Workers' Compensation. Using the outcome assessment described by Stauffer and Coventry, Zeegars et al[16]reported that 70% of patients had a good outcome at 24 months after TDR. This was despite a relatively high rate of complications and reoperations in the series of his first 50 cases.

Perhaps the most comprehensive study involving the CHARITÉ device was the FDA-regulated IDE clinical trial evaluating the safety and effectiveness of the implant.[17] The study involved 304 patients from 14 centers across the United States. Patients were randomized to either the CHARITÉ or anterior lumbar interbody fusion (ALIF) using autogenous iliac crest bone graft in BAK cages. A two-to-one ratio was used, with more patients being assigned to the CHARITÉ group (205 received the CHARITÉ Artificial Disc and 99 underwent fusion). Both surgical groups improved significantly from their preoperative status as based on Visual Analog Scale (VAS), Oswestry Disability Index (ODI), and SF-36 scores. At all postoperative follow-up periods, with the exception of the 24-month period, the CHARITÉ VAS and ODI scores were significantly less than in the fusion group. Patient satisfaction was assessed at the 12- and 24-month follow-up periods and was also high in both groups. At 24 months, the CHARITÉ group had a significantly greater satisfaction rate than did the fusion patients. In later work, Geisler et al[18] performed additional statistical analysis on the clinical outcomes of the group of patients in the IDE randomized trial as well as including the 71 training cases from the various study sites. In their analysis, a nonparametric analysis was used that was actually more appropriate after evaluating the distribution of the data and realizing that it was not normally distributed as required by the t-test analysis described in the original study protocol. Based on the new analysis and the addition of the 71 patients, increasing sample size, they found that at all study follow-up periods the VAS and Oswestry scores were significantly less in the CHARITÉ group compared to the ALIF group.

There is legitimate concern after approval is granted by the FDA for marketing in the United States that the results will decrease and the complications will increase once the devices are available for widespread use. This may be attributable to several factors, including some surgeons not being as skilled or as familiar with the required approach as those surgeons selected for the clinical trials and/or without a commitment to strict adherence to the inclusion/exclusion criteria rigorously employed during the study, results may be compromised. To address the concern over the potential for an increased complication post-approval, a registry was maintained of the CHARITÉ cases. As reported by Blumenthal et al,[19] the incidence of problems such as migration, sizing/malpositioning, subsidence, vascular injury, and death were similar in the first year after approval (approximately 4000 patients receiving the device) as during the IDE trial.

One important outcome measure that is frequently overlooked is the work status of patients. This is not only important for the patient's well-being, but is beneficial for society as well. Lemaire's study offers more than 10-year follow-up of 100 patients.[12] Of 95 work eligible patients, 91.5% returned to work. In Zeegers' study with 2-year follow-up, 81% of patients returned to work.[16] In reviewing a subgroup of patients enrolled in the FDA IDE CHARITÉ trial, the work status and length of time to return to work were compared for the TDR and fusion groups.[20] In the TDR group, the percentage of patients working improved from 42.9% to 65.7%, whereas in the fusion group, the percentage of patients working decreased from 50.0% to 41.7%. With respect to the length of time off work after surgery, the TDR group returned on an average of 105.5 days compared with 163.9 days for the patients who underwent fusion.

### Factors Related to Clinical Outcome

Perhaps one of the most important and most challenging tasks associated with spine surgery outcomes is attempting to identify factors related to outcome. Regardless of the surgical procedure or implant, there are always patients who do not do as well as desired. It is hoped that with repeated evaluation of surgery, the indications and contraindications can continually be refined to produce ever-increasing rates of favorable patient outcomes.

In a study analyzing characteristics related to the extremes of outcome, that is the 20 best and 20 worst outcomes of TDR, either with CHARITÉ or ProDisc (Synthes, West Chester, PA), Siddiqui et al[21] reported that the only factor identified that was significantly related to outcome was the length of time off work before surgery. Other variables investigated included age, gender, body mass index, device position, work status, insurance type, level operated, preoperative VAS and ODI scores, occupation type, smoking, and a history of previous lumbar surgery. None of these factore were related to the best/worst classification. Of note, when comparing the VAS and ODI scores in the subgroups of patients who were off work only a short time or none at all with those who were off work for a longer time, there was no difference. This study suggests that the patients who were off work longer and were more likely to be in the worst outcome group, were not in more pain, or have greater degree of self-report disability. This author noted that the study supported what has been previously known, that is, behavioral and psychological factors significantly affect surgical outcome.

One item related to outcome that is not generally addressed in clinical studies is the experience level of the surgeon and institution involved with the cases. In reviewing data from the FDA IDE study, it was found that high-enrolling centers had significantly reduced length of hospitalization, operating time, and adverse events.[22]

Data from the FDA trial were analyzed to determine if the device positioning (based on three subgroups of ideal, suboptimal, and poor positioning) influenced outcome.[23] The authors found that although the mean VAS and ODI scores improved significantly in all three subgroups, better device positioning was significantly related to greater improvement in outcome scores. This finding may help explain the results of the study discussed earlier[22] in that the more experienced surgeons may be more likely to position the device in the center of the disc space.

## RANGE OF MOTION

The goal of TDR is to reduce pain and allow motion. Several studies have reported the range of motion. Table 38–1 presents the ROM reported in several clinical follow-up studies. Even in the studies with more than 10 years of follow-up, the prostheses were mobile. In a review of 301 implanted prostheses in 226 patients, 87.4% of the implants were mobile at a minimum of 10 years of follow-up.[14] Various factors related to ROM have been investigated. Cinotti et al reported factors related to significantly greater ROM were initiation of rehabilitation one week after surgery, central to posterior positioning of the device in the disc space, and maximal coverage of the vertebral body end plate.[15] Based on the results of the FDA IDE study, device positioning was significantly related to ROM.[23] Among levels in which the device was implanted more than 5 mm off midline in either the AP or lateral radiographic view ($n = 18$) the mean ROM was only 3.1 degrees.

**TABLE 38–1. Reported Range of Motion Results from Various CHARITÉ Studies**

| Study | N | Follow-up | L3–4 | L4–5 (Degrees) | L5–1 (Degrees) |
|---|---|---|---|---|---|
| Cinotti et al[15] | 46 patients; 56 levels | 3.2 yr (2–5 yr) | NA | 16 | 9 |
| David et al[13] | 236 patients; 301 levels | ≥10 yr | NA | 10.2 | 7.4 |
| Lemaire et al[12] | 100 patients; 147 levels | 11.3 yr (10–13.4 yr) | 12.0 | 9.6 | 9.2 |
| | | | | **All levels combined** | |
| Zeegars et al[16] | 50 patients; 75 levels | 2 yr | | 9 | |
| McAfee et al[23] | 276 patients; 276 levels | 2 yr | | Approximately 7.5 | |

## OPERATIVE TECHNIQUE

The procedure for CHARITÉ implantation has previously been described in detail.[24] There are several technical items that can be employed for maximizing outcome and minimizing the risk of complication. One is to make sure the spine is aligned with the spinous process perpendicular to the vertebral body endplates. The implant endplates should cover as much of the vertebral body endplates as possible (Fig. 38–2 A to E). Too small an implant may result in subsidence. The implant should be positioned parallel to the endplates and as posterior in the disc space as possible. Ensuring that the anchoring teeth are engaging the bone may help prevent migration.

## POSTOPERATIVE CARE

One of the potential benefits of TDR over fusion is a more rapid participation in active rehabilitation. Like many surgical candidates, many TDR patients are deconditioned owing to months of reduced activity caused by chronic pain. Patients who undergo fusion need to reduce activities for a period of time after surgery to give the bone graft time to begin incorporation. The only restriction with TDR after healing of the incision is no extreme extension. This allows for earlier participation in a more aggressive postoperative rehabilitation program. Such a program has been outlined by Keller.[25] Patients are started with stretching and progress to more demanding strengthening exercises. Core stabilization is included in the exercise program. Also, overall physical conditioning may be helpful in many of these patients.

## COMPLICATIONS AND AVOIDANCE

### Device Migration

One potential complication of TDR is the anterior or posterior migration or displacement of the prosthesis. Anterior displacement may be more likely to occur at the L5-1 level where the disc space is more angular. Device displacement can be a serious complication potentially resulting in significant vascular or neural injury. To resist displacement, the CHARITÉ is anchored by three teeth on each of the anterior and posterior edges of both endplates. A few cases of displacement have been reported.[26] One strategy to possibly reduce the chance of migration is to coat the implant with a material that encourages boney ingrowth. The CHARITÉ implant is available with two layers of titanium coated with hydroxyapatite. The ingrowth into such a surface was investigated in a study involving seven baboons.[27] At 6 months, histopathologic evaluation found excellent bony ingrowth into the endplates with no fibrous tissue. Approximately 48% of the total endplate area had ingrowth, which was greater than seen with hip and knee implants. The authors attributed the high rate of ingrowth to the axial loading across the spinal implants.

Kurtz et al[28] analyzed 16 CHARITÉ implants retrieved from patient 3 to 16 years after implantation. Four of the 16 were porous coated, and the remaining 12 had uncoated, smooth endplated surfaces. In the groups of coated device, there was no sign of residual calcium phosphate, and one of the four had adherent bone (on less than 10% of the surface area of the endplate). In the group with a smooth coating, fibrous tissue was found. The authors supported the use of the coated implant to reduce the potential risk of migration.

### Wear Debris

Based on experience with hip and knee joints, concern has been expressed about the possibility of deleterious wear debris of the polyethylene core. However, the size, load, degree of motion, and pattern of motion are very different in the spine than in the hip or knee. The wear debris has been investigated. In a study involving baboons sacrificed 6 months after TDR with the CHARITÉ , no evidence of wear debris was identified. McAfee, Serhan, et al[29] performed biomechanical cyclical testing of the CHARITÉ using American Society for Testing and Materials (ASTM) standards. The prostheses were tested to 10 million cycles moving 7.5 degrees. They found minimal wear debris and a height loss of the implant of only 0.2 mm. With the reports of follow-up of at least 10 years now available from Europe, there were no significant problems related to wear debris reported.[12]

### Reported Complications

The anterior approach to the spine for CHARITÉ placement is the same as for anterior interbody fusion, and therefore, the potential approach-related complications are very similar. The most obvious and the most severe is vessel damage. There is also the possibility of injury to the ureters or sympathetic chain, sometimes resulting in retrograde ejaculation. As with any spine surgery, there is also great concern for the potential of neurological injuries. There is also the potential for complications related to the device itself. One study that describes the types of complications that can occur from TDR was provided by van Ooji et al,[26] who reported on a series of 27 CHARITÉ complications. Although not reported by the authors, it is estimated that the divisor was approximately 500 patients, resulting in an estimated complication rate of 5.4%. Examples of the types of complications they reported were prosthetic dislocation, broken wire around the polyethylene core, erectile dysfunction, hematomas, facet joint arthrosis, adjacent segment degeneration, spontaneous fusion at the level of the prosthesis, subsidence, anterior migration, signs of prosthetic wear, and hyperlordosis of the operated segment. As discussed by McAfee in a letter addressing the van Ooji article,[30] there were only two device-related problems in the series; these were the two cases of slow anterior migration of the implant during a 10-year period. The other complications were primarily due to poor patient selection or surgical technique, such as using too small a prosthesis, resulting in subsidence.

A comprehensive review of complications related to any surgery is usually difficult. There may be differences in how the investigators determine what qualifies as a complication. However, in the rigorously monitored prospective clinical trials in the United States, the protocol requires comprehensive capture of all adverse events and complications. This provides a thorough database for a large number of patients from which to study complications. The incidence of various neurologic complications were analyzed from the multicenter FDA-regulated clinical trial.[31] There were no significant differences in the incidence of neurological complications when comparing the

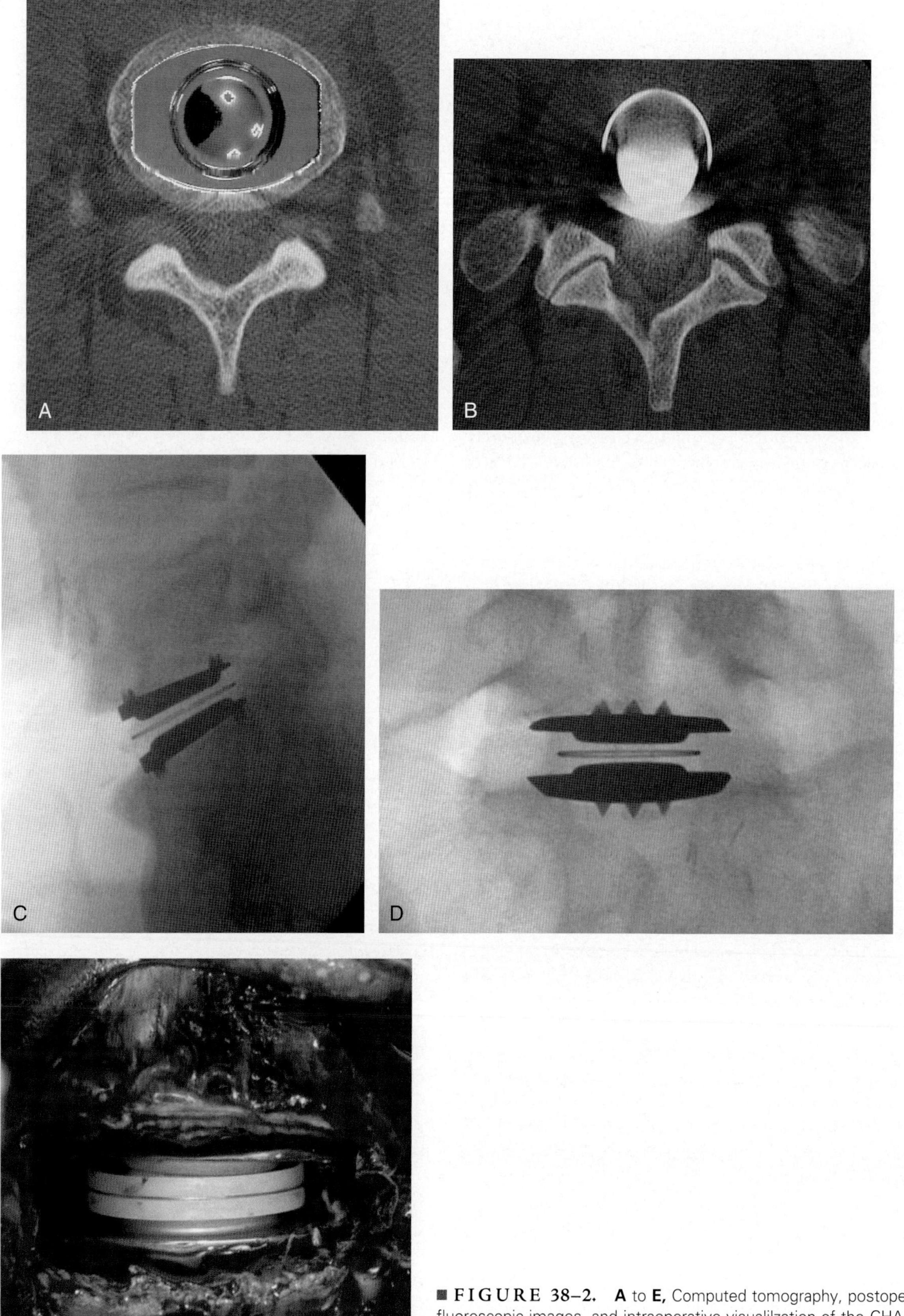


■ **FIGURE 38–2. A** to **E,** Computed tomography, postoperative fluoroscopic images, and intraoperative visualilzation of the CHARITÉ Artificial Disc demonstrating the relationship between the bony rim and the endplate size. *(Reprinted with permission from DePuy Spine, Raynham, MA.)*

CHARITÉ and ALIF groups. Major events (burning leg pain, moor deficit at index level, or nerve root injury) occurred in 4.9% of patients compared with 4.0% in the fusion group. Minor neurologic complications occurred in 9.8% of the CHARITÉ group and 8.1% of the fusion group. These included numbness in the index level and one fusion patient with numbness in the sacral nerve distribution. Other neurological problems were identified in 3.9% of CHARITÉ patients and 8.1% of the fusion group. These included numbness in a distribution other than the index level, positive Waddell signs, reflex changes, and positive straight leg raise. Among these complications, it was reported that three (1.5%) were device related in the CHARITÉ group.

Non-neurologic related complications in this study population were reported by Blumenthal et al.[17] These included 5.4% incidence of device failures requiring reoperation. There were approach-related complications in 9.8% of patients. The complication rate in the CHARITÉ group was similar to that in the ALIF control group.

Complications found during the long-term follow-up, minimum of 10 years, can be found in the European literature.[12] Lemaire found slight device subsidence in two patients who did not need to undergo additional surgery. He reported that there were no cases of device subluxation and no cases of spontaneous arthrodesis. Among the 100 patients, five required a posterior fusion during the 10-year follow-up period. Other complications in his series were painful facets (4%), ossification limiting motion (2%), adjacent-segment deterioration (2%), neurologic injury (2%), sexual dysfunction (1%), vascular injury (1%), and acute leg ischemia (1%).

In a series of 79 patients undergoing two-level TDR, Scott-Young reported no major intraoperative complications, one neurologic complication, two revision procedures, and no prosthetic failure occurred.[32]

The highest rate of reoperations was reported by Zeegers in a series of 50 patients with two-year follow-up.[16] In this series, 12 patients (24%) underwent 24 reoperations. Eleven patients underwent reoperation at an adjacent segment to treat pain, seven of which were to implant a disc prosthesis. Six patients underwent posterior spine surgery at the level of the implant, and three patients underwent seven reoperations related to complications. The most severe of these was one patient in whom an attempt was made to reposition the implant, which was later revised into a fusion and the patient required three vascular surgeries. In the same study, 44 temporary complications and eight permanent ones were reported. These occurred in 30 patients.

In a report of complications occurring in the FDA IDE trial, Holt et al[33] reported that in both the TDR and fusion groups, the incidence of approach-related complications was about 10%, neurologic complications was 16% to 17%, infections was slightly higher in the TDR group (12.7% versus 8.1%, primarily owing to a greater rate of superficial wound infections), and "other" 4%. The rate of implant-related complications was greater in the TDR group (3.9% versus 1.0%, primarily due to subsidence). The need for surgery at the index level was less in the TDR group (5.4% versus 9.1%), and 27.3% of the fusion group had fusion-related complications (pseudarthrosis 9.1% and donor site pain 18.2%).

In determining the long-term performance of the CHARITÉ, McAfee et al[34] reported a survival analysis of 359 patients with a mean follow-up of 25.4 months (range 1 to 68 months). The point of failure was defined as implant revision or a posterior surgery. In the TDR group, 4.6% failed compared with 13.0% of the fusion group. A Kaplan-Meyer survival model was created. The model forecasted a significant difference in the survival of the surgeries at 5-year follow-up. The authors also reported that incidence of reoperation at the adjacent segment was significantly less in the TDR group compared with the fusion group (0.6% versus 5.6%).

One potential concern with intervertebral implants is the risk of subsidence into the vertebrae. Several factors are thought to be related to subsidence. One important aspect is trying to cover as much of the vertebral body endplate as possible. This put the implant into the region of the more dense cortical bone on the outer perimeter of the vertebral body. This maximizes the contact area between the implant and the more dense cortical bone at the outer perimeter of the vertebral bodies. This allows for maximal loading of the stronger portion of the vertebrae. Selecting too small a prosthesis forces load transfer through the less-dense cancellous portion of the vertebrae that may result in subsidence. Similarly, positioning the prosthesis off midline may cause uneven loading of the implant and cause it to subside unevenly into the bone. Patients with osteoporosis are not good candidates for TDR because this may result in subsidence or worse, vertebral body fracture. In the FDA study group, the mean decrease in disc space height measured immediately postoperatively to 24-month follow-up was only .54 mm at L4-5 and .43 mm at L5-1.[23] Isaza et al[35] reviewed the incidence of subsidence in a series of 51 patients. They defined subsidence as migration of more than 3 mm into the vertebral body postoperatively. Subsidence was found to occur in 13.7% of the group. All cases of subsidence were identified within the first 6 weeks after surgery, and in six of the seven cases, the implant subsided into the superior vertebrae. The authors reported that positioning of the device more than 7 mm off midline was significantly correlated with subsidence.

## Facet Joints

There has been concern expressed about the effect of TDR on facet joints. Clearly, patients with significant facet joint arthrosis are not considered good candidates for TDR. One thought is that if the disc space is distracted too much, this causes the facet to be distracted. The other potential problem is that the motion and/or load on the facets may be altered by the prosthesis, resulting in degeneration or arthrosis. To date, there is no clear evidence to support these concerns. There have been several studies investigating facet joints in relation to TDR. In the study with a 10- to 16-year follow-up, facet arthrosis at the implanted level was noted in only 2.3% of patients.[13] Based on the principles that bone density increases with loading and decreases with unloading, Trouillier et al[36] investigated the facets before and after TDR using computed tomography (CT) absorptiometry in a series of 13 patients. In none of the patients did the density of the facets increase after TDR, indicating that the load on the facets was not increased. In fact, in the majority of the regions analyzed, there was a decrease in bone density, indicating unloading of the bone. The authors suggested that the decrease may be attributed to the previously overloaded bone, now being more normally loaded, may have returned to a more normal density.

## Expanding Indications

Kim et al[37] have reported on a series of five patients in whom the CHARITÉ was implanted at a level above a previous fusion. This was done to treat degeneration of the segment adjacent to the fusion at a mean of 4.9 years after the fusion. The mean ODI scores decreased from 64 preoperatively to 31 as early as 1-month follow-up after TDR. The scores improved slightly thereafter. Four of the patients had neurologic compromise before TDR, and all four had marked improvement during their hospital stay, which was maintained during the study.

Another possible use of the CHARITÉ is to combine it with a fusion procedure during the same operative setting. This "hybrid" surgery is discussed in detail in Chapter 80. This technique may be employed in patients who have two-level symptomatic degenerative disc, but in whom one level is contraindicated for TDR. Such reasons may be significant facet changes or severely collapsed disc spaces. There have been few reports on this application. In a recent presentation involving 13 patients, there was approximately a 50% reduction in Oswestry and VAS pain scores following the combined fusion-TDR procedure.[38] Geisler et al[39] also reported favorable outcomes for this hybrid procedure in a series of 36 patients from 10 centers. Similarly, Aunoble et al[40] reported on a series of 45 patients undergoing fusion at L5-1 and TDR with CHARITÉ at L4-L5 with a mean follow-up of 16 months. They noted no pseudathrosis at L5-1. The motion at L4-L5 was 8.4 degrees. ODI scores improved 29.6%. The VAS pain scores (improved 39.1%) and SF-36 mental and physical components improved significantly.

Although approved in the United States for single-level disc replacement, there is likely a role for its use in patients with painful disc degeneration at two levels. Scott-Young[32] reported on a series of 79 patients undergoing two-level TDR with the CHARITÉ. Compared with preoperative values, there was a 77.0% reduction in back pain and an 85.7% reduction in leg pain as assessed by VAS. ODI scores improved 68.1% and 87% of patients returned to work. History of previous surgery and compensation did not negatively affect outcomes, although it was noted that there was a trend for patients with compensation claims to return to work more slowly than those without.

Considering the ongoing development and use of dynamic posterior stabilization devices, the potential for combined AP motion preservation surgery has been noted. This construct has already been evaluated in biomechanical testing.[41] Use of a CHARITÉ device combined with the TOPS (Impliant Spine, Princeton, NJ) device posteriorly produced results comparable to the intact spine. To our knowledge, no clinical cases have been performed using this type of construct.

## CONCLUSIONS/DISCUSSION

The first CHARITÉ was implanted in 1984. The clinical results have been favorable for the implant. The complications have been similar to, or less than, fusion for the treatment of the same condition. There have not been reports of significant problems related to wear debris or device failure.

The role of the CHARITÉ Artificial Disc in expanded indications, such as implantation of two or more levels adjacent to a previously fused segment, combined with fusion at an adjacent segment, are being investigated in small series of patients with promising results. The ability of the device to reduce the incidence of adjacent-segment deterioration has not yet been adequately addressed. To address long-term results, likely in the 7- to 10-year range, from the randomized FDA IDE study are needed. However, it will still be several years before an appreciable number of those patients reach this long-term follow-up point.

The CHARITÉ Artificial Disc was the first TDR to be used in a large number of patients. Long-term performance as seen in the studies from Europe has generally been favorable. The results of the prospective randomized study in the United States found the procedure to be at least as good as fusion and better on some outcome parameters. The role of TDR will likely expand to be combined with other procedures, including fusion at other levels as well as dynamic posterior stabilization devices.

## REFERENCES

1. Büttner-Janz K: History and development of the LINK® SB CHARITÉ™ Intervertebral Prosthesis. *In* Büttner-Janz K, Hochschuler SH, McAfee PC (eds): The Artificial Disc. Berlin, Springer Verlag, 2003, pp 1–10.
2. Büttner-Janz K: The Development of the Artificial Disc SB CHARITÉ. Dallas, TX, Hundley & Associates, 1992.
3. Elders GJ, Blumenthal SL, Guyer RD, et al: Effect of facet joint arthrosis on outcome after artificial disc replacement. Spinal Arthroplasty Society, New York, May 2005.
4. Block AR, Gatchel RJ, Deardorff WW, Guyer RD: The Psychology of Spine Surgery. Washington, D.C., American Psychological Association, 2003.
5. Leahy M, Zigler JE, Ohnmeiss DD, et al: Analysis of total disc replacement in postdiscectomy patients and comparison to patients with no previous lumbar spine surgery. Spine (in press).
6. Buttner-Janz K: History and development of the CHARITÉ Artificial Disc. *In* Guyer RD, Zigler JE (eds): Spinal Arthroplasty: A New Era in Spine Care. St. Louis, MO, Quality Medical Publishing, Inc, 2005, pp 79–90.
7. Cunningham BW, Gordon JD, Dmitriev AE, et al: Biomechanical evaluation of total disc replacement arthroplasty. An in vitro human cadaveric model. Spine 28:S110–S117, 2003.
8. Cunningham BW, Hu N, Beatson HJ, et al: Multidirectional flexibility properties of single versus multi-level CHARITÉ total disc arthroplasty—an emphasis on revision strategies. Spine Society of Australia. Auckland, New Zealand, April 2005.
9. Serhan HA, Malcolmson G, Teng E, et al: Hybrid testing for adjacent- and other-level effects following arthroplasty with the CHARITÉ Artificial Disc vs. simulated fusion. International Meeting on Advance Spine Technologies. Athens, Greece, July 2006.
10. Liu J, Ebraheim NA, Haman SP, et al: Effect of the increase in the height of lumbar disc space on facet joint articulation area in sagittal plane. Spine 31:E198–E202, 2006.
11. Lorenz M, O'Leary P, Nicolakis M, et al: Effect of placement variability on the motion response of total disc replacement under physiologic loads. Spine Arthroplasty Society. Montreal, Canada, May 2006.
12. Lemaire JP, Carrier H, Sariali el-H, et al: Clinical and radiological outcomes with the CHARITÉ artificial disc: a 10-year minimum follow-up. J Spinal Disord Tech 18:353–359, 2005.

13. David T, Lemaire J-P, Moreno P, Bitan F: A long-term multi-center retrospective study of 226 patients with the Charite artificial disc: Minimum 10-year follow-up. International Society for the Study of the Lumbar Spine. Bergen, Norway, June 2006.
14. Putzier M, Funk JF, Schneider SV, et al: Chairte total disc replacement—clinical and radiographical results after an average follow-up of 17 years. Eur Spine J 15:183–195, 2006.
15. Cinotti G, David T, Postacchini F: Results of disc prosthesis after a minimum follow-up period of 2 years. Spine 21:995–1000, 1996.
16. Zeegers WS, Bohnen LM, Laaper M, et al: Artificial disc replacement with the modular type SB Charite III: 2-year results in 50 prospectively studied patients. Eur Spine J 8:210–217, 1999.
17. Blumenthal SL, McAfee PC, Guyer RD, et al: A prospective, randomized, multi-center FDA IDE study of lumbar total disc replacement with the CHARITÉ™ Artificial Disc vs. lumbar fusion: Part I—Evaluation of clinical outcomes. Spine 30:1565–1575, 2005.
18. Geisler FH, Hochschuler SH, Guyer RD, et al: Alternative statistical testing demonstrates superiority of lumbar arthroplasty clinical outcomes at 2 years vs. fusion for the treatment of one-level lumbar degenerative disc disease at L4-5 or L5-S1. International Meeting on Advance Spine Technologies. Athens, Greece, July 2006.
19. Blumenthal SL, Guyer RD, Geisler FH, et al: The First Year Following FDA Approval of the CHARITÉ Artificial Disc: "Real World" Adverse Events Outside an IDE Study Environment. International Meeting on Advanced Spine Techniques (IMAST). Athens, Greece, July 2006.
20. Jenis LG, Banco RJ, Tromanhauser SG, et al: Return-to-work following treatment with CHARITÉ™ Artificial Disc versus anterior lumbar interbody fusion in patients with degenerative disc disease. International Meeting on Advance Spine Technologies. Athens, Greece, July 2006.
21. Siddiqui S, Guyer RD, Zigler JE, et al: Lumbar Spinal Arthroplasty: Analysis of One Center's 20 Best and 20 Worst Clinical Outcomes. Spine Arthroplasty Society, Montreal, Canada, May 2006.
22. Regan JJ, McAfee PC, Blumenthal SL, et al: Evaluation of surgical volume and the early experience with lumbar total disc replacement as part of the investigational device exemption study of the Charité Artificial Disc. Spine 31:2270–2276, 2006.
23. McAfee PC, Cunningham B, Holtsapple G, et al: A prospective, randomized, multi-center FDA IDE study of the Charité™ Artificial Disc: A radiographic outcomes analysis, correlation of surgical technique accuracy with clinical outcomes, and evaluation of the learning curve. Spine 30:1576–1583, 2005.
24. Brau SA: Mini-open approach to the spine for anterior lumbar interbody fusion: Description of the procedure, results and complications. Spine J 2:216–223, 2002.
25. Keller J: Rehabilitation following total disc replacement surgery. *In* Büttner-Janz K, Hochschuler SH, McAfee PC (eds): The Artificial Disc. Berlin, Springer-Verlag, 2003, pp 175–182.
26. van Ooji A, Oner FC, Verbout AJ: Complications of artificial disc replacement: A report of 27 patients with the SB Charite disc. J Spinal Disord Tech 16:369–383, 2003.
27. McAfee PC, Cunningham BW, Orbegoso CM, et al: Analysis of porous ingrowth in intervertebral disc prostheses: A nonhuman primate model. Spine 28:332–340, 2003.
28. Kurtz S, van Ooij A, Ciccarelli L, Villarraga M: Analysis of textured endplates and bone ongrowth in retrieved Charité total disc replacements. Spine Arthroplasty Society. Montreal, Canada, May 2006.
29. McAfee PC, Cunningham BW, Orbegoso CM, et al: Analysis of porous ingrowth in intervertebral disc prostheses: A nonhuman primate model. Spine 28:332–340, 2003.
30. McAfee PC: Comments on the van Ooij article [letter]. J Spinal Disord Tech 18:116–117, 2005.
31. Geisler FH, Blumenthal SL, Guyer RD, et al: Neurological complications of lumbar artificial disc replacement and comparison of clinical results with those related to lumbar arthrodesis in the literature: results of a multicenter, prospective, randomized investigational device exemption study of Charite intervertebral disc. From the Joint Section Meeting on Disorders of the Spine and Peripheral Nerves, March 2004. J Neurosurg Spine 1:143–154, 2004.
32. Scott-Young M: Two level lumbar disc replacement: retrospective study of 79 patients with minimum follow-up period of 1 year. Spine Society of Australia. Auckland, New Zealand, April 2005.
33. Holt R, Majd M, Isaza J, et al: Complications of lumbar artificial disc replacement vs. fusion. Spine Arthroplasty Society. New York, New York, May 2005.
34. McAfee PC, Geisler FH, Blumenthal SL, et al: Predicted 5-year survivorship of the CHARITÉ Artificial Disc vs. anterior lumbar interbody fusion: A Kaplan-Meyer analysis. International Meeting on Advance Spine Technologies. Athens, Greece, July 2006.
35. Isaza JE, Guillory SA, Janani J: Incidence of subsidence in the Charite III lumbar disc replacement. International Meeting on Advance Spine Technologies. Athens, Greece, July 2006.
36. Trouillier H, Kern P, Refior HJ, Müller-Gerbl M: A prospective morphological study of facet joint integrity following intervertebral disc replacement with the CHARITÉ™ Artificial Disc. Eur Spine J 15:174–182, 2006.
37. Kim WJ, Lee S-H, Kim SS, Lee C: Treatment of juxtafusional degeneration with artificial disc replacement (ADR): Preliminary results of an ongoing prospective study. J Spinal Disord Tech 16:390–397, 2003.
38. Lhamby J, Guyer R, Zigler J, et al: Patients undergoing total disc replacement with spinal fusion at different lumbar levels. International Society for the Study of the Lumbar Spine. Bergen, Norway, June 2006.
39. Geisler FH, Banco RJ, Cappuccino A, et al: Lumbar total disc replacement combined with fusion at an adjacent level: Early results from a multi-center retrospective review of a hybrid procedure for multi-level degenerative disease. International Meeting on Advance Spine Technologies. Athens, Greece, July 2006.
40. Aunoble S, Le Huec J-C, Gornet M, Tournier C: Hybrid surgery for DDD: Fusion L5-S1 and disc prosthesis L4-L5. Spine Arthroplasty Society. Montreal, Canada, May 2006.
41. Cunningham BC, Hu N, Beatson H, McAfee PC: Biomechanical evaluation of a posterior dynamic stabilization system combined with total disc replacement. International Meeting on Advance Spine Technologies. Athens, Greece, July 2006.

CHAPTER 39

# ProDisc-L Total Disc Replacement

**Rick B. Delamarter** and **Ben B. Pradhan**

## KEY POINTS

- The ProDisc-L is a three-piece semi-constrained artificial lumbar disc consisting of two metallic end plates and a polyethylene inlay that is locked into the bottom end plate.
- The semi-constrained mechanics of the device allow it to share shear (translational) forces with the posterior facet joints.
- The small keels and titanium plasma-sprayed finish on the end plates allow for immediate fixation as well as longer term bony ingrowth.
- The ProDisc-L is the second artificial disc to receive U.S. Food and Drug Adminstration (FDA) approval for implantation after successfully completing Investigational Device Exemption (IDE) clinical trials: Several aspects of the clinical outcomes showed ProDisc-L actually to be superior to fusion, not simply equivalent.
- Multilevel disc replacements are possible with the ProDisc-L device, and they have been performed at two and three levels: Two-level disc replacement was part of the IDE clinical trials and will be reviewed for FDA approval.

## INTRODUCTION

Thierry Marnay created the first ProDisc-L (or ProDisc-I) prosthetic disc in 1989 at Montpellier, France. The first human implantation was in 1990. To his credit, after inserting 93 implants in 64 patients with his colleague, Dr. Louis Villette, Marnay stopped to evaluate the long-term outcomes of his implant. Finally, in 2001, he published his results after an 8- to 10-year follow-up.[1,2] All implants remained intact without any migration or subsidence. Range of motion (ROM) of the spinal segments was maintained. There was significant reduction in back and leg pain, and almost 93% of the patients were satisfied and would have the surgery again. The promising results from his experience paved the way for the pivotal clinical trials recently completed here in the United States. Since 1999, up to the time of this writing, more than 16,000 ProDisc-L devices have been implanted worldwide.

The ProDisc-L (Synthes, West Chester, PA) lumbar artificial disc received full U.S. Food and Drug Administration (FDA) approval for implantation in August of 2006. Class I data from the U.S. Investigational Device Exemption (IDE) clinical trials, a multicenter prospective randomized and controlled study, revealed that the ProDisc-L device was not only equivalent to fusion in terms of clinical results but often superior in various measures of outcome, including patient satisfaction, earlier recovery, and work status. The two largest enrolling centers, The Spine Institute, Santa Monica, and Texas Back Institute, have published their interim results ahead of the complete multicenter data.[3–6]

## INDICATIONS/CONTRAINDICATIONS

The inclusion and exclusion criteria for this device appears in Table 39–1, as listed for the pivotal FDA clinical trials. There were single-level and two-level surgical arms in the clinical trials, with one-level disc replacement having been approved and two-level disc replacement FDA approval likely to follow. The FDA has allowed some deviation from the strict requirements of the study on a carefully considered case-by-case basis, under the stipulation of "compassionate usage," such as for three-level disc replacements for disease spanning more than two levels, disc replacement next to prior fusions to avoid fusion extension, and so on.

## DESCRIPTION OF THE DEVICE

The first-generation ProDisc-L (ProDisc-I) had titanium end plates and a double keel. In 1999, it was upgraded to cobalt chrome end plates with a single keel (Fig. 39–1). The single serrated keel over each end plate, two small lateral pegs, along with the plasma-sprayed ingrowth surface give the implant immediate stability. The inlay is made of ultra-high-molecular-weight polyethylene (UHMWPE), which snap-locks to the inferior end plate, and thus has only one articulating convex side. The device is semiconstrained, allowing it to share the load with collateral structures such as the facet joints, ligaments, tendons, and muscles, especially in shear. This places more load at the device-bone interface but protects the facet joints. Axial rotation is unconstrained, and the axis of rotation of the superior end plate is angled posteriorly in the neutral position owing to the intradiscal lordosis of the prosthesis, consistent with the physiologic axis of rotation.[7]

**TABLE 39–1. Criteria for Patient Enrollment in the FDA ProDisc-L Clinical Trials**

| Inclusion criteria | Exclusion criteria |
|---|---|
| Degenerative disc disease in one or two adjacent levels between L3 and S1 | More than two levels of degenerative disc disease |
| Back and/or leg pain | End plate dimensions less than 34.5 mm ML or 27 mm AP |
| Failure of at least 6 months of conservative therapy | Known metal and/or polyethylene allergies |
| Oswestry score >20/50 (>40%) | Prior lumbar fusion surgery |
| Ability to comply with protocol and follow-up | Clinically compromised vertebral bodies due to prior trauma |
| Ability to give informed consent | Clinically significant degenerative facet disease |
| Radiographic evidence of disc degeneration includes: | Lytic spondylolisthesis and/or clinically significant stenosis |
| 1. Decrease in disc height by at least 2 mm | Degenerative spondylolisthesis >grade I |
| 2. Instability indicated by >3mm translation or >5 degrees of angulation, but less than Grade I slip | Back or leg pain of unknown etiology |
| 3. Annular thickening and disc dessication on MRI | Objective diagnosis of osteoporosis (DEXA scan) |
| 4. Herniated nucleus pulposus | Presence of metabolic bone disease (e.g., Paget's, osteomalacia) |
| 5. Vacuum phenomenon | Morbid obesity (Body Mass Index >40) |
| | Pregnancy or expected pregnancy within 3 years |
| | Active infection |
| | Medications that retard healing (e.g., steroids) |
| | Autoimmune diseases (e.g., rheumatoid arthritis) |
| | Systemic diseases (e.g., AIDS, HIV, hepatitis) |
| | active malignancy |

AP, anteroposterior; DEXA, dual-energy x-ray absorptiometry; FDA, U.S. Food and Drug Admmistration. ML, mediolateral, MRI, magnetic resonance imaging.

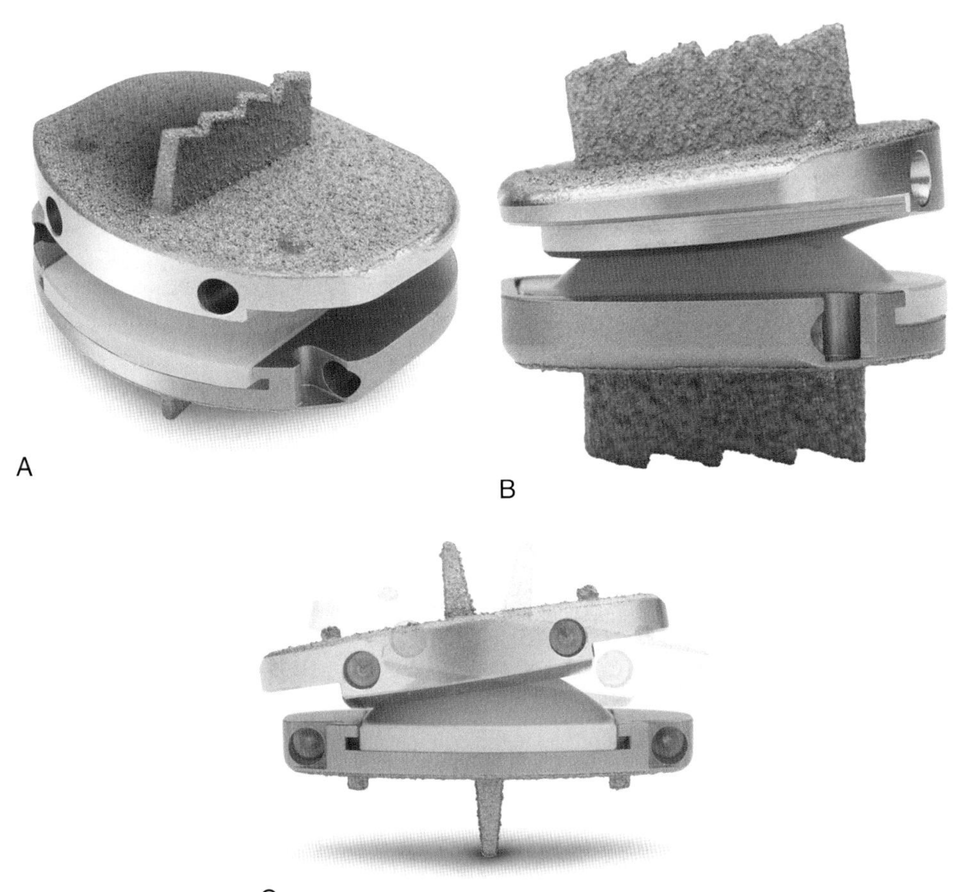


■ **FIGURE 39–1.** **A** to **C,** The ProDisc-L artificial lumbar disc. *(Synthes, West Chester, PA.)*

## BACKGROUND OF SCIENTIFIC TESTING/CLINICAL OUTCOMES

The first ProDisc-L implantation was performed in 1999. Since then, more than 16,000 prostheses have been implanted worldwide at the time of writing of this chapter. Multilevel disc replacements have also been performed (Fig. 39–2). In the original European studies, there have been no device-related failures reported. In the United States, FDA-supervised multicenter clinical trials and 2-year follow-up have been completed, culminating in full FDA approval for human implantation in the United States in August 2006.

### The U.S. Investigational Device Exemption Trial

Table 39–1 lists the eligibility criteria for the U.S. IDE study on spinal arthroplasty with the ProDisc-L device versus lumbar fusion. Table 39–2 lists some of the demographic characteristics of the patients enrolled in the U.S. multicenter IDE study. Results for the IDE multicenter study 2-year results were first reported at the American Academy of Orthopaedic Surgeons annual meeting.[8] This included 162 patients who underwent disc replacement and 80 patients who underwent fusion. Randomization was performed at a 2:1 ratio to disc replacement versus circumferential fusion. Pain, disability, and ROM were evaluated at preoperative, 6 weeks, and 3, 6, 12, 18, and 24 months follow-up visits.

Table 39–3 summarizes the results in terms defined by the FDA. Although pain on the Visual Analog Scale (VAS) decreased significantly in both disc replacement and fusion, there was no defined success criteria based on pain relief alone. Based on a 15% reduction in the Oswestry Disability Index (ODI), the success rate with disc replacement was 77% versus 65% with fusion. Although the study was designed to show at least equivalency in the two techniques, this showed that patients with ProDisc-L did significantly better. Based on a 15-point reduction in ODI, the success rate with ProDisc-L was 68% versus 55% with fusion. These showed an even greater margin of success of ProDisc-L over fusion. The failure rate, defined by reoperations, revisions, and removal or addition of devices, was low and no different between the ProDisc-L and fusion cases. Success as defined by an improvement in SF-36 showed a 79% success rate with ProDisc-L versus 70% with fusion, another benchmark that approached statistical significance. Finally, by radiographic definition (no migration, no subsidence, no loss of disc height, and ROM), the success rate in ProDisc-L was 92% versus 86% for fusion.

With this class I data showing equivalency and, in some cases, superiority of ProDisc-L over fusion, it must be kept in mind that this technology was designed to preserve motion, with the theoretical long-term benefit of retardation of accelerated adjacent-segment degeneration. Table 39–4 lists the sagittal ROM (flexion-extension) at the different follow-up time points. At 24 months, 94% of patients had motion with the physiologic range. The conclusion of the FDA IDE trial was essentially that ProDisc-L preserves ROM without compromising the results as compared with the current surgical standard of fusion, with the potential upside of decelerating adjacent-segment degeneration.

## OPERATIVE TECHNIQUE

A standard anterior left-sided retroperitoneal approach to the lumbar spine is performed. Any operating table that allows supine positioning and fluoroscopy of the lumbar spine can be used. A small bump or inflatable support may be placed under the small of the patient's back for adjustment of lordosis during surgery to open up the disc space anteriorly. In our institute, we use a mini-incision less than 6 cm for one-level cases and about 8 cm for two levels. Intraoperative fluoroscopy is used throughout the operation to verify the placement of the prosthesis. Once exposure is obtained, an anteroposterior (AP) view confirms the level and identifies the midline, which is then marked with the cautery or osteotome (Fig. 39–3A). A complete discectomy is then performed (see Fig. 39–3B, C). Cartilage is removed from the vertebral end plates. If herniated disc material is identified on the preoperative magnetic resonance imaging scan, this may be removed through the anterior approach. In some cases, the posterior longitudinal ligament may have contracted, preventing re-expansion of the disc space, so this must be released from the posterior vertebral body with a forward-angled curette. Once the normal anatomic height has been restored with distraction under fluoroscopy, a trial is placed to help select the proper disc size, angle, and height (Fig. 39–3D). A sagittal groove is then cut in the vertebral end plates in the exact midline using a chisel placed over the trial (Fig. 39–3E). This groove will accept the central keel of the implant. The trial is removed, and the final implant is then gently impacted into place with an insertion tool (Fig. 39–3F). The insertion tool allows distraction of the disc space for placement of the UHMWPE inlay, which snap-fits into position in the inferior end plate (Fig. 39–3G). After the insertion instrument is removed, gross inspection is made to ensure the UHMWPE inlay is properly flush against the inferior end plate (Fig. 39–3H), and final fluoroscopic views are taken to confirm correct position of the prosthesis.

## POSTOPERATIVE CARE

A soft back brace can be used for the first week or two to allow for wound protection. Otherwise, there is no extensive postoperative protocol. Patients can return to work as soon as they are comfortable, but they should allow 6 weeks before returning to recreational sports or full duty (if the job is physically demanding).

## COMPLICATIONS AND AVOIDANCE

No major technique- or device-related complications were observed. Table 39–5 lists the complications for both the ProDisc-L and fusion patients. There were four cases of device migration, subsidence, or loose polyethylene requiring revision surgery

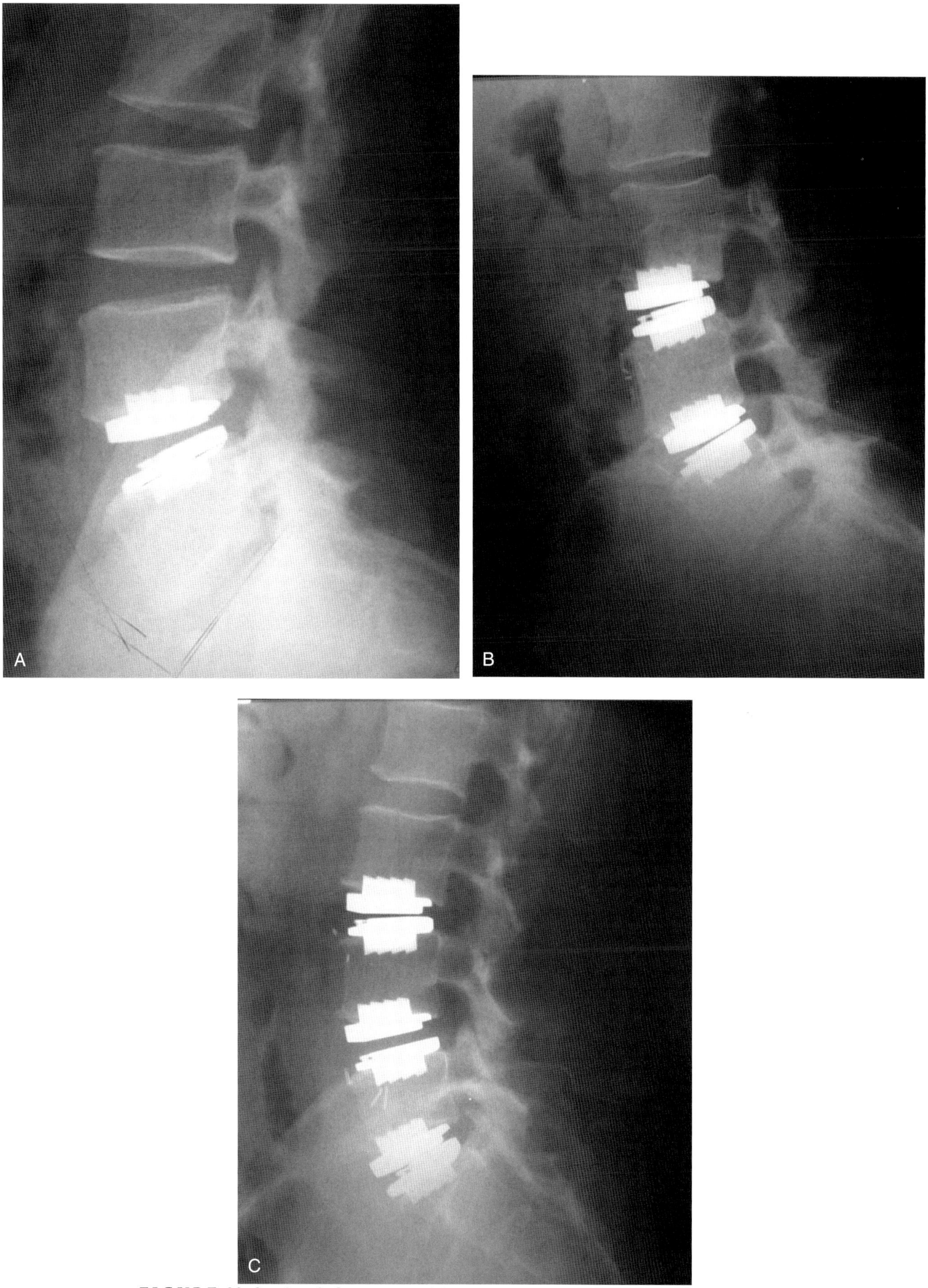

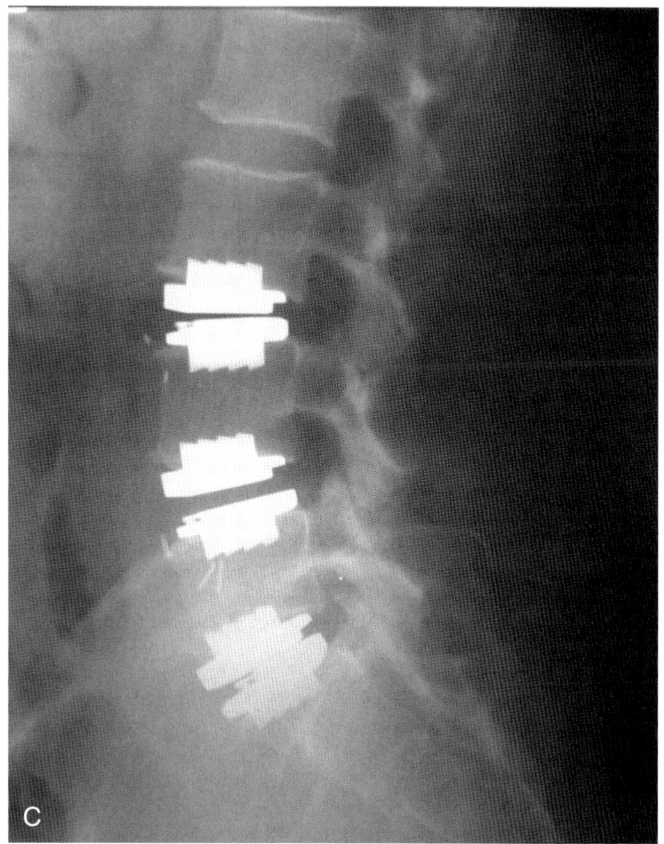

■ FIGURE 39–2. **A** to **C,** One-, two-, and three-level lumbar disc replacement with ProDisc-L.

**TABLE 39–2. Patient Demographics**

| Patient Characteristic | Fusion ($n$ = 80) | ProDisc-L ($n$ = 162) | P-value (NS is $P > 0.05$) |
|---|---|---|---|
| Average age in years (std dev) | 40.2 (7.6) | 39.6 (8.0) | NS |
| Sex (% male:% female) | 46:54 | 51:49 | NS |
| Body mass index (std dev) | 27.4 (4.3) | 26.7 (4.2) | NS |
| Preoperative Oswestry Disability Index (std dev) | 62.9 (13.4) | 63.4 (12.6) | NS |
| Target level at screening | 10.5 | 10.3 | NS |
| L3-L4 | 3 (3.8%) | 3 (1.9%) | NS |
| L4-L5 | 27 (33.8%) | 54 (33.3%) | NS |
| L5-S1 | 50 (62.5%) | 105 (64.8%) | NS |

*n*, number; NS, not significant; std dev, standard deviation.

**TABLE 39–3. Components of Overall FDA-Defined Success at 24 Months**

| | Fusion | ProDisc-L |
|---|---|---|
| ODI success | 46/71 | 115/149 |
| By 15% improvement criteria | (64.8%) | (77.2%) |
| ODI success | 39/71 | 101/149 |
| By 15-point improvement criteria | (54.9%) | (67.8%) |
| Reoperations/revisions/removal/supplemental fixation | 2/75 (2.7%) | 6/161 (3.7%) |
| Maintenance or improvement of neurologic status | 57/70 (81.4%) | 135/148 (91.2%) |
| SF-36 success (improvement over baseline) | 49/70 (70.0%) | 118/149 (79.2%) |
| Radiographic success (fusion or >5 deg ROM at L3-L4, L4-L5, and >4 deg at L5-S1) | 59/69 (85.5%) | 131/143 (91.6%) |

deg, degree; ODI, Oswestry Disability Index; ROM, range of motion FDA, U.S. Food and Drug Admmistration.

**TABLE 39–4. Time Course of Mean Flexion-Extension Range of Motion (Degrees)**

| | Month 3 | Month 6 | Month 12 | Month 18 | Month 24 |
|---|---|---|---|---|---|
| **Fusion** | 1.0 | 0.9 | 0.9 | 0.8 | 0.7 |
| **ProDisc-L** | 6.3 | 6.1 | 7.0 | 7.1 | 7.7 |

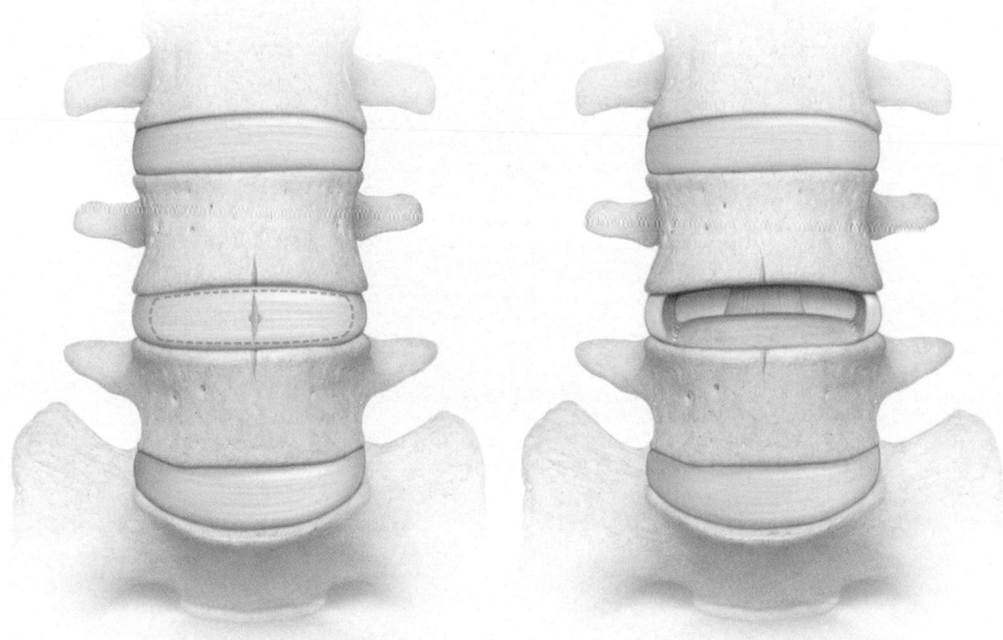


■ **FIGURE 39–3.** **A,** Marking of midline. **B,** Discectomy performed all the way back to the posterior longitudinal ligament.

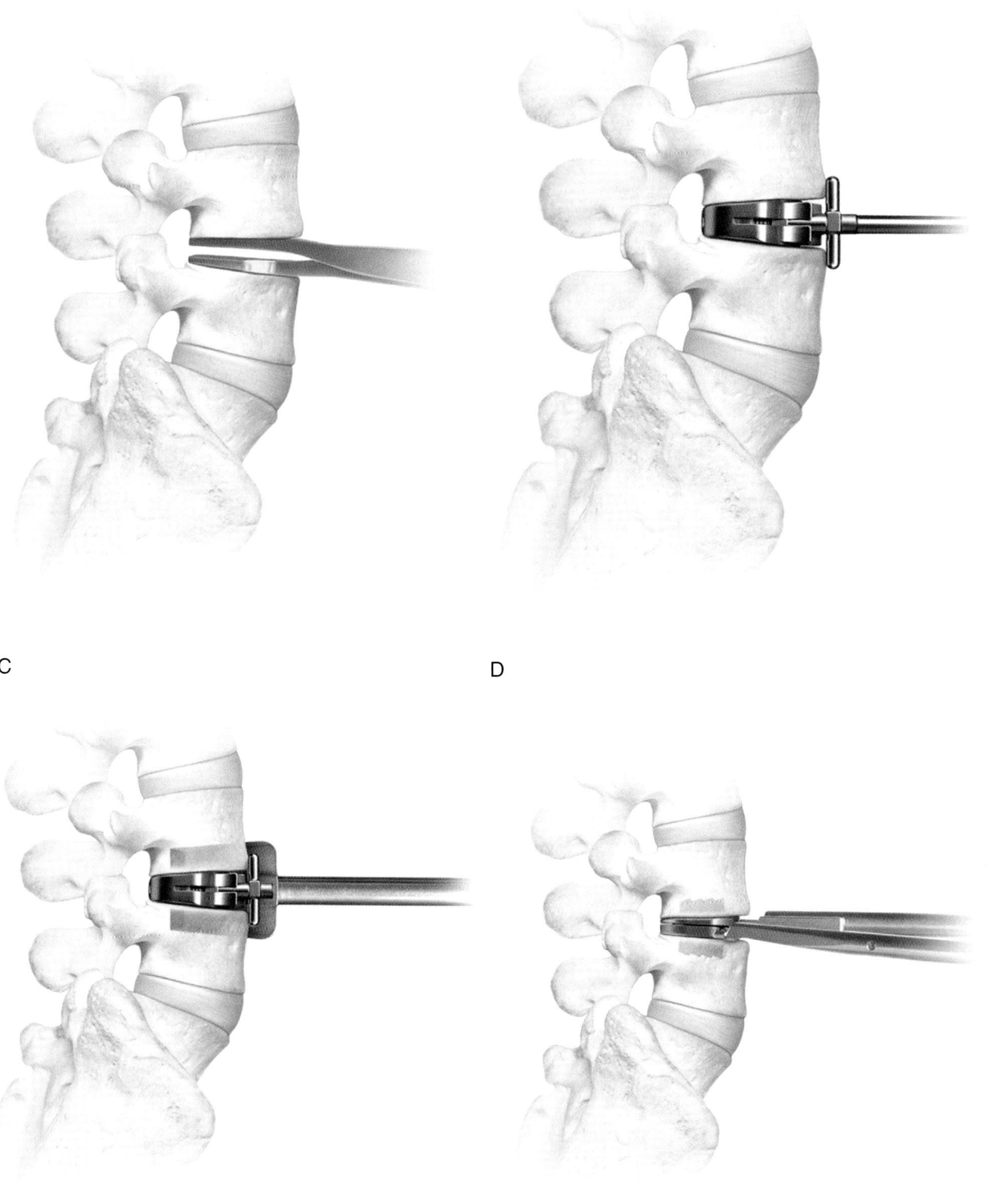


■ **FIGURE 39–3. Cont'd** **C,** Discectomy performed all the way back to the posterior longitudinal ligament. **D,** Trialing for size, height, and lordosis. **E,** Chisel cut for the keels. **F,** Placement of end plates in collapsed form.

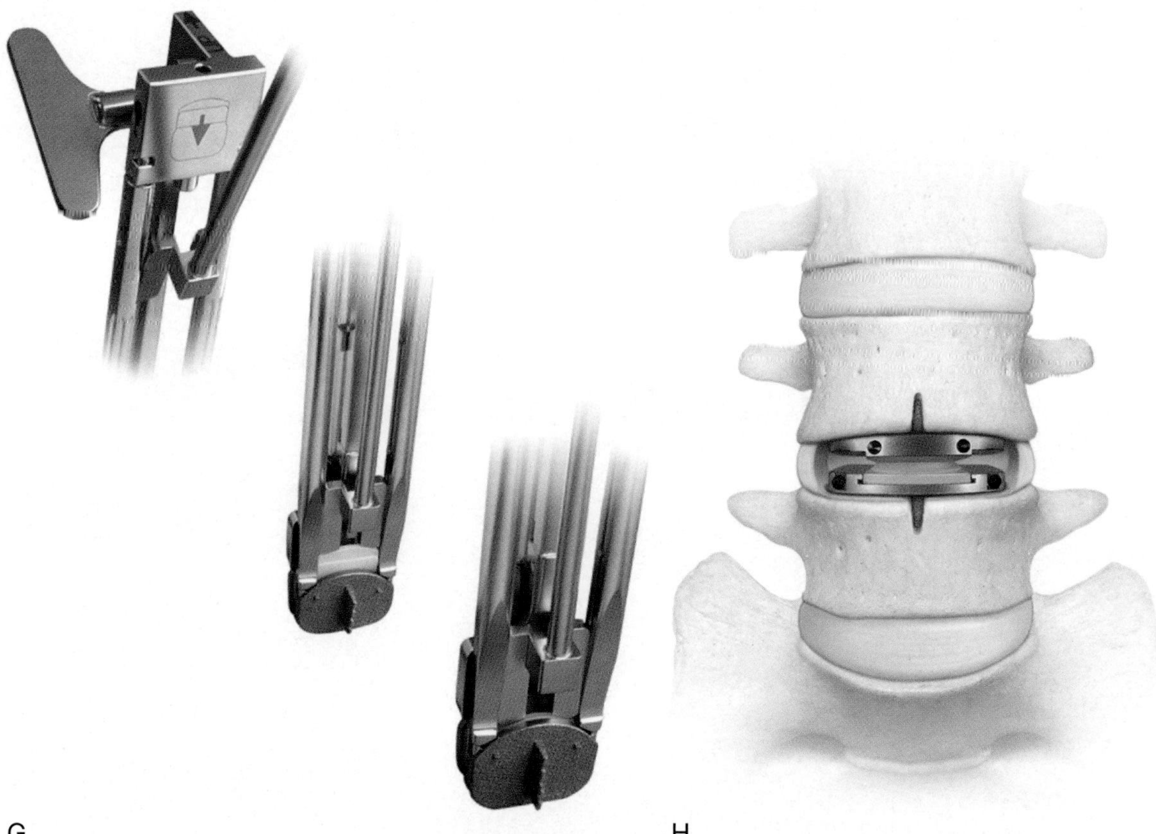

G H

■ **FIGURE 39–3. Cont'd.** **G,** Distraction of end plates and locking of the polyethylene inlay. **H,** The construct is inspected to ensure that there is no step or gap between the polyethylene inlay and the inferior end plate.

**TABLE 39–5. Complications From the U.S. IDE Trials of ProDisc-L Versus Fusion**

| Complication | Fusion | ProDisc-L |
|---|---|---|
| Clinically significant blood loss (>1,500 mL) | 2 (2.5%) | 0 (0.0%) |
| Dural tear | 2 (2.5%) | 0 (0.0%) |
| Edema | 3 (3.8%) | 8 (4.9%) |
| Gastrointestinal (e.g., ileus) | 22 (27.5%) | 32 (19.8%) |
| Genitourinary | 4 (5.0%) | 14 (8.6%) |
| Infection (all superficial) | 2 (2.5%) | 0 (0.0%) |
| Migration, not requiring surgery | 1 (1.3%) | 3 (1.9%) |
| Migration, requiring surgery | 0 (0.0%) | 4 (2.5%) |
| Motor deficit at index level | 0 (0.0%) | 4 (2.5%) |
| Numbness at index level | 1 (1.3%) | 0 (0.0%) |
| Reflex change | 0 (0.0%) | 1 (0.6%) |
| Retrograde ejaculation | 1 (1.3%) | 2 (1.2%) |
| Subsidence, not requiring surgery | 1 (1.3%) | 2 (1.2%) |
| Subsidence, requiring surgery | 0 (0.0%) | 0 (0.0%) |
| Venous thrombosis, deep | 1 (1.3%) | 2 (1.2%) |
| Vessel damage/bleeding | 6 (7.5%) | 5 (3.1%) |

IDE, Investigational Device Exemption.

in the ProDisc-L group. There were four cases of motor deficits at the index level with ProDisc-L, and this may be related to the slightly more meticulous access and retraction necessary for the device compared with femoral ring allograft insertion. There was a very low rate of retrograde ejaculation in both surgery groups.

### ADVANTAGES/DISADVANTAGES: PRODISC-L TOTAL DISC REPLACEMENT

| Advantages | Disadvantages |
|---|---|
| Semi-constrained motion is facet protective | Greater device-bone interface loading |
| Good fixation features (keels, coating)—stays where you put it, so salvage would simply need posterior fusion. | Would be difficult to remove, both from a revision approach standpoint and because of fixation |
| Familiar cobalt-chrome and polyethylene materials | Long-term data (5 to 10 years) from class I data are still pending |
| No device protrusions beyond disc space | Questionable risk of polyethylene debris |
| Class I FDA clinical data available | Anecdotal reports of vertebral fractures (in small patients) |
| Multilevel disc replacements possible and clinical data also available (2 and 3 levels) | |
| Good experience: over 16,000 implanted worldwide at time of writing (Aug 2006) | |

FDA, US Food and Drug Admmistration.

## CONCLUSIONS/DISCUSSION

This particular device has been used extensively for multilevel use, with as good or better clinical outcomes as compared to single-level surgeries, and with good preservation of motion at each replaced level, with good preservation of spinal alignment at each replaced level, and with great patient satisfaction. The technique and instrumentation are facile and streamlined.

The experience with the ProDisc-L Artificial Disc and class I data now released by the FDA suggest that lumbar disc replacement is a viable surgical alternative to fusion for disc degeneration, with preservation of motion and alignment at the treated levels, and without compromising clinical outcomes. Although it is yet too early for the U.S. clinical trials to offer any definite proof of benefit against accelerated adjacent-segment degeneration, the fact that normal intervertebral motion is preserved at the treated segment is encouraging. Longer term safety and efficacy studies are in progress.

## REFERENCES


1. Marnay T: Lumbar disc arthroplasty: 8–10 year results using titanium plates with a polyethylene inlay component. American Academy of Orthopaedic Surgeons Annual Meeting, San Francisco, CA, 2001.
2. Marnay T: Lumbar disc replacement. Spine J 2:94S, 2002.
3. Delamarter RB, Fribourg DM, Kanim LE, Bae H: ProDisc artificial total lumbar disc replacement: Introduction and early results from the United States clinical trial. Spine 28:S167–S175, 2003.
4. Delamarter RB, Bae HW, Pradhan BB: Clinical results after lumbar total disc replacement: An Interim Report from the United States Clinical Trial for the ProDisc-II Prosthesis. Orthop Clin North Am 36:301–313, 2005.
5. Zigler JE: Clinical results with ProDisc: European experience and U.S. investigation device exemption study. Spine 28:S163–S166, 2003.
6. Zigler JE: Lumbar spine arthroplasty using the ProDisc II. Spine J 4:260S–267S, 2004.
7. White AA, Panjabi MM: Clinical Biomechanics of the Spine, 2nd ed. Philadelphia, Lippincott Williams & Wilkins, 1990.
8. Delamarter RB, Zigler J, Spivak JM, et al: The US Multi-Center IDE Results of the ProDisc-L Artificial Lumbar Disc versus Fusion. American Academy of Orthopaedic Surgeons Annual Meeting, Chicago, IL, 2006.

CHAPTER 40

# Mobidisc Disc Prosthesis

**Jean-Paul Steib, Lucie Aubourg, Jacques Beaurain, Joël Delécrin, Jérome Allain, Hervé Chataigner, Iohan Bogorin, Marc Ameil, Thierry Dufour,** and **Jean Stecken**

## KEY POINTS

- Intervertebral motion results in many instantaneous centers of rotation.
- There is translation during the intervertebral rotation.
- Mobidisc is a second-generation non-constrained total disc prosthesis.
- Mobidisc has a mobile inlay.
- The surgical insertion of Mobidisc is easy and precise.

## INTRODUCTION

Lumbar disc degeneration is a major cause of back pain with huge economical consequences.[1] When all treatments have failed, fusion can be indicated, and a good result can be expected.[2] Like every treatment, arthrodesis has its specific drawbacks and its own complications. The idea to cure the pain while respecting the mobility of the joint with the help of an artificial disc is not recent.[3,4] The first clinical trials were conducted in the 1990s with the SB CHARITÉ (DePuy Spine, Raynham, MA) and ProDisc I (Synthes, West Chester, PA) prostheses.[5] Since then, many different concepts and designs were developed to address the discogenic pain.[6] Despite the available nucleus prosthesis[7] and semi-constrained[8] total disc prostheses, we believe that there is a place for non-constrained devices.[9]

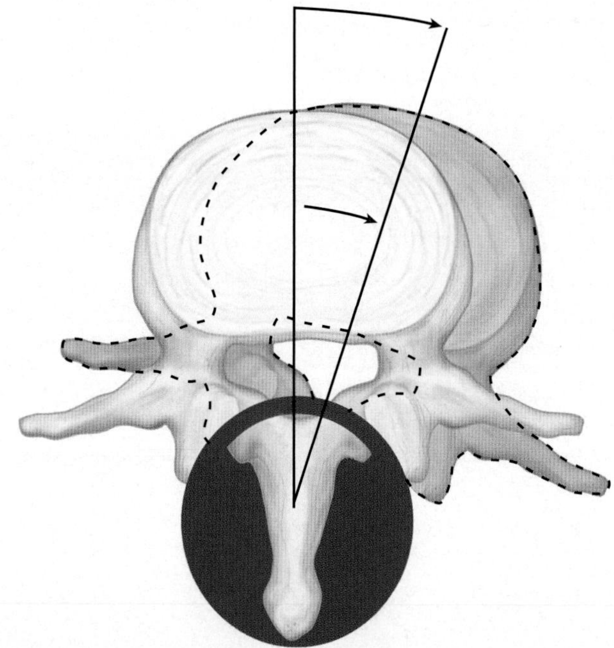

■ **FIGURE 40–1.** Intervertebral rotation is imposed by the articular processes forming a circular surface of contact.

## DESIGN THEORY

Total disc arthroplasty can be considered as a treatment when it is certain that the pathologic disc is the only cause of the pain and when all conservative treatments have failed. To be successful, the artificial disc must restore the disc height and provide physiologic movement. The centers of rotation of intervertebral movement are determined by geometric construction based on the shape of the posterior articular processes. Thus, in flexion-extension, the center of rotation is located in the posterior one third of the intervertebral space and underneath the surface of the superior plate of the inferior vertebra. This is an average center of rotation derived from many instantaneous centers of rotation. Intervertebral rotation is imposed by the articular processes forming a circular surface of contact (Fig. 40–1). The center of rotation is posterior at the level of the spinal process. Thus, there is automatically a translation of the vertebral body. In its function, an artificial disc has to respect these conditions of movement, and this is the leading concept behind the development of the Mobidisc prosthesis (LDR, Troyes, France).

## DESCRIPTION OF THE DEVICE

Mobidisc is a second-generation disc prosthesis made of two vertebral end plates and a polyethylene core (Fig. 40–2). The plates are manufactured from cobalt chrome and have a truncated elliptical form with a plasma-sprayed porous titanium coating covered by hydroxyapatite to facilitate bone integration. There are three sizes available with 0, 5, or 10 degrees of lordosis. A keel provides for primary fixation. The superior end plate has a concave inferior surface adapted to the convexity of the core. The superior side of the inferior end plate is flat to receive the polyethylene inlay captured by four stops. The stops

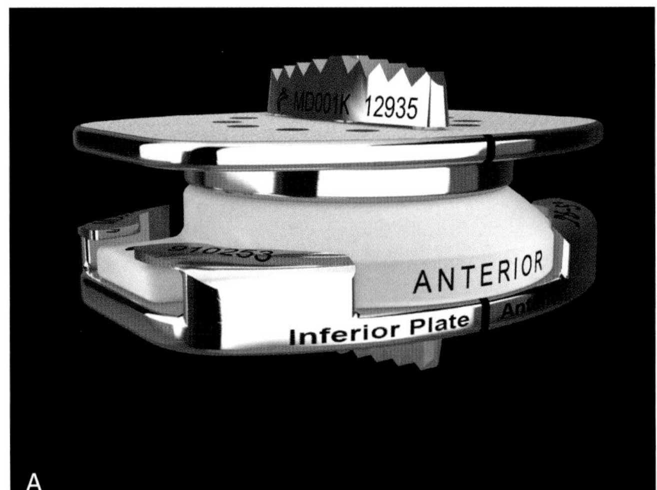


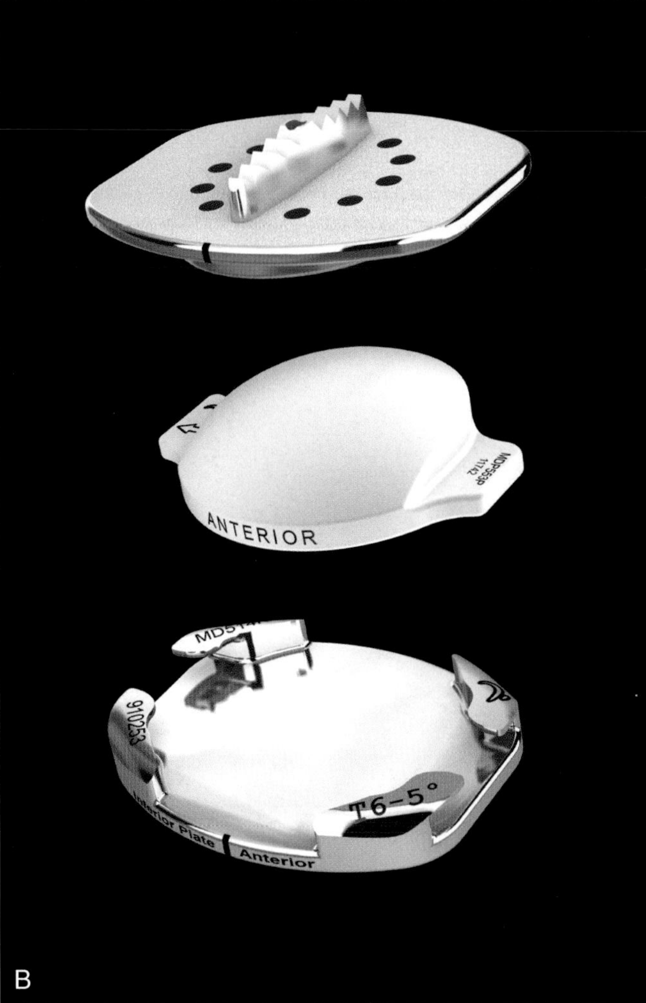


■ **FIGURE 40–2.** The Mobidisc prosthesis. **A,** Assembled prosthesis. **B,** The three components of the device: superior plate, mobile inlay, and inferior plate.

provide for controlled translation of the core on the inferior plate in all directions. The mobility of the prosthesis is physiologic and follows the instantaneous centers of rotation, allowing a translation during the intervertebral rotation. Different sizes of the polyethylene core allow for proper disc height selection.

## BACKGROUND OF SCIENTIFIC TESTING/CLINICAL OUTCOMES

During development, biomechanical tests were performed at the CRI laboratory in Charleville Mézières and at the Laboratory of Biomechanics of ENSAM (Paris, France). Repeated sliding movements of the polyethylene core on the inferior plate up to 5 million cycles did show either fracture or significant wear. The prosthesis was also tested in physiologic conditions on a cadaver to more than 15 million cycles with no or few significant modifications resulting. The first implantation was performed in November 2003.

## CLINICAL PRESENTATION AND EVALUATION

A prospective clinical case series of 149 patients were enrolled and underwent surgery by one of eight surgeons participating in the study. Demographic data and index levels are summarized in Table 40–1. The mean operative time was 161 minutes (range, 60 to 350 minutes), with a mean blood loss of 292 mL (range, 50 to 3,600 mL). Clinical endpoints are summarized in Table 40–2. After 2 years, back pain improvement on Visual Analog Scale (VAS) averaged 60%; VAS leg pain improvement was 36% on the right and 62% on the left. Improvement on the Oswestry Disability Index (ODI) was 55%. Ninety percent of patients were satisfied or very satisfied following the surgery, 77% for the back pain and 70% for the leg pain result. The mean duration of sick leave after the index surgery was 4 months (range, 1 to 11 months). The mobility of the affected level changed from 4 degrees (range, 0 to 15 degrees) preoperatively to 9.4 degrees (0 to 18 degrees) postoperatively, as observed from 76% of all prostheses had mobility at the last follow-up.

## OPERATIVE TECHNIQUE

The patient is positioned supine (Da Vinci position) and is under general anesthesia. The disc is exposed in a traditional way by a retroperitoneal approach. A pin is placed in the adjacent vertebra, which marks the midline of the disc. After discectomy, removal

TABLE 40–1. Summary of Demographic Data in 149 Patients Undergoing Mobidisc Total Disc Replacement

| | Demographic Data |
|---|---|
| Number of patients | 149 |
| **Sex** | |
| Male | 46 (31%) |
| Female | 103 (69%) |
| **Follow-up** | |
| Mean (months) ± SD | 15±6.9 |
| ≥3 months | 149 |
| ≥6 months | 142 |
| ≥12 months | 100 |
| ≥12 months | 35 |
| **Mean age** (yr) ± SD | 41.0±7.2 |
| **Age** range (yr) | 19–56 |
| **Modic Sign** | |
| Modic 0 | 26% |
| Modic I | 54% |
| Modic II | 19% |
| **Single-Level Cases** | 130 (87.2%) |
| L3-L4 | 7 |
| L4-L5 | 34 |
| L5-S1 | 89 |
| **Double-Level Cases** | 18 (12.1%) |
| L2-L3-L4 | 1 |
| L3-L4-L5 | 3 |
| L4-L5-S1 | 14 |
| **Triple-Level Cases** | |
| L3-S1 | 1 (0.7%) |
| **Previous Surgery** | |
| None | 56% |
| Discectomy | 31% |
| Fusion | 5% |

SD, standard deviation

TABLE 40–2. Summary of Clinical Scores Before and After the Mobidisc Implantation*

| | Preoperative | 3 months | 6 months | 12 months | 24 months |
|---|---|---|---|---|---|
| **VAS lumbar** | 6.7 ± 0.2 | 2.9 ± 0.3 | 2.3 ± 0.3 | 2.3 ± 0.3 | 2.7 ± 0.6 |
| **VAS left leg** | 4.2 ± 0.3 | 1.6 ± 0.2 | 1.4 ± 0.2 | 1.7 ± 0.3 | 1.6 ± 0.5 |
| **VAS right leg** | 3.8 ± 0.3 | 1.9 ± 0.3 | 1.7 ± 0.3 | 2.1 ± 0.4 | 2.4 ± 0.6 |
| **ODI (%)** | 49.7 ± 1.3 | 24.4 ± 1.8 | 23.9 ± 1.9 | 20.0 ± 2.3 | 22.5 ± 4.0 |
| **SF-36 MCS** | 31.7 ± 0.9 | 42.1 ± 1.1 | 41.7 ± 1.3 | 42.5 ± 1.4 | 41.7 ± 2.5 |
| **SF-36 PCS** | 33.9 ± 0.6 | 43.1 ± 0.9 | 44.4 ± 1.0 | 48.0 ± 1.2 | 49.2 ± 1.8 |

MCS, Mental Scale; ODI, Oswestry Disability Index; PCS, Physical Scale; VAS, Visual Analog Scale.
*Evaluation was performed preoperatively, and 3, 6, 12, and 24 months after the index surgery. Clinical endpoints are VAS (0–10 scale) for lumbar and leg pain, Oswestry and Short-Form 36 (SF-36) quality-of-life score. Results are expressed as mean ± SEM.

of osteophytes, thorough cleaning of the end plates, and the depth and the height of the disc are measured: These values are used to determine the size of the prosthesis to insert. Although the height is maintained by a spacer, a guide centered on the pin is inserted. An adapted chisel is placed in the rails of the guide to prepare the end plates for the keels. The Mobidisc prosthesis is then assembled: plates, keels, and core. The prosthesis is released in the guide and punched home with the impactor that is adjusted the same way as the chisel, using charts. Following removal of the guide, but before closing the patient, an x-ray study is performed to confirm satisfactory position of the prosthesis at the posterior wall of the vertebral body.

## POSTOPERATIVE CARE

The patient is ambulatory the following day without a corset and is discharged from the hospital as soon as possible.

## COMPLICATIONS

There have been a total of 12 reported complications resulting in three reoperations. Ten cases of subsidence (5.9%) have been reported, five were clinically satisfied, and one was converted to fusion. Additionally one laterally malpositioned prosthesis was reoperated and successfully implanted with another Mobidisc device. Finally, one improperly sized prosthesis was converted to fusion.

## CONCLUSIONS/DISCUSSION

Mobidisc is a unique second-generation disc prosthesis that includes a mobile inlay allowing maintenance of the natural movement created by the posterior articulation. When the indications and operative technique are followed, the clinical results can be very satisfying.

### ADVANTAGES/DISADVANTAGES: MOBIDISC

**Advantages**
- Non-constrained arthroplasty
- Simple, reproducible placement

**Disadvantages**
- Not indicated for:
  - instability
  - posterior arthritis

## REFERENCES

1. Rothman RH, Simeone FA, Bernini PM: Lumbar disc disease. *In* Rothman S (ed): The Spine, 2nd ed. Philadelphia, WB Saunders, 2001, pp 508–645.
2. Fritzell P, Hagg O, Wessberg P, Norwall A: Lumbar fusion versus nonsurgical treatment for chronic lumbar pain: a multicenter randomized controlled trial from the Swedish lumbar spine study group. Spine 26:2521–2534, 2001.

3. Cleveland DA: The use of methylacrylic for spinal stabilization after disc operations. Marquet Med Rev 20:62–XX, 1955.
4. Fernström U: Arthroplasty with intercorporeal endoprothesis in herniated disc and in painful disc. Acta Chir Scand 357(suppl):154–159, 1966.
5. Buttner-Janz K: Development of the Artificial Disc SB Charité. Ann Arbor, MI, Hundley & Associates, 1992.
6. Szpalski M, Gunzburg R, Mayer M: Spine arthroplasty: a historical review. Eur Spine J 11(suppl 2):S65–S84, 2002.
7. Sagi HC, Bao QB, Yuan HA: Nuclear replacement strategies. Orthop Clin North Am 34:263–267, 2003.
8. Tropiano P, Huang RC, Girardi FP, et al: Lumbar total disc replacement: seven to eleven years follow-up. J Bone Joint Surg Am 87:490–496, 2005.
9. Steib JP: A new approach to lumbar disc prosthesis. *In* Szpalski M, Gunzburg R, LeHuec J-C, Braydo-Bruno M(eds): Nonfusion Technologies in Spine Surgery. Philadelphia, Lippincott Williams & Wilkins, 2006, pp 187–190.

CHAPTER 41

# The FlexiCore® Intervertebral Disc

**Jonathan R. Stieber** and **Thomas J. Errico**

## KEY POINTS

- The FlexiCore® Intervertebral Disc is a lumbar disc replacement featuring a metal-on-metal, single-unit design.
- Tension-bearing construction is designed to prevent separation and/or dislocation.
- Fixed center of rotation is designed to minimize relative translation of implant components.
- Metal-on-metal (cobalt-chromium alloy) bearing surfaces avoid polyethylene wear and creep.
- Implantation is through anterior or anterolateral angles and intraoperative repositioning.

## INTRODUCTION

The FlexiCore® Intervertebral Disc (Stryker Spine, Allendale, NJ) is a metal-on-metal mechanical total disc replacement device designed to treat lumbar axial back pain resulting from degenerative disc disease. The implant is intended to replace the painful intervertebral disc while maintaining or restoring the motion of the diseased functional spinal unit, thus replicating the native physiology of the spine and preventing the cascade of degenerative disease.

## DESCRIPTION OF THE DEVICE

The FlexiCore® Intervertebral Disc is a single-unit, all-metal device composed of superior and inferior baseplates articulating about a centrally located, stationary center of rotation (Fig. 41–1). The baseplates are sprayed with a titanium plasma coating to promote bone ingrowth for long-term fixation and are each flanked by short spikes that promote initial stability. The baseplate morphology features a central dome that is engineered to approximate the concavity of the native vertebral body end plates in order to maximize surface area contact, minimize subsidence, and enhance stability. This design also serves to facilitate osseous fixation and to optimize the device's center of rotation. The two baseplates articulate through a central ball-and-socket joint that establishes the device's center of rotation at a midpoint between the baseplate domes. The constrained design permits a physiologic range of motion while preventing translation of the superior and inferior vertebral bodies, minimizing forces conferred on the posterior spinal elements. The joint allows ± 15 degrees of flexion and extension and lateral bending exceeding the normal physiologic range of motion of the lumbar motion segment. An internal rotational stop is designed to avoid pathologic facet loading by preventing supraphysiologic axial rotation beyond 5 degrees. The FlexiCore® is available in six disc heights (13 to 18 mm in 1-mm increments) and two baseplate footprint sizes (28 × 35 mm and 30 × 40 mm, depth × width).

The spherical metal-on-metal bearing surface of the joint, manufactured of highly polished cobalt-chromium, is intended to maximize durability, minimize wear debris, provide overall strength, and augment the life expectancy of the device. Cobalt-chromium has been shown in the orthopaedic joint replacement literature to have a lower coefficient of friction and decreased wear when compared with other bearing surfaces including polyethylene.[1,2] Moreover, metal-on-metal bearing surfaces are not subject to the "creep" phenomenon observed with metal-on-polyethylene interfaces. During manufacture, the ball of the joint is permanently captured in the socket, creating an articulating one-piece device. This prevents the device from dislocating or separating under tension loads and permits it to be held, manipulated, and inserted by the surgeon as a single unit as it is implanted in the disc space.

Specialized insertion instrumentation facilitates device implantation, and permits the device to be inserted from multiple anterior angles. The instrumentation and insertion technique minimizes implantation misalignment and other technical errors associated with modular assembly and implantation. Repositioning is possible using the dedicated repositioners after the device has been seated in the disc space. Removal is also possible using the repositioner/extractor tools.

## INDICATIONS

- Skeletal maturity
- Failure of a minimum of 6 months of conservative treatment for degenerative disc disease
- Single-level lumbar disc disease (L1-S1) resulting in axial back pain of discogenic origin
- Radiographic evidence of degenerative disc disease

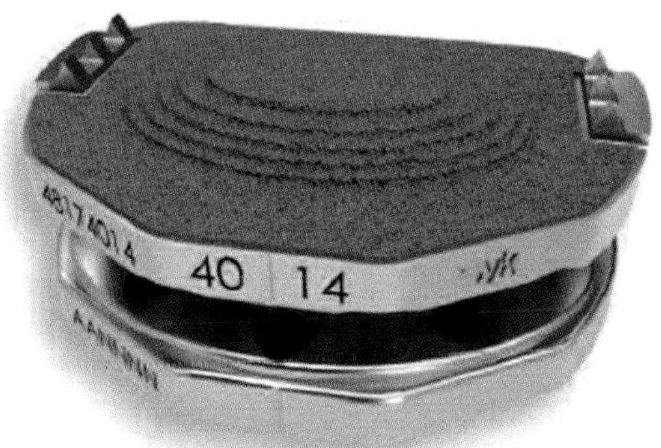

■ **FIGURE 41–1.** FlexiCore® Intervertebral Disc.

## CONTRAINDICATIONS

- History of previous lumbar fusion or bilateral open decompressive procedures
- Poor bone quality or clinically compromised vertebral body structure
- Significant end plate incompetence at the level to be treated (e.g., Schmorl's node or vertebral end plate herniation)
- Involved vertebral end plate less than 37 mm in the coronal diameter or 30 mm in the sagittal diameter
- Instability at the level to be treated (defined as any grade 1 or greater degenerative spondylolisthesis; more than 4 mm of translation [total excursion] on flexion and extension; spondylolysis, or isthmic spondylolisthesis)
- Lumbar deformity presenting as scoliosis of more than 15 degrees
- Significant facet joint disease
- Moderate to severe spinal stenosis at the level to be treated or an adjacent level
- Known infection, hepatitits, rheumatoid arthritis, autoimmune diseases, or malignancy. Patients taking medications that may interfere with bone or tissue healing.
- Morbid obesity or pregnancy
- Allergy to one of the implant materials

## OPERATIVE TECHNIQUE

### Preoperative Planning and Surgical Approach

Cross-sectional imaging on computed tomography or magnetic resonance imaging scans should be reviewed preoperatively to determine the appropriate footprint of the FlexiCore® Intervertebral Disc so that the end plate coverage does not exceed 90% of either the anterior-to-posterior depth or the lateral width of the end plate. The appropriate implant height is later determined intraoperatively with the use of distraction spacers.

Implantation of FlexiCore® Intervertebral Disc is performed with the patient under general anesthesia in the supine Trendelenburg position for an anterior or anterolateral approach to the lumbar spine. Slight elevation of the lumbar spine using an inflatable pad may be appropriate to enhance lumbar lordosis and facilitate disc space distraction, particularly in the presence of a collapsed disc space. An open or mini-open retroperitoneal approach is generally used. A Pfannenstiel mini-laparotomy transverse incision (usually 5 to 8 cm long) may be used for a single-level disc replacement from L3-S1. A midline longitudinal incision may be used if a previous midline scar is present. The necessary access to the disc space generally requires appropriate identification, ligation, and mobilization of vascular structures. For exposure of the L5-S1 interspace, the middle sacral artery and vein are identified and ligated. For exposure of the L4-L5 disc space, the iliolumbar vein should be exposed and ligated to allow the iliac artery and vein to be mobilized medially. The entire disc space must be exposed from each lateral margin, to permit centralized placement of the prosthesis.

The midline of the disc space should be determined intraoperatively and marked before commencing the discectomy by placing a metal marker in the vertebral body and verifying its location with respect to the spinous processes on an anteroposterior (AP) fluoroscopic view. For the L5-S1 disc space, the Ferguson view may allow for improved visualization.

### Discectomy and End Plate Preparation

After a localizing radiograph has been obtained to identify the proper disc space, a central annulotomy is performed approximating the width of the implant. The use of disc space distraction early in the procedure may facilitate the necessary disc removal, decompression (if indicated), and annular release to permit adequate distraction. The disc and the end plate cartilage are excised exposing subchondral bone with punctate bleeding. The lateral recesses and posterior margin of the disc space should be cleared of osteophytes or soft tissue that may prevent full distraction of the posterior disc space or proper positioning of the device. The posterior margin of the S1 end plate may exhibit an osseous ridge that may require flattening before the implant may be properly seated. The posterior longitudinal ligament and the remaining posterior annulus may be preserved so long as adequate distraction of the disc space is achieved. It may be necessary to resect the annulus and posterior longitudinal ligament in order to elevate and mobilize the posterior disc space. Loupe magnification or use of an operative microscope may facilitate disc space preparation according to surgeon discretion.

### Distraction (Disc Height Restoration)

Once the end plates have been exposed, the next step in disc space preparation is the restoration of disc space height. Adequate mobilization of the posterior intervertebral space is essential to success of the procedure. Restoration of disc space height should proceed slowly, employing suitable techniques generally used for parallel distraction of a collapsed disc space. Serial distraction may be initiated with large, thin periosteal elevators and a gentle twisting motion. When sufficient disc height has been achieved, the round distraction spacers may be used. These distraction spacers are cylindrical in shape and are available in heights ranging from 8 to 18 mm in 1-mm increments (Fig. 41–2). The round distraction spacers are used to gradually increase the height of the intervertebral space while preserving end plate integrity. The beveled geometry of the round distraction spacers coupled with the long

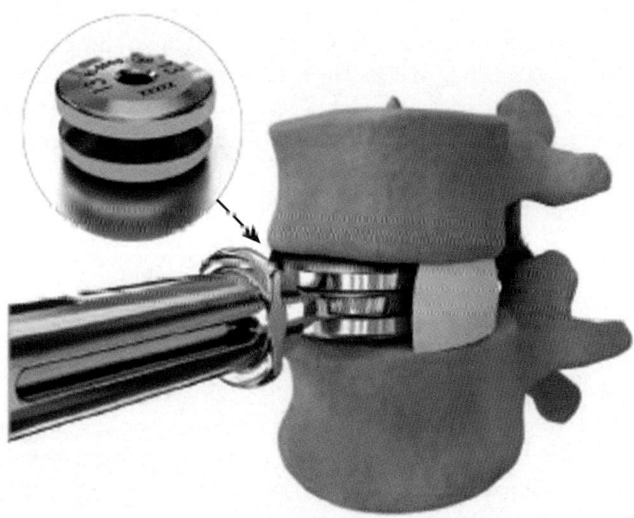

■ **FIGURE 41–2.** Insertion of the round distraction spacer with the distraction spacer handle.

lever arm of the distractor handle permits powerful but gentle distraction of the intervertebral disc space by rocking the spacer in a cephalad-caudal direction.

The FlexiCore® instrumentation set also includes distraction spacers that may be used once the disc space has been distracted to 13 mm to further distract the disc space and to determine the proper implant size (Fig. 41–3). These spacers are broader in their geometry and are shaped more similarly to the vertebral body end plates than the round distraction spacers. The design of the static distraction spacers helps to distribute the load during distraction. The distraction spacers range in height from 12 to 18 mm in 1-mm increments and are available in baseplate footprints, 28 × 35 mm and 30 × 40 mm. Each distraction spacer has a 5-degree lordotic angle such that the posterior height of the spacer is 1.8 mm less than the labeled height, and has a beveled posterior edge to ease insertion between the vertebral end plates.

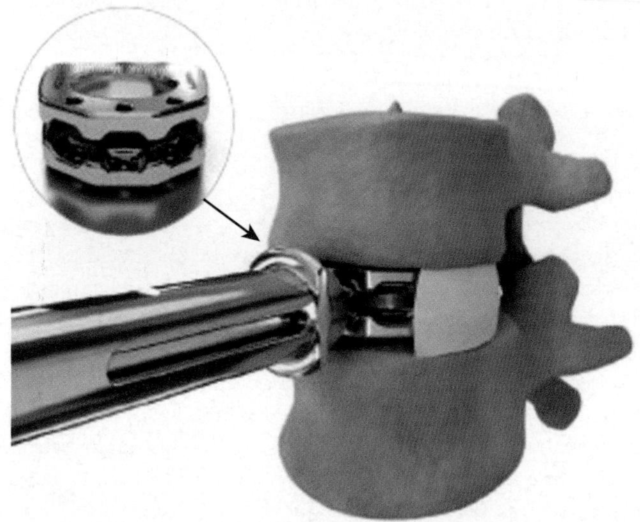

■ **FIGURE 41–3.** Insertion of the static distraction spacer with the distraction spacer handle.

The 12-mm distraction spacer is gently inserted into the disc space, rocked to loosen the surrounding ligaments, and removed. When inserted, each distractor should be centered and positioned within 2 to 3 mm of the anterior vertebral end plate margin as well as 1 to 2 mm of the posterior margin. Progressive distraction continues with sequential insertion and removal of distraction spacers of increasing size in 1-mm increments until the appropriate height of the intervertebral disc space has been restored. Resection of the remaining lateral annulus may also gradually facilitate restoration of disc space height, and this step should be performed following the removal of each successive distraction spacer. Disc space height should be maximally restored without overtensioning of the remaining annulus and ligaments or damaging the vertebral end plates.

The position of the spacer footprint in relation to the vertebral body end plates should be verified in both the coronal and sagittal planes using fluoroscopy. The static distraction spacer may be disengaged from the inserter handle in order to enhance imaging. Again, the appropriate spacer width and depth should not exceed 90% of the depth or width of the end plates. The domes of the baseplates should sit within the concavities of the vertebral end plates. In some patients, the superior end plate of the inferior vertebral body may have been flattened secondary to sclerotic changes. It is important to confirm that the inferior surface of the distraction spacer is flush with the end plate. If intraoperative imaging reveals a gap between the space and the end plate, a burr may be used to contour the end plate so that it may conform to the dome of the distraction spacer and subsequent insertion of the FlexiCore® Intervertebral Disc.

Following removal of the distraction spacer that has restored the appropriate disc space height and annular tension, the dynamic distractor (Fig. 41–4) is employed to confirm the final implant size and to ensure that the intervertebral space has sufficient height to accommodate the baseplate spikes. It is inserted between the vertebral bodies and expanded to the height of the final distractor by turning the distal knob as required. The dynamic distractor provides tactile feedback for the assessment of appropriate ligamentous laxity and confirms the optimal height of the implant. Once the optimal height has been determined, the dynamic distractor is used to further distract the disc space by an additional 1.5 to 2.0 mm in order to permit passage of the implant's baseplate spikes. This final distraction maneuver also prepares the native vertebral end plates to receive the domed baseplates of the FlexiCore® device. Care should be exercised when distracting the intervertebral disc space as excessive or aggressive distraction may result in damage to the end plates, facet joints, or soft tissues.

## Insertion of the FlexiCore® Intervertebral Disc

Once the appropriate implant size has been selected, the FlexiCore® Intervertebral Disc is secured to an impactor (Fig. 41–5). Two insertion techniques are available, each with its own impactor. The FlexiCore® may be inserted either with or without the aid of insertion ramps. For insertion of the implant without the use of ramps, the fixed-angle impactor is selected incorporating a head with a ledge that holds both baseplates of the implant firmly in a fixed angle of lordosis and prevents premature engagement of

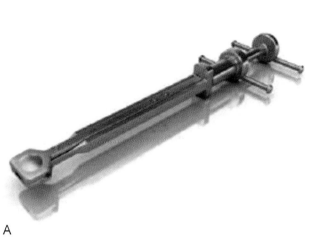

A

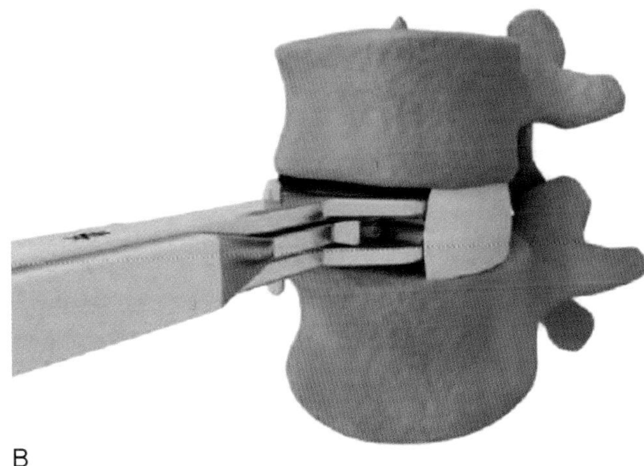

B

■ **FIGURE 41–4.** **A,** Dynamic distractor. **B,** Dynamic distractor in situ.

the baseplate spikes. The fixed-angle impactor also features a positive depth stop on both the top and bottom of the head in order to prevent overinsertion of the implant. The fixed-angle impactor should not be used with the ramps because it may result in overdistraction.

For insertion of the FlexiCore® using the insertion ramps to guide insertion, the flat plate impactor is selected. The flat plate impactor features a flat face that is held firmly in contact with the implant's lower baseplate and permits the upper baseplate to articulate during the insertion maneuver. The upper baseplate is allowed to follow the angle of the ramps during insertion, minimizing the amount of disc space distraction necessary to implant the device. The flat plate impactor has one depth stop on the bottom of the head to prevent overinsertion.

To load either of the specialized impactors, the instrument's J-hook is extended so as to engage one of the three holes in the implant's baseplate. The particular hole is selected to facilitate the desired angle of insertion. The central hole is used for a direct anterior surgical approach, whereas the offset holes are used for anterolateral approaches. When released, the spring-biased J-hook will retract to grasp the angled perimeter of the baseplates against the fitted mouth of the impactor head, preventing axial rotation during insertion. Both impactors include a locking nut on the handle shaft that is tightened to secure the implant to the impactor during insertion.

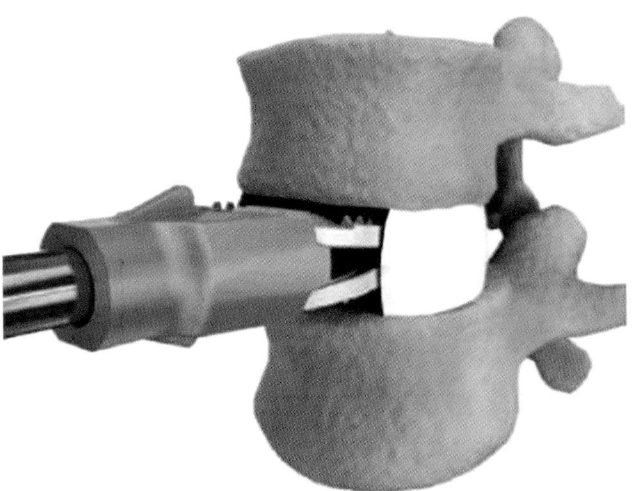

■ **FIGURE 41–5.** Insertion of the FlexiCore® Intervertebral Disc with the fixed-angle impactor.

The fixed-angle impactor can be used alone to insert the implant into the intervertebral space, similar to the manner in which a femoral ring allograft is inserted during an anterior lumbar interbody fusion procedure. The posterior edges of the baseplates are positioned between the vertebral end plates, and the implant is advanced into the space. The locking nut is loosened, and the flange is advanced to disengage the J-hook. Moderate force may then be used against the impactor handle to insert the implant to the appropriate AP depth. Excessive posterior insertion of the device is prevented by the positive stops on the impactor heads. The domes of the baseplates should be seated within the native vertebral end plate concavities. The final position of the FlexiCore® device should then be confirmed radiographically.

Alternately, the ramps may be used to distract the intervertebral space as the implant is inserted (Fig. 41–6). The ramps are provided in two sizes that correspond to the 35- and 40-mm baseplate widths. The pair of ramps is coupled at their proximal ends with a C-Clip connector. The ramps converge toward one another, such that their proximal ends are separated to receive the implant between them (previously loaded on the flat plate impactor). The distal ends converge toward one another to meet at the intervertebral space and are inserted between the vertebral end plates. The implant is inserted between the ramps and advanced into the intervertebral space. The implant spikes ride in grooves on the inner surfaces of the ramps, guiding the implant linearly. As the implant is advanced, the height of the implant forces the distal ends of the ramps to separate, distracting the intervertebral space to the requisite height for implantation of the device. As the implant is inserted using the ramps, it is important to ensure that the impactor handle is parallel to the lower map so that the locking nut has sufficient clearance as it nears the end of the ramps. Following insertion, the ramps are removed sequentially.

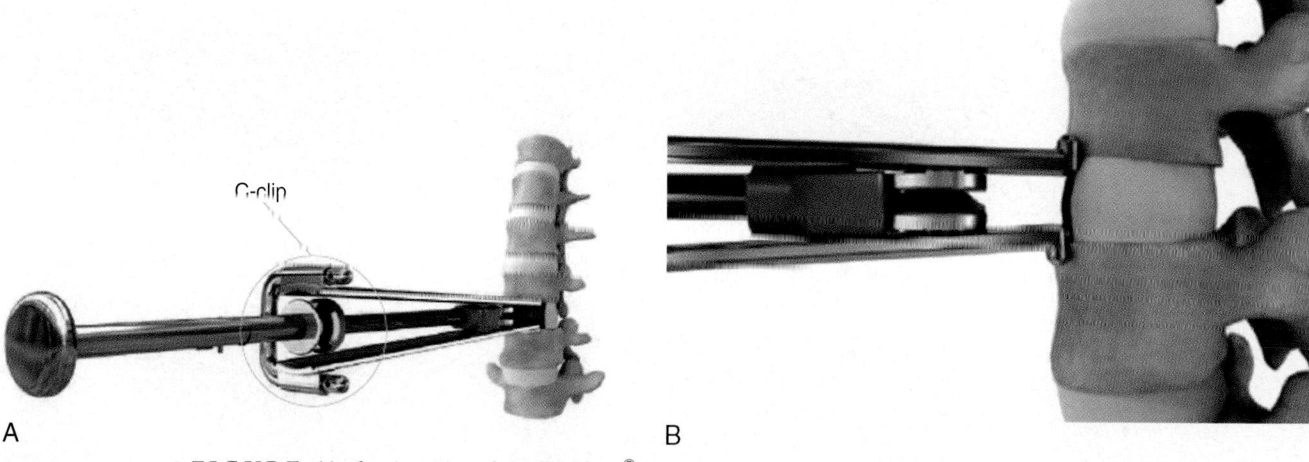


■ **FIGURE 41–6.** Insertion of the FlexiCore® Intervertebral Disc with the aid of the insertion ramps.

### Verification of Implant Size and Placement

The FlexiCore® Intervertebral Disc is appropriately positioned when the baseplate domes are seated within the concavities of the adjacent vertebral body end plates (Fig. 41–7). The implant position should be confirmed with fluoroscopy so that it is centered in the sagittal plane, and positioned 2 to 3 mm within the anterior margin and 1 to 2 mm within the posterior margin of the end plate. The implant should not protrude outside the anterior margin of the vertebral end plates. Ideal positioning entails the device being seated against the posterior annulus, parallel alignment of the baseplates with the adjacent end plates, and a central position in relation to the vertebral bodies. The end plates should be visually inspected for fractures. If fractures are present, consideration should be made of revising the surgery to fusion.

### Repositioning (or Extracting) the FlexiCore® Intervertebral Disc

If the lateral or AP images indicate suboptimal positioning of the implant, repositioning can be performed using the repositioner/extractors (Figs. 41–8 and 41–9). Anterior, right offset, and left offset instruments are available, each with a pair of pins on its distal end that can be inserted into any pair of holes in the upper or lower baseplates, thus providing multiple surgical approach angles. The repositioner/extractors may be used individually or in tandem to grasp the upper or lower implant baseplates. Once the pins are engaged, the device can be repositioned in the lateral and AP planes, as well as rotated axially. The repositioner/extractors can also be used to extract the implant by similarly engaging implant baseplates and withdrawing the handle's flange.

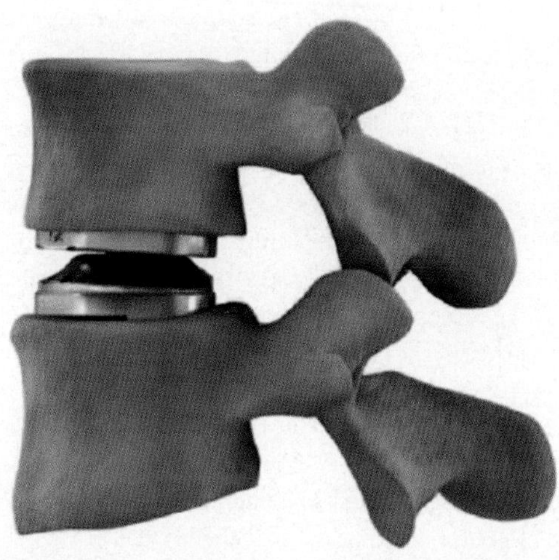

■ **FIGURE 41–7.** Lateral view of the FlexiCore® in situ.

### Closure

Standard closure procedures for anterior or anterolateral spine surgery are followed.

## POSTOPERATIVE CARE

The goal of postoperative rehabilitation is to return the patient to normal activity as expeditiously as possible without jeopardizing healing. The patient should wear a lumbar corset for 2 to 3 weeks to support healing of the abdominal incision, depending on patient comfort. The patient's rehabilitation program should be individually tailored to his or her needs, taking into account age, stage of healing, general health, and physical condition. Return to work is dependent on specific vocation. Patients should be restricted from heavy lifting until full rehabilitation has been completed, typically after 8 to 12 weeks.

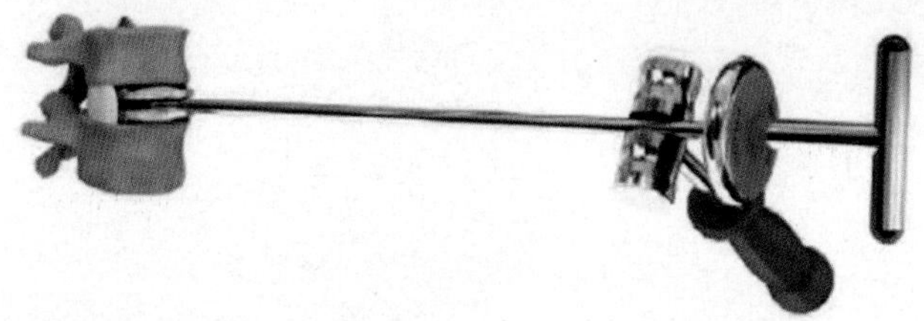

■ **FIGURE 41–8.** Extraction of the FlexiCore® Intervertebral Disc with the repositioner/extractor and slotted mallet.

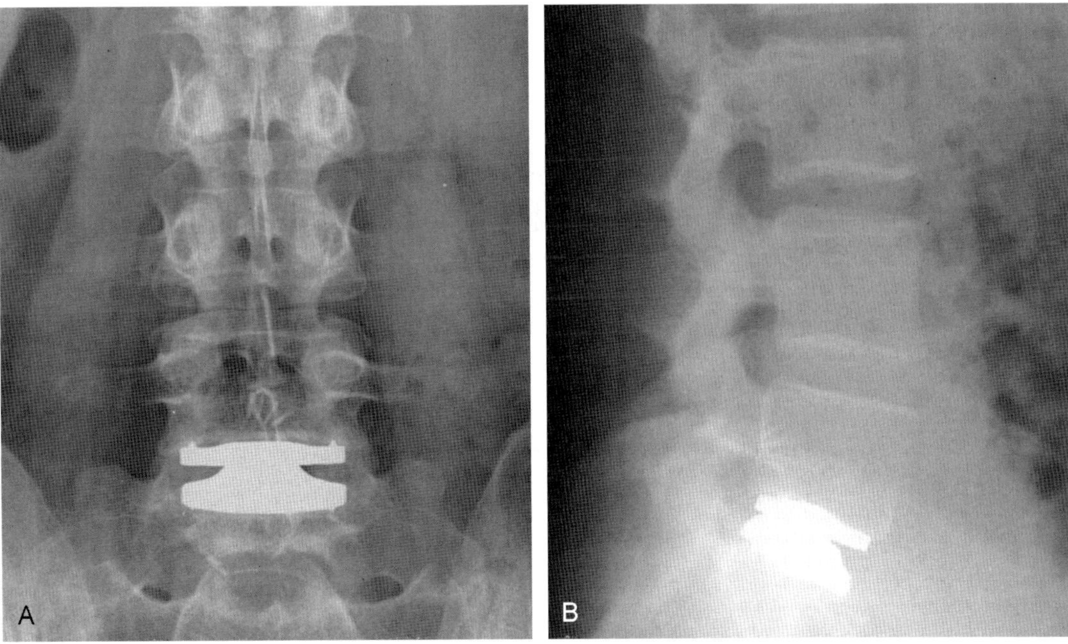


■ **FIGURE 41–9.** FlexiCore® Intervertebral Disc anteroposterior and lateral radiographs.

## CLINICAL DATA

Clinical results have been presented from four of the study sites under the IDE protocol on 103 patients of the 400 patients randomized for the treatment of symptomatic lumbar DDD. Patients were randomized in a 2:1 fashion (FlexiCore: Fusion) yielding 66 patients treated with the FlexiCore® (F) and 37 patients treated with anteroposterior fusion (C). Disability and pain were assessed using the Oswestry Disability Index (ODI) and the Visual Analog Scale (VAS), respectively (Figs. 41–10 and 41–11). Prospective data were collected preoperatively and postoperatively at 6 weeks and 3, 6, 12, and 24 months. The mean ODI scores favored the FlexiCore® at all time points, and the mean VAS score favored the FlexiCore® at both 12 and 24 months. The mean ODI scores were 60(F) and 60(C) preoperatively, 37(F) and 48(C) at 6 weeks, 29(F) and 32(C) at 3 months, 27(F) and 30(C) at 6 months, 25(F) and 32(C) at 12 months, and 22(F) and 28(C) at 24 months. The mean VAS scores were 86(F) and 83(C) preoperatively, 30(F) and 36(C) at 6 weeks, 34(F) and 29(C) at 3 months, 33(F) and 30(C) at 6 months, 28(F) and 33(C) at 12 months, and 33(F) and 37(C) at 24 months. The average operative time was 82 minutes for the FlexiCore® group and 170 minutes for the fusion group. The average estimated blood loss was 76 mL for the FlexiCore® group and 99 mL for the fusion group. The average hospital stay was 2.5 days for the FlexiCore® group and 3.3 days for the fusion group.[3]

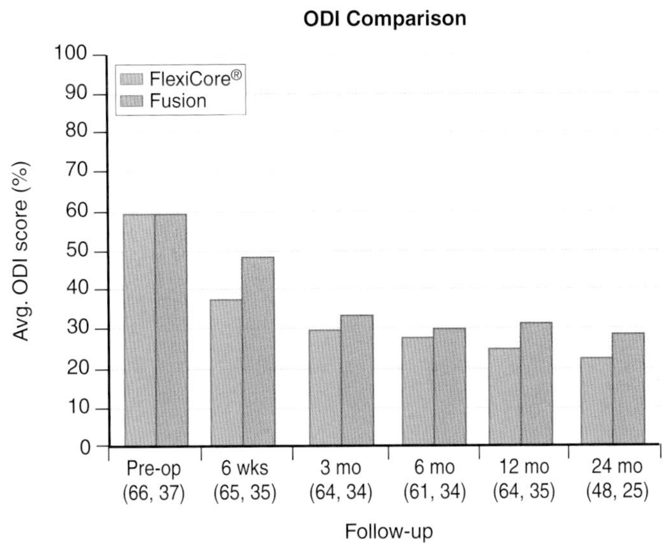


■ **FIGURE 41–10.** Oswestry Disability Index comparison.

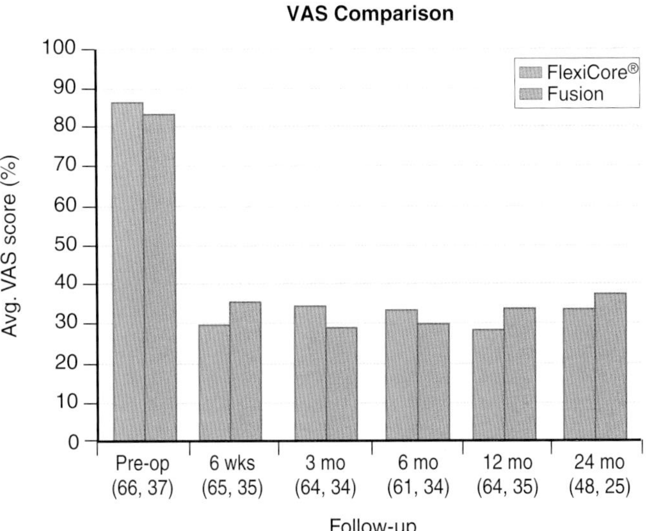


■ **FIGURE 41–11.** Visual Analog Score comparison.

## COMPLICATIONS AND AVOIDANCE

Complications can stem from inappropriate selection of a surgical candidate. Patients who do not have true discogenic back pain, who have unrecognized instability, or who suffer from multilevel symptomatic disc degeneration are poorly indicated for disc replacement surgery. Despite optimal patient selection, as with all major surgery, disc replacement is not without its own risks and concerns. Potential complications of disc replacement surgery include those traditionally associated with anterior lumbar interbody fusion. Intraoperative complications may include inadvertent peritoneum violation as well as vascular injury. The common iliac vessels, aorta, iliolumbar vein, and inferior vena cava may be at risk for injury from exposure, retraction, or loosening of the applied ligature. In a recent, large series of patients undergoing anterior lumbar spinal surgery, the risk of major vascular injury was found to be relatively low at 1.9%.[4] Deep vein thrombosis can occur from manipulation of the great vessels and requires treatment with anticoagulation. In men, injury to the superior hypogastric plexus from dissection or the use of electrocautery during the surgical approach can lead to retrograde ejaculation in a reported 0.4% to 17.5% of cases.[5–7] This can be a serious complication for a man of reproductive age, and preoperative sperm donation is often recommended. The transabdominal or retroperitoneal approach can yield a prolonged postoperative ileus necessitating insertion of a nasogastric tube. As with many abdominal surgeries, the approach also carries the risk of denervation of the abdominal wall with resulting muscular atony as well as the risk of incisional hernia. As with all surgery, especially those involving implantable instrumentation, infection can occur but can be minimized with perioperative antibiotics and meticulous sterile techniques.

In addition, device-specific complications can occur with disc replacement surgery. The importance of radiographic confirmation of final device positioning in both the AP and lateral planes cannot be overemphasized. Misplacement of the implant can disrupt the replication of normal spinal kinematics. Failure to adequately replicate the physiologic kinematics of the lumbar spine may predispose the patient to early facet joint degeneration. Anterior malpositioning can result from inadequate resection of posterior disc annulus or posterior osteophytes. Conversely, posterior malpositioning can result from excision or rupture of the posterior longitudinal ligament allowing posterior implantation. An oversized or undersized prosthesis can permit insufficient or excessive motion at the specific level. Without true motion preservation, whether due to heterotopic ossification or other causes, these devices will merely act as interbody spacers and lead to spontaneous fusion. The implant may also subside or migrate owing to overzealous end plate preparation or unrecognized instability. Prosthesis migration or extrusion, may lead to device failure and serious vascular complications.

## DISCUSSION

The FlexiCore® Intevertebral Disc incorporates a number of novel design characteristics. The single-unit design of the FlexiCore® total disc replacement has a number of advantages. The tension-bearing structure is designed to prevent separation of the bearing surfaces as well as dislocation or extrusion of the bearing surface elements. Contrary to other designs employing modular components that have exhibited the potential to dissociate, the entire device must become loosened before is likely to migrate or extrude. Implantation as a single unit facilitates proper alignment and is anticipated to reduce technical implantation error. The one-piece configuration should also serve to minimize the necessary device inventory.

The baseplate domes and the central ball-and-socket joint are designed to establish a stationary center of rotation that is centrally located between the end plates and slightly posterior to the mid line, closely matching the center of rotation of a healthy, natural, native intervertebral disc. An internal stop that limits axial rotation beyond the natural range of motion is included to prevent over-rotation and pathologic facet loading. The metal-on-metal bearing surfaces of highly polished cobalt-chromium are anticipated to maintain sphericity over the life of the device and minimize wear debris. Because the device design is free of polyethylene, the theoretical risk of osteolysis is minimized. The titanium plasma-sprayed bone ingrowth domes are engineered to fit flush within the concavities of the vertebral end plates and to assist in optimal early and late bony fixation. Initial device fixation is attained by low-profile spikes flanking the central dome. This feature is designed to maximize end plate and vertebral body preservation in order to prevent subsidence and facilitate revision if necessary.

When performed in an appropriately indicated patient, total disc replacement has a number of potential advantages over spinal fusion. Both procedures have the ability to aid or eliminate axial back pain. Disc arthroplasty, in particular, is designed to restore the functional biomechanics of the spine and to preserve spinal motion. By preserving or reestablishing motion at the functional spinal unit, the goals are twofold. Lumbar flexion-extension is preserved or improved, and the cascade of adjacent spinal segment degeneration may be impeded or possibly prevented entirely. Following implantation, a disc replacement articulates immediately, with recovery consisting of abdominal wound and tissue healing alone. This period of recovery is substantially shorter than that required for solid spinal fusion. Moreover, disc replacement surgery is a stand-alone anterior procedure compared with many spinal fusions that require a posterior approach either instead of, or in addition to, an anterior exposure. Thus, there is no additional recovery required from a posterior procedure or need for the patient to wear a postoperative orthosis. Total disc replacement is a promising development in lumbar spine surgery for the treatment of degenerative disc disease. The FlexiCore® Intervertebral Disc incorporates a number of important advances in motion preservation technology.

## REFERENCES


1. Chan FW, Bobyn JD, Medley JB, et al: The Otto Aufranc Award: Wear and lubrication of metal-on-metal hip implants. Clin Orthop Relat Res 36:10–24, 1999.
2. Dorr LD, Wan Z, Longjohn DB, et al: Total hip arthroplasty with use of the Metasul metal-on-metal articulation: Four to seven-year results. J Bone Joint Surg Am 82:789–798, 2000.
3. Tibbs R, Sasso R, Miz G, Theofilos C: Prospective, randomized trial of lumbar metal-on-metal total disc replacement: Initial treatment of

degenerative disc disease. IMAST 14th Annual International Meeting on Advanced Spinal Techniques, Paradise Island, Bahamas 2007.
4. Brau SA, Delamarter RB, Schiffman ML, et al: Vascular injury during anterior lumbar surgery. Spine J 4:409–412, 2004.
5. Flynn JC, Price CT: Sexual complications of anterior fusion of the lumbar spine. Spine 9:489–492, 1984.
6. Mayer HM: A new microsurgical technique for minimally invasive anterior lumbar interbody fusion. Spine 22:691–699; discussion 700, 1997.
7. Tiusanen H, Seitsalo S, Osterman K, Soini J: Retrograde ejaculation after anterior interbody lumbar fusion. Eur Spine J 4:339–342, 1995.

CHAPTER 42

# Kineflex

Ulrich Reinhard Hähnle, Malan De Villiers, and Ian R. Weinberg

## KEY POINTS

- The Kineflex disc is a recentering, unconstrained, metal-on-metal mechanical disc prosthesis.
- A cervical and a lumbar disc are currently Conformit Europeane (CE) certified and are also being evaluated in U.S. Food and Drug Administration (FDA) Pre-Market Approval (PMA) randomized, controlled trials.
- The Kineflex disc was designed primarily for patients with advanced motion segment degeneration using a simple insertion technique allowing powerful distraction and posterior placement within the disc space.
- The insertion of the assembled prosthesis enables free articulation of the end plates, allowing the superior and inferior end plates to be advanced independently.
- Good short-term clinical results have been achieved at a minimum follow-up of 2 years.

## INTRODUCTION

Adjacent-level degeneration is a major concern in lumbar fusion operations.[1,2] Lumbar artificial disc replacement is an alternative to arthrodesis. The purpose of the intervention is to restore the intervertebral segment stability and mobility and protect the adjacent levels against nonphysiological loading conditions. Surgical insertions of lumbar disc prostheses using a steel ball were first published by Fernström.[3] It failed clinically essentially because of subsidence of the implant into the bony end plate. Modern-type total lumbar disc replacement commenced in 1984 with the insertion of the first generation CHARITÉ (DePuy Spine Inc., Raynham, MA) disc prosthesis (CHARITÉ SB I).[4] The mechanism of the prosthesis was carried through to the third-generation device that is still being used today (CHARITÉ SB III).

Subsequently more constrained lumbar disc prostheses have been developed. Three of these prostheses are currently being evaluated in U.S. Food and Drug Administration (FDA) studies (ProDisc, Synthes, West Chester, PA; Maverick disc, Medtronic Sofamor Danek, Memphis, TN; FlexiCore disc, Stryker Spine, Allendale, NJ). Despite major advances in the disc insertion technique and design, difficulties persist with the correct midline and posterior placement of the prosthesis within the disc spaces, even in experienced hands.[5]

The Kineflex disc prosthesis was originally named Centurion disc. It was developed in Centurion, located between Pretoria and Johannesburg in South Africa. The main objectives in the development of this prosthesis were an unconstrained/semiconstrained but recentering mechanism, to facilitate reliable midline and posterior placement of the implant within the disc space in severely degenerated disc spaces and to develop a simple and safe implantation technique, with the implantation being executed through a minimal invasive approach.

## INDICATIONS/CONTRAINDICATIONS

Inclusion criteria at our center were age of 18 to 65 years, mechanical back and leg pain, symptomatic single or multilevel degenerative disc disease at the L2-L3, L3-L4, L4-L5, or L5-S1 levels confirmed on x-ray studies, magnetic resonance imaging, or provocative discography. Further inclusion criteria included recurrent disc herniation, broad-based central disc herniation without sequestration, and junctional failure after previous fusion. In all patients, supervised conservative treatment of at least 6 months had failed. Only the symptomatic levels on clinical examination and discography were replaced.

Exclusion criteria were general contraindications, such as severe obesity, osteoporosis, tumor, or infection. Spinal exclusion factors were thoracic kyphosis of more than 60 degrees, idiopathic lumbar scoliosis of more than 30 degrees, previous wide laminectomy with destabilization of the facet complex, spondylolisis or spondylolisthesis, greater than Meyerding Grade 1 of the level to be replaced, bony spinal stenosis, and sequestrated disc prolapse tracking up or down behind the vertebral body. Other contraindications were previous retroperitoneal surgery, advanced vascular pathology, and single kidney.

Advanced facet arthritis was not an exclusion criterion unless osteophyte formation from the facet resulted in bony canal or recess stenosis. Spinal or lateral recess stenosis caused by soft tissue (disc, ligamentum flavum, or joint capsule) was not considered a contraindication for disc replacement if proper decompression during surgery, by means of direct or indirect decompression, could be anticipated on preoperative imaging.

## DESCRIPTION OF THE DEVICE

The Kineflex disc (Spinal Motion, Inc., Mountainview, CA) represents a disc prosthesis with a mechanism that is unconstrained but re-centering, resulting in a mobile center of rotation. The amount of constraint lies between the CHARITÉ disc prosthesis and Mobidisc (LDR, Troyes, France) on the unconstrained side and the ProDisc, Maverick, and FlexiCore disc prostheses on the constrained side. The mechanism comprises two metal end plates congruently articulating over a sliding core that is positioned posterior to the center of and in between the end plates (Fig. 42–1). The inferior end plate has a retaining ring that limits the excursion of the inferior articulation and prevents dislodgement of the core. The superior end plate has no retaining ring. The angle of motion allowed by the articulating mechanism from the neutral position is 12 degrees into flexion-extension, left or right side bending. This is true for the lumbar as well as for the cervical disc (Kineflex|C).

The end plates and core are made of cobalt-chromium-molybdenum alloy (Biodur CCM Plus, Carpenter Technologies, Reading, PA).

The integrating side of the end plate, facing the bony end plate, is flat and oval shaped, and has a small 1.5-mm wide midline fin with an oblique leading edge and two transverse holes which follows a pre-cut insertion groove but also allows self-cutting of a groove if required. The side of the end plate has multiple machined sharp serrations for primary fixation. Only the central portion of the surface adjacent to the center fin is smooth to allow riding of the adjacent prosthesis along the 'slotted end plate distracter.' The entire leading edge of the end plates is beveled toward the bone side, to avoid cutting into the bony end plate during the insertion procedure.

Both the inferior and superior end plates are manufactured in three different sizes (small, medium, and large). The inferior end plate is manufactured in three different angles coupled with three different heights (0 degree, 5.5 mm; 5 degrees, 6.5 mm; and 10 degrees, 7.25mm). The superior end plate has no angle but two different heights (5.5 to 6.5 mm). As a result, the overall height of the prosthesis ranges from 11 mm to 13.75 mm.

## BACKGROUND OF SCIENTIFIC TESTING/CLINICAL OUTCOMES

### Preclinical Testing

Substantial preclinical mechanical testing was performed on the Kineflex arthroplasty, including static testing, monoaxial fatigue testing, and wear testing. All tests were performed using finished, sterilized devices, with the 5-×40- mm end plate size and a core. As noted earlier, there is only one core size; therefore, the size of the load-bearing area on each end plate, which conforms to the core, is the same for all end plate diameters.

#### Static Compression and Static Shear Testing

Static compression and shear testing were performed in accordance with American Society for Testing and Materials F-04.25.05.01 Draft I (February 2003) Item Z8924Z. The tests were conducted in an Instron machine, and compression of the six disc samples were increased until mechanical failure or a preset ultimate load was reached. The yield displacement, yield load, ultimate displacement, ultimate load, and stiffness were recorded. The results demonstrated that there was no height reduction in any of the samples as would be expected with a metal-on-metal construct. All loads applied to the assembled samples were in excess of 25 kN. Thus, because the maximum load-carrying capacity of vertebral bone is approximately 5 to 8.2 kN,[6] the compressive strength of the Kineflex Prosthetic Disc (KPD) substantially exceeds that of the vertebral bone.

#### Dynamic and Shear Fatigue Testing

Samples were tested under cyclic axial and shear compressive loading to assess the suitability of the fatigue resistance of the device for in vivo use. Samples were immersed in a physiologically buffered saline bath at 37°C throughout the test to simulate in vivo conditions. A test frequency of 5Hz was applied. Loads varied

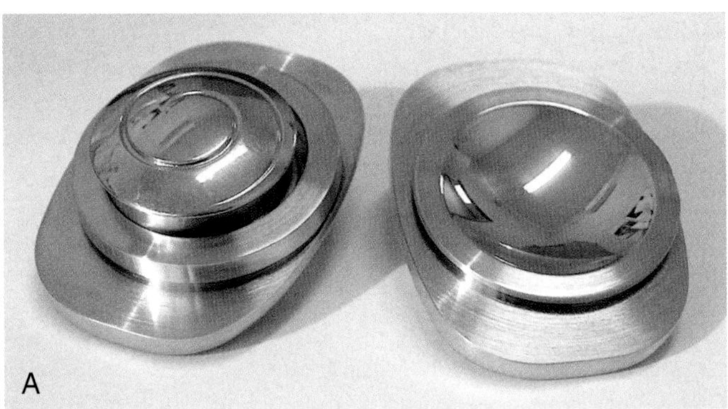

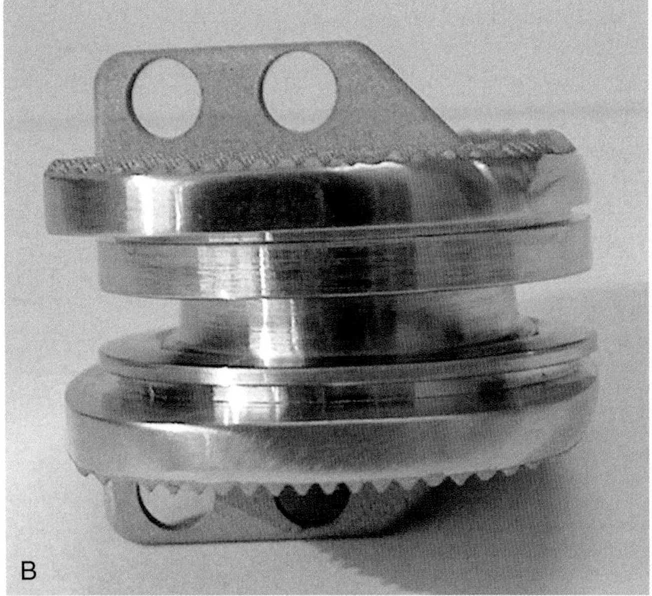

■ **FIGURE 42–1.** Kineflex metal-on-metal **(A)** mechanism. **(B)** Unit assembled.

cyclically between the maximum value of 2,000 N and 10% of the maximum, or 200 N. When viewed in terms of an average in vivo load, the results demonstrated no measurable dimensional changes in either the end plates or the core in what equates to 10 years of usage.

### Wear Testing

To evaluate the amount and size of wear particles that may be generated by the arthroplasty in vivo, five test samples were cyclically loaded in a multiaxial motion simulator for 10 million cycles. Testing was performed at a frequency of 5Hz. A constant 1,200-N load was applied throughout the wear test. A total cyclic range of motion of ± 7.1 degrees of lateral bending, a cyclic range of motion of ± 7.1 degrees of flexion-extension bending, and ± 4 degrees of axial rotation were applied.

Test specimens were immersed in a 37°C saline bath throughout testing to simulate in vivo conditions. After every 1,000,000 cycles, the disc and meniscus were weighed, and a dimensional check of height and diameter was performed. Visual inspection was also performed, and a photographic record was compiled.

Weight and dimensional measurements of the prosthesis (end plates and core) performed after every million cycles showed an average volumetric wear rate of 1.39 $mm^3$ per million cycles. Mass loss was approximately 115 mg, for an average of 11.5 mg per million cycles. This represents a loss of only approximately 0.1% of the total prosthesis mass over 10 million cycles. Dimensional changes in the core were small, with an average height loss of less than 0.3 mm; no core exhibited any change in diameter. The degree of dimensional change observed with respect to core height does not interfere with the functionality of the device.

The mean wear particle size was approximately 0.5 μm across all samples. Analysis of the form factor of the wear particles indicates that they were generally slightly elongated. Evaluation of the particles showed that they had a flake-like morphology when greater than 1 μm in size, but were granular when less than 1 μm in size.

In vivo animal data demonstrating that wear debris of this type and quantity are unlikely to generate an adverse biologic response is available. Cunningham et al[7] evaluated the neural and systemic tissue response to cobalt alloy particulate debris in an in vivo rabbit model up to 6 months. They placed 4 mg of cobalt alloy particles directly on the dura and compared the results with rabbits that had a sham procedure of dural exposure alone. All cobalt alloy particles used were less than 5 μ in diameter, and 70% of all particles were between 2 and 3 μ in diameter. It should be noted that although the majority of particles were in the 2- to 3-μ range, more than 1.03 × 1010 submicron particles were injected.

At 3 months, the number of macrophage-expressing cytokines localized within the spinal cord and overlying tissues indicated no significant differences compared with the control group.

Despite regions heavily laden with metallic particulate, histiocystic reaction, and cytokine activity, the spinal cords indicated normal distribution of myelin and the intracellular neurofibrilla network. There was no evidence of cellular apoptosis, and all specimens were characterized as without significant histopathologic changes.

The quantity of particles applied in the Cunningham study, together with the one-time application of these particles directly to the dura, represents an extreme worst-case scenario compared with the anticipated wear of the Kineflex over time. The Cunningham study used a single application of particles, compared with the gradual release of particles over time that would be expected in vivo. Based on these results, there is low risk of any adverse biologic response to the wear particles generated by the Kineflex, even under the worst-case conditions of the in vitro wear test with respect to loads, motions, and the saline lubricant environment.

### Biomechanics of the Kineflex Lumbar Disc Prosthesis

The design of the Kineflex prosthesis allows for high congruence of articulating components over its full range of articulation. However, the three-part design allows for a self-centering but relatively unconstrained motion, which enables translation of end plates with respect to each other, as opposed to ball-and-socket (two-part) designs, which are highly constrained. The instantaneous axis of rotation of the functional spinal unit (FSU) does indeed also incorporate a translating component, which is essential to allow flexion-extension motion in the three-point support structure of the FSU. The in vitro biomechanics of the Kineflex prosthesis was evaluated in harvested spines and compared with untreated harvested spines by Denis Di Angelo et al,[8] who concluded that there was no significant difference in the motion response between the Kineflex disc and the harvested spine conditions except in extension, where the motion was 73% of the untreated condition. The center of rotation of the Kineflex disc is located posterior of center, which also mimics the FSU condition.

## Clinical Testing

The primary clinical outcome measures for this study were pain relief and functional improvement as assessed by the Oswestry Disability Index (ODI) and our own questionnaire. Questionnaires (ODI and our own questionnaire) were completed by the patient preoperatively, at 6 weeks, 3 months, 6 months, and yearly in conjunction with the regular follow-up examinations. In addition to the outcome data, general demographic information, operative data, and data pertaining to radiologic examination were collected.

Our own questionnaire was designed by first and last authors and has not been validated. The patient is asked about his or her satisfaction with the outcome of the treatment operation (options: excellent, good, fair, poor) and to state if he or she would undergo the same operation again or recommend it to friends (options: yes, don't know, no). Furthermore, the patient is asked to gauge his or her pain in the last 2 weeks preoperatively and at the time of completing the questionnaire on a scale of 1(no pain) to 10 (pain as bad as it can be). No differentiation between leg and back pain is made.

### Clinical Presentation and Evaluation

Baseline characteristics of the study population are shown in Table 42–1. Our first 100 patients have reached 2-year follow-up. They constitute a heterogenous study population, with 41% having undergone previous open lumbar surgery (see Table 42–1).

TABLE 42–1. Preoperative Data of Study Population ($n$ = 100 Patients)

| Factor | Number of Patients ($n$ = 100) |
|---|---|
| Gender | |
| Male | 57 |
| Female | 43 |
| Age (years) | 44.9 (23–63) |
| Height (cm) | 174.6 ± 9.6 (154–196) |
| Weight (kg) | 81.3 ± 15.6 (47–138) |
| Pain duration (month) | 63.5 ± 74.6 (5–400) |
| Nonoperative care | |
| Physical therapy | 99 |
| Chiropractic | 61 |
| Acupuncture | 25 |
| Previous surgery | |
| Rizotomy | 15 |
| Discectomy | 32 |
| Laminectomy | 20 |
| Fusion | 13 |
| Smoking | 39 |
| Nonsmoking | 61 |

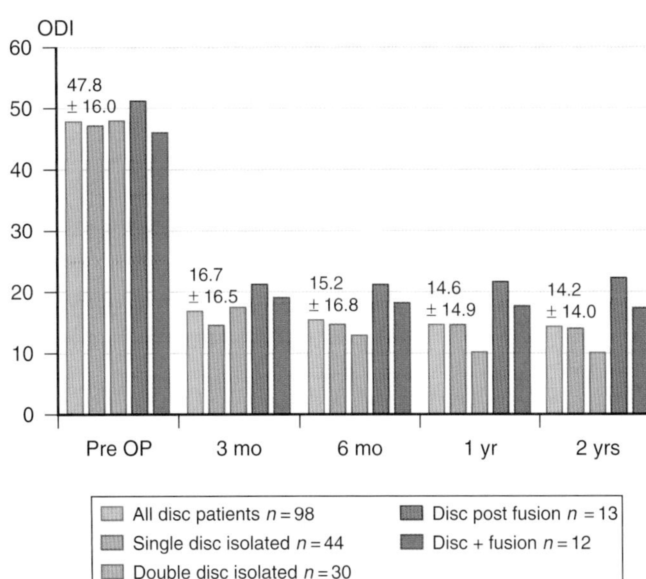


■ **FIGURE 42–2.** Oswestry Disability Index (ODI) preoperatively and at different follow-up intervals.

Clinical outcome assessment was available for 99 of 100 patients at 1 year and at 97% at 2 years.

Sixty-nine patients underwent single-level disc replacements, and 31 patients had two levels replaced. Three of the patients with single-level surgery later received a second-level lumbar disc replacement at 7, 9, and 10 months after the index procedure, respectively. Twelve patients underwent fusions at another level (hybrid cases) during the index procedure. Four of these patients had previous discectomies. Thirteen patients presented with adjacent level disc disease after previous instrumented posterolateral fusion surgery (one to seven previous operations). Another 28 patients in this series, who underwent single- or double-level disc replacements, had one to four previous discectomies or laminotomies, or both (see Table 42–1).

Operative times, estimated blood losses, and postoperative hospital stays are shown in Table 42–2.

### Recovery and Patient Satisfaction

Hospital stay averaged 2.8 ± 0.8 days (2 to 8 days). Eighty-six patients were in employment at the time of the operation (Fig. 42–2). All but one patient went back to their previous occupation at an average of 31.0 ± 16.1 days.

TABLE 42–2. Mean Operative Time, Blood Loss and Length of Hospital Stay

| Factor | Number of Patients |
|---|---|
| Operative time (minutes): all patients | 130 (45–400) |
| Operative time (minutes): single-level patients (48% at L4-L5 level) | 95.3 ± 28.3 |
| Estimated blood loss (milliliters): all patients | 282 ± 301 |
| Estimated blood loss (milliliters): single-level patients (48% at L4-L5 level) | 145.7 ± 153.2 |
| Hospital stay (days) all patients | 2.86 ± 0.8 |

The pain score (scale from 1 to 10) of all patients decreased from 9.16 ± 1.00 preoperatively to 2.88 ± 2.34 at 1-year follow-up (2.78 ± 2.2 at 2 years).

The ODI improved significantly from 47.8 ± 16 to 14.6 ± 14.9 at 1 year (14.2 ± 14.0 at 2 years) ($P$ <0.01) (see Fig. 42–2).

Patients with double-level disc replacement scored better regarding pain score improvement as well as ODI improvement at 1 year as compared with those patients with single-level disc replacements ($P$ <0.01) (see Fig. 42–2).

Patients in the isolated single- or double-level disc replacement group had poorer outcome scores if they had undergone previous discectomies and/or laminectomies ($n$ = 28) compared with patients without previous surgery (control: $n$ = 46). Their ODI improved from 50.3 ± 19.2 to 16.5 ± 17.2 (control: from 46.1 ± 15.3 to 11.0 ± 15.3 and their pain score from 9.17 ± 1.2 to 3.1 ± 1.9 (control: 9.06 ± 1.1 to 2.41 ± 2.2) at 1 year.

At 1 year, 87% (at 2 years 90%) of patients considered their result good or excellent, and 90% (92% at 2 years) would undergo the same operation again or recommend it to friends.

## OPERATIVE TECHNIQUES

In our center, all procedures are performed on an electrical radiolucent table with the patient in supine position under general anesthesia. Image control is used preoperatively to determine the level of the skin incision and to preoperatively adjust rotation of the patient's disc space to be instrumented. Cell saver, to harvest the patient's red blood cells and to re-transfuse (if necessary), is used routinely. For a right-handed surgeon, the procedure is performed from the right side of the operation table. In case of a right-sided retroperitoneal approach, the exposure is performed with the surgeon standing on the left, only to change to right side once the spine is reached. A transverse skin incision centered over the midline is used in one- to three-level exposures.

Depending on the level, a left- or right-sided retroperitoneal approach is performed along the posterior rectus sheet. For levels L4-L5 and higher, the transversus abdominis fascia may have to be incised from the arcade ligament cranially after mobilization from the peritoneum. Segmental vessels are ligated, if required, and the large vessels are mobilized off the relevant disc space. The level to be instrumented is verified under image control. Hohmann retractors are used for exposure and attached to the frame retractor throughout the insertion process. After midline annuloplasty, the nucleus, the inner layers of the annulus, and the cartilaginous end plate are removed. This is followed by sequential stretching of the disc space using wedged end plate distracters. If necessary, any sequestrated disc pieces or osteophytes are removed.

## Insertion of the Prosthesis

The disc is inserted as a single unit with a freely mobile mechanism during the insertion process to facilitate posterior placement within the vertebral disc space (Fig. 42–3). During insertion, the end plates of the prosthesis can be advanced individually, rotating

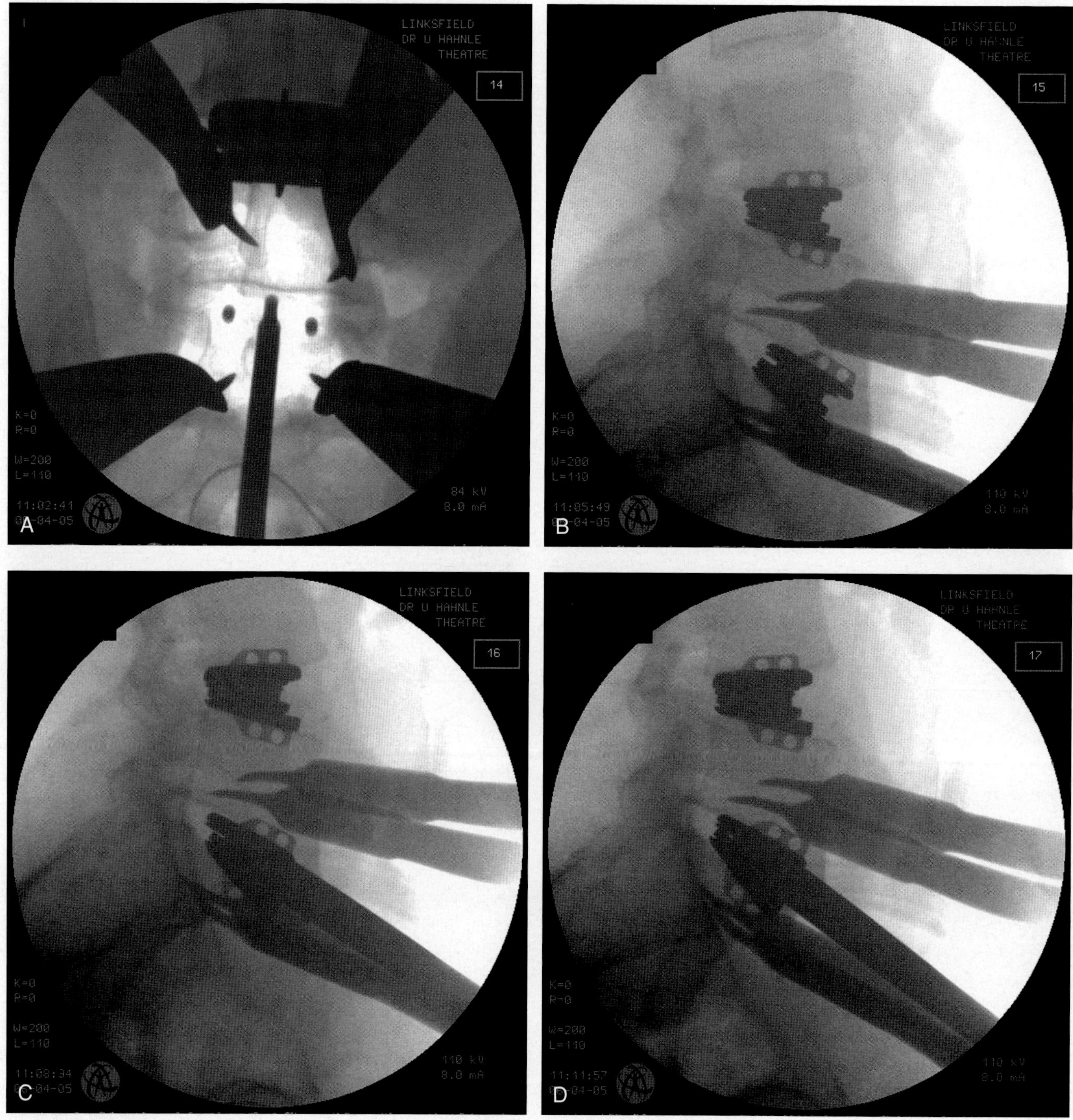


■ **FIGURE 42–3.** Insertion technique as seen on intraoperative radiographs. **A,** Midline finder in position. **B,** Initial engagement of the prosthesis into the disc space. **C, D,** Sequential advancement of the prosthesis into final position.

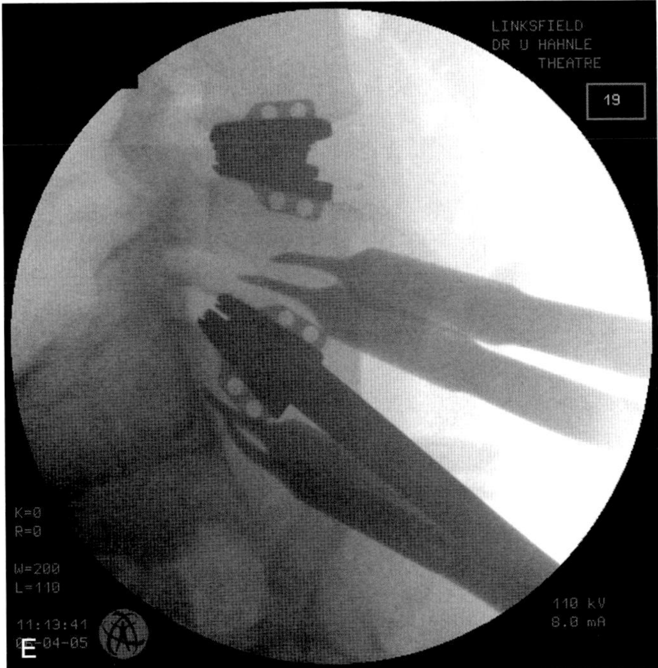


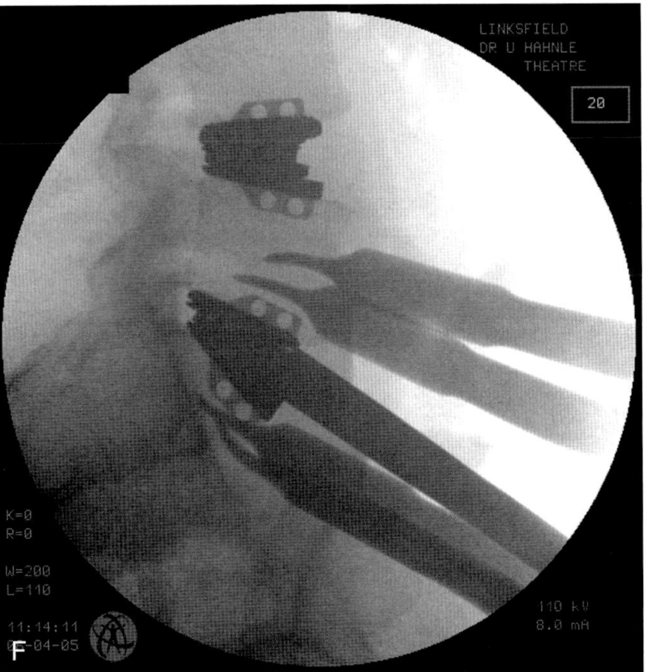


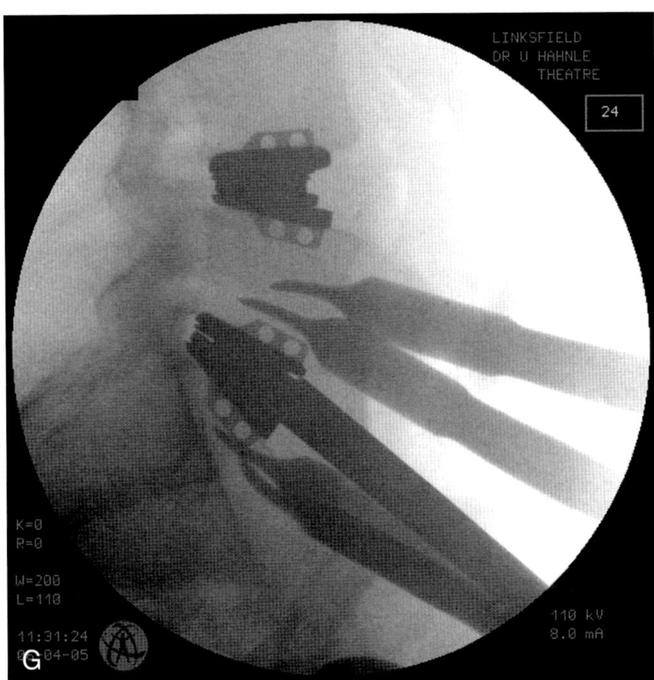


■ **FIGURE 42–3. Cont'd.** **E** to **G,** Sequential advancement of the prosthesis into final position.

in the sagittal plane around the core (see insertion video). Therefore, pressure at the bone/implant interphase at the leading edge of the prosthetic end plate is reduced during prosthetic end plate advancement. The Kineflex disc constitutes the only mechanical disc prosthesis for which final placement into the disc space is performed with a freed mechanism.

### Insertion Procedure

The insertion instruments include the following items: wedge-shaped end plate distracters (three heights), vertebral end plate seizers (three seizes), one midline finder, end plate cutters (two heights), a slotted end plate distracter including guiding plates, and an initial as well as a final implant-insertion instrument (three sizes each). It further includes an implant-removal instrument.

After the disc space is prepared as described earlier, the final end plate size of the prosthesis is determined using the end plate seizers. This is compared with the preoperatively planned seize. The angle and height of the prosthesis were determined during preoperative planning. The height and angle might be adjusted only if the ease of insertion of the wedges differs from what was expected on preoperative planning.

The exact midline is determined under anteroposterior image control after insertion of the midline finder into the disc space. The lateral border of the vertebral body and the pedicles serves as reference and is related to the outer markers of the midline finder. The midline is marked with diathermy on the vertebral body.

On the electrically motorized table, the patient's lumbar area is extended, opening the prepared disc space. The midline grooves are cut using the vertebral end plate cutter. The correct size disc prosthesis is inserted halfway into the disc space. The slotted end plate distracter should be used if the anterior entry of the disc space is tight or recollapses. Through the slotted distracter, the disc is inserted halfway into the disc space, and the slotted distracter is removed.

From here on, the open final insertion instrument of the correct size is used to advance each end plate individually into the desired position. Owing to the unconstrained nature of the mechanism, the core acts as a hypomochlion (pivot), allowing the advancing end plate to pivot over the core and thereby reducing pressure on the leading edge of the end plate at the prosthesis/bone end plate interphase. This avoids end plate violation during the insertion process with possible subsequent subsidence.

The final end plate position is controlled under fluoroscopic imaging. The annuloplasty is closed using stay sutures. A 1/8-inch closed drain is left in the retroperitoneum, if required.

## POSTOPERATIVE CARE

Postoperative mobilization: Patients are allowed to ambulate the day after surgery without bracing. Supervised gait training, isometric muscle strengthening, and stretching exercises start from day 1 postoperatively. At discharge (day 2 to 4 postoperatively), patients are instructed to walk every day and are allowed to sit as long as they feel comfortable. Cycling on a stationary bicycle, longer and faster walks, more vigorous isometric exercises, and hamstring and hip stretching exercises are encouraged after removal of stitches at 12 days after the operation. Light sports are allowed at 6 weeks. Impact sports are allowed only at 4 months in order to allow bony incorporation and remodeling at the implant bone interphase.

## COMPLICATIONS AND AVOIDANCE

In our series of 230 patients studied so far, we have had no procedure-related deaths. In general, perioperative approach-related and implantation-related complications of the first 100 patients with 2 years follow-up, including reoperations, are described as follows:

Approach-related complications included two occurences of deep vein thrombosis, four venous vascular injuries (blood loss <500 mL), two transient neuropraxia of an L-5 nerve root, six patients with postoperative warmer left leg (one permanent).

Disc level-related complications were as follows: Three patients had disc-related complications requiring reoperations. One had an incomplete decompression and was redecompressed 2 days later. The same disc was reinserted. Another patient had a traumatic partial end plate protrusion at 4 weeks. The disc was removed and converted into an anterior fusion. In a third patient, with major subsidence, the disc was removed at 2 weeks, the vertebra was bone grafted, and a larger end plate disc inserted.

Three patients underwent a second-level disc replacement procedure. All reoperated patients were followed up further, and their assessment continued to be included in the outcome results.

## DISCUSSION

The Kineflex disc prosthesis has three unique features that should be emphasized, because not all disc prostheses are the same: (1) The mechanism of the prosthesis is unconstrained and recentering, using a retaining ring on the inferior end plate to maintain the sliding core in position. (2) Two material options for the articulating surfaces are currently available (cobalt chrome on polyethylene as well as cobalt chrome on cobalt chrome). (3) It is the only mechanical disc in which the final seating into the disc space is accomplished with a fully freed articulating mechanism in order to take pressure off the implant/bone interface at the leading edges of the implant during the insertion. The aim is to minimize the danger of bony end plate violation.

The Kineflex disc is currently under evaluation by the FDA for the metal-on-metal articulation.

### ADVANTAGES/DISADVANTAGES: KINEFLEX

**Kineflex Lumbar Disc Prosthesis**
Metal-on-metal disc
Unconstrained and recentering disc mechanism
Machined pyramids of 0.6-mm height
Flat prosthetic end plates
Midline finder
Insertion technique

**Advantages**
Minimal wear
No risk of polyethylene wear particles
Motion pattern approximates natural disc motion
Translational forces are absorbed by unconstrained mechanism
Greater ROM than constrained discs
Excellent primary fixation within the disc space
Prosthetic end plates do not "rock" over bony end plates if match is not perfect
Easy to find exact midline with the help of lateral markers
As the articulating mechanism is released during the insertion process, the superior and inferior prosthetic end plates can be advanced independently during seating of the implant

**Disadvantages**
No axial shock absorption other than by coupled motion
None
None
Hypermobility can recur in preoperative hypermobile disc spaces
If cartilage is left behind during end plate preparation, the primary fixation might be insufficient
Initially, after insertion, load is concentrated on the perimeter of the prosthetic endplate
None
If disc material is left behind within the disc space, it may be carried into the spinal canal. This can be avoided by careful discectomy and end plate preparation.

More than 50% of patients in our series had advanced disc degeneration, with disc space height less than 5 mm and some with advanced facet joint arthritis.[9] In significantly collapsed and rigid disc spaces, we specifically aim to achieve a posterior position of the prosthesis within the disc space in order to unload the facets. This has been difficult with other implants owing to the rigidly held implants during the insertion process. The Kineflex disc prosthesis is disconnected from its initial insertion tool after the initial engagement into the disc space. The final placement is done with a released prosthetic mechanism that facilitates the seating of the prosthesis, avoiding excessive pressure on the bony end plate during insertion. Although the achievement of a posterior position of the prosthesis within the disc space has not yet been systematically evaluated, it seems to be much easier to achieve than with other implants.

The operative time and blood loss are higher than in other studies.[10] Twelve of our patients had additional fusion surgery, including combined posterior and anterior osteotomy surgery with operative times of up to 7 hours.[11] These cases added to operative time and blood loss. However, for single-level disc replacements, the operative time and blood loss are comparable to other studies[10] (see Table 42–2). The use of Hohman retractors for exposure causes additional bleeding from the vertebral bodies but avoids slippage of the major veins into the operative field.

Postoperative hospital stay and return to work data compare favorably with other studies.[10] Ninety-eight percent of our patients went back to work at an average of 31 days after the operation.

The ODI and pain score improvements occurred early after surgery and were maintained at the time of 2-year follow-up (see Fig. 42–2). As previously described, the patients with double-level replacement[12] scored better in their 1-year clinical outcome parameters than the patients with single-level replacement after scoring poorer results at 3 months[13] (see Fig. 42–2). We had a 6% reoperation rate within 2 years. In three of our single-level replacements, we performed a second-level replacement within the first 2 years. In all three patients, this second level had been degenerative before the first procedure. Therefore, we now tend to be more aggressive in favor of second-level replacements as compared with single-level replacements.

The improvement in the pain score and ODI scores compare favorably with the literature.[10,12,13]

## CONCLUSION

We achieved good short-term clinical results using the Kineflex disc in a heterogeneous patient group with a high number of patients with advanced disc degeneration, severe disc space narrowing, and previous fusion with lumbar flat back deformity. The independent advancement of the end plates allows seating of the prosthesis posterior into disc space with minimal trauma to the bony end plates.

## REFERENCES


1. Lehman TR, Spratt KF, Tozzi JE, et al: Long-term follow-up of lumbar fusion patients. Spine 12:97–104, 1987.
2. Park P, Garton HJ, Gala VC, et al: Adjacent segment disease after lumbar or lumbosacral fusion: Review of the literature. Spine 29:1938–1944, 2004.
3. Fernström U: Arthroplasty with intercorporal endoprosthesis in herniated disc and in painful disc. Acta Chir Scand 355:154–159, 1966.
4. Buettner-Janz K, Schellnack K, Zippel H: Eine alternative Behandlungsstrategie beim lumbalen Bandscheibenschaden mit der Bandscheiben-endoprothese Modulartyp SB Charite. Z Orthop 125:1–6, 1987.
5. McAfee PC, Cunningham BW, Holtsapple G, et al: A prospective, randomized, multicenter Food and Drug Administration Investigational Device Exemption Study of lumbar total disc replacement with the CHARITÉ artificial disc versus lumbar fusion, part II: Evaluation of radiographic outcomes and correlation of surgical technique accuracy with clinical outcomes. Spine 30:1576–1583, 2005.
6. Cunningham BW: Presentation on Charité PMA submission at FDA Orthopedic Device Panel meeting June 2, 2004.
7. Cunningham BW, Hallab NJ, Dmitriev AE, et al: Epidural application of spinal instrumentation particulate wear debris: An in vivo animal model. Spine J 4(6 suppl):219S–230S, 2004.
8. Di Angelo D, Morrow B, Gilmour L, et al: In vitro biomechanics of the Kineflex Lumbar Disc Prosthesis: Presentation at SAS6, Montreal, May 2006.
9. Hänle UR, Weinberg IR, Sliwa K, et al: Kineflex (Centurion) lumbar disc prosthesis: Insertion technique and 2-year clinical results in 100 patients. SAS Journal 1(4):28–35.
10. Blumenthal S, McAfee PC, Guyer R, et al: A prospective, randomized, multicenter Food and Drug Administration Investigational Device Exemption Study of lumbar total disc replacement with the CHARITÉ artificial disc versus lumbar fusion, part I: Evaluation of clinical outcome. Spine 30:1565–1575, 2005.
11. Hänle UR, Sliwa K, Weinberg IR, et al: Lumbar disc replacement for junctional decompensation after fusion surgery: Clinical and radiological outcome at an average follow-up of 33 months. SAS Journal 1(3):85–92.
12. Bertagnoli R, Yue JJ, Shah RV, et al: The treatment of disabling multilevel lumbar discogenic low back pain with total disc arthroplasty utilizing the Prodisc prosthesis: A prospective study with 2-year minimum follow-up. Spine 30:2192–2199, 2005.
13. Bertagnoli R, Yue JJ, Shah RV, et al: The treatment of disabling single-level lumbar discogenic low back pain with total disc arthroplasty utilizing the Prodisc prosthesis: A prospective study with 2-year minimum follow-up. Spine 30:2230–2236, 2005.

CHAPTER 43

# Activ-L Artificial Disc

**James J. Yue** and **Rolando García**

## KEY POINTS

- Biomechanically, the Activ-L implant is a semi-constrained implant.
- It permits translation in the anteroposterior direction.
- End plates are either spiked or keeled and are coated with both titanium and calcium phosphate.
- Anterior or oblique insertions are possible with a minimum disc height of 8.5 mm.
- Revision instrumentation is adapted to implant.

## INTRODUCTION

The clinical science of lumbar total disc arthroplasty continues to evolve.[1–9] From a biomechanical perspective, three main types of artificial disc replacements exist: (1) unconstrained, (2) semi-constrained without translation, and (3) the next generation, semi-constrained with translation. The Activ-L (Aesculap, Tuttlingen, Germany) (Fig. 43–1) allows for semi-constrained motion with translation in the anteroposterior (AP) direction. Other innovative features include enhanced implant stability and variability, uncomplicated prosthetic implantation, and revision instrumentation.

The next-generation implant should be optimized to minimize wear debris, allow for ease of insertion through multiple angles, and surgical revision instrumentation should be available. In addition, the implant should provide maximal end plate coverage with minimal or no end plate recontouring and be adaptable to various end plate shapes and allow ease of implant delivery at single or multiple levels. The design goals of the Activ-L prosthesis were to incorporate all of the above-mentioned next-generation requirements for lumbar artificial disc replacement.

## INDICATIONS/CONTRAINDICATIONS

The indications for Activ-L intervertebral lumbar disc arthroplasty include severe lumbar discogenic back pain as a result of lumbar spondylosis with or without radiculopathy. Clinical findings should be closely correlated with radiologic imaging findings, including magnetic resonance imaging, standing plane x-ray studies, discography, and computed tomography. Other sources of back pain such as facet disease, myofascial syndromes, inflammatory arthritic conditions, and "red flag" sources of pain should be excluded. The patient should have a mimimum trial course of 6 months of conservative treatment before total disc replacement surgery.

Contraindications to this procedure include chronic infections such as local or remote sources of infection, a body mass index of greater than 35, a bone density score of less than −1.0, active malignancy, facet degeneration, spondylolysis with or without spondylolysthesis, and circumferential spinal stenois.

## DESCRIPTION OF THE DEVICE

The Activ-L implant is composed of three components (see Fig. 43–1). The superior and inferior components are composed of a metal alloy (cobalt, chromium, and molybdenum). The superior component is composed of a one-piece design with a central keel or three anterior spikes and is available in two lordotic angles—6 and 11 degrees. The superior component has a concave polished surface that articulates with the second component an ultra-high-molecular-weight polyethylene inlay. This inlay presently is available in 8.5 mm, 10 mm, 12 mm, and 14 mm sizes. This inlay rests in the third component, the inferior component, which is composed of a solid one-piece design with a central keel or three anterior spikes (Fig 43–2). The inferior component also has a highly polished surface that permits translation in the AP direction only during flexion and extension. The "S" size permits for 1.5 mm of polyethylene inlay translation in the AP direction. The "M, L, and XL" sizes permit 2 mm of AP translation. None of the implants permit mediolateral translation of the inlay (Figs. 43–3 and 43–4). Four implant sizes are available: S, M, L, and XL (Fig 43–5). Both the superior and inferior components are plasma sprayed with a pure titanium coating as well as a thin layer (20 μm) of dicalcium phosphate dehydrate (μ-CaP).

Trial implant end plates for end plate sizing are available and can be placed directly on a mechanical distractor and interverterbal space sizer (Fig. 43–6). A midline pin marker can be placed to assist in midline accuracy (Fig. 43–7). When an oblique insertion is desired, a radiolucent marker with radio-opaque midpoint

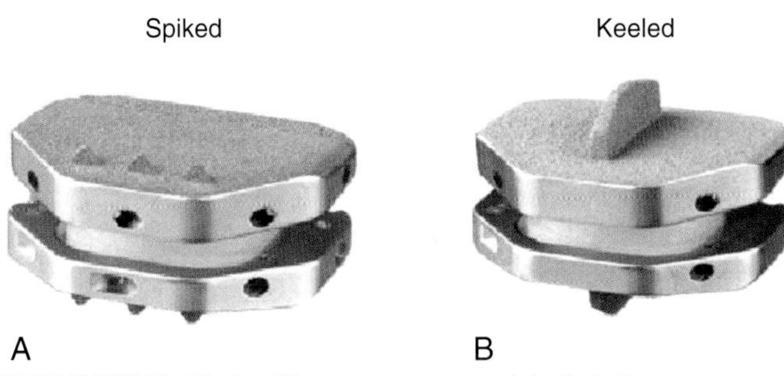


■ **FIGURE 43–1.** Three components of Activ-L disc replacement. **A,** Spiked and **B,** Keeled versions.

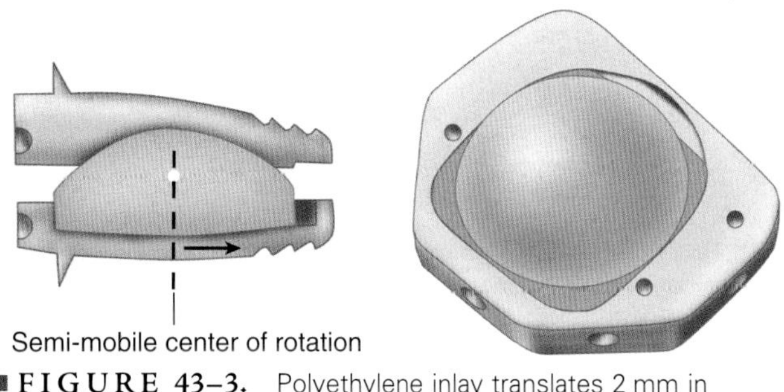


■ **FIGURE 43–3.** Polyethylene inlay translates 2 mm in anteroposterior direction, producing liberation of facet joint in flexion.

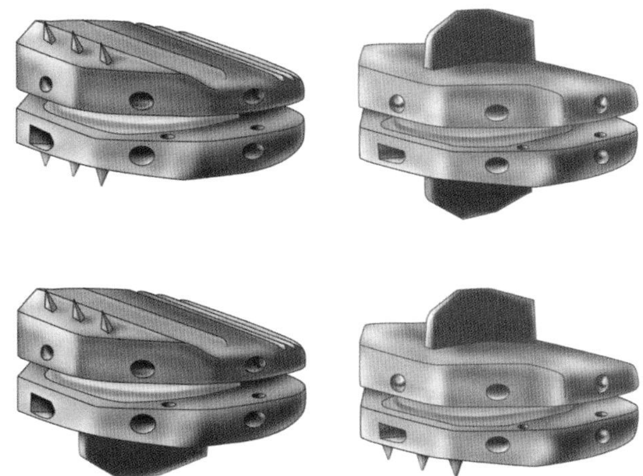

■ **FIGURE 43–2.** Activ-L lumbar disc replacement end plate fixation options.

alignment marks is available to assist in midline marking in the AP and lateral projections. When a keeled implant technique is desired, a protected chisel is available to cut the keel groove (Fig. 43–8). The chisel is available in a double- or single-chisel design. Instrumentation for the Activ-L surgical procedure also includes a set of disc space preparation instruments.

Revision instruments are included in the instrument set that permit for translation of the implant in an anterior direction if so desired (Fig. 43–9). This same set of instruments allows for complete removal of the implant. A separate revision instrument allows for removal and replacement of the polyethylene insert.

## Background of Scientific Testing/Clinical Outcomes

The Activ-L Artificial Disc has undergone comprehensive mechanical testing. In all cases, appropriate Insurance Services Office (ISO) and American Society for Testing and Materials (ASTM) standards for testing of artificial discs were followed, where available. In all tests, finished products were used. The device was tested in all of the worst-case modes and loading conditions that are anticipated in the in vivo environment.

### Static Testing

The Activ-L was tested in combined compression/shear at an angle that represents the expected loading situation in the lumbar spine, that is, device placement in lordosis with compression. The compression/shear test setup used an angulated mounting situation of 10 degrees in order to account for the resultant shear forces that, in addition to the axial forces, are applied to the prosthesis in vivo. The same test setup was also previously used to perform testing of the ProDisc-L (Synthes, West Chester, PA).

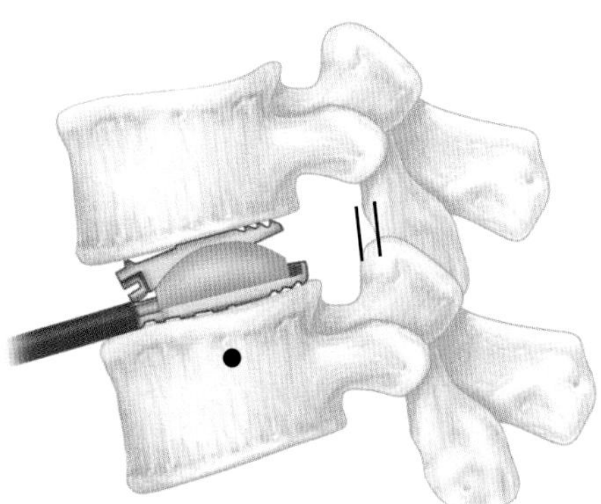


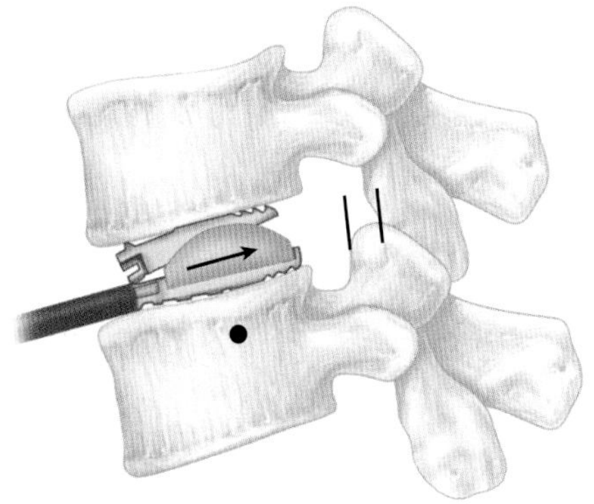


■ **FIGURE 43–4.** **A** and **B,** Combined translation and rotation equals mobilization.

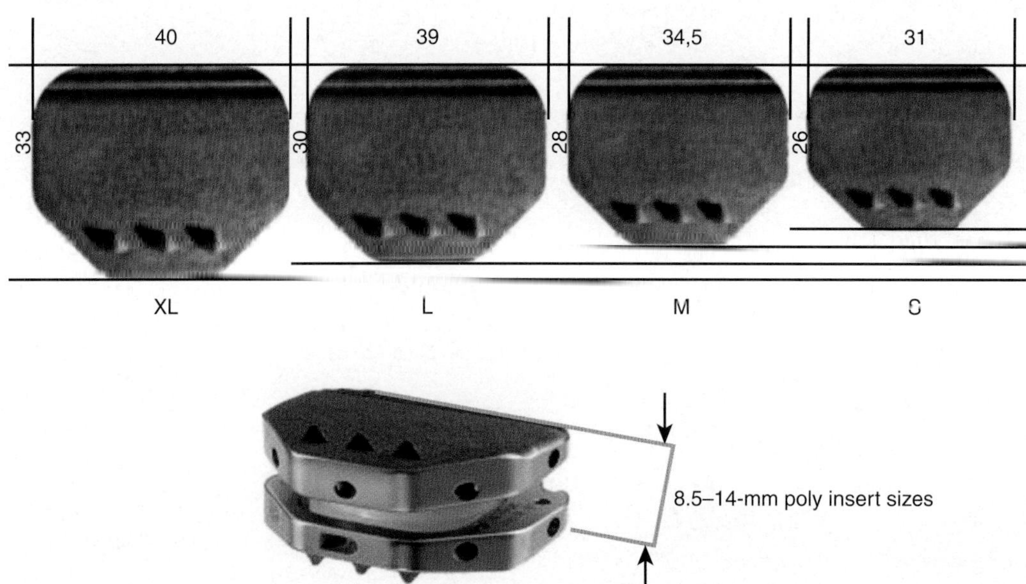


■ **FIGURE 43–5.** Available component dimensions of Activ-L prosthesis.

All devices were able to withstand compression/shear loads higher than the worst-case in vivo loads. The average yield load was 6.6 kN for the Activ-L with spikes and 6.9 kN for the Activ-L with keel. The only mode of failure observed was plastic deformation of the inlay. The yield load for the ProDisc-L was similar, 7.9 kN. This difference is not clinically significant because the yield load in all three cases exceeds the fracture load of the L-5 vertebral body, 5.5 kN, and substantially exceeds the worst-case physiologic loading conditions, with maximum reported axial compressive forces in the lumbar spine of approximately 3–3.4 kN. Thus, both configurations of the Activ-L provide adequate strength in static compression/shear to withstand worst case loads in clinical use.

Static testing was also performed to evaluate the resistance of the Activ-L end plates to dislocation under shear. A compressive load of 450 N was applied to hold the end plate against the test block to simulate the in vivo loading situation. A shear force was then applied against the end plate at 5 mm/minute.

The results demonstrated that the average maximum shear force was 1.26 kN for the Activ-L end plate with spikes, 494 N for the Activ-L end plate with keel, and 933 N for the ProDisc-L. The displacement at maximum force was similar for all three end plates, 0.33 to 0.44 mm. Both configurations of the Activ-L and the ProDisc-L exhibited sufficient shear resistance to withstand the worst-case loading conditions expected in vivo. The Activ-L has a safety factor of $d = 1.24$ to 1.98 shear resistance to avoid implant dislocation.

### Dynamic Fatigue Testing

Testing was performed according to two methods. In the first test, a single Activ-L with spikes was subjected to an initial load of 300 to 3,000 N for 5 million cycles at a frequency of 5 Hz. Temperature was monitored throughout testing to verify that this cycling rate did not cause a significant increase in temperature.

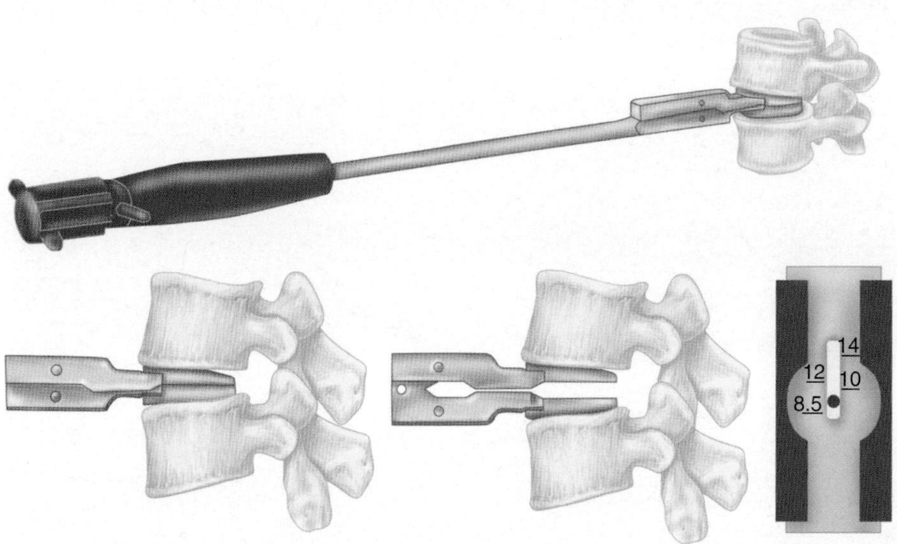


■ **FIGURE 43–6.** Parallel distraction, trial implant, and size verification instrument.

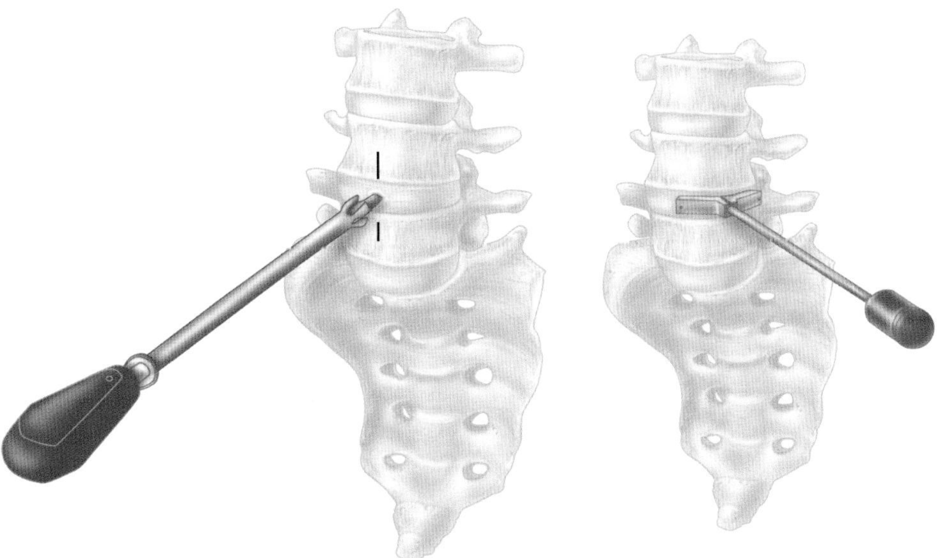

■ **FIGURE 43–7.** Midline marker for anterior and lateral approaches.

Temperature was maintained within 2°C throughout testing. The load was then increased by 1,000 N at intervals of 1 million cycles up to 8,000 N. The specimen withstood loads through 9.75 million cycles without failure but failed due to extreme creep of the polyethylene (PE) inlay following luxation of the superior plate after 757,500 cycles at the maximum load (800 to 8,000 N). This first test was also performed with a single specimen of the Activ-L with keel and produced similar results, with survival of the implant for 8.15 million cycles and failure only at a load of 700 to 7,000 N. These results were identical to the results for the ProDisc-L when tested under the same protocol, except that the mode of failure for the ProDisc-L was breakage of the inferior plate; there was no plate breakage for either specimen of the Activ-L.

In the second test, one specimen was exposed to loading at 300 to 3,000 N for 10 million cycles at 5 Hz, and four additional specimens were exposed to loading at 400 to 4,000 N for 10 million cycles. All of the specimens survived to run-out without failure. Similar results were observed for the ProDisc-L specimen, which was tested according to the same protocol at loading of 300 to 3,000 N, but a second ProDisc-L specimen tested at 400 to 4,000 N failed owing to breakage of the inferior end plate. Thus, the endurance limit of the Activ-L in compression/shear is at least 4,000 N, which exceeds the worst-case loads of 3 to −3.4 kN that are anticipated in vivo. These results are also similar to or slightly better than the corresponding results for the ProDisc-L.

### Wear Simulator Testing and Particle Characterization

Wear testing was performed in newborn calf serum (protein 30 g/L) at 37 °C at a cycling rate of 1 Hz, in accordance with ISO method

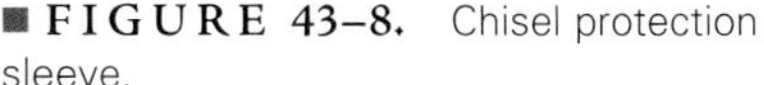

■ **FIGURE 43–8.** Chisel protection sleeve.

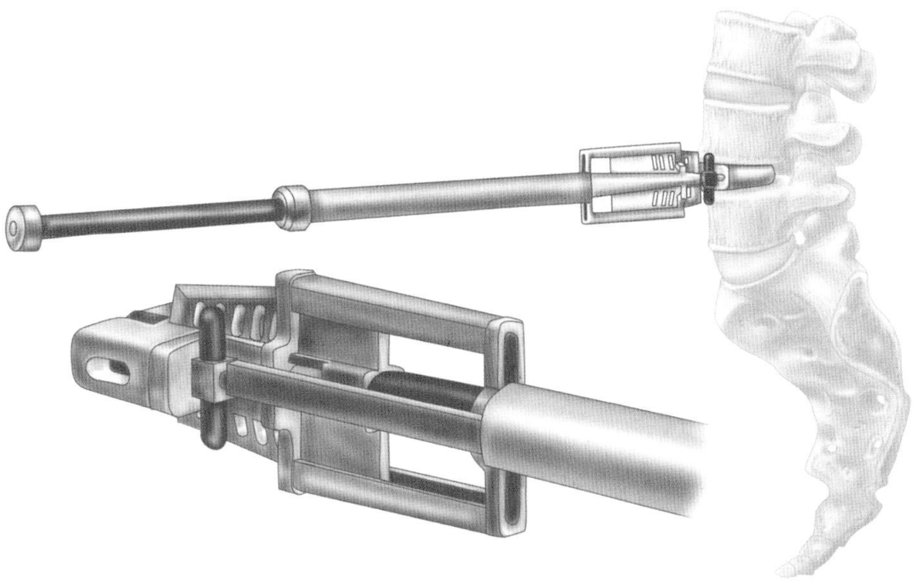

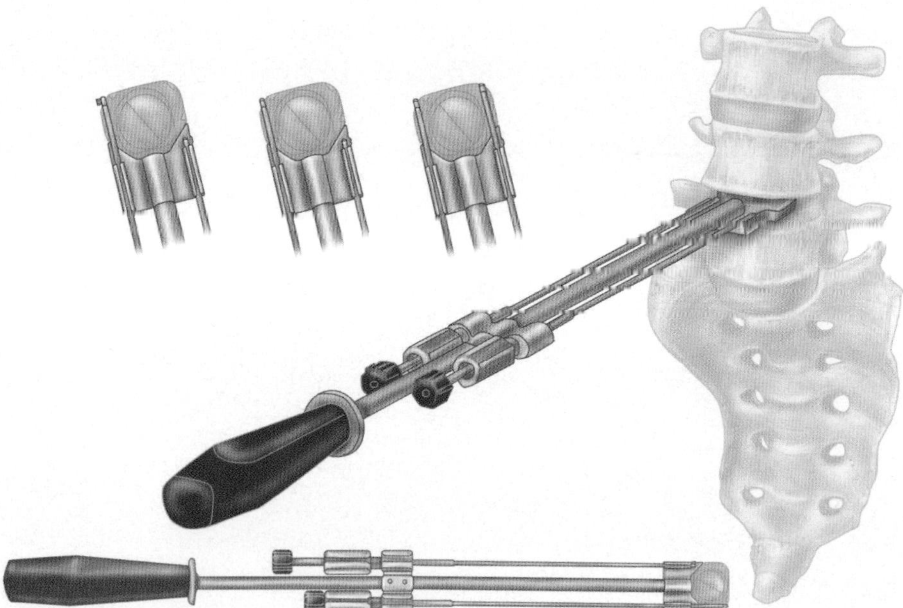

■ **FIGURE 43–9.** Revision repositioning instruments.

ISO/CD 18192-1, 2004-04-30, with combined motions in flexion-extension, lateral bending, and axial rotation. The initial period of testing was 10 million cycles. Weight loss was measured at intervals of 0.5 million cycles throughout testing.

The testing demonstrated relatively steady weight loss of 1 to 2 mg per measurement interval, averaging 2.7 (± 0.3) mg/million cycles. The total average wear over 10 million cycles was 25.3 mg, with very low variability across specimens (± 2.3 mg). Prior testing of the ProDisc-L, which also was performed by Aesculap, had exhibited a very similar wear rate with less than 1.0 mg/million cycles. The Activ-L wear rate is substantially lower than reported wear rates for hip and knee prostheses, and is similar to or lower than other artificial discs tested under similar parameters. Visual inspection of the prostheses after wear testing showed no unexpected gross damage. Abrasive wear and plastic deformation are the main wear mechanisms. There was no evidence of cracking or pitting of the inlay after 10 million cycles. The change in height of the inlay component was less than 0.5 mm after 10 million cycles, which is well below the 1.5 mm diurnal variation in height of the native disc. Thus, these results demonstrate the ability of the Activ-L to withstand the worst-case in vivo loading conditions in multiaxial motion without excessive wear.

Testing of the same prostheses continued under the conditions of ASTM guidance 2423 for an additional 5 million cycles. Compared with the wear rate in the first 10 million cycles, 2.7 mg/million cycles, the wear rate between 10 and 15 million cycles was only 0.13 mg/million cycles. Testing conditions were returned to the ISO parameters for the last 0.5 million cycles and the wear rate returned to a similar level to the initial 10 million cycles, and approximately 3.5 mg/million cycles. Thus, after a total of 15.5 million cycles of testing using both approaches, the total wear remained low, approximately 27.7 mg.

After completion of 10 million cycles, the wear particulate was characterized. The results of the particle characterization showed very similar particle size distribution and morphology for all devices. On average, the particle count ranged from $1 \times 10^7$ to $3.5 \times 10^8$ particles/mL of serum. The mean particle diameter increased slightly over the course of the wear testing, with mean diameter of 0.17 to 0.20 μ at the beginning of testing and 0.3 to 0.5 μ at the end of testing. The largest particles were approximately 5 μ in diameter, representing less than 5% of the particles analyzed. The smallest particles were approximately 0.05 μ in diameter. The particle morphology was generally granular and stable.

## Clinical Data

The Activ-L has been in commercial use in Europe since 2005, with more than 1000 discs implanted (Fig. 43–10). The commercial experience has been favorable, with a low reported complication rate. No implant-related complications or severe adverse events have been documented in the company's complaint database to date. The low rate of complaints in commercial use of the Activ-L provides further support for the safety of the device. A German clinical trial at three centers began in 2005. The study's primary efficacy endpoint is postoperative reduction in functional disability, as determined by a 15% improvement in mean total Oswestry Disability Index (ODI) score at 24 months after surgery compared with baseline. The mean ODI scores reported to date show improvements consistent with this endpoint. These results show a mean improvement of 17 points (35%) in ODI score at 3 months, and 19 points (39%) at 18 months. Patients also demonstrated substantial improvement in mean Visual Analog Scale (VAS) scores at 3 and 18 months. At 3 months, mean VAS improvement for back pain (28 mm) and leg pain (20 mm and 27 mm) met or exceeded the 20-mm improvement as hypothesized. A U.S. Investigational Device Exemption (IDE) clinical trial began in January 2007 and is comparing the Activ-L disc versus the ProDisc or CHARITÉ implant (DePuy Spine Inc., Raynham, MA).

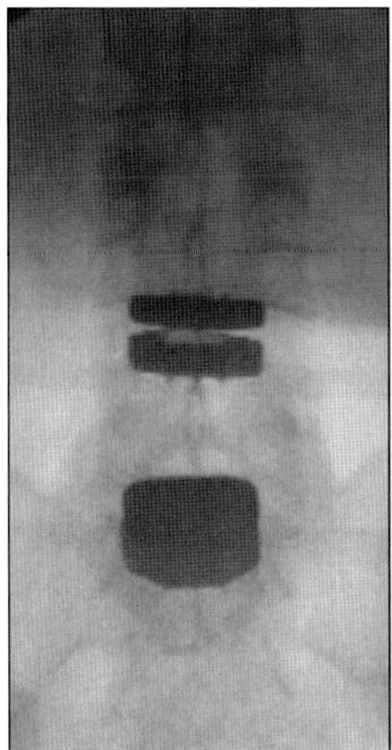

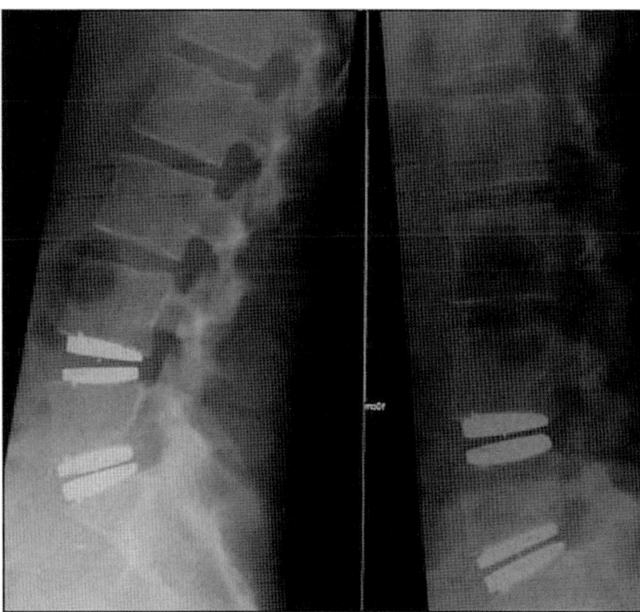

■ **FIGURE 43–10.** Two-level Activ-L in place.

## OPERATIVE TECHNIQUE

**STEP 1:** Positioning: Patients are placed on a fluoroscopic imaging table. Fluoroscopic views should be obtained such that with the C-arm in a zero degree rotation (AP view) of the spine, the spinous process should be equidistant from the medial pedicle edges. On the lateral view, the anterior and posterior vertebral body cortices should be easily identifiable.

**STEP 2:** Disc Space Preparation: Access and exposure is enhanced with the use of a self-retaining retractor. Standard retroperitoneal or transperitoneal approaches to the spine are then performed. Once the anterior disc has been exposed and the appropriate level of dissection verified, the midpoint of the disc space is marked under fluoroscopic imaging. The midline pin marker is then placed. A complete discectomy and mobilization is performed. A small curved curette should always be placed along the posterior ridge of both vertebral bodies. This palpation will aid in the release of the posterior longitudinal ligament and removal of extruded disc fragments and posterior inflammatory granulation tissue when indicated. The subchondral bone must be preserved. It is not mandatory to remove the entire posterior longitudinal ligament unless extruded disk material needs to be removed and/or greater intervertebral disc space mobilization is required.

**STEP 3:** Surgical Procedure/Technique—Trialing and Chiseling: After end plate preparation and disc space mobilization are completed, implant trialing is then performed. Disc space height and lordotic angles should be reestablished. The largest possible end plate should be chosen in all cases.

Depending on the type of end plate configuration as well as surgeon preference, the decision for a keeled or spiked implant is then made. The distractor/sizer instrument is then placed into the disc space, and the disc space is simultaneously distracted and measured by turning the handle of this instrument. If a keeled implant is chosen, the appropriate chisel trial is placed carefully in the midline of the disc space, and chiseling is then performed. Correct positioning of this trial implant is imperative. A keeled implant cannot be used for oblique insertion. Chiseling is performed under fluoroscopic imaging control. It is not necessary to perform chiseling if a spiked implant is chosen.

**STEP 4:** Insertion of Implant: Once the final implant has been chosen, it is then attached to an insertion handle. All three pieces of the implant (two end plates and PE inlay) are secured to the insertion instrument, and the implant is then inserted en bloc. If an oblique insertion is desired, several steps should be followed. First, although an oblique insertion is to be performed, vascular mobilization approximately 2 cm past the midline of the vertebral interspace is recommended. Second, the radiolucent trial is placed on the disc space before discectomy, and a small notch is made on the superior vertebra thereby defining the insertional angle for the final prosthesis.

If at all possible, complete release of the anterior annulus should be performed to allow for proper balancing of the spine to avoid causing iatrogenic scoliosis. The implant should be first positioned in the final mediolateral position. Once the implant has been positioned in the anatomic center of the interspace in the AP plane, the implant is then positioned posteriorly using lateral fluoroscopy.

## CONCLUSIONS/DISCUSSION

Early results indicate that the Activ-L implant achieves a safe and efficacious balance between intervertebral motion and implant stability. The Activ-L implant allows for semi-constrained flexion-extension, rotation, and translation. We define this combined motion as mobilization. We believe mobilization permits more physiologic motion as well as smaller disc heights in the restoration of the diseased disc space. Primary stability is achieved through the keel or spiked design of the implant, and secondary stability is achieved through the osseous integration of the titanium and dicalcium phosphate dehydrate coating. The Activ-L implant system promotes a harmonious synergy between implant design and insertional technique.

## REFERENCES

1. Tortolani PJ, Cunningham BW, Eng M, et al: Prevalence of heterotopic ossification following total disc replacement: A prospective, randomized study of two hundred and seventy-six patients. J Bone Joint Surg Am 89:82–88, 2007.
2. Siepe CJ, Wiechert K, Khattab MF, et al: Total lumbar disc replacement in athletes: clinical results, return to sport and athletic performance. Eur Spine J 16:1001–1013, 2007.
3. Tropiano P, Huang RC, Girardi FP, et al: Lumbar total disc replacement: Surgical technique. J Bone Joint Surg Am 88(suppl 1, Pt 1): 50–64, 2006.
4. Tournier C, Aunoble S, Le Huec JC, et al: Total disc arthroplasty: Consequences for sagittal balance and lumbar spine movement. Eur Spine J 16:411–421, 2006.
5. Regan JJ, McAfee PC, Blumenthal SL, et al: Evaluation of surgical volume and the early experience with lumbar total disc replacement as part of the investigational device exemption study of the Charite Artificial Disc. Spine 31:2270–2276, 2006.
6. Bertagnoli R, Yue JJ, Nanieva R, et al: Lumbar total disc arthroplasty in patients older than 60 years of age: a prospective study of the Pro-Disc prosthesis with 2-year minimum follow-up period. J Neurosurg Spine 4:85–90, 2006.
7. Bertagnoli R, Yue JJ, Kershaw T, et al: Lumbar total disc arthroplasty utilizing the ProDisc prosthesis in smokers versus nonsmokers: A prospective study with 2-year minimum follow-up. Spine 31:992–997, 2006.
8. Bertagnoli R, Yue JJ, Fenk-Mayer A, et al: Treatment of symptomatic adjacent-segment degeneration after lumbar fusion with total disc arthroplasty by using the prodisc prosthesis: A prospective study with 2-year minimum follow up. J Neurosurg Spine 4:91–97, 2006.
9. Tropiano P, Huang RC, Girardi FP, et al: Lumbar total disc replacement: Seven to eleven-year follow-up. J Bone Joint Surg Am 87:490–496, 2005.

CHAPTER 44

# Maverick Total Disc Replacement

Matthew F. Gornet

## KEY POINTS

- Motion stabilization offers documented advantages versus fusion.
- Patient selection is critical to any successful total disc replacement.
- Maverick is the first metal-on-metal, two-piece anterior lumbar total disc prosthesis.
- Fixed posterior center of rotation improves postoperative motion and limits facet loading.
- Durability, longevity, and ease of use are key characteristics of this lifetime device.

## INTRODUCTION

Spinal fusion continues to be the most frequent surgical option for patients suffering with advanced degenerative disc disease (DDD). Fusion has as its intended outcome creating stability at the diseased segment by eliminating motion in the hope of relieving the pain caused by instability at the diseased level. Meanwhile, other forms of segmental restoration continue to be developed and studied, including total disc arthroplasty, which has a history spanning 20 years with a variety of devices and insertion techniques. This construct, however, attempts to relieve pain by stabilizing the diseased level without immobilizing it, allowing the natural lordosis to return as the patient quickly heals after disc replacement. The two designs currently approved for use in the United States are discussed in Chapters 38 to 39 of this text, respectively: SB CHARITÉ III (DePuy Spine, Raynham, MA) and the ProDisc (Synthes, West Chester, PA), with both based on articulating cobalt-chromium-molybdenum (CoCrMo) on ultra-high-molecular-weight polyethylene (UHMWPE). This chapter focuses on a new entrant in this emerging category of spinal stabilization devices, the Maverick Total Disc Replacement (TDR) (Medtronic Sofamor Danek, Memphis, TN), a U.S. Food and Drug Administration (FDA) Investigational Device Exemptions (IDE) study device with a U.S. trial that started in early 2003. Readers of this chapter are asked to consider the unique design features of the Maverick TDR relative to alternative TDR prostheses, keeping in mind the natural role and functionality of a healthy intervertebral disc and the ability of the Maverick device to deliver performance comparable to that achieved with an asymptomatic disc.

## INDICATIONS/CONTRAINDICATIONS

The most important determinant of success in any spinal arthroplasty procedure is proper patient selection. As additional prosthetic devices are approved for use by the FDA, surgeons will need to be aware of the general inclusion/exclusion guidelines for TDR while also considering any device-specific factors that might influence the patient's long-term success. Patient symptoms, in conjunction with thorough magnetic resonance imaging (MRI) or computed tomography (CT) studies to determine the entire segmental pathology, both anterior and posterior, are a requisite precursor to discussions regarding suitability for total disc arthroplasty. The Maverick TDR was approved for an FDA IDE study for patients who could meet *all* of the following criteria for inclusion:

- Discogenic back pain, with or without leg pain, indicative of single-level (L4-S1) degenerative disease requiring surgery, as confirmed by patient history, including demonstrated functional or neurologic deficit, and radiographic examination that revealed one or more of the following conditions:
  - Modic changes
  - High-intensity zones in the annulus
  - Loss of disc height
  - Decreased hydration of the disc (Fig. 44–1)
- Documented annular pathology
- Intact facet joints at the involved vertebral levels as documented on MRI or CT scans
- Preoperative Oswestry Disability Index (ODI) score of 30 or more and significantly elevated back pain as evidenced by a score of 20 or more on the Back and Leg Pain Questionnaire
- Failure to respond to at least 6 months of conservative, nonoperative treatment, including bed rest, physical therapy, medications, transcutaneous electrical nerve stimulation (TENS), manipulation, or spinal injections

Just as important in the process of patient selection is adherence to the contraindications for spinal arthroplasty, which for the Maverick study included the following, any one of which disqualified an otherwise acceptable candidate:

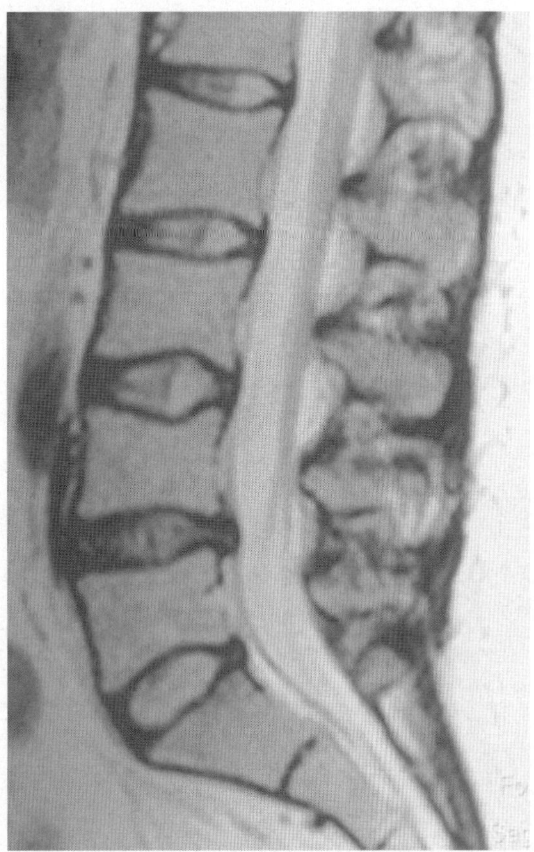

■ **FIGURE 44–1.** Thirty-eight-year old man. Magnetic resonance imaging scan reveals annular tear at L4-L5 with a central disc protrusion.

- A primary diagnosis of a spinal disorder other than DDD at the involved level
- A previous posterior lumbar spinal fusion or any previous anterior lumbar spinal surgery at the diseased level
- The need for surgical intervention at more than one level
- Severe pathology of the facet joints of the involved vertebral bodies
- Any posterior element insufficiency, for example, facet resection, spondylolysis, or pars fracture
- Spondylolisthesis, spinal canal stenosis, or rotary scoliosis at the involved level
- Risk factors that may be associated with a diagnosis of osteoporosis
- Documented metal allergy or intolerance to titanium alloy or CoCrMo alloy

## DESCRIPTION OF THE DEVICE

The Maverick TDR (Fig. 44–2) is a unique interbody prosthesis that evolved from a ceramic-on-ceramic construct developed in the early 1990s at Danek Medical by Larry Boyd, in conjunction with Richard Salib and Ken Pettine. The guiding design principles for that early concept device (posterior center of rotation, two-piece ball-and-socket construction, expulsion/dislocation avoidance) were important building blocks when, in 2001, a team of engineers and physicians began investigating the development of a disc replacement prosthesis with a posterior center of rotation for Medtronic Sofamor Danek.[1]

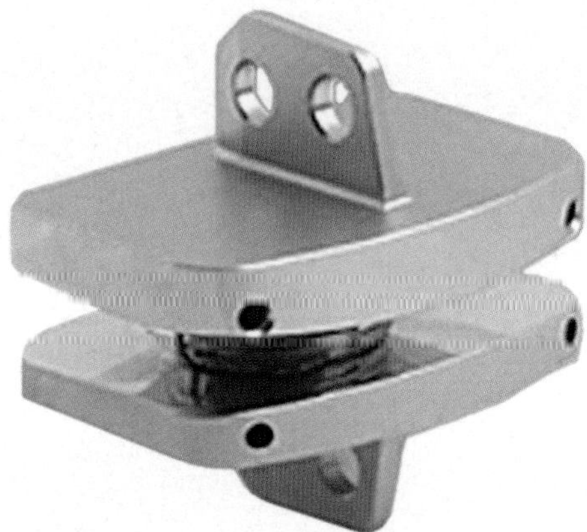

■ **FIGURE 44–2.** Maverick total disc replacement (Medtronic Sofamor Danek, Memphis, TN).

Just as the role of a healthy intervertebral disc is to stabilize the spinal unit while absorbing shock, managing load distribution, and protecting the facets, the design of an artificial disc should deliver as closely as possible the same motion stabilization and protection at the treated spinal level. With that in mind, the design rationale for this permanent implant evolved to include important biomechanical properties while not compromising on critical factors such as longevity and surgical implantation technique. The resulting Maverick TDR is a device designed to provide functional restoration with superior wear through metal-on-metal (MOM) articulation of a ball-and-socket joint with a fixed posterior center of rotation. Today, the most current design configurations of the device, the A-MAV (direct anterior approach) (Fig. 44–3) and O–MAV (oblique approach) (Fig. 44–4), have achieved clinical use.

The use of CoCrMo alloy for the two articulating surfaces is expected to deliver the same excellent wear characteristics and durability achieved with MOM total hip prostheses. Because any anterior revision of a prosthetic disc is potentially life-threatening, the overarching design consideration was to develop a device that could last a patient's lifetime while avoiding the potential complications of conventional polyethylene. When used in hip replacements, MOM produces up to two times less wear debris

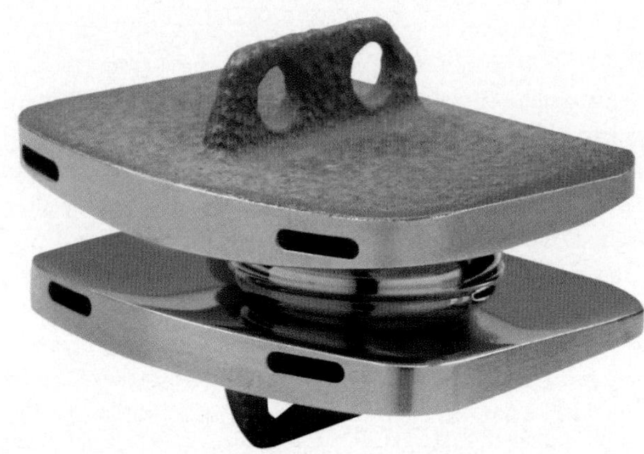

■ **FIGURE 44–3.** A-MAV, the current version for direct anterior approach total disc replacement.

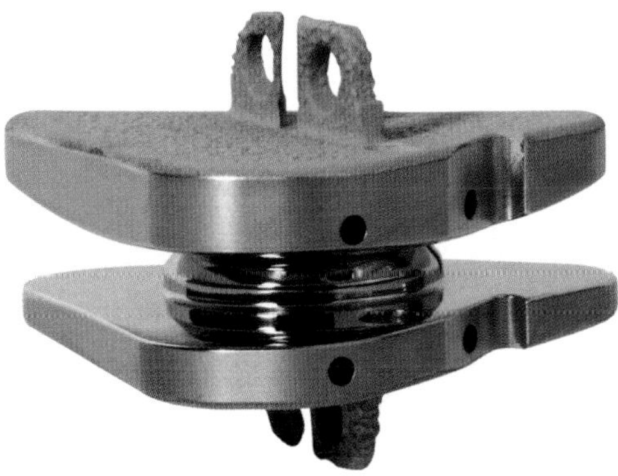

■ **FIGURE 44–4.** O-MAV, the oblique approach version of the Maverick device.

than devices with conventional UHMWPE and metal, which are associated with osteolysis and foreign body reaction issues.[2] In a disc prosthesis, MOM should be expected to exceed the high performance achieved in hip arthroplasty because of the anatomic difference in motion-generated forces on the device in daily life.[1]

Because the role of the Maverick TDR is to replace the diseased anterior column, the fixed posterior center of rotation will mimic the kinematics of a healthy disc so that the balance and load transfer points are right in the neutral axis. A TDR that delivers a center of rotation too far anterior will potentially overload the facets, causing pain and possible degeneration adjacent to the operated level.[3] With a center of rotation in the posterior third of the construct (Fig. 44–5), the Maverick TDR provides the surgeon with a placement margin of error should the device not be placed as posteriorly as desired. With translation controlled to just 3 mm or less, shear forces and the resulting potential for facet disease or translational instability syndromes are minimized.

The male end plate, available in a single height, is positioned on the superior end plate of the inferior vertebra of the involved level, whereas the female counterpart is placed in the opposing position on the superior vertebra (Fig. 44–6). A keel protrudes from the bone-abutting surface of each end plate to provide stability after placement by the surgeon in a prepared channel. In the more current A-MAV version of the original product design, the keel height is reduced to help minimize keel cut depths while delivering comparable performance. The bone-prosthesis contact surface is treated with a thermal plasma spray application of hydroxyapatite (HA), which is a highly crystalline, osseoconductive synthetic bone material used in arthroplasty for decades, after a chemical texturing process that roughens the surface to enhance friction for a press fit (Fig. 44–7). The result is excellent stability and rapid bony ingrowth.

The articulating surface of the male end plate has a protruding dome-shaped surface that mates with the concave surface of the female component, which is offered in several heights, measured from the posterior aspect of the prosthesis. Mated for a single surgical insertion, the device provides for 16 degrees of motion off the neutral position. The coupled end plates provide 6 degrees of angulation, with insertion tools that allow insertion with 6, 9, or 12 degrees of angulation. Both end plates are available in small, medium, or large sizes (Fig. 44–8) that provide flexibility in end plate coverage. The

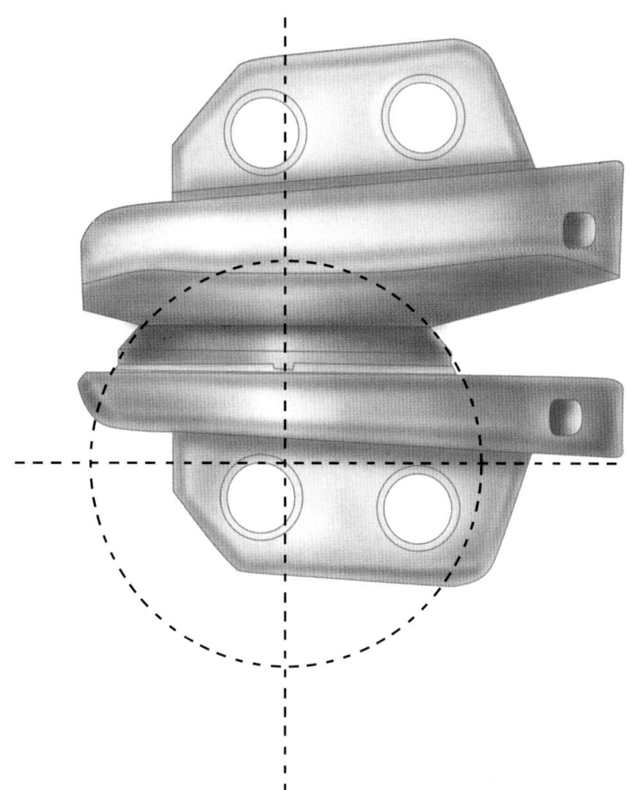

■ **FIGURE 44–5.** Posterior center of rotation corresponds closer to patient anatomy.

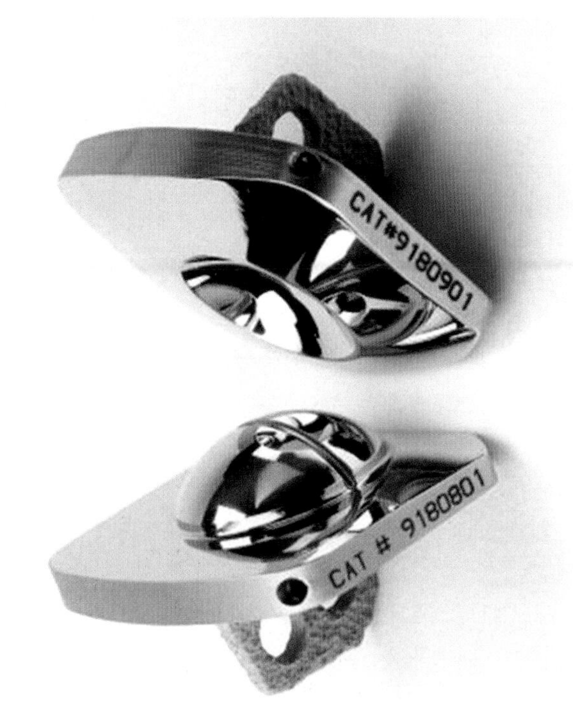


■ **FIGURE 44–6.** Maverick ball-and-socket design, metal-on-metal end plates (cobalt-chromium-molybdenum).

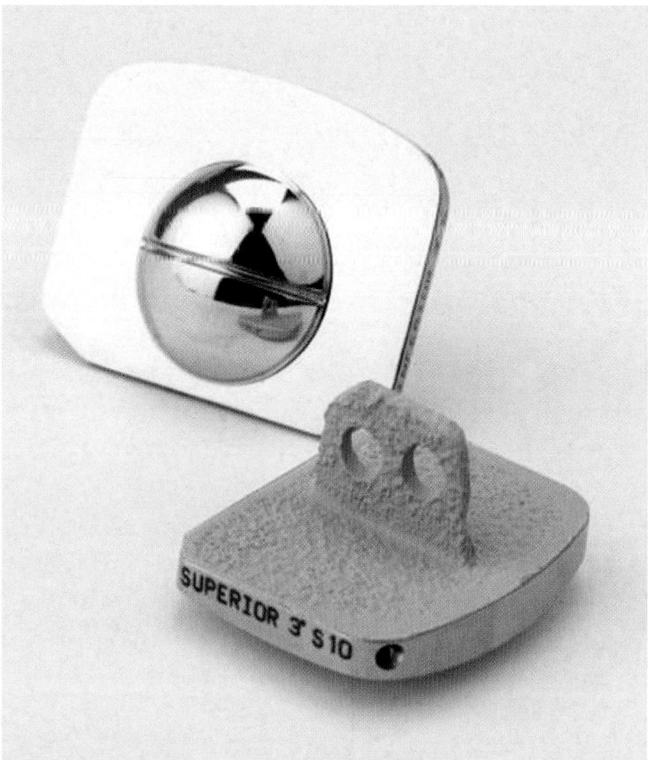


■ FIGURE 44–7. Hydroxyapatite coating and chemically roughened surface make Maverick conducive to bony ingrowth while achieving increased friction for a press-fit.

Maverick disc is designed for component interchangeability, whereby the surgeon is provided a matrix of versatile configurations to help achieve the optimal fit, balance, and lordosis. Unlike other disc prostheses, the Maverick is passive regarding lordosis; whatever lordosis the patient creates through postoperative movement is adapted by the Maverick TDR.

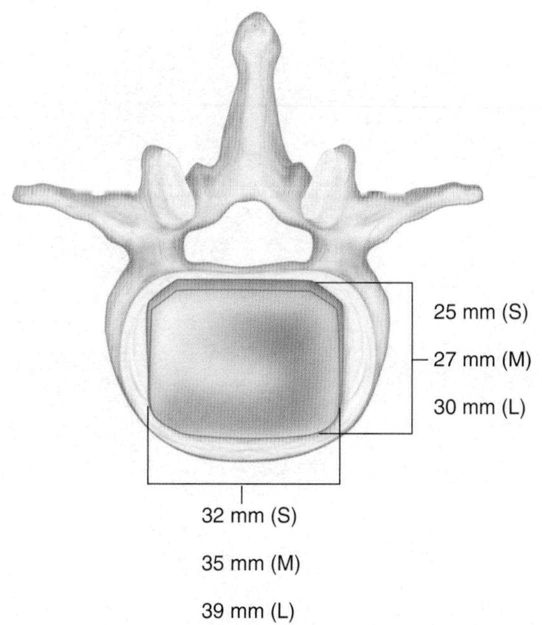


■ FIGURE 44–8. Maverick total disc replacement interchangeable end plate sizes, along with variable height and lordosis, provide the surgeon with the necessary components for a customized fit.

Developing a streamlined implantation technique that most surgeons could adopt was the final challenge in the strategic design approach of the early development team. To that end, the surgeon is provided with a complete tray for en block discectomy, and a unique All-in-1 guide that comes with the Maverick kit to promote accuracy and repeatability of results. The All-in-1 guide (Fig. 44–9A and B) promotes efficient surgical technique and maximizes the benefits of the device by assisting with measurements such as anteroposterior depth, height distraction for optimal device sizing, maintenance of proper lordosis, and keel chiseling.

In summary, the Maverick TDR was designed as a two-piece, single-insertion construct delivering restoration of normal kinematics, shear load resistance, and facet joint unloading through a fixed posterior center of rotation. This MOM, keel-anchored device with HA coating is designed to achieve optimal fixation and exceptional wear characteristics for durability and longevity.

## BACKGROUND OF SCIENTIFIC TESTING/CLINICAL OUTCOMES

In designing a prosthetic device for disc replacement, a thorough analysis of the biomechanics of the healthy spine is an essential first step.[4] The Maverick TDR is designed for permanent placement to provide optimal motion stabilization at the involved level, so exhaustive research and testing of material and design issues, including durability and wear characteristics, shear and compressive strength, shock absorbance, kinematics, biocompatibility and toxicity, were integral aspects of the product development road map.

Dooris et al[3] conducted an important analysis of the center of rotation (COR) of a ball-and-cup disc prosthesis, concluding that facet loading increased around 2.5 times with an anteriorly placed device, whereas a posterior COR device could bear a comparable load without impacting the facet load. In the same study, they also revealed that motion increased with a posterior COR device compared to an anteriorly placed ball-and-cup prosthesis.[3]

The advantages of a metal-on-metal prosthesis were confirmed by extensive 10 million load cycle wear testing, which demonstrated that the device would not fail mechanically and that wear of the Maverick is well within that reported in clinical use for total hip replacements. A typical MOM hip prosthesis would wear at a rate approximately 11 times the wear rate of a Maverick TDR.[5,6] In fact, Maverick was the subject of the only published study to compare in vitro simulated use and explanted device wear for the same type of device.[7] The results suggested that the rigorous simulated use tests may significantly overstate the wear actually generated in situ for Maverick.

In response to concerns that a lumbar disc prosthesis should possess shock absorption and vibration-dampening characteristics in addition to low wear debris levels, a test was conducted to compare the Maverick TDR and a ProDisc device, which has a polyethylene insert intended to provide those characteristics. The results indicated that there were no statistically significant differences in measured shock or vibration between the two devices.[8]

The most commonly perceived drawback of MOM use in prosthetic devices is exposure to high levels of metal ions due to device wear. In a rabbit study, CoCrMo particles were injected

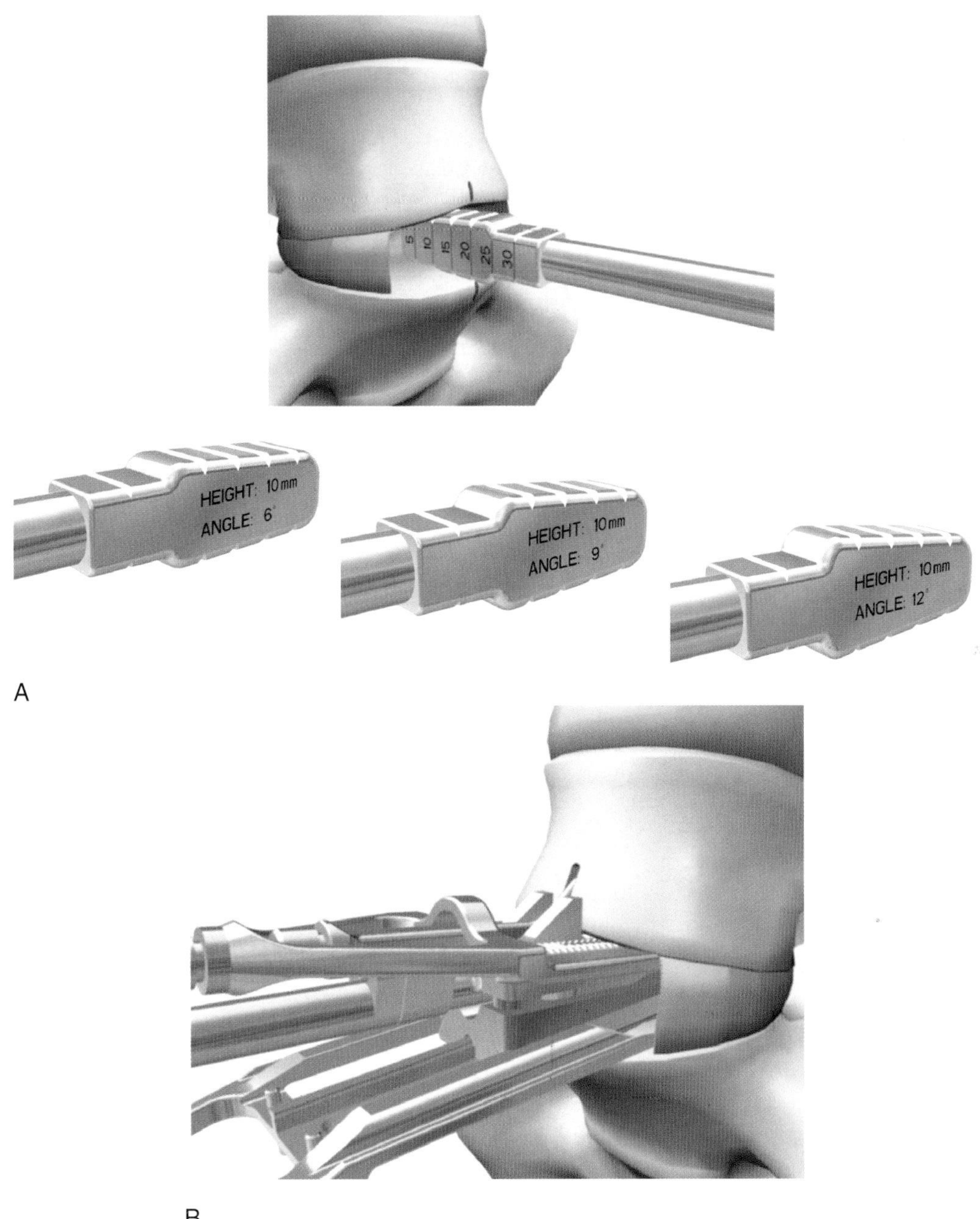


■ **FIGURE 44–9.** **A,** Templating with the all-in-1 instrument helps to establish midline, appropriate device angle, and proper footprint size. **B,** Keel cutting with the all-in-1 guide instrument for ideal midline keel placement.

into the spine at levels equivalent to estimated exposure levels based on projected Maverick wear ranging from 10 to 60 years. Upon examination of implant site, liver, kidneys, spleen, and lymph nodes, no significant histologic changes were detected between control and the investigational subjects.[9] These very encouraging results are being followed currently by human studies investigating metal ion production with Maverick.

## CLINICAL PRESENTATION & EVALUATION

In a prospective, non-randomized series by LeHuec et al[10] in Europe beginning in January 2002, more than 80% of patients achieved at least a 15-point improvement on the self-reported Oswestry Disability Index (ODI) questionnaire at 6 months and again at 24 months after surgery. This is significant because the FDA mandates 15-point improvement to be considered a success in the IDE study. In addition, there was no measurable subsidence greater than 2 mm. Mean range of motion was 6 degrees of flexion and 4 degrees of extension. Importantly, no significant change was reported in sacral tilt, pelvic tilt, or overall lordosis, indicating stable sagittal balance.[11]

The FDA IDE study enrolled 577 patients at 31 sites beginning in April 2003. In planning for this study, the decision was made to select the very best standard of care as the control treatment against which Maverick would be compared. Fusion with the LT CAGE/INFUSE bone graft (Medtronic, Memphis, TN) would represent the best anterior static stabilization for comparison with this investigational mobile stabilization device. Complete 24-month follow-up results for the IDE study are still being compiled as of this writing, but an early look at the trends suggests potentially better results than those reported in the LeHuec series. Although this might certainly be attributable to differences in patient selection, demographics, or other factors, the initial trends are positive.

In a report of 24-month outcomes for six sites participating in the Maverick IDE study,[12] 160 enrolled investigational patients (46% men, 54% women) averaged 40.1 years of age and 175.1 pounds, with 35% smokers, 51% working preoperatively, and 23% seeking worker's compensation. These demographics were statistically equivalent to the control group receiving fusion with LT CAGE/INFUSE.

Patient assessments were completed before surgery, during hospitalization, and postoperatively at 1.5, 3, 6, 12, and 24 months. Clinical outcomes were assessed using the Oswestry Low Back Pain Disability Questionnaire, neurologic status, short form SF-36, and back and leg pain questionnaires.

In this six-site report, 50 of the 160 enrolled Maverick patients had reached the 2-year follow-up. Their mean ODI score was 20.0, a 35.7-point improvement ($P$ <0.001) versus preoperative assessment (Table 44–1). ODI showed statistically significant mean improvement and sequentially better outcomes at all measured time intervals starting at 6 weeks. At 24 months, 82.0% of Maverick patients reported an ODI improvement of at least 15 points, an FDA-defined measure of success. This compares with reports in the literature of ODI success rates of 73% for patients receiving LT-CAGE with INFUSE.[13] The 24-month mean SF-36 Physical Component Score (PCS) improved 17.7 points ($P$ <0.001) to 45.1, with mean back pain and leg pain scores continuing to show significant ($P$ <0.001) improvement at 24 months. These reported outcomes suggest that Maverick TDR is a promising alternative to spinal fusion for patients meeting the strict patient screening guidelines.

## OPERATIVE TECHNIQUE

Only screened, well-qualified candidates are selected for TDR surgery, with particular attention given to the exclusion of patients with severe facet disease or significant bone abnormalities that might result in subsidence of the implanted device. During the preoperative planning process, the surgical team should attempt to match the largest disc replacement footprint possible with the patient anatomy in an effort to maximize end plate coverage. This is accomplished preoperatively by using the axial images of an MRI or CT before surgery. Once the surgeon has performed the Maverick TDR procedure often enough to gain appropriate experience, sizing can be done intraoperatively and the CT templates that are available for preoperative planning may become optional.

**TABLE 44–1. Sequential Clinical Results Compared with Preoperative Benchmark**

| Period | Variable | ODI | Low Back Pain | Leg Pain | SF-36 PCS |
|---|---|---|---|---|---|
| Preoperative | *n* | 160 | 160 | 160 | 160 |
| | Mean | 54.1 | 71.7 | 52.3 | 27.3 |
| 6 weeks | *n* | 154 | 154 | 154 | 154 |
| | Mean | 34.1 | 22.7 | 26.1 | 35.1 |
| Improvement vs. preoperative values | *n* | 154 | 154 | 154 | 154 |
| | Mean | −19.9 | −48.7 | −26.0 | 7.7 |
| | *P* value* | <0.001 | <0.001 | <0.001 | <0.001 |
| 3 months | *n* | 153 | 153 | 153 | 153 |
| | Mean | 25.7 | 19.7 | 22.8 | 39.9 |
| Improvement vs. preoperative values | *n* | 153 | 153 | 153 | 153 |
| | Mean | −28.2 | −51.7 | −30.8 | 12.6 |
| | *P* value | <0.001 | <0.001 | <0.001 | <0.001 |
| 6 months | *n* | 150 | 150 | 150 | 150 |
| | Mean | 22.3 | 19.5 | 19.1 | 42.1 |
| Improvement vs. preoperative values | *n* | 150 | 150 | 150 | 150 |
| | Mean | −31.8 | −51.9 | −34.0 | 14.6 |
| | *P* value | <0.001 | <0.001 | <0.001 | <0.001 |
| 12 months | *n* | 148 | 148 | 148 | 148 |
| | Mean | 219.8 | 17.7 | 16.6 | 43.5 |
| Improvement versus preoperative values | *n* | 148 | 148 | 148 | 148 |
| | Mean | −33.8 | −53.0 | −36.6 | 15.9 |
| | *P* value | <0.001 | <0.001 | <0.001 | <0.001 |
| 24 months | *n* | 50 | 50 | 50 | 50 |
| | Mean | 20.0 | 17.7 | 17.7 | 45.1 |
| Improvement versus preoperative values | *n* | 50 | 118 | 50 | 149 |
| | Mean | −35.7 | −54.8 | −39.5 | 17.7 |
| | *P* value | <0.001 | <0.001 | <0.001 | <0.001 |

ODI, Oswestry Disability Index; PCS, physical component score.
*$P$ values for change versus preoperative values are from paired t test.

Detailed planning must occur before anterior lumbar surgery, including operative set-up and anesthesia choice. Because skilled access by an experienced surgeon is required for this approach, appropriate complications contingency planning might include the availability of on-call anesthesia and vascular surgery expertise, as well as intensive care staff and equipment. When approaching the lumbar spine anteriorly, general endotracheal anesthesia is the norm. Foley catheterization is inserted before sterile prep and draping of the patient, and intravenous (IV) antibiotics are given prophylactically before surgery. Pneumatic sequential devices are used on the lower extremities throughout the procedure. Appropriate preparation for fluoroscopy is also required, including a high-quality C-arm, a radiolucent table, and protective wear.

Instrumentation for placement of the Maverick device includes the following:

- Centering pin for midline verification on fluoroscopy
- Template for annulotomy of the anterior longitudinal ligament
- Instruments to remove the end plate cartilage and disc material
- Posterior curettes and rongeurs
- Ligament elevators to elevate and release the posterior longitudinal ligament
- Disc space spreader
- Shim distractors
- Angle trials
- Footprint trials
- All-in-1 guide with 6-, 9-, and 12-degree plates
- Disc-shaping for superior and inferior components with keel chisels independently inserted or in conjunction with disc-shaping chisels
- Prosthesis holder for insertion and prosthesis inserter

Operating room equipment should include a multiple-position radiolucent table, which allows adequate use of the image intensifier for accurate prosthetic placement. Proper position is achieved by placing the patient supine on the operative table such that anterior or lateral fluoroscopy can be used safely. A bolster can be used under the patient's pelvis to facilitate exposure and potentially open the anterior margin to allow greater access to the disc space.

An anterior approach to the lumbar spine is then initiated, either retroperitoneal or transperitoneal, depending on anatomy of the patient and surgeon preference. The abdominal contents are retracted to gain exposure at the diseased segment. When accessing the L4-L5 level, it is important to identify any iliolumbar vessels that could limit immobilization of the left common iliac. With adequate exposure achieved, markers are placed directly anteriorly based on visual determination of the midline. The Maverick kit includes a centering pin used to identify the center of the disc space before bringing the image intensifier into AP position on a true perpendicular with the patient's spine, after which the vessels are allowed to safely retract directly over the center pin. Acquiring an AP image not only helps to confirm the midline, which is essential to successful central placement of the Maverick TDR but also provides access to any inadvertent rotation of the vertebral body, either due to the patient's position or to the surgeon's position relative to the spine of the patient. I preserve the checked and confirmed midpoint of the vertebral body with a bovie and bring the C-arm around to a lateral position to once again confirm the operative level from this viewpoint, making sure again to establish correct perpendicular position with the spine rather than external markers. Once the image is acquired, the fluoroscopy machine is removed from the immediate field up toward the head of the patient.

With the correct operative level identified and exposure established, a block discectomy is performed (Fig. 44–10), taking care to limit the size and to not remove more annulus than necessary, because the lateral fibers provide important stabilization in disc arthroplasty. Disc material is removed down to the cartilaginous end plate, although care must be taken not to violate the bony surface, which might create destabilization of the vertebral end plate and facilitate possible subsidence of the device. If necessary, the space may be mobilized after the discectomy, and osteophytes may be removed in preparation for placement of the prosthesis.

Mobilization of the vertebral space should be accomplished by progressively dilating the space; I find that using a series of central dilators typically used during anterior lumbar fusion work very well for this task. If the disc space tethers at the posterior annulus, as often occurs with a collapsed disc, first attempt additional posterior dilation until you "feel" the tether free up, or else you may use a curette to release the annulus. At that point, symmetric dilation of the segment can be achieved, and confirmed via lateral fluoroscopy imaging.

With a freely mobile segment established, trialing to establish the correct disc height is initiated, beginning 1 to 2 mm less than the snug dilator I use for lumbar fusion procedures. Care should be taken to avoid overtensioning of the facets and lateral annulus by selecting too large a disc height size, as this can lead to potential subsidence or reduced motion of the prosthesis. As a guideline, I want a snug fit, but one that is more easily removed than my standard distractors for anterior lumbar fusion. Although most surgeons will establish disc height with the all-in-1 device, I prefer the feel provided from interspace dilators.

Estimating the correct lordosis is more challenging, because patient position influences the perceived lordosis intraoperatively. Because unlike an interbody fusion, a disc prosthesis is freely mobile, the position templated and achieved during surgery will

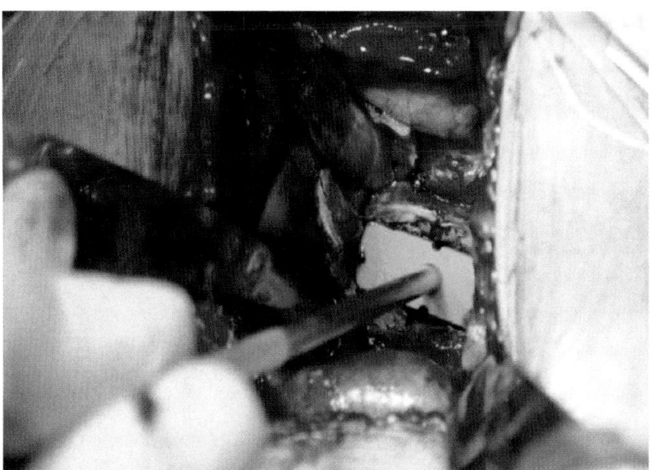

■ **FIGURE 44–10.** Block discectomy prepares the vertebral space for placement of the prosthesis.

necessarily differ from the postoperative position with the patient standing. The goal of the intradiscal trialing is to parallel the superior and inferior end plates, attempting to determine the maximum lordosis of the disc space without applying any damaging force to the vertebrae. If there are visible gaps during trialing, a larger size should be attempted until the correct angulation can be estimated, and eventually a midrange of motion between flexion and extension is determined. We then decrease the measured angle at least 3 degrees to allow segmental mobility. The L5-S1 level generally fits to an angle of 9 to 12 degrees, with less at higher levels. Whatever angle is selected during this trialing is then used to establish the appropriately angled All-in-1 guide for all remaining size parameters throughout the rest of the procedure. At this point, disc height can be reconfirmed with the all-in-1 guide in conjunction with lateral fluoroscopy.

The properly angled guide is then positioned posteriorly as far as possible in the disc space by selecting the minimum depth stops, while centering on the vertebral body AP mark. Placing the prosthesis as far posterior as possible will maximize unloading of the facets. There is not a danger of the chisel damaging the posterior wall because a 10-mm stop on the all-in-1 guide will prevent reaching that depth. The guide allows for both inferior and superior keel cuts to be made simultaneously, assuring proper device fit and alignment. Brisk bleeding typically begins with the removal of the chisel and can often be limited with the use of Flowseal and Surgiseal in the disc space.

At this point in the procedure, the surgeon has a feel for the appropriate dimensions of the required implant, including height, lordosis, and footprint. Again, the largest footprint possible should be the goal. In the author's experience, subsidence is not a significant concern with the Maverick TDR. We have most commonly selected a small 10-mm height with 6 degrees of lordosis for our previous patients, and rarely is a large prosthesis with greater than 12 mm of height required.

Early versions of the Maverick TDR offered the components in 3-degree lordotic increments, but the newer insertional tools allow the device to be inserted with 6, 9, or 12 degrees of lordosis. The ultimate lordosis will reflect the patient's natural rebalancing as he or she stabilizes the spinal unit postoperatively.

The all-in-1 guide can also be used as needed to make corner cuts where end plate morphology dictates so that the prosthesis can be evenly positioned on the end plate, although in this author's experience, this is rarely required. When corner cuts are made, special care is needed to remove all bone fragments created by the cutter.

The vertebral space is now ready for placement of the prosthesis, which should be ready to go in its inserter prior to removal of the cutting instruments so that any sinusoidal bleeding is minimized. Once inserted, the device is tamped home and the depth is verified under x-ray control with the image intensifier to ensure optimal posterior placement according to the chisel cuts for the keels. Upon tamping, the device naturally begins to dilate the space, unlike other prostheses that require distraction in order to insert a polyethylene core. This distraction creates a risk of excessive widening of the space, leading to stress risers within the end plate and opening the door to subsidence problems at some future point. The surgeon is cautioned not to overtamp the prosthesis posteriorly, because repositioning the device more anterior is difficult. In the event this is necessary, use the special guides provided that enable distraction of the device itself. The danger in overtamping is potential foramen encroachment by the lateral margins of the device. Use the image intensifier during prosthesis tamping and to acquire final confirmation of device placement in both the lateral and AP planes (Fig. 44–11). At this point, thorough irrigation is performed, the device is inspected, and radiographs are performed one last time. Closure is initiated, following the routine for anterior interbody instrumentation procedures, including antibiotic irrigation and drains, if required.

## POSTOPERATIVE CARE

Patient care following this transperitoneal or retroperitoneal approach is challenging but not unlike the stand-alone anterior fusion procedure. The use of minimally invasive techniques lessens the morbidity, whereas concerns about bowel and bladder issues and incision issues are consistent with experiences after anterior fusion surgery. The use of an abdominal binder after surgery can provide patient comfort while supporting the soft tissue. Posterior and anterior ice packs are recommended to control soreness, in particular during the mobilization process. Patients are encouraged to mobilize less than 24 hours after surgery and begin walking, although diet is restricted to ice chips until normal bowel sounds return. The catheter is removed the morning after surgery, and the patient is typically discharged if free from nausea or vomiting and if walking independently.

Walking is strongly encouraged for TDR patients as soon as tolerated, and they are advised to take the cue from their own

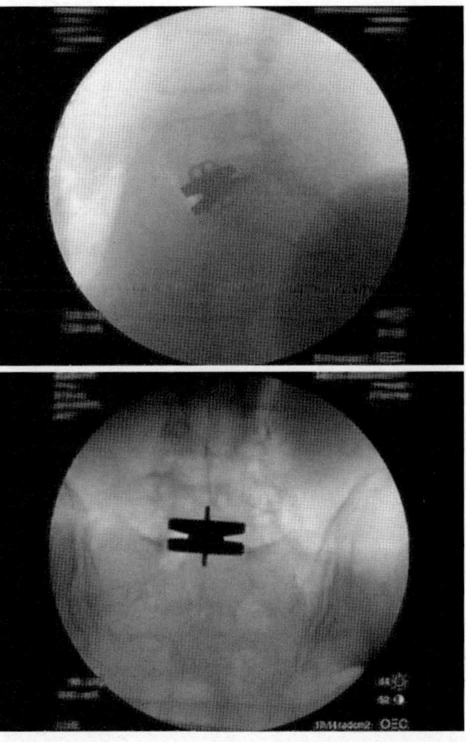

■ **FIGURE 44–11.** AP and lateral fluoroscopic images confirm proper device position.

incision pain level and to add activity if they are free of pain. To avoid the risks of an incisional hernia, patients are restricted from rigorous physical activity for the first 2 weeks, even though many patients report feeling strong enough to begin more quickly.

Activity levels are increased as tolerated from weeks 2 to 6, whereas golf, tennis, and similar impact-loading activities are discouraged for at least 6 weeks, with patient tolerance and healing of the incision determining the ultimate timetable. Likewise, patients may return to work in as little as 1 week as tolerated.

## COMPLICATIONS AND AVOIDANCE

Complications related to this anterior approach (transperitoneal or retroperitoneal) are well documented for anterior lumbar fusion surgery, and should be considered typical of what disc replacement patients might experience. The risks to this approach have been previously reported, and the need for training and expertise in anterior lumbar surgery before disc arthroplasty cannot be overemphasized.

As stated earlier, patient selection is of paramount importance in achieving successful clinical outcomes with total disc arthroplasty. Even a perfectly implanted device in a poorly selected patient runs the risk of clinical failure. Patients who have had previous anterior surgery may not be candidates for the current Maverick system. Obesity would likewise present an additional level of risk that would disqualify a potential TDR patient. Certainly, the main risk of complications would arise in a patient with bone insufficiencies, for whom subsidence is a major concern. The best way to ensure success is to be thorough in patient assessment, including the patient's need to be educated regarding the potential risks and complications.

Among the problems that have been associated with the implantation of lumbar disc prostheses are the following:

- Poor imaging studies/insufficient diagnostic rigor
- Inexperienced operating surgeon or access surgeon
- Poor disc space preparation
- Inadequate fluoroscopic visualization
- Overdistracting the disc space during preparation
- Failure to fully mobilize the disc space
- Canal encroachment/nerve injury
- Miscalculation of the midline, resulting in poor device location
- Epidural bleeding
- "Overstuffing" the disc space, leading to postoperative pain
- Improper size selection, risking subsidence
- Improper device positioning at the posterior wall (COR too anterior)
- Posterior vertebral wall fracture due to excessive force during insertion

### ADVANTAGES/DISADVANTAGES: MAVERICK TOTAL DISC REPLACEMENT

**Advantages**

Key design elements thought to represent an advantage versus other devices:

- Fixed posterior center of rotation to optimize unloading of facets
- Motion restoration with controlled translation for joint stabilization
- Two-piece metal-on-metal and longevity
- HA coating for optimal fixation and bone growth
- Single-staged insertion technique

**Disadvantages**

- No long-term studies to confirm safety and longevity

## CONCLUSIONS/DISCUSSION

At this early stage in the development of the TDR market, there is much still to be learned about the role the procedure will play as a treatment option for patients with a well-defined set of indications. Comparisons are a necessary component of the ongoing investigation into alternative treatment modalities for degenerative disc disease, helping to clearly delineate the advantages and disadvantages of techniques, devices, and instrumentation for patients in need of surgical intervention.

In this context, the debate between lumbar disc arthrodesis and disc arthroplasty continues to evolve. On the one hand, fusion provides pain relief and proven stabilization of the diseased joint. As patients are seen for long-term follow-up, questions arise about the impact of this total elimination of motion on the adjacent structure, with reports in the literature of adjacent disease and diminishing pain relief. On the other hand, a successful fusion can reasonably be expected to last a lifetime, whereas questions will remain for many years about the ultimate longevity of the disc prostheses. Although TDR provides improvements in pain relief and retained motion in the short term, longer term studies are needed to confirm what is suggested in early studies, where patient clinical outcomes reportedly may be superior for TDR patients compared with results for patients receiving fusion.

Given the FDA approvals for CHARITÉ and ProDisc and the encouraging early results with the Maverick TDR, comparisons among the devices in this rapidly growing treatment area are also increasing. Differences will be scrutinized, ultimately to the benefit of patients in need of this surgical solution. The Maverick design offers many unique characteristics intended to provide a clear differentiation from the currently available devices. A cobalt-chrome–on–cobalt-chrome construct that offers minimal wear debris, without any compromise in terms of shock absorption or vibration, provides an important foundation for this lifetime implant design. The fixed posterior center of rotation of the Maverick is intended to improve motion in the treated vertebral body while sparing the facets from any additional loading, and this design difference was a critical consideration for the engineering team. The two-piece design is easily inserted and promotes rapid ingrowth, and these characteristics will also play a role in the differentiation of the various constructs. Continued evaluation will be required for many years to fully understand the implications of differences in design, materials, implantation technique, and other factors that may influence long-term patient outcomes.

## REFERENCES

1. Mathews H, LeHuec JC, Friesem T, et al: Design rationale and biomechanics of Maverick Total Disc arthroplasty with early clinical results. Spine J 4(suppl 6):268S–275S, 2004.
2. Chan FW, Bobyn JD, Medley JB, et al: Engineering issues and wear performance of metal on metal hip implants. Clin Orthop Relat Res 333:96–107, 1996.

3. Dooris AP, Goel VK, Grosland NM, et al: Load-sharing between anterior and posterior elements in a lumbar motion segment implanted with an artificial disc. Spine 26:E122–E129, 2001.
4. Bao QB, McCullen GM, Higham PA, et al: The artificial disc: Theory design and materials. Biomaterials 17:1157–1167, 1996.
5. Chan FW, Bobyn JD, Medley JB, et al: Engineering issues and wear performance of metal on metal hip implants. Clin Orthop Relat Res 333:96–107, 1996.
6. Goldsmith AA, Dowson D, Isaac GH, Lancaster JG: A comparative joint simulator study of the wear of metal-on-metal and alternative material combinations in hip replacements. Proc Inst Mech Eng [H]; 214:39–47, 2000.
7. Chan F, Pare P, Buchholz P, et al: Is unidirectional motion clinically relevant for wear testing of artificial disc implants? International Meeting on Advanced Spine Technology, E-Poster #235, July 7–9, 2005, Banff, AB, Canada.
8. LeHuec JC, Kiaer T, Friesem T, et al: Shock absorption in lumbar disc prosthesis: A preliminary mechanical study. J Spinal Disord Tech 16:346–351, 2003.
9. Mathews H, High W, McLay C, et al: Evaluation of wear debris in the rabbit spine. Study presented at Spinal Arthroplasty Society (SAS) 3, The Journey of the Spine: Global Symposium on Intervertebral Disc Replacement and Non-Fusion Technology, May 3, 2003, Scottsdale, AZ.
10. LeHuec JC, Mathews H, Basso Y, et al: Clinical results of Maverick Total Disc Replacement: Two year prospective follow-up. Orthop Clin North Am 36:315–322, 2005.
11. LeHuec JC, Basso Y, Mathews H, et al: The effect of single-level total disc arthroplasty on sagittal balance parameters: a prospective study. Eur Spine J 14:480–486, 2005.
12. Gornet MF, Mathews H, Burkus JK, et al: Maverick Total Disc Replacement: Initial report of 24-month clinical outcomes from six investigational centers [abstract]. Spine J 6(suppl 5):66S, 2006.
13. Burkus JK, Gornet MF, Dickman CA, Zdeblick TA: Anterior lumbar interbody fusion using rhBMP-2 with tapered interbody cages. J Spinal Disord Tech 15:337–349, 2002.

CHAPTER 45

# Theken eDisc: A Second-Generation Lumbar Artificial Disc

**Richard Navarro, Randall Theken, Ravi Ananthan, Christopher Cole, James P. Price, Charles Park, Vijay K. Goel, Scott Dean Miller,** and **Hansen A. Yuan**

## KEY POINTS

- First- and second-generation total disc replacements (TDRs) differ in their ability to restore neutral position and spinal balance.
- Second-generation viscoelastic disc motion is essential to restoring load sharing among soft tissues.
- Material selection and bond joint longevity are keys to second-generation disc success.
- Theken eDisc is the first spine implant with sensors and microelectronics targeting improved patient outcomes.
- Long-term follow-up will be required to determine the importance of biomechanics and electronics to patient outcomes.

## INTRODUCTION

Lumbar artificial discs from the Fernstrom ball[1] to the discs described in Chapters 38 to 44 share a common biomechanical theme. This theme is best described by the total degrees of freedom being three to five, and a design philosophy that uses a variation of a constrained or unconstrained spheric sliding surface. Additionally, these designs constrain the spine motion segment to rotate about a fixed center of rotation, as in the ProDisc (Synthes, West Chester, PA), or allow the center of rotation to move, as in the CHARITÉ (DePuy Spine, Inc., Raynham, MA) disc. Common to this group, and to any total disc replacement (TDR), is the immediate pain relief that results from disc height restoration. Preserving disc height and restoring and/or preserving the range of motion of a spine segment are essential for long-term success.

Two important attributes of a physiologic disc are its load-deflection response curve and its ability to absorb loads owing to its viscoelastic properties (Fig. 45–1). First-generation articulating discs are capable of only restoring range of motion, and in contrast to a physiologic disc, they have no viscous properties, meaning that they do not dissipate energy and instead transmit energy to adjacent levels. Furthermore, and perhaps more importantly, first-generation discs do not provide *elastic* motion to share loads among the soft tissues, nor do they provide restoring forces to return a motion segment to its neutral or balanced position. Long-term (5 to 10 years) follow-up of these first-generation implanted patients will help determine the importance of these viscous and elastic properties as they relate to long-term pain outcomes.

## INDICATIONS/CONTRAINDICATIONS

The Theken eDisc (Theken Disc, Akron, OH) will have similar inclusion and exclusion criteria as the Synthes ProDisc and the CHARITÉ lumbar disc prostheses. The indications for use are:

- Degenerative disc disease of a single level at L-3 to S-1
- Back and/or leg pain
- Instability with 3 mm of translation; 5 degrees of angulation
- More than 2 mm loss of disc height
- Scarring/thickening of the annulus fibrosis
- Herniated nucleus or vacuum phenomenon
- Age 18 to 65 years
- Six months of conservative treatment failed to alleviate the condition
- Oswestry Disability Index of at least 20/50 or 40%

The Theken eDisc contraindications are:

- End plate size at least 36 mm mediolateral and 27 mm anteroposterior
- Titanium, polyethylene, cobalt, chromium, or molybdenum allergies
- Prior fusion at any level
- Compromised vertebra due to previous trauma
- Radiographically confirmed facet disease or degeneration
- Lytic spondylolisthesis or spinal stenosis
- Degenerative spondylolisthesis higher than grade 1
- Back or leg pain of unknown etiology
- Osteopenia or osteoporosis; dual-energy x-ray absorptiomety (DEXA) based on SCORE
- Paget's disease or any other metabolic bone disease
- Morbid obesity (body mass index [BMI] greater than 40 or weight more than 100 lb higher than normal)
- Active infection
- Rheumatoid arthritis or other autoimmune disease

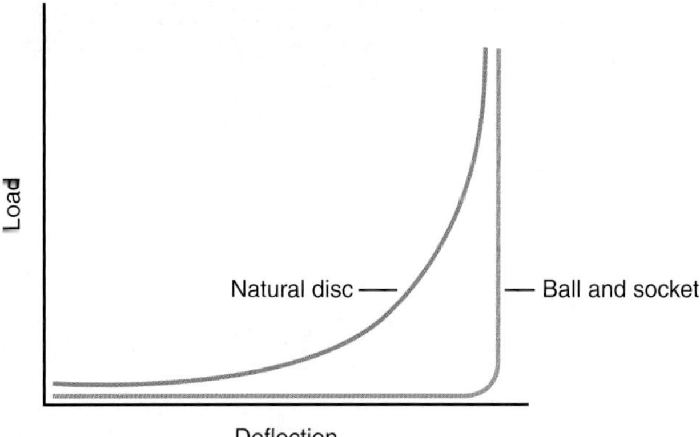


■ **FIGURE 45–1.** Simplified flexion/extension and lateral-bending response curve for a natural and articulating ball-and-socket disc.

## DESCRIPTION OF THE DEVICE

Second-generation lumbar TDRs, such as the Theken eDisc have a common attribute—elastic motion preservation and restoration. What makes the Theken eDisc design different from the first-generation TDRs is its elastomeric core bonded to titanium end plates (Fig. 45–2A and B). However, elastic core discs are not a new concept and have been attempted clinically.[2] Their lack of success as of this writing is a consequence of two factors: (1) the elastomers used were not specifically developed to withstand high-cycle, long-term biodurability loads; (2) the metal-polymer bond joint interface was incapable of withstanding in vivo loads. The Theken eDisc targets these critical factors by incorporating a patent-pending elastomer material, coupled with unique motion constraints.

The Theken eDisc is available in a range of sizes with two transverse profiles, two heights, and four lordotic angles to fit the low lumbar anatomy. The electronics feature can be ordered by the surgeon on a patient-by-patient basis as the device remains geometrically the same.

## BACKGROUND OF SCIENTIFIC TESTING/CLINICAL OUTCOMES

In order to determine the contribution of force from a natural disc, as well as implement these findings into the new Theken (TH200) elastomer, finite element modeling of a spine motion segment was performed. The results from this study (Fig. 45–3) show load sharing of the facets, ligaments, and natural disc when exercised in compression, flexion, extension, and torsion. Under a compression load of 2,600 N, the natural disc bears 99% of the load, which both first- and second-generation discs can support. Under an extension moment of 10 Nm, the natural disc carries 54.2%; facets, 26.3%; and ligaments, 19.5% of this total applied load. Only second-generation elastomer discs, such as the Theken eDisc, can replicate this 54.2% (5.4-Nm) natural disc load contribution. Although these results are based on cadaveric material properties,[3] the fundamental biomechanical goal of the Theken eDisc is to replicate the force contributions of the natural disc. Matching stiffnesses to the natural disc in six axes of motion with a homogenous material is unrealistic. Thus, the Theken eDisc focuses on matching compression stiffness and flexion stiffness, because these are the most important requirements for the lumbar spine (Table 45–1). Replicating the natural disc stiffness in the Theken eDisc prosthesis is expected to re-create the proper load sharing with soft tissues and thus improve long-term patient outcomes.

Elastomeric lumbar artificial discs developed by AcroMed in the 1980s used a vulcanized carbon black-filled polyolefin rubber originally produced by Goodyear. Ultimately, its biocompatibility and fatigue properties fell short of requirements for implantation as an artificial lumbar disc. The Theken eDisc TH200 elastomer is a thermoplastic polycarbonate polyurethane developed in-house at Theken. TH200 is optimized for biostability, crack growth fatigue, and compression set resistance. Tensile strength testing demonstrated superior in vitro hydrolytic stability compared with

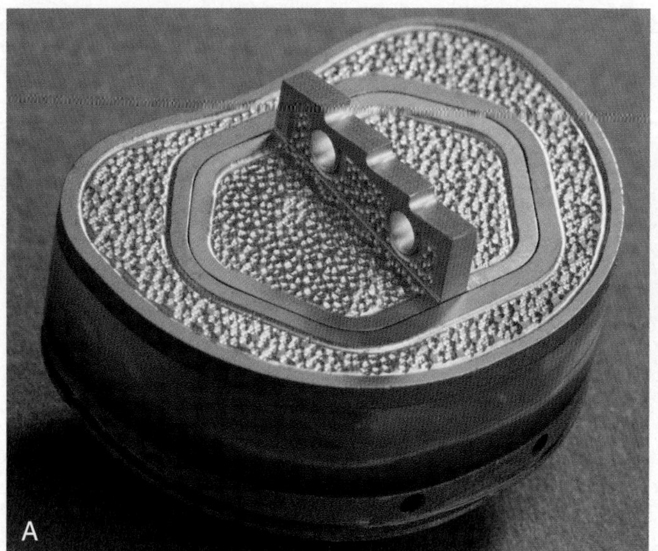


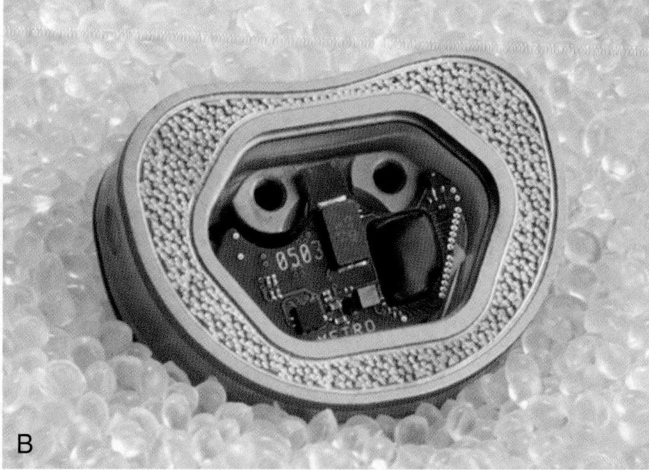


■ **FIGURE 45–2.** **A,** Theken eDisc shown with anteroposterior-oriented keel, urethane core, titanium end plates, and inductive recharging coil surrounding the lower end plate. **B,** Theken eDisc with cover removed showing microelectronics.

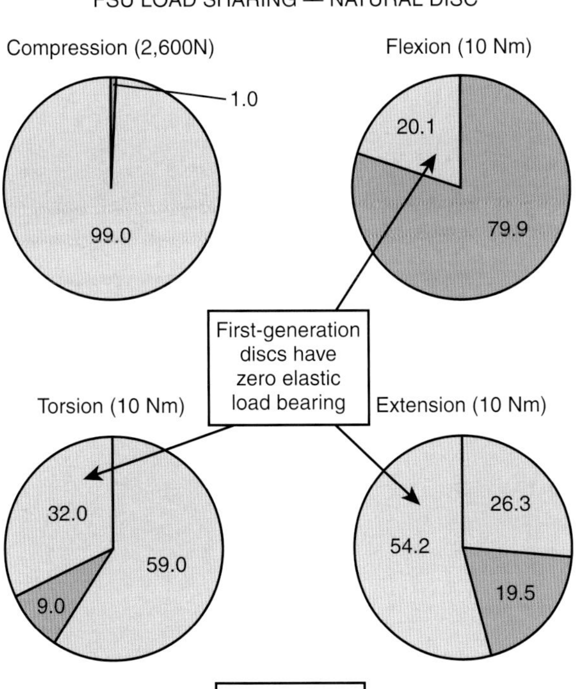


■ **FIGURE 45–3.** Finite element model of human L3-4 motion segment, showing natural disc load sharing in compression, flexion, extension, and torsion.

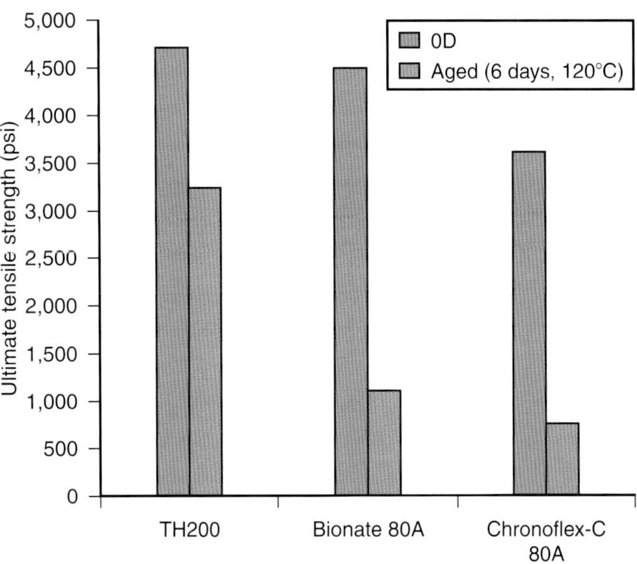


■ **FIGURE 45–4.** In vitro comparison of hydrolytic stability in Theken TH200 and commercial implant-grade polycarbonate polyurethanes.

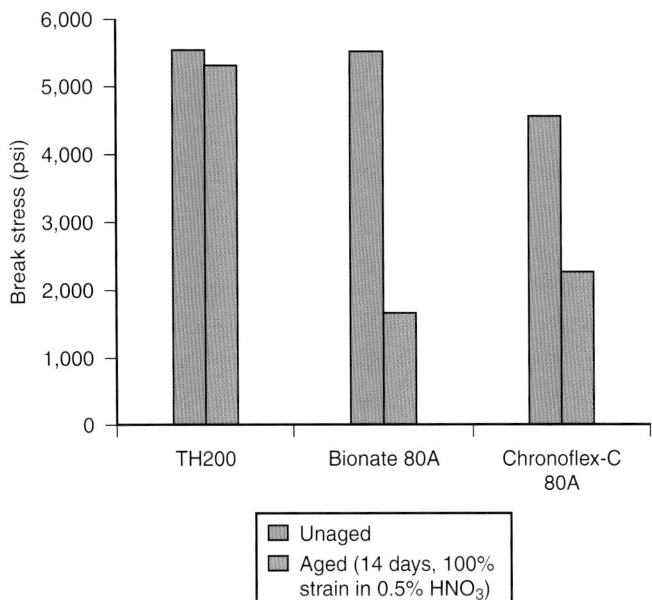


■ **FIGURE 45–5.** Retained tensile strength demonstrates oxidation resistance after nitric acid exposure. Comparison of TH200 to commercial implant-grade polycarbonate urethanes. Specimens were aged stretched over a mandrel to 100% strain.

implant-grade urethanes Bionate (Polymer Technology Group, Berkeley, CA) and Chronoflex (CardioTech International, Inc., Wilmington, MA) (Fig. 45–4). In addition, retained tensile strength in the TH200 demonstrated superior oxidation resistance after aging in nitric acid solution under 100% strain (Fig. 45–5).

The Theken eDisc has a sophisticated onboard microelectronics module that includes embedded force sensors, a 16-bit microprocessor, temperature sensor, real-time clock, nonvolatile RAM, bidirectional RF communications, and associated circuitry. This microelectronics module provides biofeedback to the patient, physician, or caregiver referencing the stresses placed on the patient's spine. The physician has the ability using either a palm or computer device to choose an appropriate peak stress level for a given patient and program this into the microelectronics after surgery. Peak load events in the patient's spine are then stored in the

**TABLE 45–1. Stiffness Comparison of Natural Discs, Articulating Polymer Core Discs, and Theken eDisc**

| | Disc Stiffness | | |
|---|---|---|---|
| **Loading Mode** | **Natural Disc** | **First-Generation Articulating Disc** | **Theken eDisc** |
| Compression (N/mm) | 500–3,214 | ~100-1,000 × natural disc | 1,600 |
| Flexion (N-m/°) | 0.9–1.9 | ~ 0 | 1.2 |
| Extension (N-m/°) | 2.1–2.6 | ~ 0 | 1.2 |
| Lateral bending (N-m/°) | 1.1–2.3 | ~ 0 | 2.7 |
| Torsion (N-m/°) | 2.0–2.7 | ~ 0 | 1.1 |

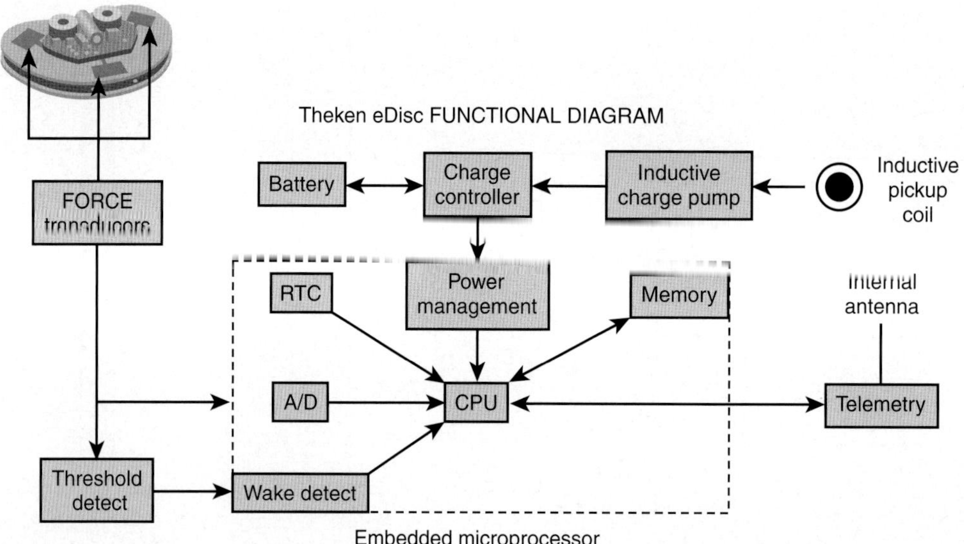


■ **FIGURE 45–6.** Functional block diagram of the Theken eDisc microprocessor, telemetry, power coupling, and FORCE sensors.

microelectronic, nonvolatile RAM memory and can be transmitted through the Internet to the physician's office by the patient, or downloaded and displayed at routine office visits.

A functional block diagram of the microelectronics module is shown in Figure 45–6. With its sensing capability, the Theken eDisc holds the promise of delivering previously unknown data on the human spine. These data may aid physicians, insurance companies, employers, therapists, and patients themselves in returning work-injured patients to function and appropriate labor more rapidly. The availability of objective data will allow more informed decisions to be made regarding suitability and timing for return to function and work. The data may also be used to alert patients of excessive loads on their spine during the early postoperative period, when migration and dislodgement are a risk.

The Theken eDisc was implanted in a baboon to demonstrate the ability of the device to:

1. Survive the shock loads of implantation,
2. Trigger on high-stress events,
3. Transmit data to an external receiver, and
4. Recharge the internal battery.

The device was implanted at L4-5 using an anterior approach in a 32-kg male baboon. A total of 56 load events were triggered and recorded to the Theken eDisc memory at a sampling rate of 30 samples per second for a duration of 2 seconds after triggering. A sample data set triggered by a 700-N load on the anterior sensor is shown in Figure 45–7. From the polarity and magnitude of the force signals from each of the three coplanar sensors, an interpretation of the bending movements can be made. In this

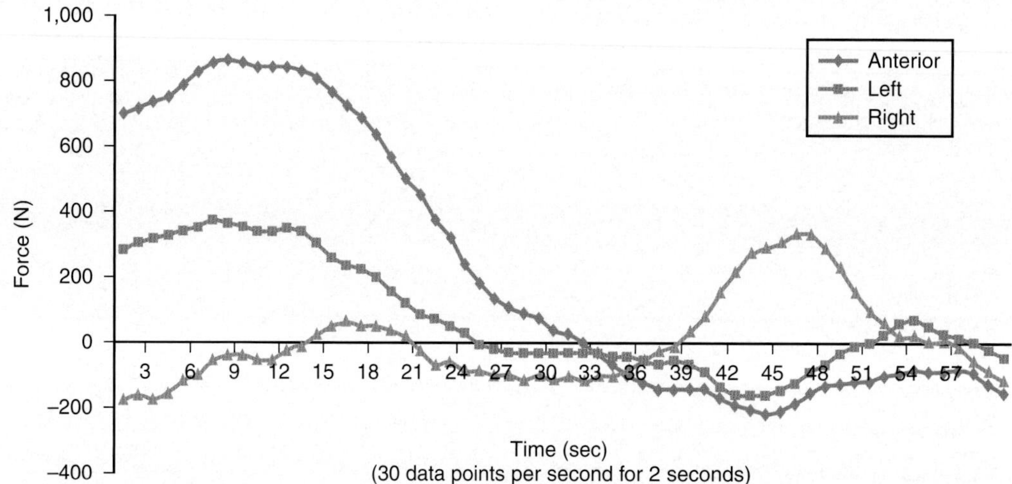


■ **FIGURE 45–7.** Primate implant of Theken eDisc at L4-5 showing event triggered recording of loads from three co-planar sensors. Event recording triggered by anterior sensor load exceeding 700 N.

example, the animal flexed forward with a slight left lateral bend, as noted by the rising positive posterior left sensor and negative posterior right sensor. In approximately 1 second, the three sensors approached roughly zero load readings, indicating a return to neutral upright posture. So not only is the Theken eDisc capable of recording a high-stress event, it is also capable of storing data to help interpret spine loading during a work task, physical therapy, or exercise. The software user interface will help interpret this data and can "play back" an animation of the recorded motion. The patient can be instructed by his or her physician to wear a pager device that has been developed in conjunction with the Theken eDisc that alerts the patient instantly if the preprogrammed physician stress value has been exceeded. This biofeedback can be used to curtail strenuous activities during the critical early postoperative period, when bone ingrowth is taking place.

## OPERATIVE TECHNIQUES

One of the concerns of surgeons implanting lumbar artificial discs is the difficulty of future revision surgeries. The anterior approach to L3-4 or L4-5 is frought with difficulty owing to the proximity of the large vessels to the disc space. Revisions at this level involve intricate dissection of scar tissue from the great vessels, with high risk to the patient for bleeding or even death. For this reason, the Theken eDisc has an optional mediolateral keel to allow a lateral approach to the disc space at L4-5 and above.

## POSTOPERATIVE CARE

The Theken eDisc with electronics offers the surgeon a tool to collect force data for evaluating a patient's recovery and level of activity. Before discharge, a patient can perform modest movements representative of activities of daily living. This allows a force threshold to be selected and programmed into a pager that can alert the patient to high loads on his or her spine. This biofeedback reminds patients to avoid strenuous activity during the early postoperative period (up to 3 months), when bone ingrowth is occurring.

### ADVANTAGES/DISADVANTAGES: THEKEN eDISC

**Advantages**

Protects facets and soft tissues
Protects adjacent level from overstress
Lateral keel option to avoid vasculature
No inherent wear debris from articulation
Mechanical stops to prevent overstressing
Electronics may reduce migration/dislodgement
Electronics may help return patients to work or function

**Disadvantages**

Less sizing options than modular discs
Electronics available at premium cost
Greater manufacturing complexity

## CONCLUSIONS/DISCUSSION

The Theken eDisc with its embedded microelectronics module will provide unprecedented data for reducing short-term migration and dislodgement complications while giving caregivers a powerful tool to aid a person's return to function and work. These data on the human spine could spawn even greater advances in artificial discs and other motion-preserving devices in the future.

## REFERENCES

1. Gerber MS, Galler RM, Papadopoulos SM: Spinal disc arthroplasty. Barrow Quarterly 19:34–38, 2003.
2. Fraser RD, Ross RE, Lowery GL, et al: Acroflex design and results. Spine J 4:245S–251S, 2004.
3. Dooris AP: Experimental and theoretical investigations into the effects of artificial disc implantation on the lumbar spin [Thesis]. Iowa City, IA, Biomedical Engineering Department, University of Iowa, 2001.

CHAPTER 46

# Lateral Lumbar Total Disc Replacement

**Luiz Pimenta, Thomas Schaffa, Juliano Lhamby, Ihab Gharzeddine,** and **Etevaldo Coutinho**

## KEY POINTS

- Surgical placement of total disc replacement (TDR) devices in the lumbar spine can be safely and effectively performed from a lateral (extreme lateral interbody fusion [XLIF]) approach.
- The lateral approach to TDR is less invasive than the traditional anterior approach, minimizing the risk of vascular and visceral complications while allowing quick patient recovery and return to normal activities.
- The lateral approach to TDR preserves the anterior and posterior longitudinal ligaments (ALL, PLL), which are known to withstand much of the torsional loads of the lumbar spine, and therefore may result in less stress on the facets than traditional anteriorly placed devices that require resection of the ALL.
- The lateral approach to TDR allows a more forgiving device placement than the traditional anterior approach because midline is easy to identify fluoroscopically. The lateral approach does require placement of the device more posterior than lateral fusion devices and, therefore, requires more caution around the nerves of the lumbar plexus within the psoas muscle. Dynamically stimulated electromyography is recommended in all cases.
- The approach to two-level L4-S1 pathology may include hybrid constructs of TDR at L4-L5 and fusion at L5-S1.

## INTRODUCTION

Lumbar total disc replacement (TDR) surgery has been proposed as an alternative to fusion procedures for the treatment of pain and instability associated with degenerative disc disease. The concept of TDR is based on the premise that stabilizing the motion segment while preserving motion will minimize biomechanical changes at adjacent levels and thereby reduce the incidence of adjacent-level degeneration. Lumbar TDR surgery has thus far been proposed only through the anterior approach. The anterior approach to place lumbar TDR devices has inherent limitations, including considerable collateral damage to surrounding tissues and risk of vascular and visceral injuries. In contrast, placement of a TDR device from a true lateral approach (extreme lateral interbody fusion [XLIF], NuVasive, Inc., San Diego, CA) allows for easier, less invasive access to the disc space, preservation of stabilizing ligaments, superior end plate support, and greater opportunity for safer revision surgery.

## CLINICAL INDICATIONS

The indications for lateral TDR are not different from those considered standard for anteriorly placed TDR devices—in general, degenerative disc disease without facet degeneration. However, placement of a TDR device laterally is limited to levels above L5-S1 due to obstruction by the iliac crest at that level. In the authors' experience, multilevel pathologies that include L5-S1 have been treated using a hybrid construct of lateral TDR at upper levels and anterior lumbar interbody fusion (ALIF) at L5-S1 (Fig. 46–1).

## RESULTS TO DATE

At the time of this writing, the authors have used the XLIF approach to implant lateral TDR devices in 36 patients with discography-confirmed one- or two-level degenerative disc disease as part of a prospective nonrandomized clinical evaluation.[1] Patients averaged 44 years of age (range: 25 to 60 years). Surgeries included 15 one-level, three two-level, and 18 hybrid TDR/ALIF procedures. The surgery was performed through a 4-cm lateral incision in an average of about an hour and 50-mL blood loss per level. There have been no intraoperative or postoperative complications. Postoperative x-ray studies show good device placement, with restoration of disc height, foraminal volume, and sagittal balance. All patients were up and walking within 12 hours of surgery, and all but nine were discharged the next day; seven of the nine patients underwent hybrid TDR/ALIF procedures. Five patients (13.8%) had psoas weakness, and three (8.3%) had anterior thigh numbness postoperatively, both resolving within 2 weeks. Four patients (11%) had postoperative facet joint pain, all in hybrid cases. Patient pain and function improved dramatically over the short term and improvements were maintained at 1-year follow-up.

## SURGICAL TECHNIQUE

**Step 1:** Surgical Exposure: The patient is placed in a lateral decubitus position on a radiolucent breaking table with the iliac crest flexed over the table break to open the space between the crest and the 12th rib (Fig. 46–2). The disc of interest is

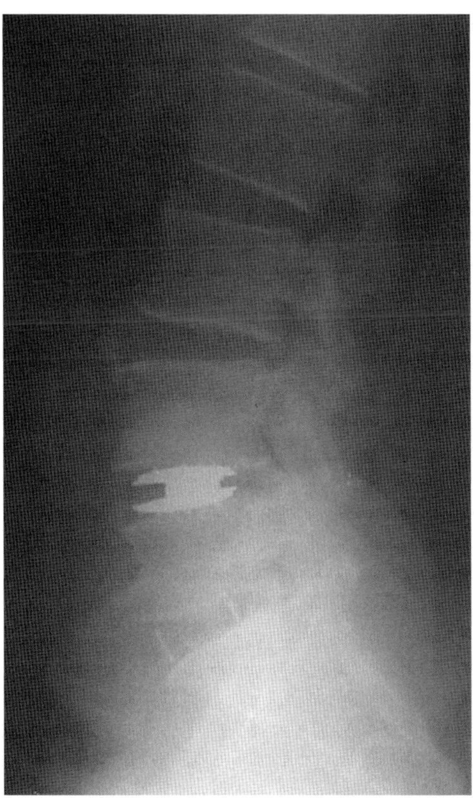

■ **FIGURE 46–1.** Lateral x-ray showing a hybrid construct of lateral total disc replacement at L4-L5 and anterior lumbar interbody fusion at L5-S1.

targeted using lateral fluoroscopy, and the skin is marked over the direct-lateral center of the disc space. A second incision is made just posterolateral to this direct-lateral marking, through which a finger is inserted to dissect the retroperitoneal space and guide dilators through the lateral incision to the surface of the psoas muscle. NeuroVision nerve avoidance (NuVasive, Inc., San Diego, CA) is used with the blunt dilators to gently split the fibers of the psoas without nerve injury (Fig. 46–3). This is an important consideration because exposure for TDR devices needs to extend further posterior than typically required for a more straightforward primary XLIF fusion procedure. The MaXcess (NuVasive, Inc., San Diego, CA) retractor is advanced over the dilators, rigidly locked to the surgical table, and expanded over the disc space (Figs. 46–4 and 46–5).

**Step 2:** Disc Space Preparation: An annulotomy is created at the lateral aspect of the disc, and conventional discectomy and end plate preparation is performed. As with the XLIF

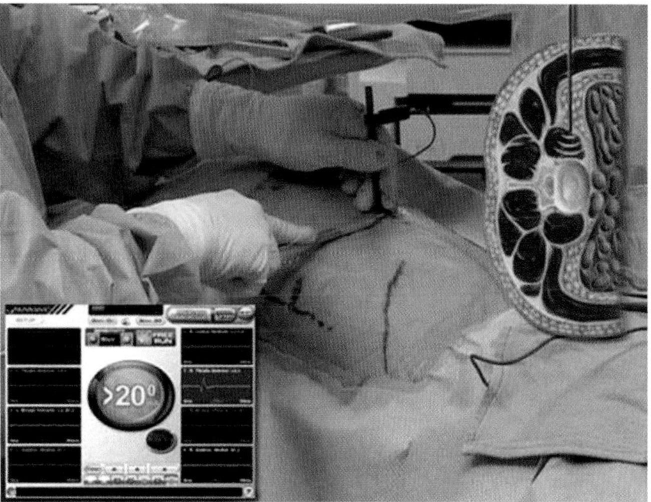


■ **FIGURE 46–3.** NeuroVision guidance uses discrete dynamic evoked electromyography to safely traverse the psoas muscle and avoid the nerves of the lumbar plexus.

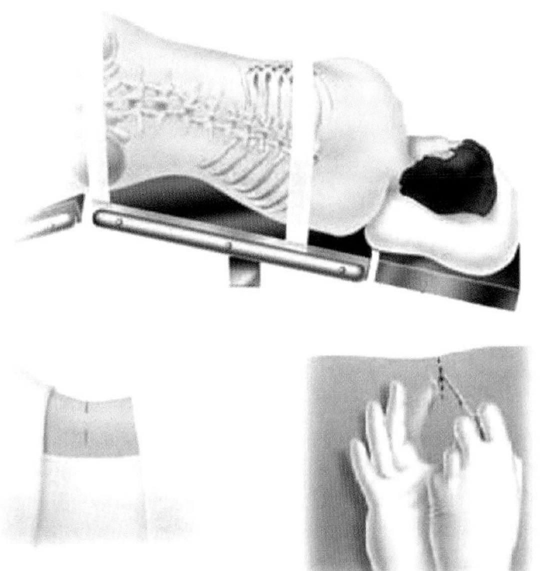

■ **FIGURE 46–2.** Patient in lateral decubitus position on breaking table and initial skin incisions. *(Illustrations provided courtesy of NuVasive, Inc., San Diego, CA).*

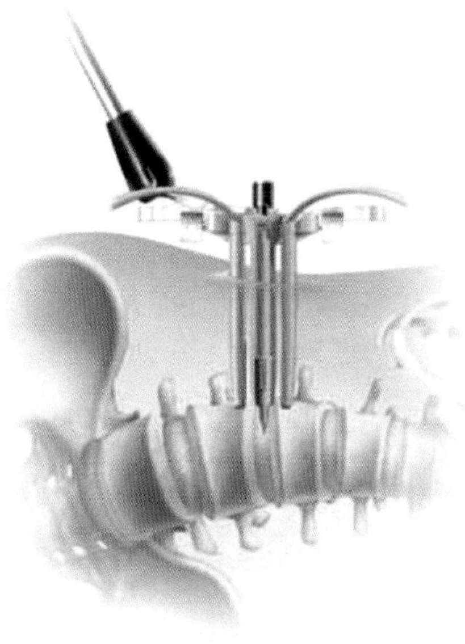

■ **FIGURE 46–4.** The MaXcess retractor is advanced over the disc space and spread to expose from superior to inferior end plates. *(Illustration provided courtesy of NuVasive, Inc., San Diego, CA.)*

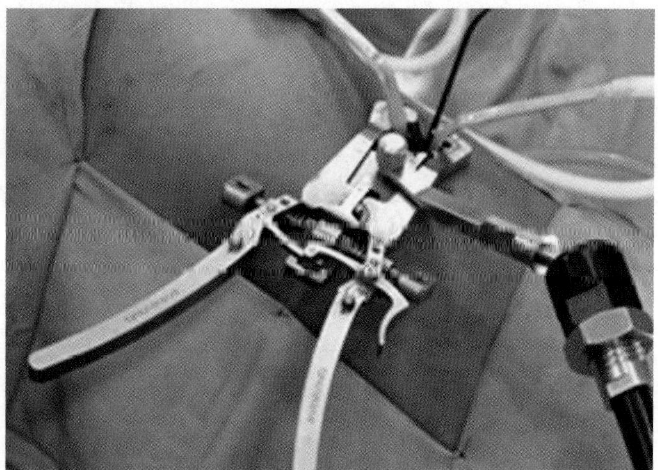

■ **FIGURE 46–5.** MaXcess retractor in place.

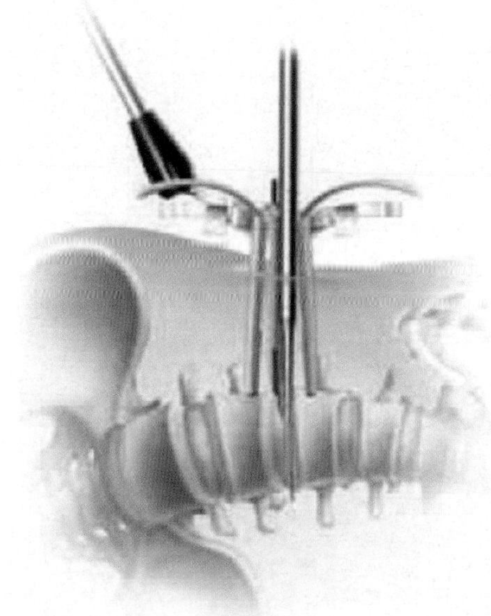

■ **FIGURE 46–6.** The contralateral annulus must be released to allow for bilateral disc distraction and insertion of the total disc replacement device across the ring apophysis. *(Illustration provided courtesy of NuVasive, Inc., San Diego, CA.)*

fusion procedure, it is important to perform a complete and thorough discectomy clear to the contralateral margin and release the contralateral annulus with a long Cobb elevator (Fig. 46–6). This step ensures parallel distraction and proper coronal alignment, and allows for the placement of the device in its ideal position spanning the ring apophysis on either side.

STEP 3: Insertion of Lateral TDR Device: After sequential sizing using device trials, the lateral TDR device (NuVasive, Inc., San Diego, CA) is inserted as one assembly such that it rests along both sides of the ring apophysis for strong end plate support. The anteroposterior (AP) midline markers should align with the spinous processes in a cross-table AP fluoroscopic view. From a lateral fluoroscopic view, the midline device markings should align with the lateral center of the vertebral bodies (Fig. 46–7).

STEP 4: Close: The retractor is closed and gently removed. The fascia and skin are closed using standard procedure.

## DISCUSSION

A laterally placed TDR may offer several theoretical advantages.

### ADVANTAGES/DISADVANTAGES: LATERAL LUMBAR TOTAL DISC REPLACEMENT

**Advantages**

- There is a lower risk of approach-related complications an morbidity. The XLIF approach has been used for anterior column arthrodesis for a number of years. Studies to date report few approach-related complications, with no visceral or vascular injuries, but a low incidence of transient postoperative hip flexor weakness and anterolateral thigh numbness.[2–5] Because the approach requires less tissue disruption to access the spine, patients are typically walking within hours of surgery and discharged to home after a single night's hospital stay, with minimal surgical pain and on minimal medications.
- It is safer to revise the procedure. The lateral approach has been used more recently as a revision strategy for primary anterior TDR surgery. Although experience to date is limited, case reports describing the successful use of the lateral approach, which does not require anterior mobilization of the major vessels, to revise anteriorly placed TDR device have been presented with encouraging results.[6]

  Primary placement of a lumbar TDR device from a lateral approach leaves multiple safer surgical approach options should removal and revision be necessary.
- It is easy to insert and place the device. The placement of a device laterally allows for easy identification of the frontal midline through cross-table AP fluoroscopy and central placement of the device through alignment of the midline device markings with the spinous processes. Additionally, the device length is designed to span the entire disc space, with easily identifiable landmarks of the lateral bodies of the vertebrae, thus easily ensuring coronal balance (Fig. 46-8). The kinematic center of rotation is located posteriorly within the device, so insertion of the device in the midline laterally provides ideal placement and rotation (Fig. 46-9).
- The approach offers stability. Although anteriorly placed TDR devices require resection of the ALL and anterior annulus, the XLIF approach to TDR placement preserves these structures and, therefore results in a construct that constrains the device from anterior expulsion, provides better ligamentotaxis and sagittal balance, and prevents excessive loading of the facet joints.
- The approach offers increased end plate support. A laterally placed TDR device, like fusion devices used laterally, too, can take advantage of the strongest regions of the vertebral end plates for initial and long-term stability. The lateral TDR device in use through the XLIF approach spans the dense ring apophysis on either side of the end plate and provides a surface area coverage of more than 50% of the end plate area (Fig. 46-10).

**Disadvantages**

- The major disadvantage of the lateral approach is inaccessibility of the L5-S1 due to obstruction by the iliac crest. Its use is only relevant for levels L4-L5 and above.

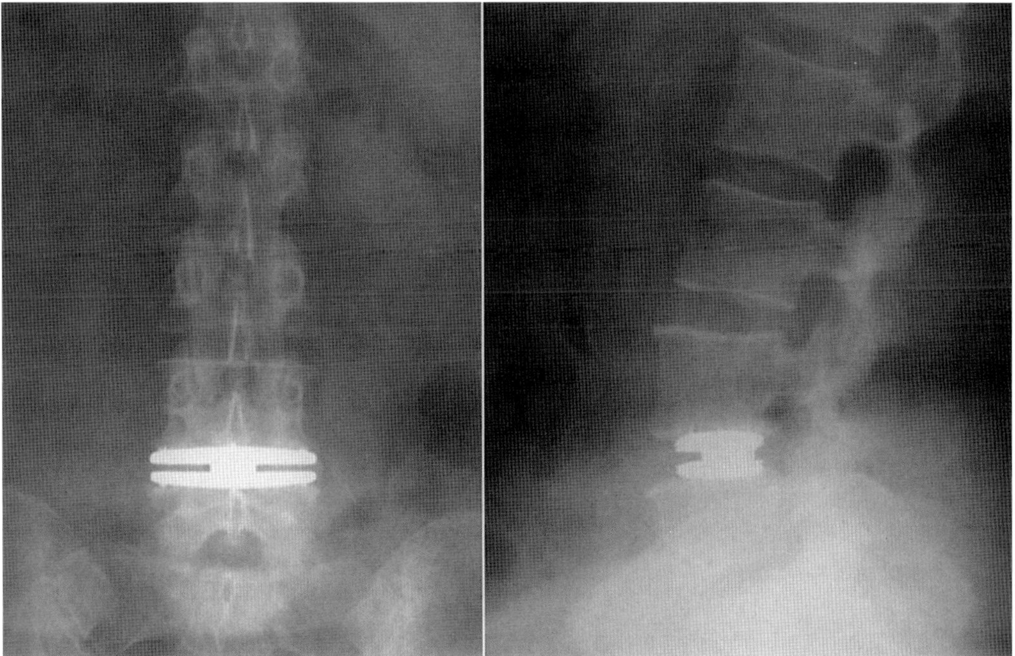

■ **FIGURE 46–7.** Postoperative x-ray studies of a lateral total disc replacement used to treat a 35-year-old woman with lower back pain that was unresponsive to medical treatment for 15 months. Patient was walking the same day of surgery and discharged to home the next day.

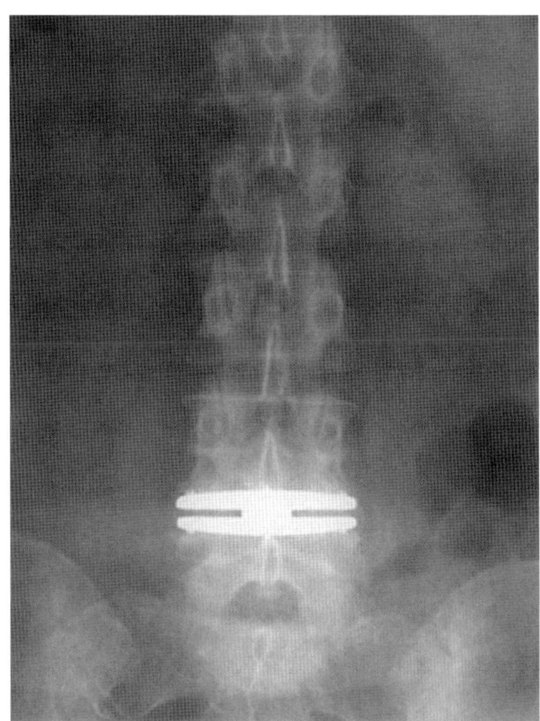

■ **FIGURE 46–8.** Anteroposterior x-ray study showing placement of a lateral total disc replacement device. Note midline and lateral margin alignments.

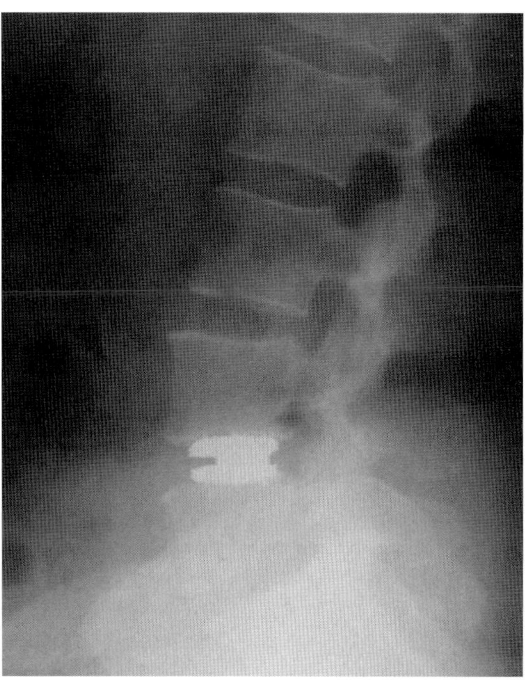

■ **FIGURE 46–9.** Lateral x-ray study showing placement of a lateral total disc replacement device. Note central position of device with rotational center located more posteriorly.

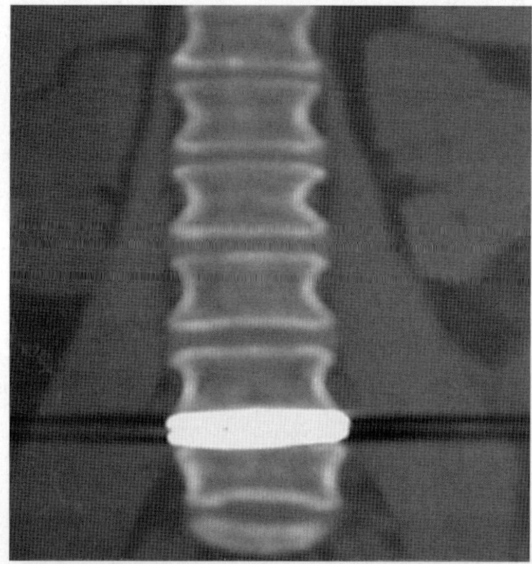

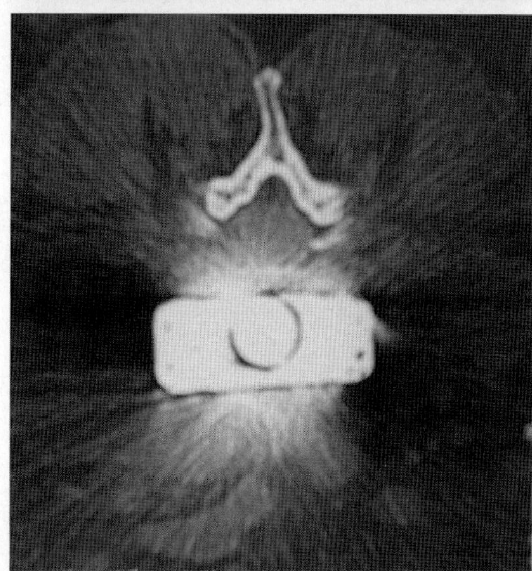

■ **FIGURE 46–10.** Coronal and axial magnetic resonance imaging scans showing the end plate coverage of the laterally placed total disc replacement device.

## CONCLUSIONS

The XLIF approach for TDR surgery offers some inherent advantages over the traditional anterior approach. Although experience to date is limited, midterm clinical results fulfill the promise of a safer and less invasive exposure, and demonstrate maintenance of pain relief and functional improvement. The benefits of this technique avoiding mobilization of the great vessels, preserving the ALL, minimal morbidity, and wider revision options—suggest a promising new direction for TDR procedures.

## REFERENCES


1. Pimenta L: Lateral TDR, Evolution, Development and Early Results. Presented at the Controversies in Motion Preservation Pre-Course, SAS7, Berlin, May 2007.
2. Diaz R, Phillips F, Pimenta L: Minimally invasive XLIF fusion in the treatment of symptomatic degenerative lumbar scoliosis. Proceedings of the NASS 20th Annual Meeting. Spine J 5(4):131S–132S, 2005.
3. Ozgur B, Aryan H, Pimenta L, Taylor W: Extreme lateral interbody fusion (XLIF): A novel surgical technique for anterior lumbar interbody fusion. Spine J 6:435–443, 2006.
4. Pimenta L, Schaffa T, da Silva Martins M, et al: Extreme lateral interbody fusion. *In* Perez-Cruet M, Khoo L, Fessler R (eds): An Anatomical Approach to Minimally Invasive Spine Surgery. St. Louis, MO, Quality Medical Publishing, 2006, pp 641–652.
5. Wright N: Instrumented extreme lateral interbody fusion (XLIF) through a single approach. Proceedings of the NASS 20th Annual Meeting. Spine J 5(4):S177–S178, 2005.
6. Pimenta L, Diaz R, Guerrero L: Charite lumbar artificial disc retrieval: Use of a lateral minimally invasive technique. J Neurosurg Spine 5:556–561, 2006.

CHAPTER 47

# Lumbar Anterior Revision: Preoperative Preparation and Approach Considerations

**Samer Saiedy** and **P. Justin Tortolani**

**KEY POINTS**

- Since the first the U.S. Food and Drug Administration (FDA) Investigational Device Exemption (IDE) studies were initiated for lumbar disc replacement, several thousand lumbar total disc replacements (TDRs) have been inserted.
- Preventing revision assumes even greater significance when we consider that revision approaches to the anterior spine have approximately six times the risk for major bleeding or thromboembolic complications as the index procedure.
- If the surgery requires a second operative procedure before 10 to 14 days, it can be performed as the index surgery. After the 10- to14-day time frame, a second procedure is considered to be a revision.
- Most failures of lumbar disc replacement can be traced to surgeon-specific factors such as incomplete discectomy, improper device insertion (location and size), or inappropriate indications.
- The approach used varies depending on the level of the index procedure and type of index incision.

## PREOPERATIVE PREPARATION

### Introduction

Since the first the U.S. Food and Drug Administration (FDA) Investigational Device Exemption (IDE) studies were initiated for lumbar disc replacement, several thousand lumbar total disc replacements (TDRs) have been inserted. Thus far, the anterior retroperitoneal approach to the lumbar spine has been used for virtually every implantation in the United States. Despite the promising results of lumbar TDR with respect to safety and efficacy, there have been failures requiring revision anterior exposures.[1,2] As more patients undergo lumbar TDR, there are bound to be greater numbers of failures, and thus, understanding the pearls and pitfalls of the revision approach to the lumbar spine will be paramount in order to reduce perioperative complications and enhance patient safety.

For these reasons, we must begin to address the concept of TDR revisions, and more important how to avoid them. Preventing revision assumes even greater significance when we consider that revision approaches to the anterior spine have approximately six times the risk for major bleeding or thromboembolic complications as the index procedure. Factors contributing to these risks include inadequate visualization of tissue planes, inability to mobilize the great vessels, and difficulty in retrieving the prosthesis due to its position (Fig. 47–1).

Despite the inherent risks in the revision scenario, the anterior retroperitoneal exposure of the lumbar spine remains an excellent first-time approach for many reasons:

1. Minimal muscle dissection reduces trunk wall morbidity, allows for short recovery times, and avoids posterior spinal muscle stripping.
2. Unobstructed visualization of the disc space allows for complete discectomy and accurate implant sizing.
3. It precludes the need to enter or retract neural structures within the spinal canal.
4. It is familiar territory for many spine and vascular surgeons.

Although the TDR approach-related risks are low for the initial procedure, in any revision situation, the opposite occurs:

1. Surgery is accompanied by a higher rate of morbidity,
2. Visualization becomes extremely difficult, and
3. Familiar territory becomes unrecognizable owing to scarring, which is characterized as dense and fibrotic.

Any discussion of revision must consider the timing of the second procedure. If the surgery requires a second operative procedure before 10 to 14 days, it can be performed as the index surgery. After the 10- to 14-day time frame, a second procedure is considered to be a revision.

As we can see, revision surgery is fraught with potential complications.[3–5] Although European surgeons have been performing TDR for 20 years, there is still no comprehensive detailed analysis regarding the percentage of revision surgeries that have taken place or the complications following the initial procedure that necessitated a revision. Some data have begun to emerge in the U.S. IDE study.[6–8]

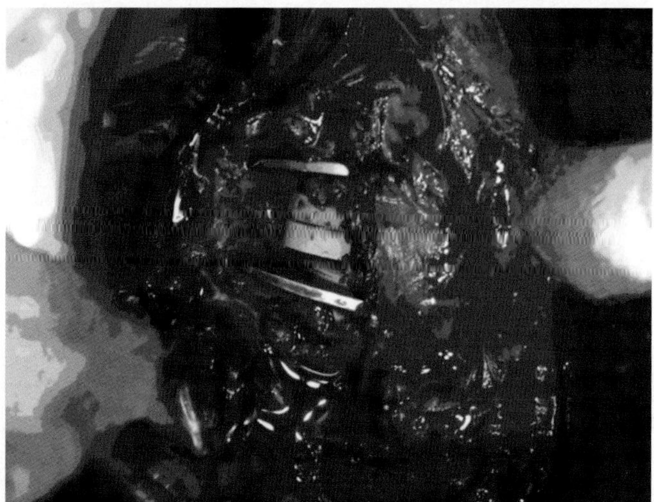

■ **FIGURE 47–1.** Intraoperative photograph identifying key structures.

## Indications for Revision

Indications for TDR revision include neurologic deficiency due to prosthetic dislodgement, resulting in nerve irritation or vascular compromise due to prosthetic or spinal cord compression. The presence of infection also necessitates revision.

## Preventing Revision

Obviously, the optimal scenario is one in which the initial surgery is also the only surgery. How then can the need for revision be prevented? Most failures of lumbar disc replacement can be traced to surgeon-specific factors such as incomplete discectomy, improper device insertion (location and size), or inappropriate indications. Our initial goal, then, is to perfect the surgical technique used, thus negating the need for further surgery. Second, if revision is indeed indicated, we must make the procedure as safe as possible. When addressing these concerns, we need to focus on preoperative and intraoperative care of the patient who requires revision.

## Patient Preparation

### Preoperative

It is paramount that a complete H&P be obtained, as well as a thorough review of the operative record from the initial surgery. The potential risks of the revision procedure need to be discussed with the patient.

When obtaining the patient history, it is important to note any previous abdominal surgeries, any complications following the initial surgery, presence of retrograde ejaculation, deep vein thrombosis (DVT), or infections.

On physical examination, the location of the previous surgical incision should be documented, as well as the presence of lower extremity edema and the quality of the lower extremity pulses, including posterior tibial (PT), anterior tibial (AT), and peroneal vessels.

Information that should be obtained from the operative report includes ligation of the iliolumbar vein in L4-L5 surgery, any damage to the vessels necessitating repair, and any unusual anatomy encountered such as low or high bifurcation of the inferior vena cava (IVC).

Regardless of the initial incision used, the surgeon performing a revision will most probably discover that the retroperitoneum and the ureters have developed an adherence that makes visualization extremely difficult. For this reason, we must prevent injury when the revision is performed. One way to avoid further injury to the area is to have a urologist insert a ureteral stent immediately before the procedure, which is most convenient for the patient, or a few days before the operation.

An angiogram and venogram may be warranted, depending on the reason for the revision. If the prosthesis has shifted anteriorly, there could conceivably be damage to either the arterial or the venous systems (Fig. 47–2). In my practice, we routinely obtain both studies so that we can determine the relationship of the disc to the great vessels. Another emerging alternative is arterial cat scan (CTA), which can give us a three-dimensional view of the disc area. At present, however, we do not have much experience with this technology.

Because of the extensive manipulation of the venous system during revision surgery, the intima of the vein suffers damage, which, in turn, creates a very high-risk situation for the development of a DVT. Because most of these clots form in the iliac vein area, an ultrasound of the leg will be negative for DVT. For this reason, it has been our routine to insert an IVC filter. A retrievable type, such as G2 (Abbott Spine, Inc., Austin, TX), may be used, which can be electively removed at a later date if the patient so desires.

Once the H&P, review of the medical records, and any indicated diagnostic studies have been obtained, then it is time to sit with the patient and explain the operative risks. He or she needs to realize that the risk is much higher than for the initial operative procedure, owing to the reasons previously discussed.

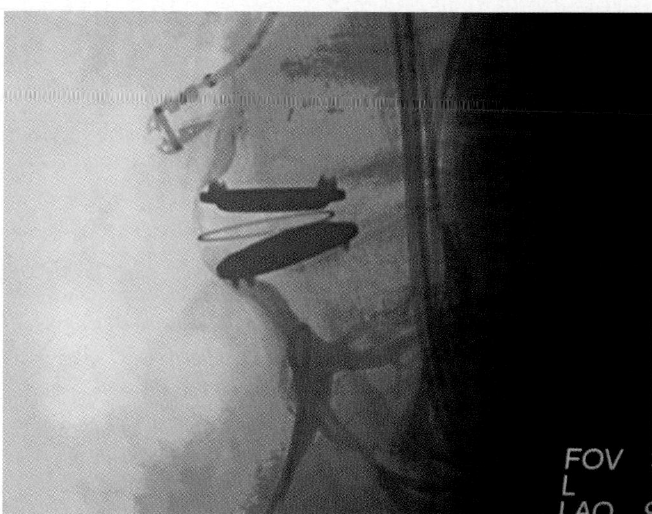


■ **FIGURE 47–2.** Venogram showing that the prothesis moved forward and interfered with the left common iliac vein with signing of early clot.

### Immediately Preoperatively

The patient should have a minimum of four units of packed red blood cells (PRBCs)s on standby. A cell saver should be in the operating room. Two large-bore intravenous lines or a central line should be placed in the patient in anticipation of the need to give large volumes of fluids, blood, or both. A Foley catheter should be inserted concurrent with the stent insertion to decompress the bladder. An nasogastric tube (NGT) must also be placed for stomach decompression.

One option that I personally do not use is that of pulse oximetry placement on the patient's great toe. Any drop in oxygen saturation during surgery indicates that there is too much retraction on the arterial system and should alert the surgeon of the need to relieve pressure. I have found that this step is not needed because our team uses hand-held retractors during surgery that we release at every opportunity to enable blood flow through the great vessels.

Draping should be done from the patient's xiphoid to the knee with access to both groins. Before the abdominal incision, I insert a guide wire in each groin, which extends up into the upper aspect of the IVC (Fig. 47–3). These wires are helpful in many ways. They are useful in identifying the vein during the surgery when it is palpated and can also be used to deploy the IVC filter before or after the procedure. In the event that a vein injury occurs causing extensive blood loss, the wire may be used as a guide to deploy a large covered self-expandable stent, which can seal the injury and halt the bleeding. With the placed wires in the venous system before surgery, you may be assured at all times that you are in the main true lumen of the vessel.

## APPROACH CONSIDERATIONS

In the previous section, we discussed the preoperative evaluation and procedures to be undertaken for the patient requiring lumbar anterior revision surgery. In this section, we focus on choosing the optimal approach for the patient and the reasons for our decisions. This type of procedure, as discussed earlier, is extremely challenging. An innovative and creative approach, along with an experienced surgical team, is critical for reducing the risks of complications and enhancing patient outcome.

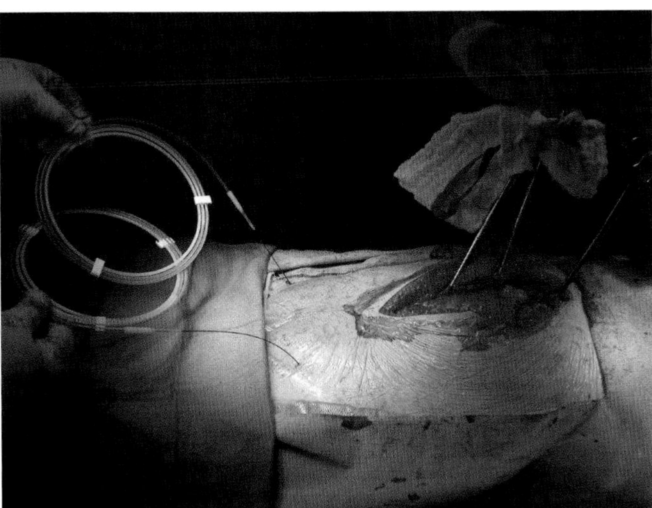

■ **FIGURE 47–3.** Intraoperative picture of guide wires inserted each in CFV.

As mentioned previously, preoperative prerequisites are two large-bore (16 gauge or larger) intravenous access lines placed in the upper extremities; four units of PBRCs must be cross-matched, with at least two on hold in the operating room; ureteral stents must be in place; and an IVC filter must be deployed. (This can be performed at the end of the procedure if desired.)

The approach used varies depending on the level of the index procedure and type of index incision.

### Revising L5-S1

Although the newest trend in Europe is to use a right paramedian as the initial incision for L5-S1 approaches, reserving the left paramedian for revison procedures, in the United States, the left paramedian approach is still used predominately as the initial incision.

If the initial incision is on the left side, then an approach with right paramedian will be best because it provides quick access to L5-S1. Despite relatively easy access to the sacral promontory, adhesions will still be encountered. However, with ureteral stents and venous guide wires (Fig. 47–4) in place, the procedure can be performed with lower risk. The position of anatomic landmarks must be known at all times.

The initial deep dissection starts at the sacrum in the midline and proceeds laterally, and the surgeon should be aware that the common or internal iliac vein can be encountered at any time and may need to be ligated. Over the sacrum in the midline, there tends to be fewer adhesions (untouched territory from the index procedure) than directly over the great vessels more proximally. I can usually get an idea of the patient's anatomy with this approach. From there, I extend my incision to the sacral bone region, using the fibrotic scar over the disc to protect the major vessels. I then advance slowly, visualizing the disc and continuing laterally on both sides while using the fibrotic scar as protection. Although a combination of both blunt and sharp dissection is needed, use of a Kittner dissector may be very helpful as it allows for blunt dissection.

Remember that if the incision extends farther laterally, the risk of encountering the great vessels increases proportionately, and consequently, the chance of injuring them also increases. A low bifurcation of the IVC poses the greatest challenges. Identifying the location of the IVC and the bifurcation with venography preoperatively helps to establish the key relationships of the veins vis-à-vis the spine.

A second viable exposure of L5-S1 is that of the transperitoneal approach; however, with this method the small bowel must be

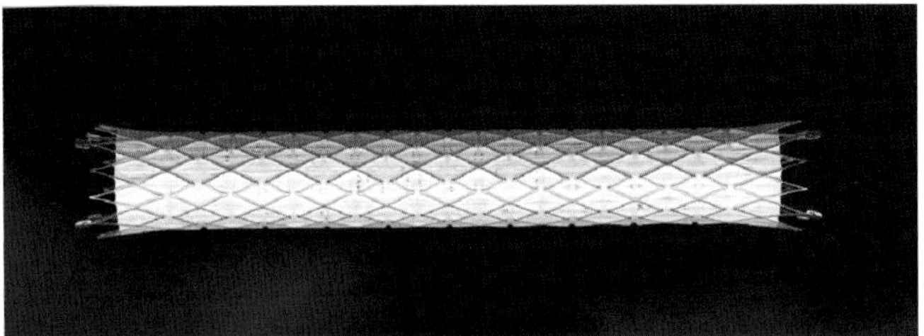

■ **FIGURE 47–4.** Stent covered with graft.

retracted. In an already difficult procedure, this can be distracting. Keep in mind that adhesions will still be encountered.

If injury to the great vessels occurs, then 6–0 prolene sutures should be used. If the injury is severe and difficult to access, the option remains for deployment of the covered stent inside the vein. This ensures that the bleeding will be controlled. If this situation arises, it is important to identify the bifurcation of the IVC so that it is not covered (see Fig. 47–4).

## Revising L4-L5

If the incision of the index procedure is on the left side (the most common surgical approach), then the approach will still be on the left, only higher, descending slowly down from the known to the unknown.

A second option is a right-sided approach. The difficulty with this approach is that the IVC will be encountered first and thus the chance of injury to it is extremely high. So my preference is still left paramedian incision.

I begin this procedure by making an incision through the initial one but extending it much higher to above the umbilicus. I then move down to the anterior fascia level. After opening it, I can move to the posterior fascia level, cutting it as far as I can. I continue the dissection very high and start to mobilize the colon to the right. This approach is more lateral than the index procedure. As the psoas muscle is approached, the iliolumbar vessels of the level above will be encountered. The psoas can be dissected from the lateral edge of L4-L5. The scar tissue above the disc can now be used as protection from injurying the great vessles. Using both blunt and sharp dissection, the disc space can be exposed. Another option that can be used is to take part of the bone with the fibrotic tissue for more protection. Both techniques are limited, however, by the degree that the LCIV and IVC can be stretched. This must be done very carefully, since stretching can cause a major venous injury and severe blood loss. As always, the ureter must be identified at all times. In this situation, placement of the ureteral stents proves to be beneficial.

## Revision at a Different Level Than the Index Level

### Descending to L5-S1 When the Index Procedure Is L4-L5

If the initial incision is on the left side, then an approach with the right paramedian incision will be best because it provides quick access to L5-S1. Despite relatively easy access to the sacral promontory, minimal adhesions will be encountered. However, with ureteral stents and venous guide wires (see Fig. 47–1) in place, the procedure can be performed with lower risk. Knowledge of the anatomic landmarks is necessary at all times.

If the index procedure was the right paramedian or intraperitoneal access, then the left paramedian approach should be used. This procedure can be done more safely if ureteral stents are inserted.

### Descending to L4-L5 When the Index Procedure Is L5-S1

If the initial incision is on the left side, then an approach with a repeat left paramedian incision will be best because it provides quick access to L4-L5. The incision must be extended higher and the dissection started lateral to the great vessel (LCIV) However, with ureteral stents and venous guide wires (see Fig. 47–1) in place, the procedure can be performed with lower risk. The location of the anatomic landmarks should be known at all times.

## REFERENCES

1. Bertagnoli R, Yue J: The treatment of disabling single level lumbar discogenic low back pain with total disc arthroplasty utilizing the ProDisc prosthesis. Spine J (in press).
2. Scott-Young M: Revision strategies for lumbar disc replacement. Spine J 4:115, 2004.
3. Matthews HH: Complications and revision considerations of total disc arthroplasty: MAVERICK metal-on-metal prosthesis. Roundtables in Spine Surgery, Complications and Revision Strategies in Lumbar Spine Arthroplasty 1:109–116, 2005.
4. David T: Revision of a Charite artificial disc 9.5 years in vivo to a new Charite artificial disc: case report and explant analysis. Eur Spine J 14:507–511, 2005.
5. Brau SA, Delamarter RB, Schiffman ML, et al: Vascular injury during anterior lumbar surgery. Spine 4:409–412, 2004.
6. McAfee PC, Geisler FH, Saiedy S, et al: Revisability of the CHARITÉ Artificial Disc Replacement: Analysis of 347 patients enrolled in the U.S. IDE Study of the CHARITÉ Artificial Disc. Roundtables in Spine Surgery, Complications and Revision Strategies in Lumbar Spine Arthroplasty 1:73–96, 2005.
7. McAfee PC, Cunningham BW, Holtsapple G, et al: A prospective, randomized, multi-center FDA IDE study of lumbar total disc replacement with the CHARITÉ™ Artificial Disc vs. lumbar fusion, part II: Evaluation of radiographic outcomes and correlation of surgical technique accuracy with clinical outcomes. Spine 30:1576–1583, 2005.
8. van Ooij A, Oner FC, Verbout AJ: Complications of artificial disc replacement: A report of 27 patients with the SB CHARITÉ disc. J Spinal Disord Tech 16:369–383, 2003.

CHAPTER 48

# Overall Revision Strategies: Lumbar

**Matthew Scott-Young** and **Frank Daday**

## KEY POINTS

- Revision procedures can be anticipated with lumbar total disc replacement (TDR) surgery.
- The revision rate of TDR is well below the revision rate of other commonly performed spinal procedures.
- Approximately 90% of revisions occur as a result of failure of indication and failure of technique.
- Patient selection and preoperative planning are essential in the execution of an effective revision strategy.
- Reliable surgical strategies can be used to provide satisfactory outcomes when revision is necessary.

## TIME, PROCEDURE, COMPLICATION SYSTEM

Reoperations with respect to TDR can be classified according to the TPC (time, procedure, complication) System. The TPC System is described in the following sections.

### Time

The occurrence of a revision procedure may be either:

E. Early (<7 days)
R. Remote (>7 days)

### Procedure

Type A. Device requiring removal
- A.1. Successful (removal of device)
  - A.1.1 Conversion to new TDR
  - A.1.2 Conversion to anterior lumbar interbody fusion (ALIF)
  - A.1.3 Conversion to posterior spinal fusion (PSF) and ALIF
- A.2. Unsuccessful (attempted removal of device)
  - A.2.1 Conversion to PSF
  - A.2.2 Conversion to posterior dynamic stabilization

Type B. Device not removed
- B.1 Decompression alone
- B.2 Decompression plus dynamic PSF
- B.3 Decompression and posterior spinal fusion
- B.4 Dynamic posterior stabilization
- B.5 PSF alone

### Complications

C.0 None
C.1 Infection
C.2 Pulmonary embolism (PE)–deep vein thrombosis (DVT)
C.3 Dislocation
C.4 Neurologic
C.5 Vascular venous
C.6 Vascular arterial
C.7 Cerebrospinal fluid (CSF) leak
C.8 Failure of fixation
C.9 Pseudoarthrosis
C.10 Ureteric injury
C.11 Other

## OVERVIEW

Revision total disc replacement (TDR) may be required for many reasons, including persistent pain, new-onset pain, progressive deformity, prosthesis subluxation, migration, unacceptable placement, neurologic sequelae, and infection. However, the underlying cause of failure of TDR generally involves failure of indication, failure of technique, or both. In my experience, these two factors account for 90% of the practical reasons that result in revision TDR.

A failed back surgical syndrome (FBSS) means that the patient has undergone spine surgery without clinical improvement. It implies the persistence of symptoms as a result of surgery, not despite surgery. The term does not always imply that the surgery was done incorrectly or that the diagnosis was incorrect. Highly experienced surgeons with good technique have patients who appear to have been a suitable candidate but end up with FBSS. This is because we are dealing with imperfect knowledge of the exact nature of the pain generators in the spine and imperfect radiologic investigations. As a result, the diagnosis and appropriate surgical solution remain an imperfect science. Inevitably there will be some results that are not ideal.

The revision surgeon needs to ensure that the patient is suffering from the ineffective application of surgical procedure (i.e., a refractory back surgical syndrome [RBSS]) that may be amenable to revision surgery. There needs to be a reasonable expectation that revision is the optimal mode of therapy for the pathologic situation. Because revision surgery at the index level can be difficult, the surgeon must be certain that no possible alternatives to an anterior revision exist. The patient needs to be informed of the advantages and disadvantages of the revision procedure so an informed decision can be made.

I have performed 12 revision TDR cases, eight women and four men. Under the TPC System, four cases were classified as R.A.1.2.C.0, one as R.A.1.2.C.2, one as R.B.5.C.0, one as R.A.1.3.C.0, one as R.B.4.C.0, and one as E.A.1.1.C.0.

## INDICATIONS

Patients who have undergone a disc arthroplasty may consult with the surgeon who performed the original procedure or another surgeon regarding new symptoms. From a patient's perspective, this is usually the result of persistent, recurrent, or new back or leg pain, or a combination thereof. At other times, they will present with radiologic findings, such as migration, subluxation, subsidence, unacceptable placement, or even wear. The specific modes of failure have previously been discussed.[1]

The rate of revision surgery following TDR has been reported to be 2.7% to 8.8%[2] and compares favorably with revision rates of other spinal procedures, such as fusion (6% to 36%),[3] decompressive laminectomy (9% to 17%),[4] and discectomy (2% to 19%).[5,6]

Revision surgery is not often successful and is indicated only if the source or type of pain can be clearly identified. In the treatment of FBSS or RBSS, accurate diagnosis of the problem is essential. The persistence of chronic low back and leg pain, despite surgery, is a therapeutic challenge. Failure of indication and failure of technique are two issues that are not mutually exclusive and are often interdependent. The challenge arises with the many possible explanations for the persistence of symptoms.

Indications can be absolute or relative. An absolute indication includes those conditions in which the patient would suffer a poor outcome without intervention. Examples of this are arterial or venous compromise, which can occur from anterior subluxation, migration, or dislocation of a prosthesis onto a venous or arterial structure. These indications dictate anterior removal of the offending device to repair the obstruction.

Neurologic compromise that results in electrophysiologic damage is another absolute indication requiring revision of the prosthesis at the nearest instance. The revision may be performed anteriorly or posteriorly, depending on the cause of the injury to the neural structures.

In most instances, deep infection (whether of early or late onset) would be an absolute indication to revise the implant. Suppressive therapy is rarely beneficial. Abscesses in the disc space tend to track into the psoas and posteriorly into the epidural space. Hence, the most appropriate revision would be a circumferential procedure, with removal of the abscess, débridement of the necrotic material, and stabilization of the motion segment.

On occasion, mechanical problems can result in an absolute indication to revise an implant, with subluxation of the whole implant anteriorly or dislocation of a core of the prosthesis (Fig. 48–1). This renders the mechanical environment unfavorable for a satisfactory outcome.

Relative indications include the various mechanical sequelae of incorrect technique. These include eccentric placement, subsidence, and migration of less than 5 mm. In these circumstances, unfavorable kinematics of the functional spinal unit are created. Neurologic symptoms, rather than overt signs, can also be a relative indication for revision. It is common for patients who have undergone disc arthroplasty to have residual symptoms, but their expectations about the outcomes may have been unrealistic. These individuals need to be carefully assessed and the options discussed. If it is agreed to proceed with revision, the patient must understand that the revision procedure is a calculated risk and not a cure for their persisting symptoms.

## CONTRAINDICATIONS

If, after considering the patient's history, performing a thorough physical examination, reviewing the radiographic evaluation, and analyzing any psychological screening results, a definitive mechanical or neurologic problem cannot be found, then revision surgery on a TDR is generally contraindicated. As with any spine surgery, the most important issue in achieving a successful outcome is related to patient selection. Bolger and Frazer attempted to aid the decision-making process and to provide some estimate of the likely outcome for repeated operations.[7] They proposed a prognostic outcome score based on the percentage reduction for a satisfactory outcome when a particular factor is present. These factors include less than 6 months without symptoms, third or subsequent operations, psychological disturbance, compensation, the type of previous surgery, and the proposed surgery, whether it is a posterior fusion, a decompression, or scar removal. They emphasize great care and caution in performing any procedure on a patient who has already undergone lumbar surgery.

An absolute contraindication would be an unfavorable psychological profile. Other contraindications include litigation or compensation problems. When significant scarring associated with prior surgery would make a vessel injury highly likely, an anterior approach would be contraindicated. However, revision is still possible through posterior approaches.

It is important for surgeons to use their expertise to identify the causes of likely failures and to resist the temptation to operate on patients because they feel compelled to offer the hope of a surgical solution to a genuinely disabled person.

## CLINICAL PRESENTATION AND EVALUATION

When considering a revision procedure on a TDR, a consensus group approach from a multidisciplinary team is advisable. Individuals with wide experience in the fields of spine surgery, pain management, and cognitive rehabilitative behavior are useful to unravel the nexus of pain and disability. If the surgery has been performed by another surgeon, it is important to ensure access to the primary clinical notes or records.

Patients who present for potential revision generally report three main problems:

1. Back and/or leg pain—radiographs show good position and movement.
2. Back and/or leg pain—radiographs show poor position and function.
3. Little or no pain or dysfunction—radiographs show poor position, and indicate that mechanical and neurologic stability may be compromised in the long term.

The more common presentation is the presence of pain despite the fact that the radiograph appears satisfactory. The origin of the

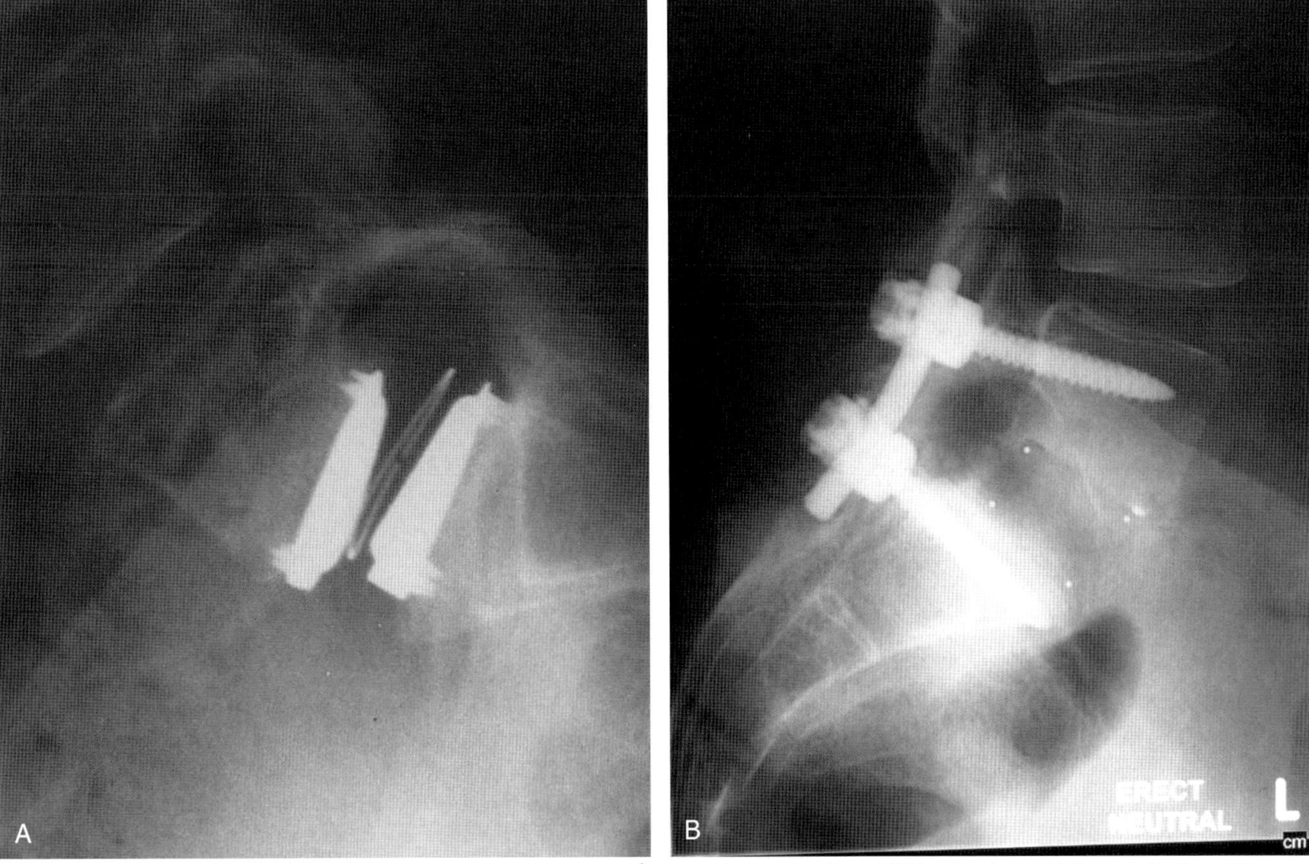


■ **FIGURE 48–1.** **A,** Patient with prior laminectomy and CHARITÉ (DePuy Spine, Raynham, MA) implant inserted. Progressive instability noted at one year after initial implantation due to incompetent posterior structures. **B,** Revision performed with removal of prosthesis and conversion to ALIF/PSF.

pain can be neuropathic, mechanical, or psychological (or a combination of these three components). Neuropathic pain, by definition, involves neural tissue injury. Mechanical pain is caused by non-neural injuries such as facet joint, disc, and muscle damage. The surgeon needs to draw on the patient history, use his clinical acumen, and additional radiologic studies. At this stage, the surgeon needs to analyze any preoperative issues, such as wrong diagnosis, wrong patient, wrong procedure, and wrong surgeon. The surgeon needs to review the patient's history to determine the evolution and type of pain. In doing so, the surgeon will ascertain whether the pain was there before surgery, whether the patient was ever symptom free, whether there is new onset of pain, and whether the pain is in the back or the leg (and in what combination).

A clinical examination is performed. The patient's overall spinal alignment is assessed both in the sagittal and coronal plane. The range of motion is noted. The examination requires observation of gait, how the patient transfers from a chair to a sitting position, how he or she undresses, how he or she bends, and a neurologic examination. Furthermore, while taking the history and performing the clinical examination, the surgeon can assess valuable aspects of the patient's psychological profile. Pain in flexion may indicate problems with the disc, perhaps instability. Extension with a staccato movement on standing indicates possible instability. Painful extension may be caused by arthritic facet joints. A neurologic examination can determine neural tension or neural loss, and its pattern may indicate a specific nerve root.

Radiologic investigations are of paramount importance. Standing anteroposterior lateral films, and flexion-extension laterals, are essential. A magnetic resonance imaging scan is inadequate for the diagnosis of neurologic problems at the surgical level due to the scatter effect of the metal. Electrophysiologic studies (electromyelograms and nerve conduction studies) can be useful in determining whether the neurologic symptoms that are referred to the leg are as a result of a radiculopathy or a referred pain. A fine-cut computed tomography myelogram would be the procedure of choice for postoperative neurologic symptoms. This will allow visualization of neural structures and elucidate their passage across the disc space and lateral recess.

## OPERATIVE TECHNIQUE

For patients who must have the same level reoperated on within 7 days after the initial surgery, the recommendation is to use the original incision and enlarge it. Dissection through the planes will not be impossible because the space has not been obliterated by fibrosis or scarring.

When revision of the TDR is carried out more than 7 days after the initial surgery, fibrosis and recognition of the vessels can make the procedure more difficult. Brau[1] has made recommendations in the past for the approaches to different levels. In my view, irrespective of whether L3-L4, L4-L5, or L5-S1 is to be revised, a midline extensile incision is appropriate. There is no role for minimally invasive surgery when revising TDR in the anterior lumbar spine. The basic principles of revision are to access virginal retroperitoneal space above or below the index level to achieve the best access possible.

## Anesthesia for Revision TDR

Preoperative evaluation is essential for the anesthesiologist to gain the patient's relevant medical and surgical history. The surgeon also needs to convey what the goals of the procedure are and any potential problems that may be encountered. General anesthesia with muscle relaxation is required. An epidural should not be used because the effects of the local anesthetic may mask potentially serious neurologic sequelae in the postoperative period. Large-bore venous access is mandatory. A reinforced endotracheal tube should be used in case the patient needs to be rolled into the prone position for a posterior stabilization procedure.

In addition to standard monitoring of vital signs, a urinary catheter is used to monitor hourly output, and bispectral index monitoring allows maintenance of adequate depth of anaesthesia. There is potential for large fluid shifts, so an arterial line and central venous line may be indicated.

A perfusionist attends for intraoperative blood salvage. Despite having cross-matched blood available for use, we are able to return approximately 60% of the blood loss through reperfusion. Use of forced-air warming blankets and warming fluids is essential during these long procedures.

Perioperative use of graduated compression stockings, sequential compression calf pumps, and low-molecular-weight heparin (I use enoxaparin [Clexane] commencing the day before surgery) are necessary, given the type of vascular handling that may be involved. Antibiotic prophylaxis with cephalothin (Keflin) is continued postoperatively. Postoperative analgesia is provided by continuous infusion of local anesthetic such as ropivacaine through a catheter into the wound and intravenous patient-controlled analgesia with an opioid.

## Type A—Device Requiring Removal

The revision approach used ultimately depends on the index surgery, the time since the index surgery, and whether the revision surgeon also performed the initial procedure.

There are three options available to the surgeon when performing an anterior revision of a TDR. They are a left retroperitoneal approach, a right retroperitoneal approach, or a transperitoneal approach. To some extent, the approach used in the prior surgery will dictate the approach used in the next procedure, but it is more important to make the decision based on the level rather than the prior scar or approach.

For L5-S1, it is customary in the index surgery for a left retroperitoneal approach to be performed. If a revision procedure is necessary at this level, a right retroperitoneal approach is straightforward, and a transperitoneal approach should be the last resort, given the high incidence of retrograde ejaculation in men. Good exposure at this level should be expected, and revision of a disc is usually able to be performed.

In regard to L4-L5, especially if the prior procedure has been performed only at that level, one is often able to get above or below the prior scarred retroperitoneum into virginal space to allow dissection up or down to the target disc. Structures at risk here are the ureter, which can be stented preoperatively, the sympathetic chain, which is sometimes difficult to discern, and the great vessels. The key to approaching L4-L5 is usually developing the interval between psoas and the anterior spine, and an exposure through this window may facilitate removal or revision of an artificial disc. Revision to an artificial disc at this level can be prohibitive if a venous tear is encountered early. In such a case, it is best to abandon the procedure and perform a posterior stabilization. Any injury to a venous structure is potentially complicated by hemorrhage or DVT and PE.

The second option at L4-L5 is to perform a transperitoneal approach. The surgeon would have to go lateral to the sigmoid colon to reenter the retroperitoneal plane through the peritoneal reflections. It is important to note that the same structures are at risk and that the adhesions following the laparotomy are not without their problems.

The third option at L4-L5 is to perform a right retroperitoneal approach; because the vein has not been exposed from the right-hand side, a slightly larger window can be accessed. Before surgery, it is important to note the vascular anatomy at this level.

For L3-L4, a left retroperitoneal approach can be used, entering the retroperitoneal space above or below the disc. Similar principles apply to locate the psoas and the anterior spine, radiographically verify where the surgery is taking place, and be aware of structures such as ureter, sympathetic chain, and so on. At this level, one is often able to mobilize the vascular structures to the right-hand side well enough to be able to revise the implant to a TDR or ALIF. I would recommend identifying and ligating the segmental vessels at L3-L4 and L4-L5 to allow retraction to the right-hand side.

As a general caveat, if the vessels are not easily mobilized, one can do a subperiosteal exposure, lifting the peritoneum and remnants of the disc annulus anteriorly as a flap from the side of least danger to the side of most danger. The principles are to stay under the flap and enter the disc space early.

In my experience, the CHARITÉ Artificial Disc is eminently revisable because it is a three-part prosthesis. Removal of the polyethylene by a piecemeal or traction technique is straightforward. An osteotome is then used to osteotomize the interval between the subchondral bone and end plate. Once the prosthesis end plates are loose within the disc space, the prosthesis can then be removed easily.

In regard to keeled devices, dedicated revision instrumentation systems are available. However, the system is dependent on the ability to retract the tissues completely across the disc. It is my experience that this is often not possible.

If a distraction system is not available, then a series of very fine osteotomes can develop a plane between the prosthesis and the bony end plate. This can lead to gradual loosening of the implant so that it can be removed. Sometimes, it requires a partial vertebrectomy from an anterolateral approach so the prosthesis can then be removed. In such cases, the area is stabilized with bone graft and then combined with a further posterior pedicular stabilization procedure.

Although it is tempting to aim for a TPC R.A.1.1, the reality is that often the revision of choice is TPC R.A.1.2 or R.A.1.3.

### Type B—Device Not Removed

In circumstances in which the device is not able to be removed, there are several options available, depending on the primary pathology. If the pathology requires decompression of the canal to remove a sequested disc fragment or a piece of bone that has been fractured off by the implant, then decompression alone may be appropriate. If a bilateral partial facetectomy is performed, the addition of posterior dynamic stabilization or a pedicle screw fusion is recommended.

Asymmetric annular resection can result in the tilt of a prosthesis in the coronal plane. This is magnified in multilevel TDR, and it has been shown that the axial rotational instability can increase significantly.[8] Generally, a minor tilt is of no significance. If multiple levels have been replaced, a segmental scoliosis can occur. It is possible that a posterior dynamic stabilization procedure can substitute for the annulus integrity by posterior dynamic stabilization.

A posterior spinal fusion can be performed for instability of a prosthesis, eccentric placement, and facet arthropathy (TPC E/R.B.5). This can be done through a minimally invasive approach with an intertransverse fusion of autograft and bone morphogenetic protein.

## POSTOPERATIVE CARE

It is advisable to manage the revision patient in a critical care unit for the first 24 hours. The patient is monitored on a continual basis by critical care specialists who must be experienced in extensive spinal reconstructive procedures. Any postsurgical complications can be recognized early and the appropriate management strategies instituted immediately.

In the postoperative phases, a pain management strategy should be initiated. This includes a local anesthetic infusion pump into the wound in conjunction with patient-controlled analgesia. It is very important to consider the pulmonary problems that can follow extensive anterior surgery. Routine intensive spirometry is generally effective. Careful monitoring of blood pressure or central venous pressure and urine output is essential in the first 24 to 48 hours following a revision procedure. Because the incidence of deep vein thrombosis following any major reconstructive procedure can be up to 10%, the use of graduated compression stockings and calf pumps in the first 24 to 48 hours is essential. A variety of gastrointestinal and nutritional problems can occur, such as ileus, constipation, and occasionally diarrhea. The net result is to leave the patient protein deficient postoperatively, which increases the likelihood of complications such as wound infection. The use of intravenous hyperalimentation is sometimes indicated.

### ADVANTAGES/DISADVANTAGES: OVERALL REVISION STRATEGIES

**Advantages**
Reduction in pain.
Functional restoration.
Return to work.
Permanent correction of pathology.

**Disadvantages**
Complex surgery.
Increased risk of complications.
Pain reduction equivocal or may be worse.
Further functional deterioration.
Unable to return to work.

In terms of rehabilitation, the constant pain and inability to maintain normal function in the preoperative phase leaves this individual physically and emotionally drained. Most patients need assistance in gaining strength and trunk mobility and cardiovascular fitness. A rehabilitation program is mandatory in the initial phases to maintain posture and balance in the sitting, standing, and lying positions; and to aid the patient in their gait cycle, up and down stairs, and to attend to their activities of daily living. On discharge, the patient then starts a rehabilitation program that focuses on core stability, flexibility, and aerobic fitness. The patient is reviewed by the surgeon at 2 weeks, 3 months, 6 months, and 12 months after surgery.

## COMPLICATIONS AND AVOIDANCE

The same complications and adverse events exist for both the primary and any revision TDR. However, the incidence is increased in revision procedures.

Closure of the wound should be done in layers to minimize the risk of hernias. With a left-sided approach, damage to the spleen, kidney, ureter, sympathetic chain, and superior hypogastric plexus should be discussed with all patients before surgical intervention. Possible injuries to the lumbar plexus by excessive retraction on the psoas muscle can also occur. Patellofemoral nerve neuromas or neuropraxia may occur. The venous and arterial vessels become fibrotic and difficult to identify, and may be stretched or torn in an attempt to gain exposure. This can lead to DVT or PE.

The vast majority of patients undergoing TDR would be relatively young and fit, and as a result, have a low level of comorbidity. Nevertheless, it is extremely important to consider these comorbidities before entertaining a revision procedure.

## CONCLUSIONS AND DISCUSSION

Knowing when to operate is a science, and knowing when not to operate is an art. Revision surgery is demanding, technically difficult, and carries a significant incidence of morbidity and an instance of mortality. It deals with neurologic and vascular structures that can be injured and result in significant morbidity to the patient. The decision process on when to reoperate can be made only after serious consideration of the alternatives to surgery and whether the patient would be likely to profit from revision. The patient needs to be aware of the risk-benefit ratio of the revision procedure.

Even with the risk that revision surgery can result in a less than favorable outcome, there will be occasions when it is mandatory or the best option for a patient. An effective revision strategy can be set into motion that can minimize collateral damage and complications, and maximize the outcome. Achieving the best outcome possible requires sufficient knowledge of the technique, meticulous planning, and an exact surgical execution of the treatment plan.

## REFERENCES

1. Brau S: Complications in revision strategies in lumbar spine arthroplasty: Roundtables in Spine Surgery 1(No. 2, Part 1):3–11, 2005.
2. McAfee P, Geisler FH, Saiedy SS, et al: Revisability of the CHARITÉ Artificial Disc Replacement: Analysis of 688 patients enrolled in the U.S.IDE study of the CHARITÉ Artificial Disc. Spine 31: 1217–1226, 2006.

3. Gillet P: The fate of the adjacent motion segments after lumbar fusion. Spine 28:338–345, 2004.
4. Hopp E, Tsou PM: Post decompression of lumbar instability. Clin Orthop 227:143–151, 1988.
5. Weir BKA, Jacobs GA: Reoperation rate following lumbar discectomy: Analysis of 662 discectomies. Spine 5:366–370, 1980.
6. Cavanagh S, Stevens J, Johnson JR: High resolution MRI in investigation of recurrent pain after lumbar discectomy. J Bone Joint Surg 4:524–528, 1993.
7. Bolger C, Frazer RD: Revisions: Outcome studies. In Marguiles JY, Aebi M, and Farcy J-P (eds): Revision Spine Surgery, St. Louis, Mosby, 1999, pp 1–10.
8. McAfee P, Cunningham BW, Hayes V, et al: Biomechanical analysis of rotational motions after disc arthroplasty: Implications for patients with adult deformities. Spine 31(19):S152–S160, 2006.

CHAPTER 49

# Revision Strategies Following Lumbar Total Disc Replacement Complications

**Luiz Pimenta, Thomas Schaffa, Juliano Lhamby, Carlos Fernando Arias Pesántez,** and **Ihab Gharzeddine**

## KEY POINTS

- Complications can arise after lumbar total disc replacement (TDR), procedures that require retrieval and revision of the TDR device to a fusion construct.
- Posterior fusion alone may not be effective with an unstable anterior column.
- Anterior revision presents significant risk to visceral and vascular structures.
- The extreme lateral interbody fusion (XLIF) approach for TDR retrieval and revision is safer and less invasive than the traditional anterior approach, minimizing the risk of vascular and visceral complications while allowing quick patient recovery and return to normal activities.
- Devices with and without end plate keels can be revised laterally with minimal vertebral body destruction.

## INTRODUCTION

Most lumbar total disc replacement (TDR) devices require an anterior abdominal approach that can be technically demanding, especially at the L4-L5 level because of the requirement to mobilize the great vessels. Given the access limitations, significant skill and experience are required to achieve optimal exposure and device placement. Inevitably, however, complications can occur, and some devices may need revision.[1–6]

In many cases, the first revision option is to leave the device in place and attempt to stabilize with a supplemental posterolateral fusion and pedicle screw fixation.[1,3,4] However, posterolateral fusion can be difficult to achieve with an unstable anterior column, and device removal is sometimes necessary. Of the 8.8% CHARITÉ TDR cases requiring reoperation in the U.S. Investigational Device Exemption (IDE) trial, approximately half required removal of the device.[3] However, anterior retrieval of a TDR device and revision to an anterior lumbar interbody fusion is difficult, particularly after the first 2 weeks postoperatively, due to scar formation and elevated risk of vascular injury.[1,3,4] The CHARITÉ U.S. IDE data showed that although the primary TDR procedure resulted in a rate of vascular complication of 3.4%, vascular injury occurred in 16.7% of the revision cases.[3]

An alternative approach to removal and revision of a lumbar TDR device that does not require anterior mobilization of the major vessels has been in recent use by the authors. The minimally invasive extreme lateral interbody fusion (XLIF, NuVasive, Inc., San Diego, CA) procedure has been performed successfully for single- and multilevel fusions above L5.[7–10] It is a direct-lateral, retroperitoneal, trans-psoas approach using blunt finger dissection of the retroperitoneal space, stimulated electromyographic (EMG) guidance (NeuroVison JJB, NuVasive, Inc., San Diego, CA) through the psoas muscle, and advancement of a split-blade retractor system (MaXcess, NuVasive, Inc., San Diego, CA) for illuminated direct visualization of the lateral portion of the spine. In addition to primary fusion procedures, the XLIF approach has more recently been used to successfully retrieve and revise failed anteriorly placed TDR devices.[11]

## ILLUSTRATIVE CASES

### Case 1—Pars Fracture

A number 5, 31-mm-wide CHARITÉ Artificial Disc (DePuy Spine, Raynham, MA) was implanted in a 39-year-old woman with degenerative disc disease at the L4-L5 level. Her back pain reappeared 15 days after surgery, and radiographs showed instability caused by an unrecognized isthmic pars defect fracture at, the implanted level. An instrumented posterolateral fusion with autologous bone graft was performed. One month later, the posterior fusion site became infected, and intravenous antibiotic therapy was administered. The patient's back pain persisted for another 18 months, and radiography revealed hardware failure of one of the fixation rods (Fig. 49–1).

TDR removal and revision were performed through a left-sided XLIF approach through a 2-inch lateral incision. The lateral aspect of the disc replacement device is easily accessed after annular discectomy. With the patient bent in a lateral decubitus position and the disc space angled open toward the access approach, the polyethylene core is easily grasped and removed using a Kocher clamp (Fig. 49–2). The device end plates are pried loose

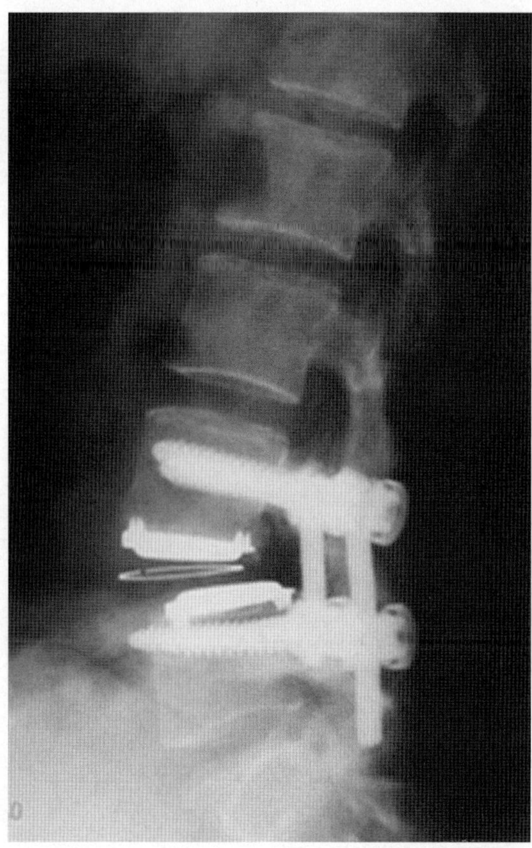

■ **FIGURE 49–1.** Case 1 pre-revision. CHARITÉ total disc replacement implantation with unrecognized isthmic pars defect requiring stabilization. A posterolateral fusion was attempted without resolution of back pain. Radiographs revealed hardware failure of right fixation rod.

from their bony attachment without much force using an osteotome. The end plates can then be grasped and removed from the disc space with a Kocher clamp (Fig. 49–3). End plate loosening and removal is repeated for the second surface (Fig. 49–4).

A 50-mm long × 18-mm wide × 12-mm tall polyetheretherketone (PEEK) cage filled with tricalcium phosphate and iliac crest bone marrow aspirate was implanted. A posterior revision was also

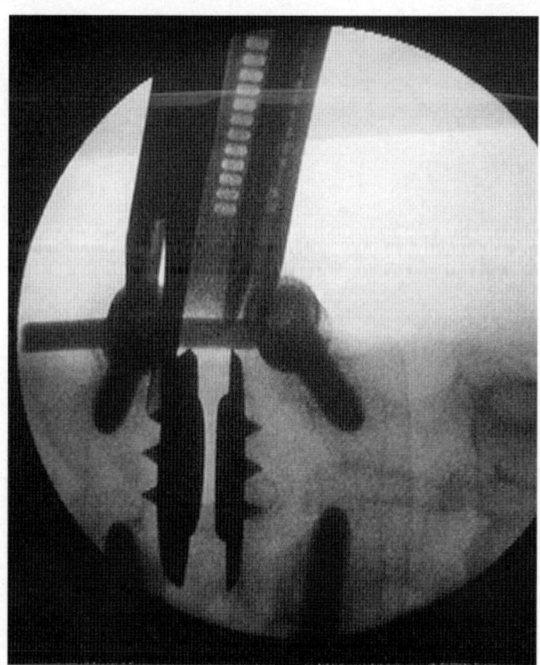

■ **FIGURE 49–3.** The metal end plates are pried loose from their bony attachment without much force using an osteotome, and they can be grasped and removed from the disc space with a Kocher clamp.

performed by open procedure with reposition of the slipped rod (Fig. 49–5). No infection or neurologic signs/symptoms were observed in the postoperative period, and the patient continued to do well at 1-year follow-up.

## Case 2—Malpositioned, Nonkeeled Implant

A 50-year-old woman with a prior L4-L5 fusion underwent a TDR with a number 4, 29-mm-wide CHARITÉ disc secondary to a symptomatic adjacent-level disease at L3-L4. Two-month postoperative radiographs showed lateral implantation of the device and iatrogenic segmental scoliosis (Fig. 49–6). At the 12-month follow-up examination, the patient reported lumbar pain, and a computed tomography scan showed left lateral disc implantation

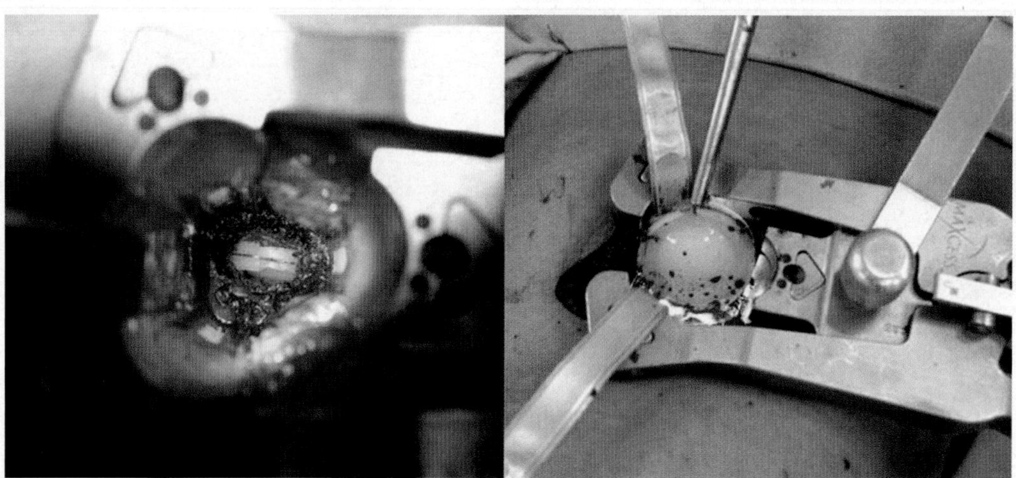

■ **FIGURE 49–2.** The polyethylene core is easily grasped and removed using a Kocher clamp.

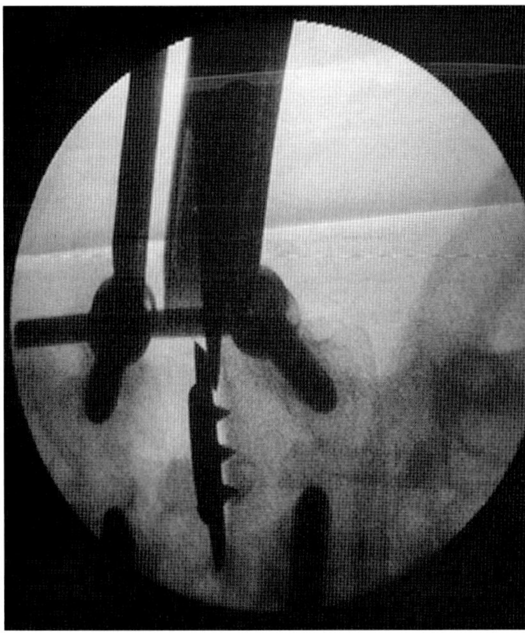

■ **FIGURE 49–4.** End plate loosening and removal is repeated for the second surface using an osteotome and Kocher clamp.

and heterotopic bone formation. She was neurologically intact at this time and was placed in medical and rehabilitation treatment without significant recovery. Artificial disc removal and revision were performed 2 years postoperatively using the XLIF technique with a PEEK cage 45 mm long × 18 mm wide × 12 mm tall, filled with iliac crest bone autograft. Supplemental posterior pedicular screws were added percutaneously (Fig. 49–7). During the postoperative period, transitory weakness (3/5) to raise the knee was observed and resolved at 3 days. No other neurologic signs or symptoms were observed. The patient did not report any symptoms at 10-month follow-up examination.

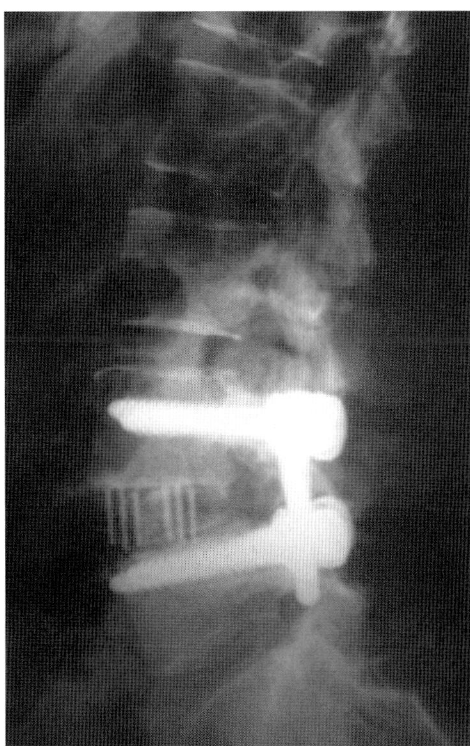

■ **FIGURE 49–5.** Case 1 post-revision. Total disc replacement removal and revision were performed via a left-sided extreme lateral interbody fusion (XLIF) approach, and the rod was repositioned posteriorly.

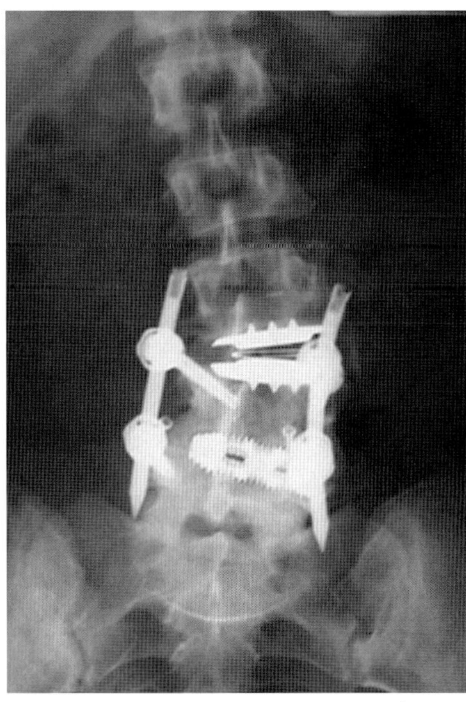

■ **FIGURE 49–6.** Case 2 pre-revision. CHARITÉ total disc replacement with lateral implantation of the device and iatrogenic segmental scoliosis and persistent pain at 2 months after surgery.

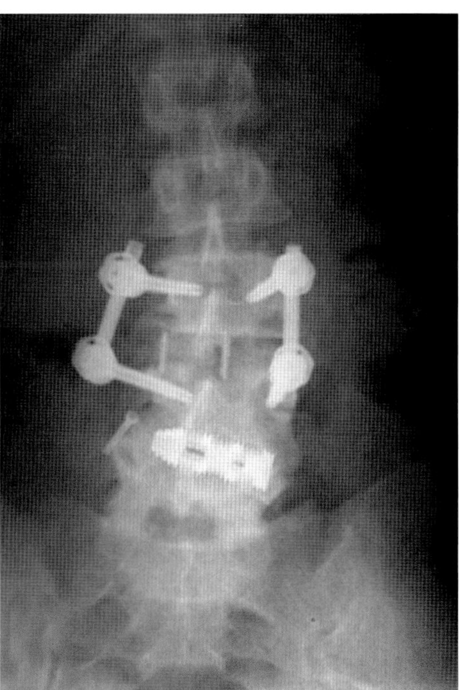

■ **FIGURE 49–7.** Case 2 post-revision. Artificial disc removal and revision were performed using the extreme lateral interbody fusion (XLIF) technique, supplemented with percutaneous pedicle screws.

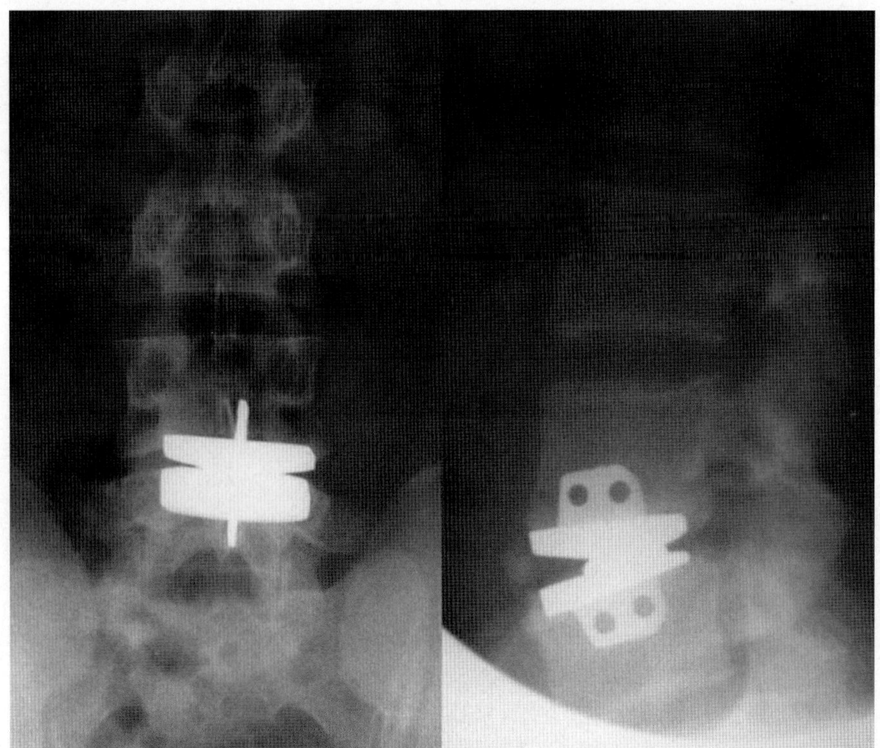

■ **FIGURE 49–8.** Case 3 pre-revision. Maverick total disc replacement implantation with device slightly off-center and anterior, causing persistent pain 1 year after surgery.

### Case 3—Malpositioned, Keeled Implant

An otherwise healthy 38-year-old man had received a Maverick TDR for L4-L5 degenerative disc disease. Postoperatively, the patient continued to have intolerable back pain. A year after the primary surgery, the patient was still disabled, unable to work, and requested removal of the device. Radiographs revealed that the device was placed slightly off-center and slightly anterior (Fig. 49–8).

Retrieval and revision were accomplished through an XLIF approach by exposing the lateral spine per the usual technique. However, removal of a keeled device requires at least partial corpectomy, and in preparation for this step, the L4 segmental vessels were clipped upon lateral exposure of the spine. An osteotome was used to selectively chisel a corner of the vertebral body to reveal the keel (Fig. 49–9). The bone fragment was removed and retained by starting a pedicle screw into it and using the screw to extract the fragment (Fig. 49–10). The superior device end plate was then pried loose (Fig. 49–11). Without the superior end plate in place, the inferior end plate then had adequate room to be pried loose. The vertebral bone fragment was reinserted by implanting it back into the defect and advancing the screw bicortically (Fig. 49–12). After implantation of a large PEEK cage in the interspace, a second screw was placed in the L5 vertebra and a rod placed for supplemental lateral fixation of the fusion construct (Fig. 49–13). The patient was walking and discharged to home the day after surgery. He returned to work 3 weeks after revision surgery and has no back pain.

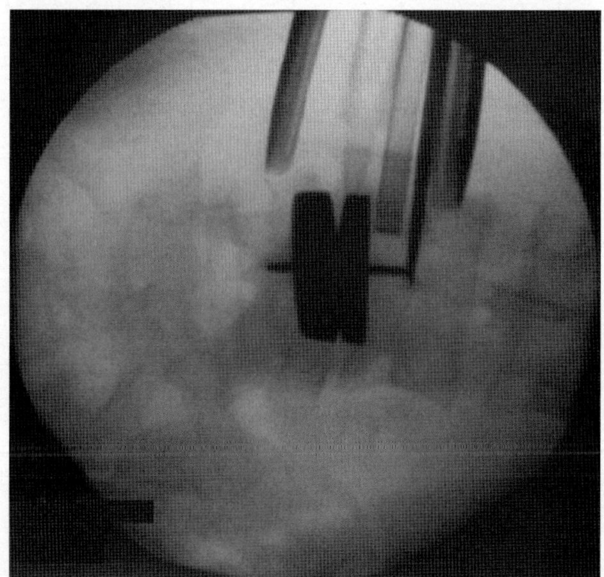

■ **FIGURE 49–9.** Removal of the keeled Maverick device required partial corpectomy. An osteotome was used to selectively chisel a corner of the vertebral body to reveal the keel.

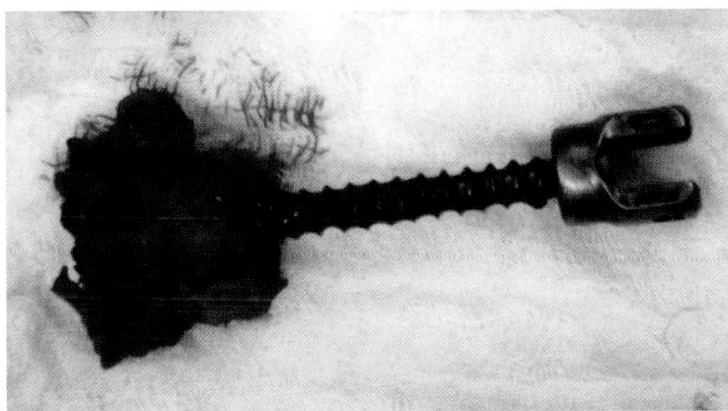

■ **FIGURE 49–10.** A pedicle screw was used to extract the bone fragment.

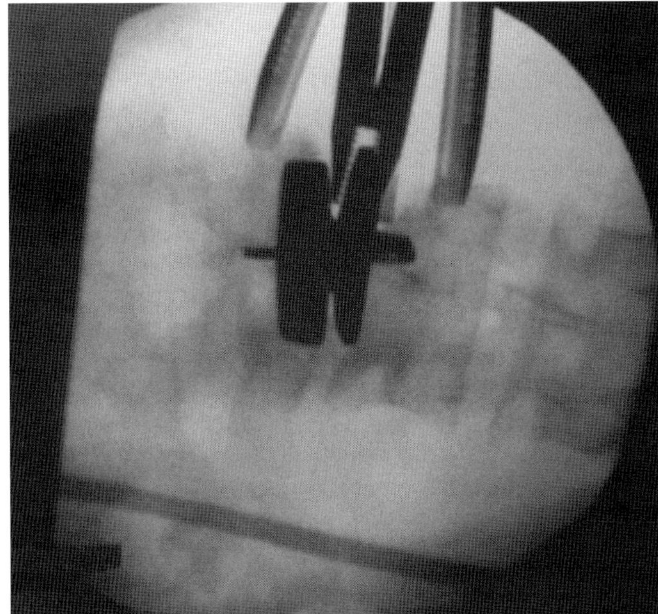

■ **FIGURE 49–11.** With the defect made in the superior vertebra, the superior Maverick end plate could be pried loose.

## DISCUSSION

The lateral retroperitoneal trans-psoas approach avoids many of the risks associated with anterior revision surgery. In no case was fibrosis or scar tissue encountered in the retroperitoneal space. Bony ingrowth onto the device end plates was superficial and sporadic such that the end plate fixations were separated from the bone using an osteotome without significant force. The fixation through the holes in the Maverick keel was fibrous rather

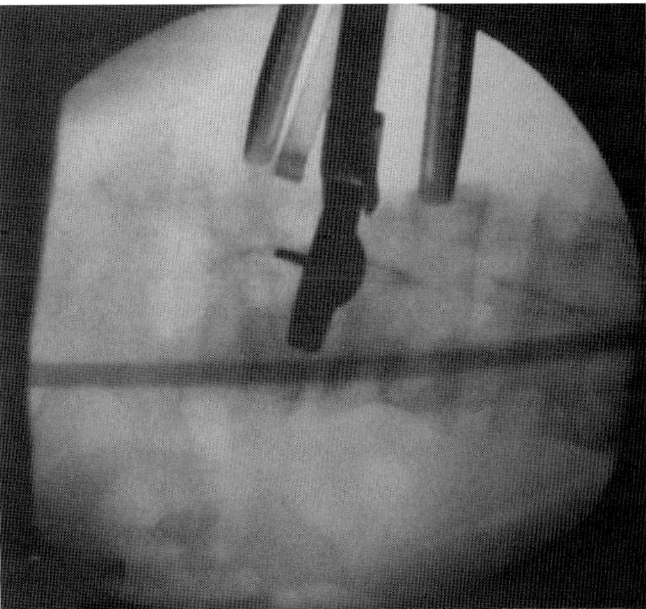

■ **FIGURE 49–12.** With the superior device end plate removed, the inferior end plate then had adequate room to be pried loose.

than osseous. Disc space preparation for fusion is uncomplicated but includes contralateral annulus release to ensure symmetric disc distraction and enable the insertion and placement of a large interbody implant across the peripheral ring apophysis, providing good end plate support and coronal and sagittal alignment.

## CONCLUSION

An anteriorly placed TDR device can be successfully and more safely revised using an XLIF approach. The direct lateral trajectory avoids anterior adhesions from the primary procedure, does not require mobilization of the great vessels, and with careful EMG-guided dilation of the psoas muscle, provides ample exposure to remove the device. A polyethylene core is easily removed upon lateral annulotomy. Keeled devices require partial corpectomy to remove the device but only at one end, and the bone can be salvaged. The limited bony ongrowth onto either type of device does not hinder revision to fusion. A large stabilizing fusion implant makes use of the more biomechanically sound ring apophysis at the periphery of the bony end plates, which is typically undisturbed by the primary procedure, with correction and restoration of proper sagittal and coronal balance. Careful and appropriate patient selection, proper surgeon training, and excellent implant technique are essential in ensuring optimal outcomes.

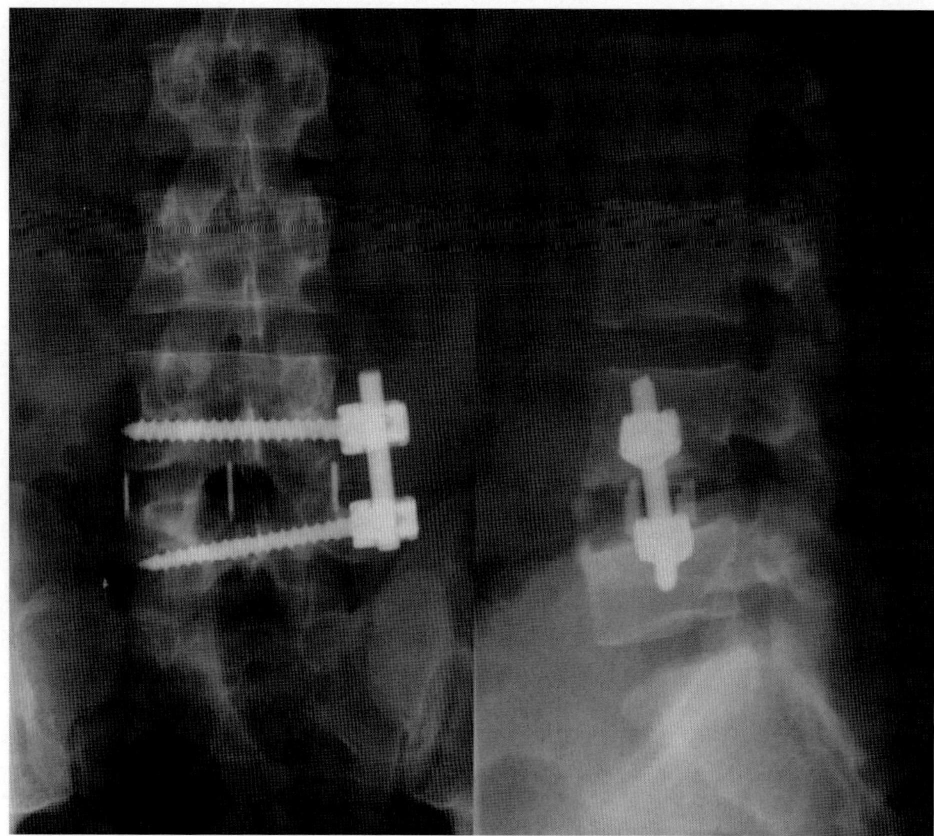

■ **FIGURE 49–13.** Case 3 post-revision. The bone fragment was re-implanted into the defect, advancing the pedicle screw across the vertebral body, an interbody cage was inserted in the disc space, and the construct was supplemented with lateral fixation.

## REFERENCES


1. Bertagnoli R, Zigler J, Karg A, Voigt S: Complications and strategies for revision surgery in total disc replacement. Orthop Clin N Am 36:389–395, 2005.
2. Kostuik J: Complications and surgical revision for failed disc arthroplasty. Spine J 4:289S–291S, 2004.
3. McAfee P, Geisler F, Saiedy S, et al: Revisability of the CHARITÉ Artificial Disc replacement: Analysis of 688 patients enrolled in the U.S. IDE Study of the CHARITÉ Artificial Disc. Spine 31:1217–1226, 2006.
4. Scott-Young M: Strategy for revision disc replacement surgery. *In* McAfee P, Geisler F, Scott-Young M (eds): Roundtables in Spine Surgery, 1(2):23–71, 2005.
5. Tropiano P, Huang R, Girardi F, et al: Lumbar total disc replacement: Seven- to eleven-year follow-up. J Bone Joint Surg Am 87:490–496, 2005.
6. van Ooij A, Oner FC, Verbout AJ: Complications of artificial disc replacement: A report of 27 patients with SB Charite Disc. J Spinal Disord 16:369–383, 2003.
7. Diaz R, Phillips F, Pimenta L: Minimally invasive XLIF fusion in the treatment of symptomatic degenerative lumbar scoliosis. Proceedings of the NASS 20th Annual Meeting. Spine J 5(4):131S–132S, 2005.
8. Ozgur B, Aryan H, Pimenta L, Taylor W: Extreme lateral interbody fusion (XLIF): A novel surgical technique for anterior lumbar interbody fusion. Spine J 6:435–443, 2006.
9. Pimenta L, Schaffa T, da Silva Martins M, et al: Extreme lateral interbody fusion. *In* Perez-Cruet M, Khoo L, Fessler R (eds): An anatomical approach to minimally invasive spine surgery. St. Louis, MO, Quality Medical Publishing, 2006, pp 641–652.
10. Wright N: Instrumented extreme lateral interbody fusion (XLIF) through a single approach. Proceedings of the NASS 20th Annual Meeting. Spine J 5:S177–S178, 2005.
11. Pimenta L, Diaz R, Guerrero L: Charite lumbar artificial disc retrieval: Use of a lateral minimally invasive technique. J Neurosurg Spine 5:556–561, 2006.

CHAPTER 50

# Persistent Pain After Lumbar Total Disc Replacement

**Jonathan R. Stieber** and **Jeffrey A. Goldstein**

**KEY POINTS**

- Pain secondary to lumbar total disc replacement (TDR) may be due to several factors:
  - Poor patient selection with incomplete diagnosis and insufficient psychometric testing.
  - Facet degeneration may continue or undiagnosed spinal deformity.
  - Surgical- or device-related causes.
  - Thorough assessment of pain generator after TDR, if necessary.

## INTRODUCTION

Persistent pain after lumbar total disc replacement (TDR) surgery may occur secondary to a variety of specific causes related to the index surgery, including poor patient selection, incorrect or incompletely diagnosed pathology, and limitations of surgical technique. Because articulating bearing surfaces are integral to arthroplasty, prosthesis-related complications may also lead to pain and inferior patient outcomes. Progressive facet disease at either the target level treated or adjacent levels, in addition to adjacent disc degeneration, may also result in continued or recurrent pain.

In order to address the problem of persistent postoperative pain, the patient must be rigorously reassessed with a thorough history, physical examination, and radiographic evaluation so that symptomatic pathology may be identified. Diagnosis of the specific pain generator or etiology may permit successful treatment of this complex clinical problem.

## POOR PATIENT SELECTION

Appropriate patient selection is paramount for the successful treatment of axial lumbar back pain with TDR. Persistent pain following surgical treatment is commonly related to underlying psychosocial or neurophysiologic factors. These may include unrealistic expectations, somatic distress, amplification of pain, chronic pain behavior, depression, and secondary gain. Poor surgical outcomes and persistent pain have been associated with abnormal pain behavior, clinical depression, and anxiety.[1,2] A variety of psychometric instruments are available for evaluating a patient's baseline psychosocial status, including the Modified Zung Depression Test, Modified Somatic Pain Questionnaire, Beck Depression Index, Fear Avoidance Beliefs Questionnaire, and the Multiphasic Personality Inventory. Psychometric testing has been shown to be predictive of inferior clinical outcomes following surgery for both herniated lumbar discs and axial back pain.[3–5] In their analysis of psychological factors associated with spine surgery outcomes, Block et al[6] reported their presurgical psychological screening to be predictive of overall outcome in 82% of patients.

Poor results are also more frequently observed in patients who may stand to benefit from a secondary gain, such as those who receive worker's compensation or who are involved in litigation.[7,8] Despite proper preoperative anticipatory guidance, some patients may maintain unreachable expectations in terms of pain relief and return to activity. Patients who are willing to embrace emerging technologies such as lumbar disc replacement may harbor some element of inherent selection bias with overly optimistic goals for surgery. Moreover, those patients who exhibit borderline personality disorder characteristics, who tend to shift from extremes of idealization to devaluation, may initially clamor for an idealized treatment but switch modes following a surgical outcome that falls short of their ideal. The psychosocial component of persistent pain, although central to treatment, is difficult to quantify and remains to be further elucidated.

## INCORRECT PROCEDURE

Persistent pain and poor clinical outcomes can ensue from misdiagnosis or failing to recognize the entirety of the spinal pathology. As with all spinal procedures, identification of the correct surgical level is central to the successful treatment of pathology. Radiographic confirmation of the correct surgical level is recommended by the North American Spine Society and has become the standard of care in nearly all cases. A failure to identify and treat all levels of symptomatic pathology may, likewise, result in persistent pain and suboptimal clinical outcomes.

An incorrect or incomplete diagnosis may result in the attribution of pain to radiographic evidence of degenerative disc disease or other age-related changes. These may include missed spinal stenosis, herniated nucleus pulposus, spondylolisthesis, spondylolysis, and advanced facet arthropathy. Although a central or paracentral herniated nucleus pulposus may be addressed through the anterior approach at the time of disc space preparation for implantation of a TDR, this pathology may be addressed only if it is recognized, and a secondary posterior procedure may also be necessary. Central and lateral recess stenosis results from a combination of processes, including disc bulging or herniation, facet hypertrophy, and infolding or hypertrophy of the ligamentum flavum. These later two entities, when not adequately addressed by the anterior procedure, may require a posterior decompression or result in persistent spinal stenosis.

Spondylolysis or significant spondylolisthesis (grade>1) decreases or eliminates the contribution of the posterior elements to the stability of the functional spinal unit (FSU). Although the devices available for TDR differ in construction, many incorporate nonconstrained or semiconstrained designs. At present, no device has been clinically evaluated in the context of a spondylolisthesis of greater than grade 1. Failure of the posterior elements may have the consequence of increasing the shear forces on the implant, which may result in increased pain from the facet joints, pars interarticularis defect (Fig. 50–1), or failure of the device either at the device–end plate junction or intrinsically.

If lumbar facet joint arthropathy is responsible for a substantial element of the patient's discomfort, treatment of the painful intervertebral disc alone will not address all pain generators. Moreover, the process of facet degeneration may continue or be exacerbated after treatment with disc replacement. For this reason, patients with advanced facet arthropathy are thought to be poor candidates for treatment with disc replacement surgery; however, concomitant posterior motion-preserving stabilization, such as facet replacement or enhancement, may ultimately expand indications to include these patients. Patients with unrecognized or untreated spinal deformity may also experience inferior outcomes when treated with disc replacement.

## TECHNIQUE-RELATED PROBLEMS

If the procedure is incompletely or incorrectly executed, the patient may experience persistent symptoms despite the correct diagnosis and choice of treatment. As previously mentioned, patients with a central or paracentral herniated nucleus pulposus may be treated with disc replacement surgery with a concurrent adequate excision of the herniated fragment. Failure to recognize the offending pathology and decompress the neural elements, however, may result in continued radiculopathy or stenosis. Similarly, among the surgical goals in treating the intrinsic disc pathology of degenerative disc disease is to remove the pain generator, that is, the intervertebral disc. Insufficient resection of the disc annulus may leave a substantial remnant of the innervated pain generator.

Care must be taken to prepare the end plates appropriately and to adequately resect posterior osteophytes. Failure to do so may result in impaction of bone fragments from the end plate or residual posterior osteophytes into the spinal canal or neural foramen leading to iatrogenic compression of the neural elements (Fig. 50–2). Inaccurate insertion of the implant out of a parallel plane with the end plates may also create this type of bony fragment and resultant problem. Implantation of an oversized prosthesis may overdistract the disc space and place the nerve roots on stretch. This can cause radiculopathic and dysesthetic pain. Furthermore, oversizing the implant may convert the articulating disc replacement into a static intervertebral spacer, which loses its ability to allow for motion.[9]

The advent of lumbar TDR has also increased the complexity of the anterior spinal procedure when compared with anterior lumbar interbody fusion. Because the disc replacement is an articulating device designed to replicate and preserve spinal motion, precision of device placement is far more integral to the success of the procedure than in fusion.[10] Device placement posterior to the posterior vertebral margin will result in spinal stenosis, but device placement too anterior will limit the range of motion (ROM) of the motion segment. Implantation of the device too lateral to midline may also result in inferior outcomes (Fig. 50–3).[11] CHARITÉ discs (DePuy Spine Inc., Raynham, MA) placed greater than 5 mm from their ideal placement in the coronal or sagittal plane had less ROM than those less than 5 mm displaced.[10] Because some of the devices currently available incorporate modular components, it is of the greatest importance that the device is assembled correctly with the components locked in place. Incorrect or incomplete assembly may result in migration or extrusion of the polyethylene component from the device and catastrophic failure.

Preoperative and postoperative disc height has been demonstrated to influence sagittal ROM following a TDR with the ProDisc-L (Synthes, West Chester, PA). Although this did not affect short-term clinical outcomes, one can only anticipate improved long-term benefit through the maintenance of intervertebral motion.

## FAILURE TO ACHIEVE SURGICAL GOALS

Among the goals of lumbar TDR are to eliminate the diseased intervertebral disc as the pain generator, to confer stability to the FSU, to restore or maintain disc height, to maintain or improve sagittal alignment, and to regain or maintain motion of the FSU. This last goal of regaining or maintaining motion differentiates TDR from our experience with spinal fusion. ROM may be limited secondary to suboptimal device placement, oversizing of the device, or autofusion.[10] Although a complete and solid spontaneous fusion is unlikely to result in pain, partial or incomplete autofusion of the segment secondary to heterotopic ossification may result in persistent pain and inferior patient outcomes.[12]

## FAILURE OF THE PROSTHESIS

Pain is likely to be the initial symptom of device failure or other device-associated complications. Various designs of TDR prostheses have been shown to migrate, disassociate, and fracture or extrude their polyethylene components. Such device migration or extrusion may place the vascular structures that lie anterior to the disc space at risk, causing pain of a vascular etiology in addition to mechanical pain.[13] Additionally, TDR designs that incorporate fins for stability have been reported to result in end plate

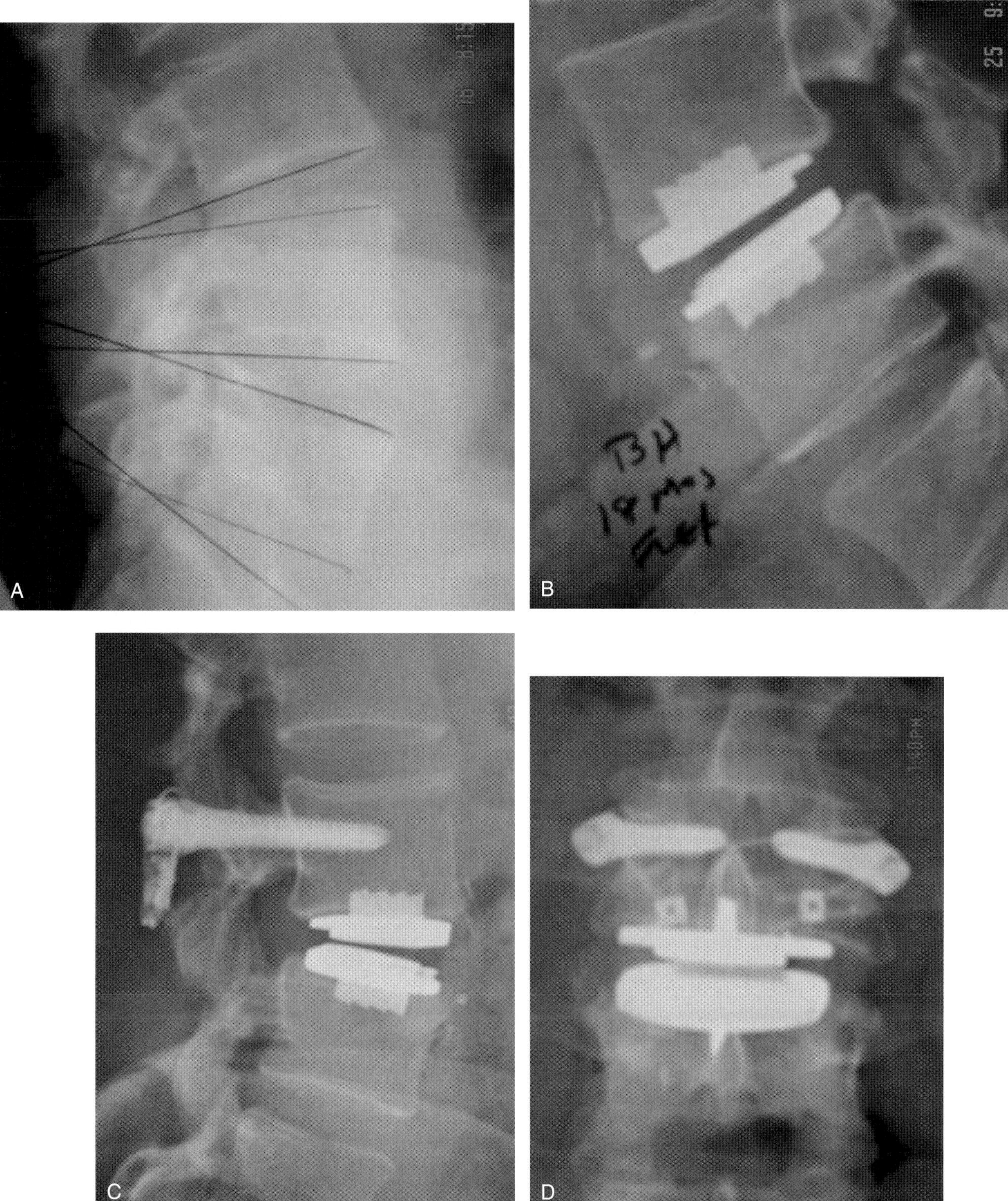


■ **FIGURE 50–1.** These radiographs are from a patient who underwent lumbar disc replacement with the ProDisc-L. **A,** The pars defect was not obvious on preoperative radiograph. The patient had complete relief of his low back pain for 18 months following surgery. The relief of pain allowed the patient to return to work with frequent heavy overhead lifting. **B,** Follow-up radiographs demonstrated the spondylolysis. Two sets of pars injections each afforded the patient complete relief of his pain. Despite the posterior column instability, the ProDisc-L did not fail. **C** and **D,** Radiographs of pars repair that subsequently afforded the patient complete pain relief and a return to his heavy lifting job.

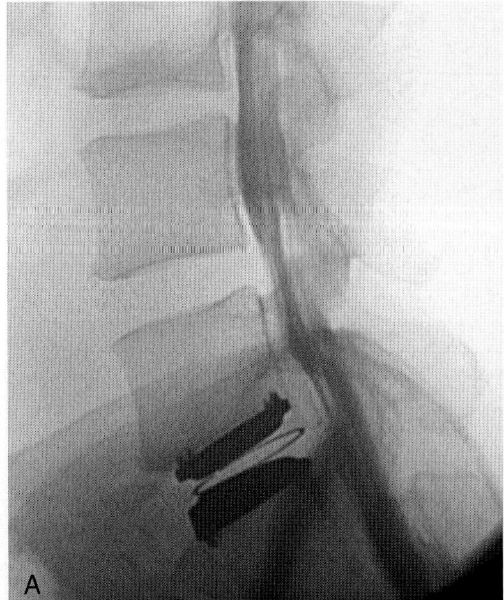


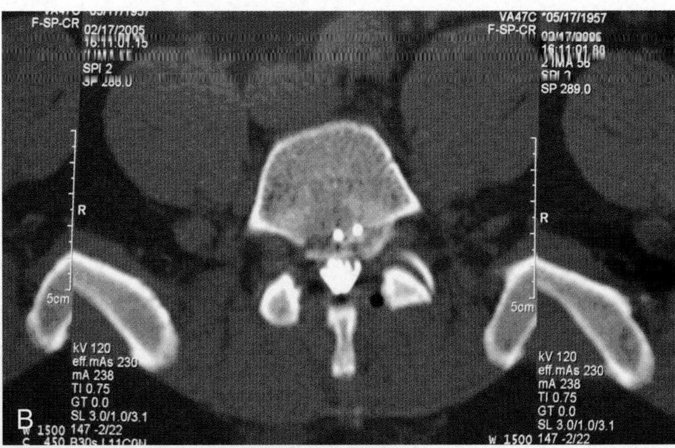


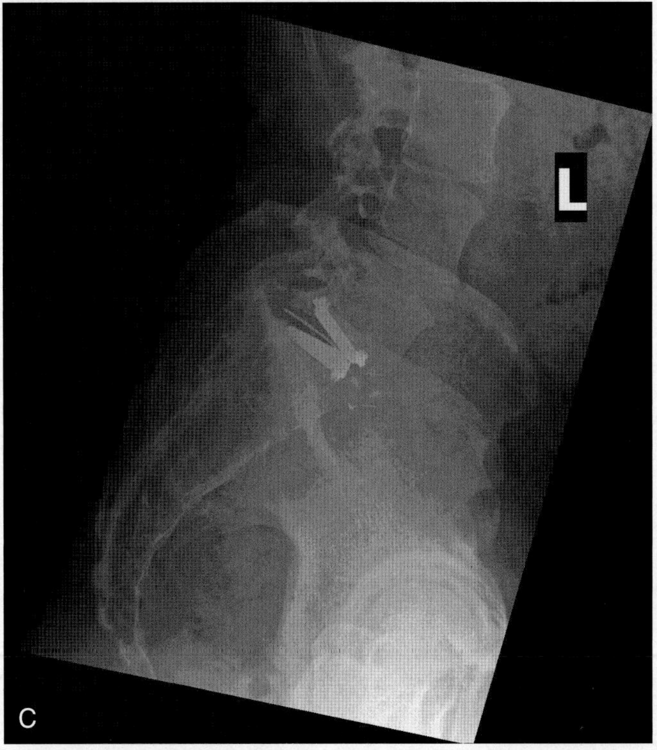


■ **FIGURE 50–2.** This patient awoke following surgery with new-onset leg pain and a neurologic deficit with a foot drop. **A,** Postoperative evaluation demonstrated that the L5 nerve root had become entrapped between a displaced fragment of the posterior inferior aspect of the L5 vertebral body and the L5 pedicle. **B,** Impaction of one of the teeth from the CHARITÉ end plate had caused the L5 end plate to fracture and a fragment to displace. Following return to the operating room, the fragment was removed and the nerve root decompressed. The postoperative leg pain as well as the preoperative low back pain resolved, but the motor deficit remained. **C,** The implant subsided and has no motion 2 years postoperatively.

fractures.[14] A case report of bilateral pedicle fracture following TDR has also been reported.[15]

## DISEASE PROGRESSION

Transition syndrome occurs when adjacent-segment disease progresses adjacent to a previous fusion due to the increased load placed on the neighboring motion segment and the consequent hypermobility of that spinal motion segment. In posterior spinal procedures, there may also exist an iatrogenic component because dissection or instrumentation may cause harm to the facet joints. Based on a Kaplan-Meier survivorship analysis, Ghiselli et al[16] concluded that 37% of the patients in their cohort would require an additional surgical procedure for adjacent-segment disease of the lumbar spine within 10 years of their index

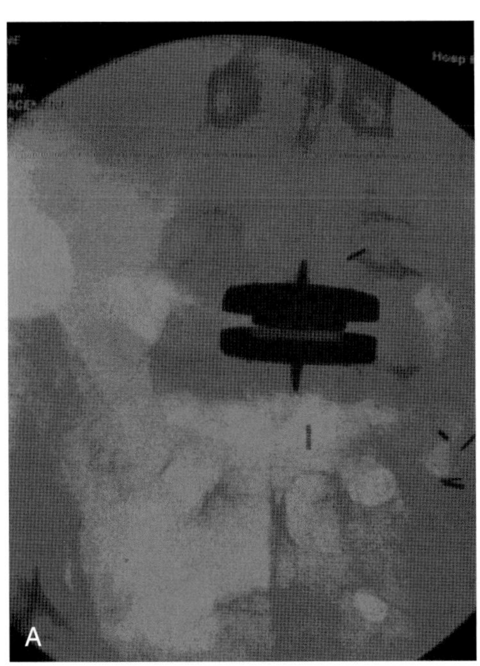

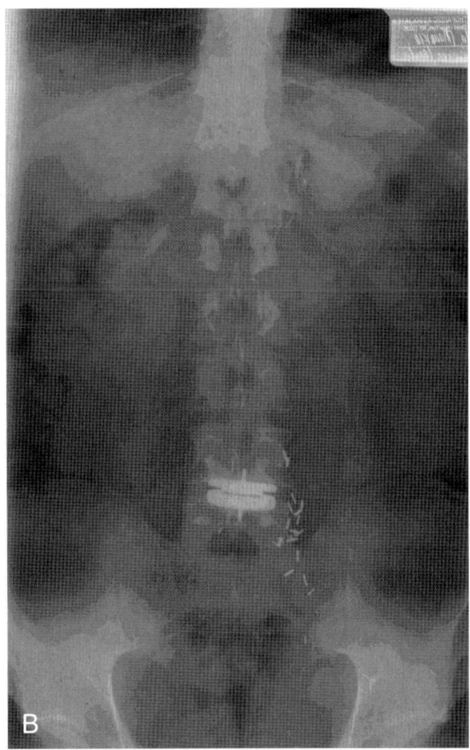

■ **FIGURE 50–3.** Failure to align the implant in the midline may lead to diminished postoperative pain scores. **A,** A well-aligned ProDisc-L. **B,** An offset from the midline and a diminished outcome.

procedure. Adjacent-segment disease may include progression of degenerative disc disease, facet arthropathy, spinal stenosis, or a new or exacerbated herniated nucleus pulposus.

Among the goals of TDR is to impede or prevent the cascade of adjacent spinal segment degeneration by normalizing the stresses placed upon adjacent motion segments when compared with spinal arthrodesis. Despite designing disc replacement prostheses to accomplish this specific goal, there is yet insufficient follow-up and data to fully support this hypothesis. Moreover, although lumbar total disc prostheses are designed to replicate the normal physiology of the intact native intervertebral disc, the complex physiology of the FSU makes achieving this task very difficult. Thus, adjacent-segment disease may still occur and serve as a source of persistent pain, especially when some element of degenerative disease is pre-existing at that level.

## EARLY-ONSET POSTOPERATIVE PAIN

Almost immediately following surgery, the patient should report some relief of axial back pain despite the expected postoperative discomfort. If the patient's symptoms are unchanged, it is possible that the symptomatic pathology was inadequately addressed due to surgery at the wrong level or, more likely, missed pathology. Unchanged or worsened axial back pain may be due to incorrect device positioning or assembly, leading to limited ROM, device migration, or device dissociation. Leg pain in the context of temperature differences between the lower extremities warrants a vascular evaluation, because it is possible that the necessary retraction during surgery may have resulted in vascular injury or occlusion. Decreased or absent pulses should trigger an examination with duplex ultrasound. More subjective patient complaints concerning temperature changes may arise from disruption of the sympathetics during the surgical exposure. In this circumstance, observation is indicated.

Following exclusion of a vascular etiology, neurogenic leg pain should be investigated. Overseating of the TDR posterior to the posterior vertebral margin may cause neurogenic claudication due to incursion into the spinal canal. Such a finding necessitates revision of the prosthesis. New-onset central stenosis may also occur due to iatrogenic retropulsion of a bone fragment into the central canal. Bilateral radiculopathic symptoms may result from overdistraction of the intervertebral disc space stretching the nerve roots. In most cases, this phenomenon is self-limiting, with resolution over weeks to months without the need for surgical revision. Unilateral radiculopathy may result from migration of either disc material or a bone fragment into the lateral recess or neural foramen. Computed tomography–myelogram may be of diagnostic utility in evaluation of the neural elements and delineation of compressive pathology.

## SUBACUTE POSTOPERATIVE PAIN

Following an initial period of postoperative improvement, a recurrence or new onset of pain may occur. It is common for patients to report new or recurrent discomfort with increased level of activity or participation in a physical therapy program. This discomfort is likely to be self-limiting and must be differentiated from more serious and persistent pathology. A history of trauma or acute onset of pain may be associated with device failure or fracture of the end plate. Such a history of acute new-onset pain requires prompt radiographic evaluation. A more insidious onset may correspond to device migration or infection. Again, evaluation with plain radiographs is indicated. Insidious pain associated with constitutional symptoms should be investigated for infection. Laboratory testing for infection markers is obligatory, including a complete blood count, erythrocyte sedimentation rate, and C-reactive protein. Nuclear imaging may also be of diagnostic use because the accuracy of magnetic resonance imaging will be degraded secondary to artifact from the implant. Combined $^{67}$Gallium citrate and technetium-99m-MDP studies are the current gold standard.

## LATE POSTOPERATIVE PAIN

Onset of pain 6 months after surgery is considered late postoperative pain. Again, infection should be excluded as a diagnosis. Late postoperative pain may be related to the implant itself. Wear and fracture of polyethylene components has been reported for certain implants, as has subsidence and migration.[17] Progression of facet disease may also be responsible for gradually progressive mechanical back pain. Continued degenerative changes of the facet joints and ligamentum flavum may lead to spinal stenosis. Adjacent-segment disease may also occur, requiring treatment of additional levels of pathology.

## SUMMARY

Preoperative psychological screening may help avoid unsuccessful surgery for patients with personality or emotional disorders that may hamper a successful surgical outcome. A vigilant and meticulous investigation and work-up is integral to the diagnosis of the cause of persistent pain after lumbar disc arthroplasty. A systematic evaluation of patients with persistent pain after disc replacement surgery should include identification of the location and character of the pain; the chronicity of the pain and any pain-free interval; and appropriate use of imaging, injections, and neurologic studies.

## REFERENCES


1. Trief PM, Grant W, Fredrickson B: A prospective study of psychological predictors of lumbar surgery outcome. Spine 25:2616–2621, 2000.
2. Waddell G, McCulloch JA, Kummel E, Venner RM: Nonorganic physical signs in low-back pain. Spine 5:117–125, 1980.
3. Carragee EJ, Lincoln T, Parmar VS, Alamin T: A gold standard evaluation of the "discogenic pain" diagnosis as determined by provocative discography. Spine 31:2115–2123, 2006.
4. Junge A, Dvorak J, Ahrens S: Predictors of bad and good outcomes of lumbar disc surgery: A prospective clinical study with recommendations for screening to avoid bad outcomes. Spine 20:460–468, 1995.
5. Spengler DM, Ouellette EA, Battie M, Zeh J: Elective discectomy for herniation of a lumbar disc: Additional experience with an objective method. J Bone Joint Surg Am 72:230–237, 1990.
6. Block AR, Ohnmeiss DD, Guyer RD, et al: The use of presurgical psychological screening to predict the outcome of spine surgery. Spine J 1:274–282, 2001.
7. Klekamp J, McCarty E, Spengler DM: Results of elective lumbar discectomy for patients involved in the workers' compensation system. J Spinal Disord 11:277–282, 1998.
8. Taylor VM, Deyo RA, Ciol M, et al: Patient-oriented outcomes from low back surgery: A community-based study. Spine 25:2445–2452, 2000.
9. DiAngelo DJ, Foley KT, Morrow B, et al The effects of over-sizing of a disc prosthesis on spine biomechanics. Spine Arthroplasty Society Sixth Annual Global Symposium on Motion Preservation Technology, Montreal, Canada, May 2006, p 97.
10. McAfee PC, Cunningham B, Holsapple G, et al: A prospective, randomized, multicenter Food and Drug Administration investigational device exemption study of lumbar total disc replacement with the CHARITÉ artificial disc versus lumbar fusion, Part II: Evaluation of radiographic outcomes and correlation of surgical technique accuracy with clinical outcomes. Spine 30:1576–1583; discussion E388–390, 2005.
11. Yaszay B, Quirno M, Bendo J, et al: Effect of intervertebral disk height on post-operative motion and outcomes following Prodisc-L lumbar disk replacement (in press) 2007.
12. McAfee PC, Cunningham BW, Devine J, et al: Classification of heterotopic ossification (HO) in artificial disk replacement. J Spinal Disord Tech 16:384–389, 2003.
13. Stieber JR, Donald GDR: Early failure of lumbar disc replacement: Case report and review of the literature. J Spinal Disord Tech 19:55–60, 2006.
14. Shim CS, Lee S, Maeng DH, Lee SH: Vertical split fracture of the vertebral body following total disc replacement using ProDisc: Report of two cases. J Spinal Disord Tech 18:465–469, 2005.
15. Mathew P, Blackman M, Redla S, Hussein AA: Bilateral pedicle fractures following anterior dislocation of the polyethylene inlay of a ProDisc artificial disc replacement: A case report of an unusual complication. Spine 30:E311–E314, 2005.
16. Ghiselli G, Wang JC, Bhatia NN, et al: Adjacent segment degeneration in the lumbar spine. J Bone Joint Surg Am 86A:1497–1503, 2004.
17. van Ooij A, Oner FC, Verbout AJ: Complications of artificial disc replacement: A report of 27 patients with the SB CHARITÉ disc. J Spinal Disord Tech 16:369–383, 2003.

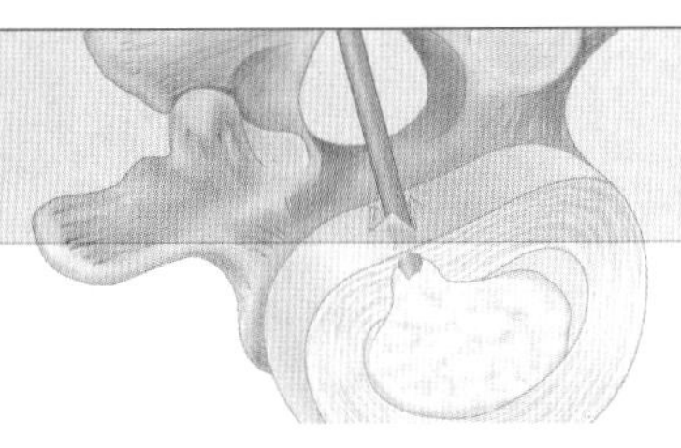

PART

# V

# LUMBAR PARTIAL DISC REPLACEMENT: NUCLEUS REPLACEMENT

CHAPTER 51

# DASCOR

Michael Ahrens, Anthony Tsantrizos, and Jean-Charles Le Huec

## KEY POINTS

- The DASCOR device is a two-part in situ–cured polyurethane injected within an expandable polyurethane balloon to form the final nucleus replacement device that conforms to the nucleus cavity created.
- Pressurized device injection in the disc space is possible using a proprietary injection system.
- Ability to verify intraoperatively the volume and size of the resultant DASCOR device before implantation using fluoroscopic imaging procedures in conjunction with a proprietary DASCOR imaging balloon.
- This catheter-based nucleus replacement technology can be used not only for minimally open procedures but also with percutaneous and endoscopic procedures.
- The technology has the capability of implanting the DASCOR device using an anterior, anterolateral, lateral, or posterolateral approach.

## INTRODUCTION

Repairing a flat bicycle tire often requires replacement of the inner tube rather than complete wheel replacement. Similarly, this analogy can extend to the intervertebral disc, depending on its degenerative condition, can be subject to different treatment options. Total disc replacement (TDR) implants have been proposed as alternatives to arthrodesis for treatment of chronic low back pain (LBP) with degenerative disc disease as the etiology. In essence, TDR implants would be analogous to removal of the complete wheel. However by replacing only the nucleus, that is, the inner tube of the disc, the clinical goals of pain relief, anatomic and biomechanical function restoration, and limiting progression of adjacent-level disease can be reestablished with less traumatic surgical techniques compared with TDRs.

Nucleus replacement techniques are rapidly reemerging as advanced treatment options for mild-to-moderate stages of degenerative disc disease since the days of the Fernstrom endoprosthesis.[1] Renewed interest in nuclear replacement, a minimally invasive treatment alternative, has resulted from novel materials and technologic innovations. Current nucleus replacement technologies can be classified as preformed or in situ–formed implants, despite the differences in materials used (Fig. 51–1). The DASCOR device (Disc Dynamics Inc. Eden Prairie, MN) is intended to alleviate discogenic pain and restore disc height and segmental mobility while preserving the patient's bony and axial connective tissue/muscular support anatomy.

The DASCOR device has received CE-Mark approval for commercial sale in the European Union in July 2005. The system has been in clinical use in trials outside the United States since 2003. The implant is also continually being used in Europe in the scope of an ongoing postmarket approval trial. The company also received approval from the U.S. Food and Drug Administration (FDA) in July 2006 to begin a clinical trial of the DASCOR device in the United States.

## INDICATIONS/CONTRAINDICATIONS

At present, the DASCOR device is advocated for implantation in patients with the following indications:

- Age between 18 and 70 years
- Single-level degenerative disc disease as confirmed by patient's history, physical examination, or computed tomography (CT) or magnetic resonance imaging (MRI)
- Persistent pain and/or symptoms after at least 6 months of non-operative care
- Leg pain, back pain, or both in the absence of nerve root compression per MRI or CT scan, without prolapse or narrowing of the lateral recess
- Minimum 5.5-mm disc height at the affected level
- Scarring or thickening of ligamentum flavum, annulus fibrosis, or facet joint capsule
- Condition involving only one lumbar disc level from L2 to the S1
- Oswestry Disability Index (ODI) score greater than 40 (based on 100-point scale)
- Back pain score of at least 5 on a 10-point Visual Analog Scale (VAS)
- Intact end plates at the affected disc level
- Positive CT discography at the affected level with concordant pain

Contraindications include the following:

- Disc herniation or reherniation with radicular pain requiring posterior discectomy

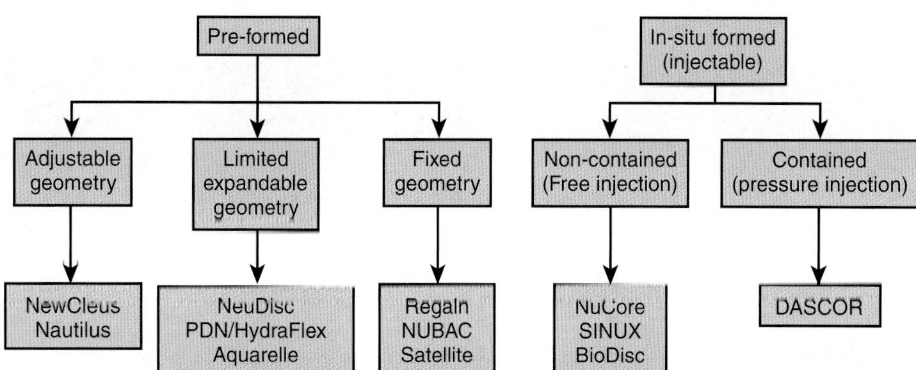


■ **FIGURE 51–1.** Classification of current nucleus replacement technologies.

- Prior invasive treatment of the disc at the implant level, such as discectomy
- Previous diagnosis of osteopenia, osteoporosis, spinal osteoarthritis, ankylosing spondylitis, advanced Scheurermann's disease, history of inflammatory bowel disease, psoriatic arthritis, Reiter's syndrome, rheumatoid arthritis or inflammatory arthritic disease, spinal tumor or other known malignancy, or arachnoiditis
- Isthmic spondylolisthesis or degenerative spondylolisthesis greater than 3 mm
- Prior lumbar fusion surgery at any level
- Moderate or severe central spinal, foraminal, or lateral recess stenosis, or cauda equina syndrome
- Facet joints that are absent, fractured, or severely degenerated
- Obesity, as defined by a body mass index of greater than 35
- Active systemic or local infection in the area of the planned surgery
- Incompetent annulus
- History of communicable disease such as human immunodeficiency virus (HIV) or hepatitis

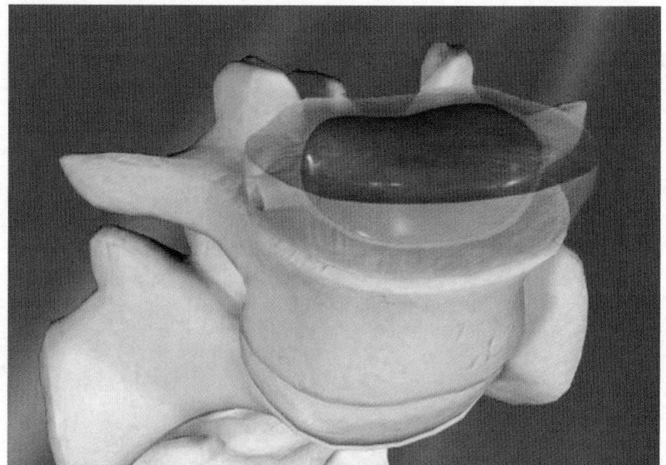

■ **FIGURE 51–2.** The DASCOR device. *(From Disc Dynamics, Inc. Reprinted with permission.)*

## DESCRIPTION OF THE DEVICE

The DASCOR device is fabricated by mixing a methylene-diphenyldiisocyanate (MDI)–based polyurethane two-part reactive system and injecting this mixture under controlled pressure while it is still liquid, through a catheter to an expandable balloon that is placed in the prepared nuclectomy space (Fig. 51–2). The polymer is contained within the expandable balloon and cures to a firm, but pliable form within minutes while concurrently bonding to the expandable balloon, forming the final device. The temperature at the interface released during the curing process is within the range of acceptable physiologic temperatures (less than 50°C) and well below typical interfacial temperatures measured with bone cements used for vertebroplasty procedures and with intradiscal electrothermal therapy (IDET) procedures.

The DASCOR device has the ability to contour and conform to any nucleus cavity created during nuclectomy because the liquid polymer is being injected under pressure using a customized injection system (Fig. 51–3). This feature creates a large implant footprint and a volume (average 4 to 5 mL) through a small annulotomy, thus enabling better axial load transfer capabilities through the implant as well as radially to the surrounding annulus. The ability to inject under pressure permits the DASCOR device to immediately distract the disc space and, on curing, obtain a final implant geometry and disc space distraction without having to rely on hydration. On the other hand, hydrogel nucleus implants do rely on the material's intrinsic swelling pressure to fully hydrate with time to attain final implant geometry and disc space distraction.

The final cured polymer inside the balloon is an incompressible isotropic aromatic polyether polyurethane with an optimal mixture of hard and soft segments to optimize resilience, flexibility, and mechanical strength. A typical compression modulus of the device per ASTM D575 ranges between 4 and 6 MPa, with an ultimate compressive stress and strain of greater than 25 MPa and 90%, respectively. The low balloon catheter profile offers the advantage for percutaneous implantation procedures. The balloon component is an aliphatic polycarbonate urethane that has excellent cavity expansion and conforming capabilities and is attached to a 5.5-mm delivery catheter. The balloon component has a large safety margin for preventing burst or leakage and is capable of holding more than 10 times the average injection volume and 2 times the maximal applied injection pressure.

## BACKGROUND OF SCIENTIFIC TESTING/CLINICAL OUTCOMES

Extensive preclinical studies have been conducted on the DASCOR device, including mechanical bench and biomechanical testing as well as biocompatibility and biologic response testing in animal models.

INJECTOR SYSTEM

Display panel
Injector head
Hand control
Cart
Foot control

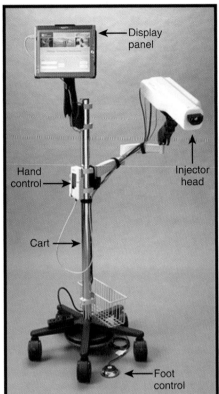

DISPLAY PANEL

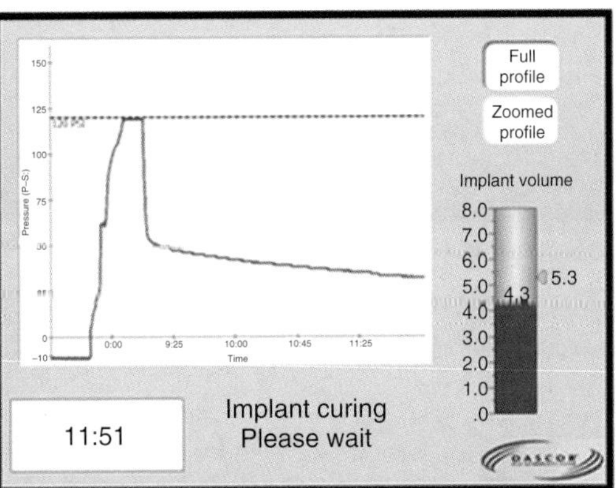


DELIVERY COMPONENTS

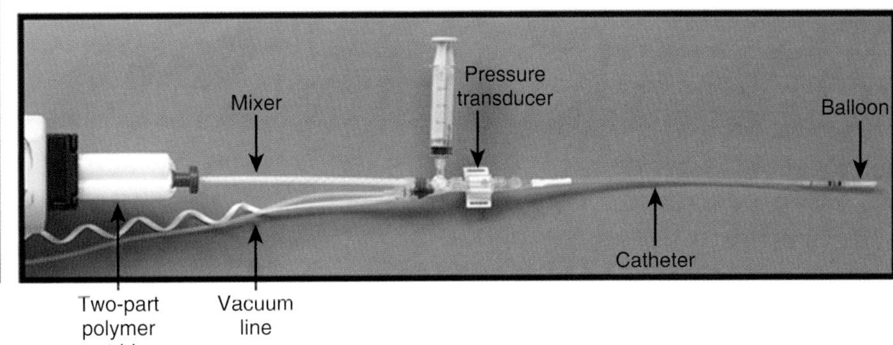


■ **FIGURE 51–3.** DASCOR-assembled injection system with injector head, polymer cartridge, mixer, and balloon catheter. The two-part liquid polymer is packaged in a dual chamber cartridge. The mixed pressurized polymer enters the containment balloon, which has been placed in the disc space, expanding the balloon to fill the entire space. *(From Disc Dynamics, Inc. Reprinted with permission.)*

## Mechanical Bench Testing

### Axial Compressive Fatigue Strength

The device's fatigue strength was investigated per American Society for Testing and Materials (ASTM) F2346 in a custom-made six-station mechanical testing apparatus using unconstrained device conditions (i.e., no simulated annulus) to create a worst-case test construct. Samples were tested using various cyclic axial compressive stress conditions ranging from 7.65 MPa to 2.0 MPa at an applied load frequency of 3 Hz. Testing was concluded once samples from a particular axial stress condition were able to sustain a 10 million cycle runout without structural deterioration leading to failure. The 10 million cycle axial compressive fatigue strength of the device after constructing an S/N plot was determined to be 2.94 MPa with a mean cyclic axial strain of 35.6% (Fig. 51–4). The axial compressive strength of the device is significantly beyond the daily axial compressive stress experienced by the lumbar motion segment.

### Durability and Particle Analysis

Similarly, the device's durability was investigated per ASTM F2346 in the same custom-made six-station mechanical testing apparatus using the same unconstrained device conditions (i.e., no simulated annulus) to create a worst-case test construct. The durability of the device was assessed for mechanical loads simulating brisk walking for testing up to 25 million cycles with concurrent 41-month device aging. Cyclic loading conditions consisted of ±5.5 degrees flexion-extension angular displacement applied at a load frequency of 3 Hz combined with 1.8 MPa axial compressive stress applied at a load frequency of 1.5 Hz. None of the DASCOR device samples tested for up to 25 million cycles showed signs of device degradation, whereas the compressive modulus did not significantly change from initial values. Aging did not influence the mechanical performance of the device. Furthermore, the average wear rates measured for devices tested during the first 10 million cycles was only 0.26 mg/million cycles, and no significant permanent set was observed (permanent set less than 3.2%). Progression of wear was slow, and the wear rates obtained were similar to those reported for other nucleus replacement devices[2] but magnitudes less than wear rates reported for TDR devices composed of polyurethanes.[3] Particle analysis of retrieved solutions conducted per ASTM F1877 using SEM demonstrated particle quantity and size, which was significantly less than what would be expected for ultra-high-molecular-weight polyethylene (UHMWPE) implants used in hips and knees.

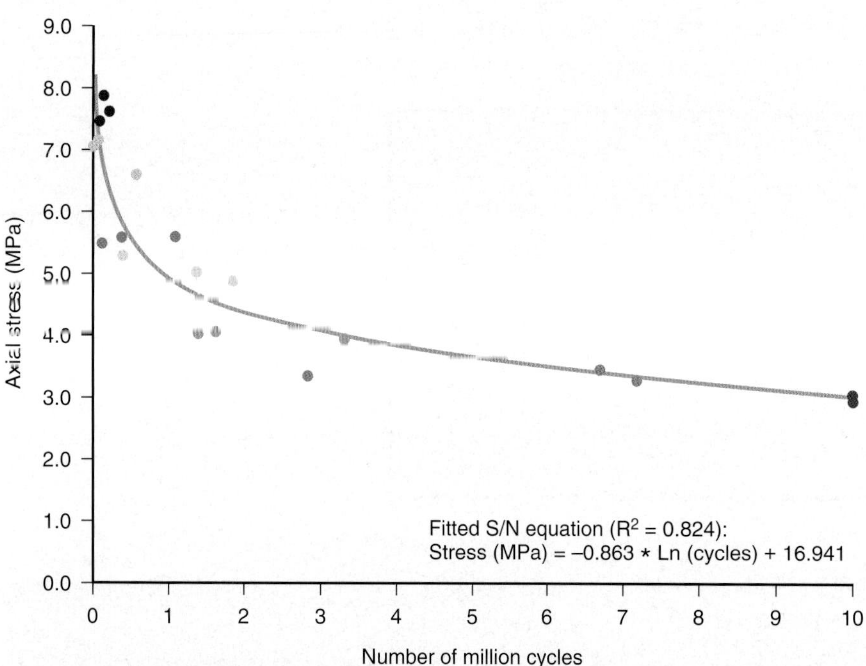


■ **FIGURE 51–4.** A plot of stress versus number of cycles (S/N plot) constructed in order to establish the endurance limit of the DASCOR device.

## Biomechanical Testing

Human cadaveric lumbar spines were used to study the biomechanics of the DASCOR device with two aims: (1) to determine the ability of the DASCOR device to restore the multidirectional segmental flexibility of a nuclectomy motion segment construct to that of an intact construct[4] and; (2) to determine and compare the end plate contact stress (Fig. 51–5) and load transfer capabilities of an instrumented DASCOR motion segment construct during multidirectional flexibility loading to motion segment constructs instrumented with a water balloon implant simulating hydrostatic conditions.[5] Axial compression (1,200 N) as well as axial rotation, flexion/extension, and lateral bending (all at 7.5 Nm combined with 500 N compression) were the loading conditions tested. The results demonstrated that the device was able to restore the segmental flexibility lost after a nuclectomy while still preserving segmental level biomechanics to within approximately ±5% of the intact motion segment behavior. Similarly, a relatively uniform contact stress distribution was observed during all segmental flexibility loads applied for both DASCOR and water balloon implanted constructs with no differences found between these constructs. The latter study results demonstrated that the modulus of elasticity of the DASCOR device was well suited to its intended purpose of nucleus replacement.

## Animal Model and Biomaterials Safety Testing

Biocompatibility performed according to an extended ISO 10993 (12 tests) demonstrated that the DASCOR device was a biocompatible material. Extensive animal model testing was similarly

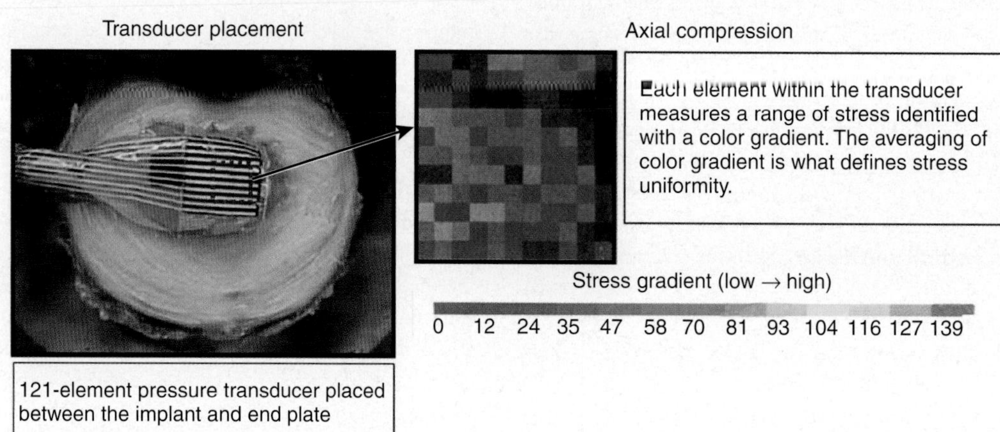


■ **FIGURE 51–5.** A pressure-sensitive transducer was placed between the implants and the end plate in order to measure end plate–implant contact stress during the multidirectional flexibility testing. The resulting stress measurements consisted of an array of color-graded stress profiles measured within various locations of the pressure-sensitive transducer.

conducted on the DASCOR device in (1) A RasH2 mouse model for carcinogenicity potential verification[6]; (2) a dorsal laminectomy rabbit model to determine the biologic response to wear debris[7]; and (3) a functional baboon model to determine the device's biodurability.[8]

## Carcinogenicity Testing

Hydrolysis of free MDI can form 4,4′-methylenedianiline (MDA), which has been reported to be a suspected carcinogen in humans. No scientific evidence has linked aromatic MDI-based polyurethanes to cancer in humans. Nevertheless, because the aromatic MDI-based polyurethane of the DASCOR device is cured in situ within the device's aliphatic balloon barrier, there is still a risk of releasing some free MDI/MDA into the surrounding tissues. Therefore, a study was undertaken to evaluate the carcinogenicity potential of the DASCOR device and its presumed byproducts using the rasH2 transgenic mouse model.

A protocol for a 26-week subcutaneous implantation was developed using seven treatment groups. Methylcellulose Millipore filter discs with 0.05-μ pores and a 20-mm$^2$ diameter were used as vehicle carriers for each test article. The treatments included (1) an uncured DASCOR polyurethane; (2) DASCOR polyurethane wear debris; (3) UHMWPE wear debris as a material control; (4) a low- and high-dose of free MDA (50 times and 1 million times the maximum amount in a DASCOR device, respectively); (5) a filter control, and (6) an ethyl carbamate–positive chemical control group. Gross necropsy observations after sacrifice included number, size, and location of tumors and histopathologic examination of implant and major visceral organ sites.

According to the gross necropsy and histopathologic findings, ethyl carbamate (positive control) demonstrated the expected carcinogenic response, supporting the validity of the mouse model. Otherwise, all other treatment groups confirmed no body weight changes, no significant clinical observations, and no organ weight differences. There was no increase in tumor incidence at the test site or in other tissues associated with the DASCOR uncured polyurethane and wear debris test treatments. Similarly, there was no evidence at the test site or in other tissues of carcinogenic changes associated with the free MDA dose treatments. Based on these experimental conditions and end points, it was demonstrated that the MDI-based nature of the DASCOR device does not cause any carcinogenic changes.

## Biologic Response to Wear Debris

The biologic response to implant wear debris is an essential element in device safety testing. A dorsal laminectomy rabbit model was used to evaluate (1) the local and systemic biologic responses to DASCOR device wear debris placed in the epidural space, and (2) the potential for DASCOR device wear debris translocation and any biologic tissue response resulting from wear debris translocation.

Seventy-two male New Zealand white rabbits were stratified into the following experimental groups: (1) two DASCOR wear debris groups (one for the balloon and one for the cured two-part polyurethane component); (2) an UHMWPE group as the material control; and (3) a sham group that had only a dorsal laminectomy performed. Dried wear debris particles were generated in vitro with a size distribution ranging between 0.1 and 100 μm. At least 50 million particles had a size distribution ranging between 1 and 15 μm. A 20-mg dose of wear debris was applied over the exposed dura mater obtained from the cured two-part polyurethane component. Similarly, a 4-mg dose was applied for wear debris obtained from the balloon component and the UHMWPE samples. At 6 weeks, 3 months, and 6 months postoperatively, six animals from each experimental group were euthanatized. All animals were immediately necropsied and histopathologically examined, and the results were compared between groups.

There were no macroscopic changes that could be attributed to wear debris. Microscopically, the local tissue reaction to wear debris was similar between the wear debris groups and consisted of a histocytic inflammatory response common to an inert, nonirritating material. Wear debris was present in all animals and wear debris groups and at all postoperative time points. There were no significant tissue alterations due to DASCOR or balloon wear debris implanted in direct contact with the spinal column and nerve roots. Most of the wear debris was located within the epidural space, with relatively less within the bone marrow and within the perivertebral region along the outer margins of the new bone formed in repair of the surgical defect. Wear debris particles were not detected internal to the dura or within the spinal cord in any of the groups. There was no evidence of neural tissue reaction to the test articles. No test article–related tissue alterations or particles were observed in distant organs that could be associated with wear debris from the implant site. Wear debris particles did not adversely affect the healing of the surgical defect. The results from the study confirmed that the DASCOR device does not pose a significant biomaterials safety concern and could be classified as an inert, non-irritant material.

## Functional Biodurability

A baboon study was designed to evaluate the biodurability and elicited histopathologic response of the DASCOR device following long-term implantation. A total of 14 mature male baboons were randomized into a 6-month ($n = 7$) and 12-month ($n = 7$) postoperative time period. Each animal underwent a lateral transperitoneal surgical approach, followed by a complete nucleotomy at the L3-L4 and L5-L6 levels with a DASCOR device implantation at the latter level. The L3-L4 served as a surgical (nucleotomy) control in each case. Postmortem analysis for each of the 6- and 12-month postoperative time points included MRI and plain radiography assessment for implant position and end plate changes, subsequent multidirectional flexibility testing and analysis on retrieved motion segments, and local or systemic histology.

All animals survived the operative procedure and postoperative interval without significant intraoperative or perioperative complications. Modic Type 1 changes were observed to a greater extent at the implanted versus control levels; however, these changes appeared to reduce from the 6- to 12-month intervals. Modic Type 1 changes observed at the implanted sites were not considered significant and have been documented in a number of other in vivo non-human primate studies. Multidirectional flexibility testing indicated trends for restoration of segmental motion for the DASCOR implanted constructs under flexion-extension and lateral bending by the 12-month time interval. Finally, the vertebral and systemic tissues indicated no evidence of significant histopathologic changes. The study demonstrated that the DASCOR device was biodurable and able to withstand physiologic loading with an insignificant elicited local and systemic histopathologic response. However, it should be acknowledged that implant volumes obtained in the baboon study were significantly less than those used in humans, a study limitation expected with such an animal model. It also was noted in these studies that significant disruption or damage to the vertebral end plate cartilage during the discectomy procedure can lead to adverse changes not related to the device itself.

The extensive preclinical testing of the DASCOR device served as the scientific basis for supporting initial and ongoing clinical investigations into the use of the device since investigations were initiated in 2003.

## CLINICAL PRESENTATION AND EVALUATION

The 2-year clinical experience of the DASCOR system evaluating safety and effectiveness is being investigated in two multicenter prospective nonrandomized European studies that use nearly identical investigational protocols.[9] Whereas the first study is already closed, the second study will close its enrollment in 2007. A standardized retroperitoneal midline or lateral approach was used to implant the DASCOR device in both studies. As of October 2006, 60 eligible patients (30 women, 30 men) with a mean age of 39±9 years meeting the specific inclusion criteria described had the DASCOR device implanted at the L3-L4 ($n = 3$), L4-L5 ($n = 26$), and L5-S1 ($n = 31$) levels. Clinical success was defined as a 2- and 15-point decrease in the respective VAS and ODI scores.

As of October 2006, of the 60 patients who underwent surgery, 44 patients were followed for up to 6 months, whereas 22 and 17 patients were followed for 1 and 2 years, respectively. Mean operating time was 89±29 minutes and average blood loss was 43.1±70.2 mL. Clinical outcome measures have been tracked from preoperative measures up through 24 months (Fig. 51–6A–C). Mean preoperative VAS and ODI scores improved significantly after 6 weeks postoperatively and throughout the 2 years. Clinical success criteria were all met at the time of write-up. Mean VAS backpain scores showed a 62% reduction from a preoperative mean of 7.5. Mean ODI results showed a 73% reduction from a preoperative mean of 58. Analgesic or narcotic drug use based on a three-point scale decreased 88% from a preoperative average of 1.7, with most patients experiencing significant improvement after 3 months. The patient analgesic medication or narcotic drug use at the 2-year follow-up was nearly none. MRI evaluations performed by an independent radiographic facility did not show any device subsidence or expulsion (Fig. 51–7). Anteroposterior and lateral radiographic films showed that disc height was improved. Overall, the 2-year clinical experience with the DASCOR device demonstrated high clinical safety based on the significant postoperative pain reduction, functional improvement, and a low complication rate.

## OPERATIVE TECHNIQUES

### Anesthesia

The anterior or lateral implantation of the DASCOR device is performed under general anesthesia. Normally, a Foley catheter is introduced into the bladder for intraoperative drainage and collapse of the bladder, especially for the L5-S1 approaches. Nitrous oxide is not recommended for general anesthesia, especially when transperitoneal access is under consideration. For intraoperative monitoring, central venous and arterial lines for continuous arterial blood pressure management have been recommended for TDR. However, because the implantation of the DASCOR device does not require a retraction of the major vessels to the degree needed in TDR procedures, the necessity for such intraoperative monitoring is less.

With the availability of the minimally invasive posterolateral procedures, the risk of bleeding might also be less; hence, normal monitoring as in any other dorsal minimally invasive surgical procedure should be sufficient. With the availability of an endoscopic implantation of the DASCOR device, even sedation without intubation seems possible, as in other endoscopic disc procedures.

### Position

Fluoroscopy is used during the surgery, and therefore, patient positioning should accommodate its use. For an anterolateral approach, the patient should be placed in a supine or lateral position. If a true lateral approach is planned, a lateral decubitus position may be used with appropriate supports. For a posterior/posterolateral approach, the patient should be placed in a prone position on a kneeling radiolucent lumbar spine frame.

### Procedure

The DASCOR prosthesis has the potential of being implanted using multiple surgical approaches (anterior, anterolateral, lateral, or posterolateral) with minimal variation in the surgical technique. Key to any approach, however, is achieving total nucleus removal (TNR) and minimizing annular and end plate cartilage disruption. The implantation of a nucleus replacement device should not be perceived to be a simple adjunct to a standard discectomy for herniated nucleus pulposus.

The initial annulotomy is created by using a 5.5-mm trephine or preferably a slit incision with a No. 11 scalpel and subsequent dilation to 5.5 mm. Care is taken to avoid damage to the annulus and cartilaginous end plates. To create a DASCOR device with the most optimal size, end plate conformity, and load transfer capabilities, TNR[10] must be attained while preserving the

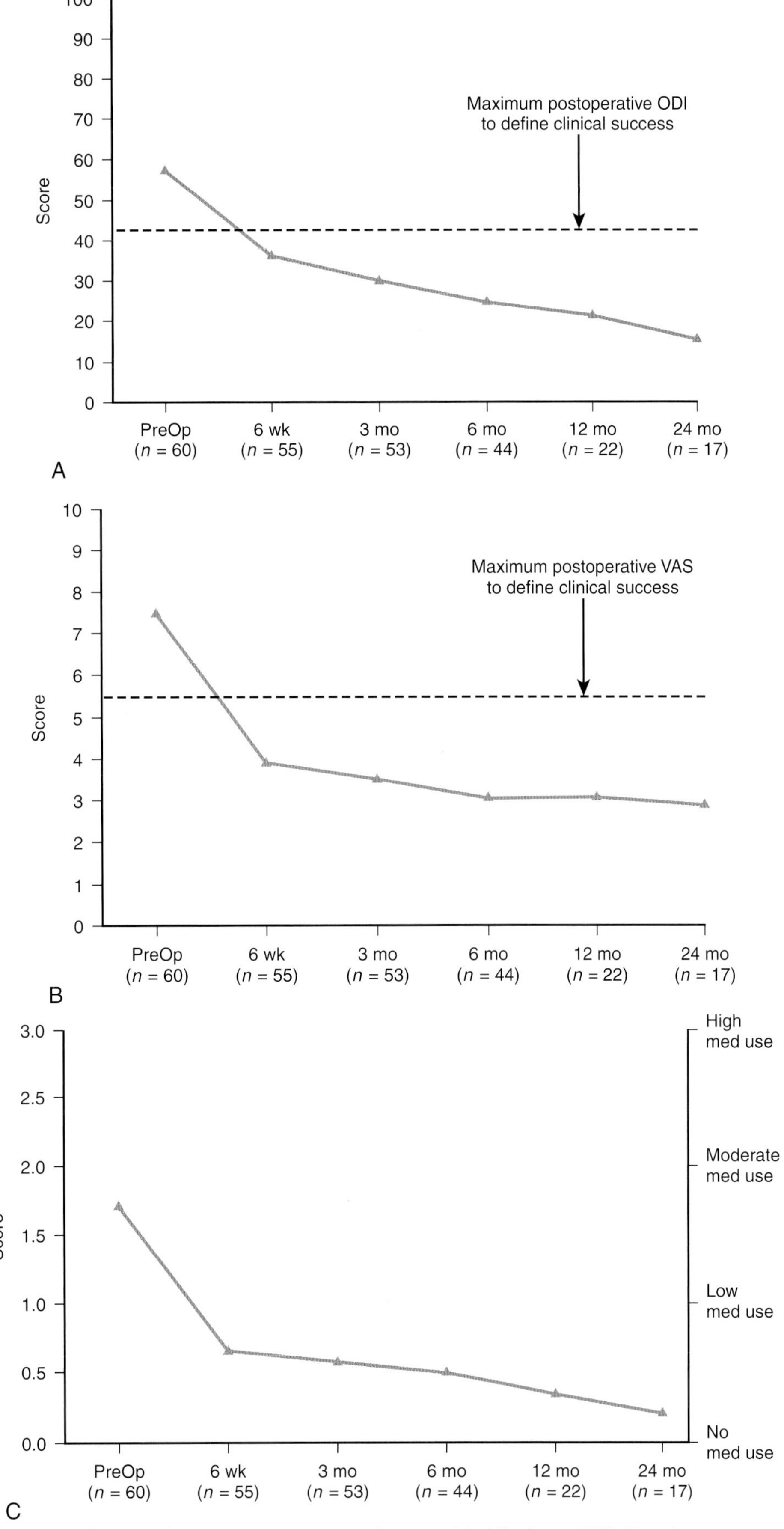


■ **FIGURE 51–6.** Clinical study results: Oswestry Disability Index (ODI) **(A)**; pain measurement on Visual Analog Scale **(B)**; analgesic medication use **(C)**.

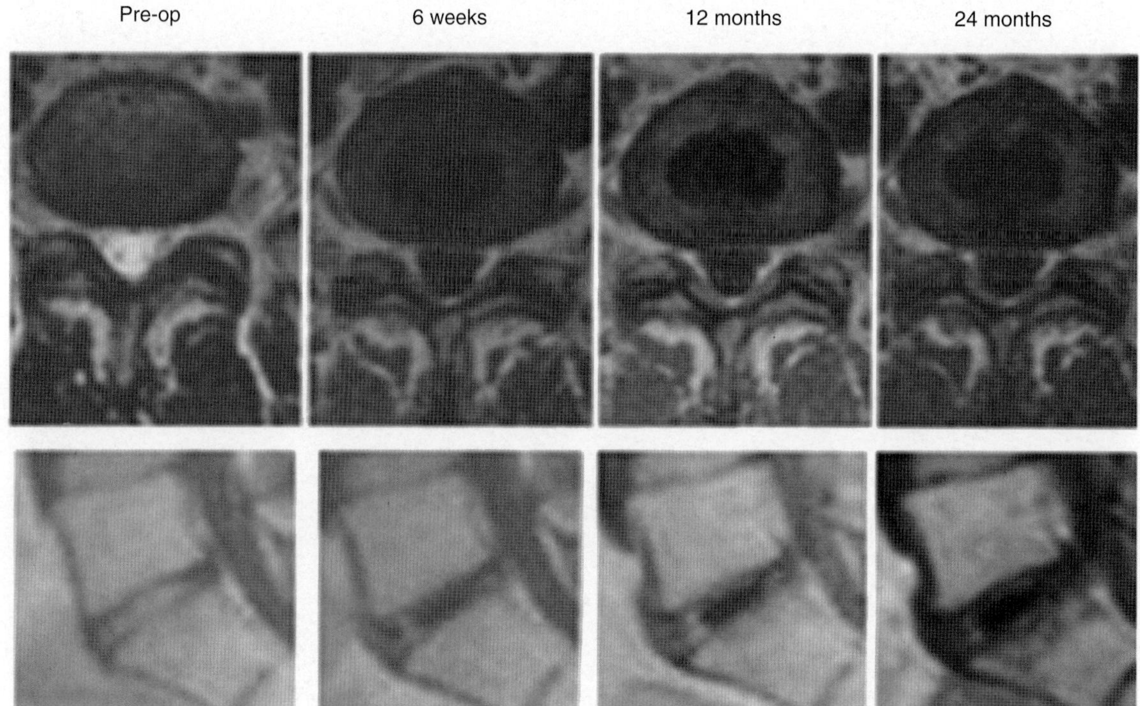


■ **FIGURE 51–7.** Magnetic resonance imaging scan of a typical implanted DASCOR device leading up to the 2-year follow-up. Images show the implant device centrally located without signs of subsidence or inflammatory reaction. *(From Disc Dynamics, Inc. Reprinted with permission.)*

annulus and end plates. Based on previous human cadaveric studies, a set of standard pituitary rongeurs were chosen and customized pituitary rongeurs were developed based on each instrument's ability to reach a particular predefined mapped region of the nucleus (Fig. 51–8). Using these instruments and a standardized method for removing tissue from predefined mapped anatomic regions, a preliminary TNR is performed until the surgeon believes that adequate nucleus has been removed.

Following the preliminary TNR, the nuclectomy performed and the tentative implant size, shape, and volume resulting from the nuclectomy created are evaluated using proprietary imaging methods developed specifically as part of the DASCOR Disc Arthroplasty System. An imaging balloon catheter is inserted in the disc space, and contrast media is injected under pressure, filling the balloon within the nucleus cavity created. Fluoroscopic images in anteroposterior, lateral, and oblique views are then taken, and a two-dimensional reconstruction of the imaged cavity is then performed in order to assess the completeness and symmetry of the nuclectomy (Fig. 51–9). If the cavity is not symmetric and centrally located, additional steps for nucleus removal and fluoroscopic imaging are conducted. Posterior annular integrity can also be assessed at this time. The contrast media and imaging balloon are then removed, and the implant balloon is inserted.

Once the balloon catheter is connected to the assembly components of the injector system, the balloon test and injection may be performed. The injection pressure profile applied by the injection

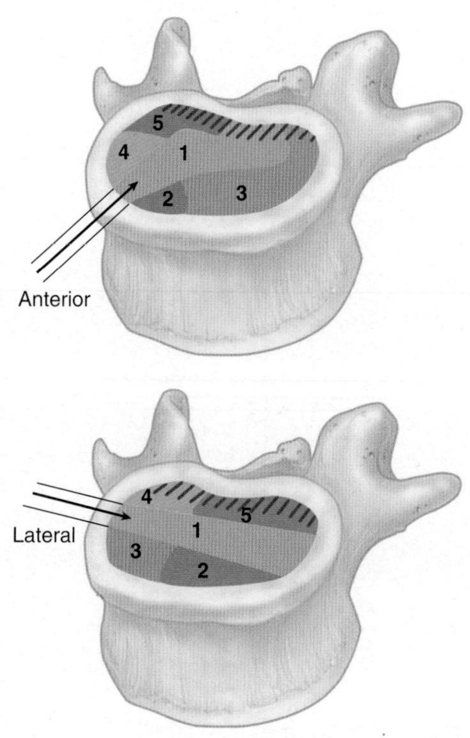


■ **FIGURE 51–8.** A step-by-step approach used to achieve a total nucleus removal (TNR) by nucleus removal of one zone at a time using specific instruments that target each anatomic zone. Specific TNR maps were created for an anterior or lateral or posterolateral approach. *(From Disc Dynamics, Inc. Reprinted with permission.)*

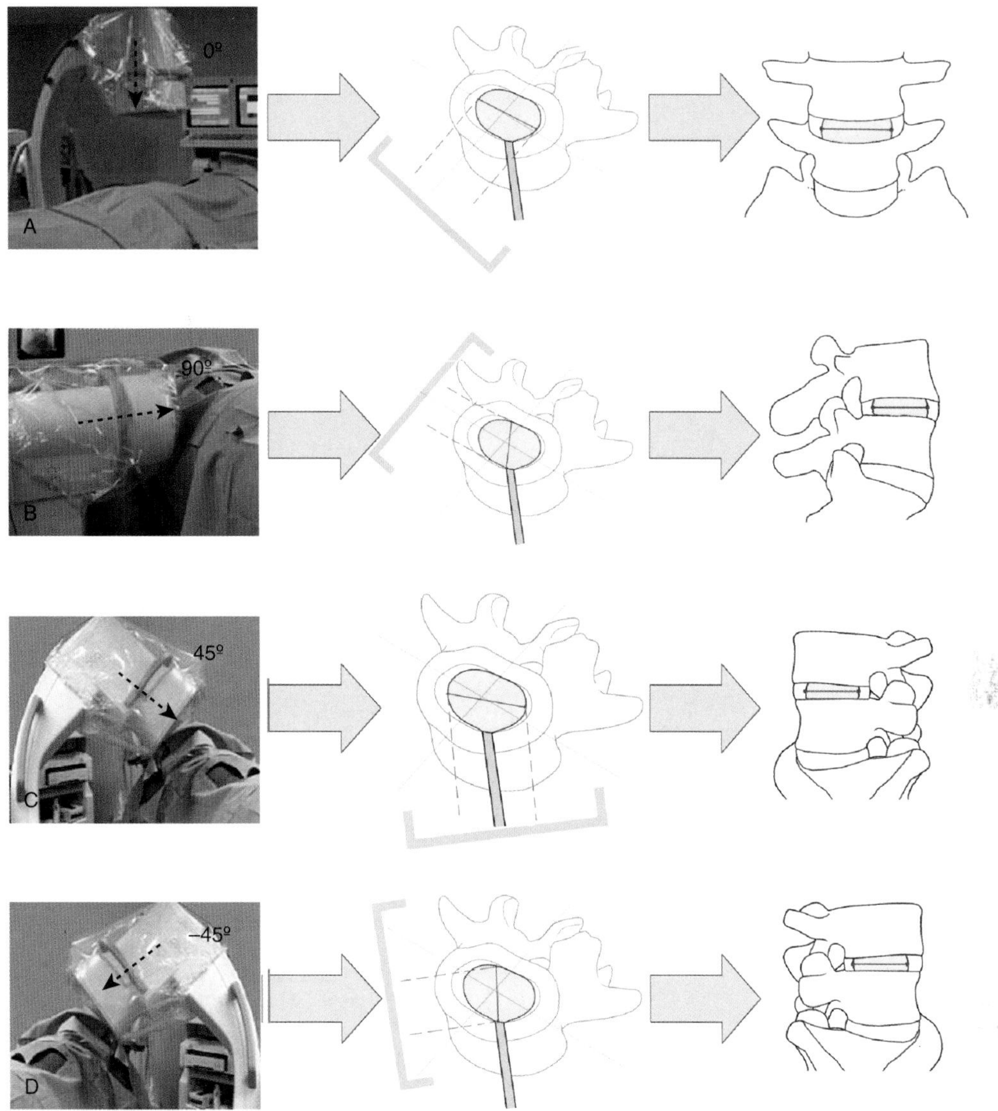


■ **FIGURE 51–9.** **A** to **D,** Intraoperative imaging steps using a proprietary contrast-filled DASCOR imaging balloon with anteroposterior, lateral, and oblique fluoroscopic C-arm positions. The procedure is used to identify remaining nucleus and anticipate the volume, position, and geometry of the actual implanted DASCOR device.

system is computer controlled and developed by the company while taking into consideration the anatomic/biomechanical limitations of a lumbar motion segment. There are several safety features to start, control, and potentially abort the injection at any time during the procedure should the surgeon feel it necessary. Once the injection is complete and the optimal filling has been achieved, the system allows for a 15-minute curing time before the catheter shaft is cut and removed from the balloon and the wound can be sutured and closed.

## POSTOPERATIVE CARE

The patients are gradually mobilized postoperatively for the first 3 weeks, but allowed to stand up the first day postoperatively for soft tissue healing. Increasing activities in the second week is advised, and sitting for long periods of time the first week should be avoided. Even during the second week after surgery, sitting is avoided for long periods of time, because this puts more stress on the spine compared with standing. Walking is recommended, but lifting should be restricted to less than 20 kg (approximately 44 lbs.) for the first 4 weeks. In some cases, wearing a soft brace might be useful, but is required only if the patient's occupation involves lifting or bending, or if the patient needs support. Braces are typically worn during daytime hours for 4 to 6 weeks after surgery.

## COMPLICATIONS AND AVOIDANCE

It is crucial that the integrity of both the annulus and end plates are in a biomechanical and somewhat viable state in order to contain the nucleus implant and avoid implant extrusions. In that respect, the preoperative assessment of annular integrity is obviously important and needs to be added to the preoperative diagnostic algorithm when nucleus replacement is chosen as the surgical treatment option. The procedure for implantation of the DASCOR device incorporates an imaging balloon step as a very important complementary test that is comparable to a dress rehearsal. This test provides feedback for positioning, volume, shape, and geometry of the final implant, and also most importantly, the annulus. Only with a satisfactory outcome of this test can the final implantation injection be conducted.

Equally important is the ability to reduce the initial implantation trauma as much as possible so that postoperative recovery time can be minimized. Therefore, minimally invasive surgery, as with a percutaneous/endoscopic implantation of a nucleus implant, should be the ultimate goal attained by nucleus replacement technologies.

## CONCLUSIONS/DISCUSSION

The concept of being able to achieve pain relief and disc function restoration using a nucleus replacement procedure is appealing. An ideal nucleus replacement technology should allow for restoration of healthy motion segment, disc height, kinematics, and load distribution. Although no perfect device has been identified for replacing the nucleus, the DASCOR device does address many, if not all, of the perceived requirements of an optimal nucleus replacement device.

There are significant differences in design features between the DASCOR device and other nucleus devices that may influence clinical results. The injectable, contained DASCOR device results in a large cross-sectional area that contours the nucleus cavity owing to its pressurized injection procedure. The favorable modulus elasticity of the device creates a more uniform load distribution across the end plates and surrounding annulus that may avoid the severe end plate reaction and device subsidence reported with other nucleus replacement devices.

The DASCOR device is introduced through a small annulotomy, creating a nucleus implant of a large volume and size, thus making device expulsion unlikely. This contrasts with the extrusion rates reported for preformed devices that require a large annular window for insertion. Appropriate patient selection is the key factor for every treatment, as is also the case with the DASCOR device. Preoperative annulus assessment is required for proper patient selection to ensure clinical successful outcomes.

## REFERENCES


1. Fernstrom U: Arthroplasty with intercorporal endoprosthesis in herniated disc and in painful disc. Acta Chir Scand Suppl 357:154–159, 1966.
2. Brown T, Bao QB, Kilpela T: Wear and mechanical durability of the NUBAC disc arthroplasty device. Spine Arthroplasty Society, 2006. Montreal, Canada, May 9–13, 2006.
3. Anderson PA, Rouleau JP, Bryan VE, Carlson CS: Wear analysis of the Bryan Cervical Disc prosthesis. Spine 28:S186–S194, 2003.
4. Ordway NR, Tsantrizos A, Yuan HA, Bowman B: Restoration of segmental kinematics following nucleus replacement with an in situ curable balloon contained polymer. North American Spine Society, 2005. Philadelphia, September 27–October 1, 2005.
5. Tsantrizos A, Ordway NR, Bao QB, Yuan HA: Endplate contact stress of the DASCOR device during segmental flexibility. North American Spine Society, 2006. Seattle, WA, September 26–30, 2006.
6. Lacy S, Streicker MA, Wustenberg W, et al: A RasH2 mouse model to study the carcinogenic potential of the DASCOR device. *In* XXX (ed): Spine Arthroplasty Society, 2006. Montreal, Quebec, Canada, May 9–13, 2006, p 46.
7. Lacy S, Johnson C, Long PH, et al: A rabbit model to evaluate the biological response to DASCOR device wear debris. Spine Arthroplasty Society, 2007. Berlin, May 1–4, 2007.
8. Cunningham BW, Hu N, Beatson HJ, et al: An investigational study of nucleus pulposus replacement using an in-situ curable polyurethane: An in vivo non-human primate model. Spine Arthroplasty Society, 2007. Berlin, May 1–4, 2007.
9. Ahrens M, Donkersloot P, Maartens F, et al: Nucleus replacement with the DASCOR Disc Arthroplasty System: Two year follow up results obtained from two prospective European multi-center clinical studies. Spine Arthroplasty Society, 2007. Berlin, May 1–4, 2007.
10. Ahrens M, Sherman J, LeHuec JC, et al: Total nucleus removal from a posterior or posterolateral approach: Technical considerations and early clinical experience. Spine Arthroplasty Society, 2006. Montreal, Canada, May 9–13, 2006.

CHAPTER 52

# PDN-SOLO and HydraFlex Nucleus Replacement System

**Reginald J. Davis**

## KEY POINTS

- One of the more unique features of the spinal disc is the ability of the nucleus tissue to hydrate and participate in the distribution of mechanical loads while providing a conduit for the transport of nutrients and waste materials.
- This hydrogel-based technology represents an optimization of the clinically proven PDN-SOLO device, with the HydraFlex device having shorter tab lengths, which allow for greater hydrogel volume, resulting in a more compliant implant.
- The HydraFlex device is indicated in skeletally mature adults between 25 and 70 years of age with symptomatic degenerative disc disease (DDD) at one level from L2-S1.

## INTRODUCTION

Replacement of the diseased nucleus pulposus portion of a spinal intervertebral disc represents a viable surgical solution to a known clinical problem. Although the concept seems straightforward, the ability to define an ideal solution has proven to be much more elusive.[1]

Many of the challenges associated with treating spinal disorders stem from the complexities of the disc itself. The disc's distinctive structure and physiology often make surgical intervention difficult. This is largely due to the fact that the disc form and function involves a combination of both biochemical and biomechanical processes.

One of the more unique features of the spinal disc is the ability of the nucleus tissue to hydrate and participate in the distribution of mechanical loads, while providing a conduit for the transport of nutrients and waste materials. The natural hygroscopic glycosaminoglycan nucleus tissue cannot be reproduced and is extremely difficult to approximate by mechanical means.[2,3]

The HydraFlex (Raymedica, Inc., Minneapolis, MN) device offers an innovative solution to address the complexities of treating degenerative disc disease (DDD). This hydrogel-based technology represents an optimization of the clinically proven PDN-SOLO device (Raymedica, Inc., Minneapolis, MN), with the HydraFlex device having shorter tab lengths, which allow for greater hydrogel volume, resulting in a more compliant implant (Fig. 52–1A and B). The implant design and material selection incorporate extensive knowledge of disc and nucleus biomechanics, physiology, and research evaluations.[4]

## INDICATIONS/CONTRAINDICATIONS

The HydraFlex device is indicated in skeletally mature adults between 25 and 70 years of age with symptomatic degenerative disc disease (DDD) at one level from L2-S1. (DDD is back pain of discogenic origin that has been confirmed by history and physical examination with degeneration confirmed radiographically.) Traditionally, such patients present with low back or leg pain, or both. Symptoms interfere with daily activities and have been present at least 6 months while not responding to conservative treatment.

Severe symptomatic central spinal, foraminal, or lateral recess stenosis are contraindications for use of the device. Other contraindications include dynamic degenerative spondylolisthesis greater than grade 1 or lytic spondylolisthesis, fractured and/or symptomatic degenerated facet joints, pronounced Schmorl's nodules at the affected level, an incompetent annulus, disc height at the affected level less than 6 mm, significant osteoporosis or osteomalacia, tumors of the spinal cord, malignant tumors of the vertebral column, malignant or benign tumors at the adjacent or affected level, and surgery at the affected or adjacent level.

Also contraindicated are symptomatic DDD requiring surgery at more than one lumbar level, active systemic or localized infection at the level where surgery will be performed, any trauma causing fracture of the bony element at the intended or adjacent level or spinal trauma leading to a neurologic deficit, congenital bony abnormalities at the affected level or congenital spinal cord abnormalities, gross obesity, disc height less than 6 mm, and allergy to polyacrylamide, polyethylene, or platinum iridium.

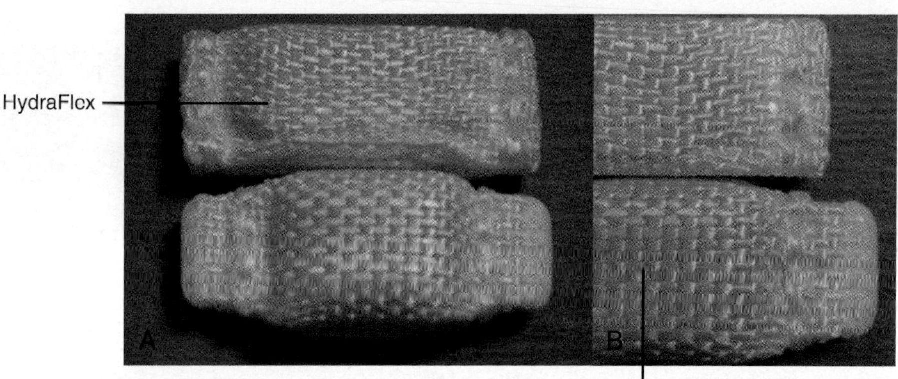


■ **FIGURE 52–1.** **A** and **B**, HydraFlex vs. PDN-SOLO. The HydraFlex device's shorter tab lengths allow for greater hydrogel volume, resulting in a more compliant implant.

## DESCRIPTION OF THE DEVICE

The HydraFlex device has three components: an inner copolymer hydrogel pellet that is designed to resume a biconvex shape once it is hydrated (Fig. 52–2A and B), an outer woven jacket of ultra-high-molecular-weight polyethylene (UHMWPE) fibers, and platinum-iridium wire markers for radiologic identification.[4]

The HydraFlex device core is formed of a physiologically inert proprietary copolymer of polyacrilonitrile and polyacrylamide. The polymer components are pressure molded into a predetermined form and then dehydrated. This controlled dehydration reduces the device profile for ease of insertion, while preserving the HydraFlex implant's shape memory. The current hydrogel polymer formulation permits the HydraFlex device to absorb up to 80% of its dry weight in water more rapidly than the PDN-SOLO device (Fig 52–3). This provides a compliant device that maintains expansion and lifting forces. Several other formulations were evaluated extensively, but none were found to have these needed abilities. This rehydration-expansion begins immediately after insertion and slows exponentially over 7 to 10 days.

The outer jacket of loosely woven UHMWPE fibers allows for rapid rehydration of the hydrogel core, while controlling device expansion to prevent possible damage to the end plates. The jacket also facilitates insertion and surgical manipulation.

Small, short platinum-iridium wires are inserted into each end of the pellet, rendering visible the position of an implant by ordinary C-arm fluoroscopic or plain x-ray scans.

When rehydrated inside the evacuated nucleus cavity, the implant properly fills the space. This process maintains or restores height and mechanical stability to the disc while maintaining reasonable segmental flexibility.

## BACKGROUND OF SCIENTIFIC TESTING/CLINICAL OUTCOMES

Extensive bench and animal testing were performed on the polymer core and jacket using scientific test methods and established U.S. Food and Drug Administration (FDA) guidelines for long-term implant materials. The HydraFlex devices and individual components passed all FDA- and ISO-required animal, cytologic, and toxicity testing. These test outcomes demonstrate biologic safety and mechanical durability, and also served as a guide to subsequent prototype improvements.

Animal studies were ethically performed in standard, approved experiments using large mongrel dogs, large goats, and transgenic mice, as well as in tissue culture preparations. In addition, a baboon study was performed to assess long-term histopathology. None of these tests or studies showed an adverse response to any of the components, the pellets and jackets, or intact miniaturized implants.

Mechanically, the pellet and jacket were subjected to standard fatigue testing for up to 50 million normal-range compression cycles and to 10 million compression-translation cycles. All components passed without demonstrated deterioration. Following prolonged cyclic tests, the terminal burst strength of intact implants exceeded the 6-kN limit of the test machine.

In cadaver segment biomechanical studies, denucleated segments showed loss of normal stiffness and decreased stability as compared with initially intact segments. Insertion and subsequent rehydration of the HydraFlex device restored normal stiffness and stability.[4–6]

## CLINICAL PRESENTATION AND EVALUATION

The clinical syndrome of the degenerating lumbar disc has gained increased recognition and significance with more precise magnetic resonance imaging (MRI) and better understanding of disc physiology. Controversy remains as to the precise nature of the disease

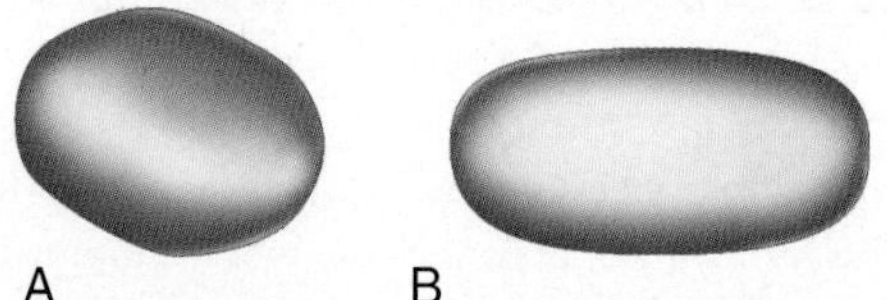


■ **FIGURE 52–2.** **A** and **B**, The inner copolymer hydrogel pellet is designed to resume a biconvex shape once it is hydrated.

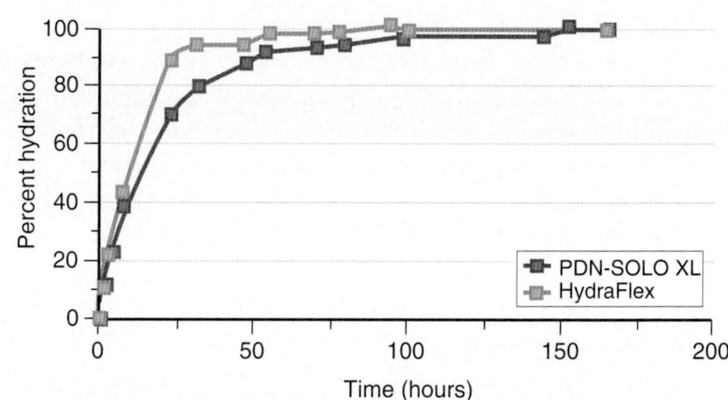


■ **FIGURE 52–3.** Hydration versus time for HydraFlex device.

with issues such as the origin of pain generators, mechanical versus chemical bases of pathology, interpretation of diagnostic data, and appropriate intervention. It is widely accepted that the degenerating disc undergoes a multifactor cascade that includes altered perfusion, loss of cellular and glycosaminoglycan components, desiccation, and compromised load transfer functions. The observed changes include the characteristic collapsed disc space with a dark or black disc on MRI and end plate changes on MRI and x-ray study. In those cases appropriate for nucleus arthroplasty, interventions occur during the mild-to-moderate phase of disease. Such patients typically present with axial back pain, with or without concomitant leg pain, which is unresponsive to conservative measures. The neurologic examination often fails to reveal discreet motor or sensory deficits. The diagnosis is confirmed on MRI demonstrating disc desiccation, loss of height, and Modic changes. Provocative discography is often used to confirm symptomatic levels.

The hallmark of clinical success is pain relief. The FDA mandates a 25% reduction in pain scores for a device to be considered effective. In a prospective multicenter international trial conducted on the PDN-SOLO device, the predicate to the HydraFlex device, there was a 74% reduction in the Oswestry Disability Index as compared with published reports of a 41% and 42% reduction with the two leading fusion cages and a 50% reduction for a leading total disc replacement. Additionally, the Visual Analog Scale declined from a preoperative level of 7.5 to 2.7 at 12 months after surgery, a 64% reduction. Finally, a patient satisfaction survey of almost 300 PDN-SOLO recipients at multiple international sites demonstrated a much better or better response in 87% of patients, and 88% of patients said they definitely would or might undergo the same surgery again.

## OPERATIVE TECHNIQUE

The surgical procedure for implantation of the HydraFlex nucleus replacement device is relatively straightforward and much less invasive than alternative treatments such as total disc replacement (TDR) or fusion. A typical procedure can be completed in as little as 1 hour.

The procedure is performed with the patient under general endotracheal anesthesia. The patient is positioned supine, with a lumbar bolster positioned to augment normal segmental lordosis. Alternatively, an operating room table with flexion and extension capability can be used. C-arm fluoroscopy is required, and this must be kept in mind during patient positioning. Nerve monitoring is optional but highly recommended if the approach truly traverses the psoas muscle.

The recommended surgical access to the disc for insertion of the HydraFlex device is accomplished using an anterior retroperitoneal approach (ARPA) and the provided HydraFlex Nucleus Arthroplasty System instrumentation. The PDN-SOLO device was also implanted using an anterolateral trans-psoatic approach (ALPA) and the traditional posterior approach. Use of the posterior approach produced a success rate that was less than optimal due to a multitude of factors addressed by use of the ARPA instrumentation and surgical technique. Instrumentation specific for use in the posterior approach is in development at this writing.

Using ARPA, the disc space is accessed by creation of a flap in the anterolateral annulus immediately adjacent to the anterior longitudinal ligament. The integrity of this flap is preserved for suture closure at the conclusion of implantation. The nucleus is totally evacuated by standard means. Care should be taken to avoid trauma to the end plates because this may lead to end plate edema, inflammation, and subsequent poor outcome. Damage or violation of the posterior annulus is to be avoided as well. Failure to preserve the integrity of the posterior annulus can lead to posterior extrusion of the device.

Once the total evacuation of the nucleus is confirmed, the internal disc space is measured using the supplied instruments. The appropriate size implant and insertion system are selected. The disc space, already positioned in lordosis, is gently distracted. The distracting tool also serves as an introducer past the outer edges of the vertebral bodies. This facilitates introduction and minimizes potential damage to the end plates and implant.

The implant is then guided into place with the introducing instruments. Proper location is in the posterior third of the space on lateral projection and in the mid-transverse portion of the space on anteroposterior projection. Rehydration of the device is initiated with saline irrigation after final positioning.

The annular flap is then reapproximated with suture.

## POSTOPERATIVE CARE

Postoperative management is critical to a successful clinical outcome and is designed to minimize potential implant migration. Device hydration in the early postoperative period results in increased device expansion in both the vertical and horizontal plane, thus accepting spinal loading. Patient activity restriction and back bracing are required for 6 weeks to allow further equilibration and healing.

## COMPLICATIONS AND AVOIDANCE

Aside from the usual complications associated with surgery, there are those specific to use of the HydraFlex device. The most significant is device extrusion. This is best avoided by strict adherence to patient selection criteria, meticulous surgical technique, and proper postoperative management and rehabilitation.[7,8]

## CONCLUSIONS/DISCUSSION

In conclusion, the PDN technologies have enjoyed increasing clinical success for more than a decade. Recent worldwide experience supports claims of clinical safety and efficacy and widespread

### ADVANTAGES/DISADVANTAGES: PDN-SOLO AND HYDRAFLEX NUCLEUS REPLACEMENT SYSTEM

**Advantages**
- Preservation of physiological motion
- Affords all secondary surgical options

**Disadvantages**
- New/unfamiliar approach
- Dependent on intact annulus

acceptance. Current improvements promise even better outcomes and are being evaluated in prospective multicenter, randomized fashion.

## REFERENCES

1. Lee CK, Langrana NA, Parsons JR, et al: Development of a prosthetic intervertebral disc. Spine 16(suppl 6):S253–S255, 1991.
2. White AA, Panjabi MM: Clinical Biomechanics of the Spine. Philadelphia, Lippincott Williams & Wilkins, 1990.
3. Pope MH: Disc biomechanics and herniation. *In* Gunzburg R, Szapalski M (eds): Lumbar Disc Herniation. Philadelphia, Lippincott Williams & Wilkins, 2002, pp 3–21.
4. Ray CD, Schönmayr RS, Kavanaugh SA, Assell R: Prosthetic disc nucleus implants. Revista di Neurorad 12(suppl 1):157–162, 1999.
5. Ray CD: The artificial disc: Introduction, history and socioeconomics. *In* Weinstein, JN (ed): Clinical Efficacy and Outcome in the Diagnosis and Treatment of Low Back Pain, pp 205–225.
6. Ray CD: The PDN prosthetic disc-nucleus device. Eur Spine J Suppl 2:S137–S142, 2002.
7. Shim CS, Lee SH, Park CW, et al: Partial disc replacement with the PDN Prosthetic Disc Nucleus Device. J Spinal Disord Tech 16:324–330, 2003.
8. Jin D, Qu D, Zhao L, et al: Prosthetic disc nucleus (PDN) replacement for lumbar disc herniation. J Spinal Disord Tech 16:331–337, 2003.
9. Bertagnoli R: Review of modern treatment options for degenerative disc disease. *In* Kaech DL, Jinkins JR (eds): Spinal Restabilization Procedures. Amsterdam, Elsevier Science, 2002, pp 365–375.

CHAPTER 53

# NeuDisc Artificial Lumbar Nucleus Replacement

**Anthony T. Yeung, Ann Prewett,** and **James J. Yue**

**KEY POINTS**

- Degeneration of the lumbar intervertbral disc, providing 80% of the support of the spinal segment, is responsible for chronic lumbar discogenic pain.
- Discectomy paradoxically induces natural and accelerated degeneration and subsequent back pain.
- The rate of degeneration may be directly related to the amount of nucleus removed.
- The nucleus pulposus is a natural hydrogel.
- NeuDisc synthetic hydrogel is a leading material for nucleus replacement.

## INTRODUCTION

Internal disruption of the intervertebral lumbar disc is a major source of back pain. Discectomy is the most frequently performed surgical procedure for back pain and sciatica. Although discectomy alone, with proper patient selection, may have a reasonably good short-term outcome in relieving radicular symptoms, less than optimal long-term relief usually results in further disc degeneration, instability, and pain. Therefore, discectomy may promote secondary sequelae, such as facet arthrosis and spinal stenosis, by altering the biomechanical properties of the intervertebral disc. Fusion has long been the standard method for treating refractory painful spinal disc disease.

Fusion, however, is a nonphysiologic solution that may cause so-called fusion disease by damaging normal muscle and spinal anatomy in addition to creating adjacent-level problems. There is a great need for more effective and longer lasting treatments for low back and radicular pain from a scientific as well as an economic point of view. The surgical focus of this chapter, therefore, is on the feasibility of surgical replacement of the intervertebral disc nucleus as a means to slow the painful consequences of the degenerative process and discectomy.

### The Clinical Challenges of Nucleus Replacement

Although it is assumed that replacement of the nucleus pulposus is desirable after nuclectomy, we must understand the natural history of discectomy for disc herniation and when it is desirable to replace the nucleus as an appropriate procedure. At present, there is evidence that adverse results of disc degeneration are directly related to the amount of disc tissue removed,[1] but there is no consensus among surgeons on how much disc to remove in a discectomy for disc herniation. The best we can assume is that the goals of disc replacement are to maintain or restore the normal height of the disc, to keep the annulus properly tensioned, and to provide shock and vibration absorption to the spinal segment. The clinical goal is to reduce or eliminate pain for as long as possible. The more realistic expectation may be for nucleus pulposus implants to maintain disc height, maintain motion, and preserve kinematics, insofar as satisfaction of these requirements is sufficient to ensure pain relief. The original concept of nucleus replacement centers on the effects that nuclectomy has on destabilizing segmental stability. Nucleus replacement, therefore, aims to reduce discogenic pain by restoring the function of a normal nucleus.

### Biomechanical Considerations of Implant Material and Design

Many biomechanical and biochemical studies have focused on various biomaterials that provide support against compression and still maintain some of the physiologic properties of the nucleus pulposus. Hydrogel, with its biocompatibility properties that mimic the function of the nucleus pulposus, a natural hydrogel, has the ability to resist deformation when jacketed or supported by a Dacron or fabric mesh.[2,3] Therefore, hydrogel is considered one of the leading materials being investigated. Implant size, the next consideration, affects the longevity of the implant. The size of the implant must be of sufficient surface area to support the spine segment and not become another loose body as residual nuclear material degenerates. The third consideration is prevention of implant migration and extrusion. If the implant is too soft, there is a greater chance of extrusion during axial loading inasmuch as the implant is able to move or migrate within the disc. Preservation of the annulus to act as a barrier to implant extrusion or reinforcement of the annulus is also an important factor, thus emphasizing the importance of a minimally invasive, tissue-sparing approach for implantation. Alternatively, there is a need to accurately access the integrity of the annulus over the long term, because success for nucleus replacement may well depend as much on the stability and integrity of the annulus as the nuclear implant itself. The size of the annulotomy or herniation defect may also affect the ability of the annulus to contain the implant. The NeuDisc (Replication Medical, Inc., Cranbury, NJ) design and configuration make the posterolateral transforaminal endoscopic approach a theoretically very desirable insertional technique. This approach is excellent both for nuclectomy and prosthesis implantation. Other approaches, such as the lateral or anterolateral approach, are also appropriate as long as a thorough nuclectomy is accomplished through the surgical approach. The ability to compress the NeuDisc implant, coupled with its rapid hydration, gives it the flexibility to be implanted from any approach as long as a thorough nuclectomy is accomplished. The final consideration is to then insert the proper size implant to provide axial support to the disc.

## DESCRIPTION OF THE DEVICE

NeuDisc by Replication Medical (Cranbury, NJ) mimics the physiologic function of the nucleus pulposus (Fig. 53–1). Its proprietary layered hydrogel structure is designed to distribute axial loads in the disc, and its hydrogel mimics osmotic properties of the nucleus pulposus. The vertically layered structure alternates soft hydrogel layers between Dacron knitted mesh to attain the proper stiffness required but should be sufficiently soft to avoid damage to the end plate. The acrylic copolymer hydrogel mimics the properties of the nucleus pulposus and allows osmotic intradiscal swelling to provide lift and shock-absorbing support.[2,3] Anisotropic swelling resists bulging as it swells, providing mostly lift support without creating undesired pressure radially. The Dacron net stabilizes the soft implant to resist extrusion. This ensures that NeuDisc can be implanted through a small incision, avoid pressure on a weakened annulus, and quickly hydrate to resume a shape that is much larger than the annular incision.

Unloaded, the NeuDisc implant expands in thickness from its desiccated, compressed state of 6.5 to 15 mm in its hydrated state (Figs. 53–2 and 53–3). Anisotropic expansion restricts lateral expansion to enlarge the footprint.

## BACKGROUND OF SCIENTIFIC TESTING/CLINICAL OUTCOMES

The NeuDisc has also undergone extensive mechanical testing to verify that its mechanical properties closely match those of the native nucleus pulposus. Biomechanical bench testing of the NeuDisc hydrogel implant tested the capability of the implant to provide axial lift force under various pressures ranging from 150 to 3,000 Newton (N). Lift force builds up to maximum lift in about 2 days, then stays constant over time, responding only to variations in temperature. When lift force is plotted for various hydration levels, at 60% to 65% hydration, it provides lift parameters similar to young nucleus pulposus at 400 N. If exposed to compression in a fully hydrated state, NeuDisc resists compression beyond the physiologic limits in the disc. Moreover, when anisotropic expansion limits radial bulging, it decreases the danger of radial expansion pushing residual disc tissue out through an annular defect created either by a surgical annulotomy incision or herniation defect.

### Endurance Testing

The endurance testing was performed in multiple motions, range-of-motion studies, expulsion testing, and fatigue testing in a cadaveric model. The testing subjected the NeuDisc implant to compression, flexion and extension combined with compression, lateral bending combined with compression, and axial torsion combined with compression. Each test was for 30 million cycles, representing a 30-year lifetime in each of the motions. No monomer elution was evident in the fluid gathered from any of the endurance-tested samples. The extensive endurance testing peformed demonstrated the device's ability to survive long-term strenuous use in multiple loading modes.

The NeuDisc implant also remained physically intact and as functional as controls after 30 million compression cycles at 150% of maximum physiologic displacement. Initial fatigue testing also included cycling the hydrogel implants in unconfined compression between load levels of 200 and 800 N. Throughout this testing, it was demonstrated that lateral expansion and deformation of the implants resulted. The implant fatigue samples completed the 30 million loading cycles intact, with only minor

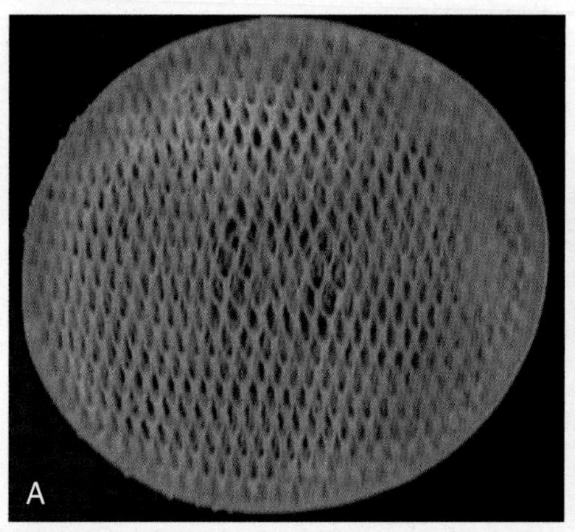


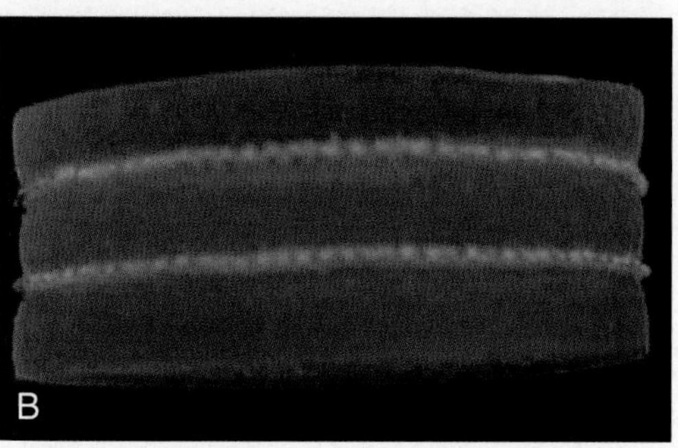


■ **FIGURE 53–1.** The NeuDisc design.

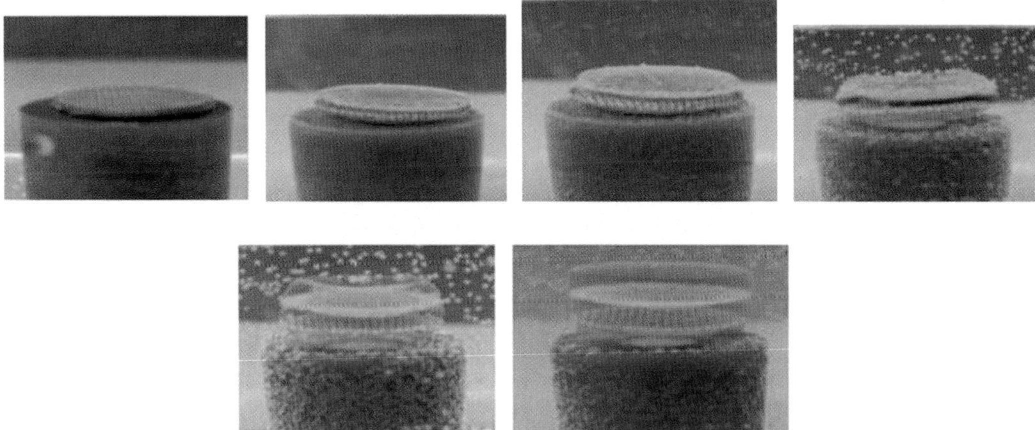

■ **FIGURE 53–2.** Anisotropic expansion from 2 to 15 mm after hydration. Anisotropic swelling, 37°C the initial thickness is 2 mm. Note that the implant expands in thickness, but the footprint size does not enlarge.

surface cracking and no loss of function or change in water uptake. Initial in vitro results of testing suggest that the NeuDisc hydrogel implant may be a suitable nucleus pulposus substitute.[2,3]

## Biocompatibiliy Testing

Short-term and long-term implantation tests in rabbits demonstrated that the acrylic copolymer hydrogel Aquacryl (Replication Medical, Cranbury, NJ) was both nontoxic and biocompatible. The long-term and chronic toxicity of the material was analyzed by implantation in rat paravertebral muscles. The results were similar to control implantations and showed no chronic cytotoxicity.

## Expulsion Testing

Expulsion testing demonstrated that the NeuDisc is unlikely to expel during normal activity. Following range-of-motion testing, 32 implanted functional spinal units were tested to failure. There were two implant expulsions. Both expulsions that were observed occurred at extremely high loads. The most common mode of failure in compression was end plate fracture. Ligament ruptures, annular tears, facet joint fractures, and vertebral compression fractures also occurred before implant failure. The average force at failure was 3,533 N, which agrees with literature values. The failures in the flexion specimens occurred at an average moment of failure of 52.2 Nm. The specimens that failed in lateral bending had five different failure modes. One specimen had an end plate fracture, three had fractures of the facet joint, six had ligament rupture, one had an annulus tear, and one implant expelled. The average moment at failure was 24.8 Nm, and the implant expulsion occurred at 47.9 Nm. The failure strengths in bending agree with published values.

## Clinical Outcomes

The 6.5-mm bullet configuration of the NeuDisc implant has been undergoing a two-arm pilot European prospective longitudindal study since June 2005. The first arm is an open approach using the anterolateral transpsoatic approach (ALPA). The second arm is a posterolateral endoscopic approach. In both arms, the primary

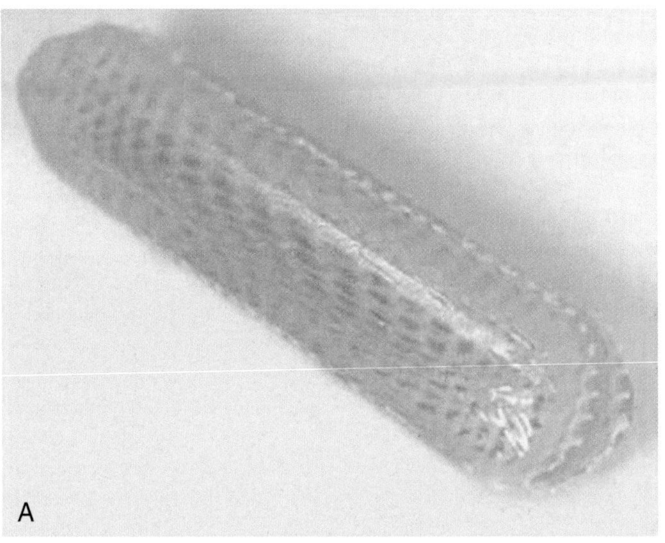

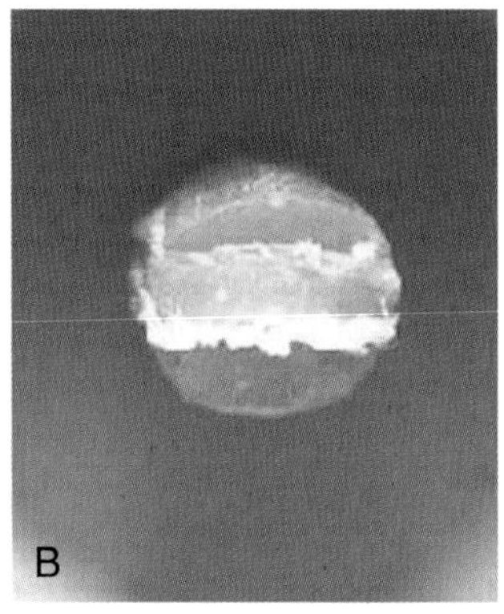

■ **FIGURE 53–3.** Bullet-shaped 6.5-mm implant.

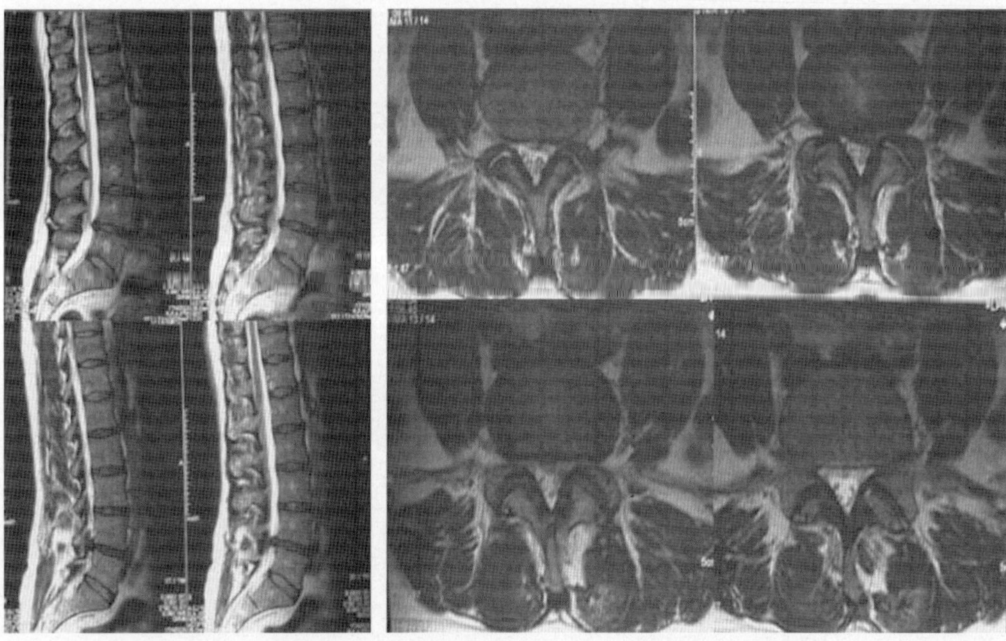

■ **FIGURE 53–4.** Preoperative images of L4-5 degeneration.

inclusion criteria is recalcitrant low back pain secondary to degenerative disc disease with or without leg pain. Disc height can be no less than 50% of normal height compared with adjacent levels. Levels of insertion have been L2-L5 for the ALPA approach and L2-S1 in the endoscopic approach. Successful insertion is dependent on complete nucleotomy and appropriate implant positioning and sizing. A total of 15 implantations have been performed. In cases of ideal disc space preparation and implant sizing, no revisions were necessary. Two revision surgeries for infection have been performed. Early clinical outcomes indicate early resolution of symptoms with mainentance of improvement at 12 months (Figs. 53–4 and 53–5).

## OPERATIVE TECHNIQUE

The ability and ease of insertion of the NeuDisc implant through a 6-mm fenestration in the annulus make this a viable implant for endoscopic as well as open use. The implant configuration makes it easy to insert through any discectomy portal, including a traditional dorsal or anterolateral microdiscectomy approach

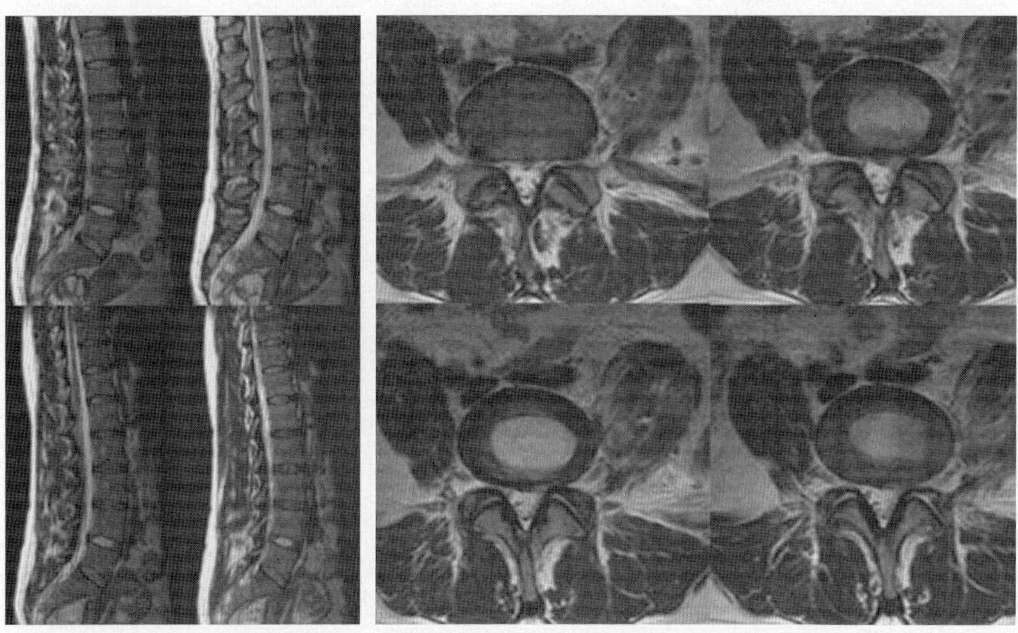

■ **FIGURE 53–5.** Six-month postoperative images.

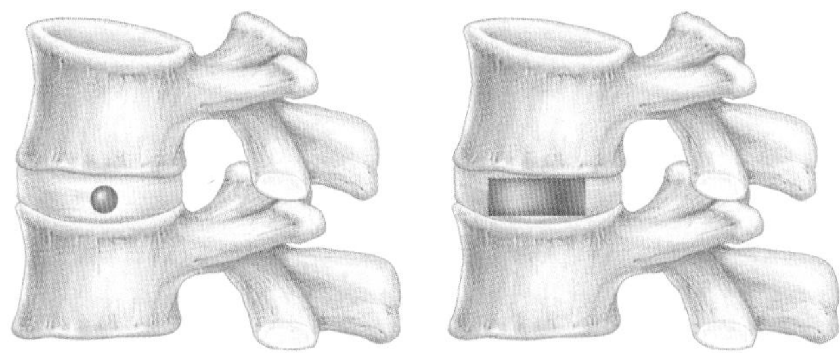

■ FIGURE 53–6. Before and after hydration.

(Figs. 53–6 and 53–7). The transcanal approach can be accomplished with a uniportal or biportal annular fenestration. The surgeon performs a nuclectomy with or without the aid of an endoscope, then measures the enucleated cavity and does a trial implantion with an implant template. A proprietary instrument to insert the NeuDisc implant is needed for the uniportal approach and facilitates the biportal approach.

Current endoscopic systems use a 6-mm inner diameter/7-mm outer diameter cannula for discectomy and a 7- to 8-mm inner diameter/8- to 9-mm outer diameter cannula for foraminoplasty. A recently developed foraminoscope has a 4.2-mm working channel that also facilitates endoscopic visualized nuclectomy. The Yeung Endoscopic Spine System (YESS) system, developed in conjunction with Richard Wolf Surgical Instrument Company, has endoscopic cannulas, discectomy instrumentation, and an introducer that is ideally suited specifically for the NeuDisc implantation.[4,5] Discectomy may be accomplished through the foraminal portal from T10-L5, with plenty of room for endoscopic instrumentation.[6] A uniportal or biportal technique may be used for nucleus implantation and has the advantage of limited annular disruption to limit implant extrusion. The further development and application of this technique have broadened application to address many concurrent painful degenerative conditions of the lumbar spine.[5,7–10] This technique is ideal for the implantation of the NeuDisc.

The implant is inserted through a standard beveled 8-mm inner diameter cannula and visualized endoscopically as the implant is seated in place. After waiting 4 hours, the implant is shown to have partially hydrated and is also demonstrated to provide vertical lift to the disc space in an unloaded cadaver trunk.

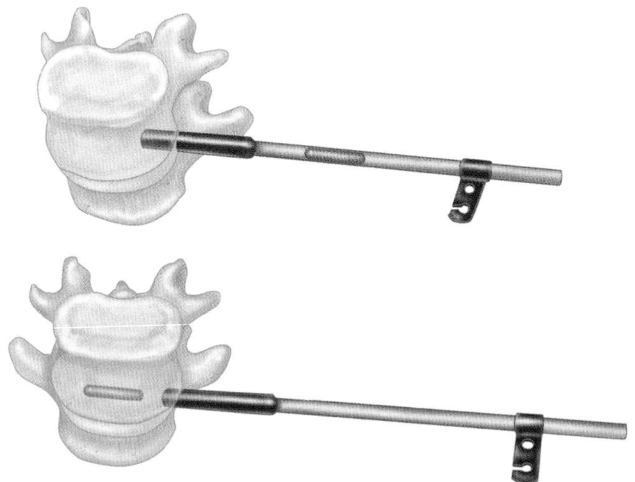

■ FIGURE 53–7. Insertion tools.

## ADVANTAGES AND DISADVANTAGES

Nucleus prosthesis replacement has obvious advantages over total disc replacement. By replacing only the nucleus, it preserves the remaining disc tissues and, therefore, preserves function. Because the nucleus has a more uniform structure and function than the annulus and end plate, the design of the nucleus prosthesis is simpler and it can be designed to be implanted by minimally invasive methods with only a small incision in the annulus. Because the implant is not fixed to the vertebrae, no fixation component is required, and the surgical time is comparable or only slightly longer than a discectomy. Although implant extrusion remains a primary concern, it is less likely to cause permanent nerve injury because of its relatively small size and modulous of elasticity. In cases of prosthesis failure, it is relatively easy to remove the implant anteriorly and convert to a total disc replacement procedure or a fusion.

The major limitation of the NeuDisc is that its application may be limited to patients with early or intermediate degeneration because it requires a relatively competent natural annulus. In a disc with severe annular delamination or loss of height, implantation of a NeuDisc may not be possible. Restoring disc height may have its own concerns if the spinal nerve and facet articulation have already adapted to its shortened state. Because of this concern, work is being considered for a less tall implant that is designed for narrowed, more degenerative discs. It is growing increasingly clear that artificial disc or nucleus implantation may become the treatment of choice for lumbar and cervical disc disease, especially if implanted in patients to mitigate the degenerative process.

It has been estimated that this technology has the potential to be part of up to 50% of future spine surgeries. The potential of disc replacement may parallel that of joint replacement for the near future and offers an exciting development in minimally invasive spine surgery.

## CONCLUSIONS/DISCUSSION

The native nucleus is composed of a hydrogel. Physiologic prerequistes for ideal functioning of the hydrogel include normal end plate metabolic diffusion and an intact annulus. The NeuDisc hydrogel implant promotes continued end plate metabolism and can be inserted with a minimal annulotomy. When it is implanted with a diameter of 6.5-mm, the implant quickly enlarges in height and width to fill the enucleated space and restore disc height. The implant can be inserted through traditional open or endoscopic techniques. Early clinical trials indicate implant stability and clinical improvement.

## REFERENCES

1. Brinkman P, Grootenbore H: Change of disc height, radial disc bulge, and intradiscal pressure from discectomy. Spine 16:641–646, 1991.
2. Stoy V, Sabatino J, Gontarz J, et al: Mechanical testing of a hydrogel nucleus replacement implant. Spine Across the Sea 2003, Maui, Hawaii, July 27–31, 2003.

3. Yeung AT: "Lumbar artificial disc nucleus." *In* Perez-Cruet, Khoo, Fessler (eds). An anatomic approach to minimally invasive spine surgery. Quality Medical Publishing, 2006.
5. Yeung AT, Yeung CA: Advances in endoscopic disc and spine surgery: Foraminal approach. Surg Technol Int 11:253–261, 2003.
6. Yeung AT: The evolution of percutaneous spinal endoscopy and discectomy: State of the art. Mt Sinai J Med 67:327–332, 2000.
7. Yeung AT: Evolving methodology in treating discogenic back pain by selective endoscopic discectomy and thermal annuloplasty. Journal of Minimally Invasive Spinal Technique 1:8–16, 2001.
8. Tsou PM, Yeung AT: Transforaminal endoscopic decompression for radiculopathy secondary to intracanal noncontained lumbar disc herniations: Outcome and technique. Spine J 2:41–48, 2002.
9. Yeung AT, Tsou, PM: Posterolateral endoscopic excision for lumbar disc herniation: Surgical technique, outcome, and complications in 307 consecutive cases. Spine 27:722–731, 2002.
10. Tsou PM, Yeung CA, Yeung AT: Selective Endoscopic Discectomy™ and thermal annuloplasty for chronic lumbar discogenic pain: A minimal access visualized intradiscal procedure. Spine J 2:563–574, 2004.

CHAPTER 54

# NuCore Injectable Nucleus: An In Situ Curing Nucleus Replacement

**Othmar Schwarzenbach, Ulrich Berlemann,** and **Thomas Wilson**

## KEY POINTS

- NuCore Injectable Nucleus is a suitable replacement for the natural nucleus pulposus.
- NuCore Injectable Nucleus treats partial nucleotomies, such as those following microdiscectomy treatment of disc herniation, and early-stage degenerative disc disease (DDD).
- Patients experience pain relief consistent with early results of standard microdiscectomy, with no extrusions or reactions to the material.
- Early data show an improvement in clinical stability in relation to predecessor implants.

## INTRODUCTION

The use of an injectable material for nucleus replacement allows the flexibility to treat partial nucleotomies, such as those following microdiscectomy treatment of disc herniation, as well as early-stage degenerative disc disease (DDD), in which complete nucleus removal and replacement may be required.

An injectable biomaterial is ideal for restoration of disc volume removed during discectomy and for preventing loss of disc height. Flowable materials may be injected through a small incision, allowing minimally invasive, even percutaneous, access to the disc space when appropriate. Fluids can interdigitate with the irregular defects and may, depending on the material used, physically bond to the adjacent tissue. The use of an injectable material allows for complete filling of the disc, a task that is not possible with preformed implants. Complete filling allows pressurization of the annulus, ensuring load transfer and load sharing between the annulus and nucleus. Injectable biomaterials allow for incorporation and uniform dispersion of cells or therapeutic agents, or both. The addition of growth factors may be valuable in enhancing the repair process. Inclusion of inhibitors of inflammatory cytokines and proteases may act to retard matrix degradation and the potential effects of these cytokines on surrounding tissue and neural structures.

Generally, these biomaterials are injected as viscous fluids and then cured through methods such as thermosensitive cross-linking, pH-sensitive cross-linking, photopolymerization, or the addition of a solidifying agent to form a gel-like substance. The setting time should be long enough to allow for accurate placement during the procedure yet short enough to not prolong the length of the surgical procedure. Any heat generated during the cure process should not cause harm to the surrounding tissue. The viscosity or fluidity of the material should balance the need for the substance to remain within the disc with the ability of the surgeon to manipulate its placement and with the need to ensure complete filling of the intradiscal space or voids. Ease in accessing the disc space also needs to be considered. For example, polymers that cure through a photopolymerization procedure could pose a problem owing to a limited ability to access the small cavities of the disc space with the light needed to initiate cross-linking.

Injectable biomaterials have been considered as an augment to discectomy for some time. As early as 1962, Nachemson suggested the injection of a vulcanizing silicone into a degenerated disc using an ordinary syringe.[1] Later, Schneider and Oyen studied the use of silicone elastomer in the intervertebral disc.[2,3] Since then, work has been put toward the development of various injectable materials, including cross-linkable silk elastin copolymer,[4,5] polyurethane-filled balloons,[6] collagen-polyethyleneglycol (PEG),[7] chitosan,[8] various injectable synthetic polymers,[9] recombinant bioelastic materials,[10,11] light-curable PEG polymers,[12] and other multicomponent polymer systems.[13] Several groups are actively pursuing the development of an injectable biomaterial for use in the intervertebral disc.[14,15]

One of those materials is a recombinant protein copolymer known as NuCore Injectable Nucleus (Spine Wave, Inc., Shelton, CT). NuCore consists of amino acid sequence blocks derived from silk and elastin structural proteins. This material appears to have ideal characteristics for the augmentation of the nucleus pulposus following discectomy procedures. Early development and characterization work on this protein polymer was performed by Cappello and co-workers.[16,17] Further clinical development of this polymer is being pursued by the manufacturer.

Successful development of these materials could drastically change the way back pain is treated in the future.

## INDICATIONS/CONTRAINDICATIONS

### Degenerative Disc Disease

Clinical symptoms resulting from herniated, protruding, and/or painful intervertebral discs are commonly treated by discectomy. Discectomy is the most commonly performed spinal surgical treatment, and is frequently used to treat radicular pain due to nerve impingement from a herniated or protruding intervertebral disc. During a discectomy, a substantial portion of the volume of the nucleus pulposus is removed and immediate loss of disc height and volume can result. This procedure is typically performed in a relatively young patient population, with a mean age between 25 and 40 years.[18–20] The impact of altered biomechanics and long-term sequelae in this young patient population may be significant.

Substantial disc height reduction following discectomy is evident soon after the discectomy procedure. Disc height loss has been found to be proportional to the amount of nucleus removed in an in vitro study.[21] Clinically, the operated disc spaces of patients postoperatively are significantly narrower following discectomy than controls.[22] Scoville and Corkill[23] found a 50% incidence of narrowing following surgery at the 3-month follow-up examination. In another study, Tibrewal and Pearcy[24] found disc space narrowing evident within 3 months following surgery as compared with control patients who had not undergone surgery.

Proper disc height is necessary to ensure proper functioning of the intervertebral disc and spinal column. On the local (or cellular) level, decreased disc height can lead to a decrease in cell matrix synthesis and an increase in cell necrosis and apoptosis. It has been shown in other cartilaginous tissues that increased static loading decreases matrix protein biosynthesis.[25–27] Animal models have shown that overloading of the intervertebral disc can initiate disc degeneration.[28,29] In addition, the change in intradiscal pressure creates an unfavorable environment for fluid transfer into the disc, which can cause a further decrease in disc height.

Decreased disc height also results in significant changes in the global mechanical stability of the spine, which may result in further degeneration of the spinal segment. With decreasing height of the disc, the facet joints bear increasing loads and may undergo hypertrophy and degeneration, which may act as a source of pain over time.[30,31] Decreased stiffness of the spinal column and increased range of motion resulting from loss of disc height can lead to further instability of the spine.[31] Excessive motion can manifest itself in abnormal muscle, ligament, and tendon loading, which can ultimately be a source of back pain.

Radicular pain may also result from a decrease in foraminal volume caused by decreased disc height. Specifically, as disc height decreases, the volume of the foraminal canal decreases. This decrease may lead to spinal nerve impingement, with associated radiating pain and dysfunction. Finally, adjacent-segment loading increases as the disc height decreases at a given level.[31,32] The discs that must bear additional loading are now susceptible to accelerated degeneration and compromise, which may eventually propagate along the destabilized spinal column.

A further issue with microdiscectomy surgery is the occurrence of reherniation. Atlas et al[33] reported a reoperation rate of 25% at 10-year follow-up of a study of patients with lumbar disc herniation, with the median time to reoperation of 24 months. Carragee et al[34] reported a 11.5% reherniation rate, with 6.5% reoperation at 5 years.

The objectives of augmentation of the nucleus pulposus following disectomy are to prevent disc height loss and the associated biomechanical and biochemical changes resulting from reduced disc height and volume. Use of an injectable biomaterial to restore disc volume and prevent loss of disc height is currently being evaluated. The ability of an injectable material to seal the disc and prevent or reduce the incidence of reherniation is also being studied.

## DESCRIPTION OF THE DEVICE

Technology has been developed for the production of synthetically designed protein polymers consisting of repeated blocks of amino acid sequence. Through a combination of biologic and chemical methods, block polymers are produced using gene template–directed synthesis. Using this method, the design and polymerization of a new polymer occurs once during the synthesis of the gene template. Through the construction of synthetic genes, it is possible to specify the sequence of protein blocks (the unit of repetition of a protein polymer) several hundred amino acids in length, many fold greater than the limit of sequence control of chemical synthesis.

Molecular architecture is critical to biologic systems. The silk fibroin portion of the polymer is a closely packed structure that serves as a reinforcing scaffold for the surrounding protein, increasing the toughness of the material. The elastin portion of the polymer is a flexible structure that winds into a spiral, functioning as a flexible molecular spring.[35] This gives the material its elastic properties.

The protein polymer used in the NuCore Injectable Nucleus is a sequential block copolymer of silk and elastin, with two silk blocks and eight elastin blocks per polymer sequence repeat. One of the elastin blocks is modified to provide for chemical cross-linking. The protein polymer is synthesized using recombinant DNA techniques through *Escherichia coli* strain K12, a nonpathogenic strain of bacterium typically used in recombinant protein expression. Following batch fermentation, the cells are ruptured by homogenization and the protein polymer is purified from the lysate using precipitation and a series of filtration and adsorption purification steps. The identity and purity of the polymer are confirmed using amino acid composition, amino acid terminal sequencing, mass spectroscopy, and other biochemical tests.

The NuCore material is composed of the protein polymer and a cross-linking agent and is formulated to closely match the properties of the human nucleus pulposus as shown in Table 54–1. The material closely mimics the protein content, water content, pH, and complex modulus of the natural nucleus pulposus. It is injected into the disc after being mixed with a very low concentration of a diisocyanate-based cross-linking agent and has approximately a 90-second working time before it becomes a viscous gel. The material reaches near-final mechanical strength approximately 30 minutes after addition of the cross-linker, but it is sufficiently gelled after 5 minutes to allow the surgery to be completed. As a consequence of the very low concentration of cross-linker used, there is no measurable temperature rise during the curing process.

**TABLE 54–1. Comparison of NuCore Injectable Nucleus and Natural Nucleus**

| Property | NuCore Injectable Nucleus | Natural Nucleus |
|---|---|---|
| Protein content (%) | 19.4 | 13.6–21.9* |
| Water content (%) | 79.1 | 74–81 |
| pH | 7.1 | 6.7–7.1 |
| Complex shear modulus, G* (kPa) | 26 | 7–21† |

*Kitano T, Zerwekh JE, Usui Y, et al: Biomechanical changes associated with the symptomatic human intervertebral disk. Clin Orthop Relat Res 293:372–377, 1993.
†Iatridis JC, Weidenbaum M, Setton LA, Mow VC: Is the nucleus puposus a solid or a fluid? Mechanical behaviors of the nucleus pulposus of the human intervertebral disc. Spine 21:1174–1184, 1996.

## BACKGROUND OF SCIENTIFIC TESTING/CLINICAL OUTCOMES

Extensive preclinical testing and characterization of the material were performed to establish its appropriateness for the intended application.

Biocompatibility and toxicology testing following the ISO 10993 guidelines were performed on the material. Acute tests include cytotoxicity, sensitization (guinea pig), intracutaneous reactivity (rabbit), systemic toxicity (mouse), pyrogenicity, muscle implant evaluation and genotoxicity testing. The material was nontoxic and nonirritating in all of these test evaluations. Chronic toxicity testing was conducted in a rat subcutaneous model and evaluated at time points beyond 1 year with no toxicity seen. Neurofunctional testing in a rat model showed no neurotoxicity of the material when placed adjacent to spinal nerve roots.

Mechanical characterization of the material was also carried out preclinically in benchtop testing. Testing of cadaveric anterior column units was done to determine how well the NuCore material resists extrusion under load. Segments were tested in axial compression and loaded to failure. In all cases, there was no extrusion unless preceded by bony failure or end plate failure of the model itself.[36] The average maximum load imparted to the spinal segments was 3,555 N, well above the loads experienced in normal daily activities. Results demonstrated that the NuCore material integrated extensively with the surrounding disc tissue and did not extrude during any of the testing (Fig. 54–1).

Human cadaveric spinal units were also tested to determine how well the NuCore material restores stability and function to a spinal unit.[37] Anterior column units (no posterior structures) were tested in compression in the intact condition, then with a partial nucleotomy, and finally with NuCore material injected. Statistical analysis using a repeated measures analysis showed that the discectomy caused a significant loss of height during the test ($P<0.05$). However, the NuCore material injection caused a restoration such that there was no significant difference ($P>0.05$) between the displacement of the intact condition and the NuCore material–treated condition.[38] Functional spinal units (anterior and posterior structures intact) were also tested in flexion/extension, lateral bending, and axial rotation with similar results.[38] This analysis indicates the NuCore Injectable Nucleus restores function and stability to the spine after being destabilized by a discectomy procedure.

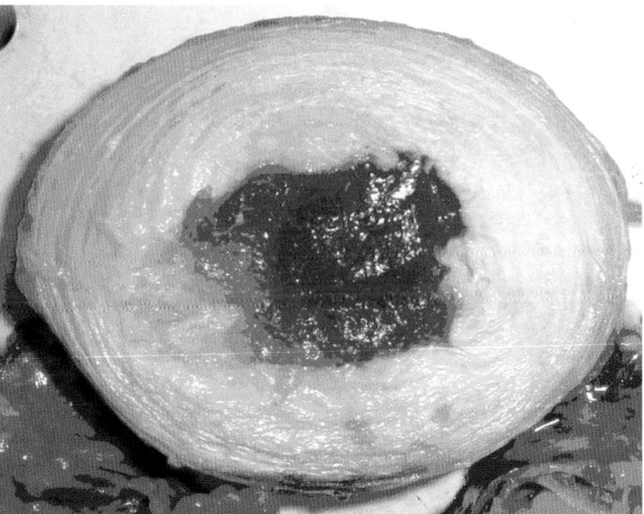

■ **FIGURE 54–1.** Sectioned test specimen showing interdigitation of NuCore Injectable Nucleus into natural intradiscal tissue.

Owing to limitations of cadaveric tissue, testing has been performed in a synthetic disc model to evaluate the effect of dynamic loading over long periods of time. The annulus fibrosus of the disc was simulated with a silicone elastomer. This silicone annulus was injected with NuCore material, and the model was subjected to cyclic physiologic loading up to 10 million cycles with no failure of the NuCore material or test model. This testing indicates the NuCore material to be durable, fatigue resistant, and capable of withstanding in vivo loads for an extended period of time.

### Early Clinical Results

As reported at the Spine Arthroplasty Society meeting in Montreal in May 2006, a nonrandomized clinical study is underway in Switzerland to investigate the use of NuCore Injectable Nucleus as a tissue replacement in cases of microdiscectomy for herniated nucleus pulposus.[39] Patients enrolled in the study suffered from a single-level symptomatic herniated nucleus pulposus in the lumbar spine that did not respond to conservative therapy. Data were collected preoperatively, postoperatively, at 6 and 12 weeks, as well as 6 and 12 months. The clinical data at each time point included a neurologic examination as well as an assessment of pain, disability, and function using Visual Analog Scale (VAS) for back and leg pain, Oswestry Disability Index (ODI), and SF-36 patient questionnaires. At each time point, standing lateral x-ray studies with a marker attached were taken. Disc height analysis was performed by an independent analysis group (Medical Metrics, Inc.) using a validated measurement method. Magnetic resonance imaging (MRI) obtained preoperatively, postoperatively, and at 6 and 12 months were qualitatively reviewed with regard to the signal in the disc and the postoperative behavior of the decompressed tissues.

Eight of 15 enrolled patients had completed 1 year of follow-up. There were no dropouts over the follow-up period. Average age of the patients was 35.9 years. Eight were male, and seven were female. Of the 15 levels treated, 11 were at L5-S1 and four were at L4-S5.

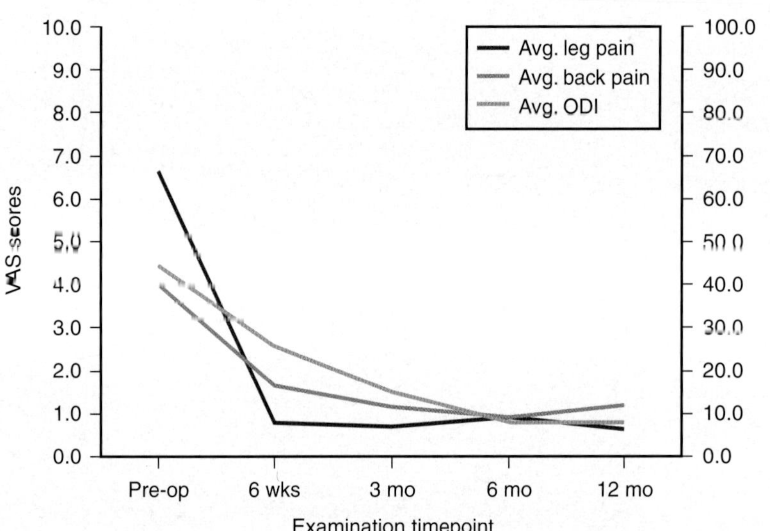


■ **FIGURE 54–2.** Average Visual Analog Scale (VAS) and Oswestry Disability Index (ODI) results from NuCore clinical study.

The mean injection volume was 1.3 mL in these 15 patients. The goal was to replace the entire amount of tissue lost to the herniation and the partial nucleotomy, thus restoring the original volume of nuclear tissue within the disc. Improvements to the injection technique led to increased injection volumes in later cases. Before the development of the improved injection technique, the injection volumes matched only the volume of tissue removed from within the disc. The improved technique resulted in complete replacement of all tissue lost in the later cases.

No device-related adverse events were reported. Results of all blood, serum, and urine tests were within normal ranges at all time points. There was no evidence of any immunologic reaction to the material.

Pain and function scores are shown in Figures 54–2 and 54–3. Mean leg pain (VAS) reduced from 6.7 at preoperative assessment to 0.6 at 1 year after surgery. Mean back pain (VAS) reduced from 4.0 at preoperative assessment to 1.2 at 1 year after surgery. Likewise, mean ODI reduced from 44.0 at preoperative assessment to 7.9 at 1 year after surgery. All of these scores were consistent with those expected in microdiscectomy patients.

Radiographic analysis of standing lateral x-ray studies showed good maintenance of disc height in the postoperative follow-up examinations. Discs treated with the early surgical technique averaged 93% of the original disc height at the 12-month follow-up. Discs treated with the improved technique showed disc height approximating 100% of the original height.

Review of the MR images showed no migration of the material and no extrusions. As can be seen in Figure 54–4, the NuCore implant appears as a hyperintense signal within the disc. Consolidation of the posterior tissue remnants from the herniation can be seen over the follow-up period.

## OPERATIVE TECHNIQUE

A typical interlaminar approach for microdiscectomy was used. The herniated tissue was removed, and the disc was further cleared of loose tissue by several washouts and gentle use of rongeurs. Following the discectomy, the amount of tissue removed was measured and used as a target volume for the NuCore material injection. The procedure was paused for 5 minutes following injection to allow the material to cure; then the wound was closed. No postoperative brace was used, but patients were reminded to restrict their activities for 6 weeks.

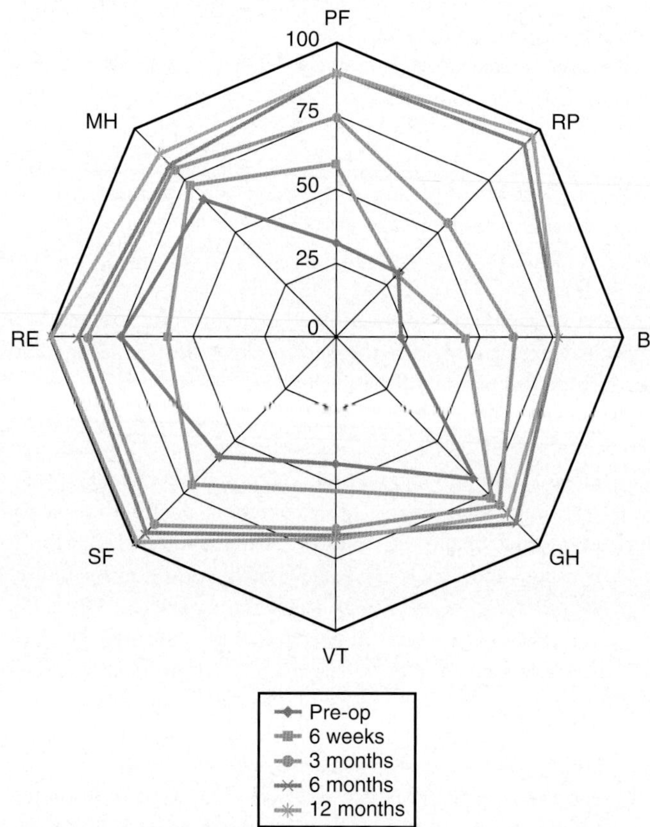


■ **FIGURE 54–3.** Average SF-36 results for NuCore clinical study.

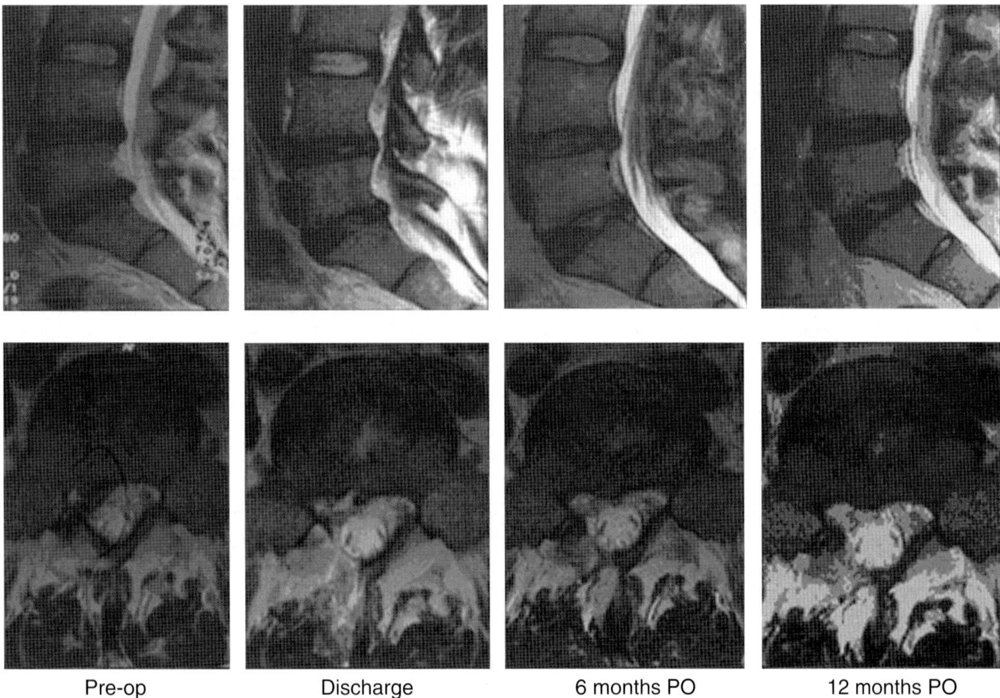


■ **FIGURE 54–4.** Representative magnetic resonance images from a NuCore clinical trial patient. Disc herniation at L5-S1, treated with microdiscectomy and nucleus replacement.

## CONCLUSIONS/DISCUSSION

Based on the preclinical and clinical data reviewed, NuCore Injectable Nucleus appears to be a suitable replacement for the natural nucleus pulposus. The preclinical characterization of the mechanical and biomaterial properties of the NuCore material is supported by the early clinical study data. Patients have seen pain relief consistent with the expected early results of standard microdiscectomy with no extrusions or reactions to the material. Disc height appears to be better maintained than that indicated by the literature. The long-term benefits will be borne out in longer term follow-up on these patients to determine whether improved biomechanics and decreased complications (reherniation, progression to fusion, recurrent pain, and so on) are indeed realized. These early data are promising at this point and show an improvement in clinical stability in relation to predecessor implants that have been tested in this application. The fact that an injectable flowable hydrogel has been successfully implanted and remained in place over considerable time is a significant step forward in the development of a viable nucleus replacement.

Additional clinical evaluation of the use of NuCore Injectable Nucleus for treatment of early-stage DDD has just recently begun. Ongoing efforts are also characterizing the use of the material as a cell delivery vehicle for disc repair and reconstruction, as well as the use of the material for repair of articular cartilage defects.

## REFERENCES

1. Nachemson A: Some mechanical properties of the lumbar intervertebral disc. Bull Hosp Joint Diseases 23:130–132, 1962.
2. Schneider PG, Oyen R: Intervertebral disc replacement, experimental studies, clinical consequences. Z Orthop Ihre Grenzgeb 112:791–792, 1974.
3. Schneider PG, Oyen R: Plastic surgery on intervertebral disc, part I: intervertebral disc replacement in the lumbar regions with silicone rubber: Theoretical and experimental studies. Z Orthop Ihre Grenzgeb112:1078–1086, 1974.
4. Cappello J, Stedronsky ER, inventors: Synthetic proteins for in vivo drug delivery and tissue augmentation. US patent 6,380,154, April 30, 2002.
5. Ferrari FA, Richardson C, Chambers J, et al, inventors: Peptides comprising repetitive units of amino acids and DNA sequences encoding the same. US patent 6,355,776, March 12, 2002.
6. Bao Q-B, Yuan HA, inventors: Implantable tissue repair device. US patent 6,224,630, May 1, 2001.
7. Olsen DR, Chang R, McMullin H, et al, inventors: Methods for the production of gelatin and full-length triple helical collagen in recombinant cells. US patent 6,428,978, August 6, 2002.
8. Chenite A, Chaput C, Wang D, et al: Novel injectable neutral solutions of chitosan form biodegradable gels in situ. Biomaterials 21:2155–2161, 2000.
9. Milner R, Arrowsmith P, Millan EJ, inventors: Intervertebral disc implant. US patent 6,187,048, February 13, 2001.
10. Urry DW, inventor: Polynanopeptide bioelastomers having an increased elastic modulus. US patent 5,064,430, November 12, 1991.
11. Urry DW, inventor: Polymers capable of baromechanical and barochemical transduction. US patent 5,226,292, July 13, 1993.
12. Hubbell JA, Pathak CP, Sawhney AS, et al, inventors: Photopolymerizable biodegradable hydrogels as tissue contacting materials and controlled-release microcarriers. US patent 5,626,863, May 6, 1997.
13. Hubbell JA, Wetering PVD, Cowling DSP, inventors: Novel polymer compounds. U.S. patent application US_2002/0177680_A1, 2002.
14. Bao Q-B, Yuan HA: New technologies in spine: nucleus replacement. Spine 27:1245–1247, 2002.
15. DiMartino A, Vaccaro A, Lee JY, et al: Nucleus pulposus replacement: Basic science and indications for clinical use. Spine 30:S16–S22, 2005.
16. Cappello J, Ferrman F: Genetically engineered protein polymers. *In* Domb AJ, Kost J, Wiseman D (eds): Handbook of Degradable Polymers. Amsterdam, Harwood Academic Publishers, 1996, pp 387–414.

17. Cappello J, Ferrari F: Microbial product of structural protein polymers. *In* Mobley DP (ed): Plastics from Microbes. Munich, Carl Hanser Verlag, 1997, pp 35–92.
18. Hermantin FU, Peters T, Quartararo L, Kambin P: A prospective, randomized study comparing the results of open discectomy with those of video-assisted arthroscopic microdiscectomy. J Bone Joint Surg 81-A:958–965, 1999.
19. Mochida J, Toh E, Nomura T, Nishimura K: The risks and benefits of percutaneous nucleotomy for lumbar disc herniation: A 10 year longitudinal study. J Bone Joint Surg Br 83:501–505, 2001.
20. Yorimitsu E, Chiba K, Toyama Y, Hirabayashi K: Long-term outcomes of standard discectomy for lumbar disc herniation: A follow-up study of more than 10 years. Spine 26:652–657, 2001.
21. Brinckmann P, Frobin W, Hierholzer E, Horst M: Deformation of the vertebral endplate under axial loading of the spine. Spine 8:851–856, 1983.
22. Frymoyer JW, Hanley EN, Howe J, et al: A comparison of radiographic findings in fusion and nonfusion patients ten and more years following disc surgery. Spine 4:435–440, 1979.
23. Scoville WB, Corkill G: Lumbar disc surgery: Technique of radical removal and early mobilization. J Neurosurg 39:265–269, 1973.
24. Tibrewal SB, Pearcy MJ: Lumbar intervertebral disc heights in normal subjects and patients with disc herniation. Spine 10:452–454, 1985.
25. Buschmann MD, Gluzband YA, Grodzinsky AJ, Huziker EJ: Mechanical compression modulates matrix biosynthesis in chondrocyte/agarose culture. J Cell Sci 108:1497–1508, 1995.
26. Ohshima H, Urban JPG, Bergel DH: Effect of static load on matrix synthesis rates in the intervertebral disc measured in vitro by a new perfusion technique. J Orthop Res 13:22–29, 1995.
27. Rand N, Juliao S, Spengler D, Dawson J: Static Hydrostatic Loading Induces In Vitro Apoptosis in Human Intervertebral Disc Cells. Orlando, FL, Orthopaedic Research Society, 2000.
28. Iatridis JC, Mente PL, Stokes AF, et al: Compression-induced changes in intervertebral disc properties in a rat tail model. Spine 24:996–1002, 1999.
29. Lotz JC, Colliou OK, Chin JR, et al: Compression-induced degeneration of the intervertebral disc: An in vivo mouse model and finite-element study. Spine 23:2493–2506, 1998.
30. Gotfried Y, Bradford DS, Oegema TR: Facet joint changes after chemonucleolysis-induced disc space narrowing. Spine 11:944–950, 1986.
31. Panjabi MM, Krag MH, Chung TQ: Effects of disc injury on mechanical behavior of the human spine. Spine 9:707–713, 1984.
32. Natarajan RN, Ke JH, Andersson GBJ: A model to study the disc degeneration process. Spine 19:259–265, 1994.
33. Atlas SJ, Keller RB, Wu YA, et al. Long term outcomes of surgical and nonsurgical management of sciatica secondary to a lumbar disc herniation: 10 year results from the Maine lumbar spine study. Spine 30:927–935, 2005.
34. Carragee EJ, Han MY, Yang B, et al: Activity restrictions after posterior lumbar discectomy: A prospective study of outcomes in 152 cases with no postoperative restrictions. Spine 24:2346–2351, 1999.
35. Urry DW, Hugel T, Seitz M, et al: Elastin: A representative ideal protein elastomer. Philos Trans R Soc Lond B Biol Sci 357:169–184, 2002.
36. Walkenhorst J, Lee D, Spenciner D: Extrusion Resistance of an Injectable Nucleus Replacement in the Human Cadaver Spine. Proceedings of the International Meeting on Advanced Spine Techniques (IMAST). Bermuda, July 2004.
37. Mahar AT, Oka R, Whitledge J, et al: Biomechanical efficacy of a protein polymer hydrogel for inter-vertebral nucleus augmentation and replacement. Proceedings of the Fourth World Congress on Biomechanics. Calgary, August 2002.
38. Walkenhorst J, Kitchel S, Spenciner D: Effect of Injectable Disc Nucleus on Function of the Human Spine. Proceedings of the Annual Meeting of the International Society for the Study of the Lumbar Spine (ISSLS), Porto, June 2004.
39. Berlemann U, Schwarzenbach O, Etter C, Kitchel S: Clinical Evaluation of an Injectable, In-Situ Curing Nucleus Replacement. Spine Arthroplasty Society Proceedings, Montreal, May 2006.

CHAPTER 55

# Aquarelle Hydrogel Disc Nucleus

**Qi-Bin Bao** and **Hansen Yuan**

## KEY POINTS

- Aquarelle was the first hydrogel nucleus device.
- Water content and swelling pressure are similar to that of the natural nucleus.
- It has low modulus yet strong mechanical strength.
- The replacement was subjected to comprehensive biocompatibility testing with favorable results.
- Implant extrusion is the main challenge due to a low elastic modulus and slippery surface.

## INTRODUCTION

The Aquarelle nucleus is the first hydrogel nucleus arthroplasty device, the development of which was started in 1990[1] by Howmedica (which was subsequently acquired by Stryker). This was almost 6 years before the development of the PDN-SOLO device by RayMedica,[2] which has the most clinical experience for hydrogel nucleus arthroplasty devices.

The definition of a hydrogel can vary slightly in different fields. According to *Dorland's Illustrated Medical Dictionary*,[3] a hydrogel is a gel that has water as its dispersion medium. From a biomaterial point of view, typically a hydrogel is a gel that has water dispersed in a polymer network. According to this definition, there is no question that the natural nucleus is a hydrogel.

The disc has a composite structure consisting of the nucleus pulposus core circumferentially surrounded by the multilayered fibers of the annulus fibrosis and superiorly and inferiorly by the cartilage end plates. The structure of a disc is analogous to that of an automobile tire. The annulus, with successive layers of collagen fibers oriented in alternating directions, surrounds the nucleus. Similar to the multilayers of a tire, these fibers have a relatively low compressive stiffness and strength but high tensile stiffness and strength. This anisotropic structure allows the tire and the disc to support the load much better when they are at a fully inflated stage than at a semiinflated stage. The nucleus is a hydrogel with 80% water in youth and gradually desiccates with age.

Water is drawn into the nucleus by the presence of hydrophilic proteins called proteoglycans (PG). Collagen fibers cross-link PG in an irregular fashion, creating a firm hydrogel matrix. It should be mentioned that the water content of the nucleus is largely dependent on the concentration of the two chemical components in the proteoglycans, chondrotin sulfate (CS) and keratin sulfate (KS), both of which carry a negative charge. Other than the hydrophilic nature of collagen and other components of the PG that can hydrate and retain a certain amount of water, these negatively charged components are especially important in regards to the amount of water the nucleus can retain. The higher the negative charge density in the proteoglycans, the higher the water content for the nucleus. In the progression of disc degeneration, the concentration of CS and KS in the PG decreases and that leads to the decrease in water content. Another interesting phenomenon for the hydration of the nucleus is called swelling pressure. In simple terms, this means that the water content of the nucleus changes with the external pressure (swelling pressure). If the nucleus is placed in a closed container with at least part of the surface allowing the permeation of water diffusion, as the external pressure on the nucleus increases and sustains at this high level, part of the water will diffuse through the permeable surface until the new equilibrium of water content is reached. After the equilibrium of water content is achieved at a high swelling pressure, if the external pressure is reduced and maintained at a lower level, the nucleus can draw the water from the external tissue through the permeable surface. For the disc, the annulus has very small water permeability. The main permeable surfaces are the two thin layers of cartilage end plates through multiple capillaries but with very low water permeability. In other words, in the short term, as the external load on the disc changes, the annulus and end plates act like a totally sealed container for the nucleus. The adjustment of water content to the new pressure can take hours to occur.

The function of the disc mirrors its compositional complexity. In a gross picture, the disc bears the load in a similar way to a tire. The annulus is inflated by the nucleus with the tire in a vertical position while the disc is in a horizontal position. Although neither the nucleus nor air has any significant mechanical strength on its own, by inflating the annulus or tire, the load on the disc or tire is supported by the radial stretch of the annulus or the tire. As mentioned earlier, because both the annulus and tire have a very high tensile (or stretching) stiffness, the inflated disc or tire becomes much stiffer than when it is less inflated. However, the major difference between the two is that instead of simply pumping a certain pressure of air into the tire, the degree of nucleus inflation is regulated by its negative charge density and the external load. A nucleus with a high negative charge density has a high swelling pressure. As the disc starts to degenerate or simply age, the negative charge density decreases and, consequently, the water content decreases. For a nucleus with a given negative charge density, there is a correlation between the swelling pressure and the equilibrium water content as shown in the solid line AB in Figure 55–1. As mentioned earlier, although the air in the tire is completely sealed, the water in the nucleus can be diffused slowly through the end plates in response to the external load change. However, the water diffusion rate of the end plates is so small that it makes the disc almost impermeable when the external load, or its corresponding swelling pressure, suddenly increases from B to D in Figure 55–1. This sudden load change creates a quasiequilibrium state. If the load is sustained, the water in the nucleus will slowly diffuse through the end plates and the water content will eventually reach the new equilibrium state of A. In the evening, when a person goes to bed and the external load decreases from point A to C, the swelling pressure and water contend again reaches a nonequilibrium state. The hydrogel nucleus will act like a water reservoir and imbibes water from the vertebrae until the new equilibrium B is reached.

Biomechanically, this water diffusion regulates the load distribution between the annulus and nucleus. Owing to the incompressible nature of the nucleus, the small diffusion rate and the high tensile modulus of the annulus, when there is a sudden load increase, the nucleus takes a large portion of the load and subsequently a high compressive stress is applied to the end plates in the nucleus region. If this high load is sustained, water gradually diffuses through the end plates and the nucleus starts to lose volume. The loss of volume in the nucleus causes a deflation of the disc, which leads to more of the compressive load being shifted to the annulus. Like the tire, the annulus is strong in tension and weak in compression. If the annulus is constantly under a high compressive load, it is more susceptible to damage.

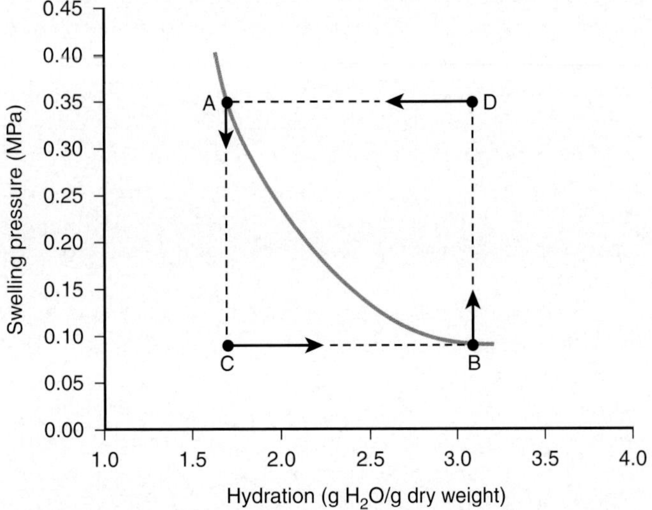


■ **FIGURE 55–1.** Expelling and imbibing of water by the hydrogel under the load change.

Other than regulating the load distribution, the water diffusion under cyclic loading provides the necessary nutrition for the disc. The intervertebral disc is the largest avascular tissue in the body, and the main cells in the disc are chondrocytes. Owing to its avascularity, nutrients for the chondrocytes and the metabolite byproducts generated in the disc must rely on the diffusion of body fluids across the disc through the end-capillaries in adjacent vertebra during cyclic loading. If this diffusion is interrupted or impaired, the disc tends to degenerate faster than the disc with proper fluid diffusion.[4]

## INDICATIONS AND CONTRAINDICATIONS

The indications for the Aquarelle nucleus should be the same as that for other nucleus devices, that is, discogenic back pain caused by degenerative disc disease (DDD), as confirmed by patient history and radiographic studies, with or without leg pain. The contraindications for the Aquarelle nucleus should also be similar to that for other disc arthroplasty devices: osteoporosis, osteopenia, scolosis, instability caused by isthmic spondylolisthesis, spondolysis, or retrolisthesis or anterolisthesis of greater than 3 mm, and so on. Because the nucleus device is more suitable for patients with early to moderated DDD, disc height less than 5 mm should also be a contraindication.

## DESCRIPTION OF THE DEVICE

From the unique characteristics of the natural nucleus and its functions, it becomes very logical to select a hydrogel material for a nucleus replacement device. The Aquarelle nucleus was the first hydrogel nucleus device. Since the Aquarelle nucleus, there are many other nucleus devices currently under development using a hydrogel as the material of choice. These hydrogel nucleus devices include PDN, or its newer version HydraFlex (Raymedica, Inc., Minneapolis, MN); NeuDisc (Replication Medical, Cranbury, NJ); NuCore (SpineWave, Inc., Shelton, CT); BioDisc (Cryolife Inc., Kennesaw, GA); Geliflex (Synthes, West Chester, PA); and SaluDisc (SpineMedica, Marietta, GA).

As mentioned earlier, hydrogel is a relatively broad term. Although the dispersion phase for these hydrogel materials is all water, the polymer network, which determines the hydrogel properties for these devices, can vary significantly from device to device. Owing to the polymer network difference, the mechanical and biologic properties for various hydrogels can be very different. What would be the optimal polymer network for a nucleus replacement device? It seems that the ideal hydrogel material for nucleus replacement should replicate all physical, mechanical, chemical, and physiologic characteristics of the natural nucleus. In reality, owing to the change in boundary conditions, it will not be the best option to choose a hydrogel with similar properties to the natural nucleus for nucleus replacement. When a patient becomes symptomatic with low back pain caused by the DDD, the annulus of the disc often has already had different degrees of damage, in addition to the dehydration of the nucleus. Even if the annulus damage is minimal, the procedure of removing the diseased nucleus and implanting the nucleus prosthesis often requires the creation of an annular window. Therefore, the annulus is no longer intact and cannot contain the loose gel under substantial pressure. If the hydrogel nucleus device is as deformable as the natural nucleus and inflates the annulus like the healthy disc, it would be easily extruded through the annular defect. If one tries to avoid the extrusion problem by substantially underinflating the disc space, it will not be able to share a substantial amount of load with the remaining annulus, restore its mechanical function, and protect the annulus from overcompression. Therefore, to minimize the risk of implant extrusion, the hydrogel nucleus implant should be much firmer, or stiffer, than the natural nucleus.

Other than the material modulus, for the same reason, the mechanical strength and durability of the hydrogel should also be taken into consideration in selecting the material for nucleus replacement. Although the natural nucleus has almost no mechanical strength by itself and can be easily fragmented, the nucleus replacement has to maintain its integrity after repeated loading cycles. If the integrity of the replacement is not maintained, the fragmented implant can be easily extruded through the annular defect. In addition to fatigue strength, the biostability of the hydrogel should also be considered. Because it is a long-term implant for patients at a fairly young age, there should be reasonable assurance that the hydrogel material selected will not degrade over time. The degradation of the material not only will deteriorate the mechanical strength but might also release toxic degradation by-products.

One of the main reasons for choosing a hydrogel elastomer over a nonhydrogel elastomer for nucleus replacement is to restore the water swelling pressure characteristics so that body fluid diffusion can be maintained. Although most hydrogel nucleus replacements do not contain living cells, it is at least a perceived benefit to restore the body fluid diffusion so that it will continue to bring nutrients for the remaining nucleus and annulus. Because a hydrogel can be made from different polymers that might have different swelling pressure characteristics, it would be desirable to use a hydrogel with a similar swelling pressure to the natural nucleus.

Last but not least, biocompatibility is a necessity for any permanent implant. If the biocompatibility of a new material has not been established yet, a series of biocompatibility tests according to the International Organization for Standardization (ISO) 10993 standards have to be conducted. Even with favorable results from these tests, the long-term stability and potential carcinogenicity issues can still be raised. If there are reasonable doubts on potential carcinogenicity, a full-scale carcinogenicity study or a relatively shorter essay using a P53 transgenic mouse model might be required.

## BACKGROUND OF SCIENTIFIC TESTING/CLINICAL OUTCOMES

The Aquarelle nucleus is made of polyvinyl alcohol (PVA) with the following chemical structure: $-[CH_2CHOH]_n-$. Chemically, PVA has a similar C-C backbone to that of polyethylene (PE), which has been widely used as a permanent implantable material due to its biocompatibility and stability. PVA itself also has a long history of being used or considered for various medical applications, spanning from contact lens to skin and cartilage replacements. Unlike PE, which is hydrophobic, the hydrophilic character of PVA is mainly from its hydroxyl group ($-OH$), and under ambient conditions, the water content is about 83%. PVA hydrogels can be formed from either chemical cross-links or physical cross-links. The Aquarelle nucleus is physically cross-linked through repetitive freeze-thaw cycles. One of the advantages of having a physically cross-linked hydrogel is that it does not include any cross-link agents, which can often be toxic if they are not fully incorporated into the polymer structure.

### Biocompatibility Testing

With the long history of PVA hydrogels for various medical applications, the full battery of biocompatibility testing per ISO 10993 standards has been performed for the Aquarelle Hydrogel Nucleus device. These tests include

- Cytotoxicity Test in L929 Mouse Fibroblast Cells PVA Hydrogel Agar Averlay Assay
- Mutagenicity Assay with a Saline Extract and a Polyethylene Glycol Extract of PVA Hydrogel
- Cytotoxicity Test on PVA Hydrogel in vitro Hemolysis in Rabbit Whole Blood
- Mutagenicity Test on Saline and PEG200 Extracts of PVA Hydrogel in the L5178Y KT+/− Mouse Lymphoma Forward Mutation Assay
- Mutagenicity Test on Saline and PEG200 Extracts of PVA Hydrogel Measuring Chromosomal Eberations in Chinese Hamster Ovary (CHO) Cells
- Genotoxicity Test on Saline and PEG200 Extracts of PVA hydrogel in the Assay for Unscheduled DNA Synthesis in Rat Liver Primary Cell Cultures
- Rabbit Pyrogen Study—Material Mediated
- Systemic Toxicity Study in Mice (Extracts)
- Intracutaneous Toxicity Study in the Rabbit (Extracts)
- Delayed Contact Sensitization Study (A Maximization Method) in the Guinea Pig (Saline Extract)
- USP Muscle Implantation Study in the Rabbit (90 days)

The Aquarelle nucleus has passed all these tests. In addition, the National Toxicology Program has conducted both 30-day and 2-year toxicology and carcinogenesis studies on PVA in mice and concluded that there was no evidence of carcinogenic activity (NTP).[5]

### Swelling Pressure Study

As mentioned earlier, swelling pressure is an important characteristic of the nucleus. Owing to its unique swelling pressure, the equilibrium water content of the nucleus changes with the external pressure on the nucleus. This water content change in response to the load change in daily activities regulates the degree of disc inflation and functions as a driving force for the body fluid diffusion, which is essential to the biologic activities of the disc.

To obtain the swelling pressure of the nucleus or a biomaterial, other than subjecting the nucleus or a biomaterial in a container with permeable membrane to various pressures, it can also be tested by subjecting the nucleus or a biomaterial in solutions to different osmotic pressures generated by different concentration of polyethylene glycol (PEG).[6] The osmotic pressure (II) of the PEG solutions was found using the following equation:

$$II/RT = c/18,500 + 2.59 \times 10^{-3} \times c2 + 13.5 \times 10^{-3} \times c^{3} \quad \textbf{55-1}$$

where c is the concentration in g PEG/mL of the solution and 18,500 is the molecular weight of the PEG.

In this study, 12 different PEG solutions of different concentrations were prepared so that a curve of PVA equilibrium water content at different swelling pressures could be obtained. For each concentration of PEG solution, five replicates of PVA hydrogel were used. Specimens were weighed and then enclosed in a 1,000 molecular weight cut off (MWCO) dialysis membrane (Spectrum Medical Industrials Inc., Los Angles, CA) and immersed in the PEG solution for 1 week to reach equilibrium. The weight of each specimen was then measured again with an analytical balance. The samples were then dried in an oven to obtain their dry weight. The equilibrium water under different swelling pressures was then calculated using the dry weight and the wet weight at a given swelling pressure. The curve of the swelling pressure of the PVA hydrogel is shown in Figure 55–2.[7] When comparing the swelling pressure of the PVA hydrogel with the swelling pressure of the natural nucleus, it was found that the PVA hydrogel has a very similar swelling pressure curve to that of the natural nucleus (Fig. 55–3).

The results of this study showed that the Aquarelle Hydrogel Nucleus would have a swelling pressure similar to that of the human intervertebral disc nucleus. It releases water under load and imbibes water when the load is released or decreased. These properties of the PVA hydrogel might bring the benefit of preventing further degeneration of the disc by providing adequate nutrition to the disc when used as a nucleus replacement. To our knowledge, this is the only study that has demonstrated the proper swelling pressure for any hydrogel nucleus devices.

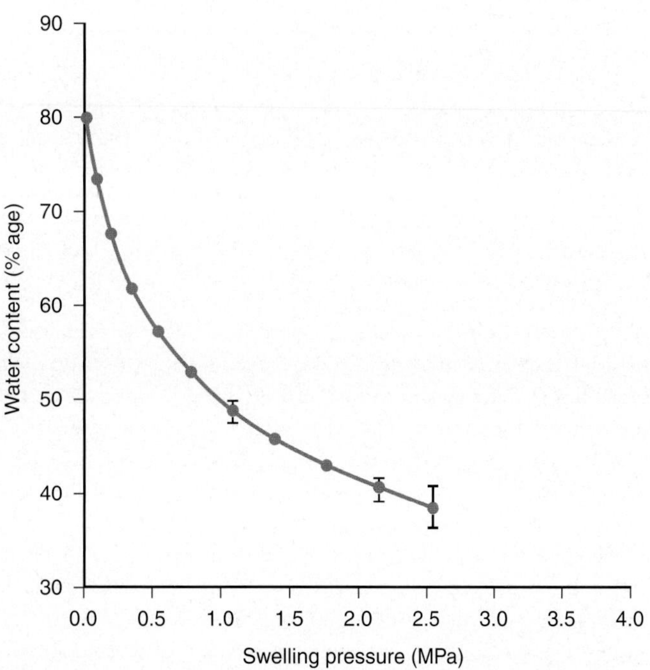


■ **FIGURE 55–2.** Swelling pressure of polyvinyl alcohol hydrogel.

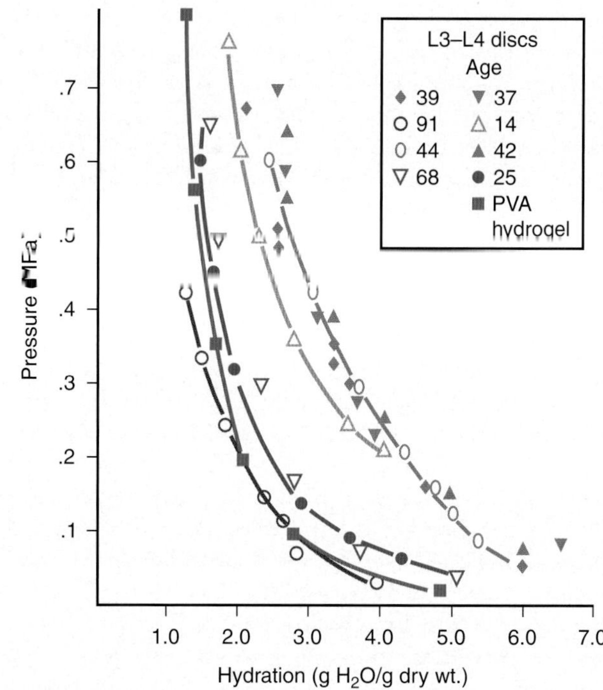


■ **FIGURE 55–3.** Swelling pressure comparison between polyvinyl alcohol hydrogel and nucleus.

## Biomechanical Test

Multiple biomechanical studies using a human cadaveric lumbar model have been conducted for the Aquarelle Hydrogel Nucleus to demonstrate the ability of the Aquarelle Hydrogel Nucleus in restoring the disc height and biomechanical function of the lumbar segment.

The first biomechanical study for the Aquarelle nucleus was presented in the 1994 annual meeting of the North American Spine Society.[8] In this study, nine fresh cadaveric lumbar functional spine units were used to assess changes in disc height, disc stiffness, facet load, and distribution of intradiscal pressure at three different stages; intact, postdiscectomy and post–Aquarelle implantation. The biomechanical tests consisted of three modes of loading: pure compression (PC), compression with 5 degrees of flexion (CF), and compression with 5 degrees of extension (CE). The maximum load applied was 1,000 N at a loading rate of 100 N/s. The intradiscal pressure was measured by inserting a strain guage pressure probe along five equidistant parasagittal paths under a constant load of 1,000 N. At the end of these three stages, the intervertebral disc was dissected and the dynamic load-displacement test was repeated between 50 N of tension to 300 N of compression on the posterior elements for each of the three loading modes.

The results of this study showed that in comparison to the intact disc height at 1,000 N, the discectomy led to a disc height loss of 12.0 ± 6.2%, 11.4 ± 5.4%, and 10.1 ± 6.1% for PC, CF, and CE, respectively. After the implantation of Aquarelle Hydrogel Nucleus, the average disc height was restored to the intact level under all the three loading modes. Stiffness, measured from 800 to 1,000 N, showed no significant difference between stages except for the implant stage in pure compression.

The stiffness for this case was about 12% lower compared with both the intact and discectomy stages ($P<0.05$). As to the facet load, no statistical differences were found among the three stages for PC and CF. However, in CE, the load through the facets measured as a percentage of the applied load averaged 13.6 ± 7.7%, 27.3 ± 15.5%, and 16.3 ± 13.4% for the intact, discectomy, and implant stages, respectively. The intact and the implant stages were not significantly different, but both were significantly different than the discectomy stage ($P<0.05$). Stress distribution plots were created from the pressure data. The magnitude of pressure within the nucleus region significantly decreased ($P<0.05$) after discectomy compared with the intact and implant stages for PC (21.5 ± 14.8%), CF (27.6 ± 23.6%), and CE (36.3 ± 24.8%). Discectomy also caused localized stress increases in the annulus. There was no significant difference in intradiscal pressure between the intact and implant stages under all three loading modes. The localized stress increase in the annulus as a result of the discectomy was reduced after the implantation of the Aquarelle Hydrogel Nucleus.

In summary, this biomechanical study demonstrated that the Aquarelle Hydrogel Nucleus could restore the disc height, the normal load sharing between the anterior column and posterior elements, and the normal load sharing between the annulus and the nucleus.

## Fatigue Test

Because nucleus arthroplasty is a relatively new technology, there is neither a guideline nor standard for testing the fatigue strength of nucleus replacement devices, especially when it was first introduced in the 1990s. The challenge for testing the fatigue characteristics of a low modulus nucleus replacement device is how to mimic the constraining effect of the annulus so that the device can be subjected to both physiologic stress and strain. Under unconstrained conditions, if a physiologic stress is applied to a low-modulus nucleus device, the strain will exceed the physiologic range. This excessive strain might cause device failure much faster than when it is used clinically. On the other hand, if the device is loaded to a physiologic strain range under unconstrained conditions, the stress will not approach the physiologic range. This low stress might not be able to detect the fatigue failure when a physiologic stress is applied. To address the limitations of unconstrained testing methodologies, a special fatigue testing apparatus was developed.

As is shown in Figure 55–4, the testing apparatus uses pneumatic pressure to provide the required stiffness. The principle of the apparatus is to seal the hydrogel nucleus device in a chamber. The implant was placed in the center of the loading piston surrounded by a sponge cushion ring. Two O-rings (dynamic, self-lubricating) on the moving piston ensure that the chamber remains sealed even under reciprocating motions. The amount of gas (air or nitrogen) inside the chamber is controlled by injecting a measured quantity of saline into the chamber. The initial pressure in the chamber is controlled by connecting it to a regulated nitrogen gas tank. There is a one-way valve between the chamber and the gas tank that keeps the sealed system above the preset low pressure limit. When the moving piston (top) comes down to compress the hydrogel implant, the volume of the chamber decreases. Because saline and the hydrogel implant are nearly incompressible, the air in the sealed chamber is compressed and pressure (also the stress on the implant) increases. By adjusting the amount of air in the system, the stress range on the implant under cyclic loading (to a predetermined strain range) can simulate the physiologic stress range on the nucleus. Based on the literature data on the physiologic stress and strain during normal activities, the stress range was set between 0.35 ± 0.05 and 0.95 ± 0.15 MPa and the strain range was set between 0% and 20%. This stress range represents the intradiscal pressure for a person jogging with hard street shoes.[9] The test apparatus was immersed in 37°C water bath and the frequency of the cyclic loading is 3 Hz.

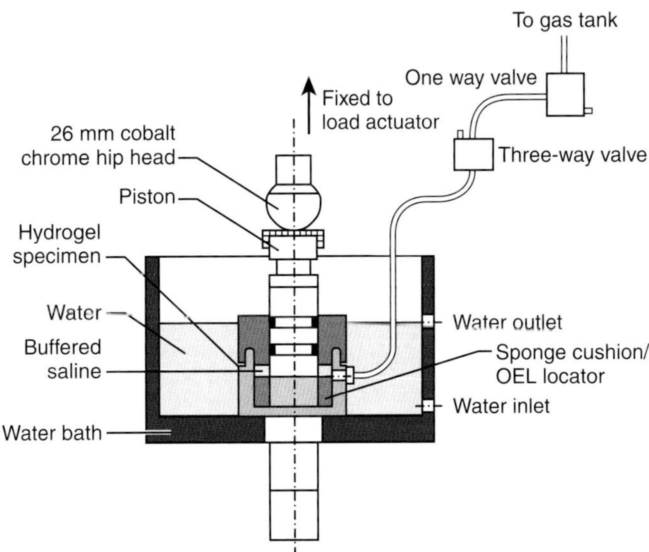


■ **FIGURE 55–4.** Fatigue test apparatus.

A total of six Aquarelle hydrogel samples were tested to 10 M cycles, and two of these samples were tested to 23.5 M cycles. Visual examination was performed, and implant modulus and water content were measured at about every 2-M cycle interval. Over this testing period, no visible implant damage was detected and the implant modulus and water content were maintained over the entire testing period.[10]

From the testing results of this study, it can be concluded that the Aquarelle Hydrogel Nucleus has adequate fatigue strength for the intended application.

## Animal Study—A Baboon Model

The primary purpose of this animal study is to determine the local and systemic safety of the PVA hydrogel for spinal implant applications using a nonhuman primate model. Twenty-eight skeletally mature male baboons were randomized to undergo either discectomy (operative control group) or discectomy followed by implantation of the Aquarelle Hydrogel Device (study group).[11] Animals were sacrificed 1, 3, 6, 12, and 24 months after surgery.

In each animal, the operation was performed on either L3-L4 level or L4-L5 level. In the first 22 animals, an anterior approach was used and the discectomy was performed through the midline annular incision with a 3-mm trephine. Fifteen of these 22 animals were implanted with Aquarelle hydrogel implants, whereas seven of them served as a discectomy control. In the second group of six animals, the surgical technique was modified so that the trephine was inserted through a percutaneous portal in the left flank, and the nucleus pulposus was removed with a 2.5-mm grasper. In the second group, five received the Aquarelle implant and one was used as an operative control. At each time interval, there were 1 to 2 control animals and 3 to 5 study animals. Animal analyses included magnetic resonance imaging, plain x-ray radiography, necropsy, and histopathology.

Six out of 20 (30%) implants extruded from the disc. Although it was difficult to visualize the implant in the MR images when it was in the disc space, it became more visible in T2-weighted images after extrusion due to the water content increase when it was no longer in a highly stressed compartment. All six extrusions were detected at 2-week postoperative MRI examinations.

Radiographic changes in the operated control group were typical of those seen after discectomy and included loss of disc height and the development of osteophytes on the anterior margins of the affected level. There was a trend for progressive osteophyte development over time, and large bridging osteophytes were seen in all of the 6- and 12-month controls. Similar trends were seen in the PVA group, although large bridging osteophytes were seen in only one of three animals in the 6-month PVA group, as compared with two of two in the operated controls.

Microscopic findings from 18 of 23 (78%) animals were unremarkable, with no significant lesions identified in either remote tissues or the spinal cord. Perineuritis was identified in one animal that displayed clinical evidence of nerve root compression, and mild to moderate sinus histiocytosis was seen in the lumbar lymph nodes from 4 animals. Three of the 4 animals had received the PVA device, but in no case was there evidence of particulate PVA debris in the sections.

The microscopic findings in the intervertebral disc were similar in both the operated control and PVA groups. The surgical site was easily identifiable as a cavity in the central region of the disc. The cavity was usually lined with a rim of apparently condensed tissue that showed increasing staining intensity. Within the disc, the fibrocartilage was often frayed in appearance, with signs of both chondrocyte death (empty lacunae) and clone formation, indicative of some form of proliferative response to injury in many specimens.

In the majority of specimens, there appeared to have been some compromise of the end plate, most likely at the time of nucleus removal. End plate damage was associated with variable degrees of cartilage loss, hemorrhage, and invasion of subchondral bone with granulation tissue. End plate damage was seen in 7 of 8 controls and six of 14 PVA specimens. The fact that these changes were seen in both control animals and in animals implanted with PVA suggests that this is not a biocompatibility issue with respect to the PVA device. In addition, the end plate response in the animals with implants was generally greater on the caudal end plate and not uniform around the implant. This suggests that the end plate response can be attributed to the procedure and limited disc height in the model.

Histologic sections from three animals showed evidence of macrophage and giant cell responses to particulate debris. This debris stained blue with Veerhof-Van Gieson stain and red with Congo Red stain, and most likely represents fragmented PVA material. The particles of hydrogel were found within the subchondral bone of the end plate, not in the disc space per se. In each of these specimens, an inflammatory reaction composed primarily of macrophages and giant cells was evident. Particles were not identified in tissues adjacent to the operative sites in any of the other PVA or control specimens. The mechanisms responsible for device fragmentation in these three cases were not apparent from review of the microscope slides alone, although it was interesting to note that the end plates in all three discs showed evidence of damage. The operative site in 6 of 8 control specimens and 12 of 14 PVA specimens demonstrated cellular debris associated with the surface of the fibrocartilage. The debris did not possess the optical properties of the PVA implant and was of uncertain origin. There was no granulation tissue associated with this cellular reaction and no evidence of acute inflammation in the adjacent bone.

The most significant postoperative complication in this study was implant extrusion. Although this high extrusion rate might be due to the limitation of the animal model (large annular window–to–disc cavity dimension ratio), surgical technique, and the high intradiscal pressure for the baboon, the low modulus and highly slippery surfaces of the Aquarelle Hydrogel Nucleus could also be the reasons for this high extrusion rate.

From the perspective of tissue compatibility, the overwhelming evidence supports the biocompatibility of the PVA material. The histopathologic data from soft tissue specimens confirmed that the PVA implant is well tolerated in vivo. There was no evidence of systemic toxicity in these animals, and the only significant microscopic finding was a mild to moderate hyperplasia in the lumbar lymph nodes of three animals from the PVA group and one animal from the operated control group. The significance of these findings is unclear because there was no evidence of PVA debris in the lymph node sections.

Inflammatory responses to particles of PVA were identified in three animals in which the PVA material had become damaged. These particles did not apparently pass to the local lymphatics but were encapsulated by a foreign body-type reaction consisting of macrophages and giant cells. The nature of this reaction was qualitatively similar to that seen associated with particles of other types of polymers currently used in orthopedic surgery, including polyethylene and silicone. There was no evidence of increased osteoclastic activity in these areas.

Microscopic evidence of end plate damage was seen in the majority of animals (13 of 22, 59%) in this study. Every effort was made to preserve the integrity of the end plates during surgery, but the identification of end plate damage in the operated controls indicates that even a simple discectomy poses a risk to the baboon end plate. Based on the histologic data, there was no evidence that insertion of the PVA device per se exacerbated the end plate damage. It should be noted that the baboon lumbar intervertebral disc measures only approximately 5 mm in height, compared with an average of approximately 10 to 12 mm in the human lumbar disc. Evidence of disc degeneration was seen in both control and PVA animals. Degenerative changes appeared to be progressive in both groups, with osteophytes becoming both larger and more common at later time points.

In conclusion, there was no evidence of local or systemic toxicity with PVA devices implanted within the intervertebral disc for periods of up to 24 months. The gross and microscopic pathology of discs implanted with the PVA device were similar to those from discs that had been subject to discectomy. Therefore, the safety of this device has been established.

## CLINICAL PRESENTATION AND EVALUATION

Although Aquarelle was the first hydrogel nucleus device developed by Howmedica, and subsequently by Stryker, which had conducted very extensive preclinical studies on this device, there has been only very limited clinical experience on Aquarelle Hydrogel Nucleus. Although many factors, such as the company's strategy and vision on the motion preservation technology at that time and resource limitations, could be attributed to this slow advancement, implant extrusion in the early clinical trial is undeniably a major reason the company halted further development. Whether this early clinical failure should be considered as a part of the learning curve due to nonoptimized instrument or surgical technique, or is a fatal fundamental design deficiency, remains debatable. Unforturnately, without extensive clinical data, it is difficult to assess the efficacy, especially the benefits of its swelling pressure characteristics, of the Aquarelle Hydrogel Nucleus. However, based on the preclinical data, it is expected that the Aquarelle Hydrogel Nucleus should perform at least the same, if not better, as other nucleus devices.

## OPERATIVE TECHNIQUES

Being a hydrogel with high-equilibrium water content, the Aquarelle device has several options on how it can be implanted. It can be implanted either as a deformable elastomer (fully or semihydrated) or as rigid plastic at fully dehydrated stage. Because for a given size implant the volume is proportional to its water content, it is generally advantageous to implant a hydrogel nucleus device at the fully dehydrated stage or semihydrated stage so the implant has a smaller volume during implantation than later, when it is more hydrated. For a hydrogel with high water content, such as the Aquarelle hydrogel, the volume difference between the fully dehydrated stage and the hydrated stage can be significant. For a 75% water content hydrogel, an implant with 4 mL volume at the hydrated stage has only 1 mL at a fully dehydrated stage. It would be much easier to implant a dry implant with a small volume through a small annular window. Alternatively, the hydrogel nucleus can also be implanted at the semihydrated stage. When implanting at the semihydrated stage, the implant will immediately start sharing load with the annulus and avoid the hydration time, which could be several days. At the semihydrated stage, the implant can be fairly very deformable and inserted through a tapered cannula.

The Aquarelle nucleus was implanted at water content close to its physiologic equilibrium water content. The implant was inserted through a tapered metal cannula with a distal diameter less than 6 mm using a specially designed injector. With such a small distal tip cannula, the Aquarelle can be implanted through the posterior approach, as well as through the lateral or anterolateral approaches.

## POSTOPERATIVE CARE

General postoperative care for the Aquarelle nucleus should be similar to other nucleus devices. Because it is implanted at a semihydrated stage and carries its mechanical function immediate postoperatively, it does require the patient to be on bed rest for a few days for the device to be hydrated.

## COMPLICATIONS AND AVOIDANCE

From the limited clinical experience, the only complication encountered by the Aquarelle nucleus was implant extrusion. A small annular window or a more competent annulus might be important in reducing the implant extrusion.

**ADVANTAGES/DISADVANTAGES: AQUARELLE HYDROGEL DISC NUCLEUS**

| Advantages | Disadvantages |
|---|---|
| Low modulus for uniform load distribution | Highly deformable—high risk of extrusion |
| Swelling pressure similar to the nucleus | Slippery surface—high risk of extrusion |
| Potentially prevent further degeneration | |
| Well-established biocompatibility | |
| Excellent mechanical strength | |

## CONCLUSIONS/DISCUSSION

Compared with other material choices for nucleus replacement, the Aquarelle nucleus has an almost "ideal" material, PVA, for its intended application. The biocompatibility of the PVA hydrogel has been well established through a series of biocompatibility testing, including the carcinogenicity study and the animal study. Although it has a low modulus, the PVA hydrogel has an excellent mechanical strength. The low modulus of the Aquarelle also allows the device to be implanted through a tapered cannula with a distal diameter less than 6 mm. This small cannula makes it feasible to implant the Aquarelle hydrogel from all three major surgical approaches—posterior, lateral, and anterolateral—with the possibility of even posterolateral percutaneous surgery. The water content and the corresponding swelling pressure of the PVA hydrogel are almost identical to that of the natural nucleus. Although many other nucleus replacement devices are composed of different hydrogel materials, to our knowledge, the Aquarelle is the only hydrogel nucleus that has characterized its swelling pressure. Unless the swelling pressure of a hydrogel nucleus has been characterized, the perceived benefit of using a hydrogel to restore the body fluid diffusion remains questionable.

However, sometimes an "ideal" design can also bring more challenges and might take longer to develop compared with some less "ideal" designs. For example, in total disc replacement development, a disc with shock-absorbing capabilities, such as the design of a metal-elastomer-metal, is more "ideal" than a disc without shock-absorbing capabilities, such as the design of a metal-on-metal or metal-on-PE ball-and-socket. Although the development of both of these designs started in the mid 1980s, several of the less ideal total disc designs (ball-and-socket) have either gained premarket approval or been in Investigational Device Exception (IDE) clinical studies, while the discs of the metal-elastomer-metal design are still at the preclinical stage owing to the challenges of debonding of the elastomer-metal interface or the fatigue failure of the elastomer core. The Aquarelle Hydrogel Nucleus has also faced some challenges; mainly implant extrusion, in the early clinical trials. It is believed that this issue will eventually be resolved, maybe with the technology of annular repair or annular retaining devices.

## REFERENCES


1. Bao Q-B, Higham PA, inventors: Hydrogel intervertebral disc nucleus. US patent 5,047,055, September 10, 1991.
2. Ray CD, Dickhudt EA, Ledoux PJ, Frutiger BA, inventors: Prosthetic spinal disc nucleus. US patent 5,674,295, October 7, 1997.
3. Dorland's Illustrated Medical Dictionary, 31st ed. Philadelphia, WB Saunders, 2007.
4. Urban JPG, Smith S, Fairbank CT: Nutrition of the intervertebral disc. Spine 23:2700–2709, 2004.
5. National Toxicology Program TR 474, 1998. http://ntp.niehs.nih.gov/ntp/htdocs/LT_rpts/tr474.pdf
6. Urban JPG, McMullin JF: Swelling pressure of the lumbar intervertebral discs: Influence of age, spinal level, composition and degeneration. Spine 13:179–187, 1988.
7. Bao Q-B, Bagga CS, Higham PA: Swelling Pressure of Hydrogel: A Perceived Benefit for a Spinal Prosthetic Nucleus, 10th Annual Meeting of International Intradiscal Therapy Society, Naples, FL, 1997.
8. Ordway NR, Edwards WT, Han ZH, et al.: Biomechanical Evaluation of the Intervertebral Disc with a Hydrogel Nucleus, 9th Annual Meeting of the North American Spine Society. Minneapolis, MN, 1994
9. Wilke H-J, Neef P, Caimi M, et al: New in vito measurement of pressures in the intervertebral disc in daily life. Spine 24:755–762, 1999.
10. Bagga CS, Williams P, Higham PA, Bao Q-B: Development of Fatigue Test Model for a Spinal Nucleus Prosthesis with Preliminary Results for a Hydrogel Spinal Prosthetic Nucleus. 1997 ASME/AIChE/ASCE Summer Bioengineering Conference, Sunriver, OR.
11. Allen MJ, Schoonmaker JE, Bauer TW, et al: Preclinical evaluation of a poly (vinyl alcohol) hydrogel implant as a replacement for the nucleus pulposus. Spine 29:515–523, 2004.

CHAPTER 56

# BioDisc Nucleus Pulposus Replacement

Douglas Wardlaw

## KEY POINTS

- Biocompatible hydrogel prepared for immediate injection.
- Ideal patient has sciatica due to a soft disc herniation at L4-L5 or L5-S1.
- Repairs the disc following discectomy.
- No immediate complications.
- Mobilization immediately without changing practice.

## INTRODUCTION

Low back pain (LBP) is very common in Western societies, with the majority of disc herniations occurring in the L4-L5 and L5-S1 segments of the spine. Sciatica caused by lumbar disc herniations is the most common cause of radicular pain. The majority of patients with herniations recover with a course of nonsurgical treatment involving physical therapy and analgesics within 4 to 6 weeks, but in some patients, surgery is required for persistent and severe symptoms. Standard open or microdiscectomy is usually the preferred surgical treatment for lumbar disc herniations. Favorable outcomes have been reported in the literature ranging from 49% to 90%, although residual LBP and recurrent herniation are still problems for some patients following a discectomy.[1] The residual disrupted discs must continue to endure the weight of the patient for the remainder of his or her life.[2] A discectomy changes the mechanics of the disc with the removal of the nucleus pulposus. Several studies have demonstrated that 20% to 40% of patients who have had a lumbar discectomy have persistent or recurrent sciatica, intractable back pain, or recurrent disc herniation.[3] Carragee et al[1] reported reherniation rates at 6 months, 1 year, 2 years, and 5 years were 0.7%, 5.2%, 7.7%, and 11.5%, respectively.

While taking into account the functions of the normal nucleus, investigators have been drawn to the use of hydrogels as a nucleus replacement. Hydrogels closely mimic the functions of a normal nucleus because their water content mimics the hydrostatic load-bearing and load distribution properties of an intact disc.[4] An in situ curable implant can be implanted through a small annulotomy as opposed to a preformed implant, which requires a larger annular incision. The smaller annulotomy could reduce the risk of extrusion of the implant.[4] BioDisc Nucleus Pulposus Replacement (CryoLife, Inc., Kennesaw, GA) is an in situ polymerizing protein hydrogel proposed as an adjunct for in-patients undergoing discectomy. BioDisc is intended to fill the void space within the disc nucleus and repair the annulus following removal of the herniation and part of the nucleus pulposus in the treatment of lumbar intervertebral disc herniations. It is designed to prevent or reduce the incidence of instability and long-term LBP.

## INDICATIONS AND CONTRAINDICATIONS

BioDisc is intended to fill the void space within the disc annulus following discectomy to treat patients undergoing surgery for sciatica due to acute disc herniation. It is recommended as an addition to the standard surgical procedure with the partial replacement of the nucleus pulposus and repair of the annulus. BioDisc is designed to preserve disc height, reduce lumbar motion segment instability, and reduce recurrent disc herniation.

BioDisc is contraindicated in any patient with a known sensitivity to materials of bovine origin and glutaraldehyde. Additionally, BioDisc is contraindicated in any patient with large annular tears or rents, recurrent disc herniation, herniation in association with spondylolisthesis, dominant LBP, presence of infection, and disc narrowing greater than 60%.

## DESCRIPTION OF THE DEVICE

BioDisc is a biopolymer consisting of a protein-based hydrogel. The solutions are dispensed by a controlled delivery system composed of a delivery device and delivery tips (Fig. 56–1). On dispensing, the solutions (in a predefined ratio) are mixed in the delivery tip, where cross-linking begins. The glutaraldehyde molecules cross-link the BSA molecules to each other and to the recipient's proteins at the repair site by covalent bonds, creating a flexible, viscoelastic hydrogel implant that is chemically bonded to the patient's tissues. The delivery device–mediated implantation is designed to provide reproducible mixing of the components in vitro. Surgery is carried out with the patient in the prone

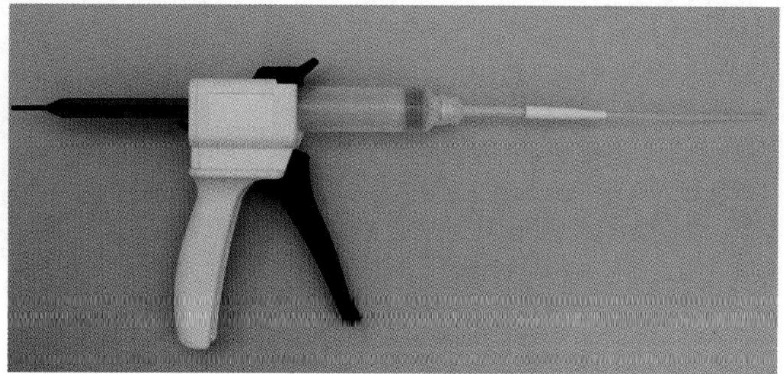

■ **FIGURE 56–1.** BioDisc assembled delivery device.

position, and the mixed components of BioDisc are injected through the annulotomy until the material is seen to fill the void. Polymerization begins immediately, and setting occurs in 20 to 30 seconds. Full strength is reached within 2 minutes (Fig. 56–2).

## BACKGROUND OF SCIENTIFIC TESTING/CLINICAL OUTCOMES

The full battery of International Organization for Standardization (ISO) 10993 biocompatibility studies has been performed for the BioDisc implant material. Additionally, all product-contacting components of the BioDisc delivery system have passed USP Class VI testing.

BioDisc is a biopolymer consisting of a protein-based hydrogel. Axial compression and creep tests determined the biopolymer has reproducible modulus and yield point, and that the material achieved 100% height recovery upon removal of the load. Cyclic axial compression (fatigue test) run out to 10 million cycles (10 Mc) has been completed for unconstrained coupons of the biopolymer and a stress-durability curve constructed indicating durability.

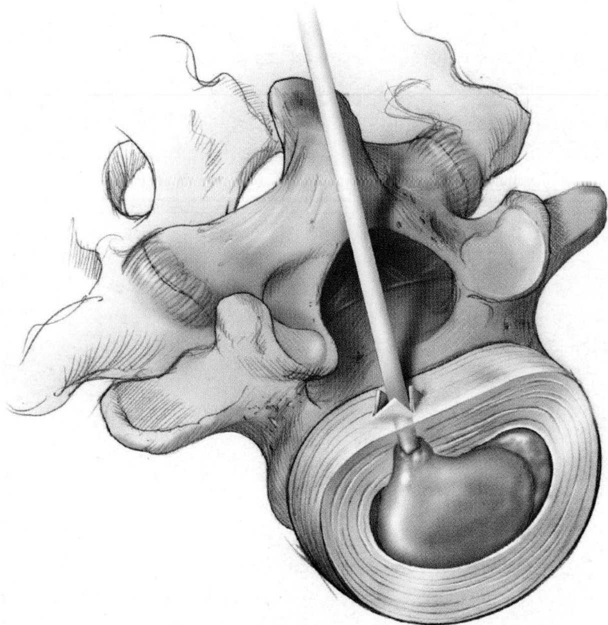

■ **FIGURE 56–2.** BioDisc.

Because BioDisc polymerizes in situ within the denucleated disc cavity, the BioDisc implant, the disc annulus, and the adjacent vertebrae were considered a construct, and were tested as a single unit. The noncyclic properties of the construct were evaluated in vitro with a BioDisc implant in calf spine bone-disc-bone motion segments, with the posterior elements removed. In motion segments without the posterior elements, the axial load is carried only by the annulus and nucleus, and the angular motion (flexion/extension, lateral bending, and torsion) is limited only by the elasticity of the fibers of the annulus. These data suggest that the BioDisc implantation restored the biomechanical properties of the motion segments that were compromised on denucleation.

The calf spine bone-disc-bone motion segments were also used to evaluate the fatigue properties of the construct. After more than 10 Mc cyclic axial compression, the BioDisc construct ($n = 18$) and native motion segments showed no statistical difference in moduli (analysis of variance [ANOVA], $P > 0.05$). Run out of the construct, samples in flexion/extension ($n = 6$) and lateral bending ($n = 7$) has been restricted by tissue decay experienced during testing. After 5 Mc of fatigue, there were no statistical differences (ANOVA, $P > 0.05$) between the range of motion of the native motion segments and the BioDisc constructs.

Wear debris generation and expulsion are common concerns for devices implanted into motion segments. Because the BioDisc implant is strictly a nucleus repair, has no moving parts, and covalently binds to the disc annulus, no wear debris generation from the implant is anticipated. Filtrates from the motion segments used for fatigue testing ($n = 21$), examined using up to 20× magnification, have not shown any wear particles. Potential expulsion was also addressed during compressive and angular load fatigue testing, in addition to a specifically designed extrusion test. In the latter model, an impact load capable of generating vertebral fractures was applied to motion segments that were denucleated, and then implanted with gelatine (positive control), epoxy resin (negative control), or BioDisc (test article). Results have demonstrated no extrusion of BioDisc in any of the motion segments tested.

Aged human cadaver lumbar spines were studied using manually pressurized contrast discography and computed tomography (CT) scanning to demonstrate naturally occurring degenerative radial and circumferential lamellar tears. Contrast was removed by saline perfusion using the same technique as discography. These segments were then discectomized using a standard posterolateral laminotomy approach. The nuclear void was filled with BioDisc under direct visualization through the surgical annulotomy using minimal delivery pressure (Fig. 56–3).

The morphology of BioDisc was compared with the annular defects demonstrated on discography, CT, or both. Additionally, iatrogenic annular defects were created with a #2 straight curette and studied using the same techniques to determine if surgical error could lead to escape of the implant material. The implanted discs were imaged using magnetic resonance imaging (MRI) and CT, and then sectioned to observe the morphologic characteristics of the implant. BioDisc was noted to completely fill the center of the discectomy void, as well as the peripheral interstices, and appeared to bind firmly to the surrounding nuclear and annular

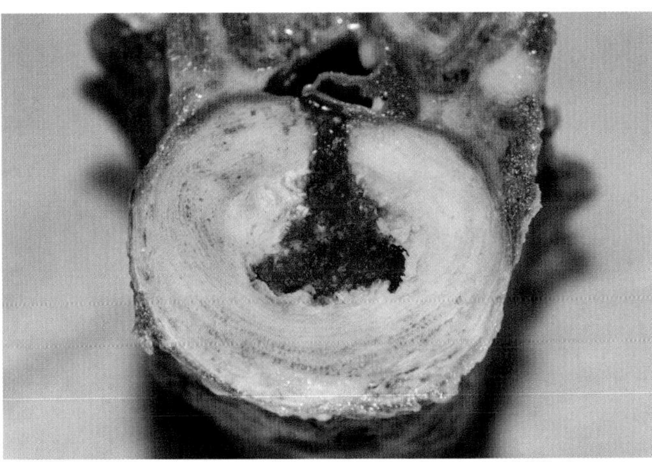

■ FIGURE 56–3. Cadaver spine.

tissue. No inadvertent, extra-annular leakage was observed through natural or iatrogenic annular defects, presumably due to the slowing of hydrogel flow by its rapid polymerization (Fig. 56–4).

Eleven patients have now had surgery in a safety study. No intraoperative or immediate postoperative complications have been encountered, and all patients had relief of their leg pain immediately on recovery from the anesthetic. The follow-up data will be presented and published when available following follow-up.

## CLINICAL PRESENTATION AND EVALUATION

Suitable patients for BioDisc have an intervertebral disc herniation of a lumbar spinal disc causing radicular pain, with or without LBP. Therapy with at least 6 weeks physical therapy with a course of drugs/analgesics should have been ineffective to resolve the patient's pain. There should be a proven disc herniation on CT or MRI with no more than mild disc narrowing (Fig. 56–5A and B).

## OPERATIVE TECHNIQUES

General anesthesia with induced hypotension is recommended to minimize bleeding. Position the patient in the standard prone position, preferably on a frame that avoids abdominal compression to reduce bleeding.

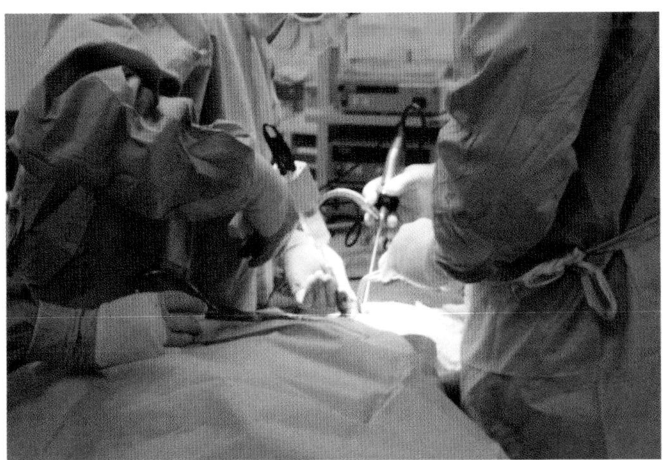

■ FIGURE 56–4. Surgical procedure.

### The Surgical Procedure

BioDisc implantation uses the standard technique for open standard discectomy or microdiscectomy for surgical treatment of lumbar disc herniations. Perform a standard exposure for an open discectomy at the level of herniation. Mobilize and retract the paraspinous muscles to expose the interlaminar space and ligamentum flavum. Remove bone of the laminar edges and facet joint as needed. Reflect or remove the ligamentum flavum to expose the dura and nerve root. Carefully mobilize the root and dura of the cauda equina medially and maintain retraction. Incise the herniation with a cruciate incision, and carefully remove the herniation with a MacDonalds dissector and pituitary rongeurs. If necessary, further incise the annulus to create a cruciate-type incision and fold the corners back to create a clear opening. It is important to remove as much of the nucleus material as possible, while preserving the integrity of the cartilaginous end plates and annulus. Enlarge the "shoulders" of the cavity laterally and medially to produce a mushroom-shaped cavity. Dry out the nuclear void and protect the surrounding tissues, nerve roots, and dura, if necessary, with moist cottonoids to prevent BioDisc from adhering to these tissues. Prime the delivery tip by depressing the syringe, and start the flow of components onto a dry cottonoid positioned next to the hole in the annulus (according to the instructions for use). Without interrupting the flow, transfer the delivery tip into the annulotomy. Fill the nuclear void under direct visualization, with a smooth consistent delivery. Watch the level of the BioDisc implant rise within the annular defect to the level of the annulus. Fold the corners of the annulotomy over the BioDisc material. After 2 minutes, the implant is firm and secure. Inspect the site and carefully remove any excess BioDisc material to ensure that the implant is level with the posterior annulus. Release neural retraction, and allow nerve structures to return to their anatomic positions and ensure that they lie freely within the spinal canal. Inspect all areas closely for any BioDisc material outside the disc space, especially the adjacent root canal, before wound closure. Any extraneous material should be carefully removed. Release the ligamentum flavum and place into natural position. Inspect the wound to ensure that there is no significant bleeding and no cerebrospinal fluid leakage. Close wound in the standard fashion.

## POSTOPERATIVE CARE

Postoperative care for a patient with BioDisc is no different from the standard of care for a discectomy patient. Patients can be mobilized as soon as comfortable later the same day. A lumbar support is recommended to discourage lumbar flexion for the first 6 weeks.

## COMPLICATIONS AND AVOIDANCE

A similar material has been used in vascular and neurosurgery for about 10 years without encountering any adverse reactions due to the material. BioDisc is in the early stages of clinical investigation as a partial disc or nuclear replacement in patients with disc herniation with mild loss of disc height.

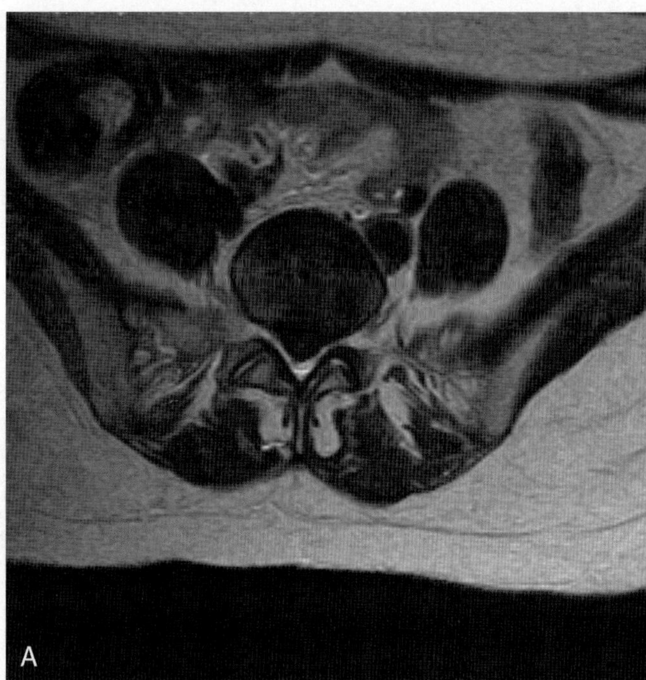


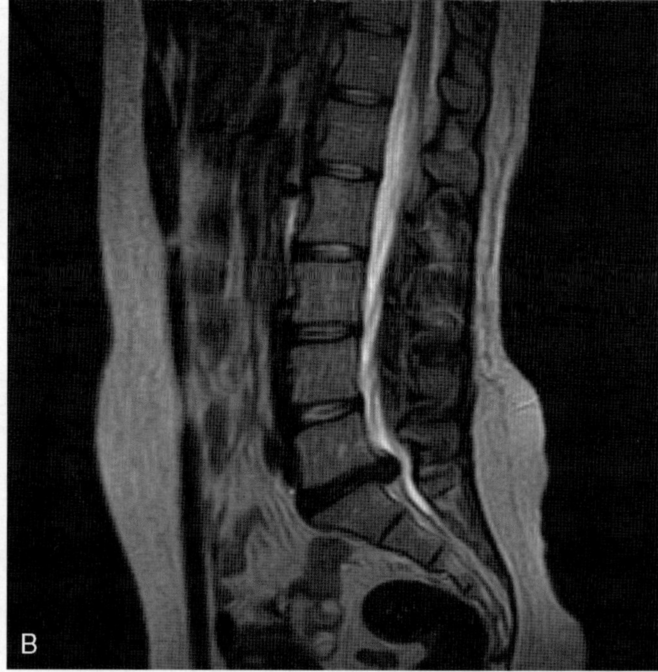


■ FIGURE 56–5. **A,** Axial view of the spine. **B,** Parasagittal view of the spine.

**ADVANTAGES/DISADVANTAGES: BIODISC NUCLEUS PULPOSUS REPLACEMENT**

- BioDisc provides an immediate intraoperative nuclear repair for patients with a herniated lumbar intervertebral disc. It can be inserted at routine disc surgery with little modification of the surgical procedure. The procedure adds very little to the surgery time, and routine postoperative care is followed.
- There are no evident disadvantages to its use.

## CONCLUSIONS/DISCUSSION

Recurrent disc herniation and continuing leg and LBP following surgery are relatively frequent short-term and long-term complications and a source of continued morbidity for patients. Any material that can potentially prevent or significantly reduce these complications must merit study. BioDisc is one such material and has great potential as an addition to routine surgery. It requires little additional expertise and appears to have no significant complications. Two-year follow-up of the safety study is under way, and a multicenter prospective randomized study comparing routine surgery with the addition of BioDisc to surgery alone is being organized.

## ACKNOWLEDGMENTS

I wish to acknowledge the contribution of Linda Tedder, Cryolife, Inc., for photographs, description of the device, and background of scientific testing, and Rachel Venables for her assistance with the general preparation of this chapter.

## REFERENCES

1. Carragee EJ, Han MY, Yang BS, et al: Activity restrictions after posterior lumbar discectomy. Spine 24:2343–2351, 1999.
2. Yorimitsu E, Chiba K, Tayaama Y, Hirabayashi K: Long-term outcomes of standard discectomy for lumbar disc herniations: A follow-up study of more than 10 years. Spine 26:652–657, 2001.
3. Carragee EJ, Han MY, Suen PW, Kim DH: Clinical outcomes after lumbar discectomy for sciatica: The effects of fragment type and anular competence. J Bone Joint Surg Am 85A:102–108, 2003.
4. Goins ML, Wimberley DW, Yuan PS, et al: Nucleus pulposus replacement: An emerging technology. Spine 5(6):317S–324S, 2005.

CHAPTER 57

# TranS1 Percutaneous Nucleus Replacement

Roberto Díaz, Luiz Pimenta, Hazem Nicola, Larry T. Khoo, Rick Sasso, Bradley J. Wessman, and Andrew H. Cragg

## KEY POINTS

- The Percutaneous Nucleus Replacement (PNR) is intended to restore the function of the intervertebral disc by restoring disc height and internal disc pressure via a transsacral approach.
- The nuclectomy, mechanical distraction, and PNR insertion are accomplished through a single small incision.
- Proper tensioning of the preserved annulus fibrosis allows distribution of loads across the vertebral end plates using a load-bearing elastomeric polymer.
- The PNR is contained by the annulus and thus functions biomechanically in a similar manner as the intact disc.
- Early results indicate that the TranS1 PNR provides safe and reliable relief of discogenic pain at L5-S1.

## INTRODUCTION

Recently, Cragg et al[1] described the technique of minimally invasive axial access to the L5-S1 disc space. In this technique, a small incision is made in the paracoccygeal region and a probe is advanced through the presacral space until it is aligned on the anterior sacrum with a point in the middle of the L5-S1 interspace. An axial working channel is created into the disc space that allows passage of instruments for discectomy and, in the case of fusion, osseous filler, and an axial distraction and fixation rod.

This approach to the spine for fusion has been validated both experimentally and clinically. Tobler[2] evaluated 25 initial patients. The mean preoperative score on the Visual Analog Scale (VAS) was 66 mm, with a mean preoperative Oswestry Disability Index (ODI) of 49%. By the 3-month follow-up visit the mean VAS was 42 mm, with a mean ODI of 30%. At 6 months, the VAS and ODI continued to decrease to 35 mm and 29%, respectively. The investigator reports that of 19/21 subjects that have 6-month CTs, are fused or are in stages of fusion, for example, bridging and/or developing bone.

For lumbosacral fusion, axial disc access has provided several distinct benefits over posterolateral or anterior minimally invasive approaches.

The TranS1 Percutaneous Nucleus Replacement (PNR) (TranS1, Wilmington, NC) is inserted in the same axial fashion as the fusion construct. This motion-preserving device is intended to restore the function of the motion segment complex by restoring disc height and internal disc pressure, resulting in proper tensioning of the disc annulus, allowing normal loading patterns and motion segment mechanics.

By preserving the integrity of the annulus, there may be less morbidity with insertion, less risk of extrusion with use, and no destabilization of the disc complex. Radial disc removal through a transsacral access may also allow for more complete nucleus removal than can be achieved with minimally invasive posterolateral approaches. The ability to produce disc height distraction during deployment of the device may allow placement of appropriately sized more efficacious nucleus replacement devices.

This chapter discusses our initial experience with the TranS1 PNR (Fig. 57–1).

## INDICATIONS/CONTRAINDICATIONS

The PNR is indicated for spinal arthroplasty in skeletally mature patients with degenerative disc disease (DDD) of the L5-S1 level alone or both the L5-S1 and L4-L5 levels. DDD is defined as discogenic back pain with degeneration of the disc confirmed by patient history and radiographic studies. These patients with DDD should have more back pain than leg pain, and at least six months of conservative treatment should have been ineffective in relieving the pain.

Use of the PNR is contraindicated when the patient is diagnosed with spondylolisthesis higher than grade 1 or scoliosis greater than 10 degrees. The PNR should not be used with degenerated facets or nerve root impingement due to disc herniation, and it should be used cautiously on patients with a ruptured annulus. Patients with known allergy or sensitivity to implant materials are also contraindicated.

## DESCRIPTION OF THE DEVICE

The PNR consists of two threaded titanium vertebral body anchors connected by a cylindrical, silicone rubber membrane

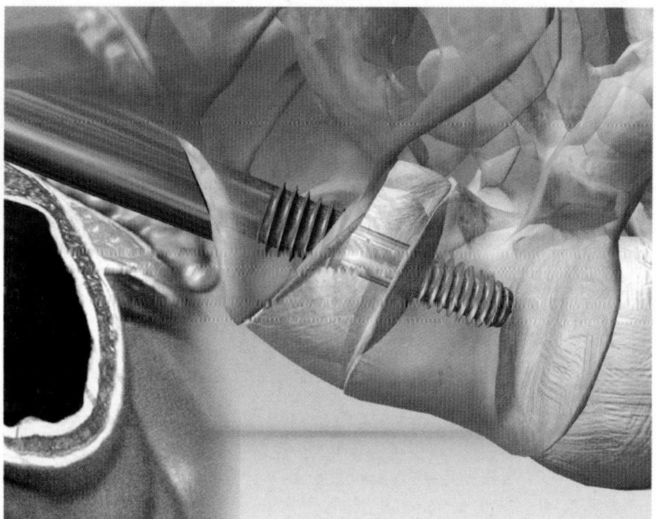

■ **FIGURE 57–1.** TranS1 Percutaneous Nucleus Replacement (PNR) at L5-S1.

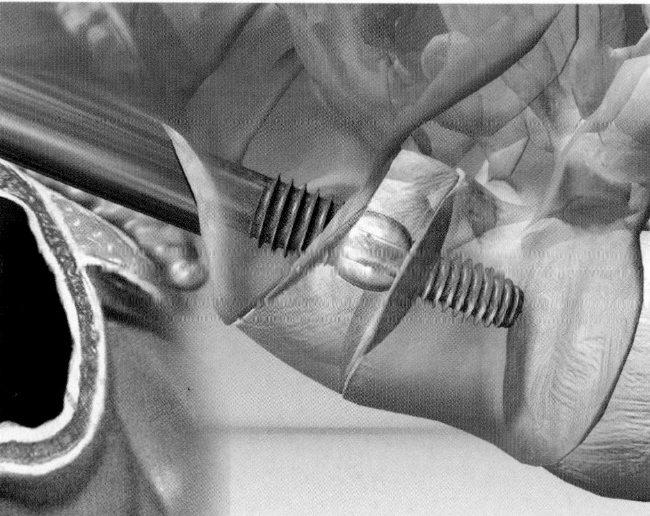

■ **FIGURE 57–2.** Image of TranS1 Percutaneous Nucleus Replacement (PNR) with unexpanded nucleus replacement.

(Table 57–1, Fig. 57–2). Following an end plate–sparing discectomy using the PNR access and discectomy instrumentation, this construct is mounted on a stainless steel and titanium delivery device for axial implantation using the same techniques as the approved AxiaLIF fusion construct.

The delivery device holds the anchors in fixed axial and radial position and simultaneously transmits torque to advance the anchors for positioning within the vertebral bodies. Distraction of the disc space is achieved through a differential thread pitch between the proximal and distal vertebral body anchors.

The delivery device is cannulated and the driver tip is fenestrated, thus allowing infusion of flowable, in situ curing silicone rubber into the expandable silicone membrane within the disc space (Fig. 57–3). This in situ curable silicone rubber consists of two separate polymers and a catalyst to initiate cross-linking of the polymers into a permanently elastic silicone rubber. The materials are low viscosity and delivered to the expandable membrane within the disc through the delivery device until the denucleated, distracted disc space is filled.

The mixed materials cross-link to form elastomeric silicone rubber in approximately 5 minutes at body temperature. The cross-linking reaction is nonexothermic, does not result in the production of other materials (non–out gassing). The material produced is a radiopaque, low-durometer rubber with high mechanical properties (tensile strength, elongation, and tear strength) and excellent resistance to flattening and permanent deformation.

Once the device is implanted, the vertebral body anchors are load-bearing only to the extent of the equivalent cross-sectional area of the end plate. There is no fixed shape or size for the silicone implant, the material fills all of the volume created during the discectomy and subsequent distraction, regardless of shape. The silicone material has a low durometer and acts as an incompressible fluid within the intact annulus. This material transfers compressive loads on the disc into tensile loads (hoop stress) on the annulus, resulting in even distribution of loads across the vertebral body end plate. This was the function of the natural annulus, but loss of hydration in the disc decreases the volume of the nucleus and requires that the annulus bear more axial load than in a healthy disc.

**TABLE 57–1. Percutaneous Nucleus Replacement (PNR) Device Description**

| |
|---|
| The PNR implant consists of two titanium vertebral body anchors connected by a silicone membrane, available in overall lengths of 40, 45, and 50 mm. |
| The diameter of the distal and proximal vertebral body anchors is 11 and 14 mm, respectively, with the proximal vertebral body anchor available with either 9 or 10 threads per inch (TPI). |
| The distal vertebral body anchor is available with thread pitches of 10, 11, and 12 TPI. |
| By using an implant with a differential thread pitch, disc space distractions can be attained during implant insertion. |
| The implant is available in nine configurations of varying lengths and thread pitch differentials. |

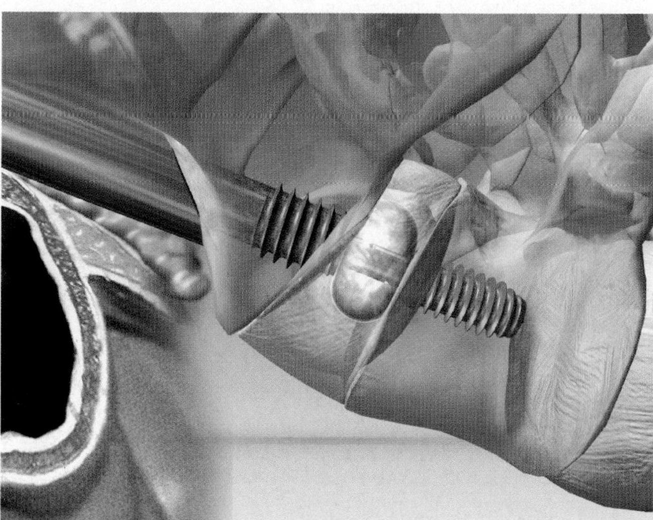

■ **FIGURE 57–3.** Infusion of flowable, in situ curing silicone rubber into the expandable silicone membrane within the disc space.

## BACKGROUND OF SCIENTIFIC TESTING

A biomechanical study was performed to evaluate the effect of the PNR implant on the kinematics of the L5-S1 spinal motion segment. Human cadaveric lumbar spine segments (L4-S1) were mounted in custom-made, six degrees of freedom spinal motion test fixture, and preloaded to 400 N of axial compression using a follower load. Test specimens were loaded to 7.5 Nm in axial torsion, lateral bending, and flexion extension. Spine specimens were initially tested intact to establish a baseline for disc height and range of motion (ROM) and to characterize the neutral zone. The specimens were then tested after discectomy to simulate degenerative disc disease. Finally, the specimens were tested after implantation of the PNR. This testing demonstrated the ability of the PNR to restore intact disc height and motion kinematics.

Fatigue testing was performed on the nucleus replacement material to evaluate the durability of this material under physiologic loading conditions. The PNR is intended to function constrained within an intact annulus with a maximum axial compression of approximately 2 to 3 mm. In order to simulate the worst-case scenario, the samples were tested unconstrained to 50% axial compression (i.e., 5 mm) for 10 million cycles in physiologic saline.[3–5] This testing is intended to simulate at least 10 years of normal activity. No material failures resulted from this fatigue testing.

Biocompatibility testing is being conducted per International Organization for Standardization (ISO) 10993 guidelines. The PNR is considered a class III spinal implant device for long-term implantation (i.e., >30 days) in contact with tissue and bone. Tests include cytotoxicity, acute systemic toxicity, subchronic toxicity, chronic toxicity, sensitization, irritation, genotoxicity, and implantation.

In addition to the ISO 10993 testing requirements, the silicone materials are being tested for extractable and leachable components using saline, isopropyl alcohol, and bovine serum as extract media.

Owing to the proximity of this device to the spinal canal, animal studies will be conducted to evaluate the response to particulate wear debris in contact with the dura. Because this device has no articulating surfaces, the quantity and size distribution of particles chosen for this study is consistent with studies conducted on other spinal devices.[6–8]

## CLINICAL OUTCOMES

### Methods

Twenty-six consecutive partial lumbar disc arthroplasty in patients ($n = 26$) were performed with use of the PNR between 2005 and 2006. Careful review of the charts, operative notes, preoperative and postoperative radiographs, magnetic resonance images, and follow-up records of all patients was performed. VAS, Sf-36, and ODI were performed to determine clinical outcome and radiologic follow-up. Patients were reviewed at 1-, 3-, 6-, 9-, and 12-month intervals after the surgery. An independent radiologist evaluated all radiologic control studies. Data were analyzed using unpaired Student's t-test. *P* values less than 0.05 were considered statistically significant.

### Results

Between September 2005 and June 2006, 26 subjects who were radiographically and clinically confirmed with a diagnosis of DDD were implanted with the PNR. All patients had clinical, functional, and radiographic follow-up examinations. The study subjects (12 women and 14 men) averaged 43 years, ranging from 29 to 62 years of age. Mean operative time was 78 minutes, with average blood loss of less than 50 mL. Subjects were able to take their first unassisted walk in an average of 11 hours (7 to 13 hours) after implantation.

Clinical outcomes measured pain (VAS) and disability related to pain (ODI). All subjects had a decrease in the severity of pain (89 mm to 52 mm) at the time of hospital discharge. At the 3-week follow-up, their mean VAS had decreased to 31 mm and ODI had improved from a preoperative average of 56% to 27%.

The results demonstrated that the PNR device was effective in most of the patients who underwent surgery. After implantation, most patients experienced relief of pain. Five patients had persistent pain after implantation of the PNR and underwent uneventful anterolateral or posterolateral interbody fusion. Improvements were noted in pain intensity, walking distance, lumbar mobility, and neurologic weakness, ODI scores, intervertebral disc height, and segmental ROM. No difference in work status after PNR implantation could be detected. Compared with the preoperative height, the patients who had the intervertebral disc had gained 18.3% ($P < 0.05$). In contrast to other nucleus replacement technologies, no Modic changes were observed radiographically at 12 months.[9] However, long-term follow-up of PNR implantation needs to be studied further. A representative case study is illustrated in Figure 57–4.

## PATIENT PREPARATION AND OPERATIVE TECHNIQUE

The following steps should be followed in addition to standard spine surgery preparation and standard bowel preparation for barium enema. The procedure is undertaken with the patient under general anesthesia, and the patient is positioned prone on a radiolucent operative table. A 20-French catheter is optionally inserted into the rectum, and the rectum is insufflated with 30 mL air to provide for visualization of the rectum during lateral fluoroscopy. This tube is isolated with an occlusive dressing that is placed to separate it from the paracoccygeal working area.

A fluoroscopic C-arm is then brought into the surgical field to provide for real-time lateral and anteroposterior imaging during the entire procedure. The operative area is prepped and draped in the usual sterile fashion. An adhesive barrier dressing is applied to the skin. A 15-mm incision is made on the skin 20 mm caudal to the left or right paracoccygeal notch. After a local anesthetic containing 25% bupivacaine (Marcaine) with 1:200,000 epinephrine has been applied to the area, a No. 15 blade is use to incise the skin and underlying fascia. Blunt finger dissection is used to enter through the opening to ensure that the fascia is appropriately opened. The remainder of the access approach is followed similar to the AxiaLIF technique, as described by Pimenta and Khoo.[10]

Next, the surgeon performs a partial volumetric discectomy using a variety of proprietary cutting-loop devices and disc extractors specially designed for a transsacral approach. These

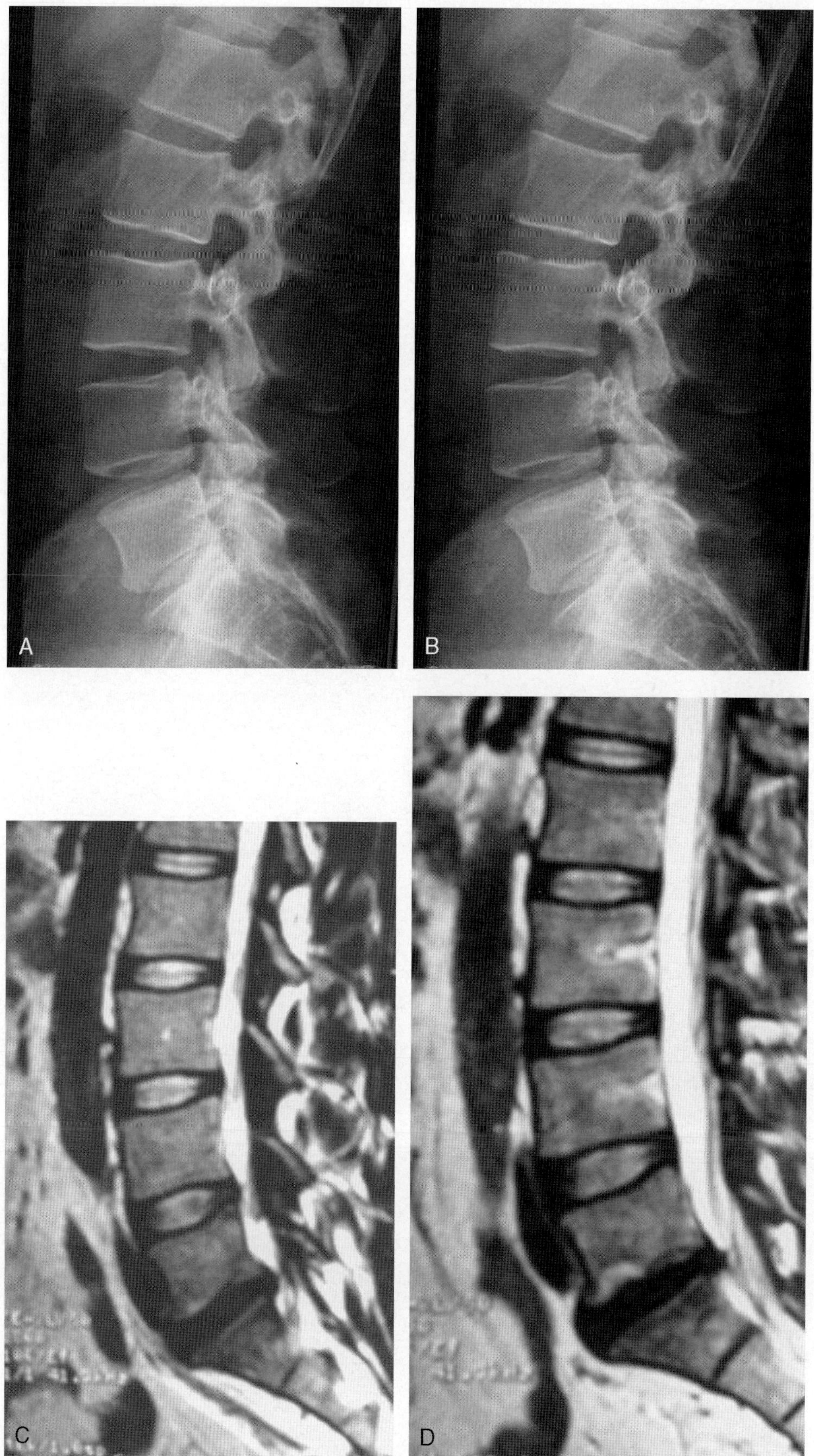

■ **FIGURE 57–4.** Case study: 37-year-old man who underwent discectomy at L5-S1 1 year ago for persistent low back pain. **A–D,** Preoperative images.

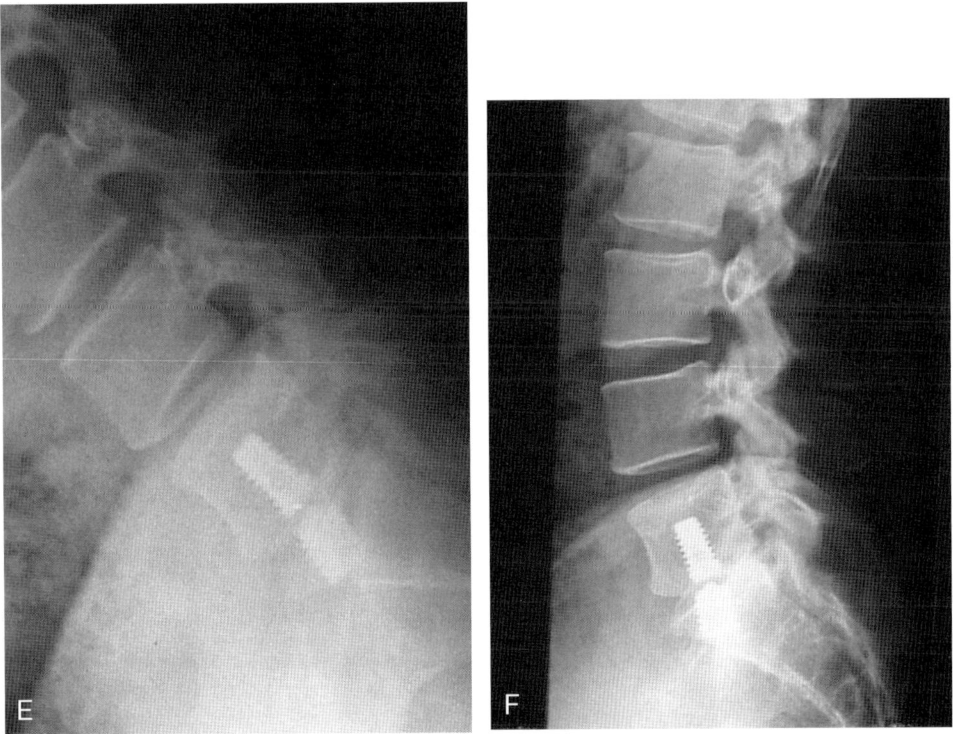


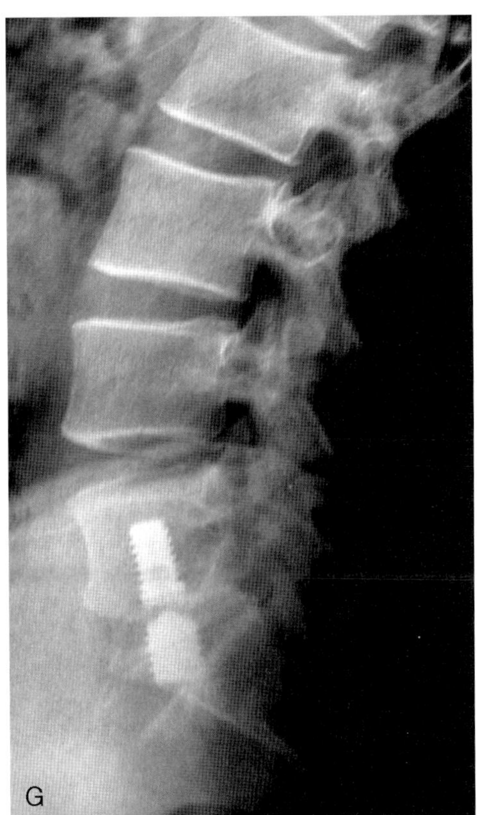


■ **FIGURE 57–4. Cont'd.** **E–G,** Six-week postoperative images with implanted PNR.

devices are composed of cutting-loops made from nitinol memory metal that allows for introduction through a working sheath in a straight coaxial fashion. Once it is advanced out of the introducer sheath, however, the loop will return to a preset angle and curvature to allow a variety of cutting angles and length. These cutting loops are passed into the L5-S1 disc space sequentially under fluoroscopic guidance to complete a rotation-type discectomy. In addition, these cutting loops are designed to cut only disc material, leaving an intact end plate in order to maintain the integrity of a major part of the disc and restore the natural biomechanics of the spine segment. After volumetric discectomy has been completed, a 7.5-mm diameter drill is inserted through the working sheath and intervertebral space, penetrating directly into the L5 vertebral body under biplanar fluoroscopic guidance. Once the trajectory has been reconfirmed, the 7.5-mm bit is rotated and advanced to within 1 cm of the superior L5 end plate. The reamer is then removed, and a final guide pin is inserted through the dilator sheath that is then removed. A larger introducer cannula is inserted over the final guide pin to permit placement of the PNR.

Before advancing the implant into the sacrum and then through the L5-S1 disc space, an 11-mm dilator is advanced through the sacral tract. The implant thread differential will cause the vertebral bodies to distract as the implant is threaded into position. The PNR implant is advanced under fluoroscopic guidance until the membrane is centered within the L5-S1 disc space. The guide wire is removed, and the distal anchor plug is introduced.

The nucleus replacement material is delivered through the PNR Delivery Device into the expandable membrane of the PNR within the denucleated L5-S1 disc space. The material will expand the membrane and fill the entire denucleated and distracted volume of the disc space through a 50-mL side-by-side double-barrel syringe.

## POSTOPERATIVE CARE

Return to walking is indicated after 4 hours of surgery and an unrestricted diet is started 8 hours postoperatively. The patient is observed in the hospital for 24 hours. Medications include antibiotics and analgesics. Front and lateral standing x-ray studies are made after 12 hours.

Patients are discharged with nonsteroidal anti-inflammatory drugs per mouth for 1 week, with some activities, like driving a car and lifting heavy weights, being restricted for 10 days.

Follow-up visits at 1 and 3 weeks, 3, 12, and 24 months, with front, lateral, Fergusson view, and flexion-extension x- ray studies are requested.

## COMPLICATIONS AND AVOIDANCE

Appropriate selection of a patient with DDD should be verified for discogenic pain at operative level through provocative discography. One may consider facet block to eliminate the facet joints as primary pain generators. Evaluate magnetic resonance images and patient history to eliminate the risk of ruptured annulus or prior discectomy and to assess the relative degree of back pain versus leg pain.

Liberal use of fluoroscopic guidance during midline access steps should mitigate nerve, vessel, or bowel damage during access. Use extra caution when performing access steps on very thin patients.

To reduce the possibility of infection, perform a preoperative bowel preparation and consider use of prophylactic antibiotics to lavage the denucleated disc space and presacral space. Do not reuse instruments in the same procedure for any other access approach.

During the nucleus removal step, maintain a 6-mm annulus margin anteriorly and a 3-mm margin posteriorly. Do not cut end plates down to the bone; use only PNR end plate sparing and serrated cutters. Properly size the implant per the technique indicated and distract to achieve the disc height equivalent to that of the next adjacent healthy segment.

**ADVANTAGES/DISADVANTAGES: TRANS1 PERCUTANEOUS NUCLEUS REPLACEMENT (PNR)**

**Advantages**

- Full volume discectomy
- Soft tissue and annular sparing
- Restore disc height, neural foramen, and facet alignment
- PNR allows full physiologic L5-S1 ROM
  - 15 degrees of flexion
  - 10 degrees of extension
  - 5 degrees of L/R Lateral Bending
  - 2 degrees of L/R Axial Rotation
  - Mobile IAR
- Provides cushioning of the motion segment
  - Transfer hydrostatic pressure within the nuclear space into tensile "hoop stresses" in the annulus.
- Does not adversely affect the stiffness of the motion segment or adjacent levels
- PNR is revisable, removable, and convertible to fusion
- Material is safe, free of wear debris, and has a modulus of elasticity that mimics the native nucleus

**Disadvantages**

- Not suitable for stenosis, instability, or facet arthrosis
- Not suitable for patients who have a disrupted annulus
- Cannot perform isolated L4-L5
- Does not relieve facet disease
- Known allergy or sensitivity to implant materials

## CONCLUSIONS/DISCUSSION

The insertion of the TranS1 PNR is feasible because of the novel axial transsacral access to the lumbar spine. The access has been used in a large population of patients who have undergone fusion, and it has been found to be safe and reproducible.

The TranS1 PNR is a unique motion preservation device that can restore height and function to a diseased motion segment without violating the paraspinal tissues and annulus, and is intended for use at L5-S1 alone, at both L5-S1 and L4-L5, or at either level in conjunction with a transsacral fusion.

The PNR is intended for patients with discogenic back pain due to DDD or patients with both back and leg pain in whom the back pain is more severe than the leg pain, not for patients whose primary symptom is leg pain, patients who have experienced a disc herniation with nucleus extrusion, or patients who have previously undergone a discectomy.

The PNR instrumentation system permits a reproducible, transsacral approach that is key to enabling the complete reconstruction of the lumbar disc complex. Proprietary nucleus removal tools efficiently release and remove nucleus pulposus without damaging the cartilaginous end plates. The degree of nucleus removal is controlled by the surgeon through fluoroscopic guidance.

A key benefit of the implant is the ability to mechanically restore disc height and, therefore, proper foraminal and facet alignment as well as annulus tension, before the introduction of the in situ curing elastomeric nucleus replacement material.

During the pilot study experience, the authors also found the implant to be completely revisable and convertible to a lumbar fusion without the common morbidities of traversing a previous surgical approach, for example, ALIF, PLIF, or TLIF.

Finally, the PNR is unique among all disc arthroplasty devices in the ability to completely restore a degenerated lumbar motion segment complex. The PNR results in normal disc motion mechanics; physiologic loading of end plates, annulus, and facets; and restoration of motion control limits to the anterior longitudinal ligament, posterior longitudinal ligament, annulus, and facet joints.

To date, the clinical function of the PNR has been validated in a small group of patients. Initial experience has been associated with a relatively low complication rate, significant improvements in VAS and ODI scores, early ambulation, and a high level of patient satisfaction in an outpatient setting. Further clinical experience and randomized studies are warranted.

## REFERENCES


1. Cragg A, Carl A, Casteneda F, et al: New percutaneous access method for minimally invasive anterior lumbosacral surgery. J Spinal Disord Tech 17:21–28, 2004.
2. Tobler WT: AxiaLIF: A percutaneous, minimally invasive fusion technique for anterior interbody fusion at L5-S1. J Neurosurg (in press).
3. Crawford NR, Dickman CA, Sonntag VKH: Principals of spinal biomechanics. *In* Crockard A, Hayward R, Hoff JT (eds): Neurosurgery: The Scientific Basis of Clinical Practice. 3rd ed. Oxford, England, Blackwell Science Ltd., 2000, pp 1073–1092.
4. Eijkelkamp MF, van Donkelaar CC, Veldhuizen AG, et al: Requirements for and artificial intervertebral disc. Int J Artif Organs 24:311–321, 2001.
5. ASTM F2346-05: Standard Test Methods for Static and Dynamic Characterization of Spinal Artificial Discs.
6. Cunningham BW: Basic scientific considerations in total disc arthroplasty. Spine J 4:219S–230S, 2004.
7. Rivard CH, Rhalmi S, Coillard C: In vivo biocompatibility testing of PEEK polymer for a spinal implant system: A study in rabbits. J Biomed Mater Res 62:488–498, 2002.
8. Claes JE, Ludwig J, Margeviciu KJ, Durselen L: Biological response to ligament wear particles. J Appl Biomater 6:35–41, 1995.
9. Bertagnoli R, Schonmayr R: Surgical and clinical results with the PND prosthetic disc-nucleus device. Eur Spine J 11(2):S143–S148, 2002.
10. Khoo L, Marotta N, Cosar M, Pimenta L: A novel minimally-invasive presacral approach and instrumentation technique for anterior L5-S1 intervertebral discectomy and fusion: Technical description and case presentations. Neurosurg Focus 20:E9, 2006.

CHAPTER 58

# NUBAC Disc Arthroplasty

**Qi-Bin Bao, Matthew N. Songer, Luiz Pimenta, Hansen A. Yuan,** and **Domagoj Coric**

## KEY POINTS

- Unique inner articulation design for uniform stress distribution under all physiologic loading conditions.
- Made of PEEK-OPTIMA, which has an established history of biocompatibility and superior biodurability.
- Novel articulating surface material with superior wear characteristics to conventional metal-ultra-high-molecular-weight polyethylene (UHMWPE) wear surfaces.
- Easy surgical procedure for all surgical approaches.
- Less invasive and reversible option for degenerative disc disease.

## INTRODUCTION

The design rationale of the NUBAC (Pioneer Surgical Technology, Marquette, MI) disc arthroplasty device was largely based on the intended clinical objectives of a disc arthroplasty device and the clinical history of disc arthroplasty devices. Clinically, a disc arthroplasty device is mainly used to treat patients with discogenic back pain caused by disc degenerative disease (DDD). Because discogenic back pain can be caused by a chemical origin or mechanical irritation or instability, without yet a definite diagnostic method to determine exact pain mechanism, a disc arthroplasty procedure must address both potential pain mechanisms. To eliminate the potential chemical pain, the "diseased" nucleus needs to be removed in the disc arthroplasty procedure. It is well known that removal of the nucleus will cause collapse of the disc height and lead to further instability of the index segment, which, in turn, can cause mechanical pain. Therefore, a disc arthroplasty device should maintain or restore the disc height and mechanical function of the natural nucleus. Mechanically, in a healthy disc, the nucleus shares the compressive load with the annulus, taking about half of the total load passing through the anterior column.[1] Owing to its hydrostatic nature, the nucleus distributes the load evenly over the end plates under all physiologic loading conditions[2] and presents no restriction to the rotational motion by itself. The resistance to rotation relies mainly on the annulus and the facet joints.

## INDICATIONS/CONTRAINDICATIONS

Before the safety and efficacy of the NUBAC disc arthroplasty device can be analyzed, we must establish the indications and contraindications for the device. The main indication for this device is discogenic back pain caused by disc degenerative disease (DDD) with and without leg pain, similar to that for interbody fusion and total disc arthroplasty devices. The contraindications for the NUBAC are also similar to that for total disc and interbody fusion, with the exception of a disc height requirement of 5 mm for the NUBAC. The main reason for a minimal height disc requirement for disc arthroplasty is the aforementioned objectives of restoring and maintaining disc height and natural load sharing between the nucleus and annulus in order to achieve mechanical stability. If the disc is already severely collapsed, a nucleus replacement device must stretch the annulus in order to regain the normal disc height, which leads to high tension and having the disc arthroplasty device take all or the majority of the compressive load. By doing that, the contact stress between the device and the end plates would be unphysiologically high and lead to subsidence. If one uses disc height as an indicator for the stage of disc degeneration cascade, significant disc height loss typically represents the late stage of disc degeneration. Therefore, disc arthroplasty is indicated more often for patients at the early-to-moderate stage of the disc degeneration cascade, whereas fusion and total disc arthroplasty, due to their invasiveness and nonreversible nature, are recommended for patients at the late stage of the cascade. The stage of degeneration should not be confused with the degree of pain. The early-to-moderate stage in the degeneration cascade does not equal to less pain than the late stage of the cascade. Patients with early to moderate disc degeneration can have as much pain, if not more, as patients at the late stage of degeneration.

Owing to the less invasiveness, reversible nature and compatibility with a posterior approach, the NUBAC may be further indicated for patients with disc herniation without significant back pain, after the safety and efficacy of the NUBAC have been established in clinical trials. For this patient population, the NUBAC system will be used as an adjunctive device to the discectomy with the same surgical approach. The main benefit of the NUBAC here is to prevent discogenic back pain secondary to the discectomy surgery. This is a distinguishing difference between the total disc arthroplasty devices and the NUBAC disc arthroplasty device. Because of its invasiveness, need for the anterior approach in surgery, and high revision risk, total disc arthroplasty will probably never be justified for patients with only leg pain due to disc herniation.

## DESCRIPTION OF THE DEVICE

For total disc arthroplasty, the ball-and-socket articulation has become the most popular design and has shown its ability to restore the physiologic range of motion (ROM) in flexion/extension and lateral-bending directions. Clinically, total disc replacements incorporating a ball-and-socket design have shown reasonably good results, in both relieving pain and maintaining ROM. The designs and materials for nucleus arthroplasty, however, vary from different types of hydrogel or nonhydrogel elastomers, which are either preformed or formed in situ, to nonelastomeric materials, such as metal, polymethyl methacrylate (PMMA), and pyrolytic carbon. None of these nucleus devices has yet to incorporate an inner articulation design. Clinically, the early Fernstrom ball, which has bipolar articulation with the end plates, showed fairly good short-term and long-term results.[3,4] The main issue and criticism of the Fernstrom ball were its high rate of implant subsidence. This was due to the obvious reason that the implant has an initial point contact with the end plates, leading to a high contact stress and, therefore, inevitably some subsidence. As the implant subsides into the vertebrae, the contact area increases and the contact stress decreases. Eventually, the contact stress will reach a point that is below the critical stress and subsequently the subsidence risk becomes relatively low. It has been reported that most of the Fernstrom devices had 1 to 3 mm of subsidence on each side.[4] Taking a 12-mm diameter Fernstrom device (the diameter range of Fernstrom is 10 to 16 mm) as an example, the projected contact cross-section area is 85 mm$^2$ after 3 mm subsidence. Therefore, if a device with an initial contact area is larger than this value, the subsidence risk should be relatively low if the implant height is properly chosen to achieve adequate load sharing between the nucleus device and the annulus. It should be pointed out that regardless of the amount of subsidence, the clinical outcome for the Fernstrom device, in both the short term and long term, was fairly good, with more than 75% of patients reporting good to excellent.[3,4] It was also reported that ROM was observed after the implantation of the Fernstrom ball. This favorable clinical outcome as compared with other intradiscal devices, such as PMMA, should be largely due to its biconvex feature that allows more uniform stress distribution under various physiologic rotational motions.

Based on the design objectives and the lessons learned from various previous disc arthroplasty devices, the design of the NUBAC includes all the major benefits of both total disc arthroplasty and nucleus arthroplasty while eliminating the major pitfalls of these designs (Fig. 58–1). It has a unique two-piece design with an inner ball-and-socket articulation. The implant is made of polyetheretherketone (PEEK)–OPTIMA, which has well-established biocompatibility, superb biodurability, and a history of being used as a permanent spinal implant.

The outer surface of each piece has racetrack geometry to mimic the general shape of the nucleus and a large contact surface for the end plates. This large contact area is designed to distribute the load, reduce the contact stress, and, subsequently, mitigate the risk of subsidence. For example, the smallest footprint available has a contact surface area 2.2 times that of the contact area of a 12-mm Fernstrom ball device after 3 mm of subsidence. Therefore, the risk of subsidence of the NUBAC should be relatively low.

The NUBAC disc arthroplasty device retains the advantages of nucleus devices of being less invasive and a more reversible procedure than total disc devices. However, like many total discs, it has an inner articulation, which has several advantages over nonarticulating nucleus arthroplasty devices, as outlined later. Therefore, the NUBAC to some degree is a hybrid device and forms a unique category—intradiscal arthroplasty. First, like the natural nucleus tissue, it does not restrict any physiologic rotational motions. It should be pointed out that, unlike total disc replacement, the constraint, or the stability, of the motion segment after a nucleus arthroplasty procedure is largely determined by the surrounding tissues, such as the annulus and ligaments. Because most of these surrounding tissues are preserved in the disc arthroplasty procedure and the annulus is restored to the normal tension stage, the segment mobility and stability after the NUBAC implantation will be maintained. Second, it allows more uniform stress distribution on the end plates under all physiologic rotational motions as compared with nonarticulating intradiscal devices (Fig. 58–2). Last, it should reduce the risk of implant extrusion because as the segment bends opposite to the annular window, which is required for implant insertion, the dimension of the NUBAC near the annular window increases and makes extrusion more difficult (see Fig. 58–2).

In selecting the proper material for the NUBAC, a novel articulating material combination of PEEK on PEEK was chosen. Historically, metal (CoCr) on ultra-high-molecular-weight polyethylene (UHMWPE) has been the predominating articulating material combination for orthopaedic load-bearing arthroplasty devices, followed by metal-on-metal and a few other less frequently used material combinations, such as ceramic on ceramic. The wear and durability of UHMWPE for the total joint applications, which are typically used for the elderly population, have been well studied, but the limiting factor has been osteolysis leading to early implant failure. Although osteolysis has yet to become a major clinical problem in total disc arthroplasty, the long-term wear and durability of UHMWPE have not been well established for disc arthroplasty applications, and this is especially important considering that the patient population for disc arthroplasty is much younger than that for total joints. Although metal-on-metal has better durability, long-term metal ion data have not been fully studied. For disc arthroplasty devices, it is beneficial that they be manufactured from nonmetallic materials so as not to interfere with conventional radiographic images, such as magnetic resonance imaging (MRI) and computed tomography (CT). PEEK-OPTIMA is one of the best thermoplastic materials with well-established biocompatibility and superb mechanical and biostability

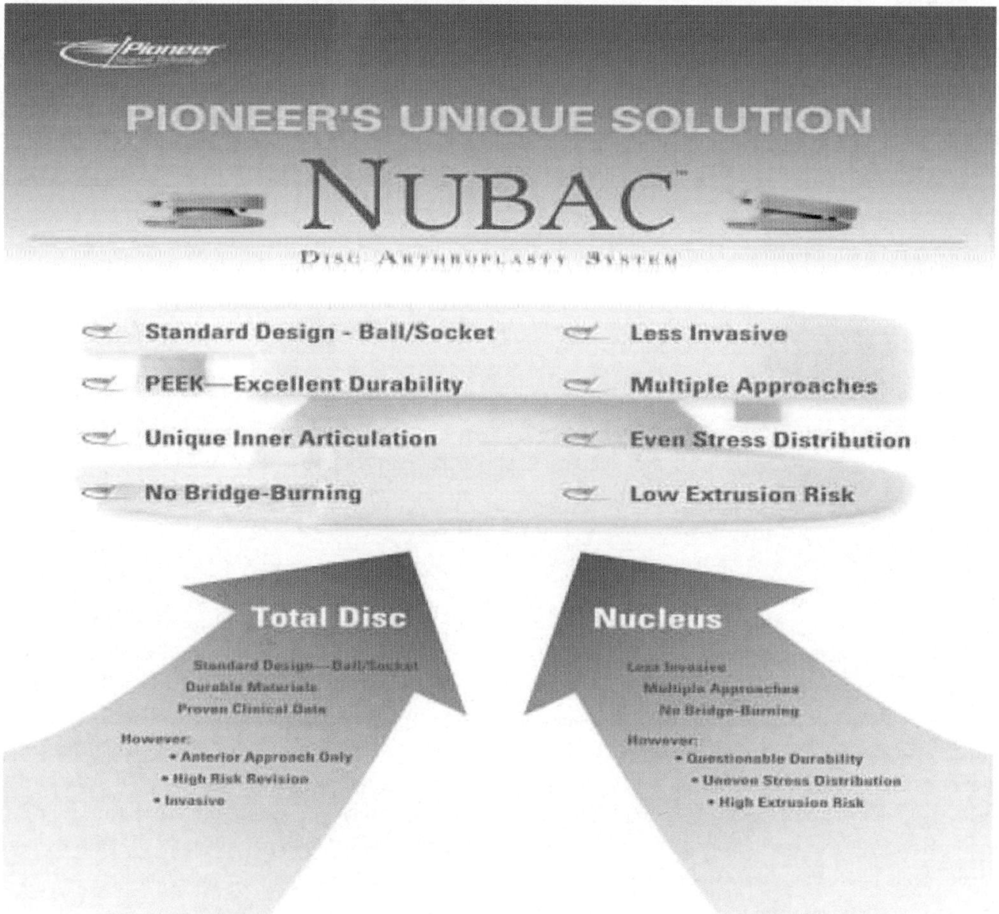


■ **FIGURE 58–1.** Key feature comparison of NUBAC disc arthroplasty with total disc arthroplasty and nucleus arthroplasty.

characteristics. Because most patients with DDD are in their 30s or 40s, it is especially important to use a material that has exceptional durability.

## BACKGROUND OF SCIENTIFIC TESTING/CLINICAL OUTCOMES

### Biocompatibility and Biodurability

Since its introduction to the medical market in 1999, PEEK-OPTIMA has quickly gained the confidence and acceptance of the medical community as a highly reliable implantable material. Independent laboratories have performed biocompatibility and biostability testing on PEEK-OPTIMA relevant to ISO 10993 and USP Class VI procedures, which have shown excellent results. Device (MAF) and Drug (DMF) Master Files are on file with the Food and Drug Administration (FDA) containing these results, as well as additional testing and extensive data concerning the polymer and its manufacturing methods.

Biodurability requirements for a permanent implantable device are largely dependent on its application. For implants primarily used for older patients, such as total joints, a biodurability of 15 years would most likely be adequate, although with an increasing life expectancy and a progressively younger age group receiving these implants, the biodurability requirements for these implants are likely to increase as well. However, for disc arthroplasty devices, which are used for much younger patients, the biodurability requirement should be much higher than that for total joints. Invibio (Greenville, NC), the manufacturer of PEEK-OPTIMA, has conducted extensive biodurability studies. In a study subjecting PEEK-OPTIMA to 200 kGy gamma irradiation and then followed with accelerated aging in oxygen (40 days at 5 bar at 70 °C), it was found that there was no significant change in material, chemical, and mechanical properties, as verified by Fourier transform infrared spectroscopy (FTIR), gel permeation chromatography (GPC), and differential scanning calorimetry (DSC).[5] In an in vivo biodurability study, samples of PEEK-OPTIMA extruded rod were gamma sterilized with a dose of 73.2 kGy and then incubated in physiologic saline for 3 months at 90 °C (simulation of 10 years real-time aging at 37 °C). The PEEK-OPTIMA samples were implanted in an animal model for a period of 12 months and subjected to cytotoxicity testing (ISO 10993–5), chemical analysis (ISO 10993–18), and histopathologic examination. These tests confirmed the material to be noncytotoxic, and histopathology found no muscle degradations, necrosis, marked inflammatory responses, or any other significant changes.[5]

### Kinematic Test

Two separate kinematic tests, each with somewhat different emphases, were conducted using a human cadaveric model. The

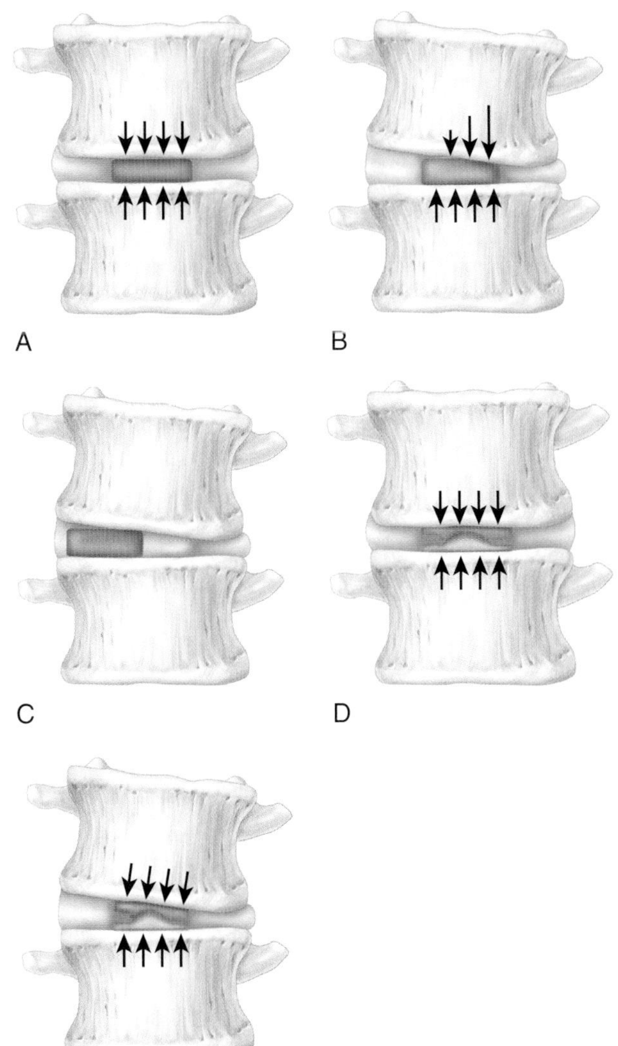


■ **FIGURE 58–2.** Schematic drawings of stress distribution under compression and bending. **A,** Bulk polymer nucleus implant under compression. **B,** Bulk polymer nucleus implant under bending. **C,** Partial extrusion of bulk polymer nucleus implant under bending. **D,** NUBAC nucleus device under compression. **E,** NUBAC nucleus device under bending.

first study conducted by Cunningham (Union Memorial Hospital, Baltimore, MD) emphasized the effect of the NUBAC on the multidirectional ROM and neutral zone (NZ), and the second study conducted by Ordway (SUNY-Syracuse, NY) emphasized more the effect of the NUBAC on the disc height change and fatigue/extrusion behavior.

## Multidirectional Flexibility Study

An in vitro biomechanical study was undertaken to compare the multidirectional flexibility kinematics of the articulating NUBAC disc arthroplasty device for single-level reconstruction. A total of eight human cadaveric lumbar spines (L2-L3 and L4-L5 segments) were used in this investigation and nondestructively evaluated under the following conditions: (1) intact spine, (2) nucleotomy alone, and (3) reconstructed with the NUBAC implant.

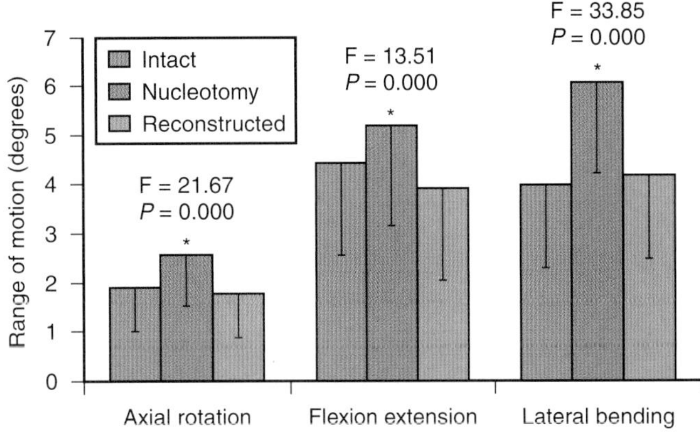


■ **FIGURE 58–3.** Operative-level range of motion. *Indicates statistical difference between the nucleotomy condition and the intact and reconstructed conditions at $P<0.05$. No other differences were observed. Error bars indicate one standard deviation.

Unconstrained intact moments of ±7.5 Nm were used for axial rotation, flexion-extension, and lateral-bending testing, with quantification of the operative-level ROM (degrees) and NZ (degrees).

Multidirectional flexibility testing indicated significant increases in the segmental ROM and NZ secondary to the annulotomy/nucleotomy procedures according to repeated measures ANOVA. For both calculated parameters, the segmental rotation increased for the destabilized condition versus the intact and reconstructed specimens ($P<0.05$). Importantly, the NZ, an indicator of spinal stability, for the NUBAC reconstructed condition returned to levels not statistically different from the intact condition. Overall, the use of the articulating NUBAC device re-established the operative level kinematics to the intact condition (Figs. 58–3 and 58–4).

## Disc Height and Biomechanical Assessment

The purpose of this study was to examine the following performance characteristics of the NUBAC device: ROM, disc height, and stiffness. Six adjacent pairs of human cadaver lumbar

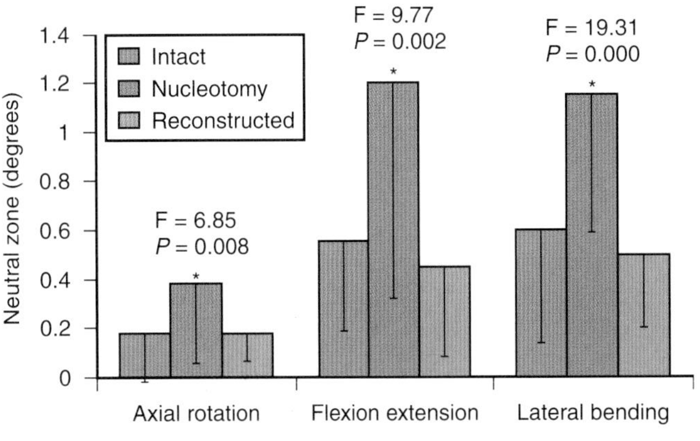


■ **FIGURE 58–4.** Operative-level neutral zone. *Indicates statistical difference between the nucleotomy condition and the intact and reconstructed conditions at $P<0.05$. No other differences were observed. Error bars indicate one standard deviation.

functional spine units (FSU) (L3-L5) were tested at three different stages (intact, after discectomy, and after the NUBAC implant) under various physiologic loading conditions. One disc level of each specimen was left intact and served as a control level. The second level served as the surgical level. A 6 mm × 10 mm annular window using a right lateral approach was created in each specimen followed by a complete nucleotomy and insertion of the NUBAC device. A 7.5-Nm moment was applied to evaluate the ROM and stiffness (sagittal, coronal, and axial rotation).

Insertion of the NUBAC significantly increased the construct height under load in comparison to the discectomy condition. The disc height after discectomy significantly decreased ($P<0.05$) for all specimens in comparison to the intact condition under 1.2 kN of compressive loading. Implantation of the NUBAC disc arthroplasty device significantly increased ($P<0.05$) the disc height compared with the discectomy condition. There was no significant difference between the intact and implanted conditions (Fig. 58–5). Maintaining or restoring the disc height at the index level is important for balancing the load distribution between the anterior column and posterior column and maintaining the opening of foramen space.

For ROM testing, the control levels displayed consistent motion for all modes throughout the testing. There were no significant differences in torsional motion for any disc condition. The surgical levels showed increased flexion motion following discectomy, but this was not statistically significant. For extension, the motion was significantly reduced ($P<0.05$) following discectomy and the motion was restored to intact status ($P<0.05$) following insertion of the implant. There were no significant changes in left or right bending after discectomy or following insertion of the implant. Overall, the in vitro biomechanical function of the FSU with the NUBAC was similar to that of the intact FSU.

From these two studies, it is clear that the NUBAC was able to restore the normal ROMs and NZs in all three major rotational motions and restore the normal disc height in a human cadaveric spine model.

## Expulsion Test

Because a nucleus arthroplasty device is typically not fixed to the end plate, the potential for implant extrusion has become a significant concern for this type of device. The only modern nucleus replacement with a fairly large number of clinical cases is RayMedica's PDN-SOLO. Its initial poor clinical experience was due to an implant extrusion rate ranging from 8% to 36%.[6] This has heightened the concern on implant extrusion for all other nucleus replacement devices.

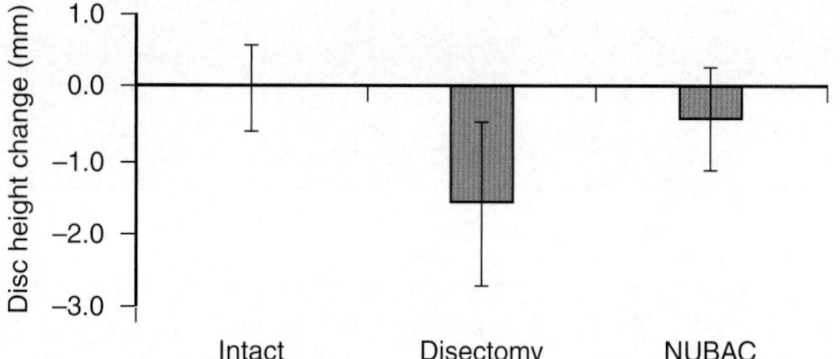

■ **FIGURE 58–5.** Disc height change after nucleotomy and NUBAC implantation.

Because expulsion was recognized as a potential risk at the very beginning of the development of the NUBAC device, several human cadaver studies have been conducted for the NUBAC. It should be realized that owing to the limited clinical experience with nucleus devices, there have not been any clinically validated standards for assessing the risk of nucleus implant expulsion. Although not clinically validated, it is believed that an in vitro cyclic bending test under physiologic ROM is clinically relevant in assessing the implant expulsion risk. Unilateral bending opposite the annular window, through which the NUBAC was inserted, was selected as the worst-case expulsion scenario.

Six adjacent pairs of human cadaver lumbar FSUs (L3-L5) were tested at the postnucleus implant conditions. One disc level of each specimen was left intact and served as a control level and the second level served as the surgical level. A 6 mm × 10 mm annular window using a right lateral approach was created in each specimen, followed by a complete nucleotomy and insertion of the NUBAC device. After some initial nondestructive tests under pure compression, axial rotation, lateral bending, and flexion/extension, each specimen was then tested for 100,000 cycles of unilateral left bending opposite to the annular window ranging from 2.5 to 7.5 Nm at 2 Hz with the compressive load ranging between 250 and 750 N. Under this loading condition, the average bending angle was 4.4 degrees at the beginning of the test and 9.2 degrees at 100,000 cycles. Implant expulsion did not occur for any of the six samples. Therefore, the NUBAC expulsion risk was estimated to be relatively low.

In addition to these two cadaver studies, another cadaver study was conducted in Goel's laboratory at the University of Toledo. As part of assessing the risk and benefit of different outer surfaces for the NUBAC implants, implant extrusion risk was assessed. This started from hand bending the implanted FSUs following a normal surgical procedure. Then all of the annulus was removed and it was tested in the MTS machine with lateral bending with an angle of approximately 7 degrees. A total of five human cadaver lumbar FSUs were used. No implant extrusion occurred during hand bending with an annular window of 8 × 10 mm. After dissecting all of the annulus and lateral bend testing on the machine for at least 8,000 cycles, no implant extruded. This test demonstrated that the inner articulation design of the NUBAC allowed for the two plates to rotate along with the segment during rotation, and allowed both plates to maintain full contact with the end plates. The inner articulation design also helped the implant remain in the center of the disc even without annular constraint. However, it also should be noted that from the two cadaver studies discussed earlier, the worst-case scenario for extrusion of this implant may be in a situation in which there is a large annular window with excess nucleus tissue at the distal end, instead of having all the annulus removed.

## Wear Test

Because the NUBAC has a ball-and-socket articulating joint and consists of a novel PEEK-on-PEEK self-mating material couple for load-bearing arthroplasty application, extensive wear testing has been conducted. To understand the wear characteristics of PEEK-on-PEEK as a self-mating material couple and be able to compare it with the wear characteristics of other bearing materials, several wear tests with different methodologies have been conducted. Owing to the relatively short history of disc arthroplasty, there is no established testing standard or guidelines in place to give an accurate and clinically validated kinematic and wear assessment of the functionality of nucleus replacement devices. For this reason, at best, an educated, realistic assumption can only be made given the lack of clinical retrievals. Because a nucleus device is designed to share the compressive load with the remaining annulus, a dynamic compressive load representing the range of loading according to the literature based on the nucleus supporting about one-half of the compressive load was used in all testing methodologies.[1]

In the first test, six small NUBAC implants, which have the smallest contact area and therefore the highest contact stress, were used. The samples were subjected to dynamic axial load between 225 and 1024 N at 4 Hz coupled with a flexion/extension rotation with a total of 15 degrees at 2 Hz in such a way that peak load coincided with the maximum rotation angle. The load magnitude was chosen based on the design goal of having the disc arthroplasty device to share the compressive load with the annulus. The ROM of this test represents the high end of the physiologic flexion/extension for the lumbar discs. The test samples were bathed in 37 ± 3 °C newborn calf serum and the test was conducted to 10 million cycles. At approximately every 500,000 cycles, the test was stopped, all components were cleaned, and the specimens were weighed to assess the mass loss and wear rate. The test fluid was also changed at this time and stored at −20 °C for particle analysis.

The results of the test showed an average total mass loss of 2.79 ± 0.14 mg at 10.35 million cycles. The corresponding average wear rate was 0.28 ± 0.07 mg/million cycles. There were no failures of the test specimens throughout the duration of the test period and all specimens functioned according to their design under the tested conditions in this study.

To allow for a more comprehensive assessment of the wear and mechanical durability under coupled motion, the devices were rotated 90 ° to simulate a lateral bending profile and tested under the same load magnitude and ROM for an additional 10 million cycles.

The wear rate was 0.27 ± 0.09 mg/million cycles, similar to what was found in the flexion/extension test. The total mass loss was 5.5 mg at 20.5 million cycles for both the flexion/extension and lateral bending tests. Overall, the wear rate for each individual sample over the entire testing period was consistent, suggesting that there was only a small variation between the samples. This test also demonstrated that the wear rate is relatively insensitive to bi-directional motion.

To address the long-term wear durability for the disc arthroplasty devices, the wear test for the NUBAC has been further extended to a total of 40 million cycles with alternating flexion/extension and lateral bending. Over the entire period, the wear rate remained fairly consistent. To our knowledge, the NUBAC is the only disc arthroplasty device with a ball-and-socket articulation that has been tested to 40 million cycles while maintaining full functionality.

The size and morphology of the wear debris for every sample were analyzed using enzymatic digestion of the testing fluid and then subjected to laser diffraction at 0.5 million cycles and at every million cycles thereafter (1.0, 2.0, and so on). The results of the laser diffraction analysis for flexion/extension showed a volumetric diameter mean of 17.5 μm and a number diameter mean of 0.86 μm. For lateral bending, the results showed a volumetric diameter mean of 37.3 μm and number diameter mean of 0.48 μm. Scanning electron microscopic (SEM) analysis was also performed on some representative samples at 0.5 million cycles and at every odd million-cycle count thereafter (1.0, 3.0, and so on). The results of the SEM analysis showed an average diameter size of 0.78 μm and an aspect ratio of 1.34 for flexion/extension.

To assess the coupled motion effect on the wear characteristics of the NUBAC device, a second wear test using conditions the same as the ISO standard[7] for total disc arthroplasty was conducted by Rush University Medical Center (Chicago, IL) using an Endolab spine testing machine, except the dynamic compressive magnitude was adjusted to 225 to 1,024 N in order to reflect the load-sharing mechanism for a nucleus device. Again, six small NUBAC implants were used. The wear rate for this test was 0.5 mg/M cycles, which compares very favorably to the wear rate of 10 mg/M cycles for ProDisc using the same ISO standard.[8]

### Static and Fatigue Strength Test

Six small NUBAC implants, which represent the worst-case scenario, were tested in an axial static compressive mode. The results showed a mean axial static load at offset yield of 10,427 N, which is well beyond the static failure strength of the human vertebral body or end plate. The failure mode was excessive plastic deformation of the top shell in all specimens.

A total of six specimens were tested in axial dynamic fatigue mode at 10 Hz. The results of the dynamic axial fatigue test show that the device has excellent axial fatigue strength. There was no specimen failure at 80% (8,342 N) and 90% (9,384 N) of the average static offset yield load of 10,427 N. At offset yield, one specimen ran out to 10 million cycles while one specimen failed immediately. The failure mode was excessive plastic deformation of the top shell. These static and fatigue failure loads are much higher than the static and fatigue strengths of the vertebrae. Therefore, the results of these tests suggested that the NUBAC has sufficient static and fatigue strengths for the intended application.

### Animal Study

An animal study using a baboon model was conducted by Cunningham (Union Memorial Hospital, Baltimore, MD) to assess the safety and limited efficacy of the NUBAC device. Although there are still limitations to using a baboon model to assess disc arthroplasty devices, the baboon is considered to be one of the best models.

The study consisted of 14 mature male baboons that were randomized into two postoperative time periods of 6 months ($n = 7$) and 12 months ($n = 7$). Comprehensive analyses, which include gross necropsy, MRI, plain x-ray study and microradiographies, multidirection biomechanical test, and biocompatibility assays with local and systemic histology and immunohistochemistry, were performed at 6 and 12 months after surgery.

Each animal underwent a lateral transperitoneal surgical approach, followed by complete nucleotomy at L3-L4 and L5-L6 levels. The L5-L6 level was reconstructed using the NUBAC device. The L3-L4 served as a surgical (nucleotomy) control in each case.

A limitation of this study was the use of a single NUBAC height of 6 mm for all treated discs, which lead to a significant increase of the disc heights. The mean preoperative height of 5.61 ± 0.88 mm was significantly increased to 6.41 ± 0.83 mm at the postoperative interval ($P<0.05$). There was no significant change in disc height between the preoperative and postoperative conditions for the control level. For the 6- and 12-month treatment groups, the operative and control-level intervertebral disc space heights were compared before surgery and at sacrifice. For the 6-month group, the preoperative disc height at L3-L4 and L5-L6 levels averaged 4.5 ± 0.62 mm and 5.6 ± 0.73 mm, respectively. At 6 months postoperatively, the L3-L4 level decreased to 2.9 ± 0.15 mm and the L5-L6 level decreased to 3.7 ± 0.66 mm, both of which were statistically less than the preoperative condition ($P<0.05$). At 12 months postoperatively, the L3-L4 and L5-L6 levels decreased to 2.7 ± 0.28 mm and 3.5 ± 0.92 mm, respectively, which were statistically less than the preoperative conditions ($P<0.05$). The overdistraction resulted in difficulties for insertion and placement of the device. This may have resulted in the use of more force for proper placement and potentially induced end plate damage, Modic changes, and a corresponding decrease in disc height at the treated disc levels.

Multidirectional flexibility testing indicated diminished segmental motion for the NUBAC under all loading modes; however, these findings were also noted in the operative control levels, demonstrating the effect of surgical intervention itself on segmental stability. By 12 months postoperatively, flexion/extension motion returned to the intact levels (Fig. 58–6).

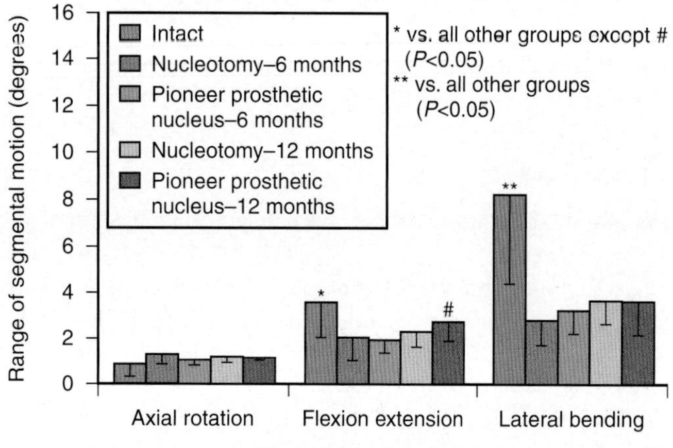


■ **FIGURE 58–6.** Range of motion of implant and control levels in baboon study.

All treatments containing the NUBAC exhibited increased densification of trabeculae along the end plate periphery, which corroborated with Modic type I changes observed radiographically. These patterns of trabecular densification are considered normal and have been documented in a number of in vivo nonhuman primate studies investigating total disc arthroplasty devices. Evidence of mild implant subsidence was noted in five of seven cases, which correlated with the absence of articular cartilage in subsidence regions. This may have been caused by overdistraction of the disc space, leading to higher end plate stress. No change in densification or end plate sclerosis was observed at the L3-L4 surgical control levels. In the histological analyses, there was no detectable wear debris from the NUBAC device and no evidence of macrophage activities or osteolytic response.

Pathologic assessment for all undecalcified tissues assessed the following factors: tissue architecture, presence of debris, signs of foreign body giant cell/granulomas inflammatory reactions, degenerative changes, or autolysis. The histology demonstrated no significant evidence of any inflammatory reaction along the vertebral end plate. Pathologic assessment characterized all systemic organs and organ systems as having normal tissue architecture, without the presence of foreign body material, foreign body giant cell/granulomas inflammatory reactions, degenerative changes, or autolysis. Plain and polarized light microscopy of local tissues overlying the operative sites from both the experimental and control levels indicated a chronic inflammatory reaction, with evidence of fibrous connective replacement and infiltration of mononuclear cells. These observations were considered secondary to the surgical procedure and, more importantly, occurred at both the control and experimental operative levels.

A cytokine analysis showed that there was no evidence of cellular apoptosis, giant cell reaction or other significant pathologic changes. Analysis of the immunohistochemical antibody stains for the local tissues overlying the experimental and control levels was negative in each case. There was no evidence of a proinflammatory cytokine reaction at any of the experimental or control levels. The study serves as a basic scientific basis for ongoing clinical investigations into the use and efficacy of the NUBAC for replacement of the intervertebral nucleus pulposus.

## CLINICAL PRESENTATION AND EVALUATION

The extensive preclinical studies and design verifications and validations led to the CE mark approval of the NUBAC in July 2005. A multicenter prospective clinical study outside of the United States was then initiated. Although there has been limited experience, the initial clinical results were very promising. Figures 58–7 and 58–8 summarize the ODI and VAS improvement of these early patients. In July 2006, the Investigational Device Exemption (IDE) study of the NUBAC device was initiated. This IDE study will allow the full assessment of safety and efficacy for the NUBAC disc arthroplasty in a level-one study.

## OPERATIVE TECHNIQUES

In addition to being less invasive and more reversible than total disc arthroplasty, the NUBAC disc arthroplasty has another

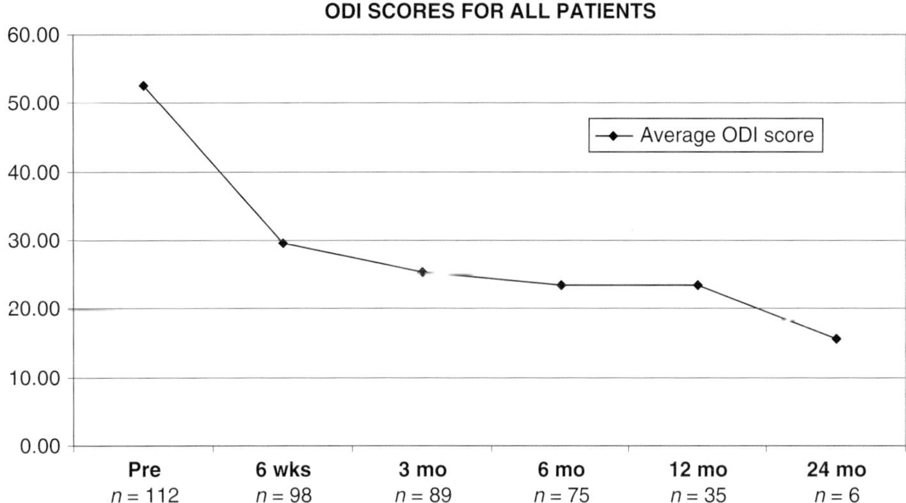


■ **FIGURE 58–7.** Oswestry Disability Index (ODI) score improvement after the NUBAC procedure.

advantage of being compatible with different surgical approaches. In the limited clinical experience so far, the NUBAC has been successfully implanted through all three common surgical approaches: posterior, straight lateral (ALPA), and retroperitoneal anterolateral. Other than the differences in patient position, tissue dissection, and retraction for these three different approaches, the general surgical procedure for the NUBAC for the three approaches is very similar. General anesthesia is required for the patient in all three of these approaches. The following highlights some key steps related to each approach.

The posterior approach is often used for patients with sequestrated or large contained disc herniation. Patient position, skin incision, and the approach to the disc are the same as that for discectomy. Depending on the pathology, the surgeon can approach the disc from either the left side or right side. Like a discectomy procedure, a partial laminectomy is often required, so that there will be enough window to conduct the discectomy and laminectomy. Although it is acceptable to remove a small edge of the facet in the medial side, care should be taken not to dissect too much facet. A nerve retractor should be used during the discectomy and device implantation.

For discs at L4-L5 or above, the straight lateral approach can be used. After positioning the patient in a lateral position, the disc is approached through a lateral retroperitoneal, transpsoas pathway. Although this is not a conventional approach in the past for discectomy and interbody fusion, this approach has gained some popularity recently for implanting both nucleus devices[9] and interbody fusion.[10] Compared with the conventional retroperitoneal anterolateral approach, this approach has the advantages of allowing for anterior access to the disc space without the need for an approach surgeon or avoiding the potential complications of an anterior intra-abdominal procedure. For a disc arthroplasty device, this approach also has the advantage of easy cleaning of the nucleus space.

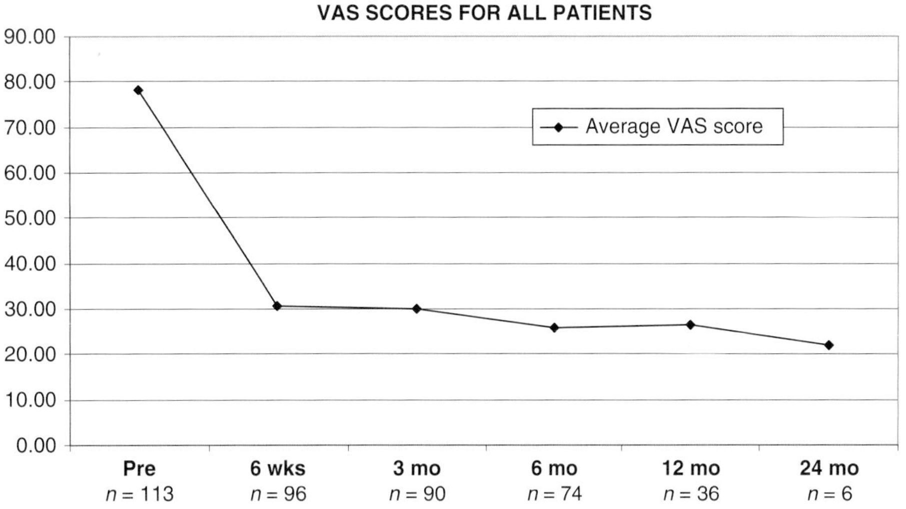


■ **FIGURE 58–8.** Visual Analog Scale (VAS) score improvement after the NUBAC procedure.

Alternatively, the conventional retroperitoneal anterolateral approach can be used. The patient will be in a supine position. The disc can be approached from either the left or right side. Although the surgical approach is similar to that for total disc implantation and anterior interbody fusion, due to the small size of the NUBAC implant, the area of disc exposure is much less than that for fusion and total disc replacement. With less tissue retraction and less bleeding than with fusion and total disc replacement, the risk of vascular injury and scar tissue formation should also be less.

Because the NUBAC procedure requires smaller disc exposure, less tissue dissection, and no end plate preparation, the surgical procedure and instrumentation for the NUBAC are relatively simple and straight forward. After the disc exposure with one of these three approaches, a small 6 mm × 6 mm annular window is cut using a parallel cutter with #11 blade. In cutting the annular window, care should be taken not to cut into the end plates. For a relatively narrow disc or during the posterior approach, the parallel cutter might be only used to cut the width of the annular window. The two vertical annular slits can then be connected by cutting two horizontal lines adjacent to the superior and inferior vertebrae. The box annular plug is then removed by pituitary rongeur. A complete nucleotomy is then performed with care not to damage the annulus and end plate. Up-angle, down-angle, and curved rongeurs are helpful to remove the nucleus in the corners or in the area that cannot be reached by a straight rongeur. After the discectomy, the annular window is then dilated with an annular dilator. The cavity size and location is then assessed with specially designed trials with different footprints, heights, and lordotic angles using a fluoroscope. Care should be taken to make sure that the trial is positioned in the center of the disc in the anteroposterior (AP) fluoroscopic image. Because the trials may pack some loose nucleus toward the distal end of the cavity, it is advised to use the rongeur again to remove the packed nucleus material. The final implant size is then chosen based on the size and lordotic angle of the last trial. The NUBAC implant is held by the implant inserter with a wedge angle in the distal end to facilitate the entry of the implant into the annular opening. After inserting the NUBAC implant into the disc cavity, the AP and lateral fluoroscopic images should be taken to verify the implant position using the radiopaque markers before disengaging the inserter from the implant.

## POSTOPERATIVE CARE

Owing to the less invasive nature of surgery for the NUBAC device, patient recovery normally is much faster than that for total disc arthroplasty and fusion procedures. Many of the patients who had the NUBAC device inserted were discharged the day after the surgery. Patients are encouraged to ambulate but to increase activity slowly. The main reason for this slow activity increase is to allow the end plates to adjust the contact stress increase slowly. For patients with chronic discogenic back pain, typically the contact stress in the nucleus region has been low for a while owing to the disc desiccation. Because the objective of the NUBAC disc arthroplasty is to restore the normal load sharing between the nucleus region and the annulus, the contact stress in the nucleus region will be increased after the NUBAC surgery. The slow activity increase would allow the end plates to adjust to the sudden stress increase and avoid subsidence. A corset back brace is recommended for the first 6 weeks to avoid extreme bending motions.

## COMPLICATIONS AND AVOIDANCE

Because the procedure for the NUBAC device is less invasive than the procedure for total disc or fusion, the intraoperative vascular and neurologic risks should be less for the NUBAC device. Although the inner articulation design for the NUBAC would reduce the risk of implant extrusion as compared with other nucleus arthroplasty devices, the potential postoperative complication of implant extrusion still exists for the NUBAC device because it is not fixed to the end plates. A good surgical technique should further help to reduce this risk. First, cutting too large of an annular window should be avoided. A large annular window will increase the risk of implant extrusion. In the NUBAC instrument set, a parallel cutter is provided to help surgeons to create a defined size (6 mm × 6 mm) annular window. An annular dilator is provided to dilate the annular window to facilitate the trial and implant insertions without a large annular window. Second, a complete nucleotomy should also help to reduce the extrusion risk. Too much remaining nucleus will act as a hydrolytic pump, which will push the implant out. Third, while completing the nucleotomy, one should avoid damaging the annulus. Any disc arthroplasty device relies on the competent annulus to confine the device in the disc space.

Another potential complication for the NUBAC is subsidence. Proper patient selection is a key to minimize this risk. In order for the NUBAC to function properly, it is expected to carry certain percentages (roughly 50%) of the load passing through the anterior column. Patients with contraindications, such as osteoporosis and Schmorl's nodes, should be excluded. The presence of both osteoporosis and Schmorl's nodes suggests a weak vertebra, which might not be able to support the expected load. Because one of the objectives for the NUBAC disc arthroplasty device is to restore the normal load-sharing mechanism between the annulus and nucleus, a disc height of greater than 5 mm is required. In total disc procedures, most of the annulus and ligaments are dissected, and therefore, it becomes very easy to distract the disc space. However, most of the annulus and all the ligaments are preserved in the NUBAC procedure. Distraction of a disc with a height less than 5 mm to a normal disc height and the subsequent implantation of the NUBAC will lead to unphysiologic stress in the contacting end plate and, therefore, increase the risk of subsidence. From a surgical technique point, one should avoid damaging the end plates during the surgery. End plate damage will also increase the risk of subsidence.

## ADVANTAGES AND DISADVANTAGES

Like any device, the NUBAC has its advantages and disadvantages, some of which are more real and some of which are perceived. Although it might be impossible to design an ideal device, it is important to capture as many real and critical advantages/features as possible and, if needed, sacrifice some less important or perceived benefits in exchange for more important ones. The following table summarizes the advantages and disadvantages as compared with total disc replacement, fusion, and other nucleus devices.

**ADVANTAGES/DISADVANTAGES: NUBAC DISC ARTHROPLASTY**

| Advantages Over Total Disc and Fusion | Advantages Over Other Nucleus Devices |
|---|---|
| Less invasive and less surgical risk | Established biocompatibility/biodurability |
| Less revision risk and less bridge-burning | Excellent fatigue strength |
| Radiolucency | Excellent wear resistance |
| Less surgery time and fast recovery time | Less extrusion risk |
| Compatible with lateral and posterior approaches | More uniform stress distribution under bending |
| Easy to restore normal load distribution between anterior column and facet joint—avoid facet degeneration | Simplicity in implant and instrument |
| **Disadvantages Over Total Disc and Fusion** | **Disadvantages Over Other Nucleus Devices** |
| More risk of extrusion | Lack of device shock absorption |
| Not indicated for late-stage degenerative disc disease | Lack of device swelling pressure |
| More risk of subsidence | |

## CONCLUSIONS/DISCUSSION

The design of the NUBAC is based on lessons learned from the successes and failures of various disc arthroplasty devices and a clear understanding of the objectives of an disc arthroplasty. A novel self-mating material, PEEK-on-PEEK, articulation was chosen to capitalize on its well-established biocompatibility and superb biodurability, which are critical for any disc arthroplasty devices. The unique inner articulation distinguishes it from other nucleus arthroplasty devices and brings the advantages of uniform stress distribution under all physiologic motions and low risk of implant extrusion. The extensive preclinical tests and favorable results have led to rapid CE mark and the IDE approval. The early clinical data suggested that the NUBAC provides discogenic back pain relief that is similar to other more invasive and nonreversible procedures, such as fusion and total disc. There is no question that if the safety and efficacy the NUBAC are further established in the future OUS clinical trials and the U.S. IDE study, the NUBAC should become a better option for this subset of discogenic back pain patients than fusion and total disc.

## REFERENCES

1. Nachemson A: The load on lumbar disks in different positions of the body. Clin Orthop 45:107–122, 1965.
2. Brinckmann P, Grootenboer H: Change of disc height, radial disc bulge, and intradiscal pressure from discectomy. Spine 16:641–646, 1991.
3. Fernstrom U: Arthroplasty with intercorporal endoprothesis in herniated disc and in painful disc. Acta Scand Suppl 357:154–159, 1966.
4. McKenzie AH: Fernstrom intervertebral disc arthroplasty: A long-term evaluation. Ortho Int Ed 3:313–324, 1995.
5. Cartwright K, Devine J: Investigation into the effect of gamma sterilization (200 kGy) and accelerated aging on the properties of PEEK-Optima. Invibio (Greenville, SC), InvibioTechnical Report, 2005.
6. Klara P, Ray C: Artificial nucleus replacement: Clinical experience. Spine 27:1374–1377, 2002.
7. ISO/DIS 18192-1 Implants for surgery: Wear of total intervertebral spinal disc prostheses, Part 1: Loading and displacement parameters for wear testing and corresponding environmental conditions for tests.
8. Wright TM, Cottrell JM, Punga K, et al: Retrieval and wear analyses of ProDisc lumbar disc implants. Annual Meeting of Spine Arthroplasty Society 2006, Montreal, Quebec, Canada.
9. Bertagnoli R, Vazquez RJ: The anterolateral transpsoatic approach (ALPA): A new technique for implanting prosthetic disc-nucleus devices. J Spinal Disord Tech 16:398–404, 2003.
10. Ozgur BM, Aryan HE, Pimenta L, Taylor WR: Extreme lateral interbody fusion (XLIF): A novel surgical technique for anterior lumbar interbody fusion. Spine J 6:435–443, 2006.

CHAPTER 59

# Satellite: Spherical Partial Disc Replacement

**Robert S. Biscup** and **Vinod K. Podichetty**

## KEY POINTS

- Motion preservation surgery of the spine is becoming increasingly studied as an attractive alternative to fusion procedures.
- Disc stabilization arthroplasty with spherical prostheses has a long clinical history, and modern short-term data are showing very promising results.
- This is a promising indication for current arthroplasty procedures for disc herniation patients with elements of both leg and back pain. Nonetheless, certain contraindications, such as poor bone quality, can affect outcomes.
- The design rationale for spherical prosthesis is to mimic the natural nucleus under compressive load at the center of rotation of the intervertebral disc. It is intended to achieve this by using the end plate geometry for proper placement.
- Within the United States, the Satellite device is intended to be used to provide stabilization and help promote intervertebral body fusion.

## INTRODUCTION

The degenerative spine cascade of segmental spinal injury, instability, and spontaneous stabilization has been well studied and documented. This multiyear pathologic process occurs in a majority of the population, with the large majority being asymptomatic. There is a clear natural history to this condition, with the end stage being spontaneous stabilization. However, it is the early injury and instability phase of the spinal motion segment that most believe can be problematic with any combination of disabling symptoms including (1) mechanical back pain, (2) discogenic back pain, (3) inflammatory facet pain, and (4) sciatic-type pain.

Failing conservative management, traditional surgical approaches include decompression and discectomy, spinal fusion, and, more recently, artificial disc replacement. For a long time, spinal fusion has been considered the surgical treatment for degenerative disc disease (DDD). However, this technique has been associated with a range of adverse effects, including increased morbidity, pseudoarthrosis, infection, failed back syndrome, and acceleration of degenerative changes in the adjacent intervertebral discs.[1–3] There has been much interest in artificial discs and motion preservation over the past decade, and the potential for clinically effective disc replacement surgery is now becoming a reality.

The first study on disc replacement was in 1955 by David Cleveland.[4] He injected methyl methacrylate into the evacuated disc space of 14 patients at the time of discectomy, yielding acceptable results. Wallace Hamby and Glaser (1959)[5] presented his results of disc replacement with locally polymerizing methyl methacrylate. They compared discectomy alone with discectomy with methyl methacrylate and found no significant difference in the outcomes 1 year after surgery. However, van Steenbrugghe[6] was the first to establish the concept of disc prosthesis in 1956 in a French patent.

In 1959, Paul Harmon devised Vitalium spheres and implanted these in the lumbar spine in 13 patients between 1959 and 1961.[7] In New York in 1962, Nachemson[8] reported the study of silicone rubber implants and their mechanical properties when injected into the disc space. However, this study was carried out in vitro using autopsy specimens and could not be proven in vivo. In 1964, Reitz and Joubert[9] in South Africa reported the treatment of intractable headache and cervicobrachialgia in 19 patients by implanting a steel ball prosthesis in cervical discs after discectomy yielding good results.

Fernström[10] in Sweden also implanted stainless steel spheres in the cervical and the lumbar spine after discectomy in two separate treatment groups. Group one was composed of patients with herniated discs, and group two included patients with painful degenerative discs. The endoprosthesis was oxygen-resistant and was inserted into the center of the evacuated disc. Between 1962 and 1964 he inserted the ball into 191 lumbar discs in 125 cases and 13 cervical discs in eight cases. His follow-up results demonstrated a better surgical result when excision of a disc herniation was combined with an intercorporal endoprosthesis. These results were similar to the results obtained with fusion.[11–13] Reported complications included a displacement of the endoprosthesis into the spinal canal as well as a temporary paresis of the peroneus nerve. In 1995, Alvin McKenzie[14] described his series of 103 patients who underwent Fernström's intervertebral disc arthroplasty with an average follow-up of 17 years in 67 patients. Excellent or good results were obtained in 75% (patients treated for DDD) and 83% (treated for disc protrusions).

Following these breakthrough innovations, numerous other mechanical disc designs were introduced in the 1970s and 1980s.[15–19]

Many of these discs never made it to clinical applications due to their limited quantifiable use. Currently the FDA approved total disc replacement implants include: The SB CHARITÉ (DePuy Spine Inc., Raynham, MA) and the ProDisc (Synthes, West Chester, PA). It is important to note here that they have been developed and introduced within the last decade.[20,21]

Basic design concepts and component material(s) have been built on three fundamental groups: metal, nonmetal, and composite. Implants are placed into subgroups based on the type of disc replacement, i.e. (1) total disc replacement and (2) nucleus pulposus replacement. Other emerging technologies include facet joint resurfacing, facet replacement, and cervical intervertebral disc replacement. The main advantage of a disc prosthesis design using metal alone is its inherently high fatigue strength in comparison with a nonmetal design. Four prosthetic models have been proposed, which include hydraulic, elastic, composite, and mechanical.[22]

Basic design concepts and component materials have been built on three fundamental groups: metal, nonmetal, and composite. Implants are placed into subgroups based on the type of disc replacement: (1) total disc replacement and (2) nucleus pulposus replacement. Other emerging technologies include facet joint resurfacing, facet replacement, and cervical intervertebral disc replacement. The main advantage of a disc prosthesis design using metal alone is its inherently high fatigue strength in comparison with a nonmetal design. Four prosthetic models have been proposed that include hydraulic, elastic, composite, and mechanical.[21]

Building on the early work of Paul Harmon, Ulf Fernström, and Alvin McKenzie, a revised procedure has been developed by the lead author from a posterior approach using minimally invasive techniques that inserts an appropriate-sized implant into the nuclear recess of the lumbar intervertebral disc to help stabilize the segment while preserving motion with effective surgical and clinical outcomes. The concept is to assist the natural history of the degenerative spine cascade process by stabilizing rather than replacing the intervertebral disc space. The technique and implant are an effective alternative to the discectomy procedure, which has a documented history of disc height loss, reherniations, and adjacent level breakdowns.

## INDICATIONS, CONTRAINDICATIONS, AND POSSIBLE ADVERSE EVENTS

### Indications

At the time of this writing, the Satellite spinal system (Medtronic Sofamor Danek, Memphis, TN) has been approved by the Food and Drug Administration (FDA) and is intended to be inserted between the vertebral bodies into the disc space from L3-S1 to help provide stabilization (and to help promote intervertebral body fusion). This internal device is intended for and designed to hold bone parts separated and in alignment. It is intended to be used with bone graft, bone substitute, or other osteobiologics. Indications include primary symptomatic DDD, primary disc herniations with symptomatic DDD (50% back and 50% sciatica), midline disc herniations, recurrent disc herniations, and mild translational deformities with instability. Additionally, the spherical implant can be inserted through a variety of approaches including posterior, posterolateral, extreme lateral, or anterior using standard or minimally invasive procedures. When used as a disc spacer for motion preservation surgery, the implant is considered an off-label device. The primary difference between the on-label construct and the off-label construct is the addition of bone graft material for the promotion of intervertebral fusion.

**TABLE 59–1. Contraindications for Use of the Satellite Spinal System**

| |
|---|
| Active infectious process or significant risk of infection (immunocompromised patients) |
| Signs of inflammatory parameters |
| Pregnancy due to use of fluoroscope |
| Mental illness/mental attitude |
| Grossly distorted anatomy caused by congenital abnormalities to allow precise positioning of implant |
| Rapid joint disease, bone absorption, osteopenia, osteomalacia, and osteoporosis (osteopenia is a relative contraindication because this condition may limit the degree of obtainable correction and stabilization and the amount of mechanical fixation that can be used to prevent subsidence of implant) |
| Suspected or documented metal allergy or intolerance (people are sensitive to nickel, cobalt, or chromium 11) |
| Any case in which the implant components selected for use would be too large or too small to achieve a successful result |
| Coexistence of dissimilar metals, specifically cobalt and stainless steel, that can lead to a battery effect, corrosion, and failure of the hardware |

### Contraindications

A summary of the contraindications for placement of the Satellite system are listed in Table 59–1.

### Adverse Events

A summary of the possible adverse effects from placement of the Satellite system are listed in Table 59–2.

### Patient Selection

Selection of patients is based on several criteria.

#### Age Versus Bone Quality

The patient's age is not a strong indication or contraindication for disc stabilization arthroplasty. Relatively good bone quality is a major factor for success, so use of computed tomography scan and a bone density determination by a DEXA scan should be performed. In addition, care must be taken when selecting patients with a history of chronic steroid use. This is to prevent subsequent end plate fractures around the device. Furthermore, patients who have disc end plate herniation (Schmorl's node) have the theoretical possibility of subsidence into the vertebral body. Careful evaluation of the preoperative magnetic resonance imaging scan should be performed to avoid placing the sphere at a level with Schmorl's nodes.

#### Spondylolisthesis

Spinal instability is to be assessed before disc stabilization arthroplasty. Although degenerative spondylolisthesis is not a contraindication for implantation of the device, flexion/extension radiographs are necessary to confirm lack of pathologic spinal motion. For this reason, we do not recommend disc stabilization arthroplasty for patients with previous facetectomies.

| TABLE 59–2. Adverse Effects Associated with the Satellite Spinal System |
|---|
| Loosening of the device and migration |
| Breakage of the device |
| Foreign body (allergic) reaction to implants, debris, corrosion products (from crevice, fretting, and general corrosion), including metallosis, staining, tumor formation, and/or autoimmune disease |
| Pressure on the skin from the device in patients with inadequate tissue coverage over the implant possibly causing skin penetration, irritation, fibrosis, necrosis, or pain; bursitis; tissue or nerve damage caused by improper positioning and placement of implants or instruments |
| Postoperative change in spinal curvature; loss of correction, height, or reduction |
| Dural tears, pseudomeningocele, fistula, persistent cerebrospinal fluid leakage, meningitis |
| Loss of neurologic function (e.g., sensory and/or motor), including paralysis (complete or incomplete) (dysesthesias, hyperesthesia, anesthesia, paresthesia), appearance of radiculopathy, and/or the development of pain, numbness, neuroma, spasms, sensory loss, tingling sensation, and/or visual deficits |
| Cauda equina syndrome, neuropathy, neurologic deficits (transient or permanent), paraplegia, paraparesis, reflex deficits, irritation, arachnoiditis, muscle loss, and loss of bowel and bladder control |
| Fracture, microfracture, resorption, damage, or penetration of any spinal bone |
| Cessation of any potential growth of the operated portion of the spine; loss of or increase in spinal mobility or function |
| Hemorrhage, hematoma, occlusion, seroma, edema, hypertension, embolism, stroke, excessive bleeding, phlebitis, wound necrosis, wound dehiscence, damage to blood vessels, or other types of cardiovascular system compromise (shorter) |
| Reproductive system compromise, including sterility, loss of consortium, and sexual dysfunction |

### Surgical History

Patients who have had a prior discectomy with a recurrent herniation are still candidates for a disc stabilization arthroplasty. However, active infection or a history of a discitis or bacterial spinal meningitis is a strong contraindication. Transition syndrome above or below a lumbar fusion is effectively treated with a disc stabilization arthroplasty.

### Spinal Stenosis

The majority of these spinal stenosis patients are elderly. However, the young healthy patient with a central stenosis from a central herniation, ligamentous hypertrophy, or a stable grade 1 anterolisthesis is effectively treated with disc stabilization arthroplasty. This also applies to lateral recess stenosis from a far lateral disc herniation. Foraminal stenosis with DDD can also be effectively treated with a foraminotomy and disc stabilization arthroplasty.

### Trauma

Disc stabilization arthroplasty has not been used in a spinal trauma patient.

## Description of the Device

The Satellite is a spherical implant designed to hold vertebrae in alignment. It can be used as a stand-alone device or in conjunction with pedicle screws with plates or rods. These spheres are placed into the disc space between two vertebral bodies. Currently, the system is limited to the L3-S1 levels. The device is fabricated from cobalt-chromium-molybdenum (CoCrMo) or polyetheretherketone (PEEK) and serves as a single-use implant. It is dependent on surgeon preference as to which implant is used (CoCrMo or PEEK), and their perceived features and benefits are not unlike those of other PEEK and metallic intervertebral cages or vertebral body spacers. Regardless of the material, the Satellite implants are indicated for the same patient in the same manner. The use of the device is restricted to surgeons trained and familiar with the surgical aspects involved in arthroplasty with in-depth knowledge of disc mechanics and material applications.

## Biomechanics of Disc Stabilization Arthroplasty

A partial disc replacement or disc stabilization arthroplasty maintains the annulus fibrosis but replaces the nucleus pulposus. The normal nucleus pulposus is a remnant of the notochord composed of proteoglycans and type I collagen. It functions to resist compressive loads. Partial disc arthroplasty resists compressive loads while allowing for motion in rotation, flexion, extension, as well as side bending. End plate sclerosis and partial subsidence maintain the implant between the vertebral bodies, thus allowing it to act as a fulcrum for spinal motion. The implant has been observed to nest in the nuclear recess and finds its own center of rotation based on the disc level and morphology of the intervertebral disc space (Fig. 59–1A–E).

## BACKGROUND OF SCIENTIFIC TESTING

Motion preservation and restoration of the stability of the spine at the intervertebral level have been discussed extensively in the literature. The ultimate objective is to implant a safe device that functions similar to a normal intervertebral disc, specifically allowing motion while stabilizing the motion segment (see Introduction).

Fernström concluded that the results obtained in his follow-up studies as a result of disc replacement were better than those achieved as a result of discectomy alone and that these results were similar to the results of discectomy combined with fusion (Table 59–3). However, biomechanical testing, clinical utility in terms of indications and contraindications remained inadequate. Although the procedure of inserting a spherical endoprosthesis (*intercorporal endoprosthesis*) into the center of the evacuated disc produced satisfactory clinical results with few complications, it was abandoned because of subsidence of steel balls into the adjacent vertebral bodies. Enker et al[18] reported a 3-year follow-up study in 1993 of intervertebral disc replacement using the Acroflex prosthesis, comprising of a rubber core vulcanized to titanium end plates. Four of the six patients studied had a satisfactory outcome at follow-up. Additionally, McKenzie's[14] report on his experiences with patients who underwent Fernström intervertebral arthroplasties (see introduction) credits the Fernström procedure as probably ahead of its time. The results in his series were somewhat better in patients who had disc protrusions in otherwise intact spines, but a high percentage of good and excellent results were seen in patients with moderate degenerative spinal alterations and instability. There are several other discs that have been designed and are in various stages of scientific testing in the United States and in Europe. Although clinical trials have not yet been initiated in the United States for implants and uses being discussed specific to this chapter, at the time of this writing, unpublished data collected from outcomes registry of using spherical disc arthroplasty to help stabilize the motion segment indicate potentially encouraging outcomes (Fig. 59–2A–C).

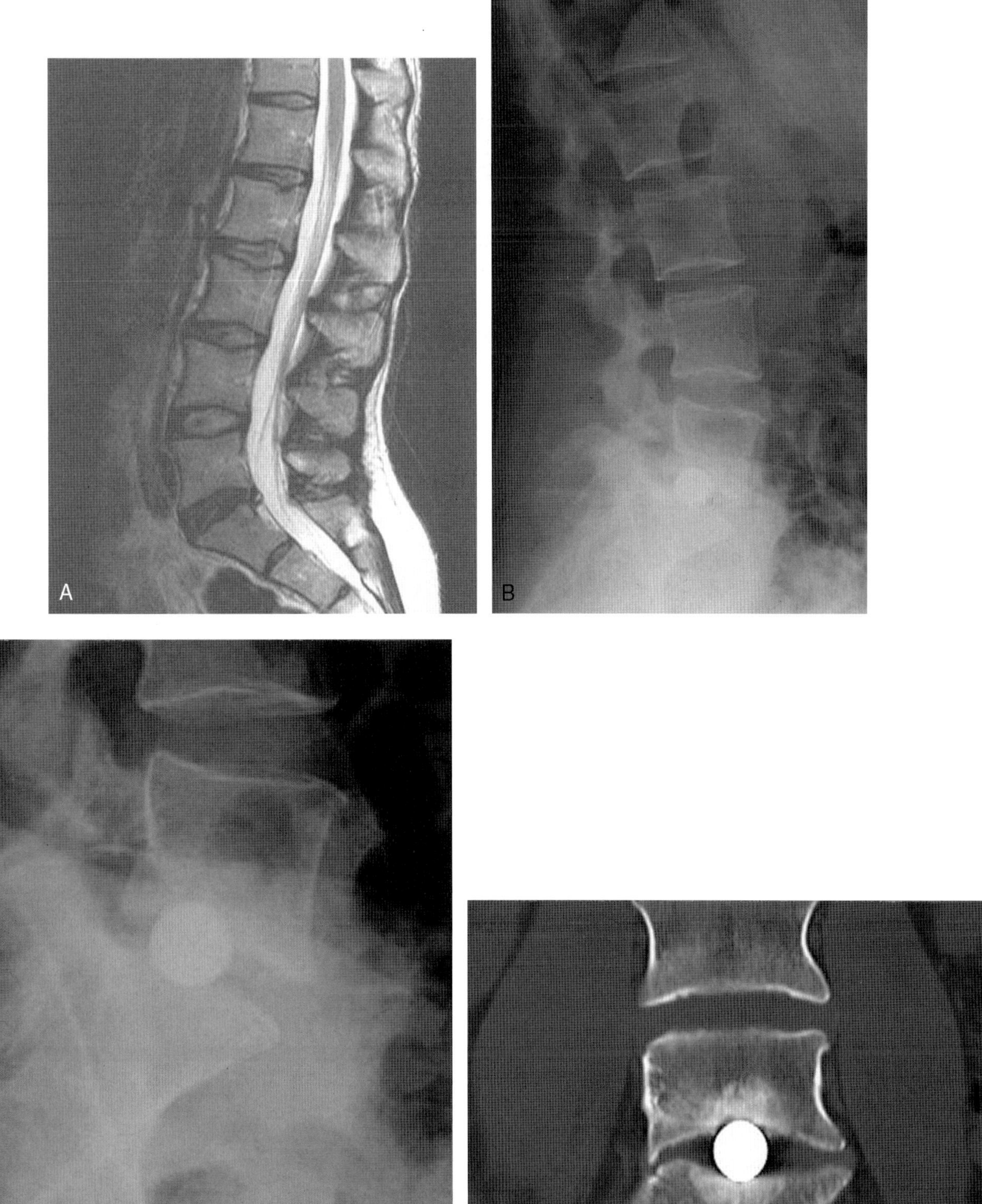


■ **FIGURE 59–1.** **A,** Preoperative symptomatic degenerative disc disease at L5-S1 as shown on lateral computed tomography (CT) scan. **B,** A 12-month postoperative lateral x-ray study of the same patient. Implant sitting in the center to posterior third of the disc space in line with the center of rotation. Implant enclosed by the nuclear recess of the vertebral body end plates. **C,** Close-up view of the implant. **D,** A 12-month follow-up anteroposterior CT scan of the same patient. Implant shows good mediolateral placement, with Wolff's law cortication around the device.

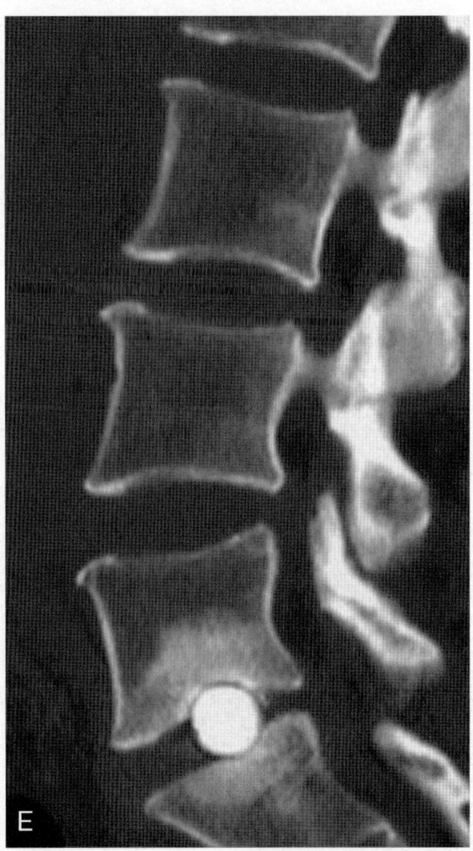


■ **FIGURE 59–1. Cont'd.** **E,** Lateral 12-month CT scan (midline) of the same patient. The scan shows implant sitting toward the posterior third of the disc and placement within the nuclear recess of the end plates.

**TABLE 59–3. Fernström's Two-Year Follow-Up Results of Replacing a Disc with a Mechanical Prosthesis**

| | Two-Year Follow-Up Results | |
|---|---|---|
| | **Group I Herniated Disc** | **Group II Degenerative Disc** |
| Patients undergoing disc replacement surgery | 12% reported back pain<br>14% reported sciatica | 40% reported back pain<br>47% reported sciatica |
| Patients undergoing a discectomy | 60% reported back pain<br>50% reported sciatica | 88% reported back pain<br>80% reported sciatica |

## Operative Technique

### Preoperative Planning and Patient Positioning

The patient is placed on a Wilson frame in the prone position, making sure to allow enough room for lateral fluoroscopy (see Fig. 59–3). A midline incision provides the approach and unilateral exposure of the interlaminar space and facet joints at the affected level. A hemilaminotomy is performed to expose both the dura and annulus lateral to the dura (Fig. 59–4). If needed, the spinous process can be undercut to gain access. The lateral half of the ligamentum flavum is thoroughly removed in order to explore the spinal canal and its contents. Care should be taken to identify the lateral dura and traversing nerve root at the affected level. The epidural veins are coagulated over the annulus, and any other tethering of the traversing root is dissected to allow for sufficient retraction of the dura and root.

### Distraction and Disc Removal

Distraction can be achieved with a lamina or interspinous spreader. Using the table frame to place the patient in a kyphotic position may help to provide an adequate opening of the disc space (Fig. 59–5). While protecting the dura and nerve root, a discectomy is performed by incising the annulus lateral to the dura. A pituitary rongeur removes the excised annulus and nuclear material. Extruded fragments are removed to decompress the neural elements and provide entry to the disc space for distraction with minimal or no nerve root retraction.

### Trial

Trials are used to confirm the appropriate final sphere diameter. The trials are tapered on the leading and trailing edge for easier insertion and removal from the disc space. Align the flat ends on the trial parallel to the end plates (Fig. 59–6A–C). Lightly tap

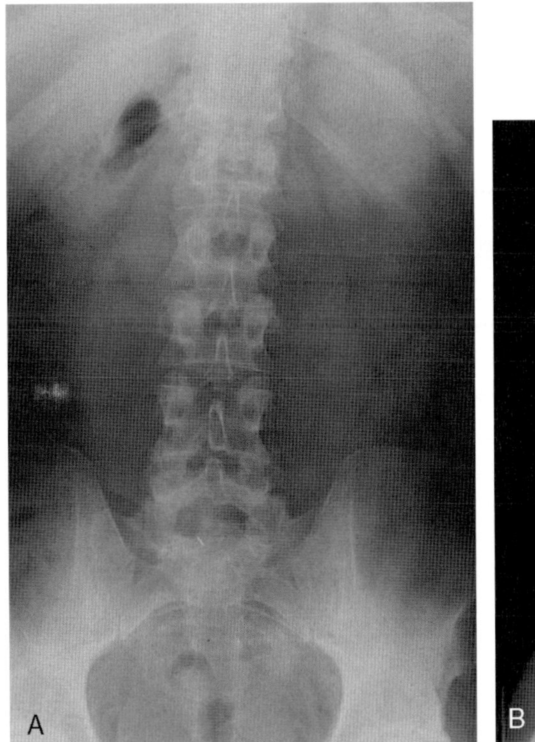


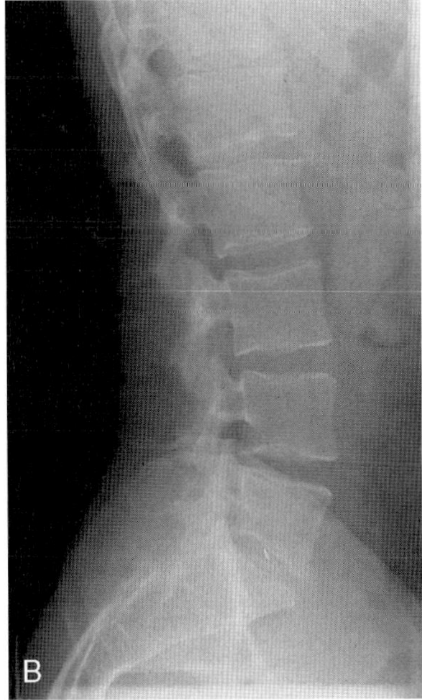


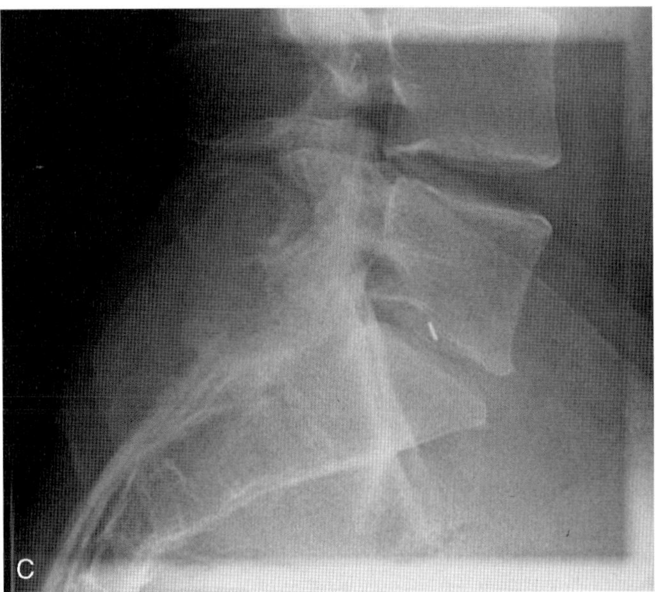


■ **FIGURE 59–2. A,** One-month postoperative anteroposterior (AP) film of a Satellite PEEK device implanted. Tantalum marker allows for AP visualization and determination of positioning on x-ray. **B,** One-month postoperative lateral film of a Satellite PEEK device. Tantalum marker can be seen clearly. **C,** Close-up lateral film of the same patient.

the trial into the disc space and turn the handle 59 degrees to assess the fit. The trial should fully engage the end plates and restore the disc space to its normal height (see Fig. 59–6A–C). Lateral fluoroscopic imaging is helpful to assess the fit of the trial. To remove the trial, turn the handle 59 degrees, attach the slap hammer to the extension handle, and gently tap it to remove the trial from the disc space. Continue to use sequentially larger trials until the final sphere diameter is determined (Fig. 59–7).

### Final Preparation

The sphere curettes can be used to remove any excess nucleus material. Using a curette equal to the final trial diameter, the curette is inserted into the disc space, with the smooth side oriented toward the surrounding neural structures (Fig. 59–8). Position the curette at the desired location of the implant. Generally, this is in the center of the disc space and slightly posterior to midline (Fig. 59–9A). Turn the curette 360 degrees to remove excess

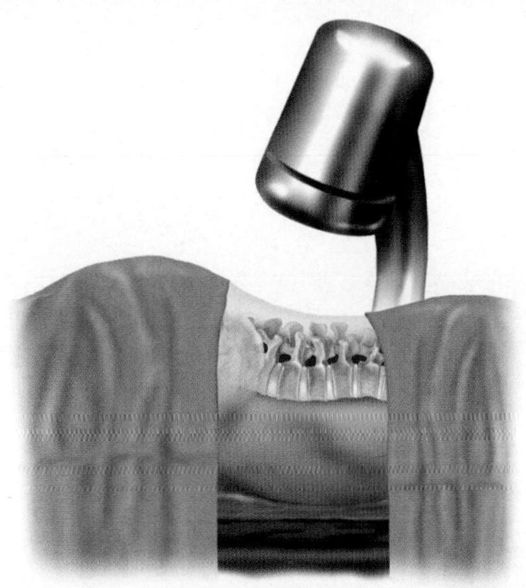

■ **FIGURE 59–3.** Patient positioning for implanting the Satellite device.

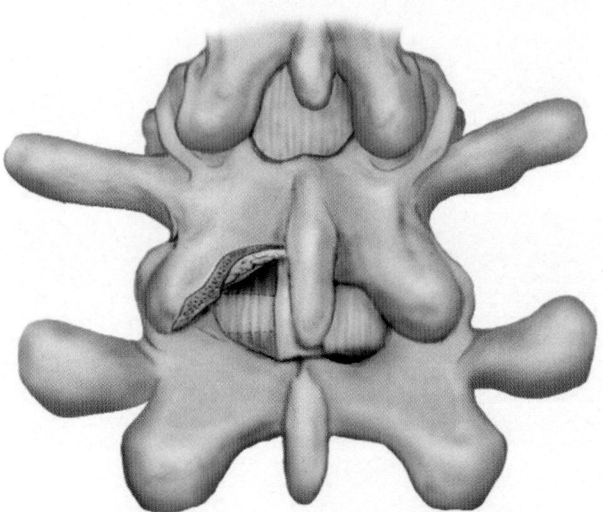

■ **FIGURE 59–4.** A hemilaminotomy is performed to expose both the dura and annulus lateral to the dura.

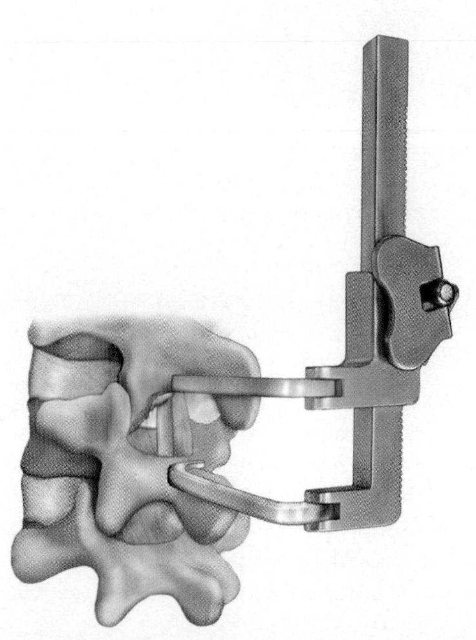

■ **FIGURE 59–5.** Distraction and end plate preparation.

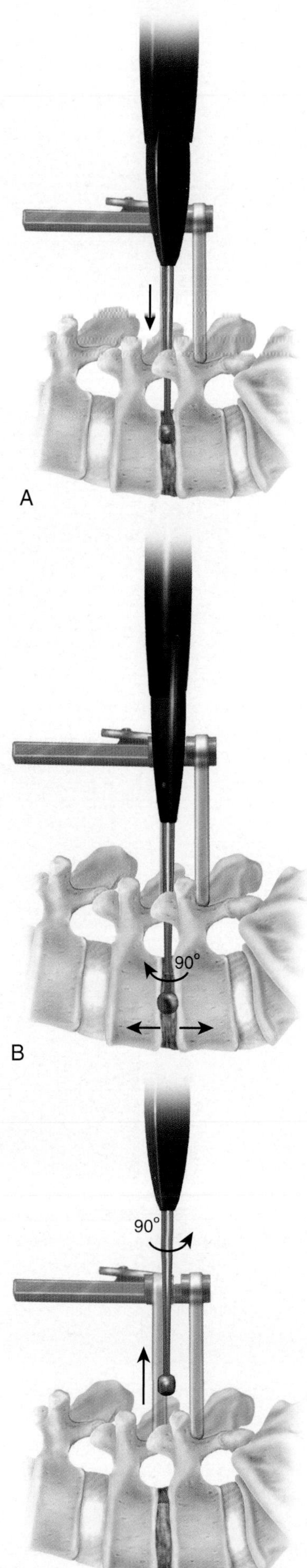


■ **FIGURE 59–6.** **A** to **C,** Trials are used to confirm the appropriate final sphere diameter.

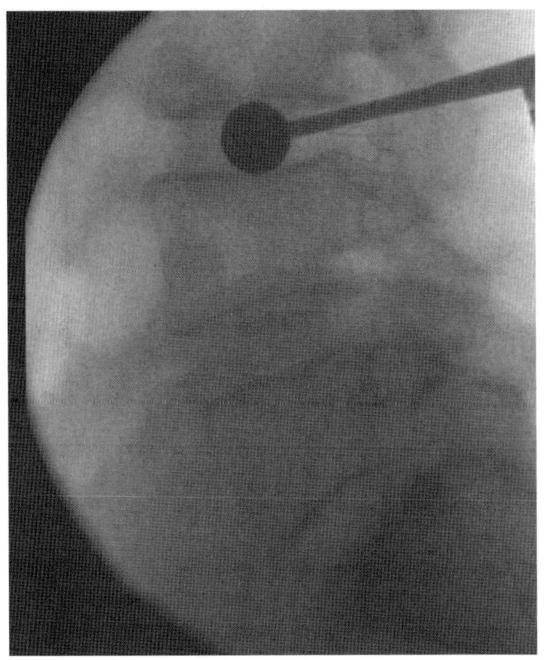

■ **FIGURE 59–7.** Trial of the Satellite implant. The trial is placed in a flat orientation, with tapered front and back edges for easier insertion into the disc space. Once inserted, the trial is rotated 90 degrees to assess proper fit within the nuclear cavity.

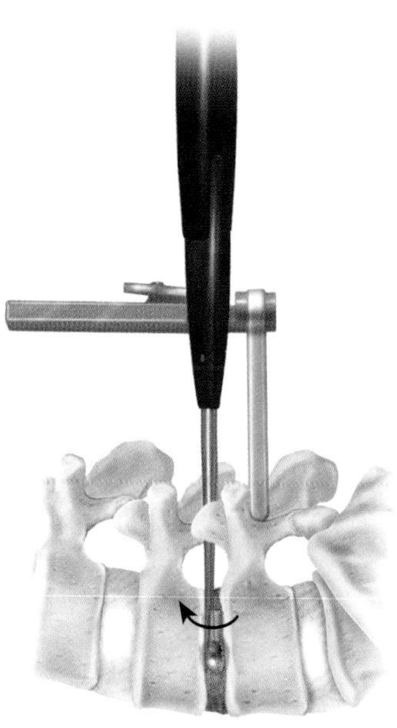

■ **FIGURE 59–8.** Using a curette equal to the final trial diameter, the curette is inserted into the disc space, with the smooth side oriented toward the surrounding neural structures.

A

B

C

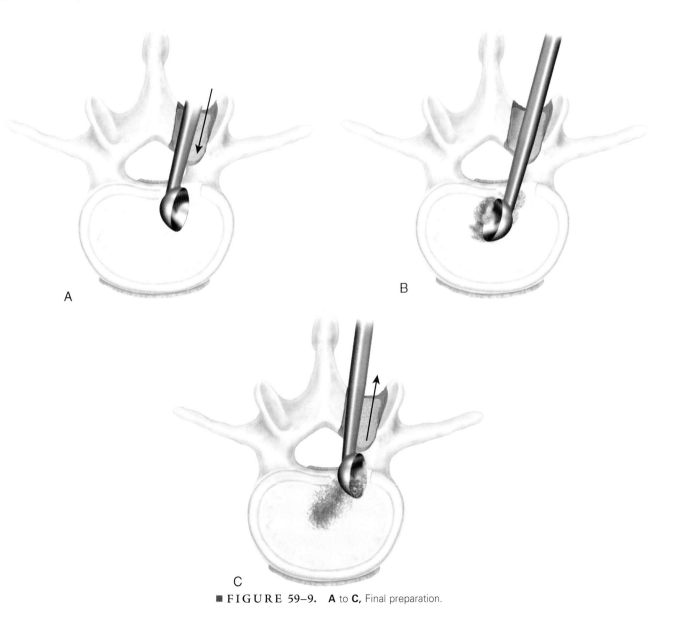

■ **FIGURE 59–9.** **A** to **C,** Final preparation.

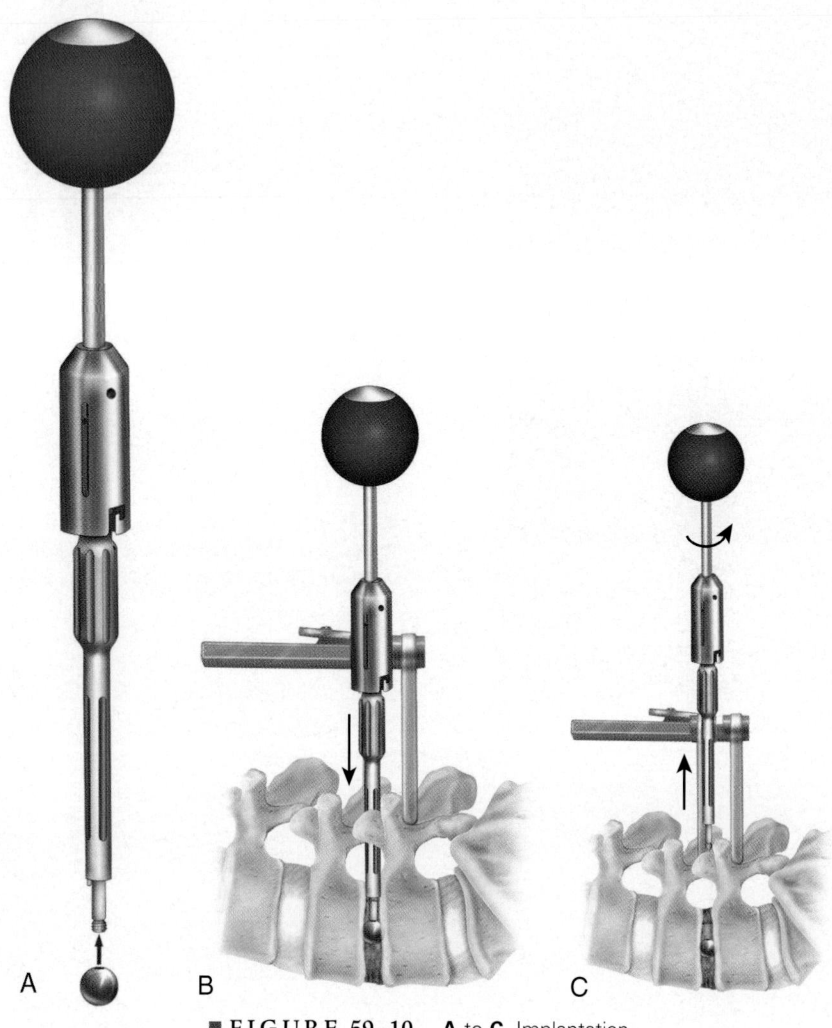


■ **FIGURE 59–10.** **A** to **C,** Implantation.

nucleus (Fig. 59–9B). Remove the instrument by orienting the smooth side of the curette toward the neural structures and gently removing it from the disc space (Fig. 59–9C).

### Implantation

Thread the appropriately sized sphere onto the inserter (Fig. 59–10A). Slide the inserter's outer sleeve forward so the pin engages the small antirotation dimple on the sphere and tighten the wingnut to lock into place. Gently impact the sphere into the disc space by orienting the sphere toward midline of the disc space (Fig. 59–10B). Once the sphere is fully seated, turn the inserter's handle counterclockwise to disengage the implant (Fig. 59–10C). The angled graft impacter can be used to achieve the desired position of the implant. In the event that the implant needs to be removed, thread the inserter into the implant and remove.

### Closure

The wound is closed in a routine manner. Ambulation begins the day of surgery, and patients are generally discharged the following day.

## POSTOPERATIVE CARE

Extensive preoperative education about the expected postoperative course and expectations is required. We follow patients 1 week, 1 month, 6 months, and 1 year postoperatively with serial radiographic evaluations. A 24-month outcome evaluation is also preferred. Patients are allowed to stand immediately with the use of a lumbar-sacral orthosis (LSO). Patients are advised to avoid driving and prolonged sitting for the first week, and extremes of lumbar flexion or extension within the first 6 weeks. This is the major function of the LSO. Because reherniation at the operative level is not a major concern, we instruct patients not to lift heavy objects as a matter of patient comfort as well as to maintain wound integrity. In addition, clinical outcome measures (ODI, SF-36, etc.) should be obtained on all patients preoperatively as well as during the postoperative follow-up visits.

## ADVANTAGES/DISADVANTAGES

The Satellite spinal system is a pioneering development in technology that will change the way patients with DDD are treated. In the midst of current and evolving modern surgical techniques,

**ADVANTAGES OF THE SATELLITE**

**Featured Advantages**

- Inserted through a minimally invasive posterior approach
- Highly polished cobalt-chromium-molybdenum implant or PEEK
- Maintains disc height and sagittal balance
- Less patient morbidity; faster recovery
- Smooth surfaces for minimization of wear and friction with vertebral end plates
- To match varying anatomy, the Satellite device can be customized with ranges between 9 mm and 16 mm diameter

**Stabilization Advantages**

- Intradiscal stabilization
- Satellite restores disc space height and sagittal balance
- Fits within the natural concavity of the vertebral bodies
- Rests in the anatomic center of rotation

nucleus replacement with a metallic sphere is a successful and viable procedure, owing to its biomechanical uniqueness, and is the result of early progressive thinking, years of prospective clinical trials, and the Satellite spinal system's unique capabilities to restore normal kinematics.

## CONCLUSIONS

We are only in the infancy of understanding and comprehending the implications of the spine arthroplasty and nonfusion techniques. Consequently, the next decade will see new growth in innovation and undiscovered frontiers of treating back pain patients, particularly DDD. Nonetheless, with the advent of new technology innovation and possible alternatives for the treatment of patients worldwide, there is clear skepticism. Surgical technique training and education, thorough clinical trials, and comprehensive clinical testing continue to become critical to successfully guide the new era of spine arthroplasty surgery. From our experiences we can conclude that mechanical articulated devices such as the Satellite system to replace the diseased nucleus pulposus as a treatment for low back pain secondary to disc degeneration have emerged as promising tools for selected patients.

## REFERENCES


1. Stambough JL: Lumbosacral instrumented fusion: Analysis of 124 consecutive cases. J Spinal Disord 12:1–9, 1999.
2. Kumar MN, Jacquot F, Hall H: Long-term follow-up of functional outcomes and radiographic changes at adjacent levels following lumbar spine fusion for degenerative disc disease. Eur Spine J 10:309–313, 2001.
3. Phillips FM, Reuben J, Wetzel FT: Intervertebral disc degeneration adjacent to a lumbar fusion: An experimental rabbit model. J Bone Joint Surg Br 84:289–294, 2002.
4. Cleveland DA: The use of methylacrylic for spinal stabilization after disc operations. Marquette Med Rev 20:62–64, 1955.
5. Hamby WB, Glaser HT: Replacement of spinal intervertebral discs with locally polymerizing methyl methacrylate. J Neurosurg: 16311–16313, 1959.
6. van Steenbrugghe MH, inventor: Improvements in joint prosthesis. French patent 1,122,634, May 28, 1956.
7. Harmon PH: Anterior excision and vertebral body fusion operation for intervertebral disk syndromes of the lower lumbar spine. Clin Orthop Relat Res 26:107–127, 1963.
8. Nachemson A: Some mechanical properties of the lumbar intervertebral disc. Bull Hosp Joint Dis 23:130–132, 1962.
9. Reitz H, Joubert MJ: Intractable headache and cervicobrachialgia treated by complete replacement of cervical intervertebral discs with a metal prosthesis. S Afr Med J 38:881–889, 1964.
10. Fernström U: Arthroplasty with intercorporal endoprosthesis in herniated disc and in painful disc. Acta Chir Scand (suppl) 357:154–159, 1966.
11. Cloward R: Lesions of the intervertebral disks and their treatment by interbody fusion methods. The painful disk. Clin Orthop Relat Res 27:51–77, 1963.
12. Harmon PH, Abel MS: Correlation of multiple objective diagnostic methods in lower lumbar disk disease. Clin Orthop Relat Res 28:132–151, 1963.
13. Kristionsen K, Eie N: The surgical treatment of low back pain and sciatica. J Oslo Cy Hosp. 7, 133, 1957.
14. McKenzie AH: Fernström intervertebral disc arthroplasty: A long-term evaluation. Orthop Int 3:313–324, 1995.
15. Froning EC: Intervertebral disc prosthesis and instruments for locating same. US patent 3,875,595;1975.
16. Fassio B, Ginestie JF: Discal prosthesis made of silicone: experimental study and 1st clinical cases. Nouv Presse Med 7:207, 1978.
17. Hedman TP, Kostuik JP, Fernie GR, Maiki BE: Artificial spinal disc. US patent 4,759,769;1988.
18. Enker P, Steffee A, McMillin C, Kedppler L, et al: Artificial disc replacement. Preliminary report with a 3-year minimum follow-up. Spine 18:1061–1070, 1993.
19. Büttner-Janz K: The development of the artificial disc: SB CHARITÉ. Dallas: Hundley and Associates, 1992.
20. Marnay T: Prothèse pour disques intervertébraux et ses instruments d'implantation. French patent FR2,659,226;1990.
21. Ray CD, Dickhudt EA, Ledoux PJ, Frutiger BA: Prosthetic spinal disc nucleus. US patent 5,674,295;1997.
22. Lemaire JP, Skalli W, Lavaste F et al: Intervertebral disc prosthesis. Results and prospects for the year 2000. Clin Orthop 337:64–76, 1997

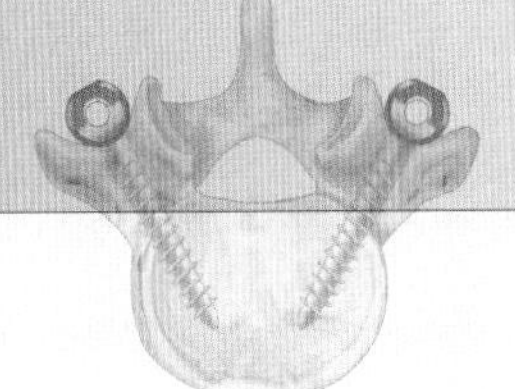

PART

# VI

# Lumbar Posterior Dynamic Stabilization: Pedicle Screw Based

CHAPTER 60

# Dynesys Dynamic Stabilization System

Reginald J. Davis

### KEY POINTS

- Dynamic stabilization is a rapidly evolving philosophy in spine surgery.
- The Dynesys Spinal System is the most widely used dynamic stabilization device.
- Dynesys is composed of titanium screws, PCU spacers, and PET cords.
- The posterior approach minimizes the learning curve in Dynesys surgery.
- The Dynesys actively shares load and delivers energy to the spinal segment.

## INTRODUCTION

The Dynesys (DYnamic NEutralization SYStem) Spinal System (Zimmer Spine, Inc., Warsaw, IN) is a pedicle screw–based system for dynamic stabilization of the lumbar spine. Dynamic stabilization is an evolving philosophy in the treatment of back and leg pain. It employs the familiar surgical approach of traditional pedicle-based systems while using flexible materials and preserving anatomic structures. The goal is restoration of stability and improved clinical outcomes without traditional rigid fixation.

Dynesys was invented and developed by Dr. Gilles Dubois.[1] It was first implanted in 1994 and received Conformité Européene (CE) mark in 1999 as a nonfusion stabilization system. It received 510(k) clearance by the U.S. Food and Drug Administration in 2005 as a substantially equivalent pedicle screw system and is being evaluated in a U.S. Investigational Device Exemption (IDE) study as a nonfusion stabilization system. There have been more than 25,000 devices implanted worldwide.

## INDICATIONS/CONTRAINDICATIONS

The Dynesys Spinal System is generally indicated to treat conditions of the lumbar spine characterized by mild to moderate segmental instability. Specifically, five indications have been reported globally: spinal stenosis with moderated instability, spondylolisthesis grade 1, adjacent-segment degeneration after previous fusion, recurring disc herniation or herniation associated with disc degeneration, and degenerative disc disease (DDD).[2–9]

Lumbar spinal stenosis can be associated with degeneration and laxity of supporting ligaments. Patients will have not only characteristic neurogenic claudication but significant mechanical back pain as well. The resulting instability will not be addressed with decompression alone. Further stabilization is needed as well. Stabilization with the Dynesys Spinal System, combined with surgical decompression of lumbar stenosis with moderate instability, results in statistically significant clinical improvements (Fig. 60–1). Patients demonstrated improvements in Oswestry Disability Index (ODI) and Visual Analog Scale (VAS) scores for back pain and leg pain, as well as Prolo functional and economic categories.[10]

Grade 1 lumbar spondylolisthesis is usually indicative of mild instability of lumbar supportive ligaments. In such cases, the additional increment of stability afforded by the Dynesys Spinal System can result in significant pain reduction and functional improvement.[10]

The spinal segment adjacent to a previous fusion sometimes undergoes destabilization and further degeneration. In instances of mild to moderate symptomatic adjacent-segment degeneration, Dynesys stabilizes the affected joint. By using flexible materials and preserving much of the normal anatomic structure, the Dynesys Spinal System avoids the impact of traditional rigid fixation on the next segment.

Recurrent disc herniations and herniations associated with degeneration are complex in presentation and clinical resolution. Routine acute disc herniations are well treated with simple decompressive procedures. The more complex presentations are rarely treated effectively with simple discectomy techniques alone. Simple discectomy in these cases often results in progression of disease and reccurrence of symptoms. Stabilization with Dynesys following discectomy resulted in better long-term maintenance of clinical improvement (Fig. 60–2). The ODI was significantly better, as were the VAS and radiographic parameters. No progression of DDD, fatty degeneration or sclerotic bone reaction, or spondylarthrosis was seen.[5]

DDD remains a controversial entity. Although individual opinions may vary, it is broadly accepted that abnormal load-handling characteristics of the degenerating disc represent a key component of this clinical syndrome. This defines a relative instability of the motion segment that is painful. This observed instability is treated

CASE 1

- 63 y. o. male
- L3-L5 stenosis
- 1 block claudication
- Laminectomy and Dynesys stabilization
- Resolution of clinical syndrome

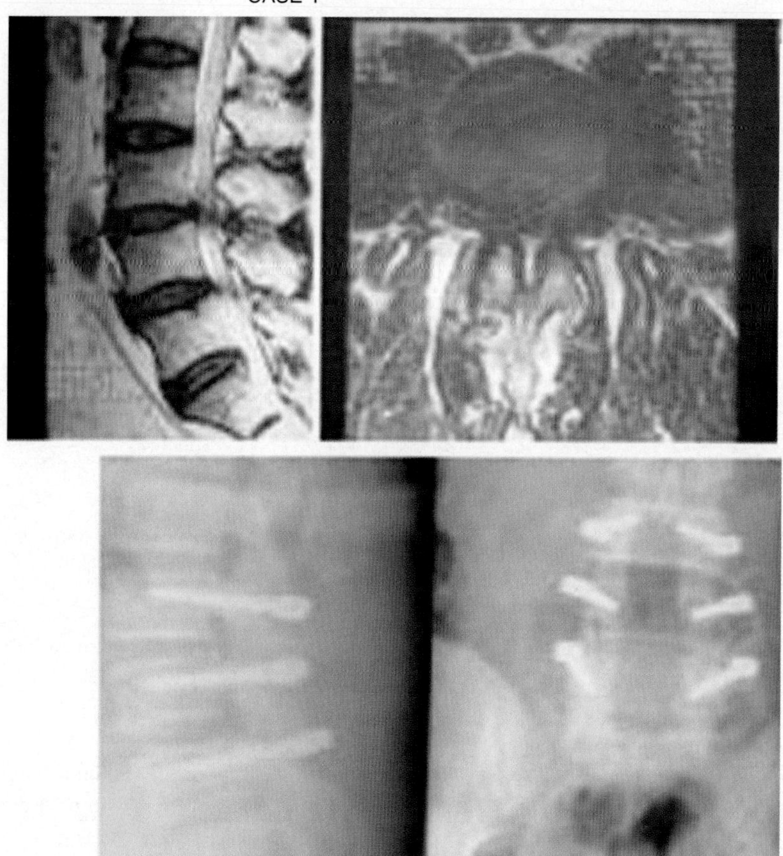

■ **FIGURE 60–1.** Case of lumbar stenosis treated with laminectomy and Dynesys stabilization.

CASE 2

- 43 y. o. F
- L4-L5 DDD, HNP
- LBP, sciatica
- L4-L5 discectomy and Dynesys
- Resolution of clinical syndrome

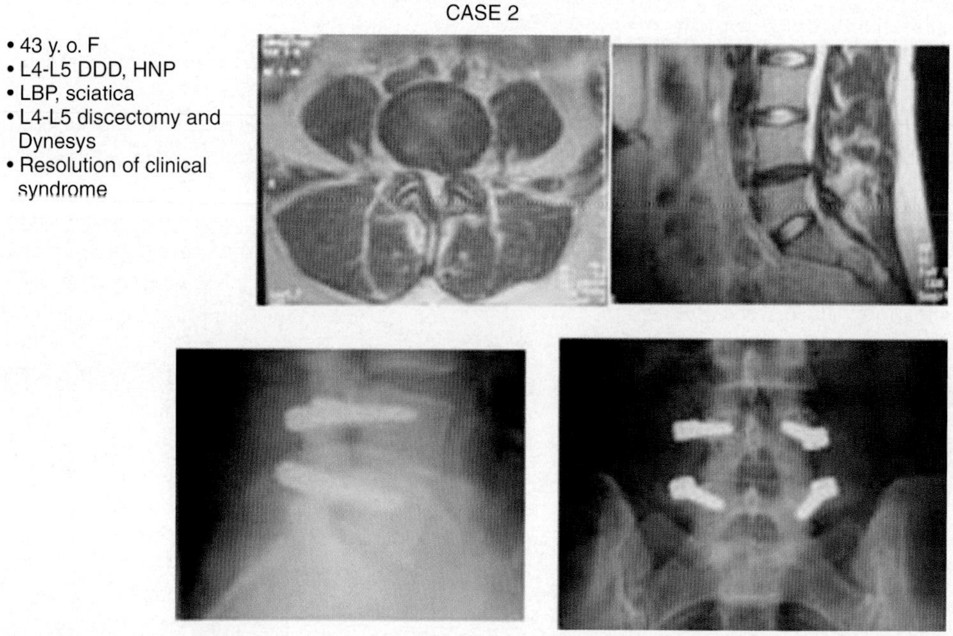

■ **FIGURE 60–2.** Case of disc herniation and degeneration treated with discectomy and Dynesys stabilization.

with clinical success using the Dynesys Spinal System to unload the failing disc.

The Dynesys Spinal System is not indicated for all patients. Contraindications include active systemic or local infection; severe osteomalacia, osteoporosis/osteopenia, metabolic bone disease; chronic steroid use; spondylolisthesis higher than grade 1; isthmic spondylolisthesis or spondylolysis; pedicle fracture; total facetectomy; skeletal immaturity; scoliosis greater than 10 degrees; and allergy to metals, polymers, polyethylene, polycarbonate urethane, and polyethylene terephthalate.

## DESCRIPTION OF THE DEVICE

The Dynesys Spinal System consists of three components; pedicle screw, cord, and spacer (Fig. 60–3).

The pedicle screw is composed of the titanium alloy Protasul 100. The tapered minor diameter shank and constant major diameter threads afford a press fit in the pedicle when fully seated. The surface is textured or optionally HA coated to maximize osseous incorporation. It is a closed-head fixed screw with a top-loaded set screw.

The cord is composed of Sulene-polyethylene-terephalate (PET). It is divided into three zones. The introductory zone is narrow, tapered, and malleable. It affords easy insertion into the spacers and screws. The working zone is marked by green bands and is meant to be manipulated during insertion. The functional zone is that portion that remains in the patient and is not meant to be damaged by manipulation.

The spacer is composed of Sulene-polycarbonate-urethane (PCU). The spacers are universally sized and need to be cut to patient-specific dimensions.

When the system is implanted, the screws are securely anchored in the pedicle. The spacer is compressed between the screws and thus exerts a flexion moment. The cord, spanning the screws and threading the spacer, is under tension and exerts an extension moment. The resultant equilibrium affords dynamic stabilization to the motion segment. The tensioned cord also acts to restrict excessive flexion much as the compressed spacer acts to block excessive extension. This helps to maintain neutral position of the spinal segment.[3]

## BACKGROUND OF SCIENTIFIC TESTING/CLINICAL OUTCOMES

The goal of biomechanical testing was to demonstrate that the system will perform and survive under conditions simulating clinical use. Components were tested individually, and assemblies and constructs were tested to verify in vitro performance.

The pedicles screws were subjected to cyclic loading between 100 and 800 N. The smallest screw size (5.2 mm × 35 mm) successfully passed 5 million loading cycles without fatigue breakage.

The PET cord passed 5 million cycles of loading between 100 N and 800 N. Creep elongation at 20 hours was 1.24% of the initial cord length, and static tensile strength was approximately 3,000 N. No rupture occurred.

The PCU spacers were tested under conditions simulating an in situ environment. No appreciable creep deformation was observed. Stiffness was 243 N/mm at room temperature and 136 N/mm at body temperature.

Screw/cord constructs were tested with static tensile loads to quantify the pullout strength of the cord. Static pullout strength was 1,060 N at nominal set screw torque (4 Nm). Screw/cord assemblies were cyclically loaded between 100 and 800 N. No slippage was observed past 5 million cycles.

Screw/cord/spacer assemblies passed 10 million cycles of 5 mm of shear displacement or 3 degrees of axial rotation in a

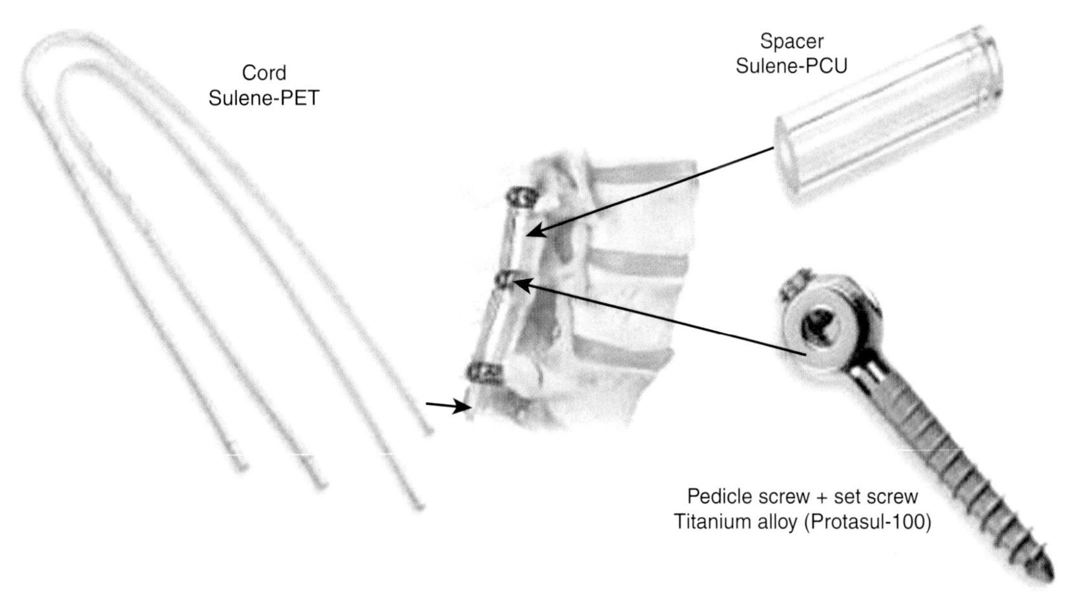


■ **FIGURE 60–3.** Dynesys Spinal System materials.

lipid environment at body temperature without any instances of cord failure. Cord abrasion after 10 million cycles was inconsequential.

In summary, the screws and cords have adequate static and cyclic strength. The cords and spacers have adequate creep and stress-relaxation characteristics. The assembled system exhibits robust static and cyclic interconnection strength yielding initial and long-term stability in assembly tests.

## Clinical Experience

Significant clinical experience has been gained from more than 25,000 Dynesys implantations worldwide. In the vast majority of patients, an element of segmental instability is a component of the clinical syndrome leading to surgery. Most cases treated to date and reported scientifically fall into one of several categories.

Lumbar stenosis (case 1) is a frequent condition treated with Dynesys. In an initial series of 83 patients subsequently expanded to 150 patients with 4-year follow-up, Stoll et al[10] reported significant clinical success. Patients receiving dynamic stabilization following decompressive laminectomies showed statistically significant improvements in VAS for back and leg pain, ODI, and Prolo functional and economic catagories. Overall complication rates, especially screw loosening, were less than prevailing rates for traditional rigid fixation.

Degenerative spondylolisthesis of grade 1 or less is another condition frequently addressed with Dynesys stabilization. This diagnosis has traditionally required fusion to treat cases refractory to nonsurgical interventions. Dynesys offers a viable nonfusion option. In the preliminary results of the U.S. IDE trial comparing Dynesys dynamic stabilization to rigid posterior instrumented fusion, these patients enjoyed high rates of patient satisfaction in association with improvement in all clinical parameters.[11]

Lumbar DDD is increasingly treated successfully with the Dynesys Stabilization System. Disc degeneration can lead to vertical and translational instability amenable to stabilization. Both pure DDD and that associated with herniated nucleus pulposus (HNP), previous surgery, and adjacent-segment breakdown have been addressed with good clinical outcomes (case 2). Putzier[4] reported on 35 patients with HNP associated with symptomatic DDD. When compared with a cohort treated with discectomy alone, those patients undergoing dynamic stabilization in addition to discectomy did statistically clinically better after 34 months. VAS pain scores and ODI scores were significantly better, and no progression of spondyloarthrosis or sclerotic bone changes was seen. This was not true for the control group.

Successful intervention with Dynesys implantation has also been reported in cases of adjacent segment disease and previous surgery.[2,6,7]

## OPERATIVE TECHNIQUE

The Dynesys Spinal System is placed through the posterior or posterolateral approach. This approach is very familiar to all spine surgeons and thus minimizes the learning curve. General endotracheal anesthesia is used, and neurophysiologic monitoring is recommended.

The patient is positioned prone, and normal lordosis should be maintained. This can be accomplished with the Andrew's frame, Jackson table, Wilson frame, or rolls. The use of fluoroscopy or other navigation assistance is strongly recommended to ensure accurate and efficient screw placement.

The pedicles can be accessed by any standard approach. The single midline incision with lateral tissue retraction is most common. The exposure should extend to the tips of the transverse processes to ensure proper entry and trajectory. Paired paraspinal incisions as with the Wiltse approach offers advantages of minimal surgical trauma and more convergent trajectory through the pedicles. Less invasive techniques with tubular retractors or expandable retractors are also possible. Surgeon preference and experience should be the determining factor in choosing a surgical approach. Whatever the approach, the desired entry point into the pedicle is lateral to the facet. The facet capsule is spared during the exposure.

The pedicle screws should be placed lateral to the facets on a convergent path to the midline of the vertebral body (Fig. 60–4). Not only does this lateral placement avoid trauma and impingement on the facets, it also places the force vectors closer to the axis of rotation. The convergent trajectory ensures the longest path possible to maximize screw length and purchase. The facets should not be disrupted. Competent facets and capsular ligaments ensure maximal posterior stability. The spacer-template tool allows determination of the correct angle of the pedicle screws and ensures that the spacer will lay in the lateral gutter without impingement on the facet.

Once the proper entry and trajectory are confirmed, the pedicle is opened. This can be accomplished with high-speed burr or awl. The pedicle screw channel is made with the pedicle probe. Curved probes should be avoided because the resulting channel may be excessive, thus compromising screw purchase. Fluoroscopy or other imaging assist is strongly recommended. The integrity of the pedicle channel is confirmed with the pedicle sound. Neuromonitoring is also useful at this juncture.

The longest screw of the largest diameter feasible is selected. All screws are inserted (Fig. 60–4A). The screws are advanced until the screw heads abut the bone. The screw-head eyelets must align parallel to the spine and face one another. This ensures proper passage of the cord. It is recommended to leave the screws "proud" on initial insertion. Final positioning can then be fine-tuned by advancing the screws forward. Backing the screws out will result in loss of purchase and can lead to screw loosening. When ideally placed, the screws will occupy two-thirds of the vertebral body on lateral x-ray study, converge toward the midline on anteroposterior (AP) x-ray study, and be parallel with its contralateral partner.

The spacer length is now determined for all interspaces (Fig. 60–4B). The pedicle-distance gauge is placed between the pedicle screw heads near the center of the eyelets. Distraction force is applied, and the distance is measured. Reasonable force is applied to create parallel end plates or neutral facet joint position. Caution should be exercised not to induce kyphosis. Spacer length measurement must be performed for both sides prior to implantation. The spacers are cut to proper length using the spacer cutting tool.

The PET cord is selected. The 100-mm cord is used for one or two levels, and the 200-mm length for two or more levels.

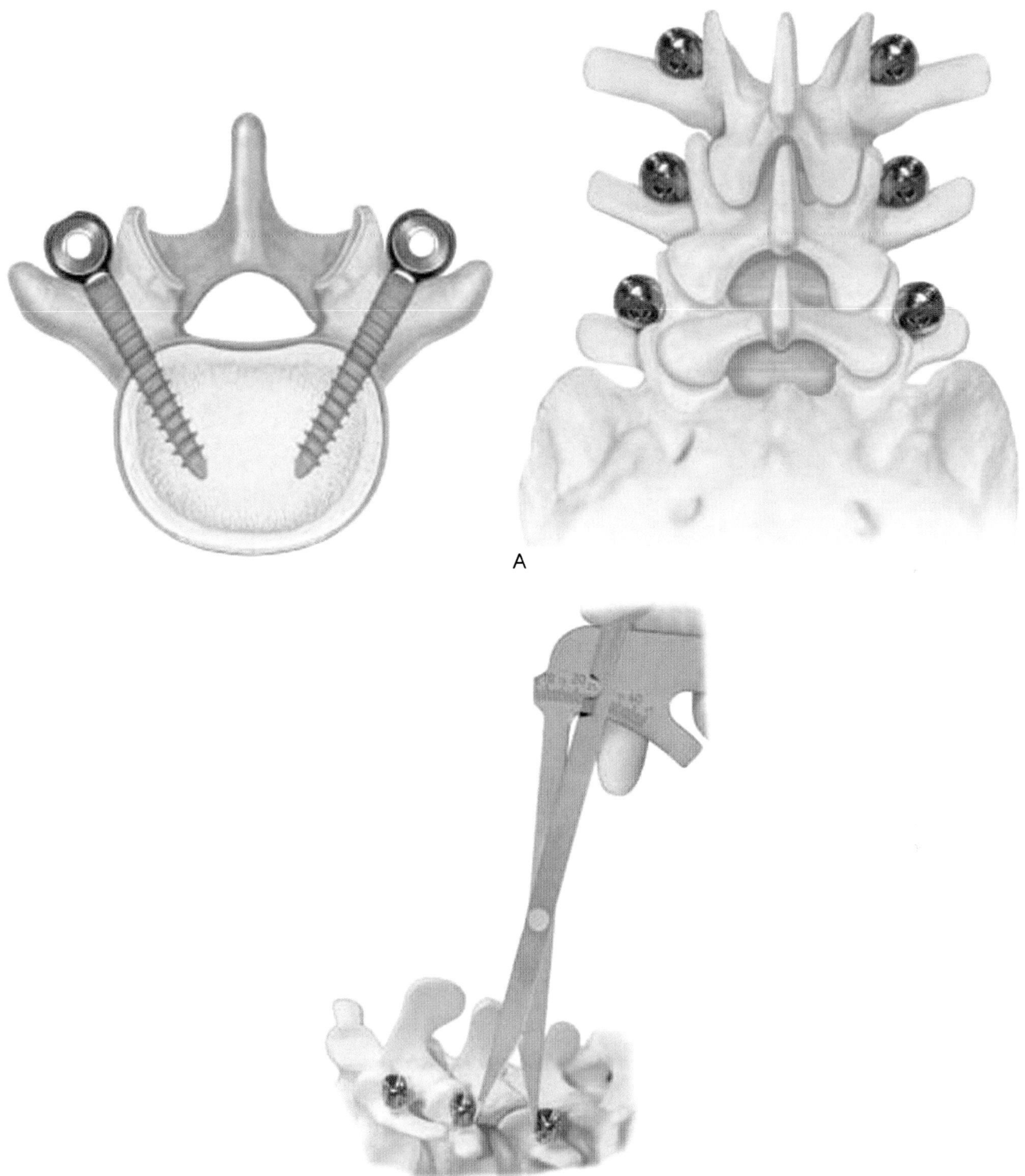

■ **FIGURE 60–4.** The Dynesys pedicle screws should be placed lateral to the facets leaving the facet joints intact. **A,** All screws are properly placed and aligned. **B,** Spacer lengths are determined.

The 200-mm length has two introductory zones allowing passage from both ends. The cord is inserted through the caudal screw in one- and two-level cases, and through the middle screw in cases with two levels or more. It is passed up to the middle of the functional zone. The cord is then passed through the appropriately sized spacer and through the eyelet of the next screw. The cord-tensioning instrument is used to pull the spacer into position (Fig. 60–4C). The cord is fixed at the caudal screw with the set screw. Appropriate tension is applied while the cord is fixed at the next screw (Fig. 60–4D). The procedure is repeated for the contralateral side, and then the next level until the system is fully implanted and tensioned (Fig. 60–4E).

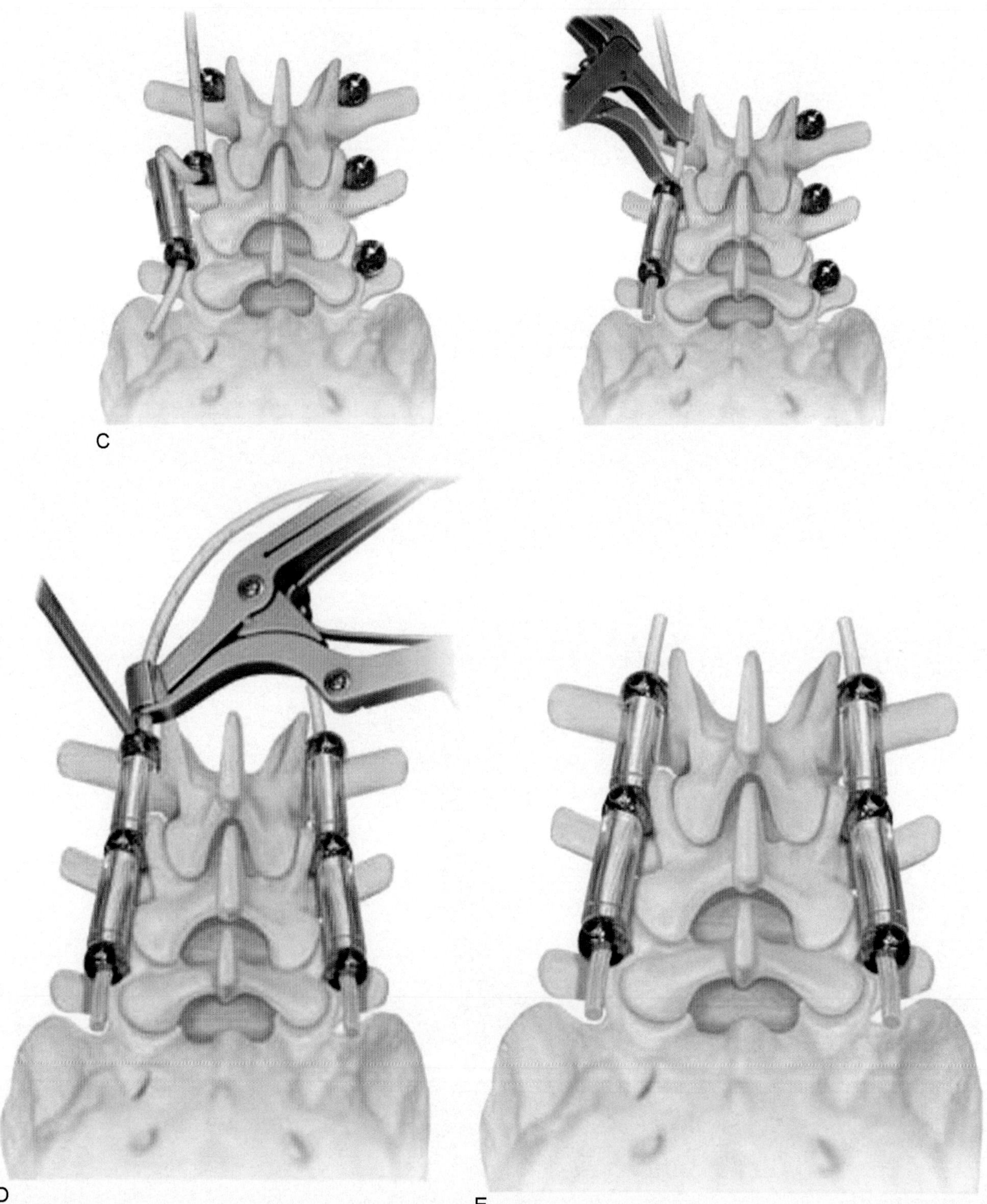


■ **FIGURE 60–4 Cont'd.** **C,** The cord is tensioned, thus properly positioning the spacer. **D,** The set screws are sequentially tightened while the cord is being tensioned. **E,** Fully tensioned implant

## POSTOPERATIVE CARE

Postoperative management follows the usual guidelines for pedicle screw fixation. Analgesics, antibiotic prophylaxis, and prophylaxis against thromboembolism are applied as indicated. In the case of Wiltse approaches, increased muscle spasm should be anticipated and treated. Early physiotherapy is recommended, and a lumbosacral brace should be used to protect the healing bone-screw interface.

## COMPLICATIONS AND AVOIDANCE

As with any surgical procedure, complications can occur. The general issues associated with all posterior approaches and placement of pedicle screws are observed with Dynesys procedures and with similar frequency.

Screw loosening is a particular concern when using the Dynesys Spinal System. Pedicle screw fixation in the absence of solid fusion of a motion segment leads to a high percentage of instrument failure when using traditional systems. Extrapolating this experience to Dynesys, one would anticipate frequent instrument failure. The overall reported screw loosening rate is 3.6%. This is well below the reported screw loosening rate of rigid systems, which ranges from 5.7% to 27.5%.[2] Screw loosening is avoided by strictly adhering to surgical guidelines. In particular, proper screening of potential osteomalacia, use of the largest screw available along the longest trajectory possible, fluoroscopic guidance of screw placement, and avoidance of backing out of screws will enhance success. Other risk factors include smoking, obesity, diabetes, immunosuppresion, and congenital anomaly.

Another concern with the Dynesys Spinal System is the possible increased infection rate or system failure due to the PET cord. The observed infection rate is comparable to other instrumented spinal procedures, and no instances of cord rupture or failure have been reported.

### ADVANTAGES/DISADVANTAGES: DYNESYS DYNAMIC STABILIZATION SYSTEM

**Advantages**

- Preservation of facet capsules and normal anatomic structures renders the procedure reversible. The system can be removed without significant sequelae, or it can be converted to more traditional rigid fusion.
- The system is versatile. It is indicated across a broad spectrum of lumbar ailments. It is effective as an adjunct to fusion and can be used in conjunction with posterior lateral and interbody fusions. Thus, different segments of the same spine can be managed independently using one system.
- The use of flexible materials lessens the impact of stabilization with regard to adjacent segments.
- Avoidance of fusion lessens the surgical trauma and overall physiologic impact.

**Disadvantages**

- The system has limitations owing to the use of flexible materials. It is not indicated in trauma, complete facetectomy, isthmic spondylolisthesis, or high-grade spondylolisthesis.

## CONCLUSIONS/DISCUSSION

The Dynesys Spinal System affords statistically significant pain reduction and functional improvement in a broad range of clinical syndromes. Implantation can be done with little surgical morbidity and little instrument failure. But with Dynesys, as with all motion-preserving technologies, crucial questions remain unanswered. Does avoidance of rigid fusion result in less adjacent-segment disease? Is there a demonstrable long-term advantage conferred by not fusing the discs? What is the impact of restoring or maintaining motion on the aging and stiffening spinal column? Does one device adequately address the varying needs of a broad spectrum of patients, or is customization necessary?

These and other issues will be addressed only with the scrutiny of time, clinical experience, and further study.

## REFERENCES

1. Dubois G, de Gemany B, Schaerer N, Fennema P: Dynamic neutralization: A new concept for restabilization of the spine. *In* Szpalski M, Gunzburg R, Pope MH (eds): Lumbar Segment Instability. Philadelphia, Lippincott Williams & Wilkins, 1999, pp 233–240.
2. Cakir B, Ulmar B, Koepp H, et al: Posterior dynamic stabilization as an alternative for instrumented fusion in the treatment of degenerative lumbar instability with spinal stenosis. Z Orthop 141:418–424, 2003.
3. Schmoelz W, Huber JF, Nydegger T, et al: Dynamic stabilization of the lumbar spine and its effects on adjacent segments: An in vitro experiment. J Spinal Disord Tech 16:418–423, 2003.
4. Putzier M, Schneider SV, Funk J, Perka C: [Application of a dynamic pedicle screw system (DYNESYS trade mark) for lumbar segmental degenerations—comparison of clinical and radiological results for different indications]. Z Orthop Ihre Grenzgeb 142:166–173, 2004.
5. Putzier M, Schneider SV, Funk J, et al: The surgical treatment of the lumbar disc prolapse: Neucleotomy with additional transpedicular dynamic stabilization versus nucleotomy alone. Spine 30:E109–E114, 2005.
6. Grob D, Benini A, Junge A, Mannion AF: Clinical experience with the Dynesys semirigid fixation system for the lumbar spine: Surgical and patient-oriented outcome in 50 cases after an average of 2 years. Spine 30:324–331, 2005.
7. Nockels R: Dynamic stabilization in the surgical management of painful lumbar spinal disorders. Spine 30:S68–S72, 2005.
8. Schwarzenbach O, Berlemann, Ustoll T, Dubois G: Posterior dynamic stabilization systems: Dynesys. Orthop Clin North Am 36:363–372, 2005.
9. Bordes M, Bordes V, Rodrigo F, Saez D: A dynamic neutralisation system for the spine: Dynesys System: Experience in 94 cases. Neurocirugia 16:499–506, 2005.
10. Stoll TM, Dubois G, Schwarzenbach O: The dynamic neutralization system for the spine: A multi-center study of a novel nonfusion system. Eur Spine J 11(2):S170–S178, 2002.
11. Davis R, Delamarter RB, et al: Dynesys US Clinical IDE: Preliminary data From Six Investigative Sites. Podium presentation at CNS, 2006.

CHAPTER 61

# Dynamic Stabilization System

**Dilip K. Sengupta**

## KEY POINTS

- Load sharing of the device with the disc and the facet joints should be uniform throughout the normal range of motion.
- The device and design rationale: The load-deformation characteristics of the Dynamic Stabilization System restrict the range of motion uniformly in flexion-extension, right and left lateral bending, and also rotation.

## INTRODUCTION

The rationale of dynamic stabilization in the treatment of activity-related mechanical low back pain is to unload the disc and the facet joint by load sharing with these anatomic structures while preserving motion.[1] Most dynamic stabilization systems result in some degree of restriction of range of motion.[2] This is not the aim but a side effect. The aim is to preserve as much motion as possible within the normal range but to stop any abnormal motion.

It remains unclear how much of unloading or load sharing is ideal, but possibly the ideal magnitude of load sharing is variable, depending on the degree of degeneration or collapse of the motion segment. Load sharing and motion restriction are related to each other. The greater the unloading, the larger is the motion restriction.

The load sharing of the device with the disc and the facet joints should be uniform throughout the normal range of motion. The total load that passes through a motion segment is the sum of the body weight cranial to and the muscle action across the motion segment. This load is shared between the device and the spine. If the device unloads predominantly in one direction, for example, in flexion, it will also have to bear more load in flexion, and may eventually lead to fatigue failure. The fulcrum assisted soft stabilization (FASS) system, described by the author previously in the literature, (and not in any previous chapter of this book)[3] is an ideal example of such concerns.

## DESCRIPTION OF THE DEVICE

The Dynamic Stabilization System (DSS) (Abbott Spine PLC, Austin, TX) was developed with the above-mentioned objectives in mind. This is essentially a titanium spring. The first generation of the DSS device looked like a C-shaped spring (DSS-I), with straight ends that attached to the pedicle screws. This device was tested extensively in the biomechanics laboratory, with particular attention to its effect on load-sharing and motion-sparing properties in cadaver lumbar spine (Fig. 61–1). DSS-I permitted approximately 70% of normal range of motion in flexion-extension, and the restriction of motion was uniform. The device also off-loaded the disc in flexion by about 30%, which was thought favorable. However, in extension, the device appeared to off-load the disc completely, taking 100% load on itself and permitting no load to be shared by the disc. It was anticipated that the device would fail in extension, because it was not strong enough to take full load off the lumbar spine (Fig. 61–2).

The next generation of the device was DSS-II, which looked like an alpha-shaped spring (see Fig. 61–1). This is made of 4-mm diameter spring-grade titanium. The load-deformation characteristics of this device show that it restricts the range of motion uniformly in flexion-extension, right and left lateral bending, and also in rotation. At physiologic loading, it restricts flexion-extension of a lumbar motion segment by 30% and lateral bending by 20%, and it has minimal effect on rotation movement. The disc pressure studies showed that unlike the previous design, the DSS-II device off-loaded the disc by around 25% both in flexion and in extension.[4] Therefore, it was anticipated that the device will never be subjected to the full load of the spine and will always act as a load-sharing device together with the disc and the facet joints.

The DSS II device survived 10 million cycles of flexion-extension when tested in the range of 15 degrees of motion. The fatigue testing was performed with the device applied between two poly-blocks, where the cyclical motion is not interfered with or influenced by the disc or the facet joints. It is nearly impossible to re-create the real-life stress pattern for proper fatigue testing of the device. True information of the fatigue life may be available only from clinical use of the device.

## BACKGROUND OF SCIENTIFIC TESTING/CLINICAL OUTCOMES

Following the bench testing as noted above, a pilot clinical trial was conducted. The primary aim of this clinical study was to determine whether the application of this device can relieve

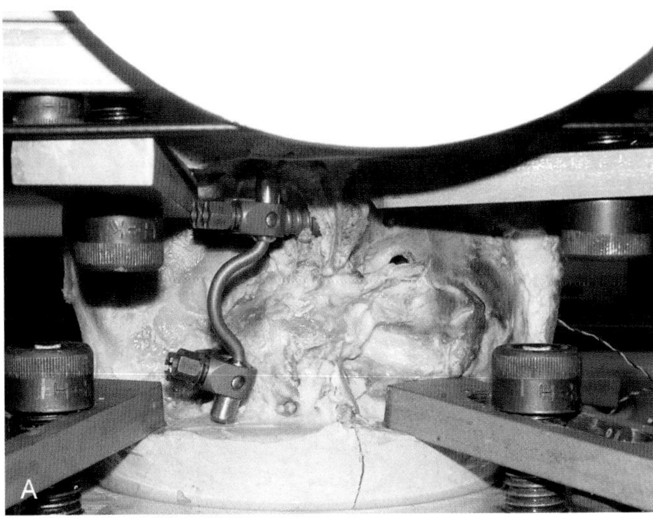


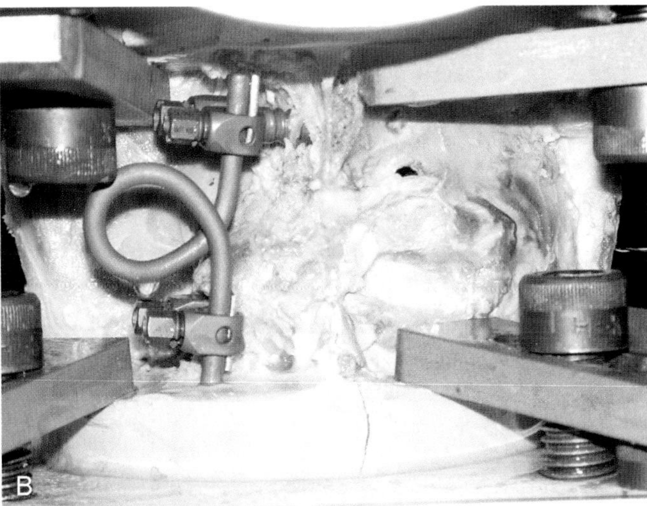


■ **FIGURE 61–1.** The DSS-I (**A**) and DSS-II (**B**) titanium-spring device implanted in cadaver spine for biomechanical testing.

mechanical low back pain. The secondary aim was to determine the limitation of the device, particularly device failure, or loosening. Because decompression or discectomy has a very high success rate in relieving radicular symptoms, which may confound the real efficacy of the DSS-II device, it was decided to exclude these cases. The outcome may also have been influenced by any concomitant fusion or other surgery. Therefore, the study included only those cases in which the patient had mechanical low back pain but did not have radicular pain or claudication symptoms and did not

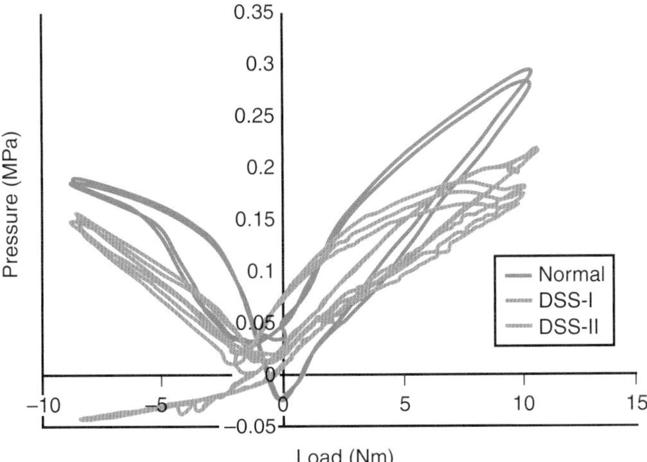


■ **FIGURE 61–2.** Disc pressure tracing from the center of the disc in a cadaver lumbar spine during flexion-extension movement, with 10 Nm pure moment, in a spine tester with 6 degrees of freedom. Normally, the pressure rises in both flexion and extension and is lowest during the early phase of extension. Following stabilization with the DSS-II system, the disc was partly unloaded in both flexion and extension because of uniform load sharing with the disc. Following DSS-I, stabilization of the disc was partly unloaded in flexion but fully unloaded in extension, which indicates that the implant becomes a fully load-bearing structure in extension. *(Modified from Sengupta DK: Dynamic stabilization of the treatment of low back pain due to degenerative disorders. In Herkowitz HN, Dvorak J, Bell GR, et al (eds):* The Lumbar Spine: Official Publication of the International Society for the Study of the Lumbar Spine, *3rd ed. Philadelphia, Lippincott Williams & Wilkins, 2004. With permission.)*

require any concomitant surgery like decompression or adjacent-segment fusion. During 2002 to 2004, 19 cases were treated with the DSS device. One patient had persistent pain following disc replacement, and two other patients had failed nuclear replacement, leaving 16 patients who had DSS-II stabilization for mechanical low back pain secondary to degenerated disc/facet joint complex. The mean age of the patients was 52 years (range 42 to 58 years). Eleven patients underwent surgery for disc degeneration with back pain, and five patients had degenerative spondylolisthesis without significant stenosis. Single-level stabilization was performed in 14 cases (L4-L5, 6; L5-S1, 8), and two-level stabilization (L4-S1) was performed in two cases. Preoperative discogram was performed in all the cases.

At 2-year follow-up, mean Visual Analog Scale (VAS) was reduced from 7.3 to 3.5, and mean Oswestry Disability Index (ODI) was reduced from 65 to 27. Fourteen of the 16 cases improved significantly from the preoperative pain and functional status; 12 returned to their original jobs, and the other two returned to sedentary jobs. Postoperative flexion-extension radiographs showed mean 7.5 degrees of motion at the operated segment, which was equivalent to 68% of the motion observed in the proximal adjacent segment (Fig. 61–3). More important, the quality of flexion and extension was comparable to a normal motion segment, that is, the anterior edges of the end plate apposing each other in flexion and posterior edges in extension (Fig. 61–4). This indicated that the device was sharing the load with the disc in both flexion and extension, allowing the remaining load to be transmitted through the disc. No radiographic loosening or implant breakage was seen.

## OPERATIVE TECHNIQUE

The patients were positioned prone, with the lumbar spine in desired lordosis. Pedicle screws were inserted using minimally invasive pedicle screw insertion technique over guide pins and using the dilators. The pedicle screw heads were connected to slotted outriggers, which extended outside the skin. Once the screws were inserted, the DSS-II system was inserted along the groove of the outriggers, to guide them into the slot of the pedicle screw head,

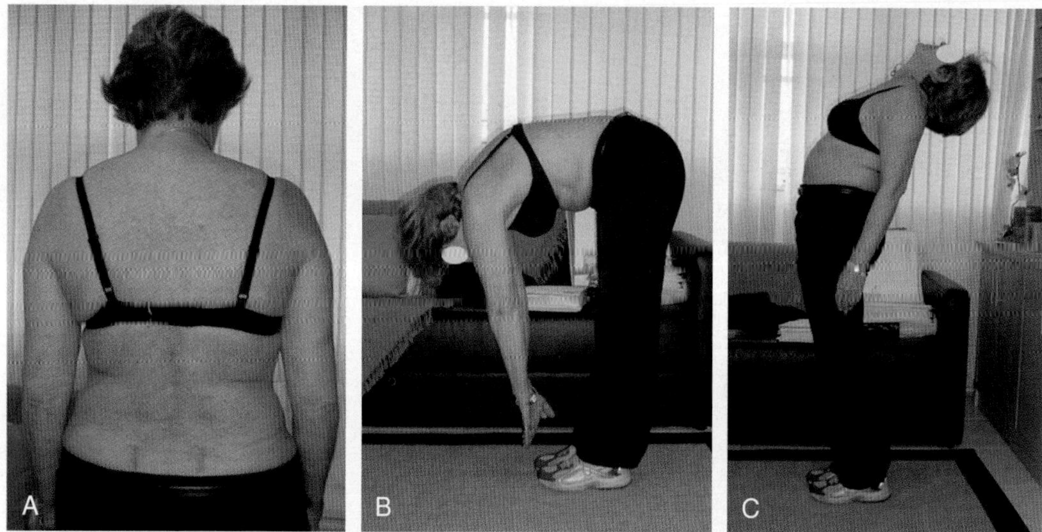

■ **FIGURE 61–3.** Example of one patient in 3-month follow-up with good range of flexion-extension motion.

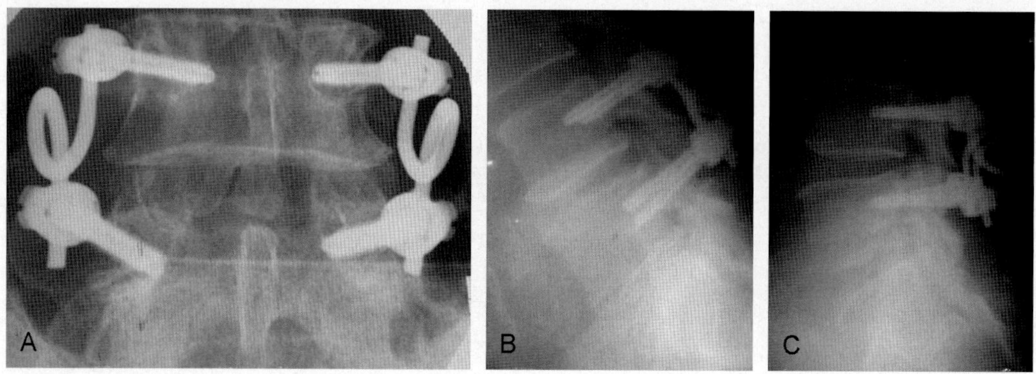

■ **FIGURE 61–4.** **A,** Postoperative anteroposterior radiograph. The lateral radiographs in flexion (**B**) and extension (**C**) show that the anterior vertebral margins come closer to each other during flexion and the posterior margins in extension, indicating the device permits load sharing to the disc in both flexion and extension.

and secured into position. Because lordosis was achieved by patient positioning, no compression or distraction was applied (Fig. 61–5). In the two patients who had two-level fixation, pedicle screws were placed only at L4 and S1 vertebrae, and one device was placed across two motion segments on each side. Postoperatively, the patients were mobilized out of bed within a few hours of surgery. Postoperative morbidity was minimal because the soft tissue dissection was minimal, and there was no need for exposure of bone or decortication or bone graft harvesting.

## CONCLUSIONS/DISCUSSION

The development of the DSS system is still in its early stage. The preliminary clinical study shows that the device can relieve mechanical low back pain secondary to degenerative disc and facet disease. The device also survived fatigue failure in 2-year follow-up. There was no screw-bone loosening. Further development of the device may be necessary to determine the ideal diameter and thickness of the DSS spring suitable for patients with body weight below or above average. The system must be adapted for multiple-level stabilization or stabilization of a segment adjacent to fusion with standard instrumentation.

The advantage of a titanium spring device is that it may be inserted with a minimally invasive approach, when no decompression is necessary. In addition, the metal device makes it possible to identify any fatigue failure or permanent deformation in vivo radiologically. Radiolucent devices may deform or stretch and, therefore, may lose their effects over time. But these problems may go unrecognized in postoperative follow-up radiographs. The most important disadvantage of a metal device is that it may interfere with subsequent magnetic resonance imaging.

There is no set duration or life span for the dynamic stabilization device. Ideally, it should survive for a lifetime. The fatigue life of the device will depend on the stress or the load that the device is subjected to. This may vary over time after implantation of the device in vivo. The disc and the facet joint may undergo changes as the load is shared by the device and abnormal movement and stresses are removed. It may be wishful thinking that such changes may be favorable and that the disc/facet joints may be able to repair themselves, and the device may be removed after serving its job for a period.

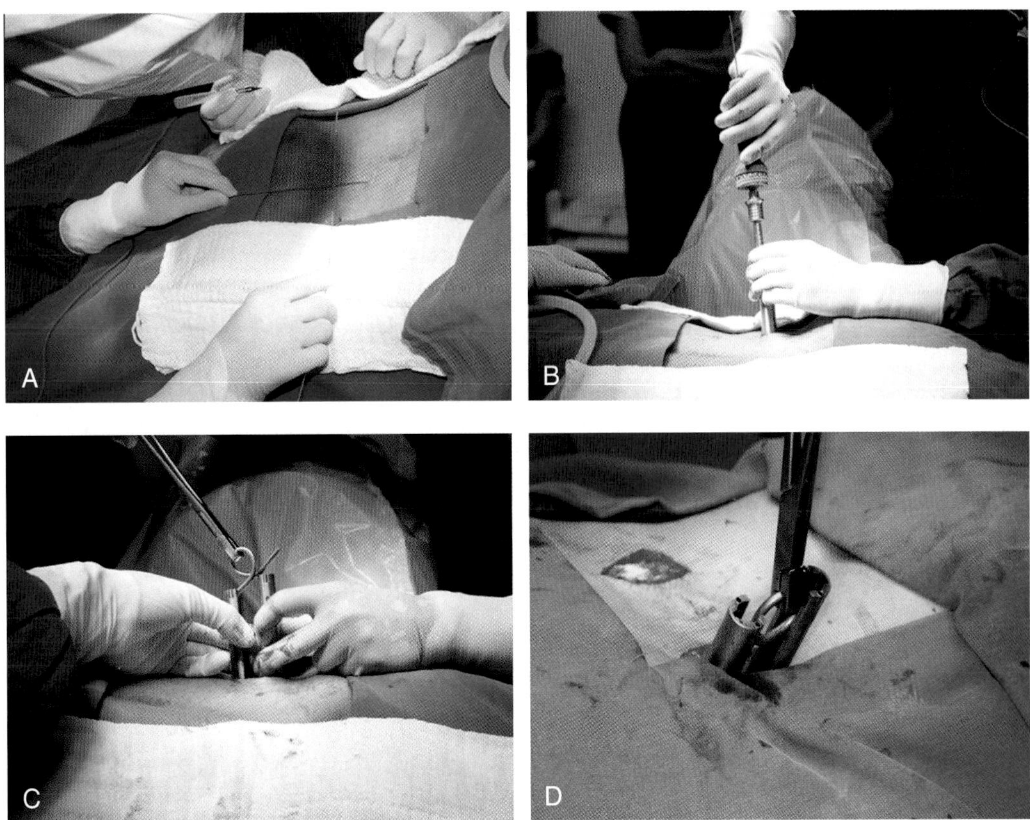

■ **FIGURE 61–5.** Surgical technique. **A** and **B,** The pedicle screws are inserted through two separate paramedian incisions, using a minimally invasive technique. **C** and **D,** The screw heads are attached to slotted outriggers, and the DSS-II device is inserted along the slots into the screw head. Finally, the device is secured into the screw head under fluoroscopic guidance to achieve proper positioning and alignment. The patients are mobilized within hours after surgery, because the postoperative morbidity is minimal.

On the other hand, if the motion segment should continue to deteriorate, the dynamic stabilization may be revised to fusion.

The pilot clinical trial was performed for isolated mechanical low back pain, without decompression or concomitant fusion of another segment, for a specific purpose. It does not limit the use of this device. The other indications for use of a posterior dynamic stabilization device may include stabilization after decompression, or a segment adjacent to fusion, and also to salvage other failed motion preservation procedures. The DSS-II system has been used to stabilize one patient with prosthetic disc replacement with good relief of persistent pain. Ideally, the device needs to be tested together with a prosthetic disc device in the cadaver spine to ensure that their combined biomechanical effects are complementary to each other.

## REFERENCES


1. Mulholland RC, Sengupta DK: Rationale, principles and experimental evaluation of the concept of soft stabilization. Eur Spine J 11(suppl 2):S198–S205, 2002.
2. Sengupta DK: Dynamic stabilization devices in the treatment of low back pain. Orthop Clin North Am 35:43–56, 2004.
3. Sengupta DK, Mulholland RC: Fulcrum assisted soft stabilization system: A new concept in the surgical treatment of degenerative low back pain. Spine 30:1019–1029; discussion 1030, 2005.
4. Sengupta DK: Dynamic stabilization in the treatment of low back pain due to degenerative disorders. *In* Herkowitz HN, Dvorak J, Bell GR, et al (eds): The Lumbar Spine: Official Publication of the International Society for the Study of the Lumbar Spine, 3rd ed. Philadelphia, Lipppincott Williams & Wilkins, 2004.

CHAPTER 62

# The Stabilimax NZ Posterior Lumbar Dynamic Stabilization System

**James J. Yue, George Malcolmon,** and **Jens Peter Timm**

**KEY POINTS**

- Lumbar posterior dynamic stabilization device is designed to specifically address pathologic alterations in the neutral zone.
- Dual-spring mechanism permits controlled motion in flexion and extension.
- Ball-and-socket pedicle screw–based system permits rotation.
- Single-level or multilevel application.
- The device can be combined or used primarily as fusion device using nondynamic connectors.

## INTRODUCTION

One potential source of low back pain is the alteration of the normal kinematics of a given lumbar spinal motion segment or segments. Panjabi et al[1–5] have developed the principle of the neutral zone (NZ), a region of high flexibility in either flexion or extension around the neutral posture position in which there is little resistance to motion (Fig. 62–1). A component of spinal range of motion (ROM), the NZ is a region of high spinal flexibility around neutral posture. Spinal degeneration or injury increases the NZ, causing pain. Dynamic stabilization systems are designed to support and stabilize the spine, ideally while maintaining ROM.

To understand the NZ principle, it is necessary to understand the three subsystems of spinal stability. The stabilizing systems of the spine are the active subsystem (musculoskeletal system), the passive subsystem (the spinal column), and the neural system (activation of the active system through neurologic control). Under normal conditions, the three subsystems maintain mechanical stability. Damage or dysfunction of one subsystem requires the other two systems to compensate.

Panjabi determined that removal of a disc's nucleus produced an increase in flexion, lateral bending, and axial rotation.[6] Other researchers, using similar models of spinal injury, have also observed that degeneration and trauma produced multidirectional laxity in the spinal column (Fig. 62–2).[7–14]

Panjabi also investigated the contribution of the spinal muscles (active subsystem) to the stability of the spine. After each injury, simulated muscle forces applied to the spinous process reduced the NZ almost to its intact value, without significantly affecting the ROM. These results suggest that the extra work muscles perform in an injured spine is predominately to restabilize the NZ, not to restrict the overall range of motion.

The interconnection of the third spinal stabilizing subsystem (neural control system) has been evaluated by comparing cohorts of patients with back pain to patients without back pain. Marras[15] has demonstrated that there is a higher level of muscle activity in those patients experiencing back pain. This increase in muscle activity is triggered by the neural subsystem's responsibility to maintain the mechanical stability, which is not being provided by the degenerated passive subsystem.

Recent research in the field of spine biomechanics examined the contribution of the musculoskeletal and neural elements to maintaining stability of the spine. The most important observation yielded by these studies is that degeneration or injury of the spinal structures results in an increase of the NZ. When muscles are recruited to compensate for the laxity of the spine, dysfunction and low back pain result.[16–19]

The Stabilimax NZ (Applied Spine Technologies, New Haven, CT) was designed to complement Panjabi's principles of spinal biomechanics. The Stabilimax NZ, a posterior pedicle screw–based dynamic stabilization system, features dual concentric springs combined with a ball-and-socket joint, all to enhance spinal stability around neutral posture (Fig. 62–3). The Stabilimax NZ is designed to increase the resistance of the passive spinal system around neutral posture (the NZ) while maintaining the maximum range of motion. As is discussed in subsequent sections, the essential components include the pedicle screw, a single-level or multilevel dynamic connector, and an end connector. The system is designed to be used from L1-S1 in either single-level or multilevel configurations.

## DEVELOPMENT AND BIOMECHANICAL TESTING OF THE STABILIMAX NZ

The initial development testing of the Stabilimax NZ was conducted by Panjabi to determine the optimal device parameters for spring

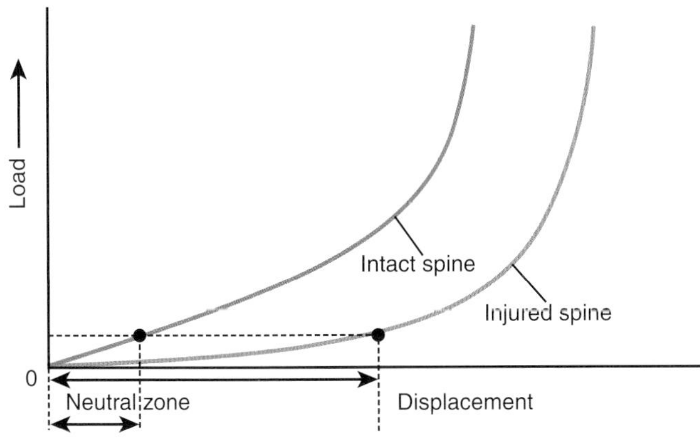


■ **FIGURE 62–1.** Change in load displacement curve and neutral zone with injury to spine.

stiffness and interpedicular travel. Subsequent studies were conducted to verify that the load placed on the bone/screw interface by the Stabilimax NZ was less than that of other systems. Additional investigations were performed to measure the effect of the device on NZ and ROM following progressive destabilization procedures.

Regarding optimization of the device characteristics, a study was undertaken to determine the optimum spring stiffness of the device in intact and destabilized spine preparations. Optimal spring stiffness for the device was evaluated in intact spines and in destabilized by nucleotomy and laminectomy with partial facetectomy (LPF). Optimal interpedicular travel of the device was obtained for both compression (spinal extension) and extension (spinal flexion). Wear testing and in vivo animal testing have also been performed verifying biocompatibility.

A verification study was performed to evaluate the device on NZ and ROM in intact and destabilized spines. In this study, NZ and ROM were measured during spinal loading, before and after the device was attached to the lumbar vertebrae. Implantation of the Stabilimax NZ decreased the NZ during flexion-extension and lateral bending in all states. The study also included measurement of the NZ and ROM in progressive spinal destabilization produced by nucleotomy and LPF. Both nucleotomy and LPF increased the NZ and total ROM of the spine, indicating spinal injury/degeneration. Attachment of the Stabilimax NZ to the spine diminished the NZ while having only a minimal effect on ROM. The results confirm that both the ROM and the NZ increase with progressive spinal injury and that implantation of the Stabilimax NZ shrinks the NZ while maintaining overall ROM, meeting a critical design objective.

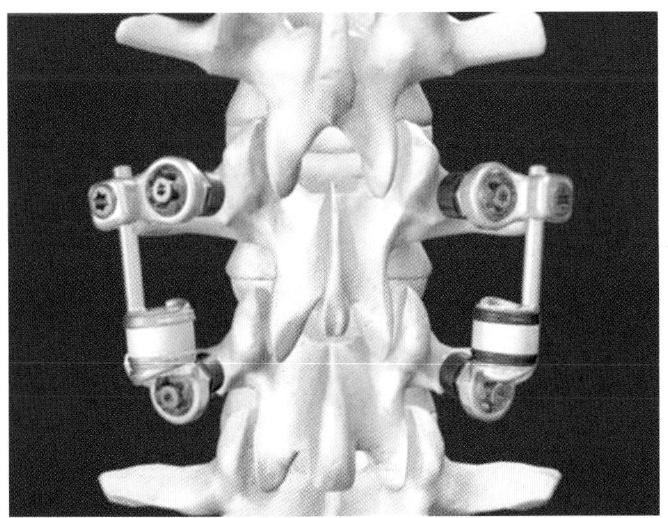

■ **FIGURE 62–2.** Stabilimax NZ system.

## INDICATIONS/CONTRAINDICATIONS

The Stabilimax NZ system is currently undergoing an Investigational Device Exemption clinical trial by the U.S. Food and Drug Administration. Indications include moderate to severe degenerative spinal stenosis of the lumbar spine associated with neurogenic claudication. A discogenic low back pain indication is also being currently assessed in clinics outside the United States. Contraindications include spondylolisthesis or retrolisthesis beyond grade 1; scoliosis or degenerative scoliosis of more than 10 degrees; osteoporosis with a T score of less than 2.5; fracture or comorbidity at the treated levels that would compromise bone integrity; gross instability, defined as greater than 3 mm motion on flexion/extension studies; or spondylolysis.

## DESCRIPTION OF THE DEVICE

The Stabilimax NZ system is composed of pedicle screws, either a dynamic or single-level dynamic connector, and an end connector (Figs. 62–3 to 62–6). The pedicle screws range from 35 to 50 mm in length and 5.5, 6.5, and 7.5 mm in width. The screws are composed of a titanium alloy ($Ti^6Al^4V$). The solid portions of the dynamic connector are composed of a cobalt-chromium-molybdenum alloy. The spring component of the dynamic connector is composed of Elgiloy. The end connector is composed of a cobalt-chromium-molybdenum alloy.

## OPERATIVE PROCEDURE

**STEP 1—POSITIONING:** The patient is placed in the prone position on a fluoroscopic imaging table. The patient's spine should be positioned in a neutral position, limiting the amount of kyphosis. After positioning, fluoroscopy should be used to verify level of surgery and to ensure adequate visualization of the vertebral elements.

**STEP 2—EXPOSURE:** Placement of the pedicle screws can be done through either a midline exposure or a paramedian approach, using right and left incisions and an intermuscular approach. The use of fluoroscopic imaging is mandatory to ensure proper levels of insertion and to ensure proper alignment of the pedicle screws in the anteroposterior and lateral projections.

**STEP 3—PLACEMENT OF DEVICE:** The starting holes for the pedicle screws should be lateral to the facet joints at each starting hole (Fig. 62–7). The screws should be positioned as parallel as possible in the lateral projection (Fig. 62–8). Standard

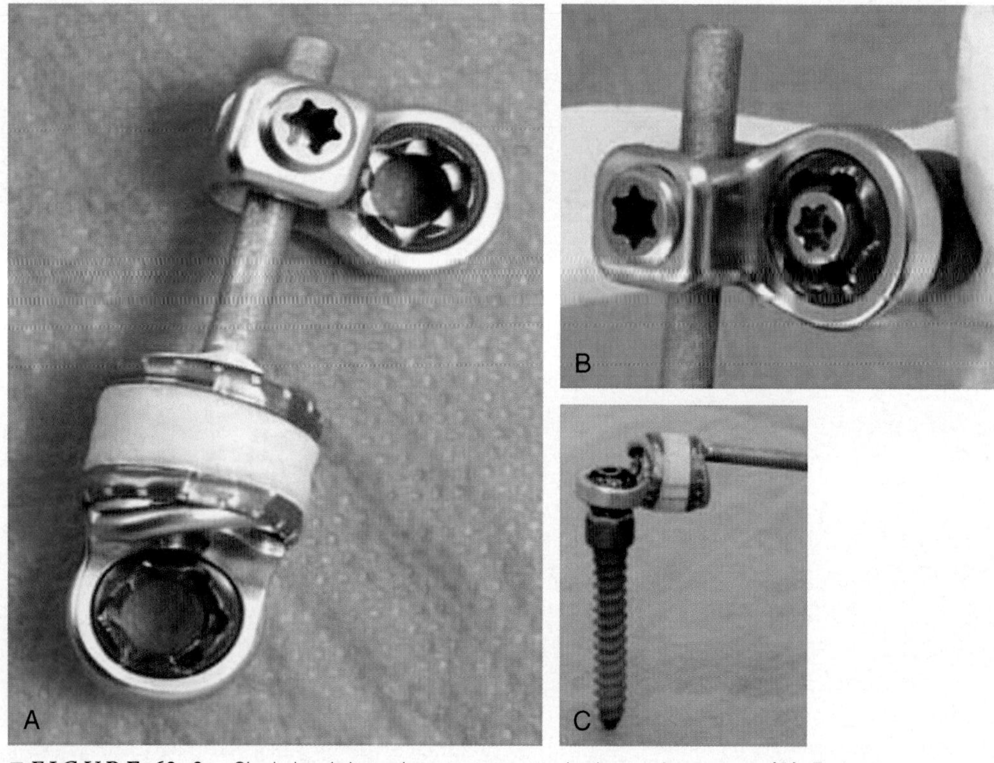

■ **FIGURE 62–3.** Single-level dynamic connector attached to end connector **(A)**. End connector **(B)**. Dynamic connector attached to pedicle screw **(C)**.

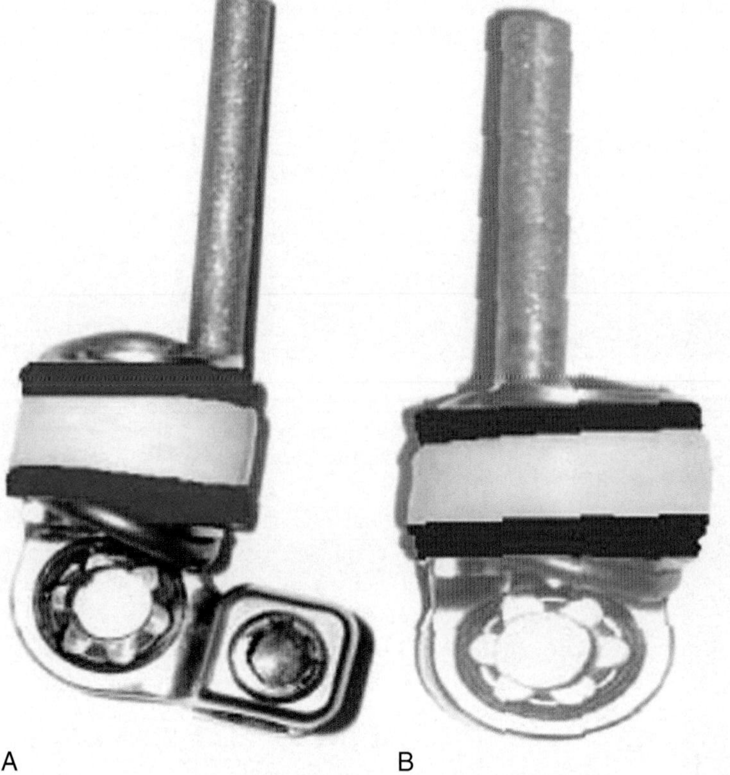

■ **FIGURE 62–4.** Double- **(A)** and single-level **(B)** dynamic connectors.

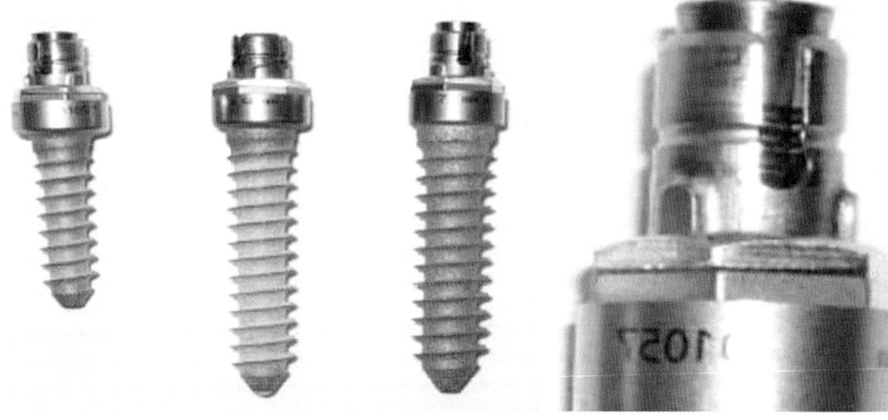

■ **FIGURE 62–5.** Pedicle screws 5.5, 6.5, and 7.5 mm from 35 to 50 mm.

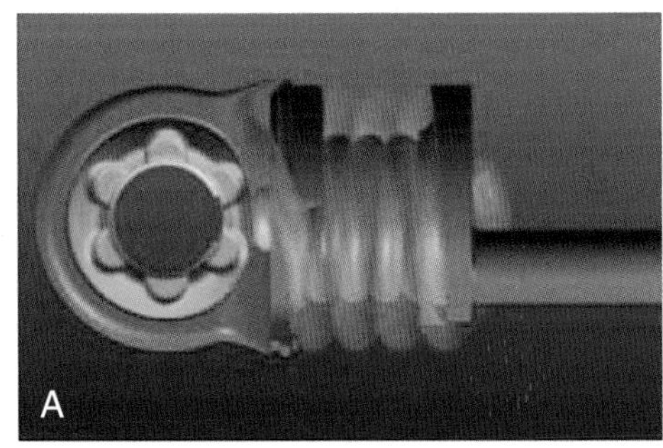


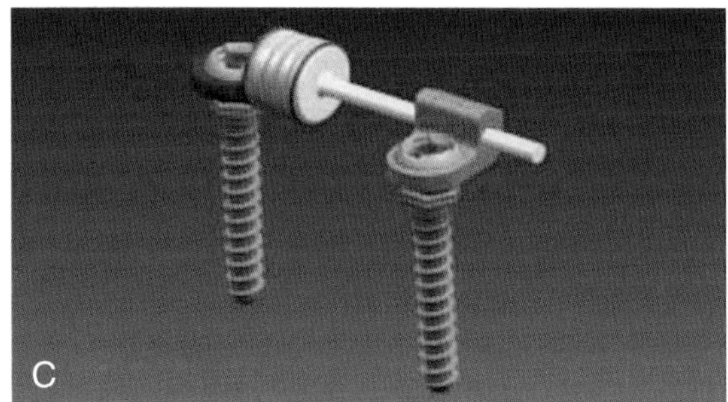


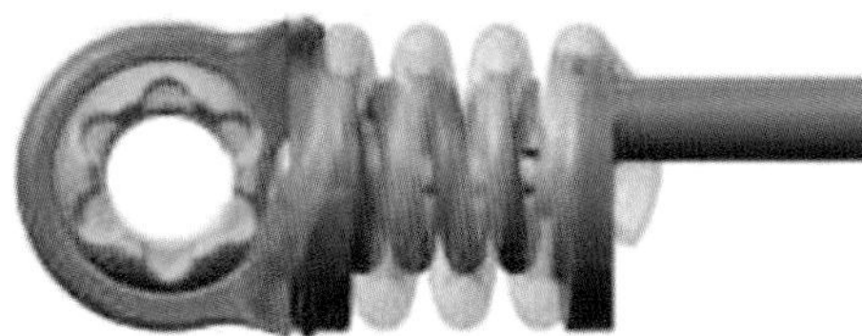


■ **FIGURE 62–6.** Dual-spring mechanism. **A,** Extension. **B,** Flexion. **C,** Neutral.

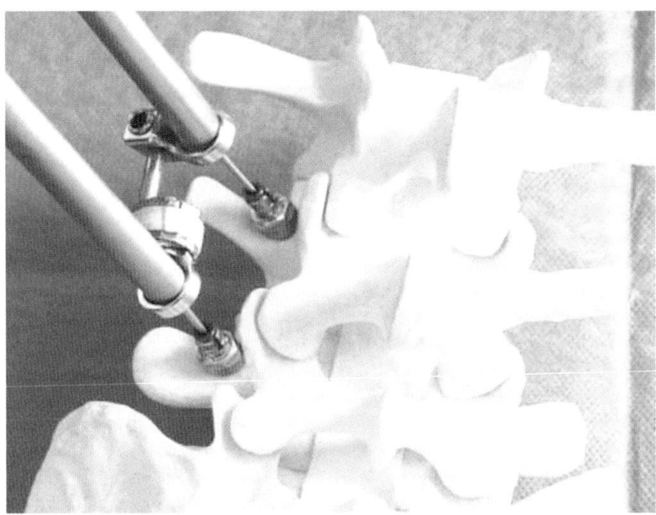

■ **FIGURE 62–7.** Application of connectors to pedicle screws.

pedicle canal formation is performed with either a solid pedicle probe or a cannulated probe. The outer cortex is tapped, and the screw is placed. The L5 screw should be placed first, and then either the S1 or L4 screw should be placed using the interpedicular spanner to ensure at least 30 mm in distance. After all screws are placed, the distance between the screws is measured, and the rod on the dynamic connector is cut to an appropriate length. The end connector is placed onto the dynamic connector rod, and the construct is then placed onto the pedicle screws (Figs. 62–8 and 62–9).

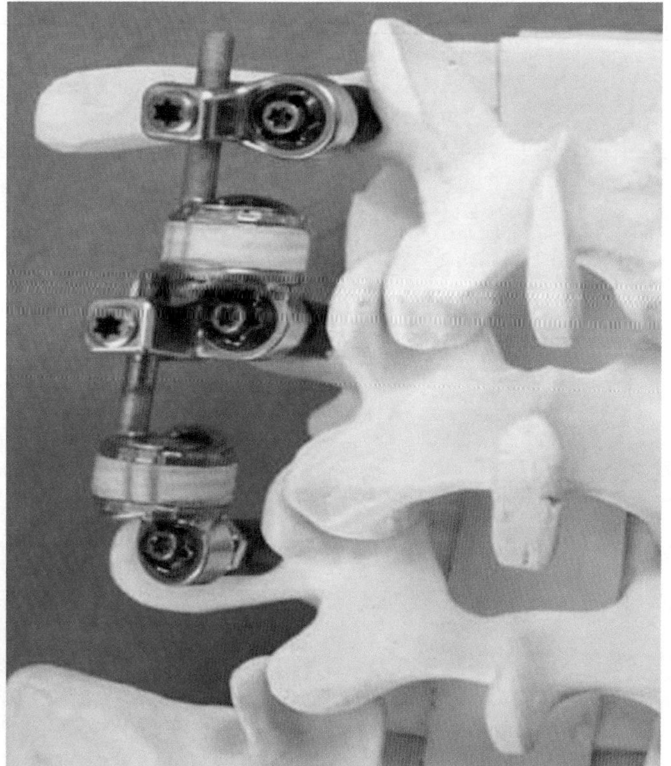

■ **FIGURE 62–9.** Final positioning of L3-L5 construct.

## CLINICAL DATA

At the time of preparation of this manuscript, both the European and U.S. trials had been initiated. This initial evaluation of the Stabilimax NZ device appears to show early validation of the intraoperative process and nascent postoperative results in our two patients. Further evaluation will be necessary to validate early and midterm results of the device from a clinical standpoint (Figs. 62–10 and 62–11).

## DISCUSSION

Alterations in the NZ have been associated with the presence of low back pain. Correction of excessive motion as a result of an increase in the NZ may theoretically decrease the associated symptoms of low back pain. The Stabilimax NZ device is designed to remodulate the NZ, thus providing a more normal ROM around the neutral posture position. Multiple laboratory results indicate correction of abnormal motions and biocompatibility. The U.S. Food and Drug Adminstration Investigational Device Exemption clinical trials are currently being performed.

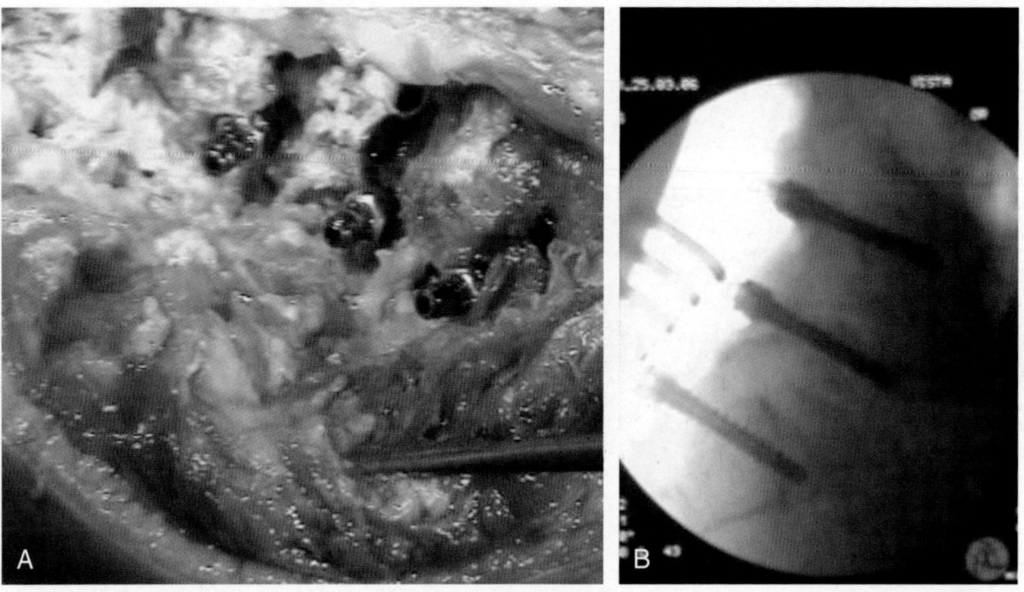


■ **FIGURE 62–8.** Pedicle screw placement lateral to facets **(A)** and parallel in sagittal plane **(B)**.

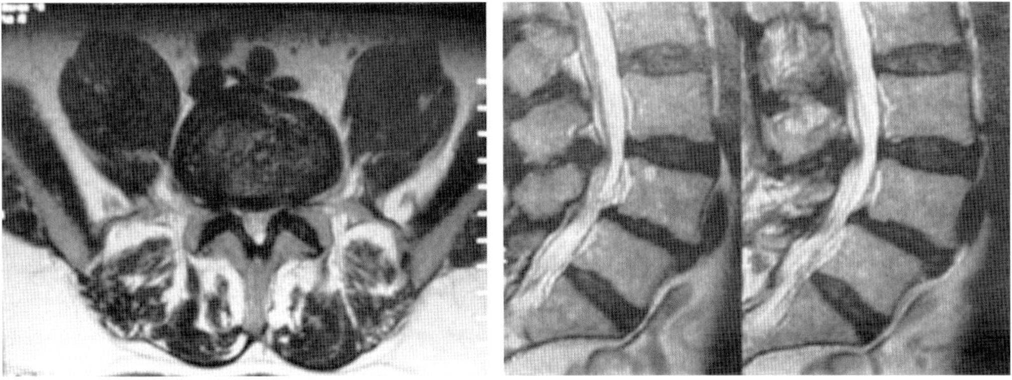

■ **FIGURE 62–10.** Preoperative magnetic resonance images of patient with L4-L5 stenosis.

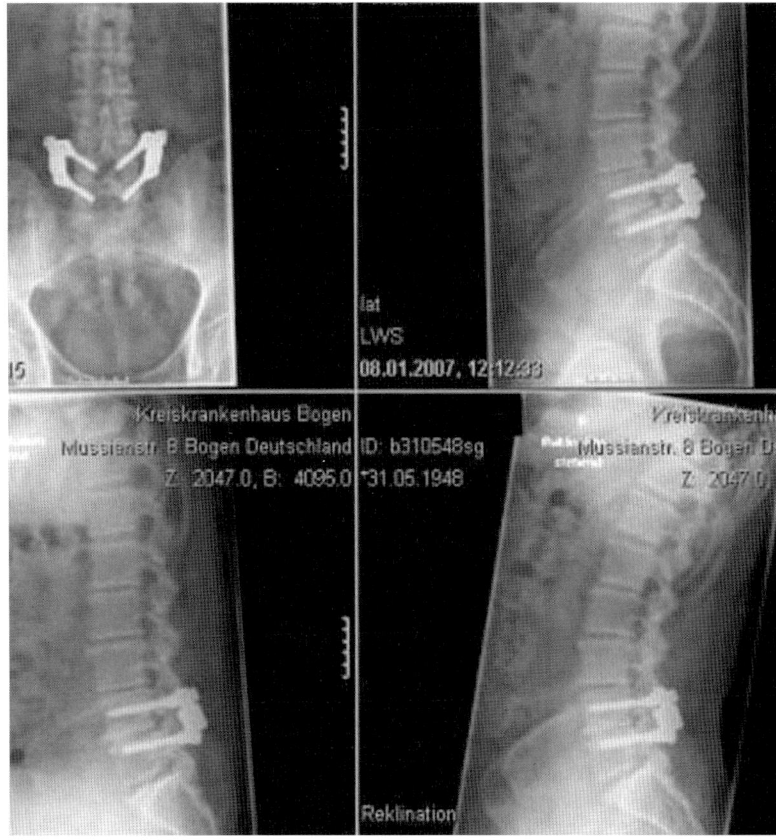


■ **FIGURE 62–11.** Postoperative radiographic images.

## REFERENCES

1. Panjabi M, Abumi K, Duranceau J, et al: Spinal stability and intersegmental muscle forces: A biomechanical model. Spine 14:194–200, 1989.
2. Panjabi MM: The stabilizing system of the spine, Part II: Neutral zone and instability hypothesis. J Spinal Disord 5:390–396; discussion 397, 1992.
3. Panjabi MM: The stabilizing system of the spine, Part I: Function, dysfunction, adaptation, and enhancement. J Spinal Disord 5:383–389; discussion 397, 1992.
4. Panjabi MM: Clinical spinal instability and low back pain. J Electromyogr Kinesiol 13:371–379, 2003.
5. Panjabi MM: A hypothesis of chronic back pain: Ligament subfailure injuries lead to muscle control dysfunction. Eur Spine J 15:668–676, 2006.
6. Panjabi MM, Krag MH, Chung TQ: Effects of disc injury on mechanical behavior of the human spine. Spine 9:707–713, 1984.
7. Abumi K, Panjabi MM, Kramer KM, et al: Biomechanical evaluation of lumbar spinal stability after graded facetectomies. Spine 15:1142–1147, 1990.
8. Ahlgren BD, Lui W, Herkowitz HN, et al: Effect of anular repair on the healing strength of the intervertebral disc: A sheep model. Spine 25:2165–2170, 2000.
9. Ahlgren BD, Vasavada A, Brower RS, et al: Anular incision technique on the strength and multidirectional flexibility of the healing intervertebral disc. Spine 19:948–954, 1994.

10. Atlas OK, Dodds SD, Panjabi MM: Single and incremental trauma models: A biomechanical assessment of spinal instability. Eur Spine J 12:205–210, 2003.
11. Kato Y, Panjabi MM, Nibu K: Biomechanical study of lumbar spinal stability after osteoplastic laminectomy. J Spinal Disord 11:146–150, 1998.
12. Mimura M, Panjabi MM, Oxland TR, et al: Disc degeneration affects the multidirectional flexibility of the lumbar spine. Spine 19:1371–1380, 1994.
13. Osman SG, Nibu K, Panjabi MM, et al: Transforaminal and posterior decompressions of the lumbar spine: A comparative study of stability and intervertebral foramen area. Spine 22:1690–1695, 1997.
14. Oxland TR, Crisco JJ 3rd, Panjabi MM, et al: The effect of injury on rotational coupling at the lumbosacral joint: A biomechanical investigation. Spine 17:74–80, 1992.
15. Marras W: Spine loading charactertistics of patients with low back pain compared with asymptomatic individuals. Spine 26:2566–2574, 2001.
16. Cholewicki J, Crisco JJ 3rd, Oxland TR, et al: Effects of posture and structure on three-dimensional coupled rotations in the lumbar spine: A biomechanical analysis. Spine 21:2421–2428, 1996.
17. Dvorak J, Panjabi MM, Chang DG, et al: Functional radiographic diagnosis of the lumbar spine: Flexion-extension and lateral bending. Spine 16:562–571, 1991.
18. Dvorak J, Panjabi MM, Novotny JE, et al: Clinical validation of functional flexion-extension roentgenograms of the lumbar spine. Spine 16:943–950, 1991.
19. Dvorak J, Vajda EG, Grob D, et al: Normal motion of the lumbar spine as related to age and gender. Eur Spine J 4:18–23, 1995.

CHAPTER 63

# Scient'x IsoBar TTL Dynamic Rod Stabilization

**Antonio E. Castellvi** and **S.A. Andrew**

## KEY POINTS

- Dynamic stabilization is defined as a system that would alter the movement and load transmission of the spinal motion segment in such a way as to favor protective physiologic motion and load through that segment without producing a fusion.
- Recent literature suggests that there may be a window of opportunity in which the functional spinal unit may be spared the degenerative cascade if the mechanical loads on it return to within the physiologic range.
- The IsoBar system is denoted IsoBar TTL and consists of a 5.5-mm-diameter rod with an integral dampener element; the dampener element contains stacked titanium alloy disc-shaped elements that allow linearly elastic controlled axial and angular motions.
- Early overall radiographic results demonstrated no lucency at the bone/screw interface, no breakage of the rods or screws, no increase of translation, preserved disc heights, and no pseudoarthrosis.

## INTRODUCTION

The intervertebral disc is a vital component of the functional spinal unit. Anatomically, the disc is structured such that the outer fibrous layer (annulus) surrounds and contains a highly viscous, gelatinous inner core—the nucleus pulposis. This inner core is composed of proteoglycans and water, which has a great capacity to absorb shock and distribute loads to the end plates of the vertebrae. Over time, as degeneration occurs with advancing age, the water content of the nucleus decreases, and the disc becomes fibrotic and becomes less able to absorb shock and distribute loads. As a consequence, the loads are then distributed to the vertebral end plates and the annulus of the disc, leading to end plate changes and annular fissuring.[1]

At this point, on a magnetic resonance image (MRI) of the spine, the disc will appear dark. As the degenerative process progresses, the functional spinal unit becomes unable to withstand physiologic loads, and instability develops. Instability in the spine is defined as greater than physiologic displacement of the functional spinal unit under physiologic loads.[2] With instability, the neurologic structures are more prone to impingement and injury. Instability of the intervertebral disc shifts greater-than-normal motion and loads to the facet joints and ligamentum flavum. Under greater stresses, these structures then undergo hypertrophy and narrow the vertebral canal and foramina. This process is known as degenerative disc disease (DDD) or, as Crock put it, "internal disc disruption."[3] Acute back pain can present at any stage of this degenerative process. However, not all individuals with DDD develop incapacitating axial back pain. It is unknown why some individuals proceed to become symptomatic and others appear to be spared this fate.

Kirkaldy-Willis clearly categorized this degenerative cascade into three stages. Stage one begins with the initiating event, which is generally unknown, and progresses to end plate calcification, which limits nutrient diffusion into the disc. The biochemical and physiologic status change in the intervertebral disc during this stage. Again, this corresponds to a dark disc on MRI. The second stage develops as the functional spinal unit becomes unstable. The third and last stage is noted as hypertrophic tissues attempt to stabilize the unstable spine.[4]

Fusion has long been the traditional mainstay of surgical treatment for DDD and other degenerative conditions of the spine. As technology has advanced, so, too, have the instrumentation and devices available to the spine surgeon to produce a successful fusion. Screws, rods, plates, and intervertebral cages in their various forms have increased the odds of producing a solid fusion mass. However, these advancements in technology and surgical techniques have not always provided better odds of achieving good to excellent clinical results.[5] There are several potential postoperative complications when fusing the spine to treat spondylosis or DDD. Pseudoarthrosis, flat back syndrome, adjacent-level degeneration, adjacent-level kyphosis, juxtafusion scoliosis, failures under fusion (herniated disc/spinal stenosis after fusion), and implant failures are commonly reported after a lumbar fusion, leading to the "failed spine."[6] It has been recognized that rigid immobilization of the spine tends to increase motion of adjacent segments (especially those above the levels fused), which may lead to rapid progression of DDD and spondylosis at those levels. As a result, any one or more of the myriad of degenerative complications of having a solid fusion may occur. Recent attention has focused on these postoperative complications with attempts at creating new and innovative surgical techniques to minimize or avoid these altogether.

Because rigid fusion of the spine appears to propagate adjacent-level degeneration in its various forms, numerous newimplants have been developed with the aim of maintaining physiologic motion while sharing physiologic loads at the surgical levels. Theoretically, this would prevent the problems seen with the adjacent levels. Dynamic stabilization, total disc replacement, nucleus pulposis replacement, and total facet arthroplasties, among others, are currently being studied as alternatives to fusion.

Dynamic stabilization or "soft stabilization" is defined as a system that would alter the movement and load transmission of the spinal motion segment in such a way as to favor protective physiologic motion and load through that segment without producing a fusion. By accomplishing this goal, the hope is that not only will there be pain relief, but the body's reparative processes will reverse the underlying damage to the intervertebral disc and surrounding tissues.[7] Recent literature suggests that there may be a window of opportunity in which the functional spinal unit may be spared the degenerative cascade if the mechanical loads upon it return to within the physiologic range.[8] The early results from the European experience with dynamic stabilization are thought to be not only safe but effective.[9]

Any attempt to preserve motion of the functional spinal unit must keep the physiologic instant axes of rotation in mind. The axes of rotation the implant provides should be the same or close to that of the normal functional spinal unit. If not, then failure of the system will surely result. An example of this system failure is the Graf ligament replacement system pioneered by Henry Graf. The implant was a pedicle-based system with nonelastic braided polyester ligament replacements placed between the pedicle screws. The clinical results were fair, with results similar to fusion. The problem with the Graf ligamentoplasty was that if any facet hypertrophy was present, then lateral recess stenosis resulted after placement of the implants. This was due to nonphysiologic loading of the functional spinal unit instrumented. Because the disc was loaded in a nonphysiologic manner by which the posterior aspect of the disc was loaded instead of the anterior portion, DDD developed at an accelerated rate, and eventual failure of the surgery resulted.[1,10]

Thus, the ideal dynamic stabilization system would incorporate the following characteristics: (1) have the ability to unload the disc, (2) distribute loads, (3) preserve physiologic relevant motion, (4) provide stability, (5) maintain lordosis (in the lumbar spine), (6) maintain the instaneous axis of rotation (IAR), and (7) have long in vivo longevity of the implants without failure. Additionally, these systems should not eliminate the possibility of using more traditional methods of providing a fusion should it be needed at a future date.

## INDICATIONS/CONTRAINDICATIONS

Indications for the use of the IsoBar dynamic instrumentation in the lumbar spine are:

1. Internal disc derangement
2. Grade I or II degenerative spondylolisthesis
3. Recurrent disc herniations
4. Massive discectomies
5. Iatrogenic instability (decompressive laminectomy or unilateral facetectomy)
6. Adjacent-level degeneration prophylaxis

The contraindications for use of the IsoBar device are:

1. Bilateral spondylolysis
2. Bilateral facetectomies
3. Grade III or IV spondylolisthesis
4. Greater than 50% disc space narrowing
5. Fracture
6. Scoliosis
7. Crossing the thoracolumbar junction
8. Osteoporosis

## DESCRIPTION OF THE DEVICE

The Scient'x USA IsoBar (Scient'x USA, Maitland, FL) dynamic rod stabilization system was based on the work of French scientist Albert Alby and then refined in design and materials. At present, the device is produced from titanium alloy (Ti6Al4Va). The system is denoted IsoBar TTL and consists of a 5.5-mm-diameter rod with an integral dampener element (Figs. 63–1 and 63–2). The dampener element contains stacked titanium alloy disc-shaped elements that allow linearly elastic controlled axial and angular motions. Each of these discs has a nitrogen ion surface treatment intended to substantially increase its wear resistance. This dampener feature of the rod results in a design-allowable 0.75 mm of maximum axial compression or distraction, as well as maximal allowable 4 degrees of angular motion (in flexion-extension and lateral bending). Finally, the dampener feature also serves as a linearly elastic "shock absorber." In an assembled instrumentation system applied to a nonfused segment, only flexion-extension bending and axial motions are permitted (lateral bending is restricted due to the bilateral geometry of the device). This system also includes an approximate 15 degrees of lordosis built into the device.

## BACKGROUND OF SCIENTIFIC TESTING/CLINICAL OUTCOMES

Biomechanical testing of the IsoBar TTL system was performed using Cunningham models as well as a finite element analysis. Twelve models of the lumbar spine from L1-L5 were created after the manner described by Cunningham,[11] which has been formalized by the American Society for Testing and Materials in the form of a protocol (F1717). The 12 models were then split evenly into test and control groups, with six being instrumented with the

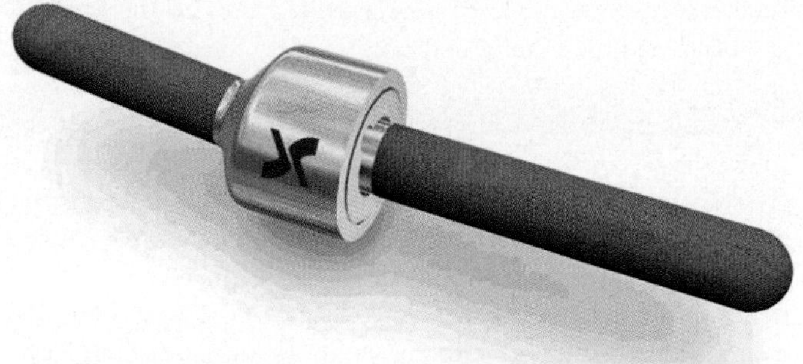

■ **FIGURE 63–1.** IsoBar TTL dynamic rod.

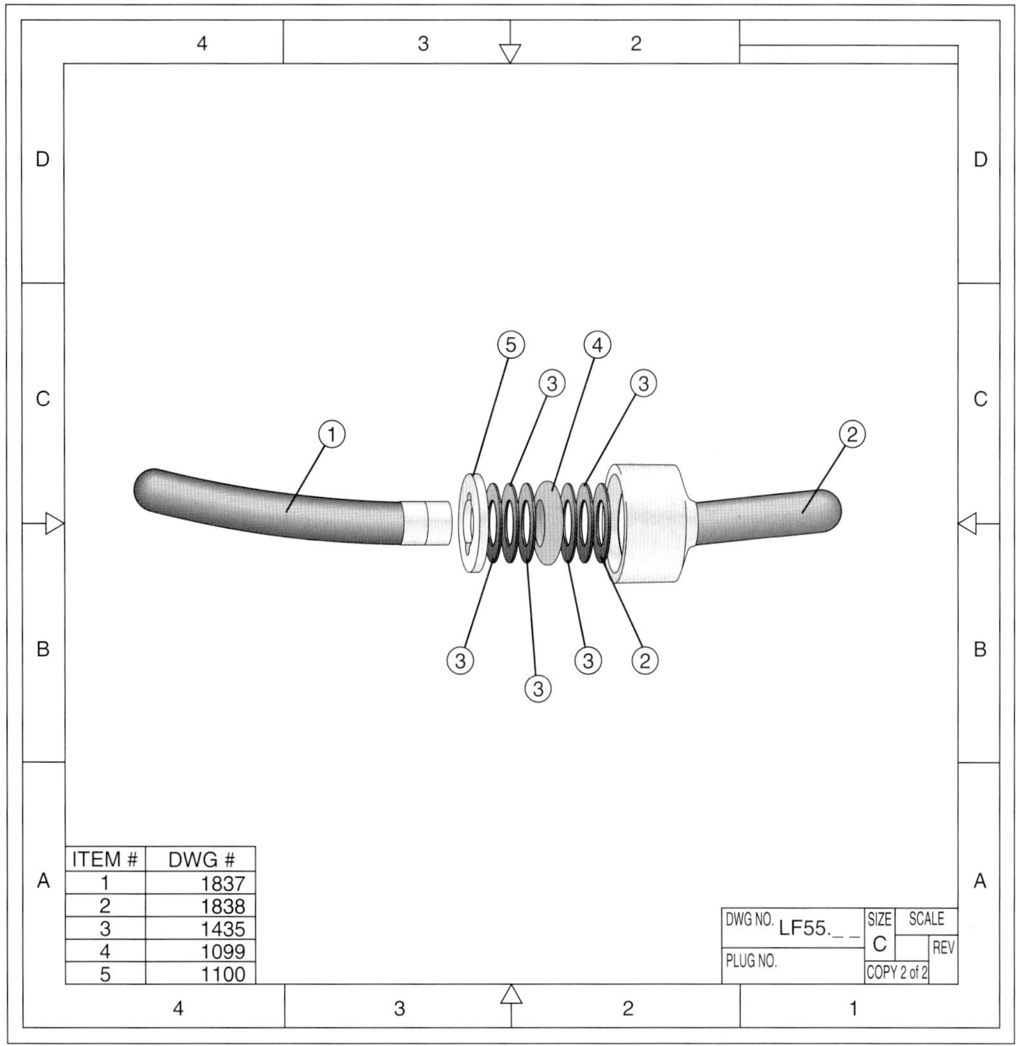


■ **FIGURE 63–2.** Design schematic of IsoBar TTL dynamic rod.

IsoBar TTL system from L4-L5 and the other six with rigid instrumentation. The models were then subjected to axial compression, and load-deformation data were collected and recorded. The IsoBar TTL system was 3.6 times less rigid in axial compression than the rigid constructs[12,13] (Fig. 63–3).

Finite element analysis was performed after producing wire-mesh mathematical lumbar spine models with both the IsoBar TTL system and rigid instrumentation at L4-L5. In vivo measurements of stresses at adjacent levels are not possible at this time; therefore, these computer models were produced to replicate the spine in vivo. The model was constructed based on the computed tomographic scans of the spine of a 44-year-old man without spinal pathology (Fig. 63–4). The biomechanical properties of the bone and each instrument system obtained with the Cunningham models were factored into the equation. Additionally, mathematical entries representing an intervertebral disc and the annulus fibrosis between the adjacent level and the instrumented level were also factored in. The models were tested in flexion and extension combined with axial loading. Simulated models were taken through 15, 30, and 45 degrees of flexion and extension at 15 degrees. An axial compressive load was combined with these flexion and extension moments of 400 Newton's amplitude. The characteristics of the IsoBar TTL system were entered with 3.6 times less stiffness than the rigid construct and allowed for micromotion of 0, 0.4, 0.6, and 0.8 mm axial compression. Using these two variables, the dampener mechanism of the TTL system was simulated and tested. The L5-S1 vertebral level was considered fixed, and the loads were transferred through the superior end

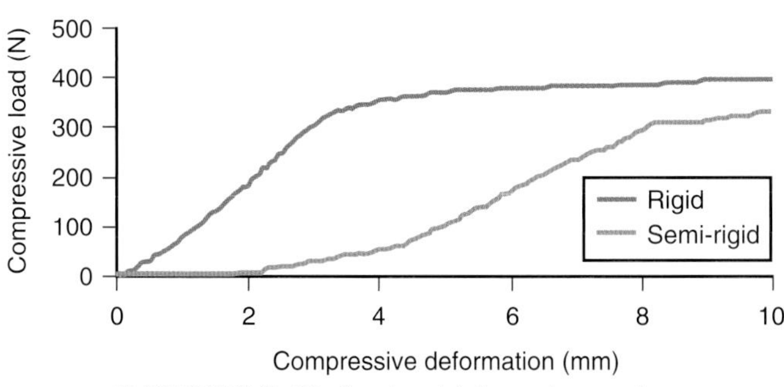


■ **FIGURE 63–3.** Load deformation results.

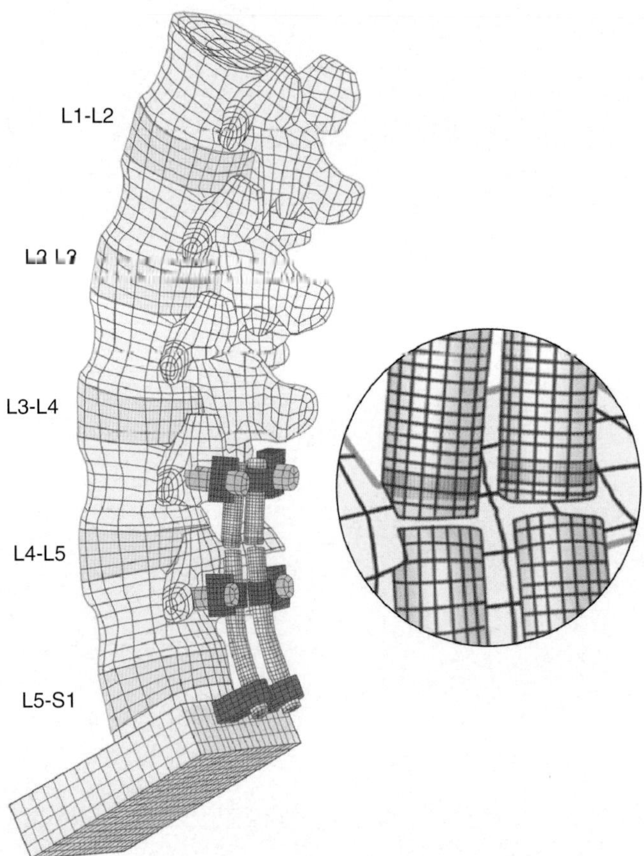

L1-L2
L2-L3
L3-L4
L4-L5
L5-S1

■ **FIGURE 63–4.** Isometric view of the finite element mesh of the lumbar spine and dynamic rods.

plate of L1. All components were modeled by using linearly elastic materials; each was assigned standard material properties according to Young's modulus and Poisson's ratio (Table 63–1). Data collected included:

- Kinematics
- Maximum stress amplitudes induced in the discs
- Distribution of stresses within the discs
- Instantaneous IAR

Kinematic data showed that allowing two degrees of rotation at L4-L5 generates less stress and angular deformity at the L3-L4 disc (see Fig. 63–5). By allowing axial compression and distraction and moving the IAR to physiologic norms (near the center of the disc), smaller loads are needed to create the 2 degrees of rotation (see Fig. 64–4).

**TABLE 63–1. Young's Modulus and Poisson's Ratio**

| Material | Young's Modulus, GPa | Poisson's Ratio |
|---|---|---|
| Cortical Bone | 3 | 0.2 |
| Cortex | 12 | 0.3 |
| Cancellous Bone | 0.5 | 0.2 |
| Fibrous | 0.03 | 0.45 |
| Nucleus | 0.001 | 0.49 |
| Steel | 190 | 0.3 |
| Titanium | 116 | 0.33 |

Von Mises' stress values (combined stresses in all three dimensions) were decreased at the L3-L4 disc in simulated models with dynamic instrumentation at L4-L5 as compared with rigid instrumentation. Volumetric distribution of maximum stresses was decreased by 40% at this same level in the dynamic model.

Testing also revealed that allowing more axial displacement through the dampener had a greater impact on stresses at the L3-L4 disc space than decreasing the stiffness of the dampener. This displacement also decreased the force necessary to produce 2 degrees of rotation and maintained a more physiologic IAR.

Based upon the results from biomechanical testing, the values of axial displacement and stiffness for both constructs were calculated and are shown in Figure 63–5. Additionally, there was a 47% reduction in disc volume subjected to maximum stresses at the L3-L4 level in the dynamically instrumented simulation as compared to the rigid construct. This effect was maximal at 45 degrees of forward flexion; however, it was observed at magnitudes of flexion and extension (Figs. 63–6 to 63–8).

## Clinical Outcomes

Clinically, our experience consists of 64 patients with a mean age of 52.1 years. There were 28 men and 36 women in the study. The subjects were operated on for single-segment stenosis, spondylolisthesis, postlaminectomy syndrome, and DDD. The patients were followed up at 6 weeks; 3, 6, and 12 months; and then yearly thereafter. The study length ultimately will be 10 years. At present, data have been collected at an average follow-up time of 18 months. Functional outcomes (Oswestry Disability Index [ODI] and Short Form-36 [SF-36]) as well as radiographic (plain film, flexion and extension films, MRI, and computed tomography) data were collected. Twenty-eight patients had a combination fusion/dynamic stabilization procedure consisting of L5-S1 fusion with dynamic instrumentation at L4-L5 or fusion at L4-L5, L5-S1 with dynamic instrumentation at L3-L4. Thirty-six patients underwent dynamic stabilization without fusion. Adjacent levels will be evaluated at each visit for up to 10 years.

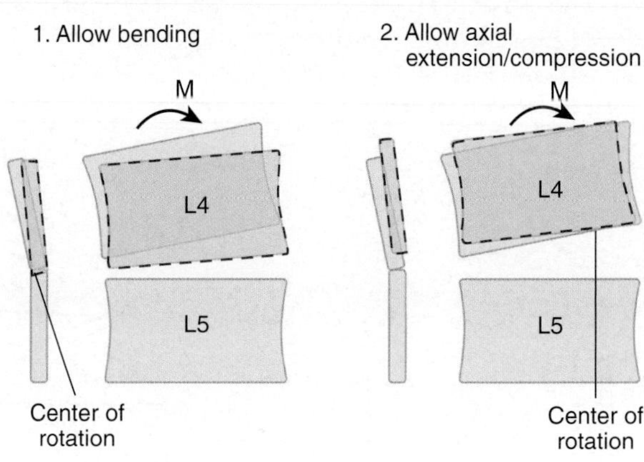

1. Allow bending
2. Allow axial extension/compression
M
M
L4
L5
L4
L5
Center of rotation
Center of rotation
Note: 1. It is easier to rotate L4 if the COR is closer to the center of the cross-section.
2. The material farthser from the COR plays a larger role on resisting rotation.

■ **FIGURE 63–5.** Centers of rotation.

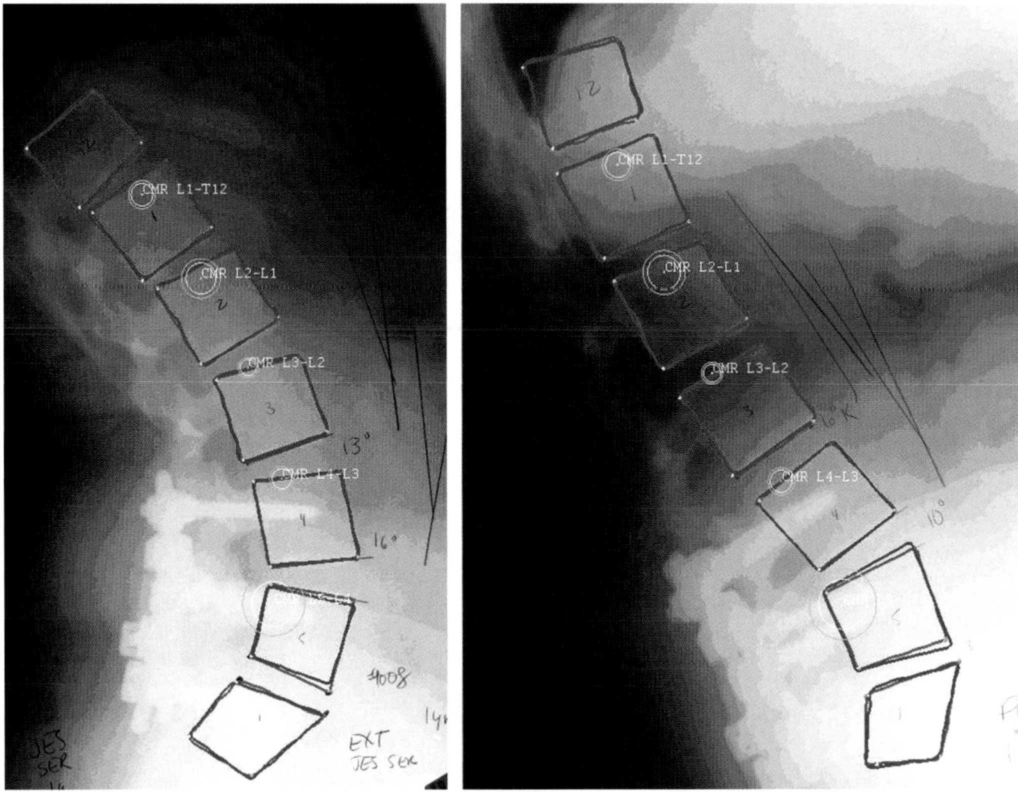


■ **FIGURE 63–6.** Computer-assisted analysis of the in vivo dynamic (flexion-extension) radiographs shows that motion is preserved at the dynamic level; there is no pathologic motion at the adjacent level, and the instantaneous angle of rotation (IAR) at the dynamic level is at a more physiologic position. The IAR of the adjacent level is preserved in its physiologic location.

The results of the ODI demonstrate 45% absolute improvement when a hybrid fusion/dynamic stabilization procedure is mixed and 83% improvement with dynamic stabilization alone. SF-36 scores also improved in all groups over 18 months.

Early overall radiographic results demonstrated no lucency at the bone/screw interface, no breakage of the rods or screws, no increase of translation, preserved disc heights, and no pseudoarthrosis.

## OPERATIVE TECHNIQUE

This system is one that is pedicle based, and the approach is best left to the treating physician. Our approach has been a typical midline skin incision over the segments to be dynamized. The incision is then carried down to the fascia, which is also incised in line with the skin incision. The posterior elements (spinous process, lamina, and pars interarticularis) are then subperiosteally

■ **FIGURE 63–7.** Finite element analysis (FEA) of stress distribution of L3-L4 demonstrating increased stress when using the rigid rod. Note the intensity of color.

STRESS DISTRIBUTION OF L3-L4 DISC (45° FLEXION)

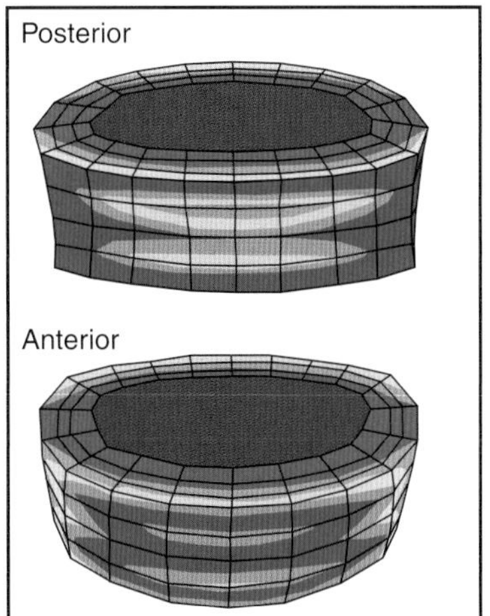


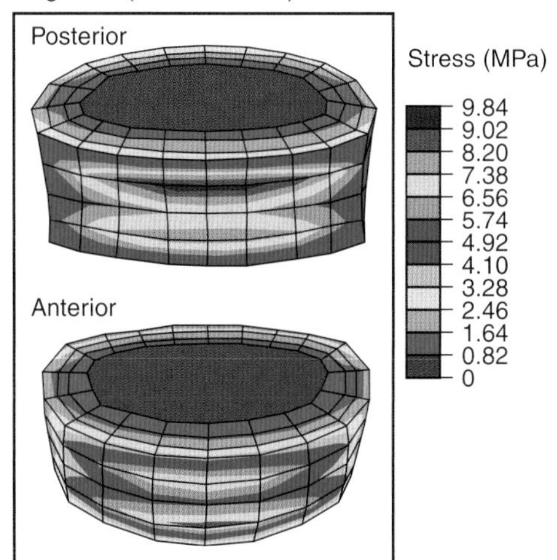

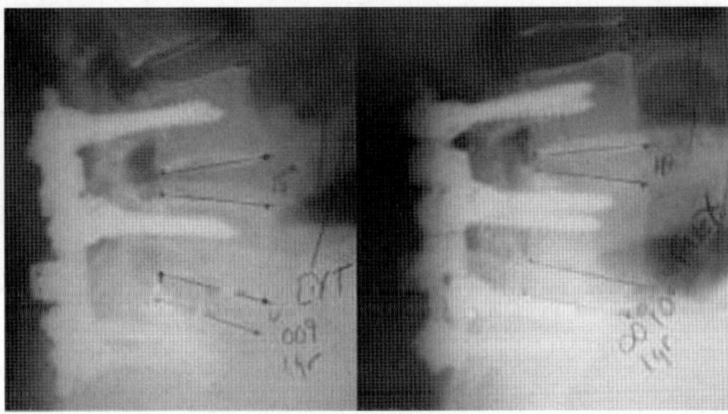

■ **FIGURE 63–8.** Four degrees of motion in flexion and extension, and 0.75 mm of axial motion.

exposed except for the facet joints. Care should be taken not to violate the facet joint capsules during the exposure.

Technical points for placement of the IsoBar TTL dynamic rods are as follows:

1. Use a lateral starting point for the pedicle screw placement.
2. Maintain lumbar lordosis and connect the rods to the screws in situ. Be sure the writing on the rod and dampener are aligned and that this portion of the rod construct faces dorsally.
3. Do not place rod connectors against the caudal aspect of the rod dampener—doing so will prohibit motion within the dampener. Use of offset rod connectors with screws that are closely placed may help avoid this problem.
4. Do not place a flexion or extension moment on the construct because this will lead to nonphysiologic loading of the disc with neuroforaminal stenosis (with extension moment) and potential accelerated degeneration of the disc (from increased load anteriorly or posteriorly).

## POSTOPERATIVE CARE

Postoperatively, the patients are placed on bed rest the day of surgery, followed by an active physical therapy program beginning postoperative day one. This consists of ambulation and activities of daily living routines. No bracing is required. By postoperative day three to four, patients are discharged from the hospital and restricted to light duty–type work (no heavy lifting, bending, or twisting). They are followed in the clinic at 1 week for wound check and staple removal, then 6 weeks, 3 months, 6 months, and 1 year.

## COMPLICATIONS AND AVOIDANCE

There were complications related to the implant and those unrelated to the implant (infection, dural tears, chronic regional pain syndrome [CRPS], herniated disc, and seromas). There were two complications related to the implant itself; one was a segmental kyphosis that was secondary to error of implantation. The synovial cyst developed as a result of iatrogenic injury to the facet joint with pedicle screw placement. Additionally, unrelated to the implant, there were two dural tears, two cases of CRPS that resolved less than 6 weeks postoperatively, two seromas, two infections, and one recurrent herniated disc.

## CONCLUSIONS/DISCUSSION

Adjacent-level degeneration in its many forms has become the subject of much research and debate in recent years. The IsoBar system of soft stabilization has some ideal characteristics to help prevent these phenomena. Perhaps the most important is maintenance of a more physiologic IAR. This is achieved through allowing axial motion in the stabilized segments, which shifts the IAR toward the midportion of the disc, thereby creating a more physiologic IAR. Consider a single-segment instrumentation between two vertebrae (L4-L5). If dynamized and no axial compression is allowed to occur through the disc space, then the resultant extension moment is centered posteriorly near the facet joints (see Fig. 64–4). However, when axial motion is allowed through the instrumented level, then the IAR moves anteriorly into the disc space, more closely mimicking the natural physiology of the functional spinal unit. This more anteriorly situated IAR reduces the moment arm for the L4 level, with a subsequent reduction of stress placed on the L3-L4 disc space. The results from the finite element analysis demonstrate that allowing greater axial compression and subsequent anteriorization of the IAR is more effective in reducing the adjacent-level stresses than simply reducing the rigidity of the construct.

Owing to the reduced stiffness, increased axial movement, and anterior IAR of the IsoBar dynamic stabilization system, some small degree of rotation is allowed across the instrumented segment. This equates to decreased stress of rotation at the adjacent segments when the spine flexes and extends at these levels. Rotation is not allowed by the posterior hinge designs of dynamic instrumentation; therefore, there is a corresponding increased stress across the adjacent segments.

The tradeoff in using dynamic stabilization is the remaining stresses across the instrumented disc. There may be up to 28% greater maximum stress amplitude in the L4-L5 disc. However, in consideration, the overall maximum stress in the L4-L5 disc must be taken into account. The stress amplitudes at this level were only one half to one third that of the amplitudes noted in the L3-L4 level.

In addition to preserving some limited motion in the functional spinal unit, this system distributes loads and is able to decrease pain through these capabilities. Sagittal alignment is also maintained due to the 15 degrees of lordosis built into the system. The stabilizing effect of this device prevents abnormal motion across the instrumented segment yet preserves the physiologic instant access of rotation of the unit. It can be likened to the hip replacement data and theory in which the desired goal is motion (functional range of motion) centered in the middle of what is considered physiologic or normal range of motion. When the functional range of motion is skewed to one side or the other of physiologic motion, then dislocation (either anterior or posterior, depending on the placement of components) is the likely result. Likewise, in the functional spinal unit, our goal is to center the constrained IAR of the instrumented segment in or near the middle of the physiologic range of motion or IAR of the healthy spine. If this is accomplished, then pain relief can be accomplished without sacrificing the result due to placing a greater extension or flexion moment through the device and subsequent spinal segment. In the spine literature, we have seen that skewing the IAR (usually posterior) will result in increased rate of disc degeneration. Additionally, by maintaining a near physiologic IAR, this device may be a potentially valuable adjunct with total disc replacement technology.

The Scient'x TTL instrumentation meets the "ideals" noted earlier because it:

- Provides easy implantation
- Is reversible
- Provides longevity
- Preserves motion
- Stabilizes the motion segment
- Shares the stresses or loads
- Preserves the IAR
- Maintains sagittal alignment-lordosis of the functional spinal unit

## ACKNOWLEDGMENTS

I want to thank Deborah H. Clabeaux RN for assistance with this chapter.

## REFERENCES

1. Mulholland RC, Sengupta DK: Rationale, principles and experimental evaluation of the concept of soft stabilization. Eur Spine J 11 (suppl 2):S198–S205, 2002.
2. Frymoyer JW: The Adult Spine: Principles and Practice, 2nd ed. Philadelphia, Lippincott-Raven, 1997.
3. Crock HV: Internal disc disruption: A challenge to disc prolapse fifty years on. Spine 11:650–653, 1986.
4. Kirkaldy-Willis WH, Farfan HF: Instability of the lumbar spine. Clin Orthop Relat Res 165:110–123, 1982.
5. Gibson JNA, Waddell G: Surgery for degenerative lumbar spondylosis (Cochrane Review). *In* The Cochrane Library, Issue 1, 2006. Oxford: Update Software.
6. Boden SD, Bohlman HH: The Failed Spine. Philadelphia, Lippincott Williams & Wilkins, 2003.
7. Sengupta DK: Dynamic stabilization devices in the treatment of low back pain. Orthop Clin North Am 35:43-56, 2004.
8. Stokes IA, Iatridis JC: Mechanical conditions that accelerate invertertebral disc degeneration: Overload versus immobilization. Spine 29:2724–2732, 2004.
9. Perrin G: Prevention of adjacent level degeneration above a fused vertebral segment. Presented at the International Meeting for Advanced Spine Techniques. Rome, Italy, 2003.
10. Gevitt MP, Gardner AD, Spilsbury J, et al: The Graf stabilisation system: Early results in 50 patients. Eur Spine J 4:169–175; discussion 35, 1995.
11. Cunningham BW, Sefter JC, Shono Y, McAfee PC: Static and cyclical biomechanical analysis of pedicle screw spinal constructs. Spine 18:1677–1688, 1993.
12. Huang H, Pienkowski D, Saijal S, Castellvi AE: Finite element analysis of dynamic instrumentation demonstrates stress reduction in adjacent level discs. Presented at the 51st Annual Meeting of the Orthopaedic Research Society. Washington, DC, 2005.
13. Castellvi AE, Huang H, Vestgaarden T, et al: Stress reduction in adjacent level discs via dynamic instrumentation: A finite element analysis. SAS Journal, Vol 1, Issue 2, Spring 2007.

CHAPTER 64

# Cosmic: Dynamic Stabilization of the Degenerated Lumbar Spine

**Archibald von Strempel**

## KEY POINTS

- Cosmic is a dynamic nonfusion pedicle screw rod system for the stabilization of the degenerated lumbar vertebral column.
- The hinged pedicle screw provides for the load being shared between the implant and the vertebral column and allows a high stability in relation to the rotational forces.
- Load sharing and axial displacement preserve the shock-absorbing function of the disc and protects the implants from breakage or loosening.
- Bone ingrowth into screw is enhanced with Bonit coating.

## INTRODUCTION

The degeneration of the lumbar motion segment often starts with disc height loss caused by dehydration and other internal changes within the nucleus pulposus and annulus fibrosis. The facet joints lose their congruence, which may result in arthrosis.[1] The fibers of the annulus fibrosis and the vertebral column ligaments lose tension so that a structural loosening occurs including an increase in rotational instability.[2–4] A compensatory hypertrophy of the ligamentum flavum as well as the facet joints occurs frequently, leading to a reduction of the cross-sectional area of the central as well as lateral spinal canal. At the same time, the motion segment may lose its original position, and scoliosis, flat back, rotation, and rotational sliding may develop. During the course of the degeneration, lateral and anterior spondylophytes up to and including syndesmophytes may form, which, in turn, may lead to a spontaneous stiffening of the segment.

Reported symptoms depend on the respective stage of the vertebral column degeneration. In the initial stage of lumbar spondylosis, recurrent episodes of lumbago may occur that increase under load stress. When the stenosis of the spinal channel increases, additional symptoms such as neurogenic claudication may occur. If a spontaneous ankylosis of the segment occurs before a symptomatic spinal channel stenosis, the frequency and intensity of lumbago decrease.

The cause of the leg symptoms can be explained by the compression of the nerve structures caused by a narrow spinal channel, lateral recess, or neuroforamen. As a rule, adequate decompression of the neural structures leads to good clinical success. The etiology of the lumbago is less clear, and clinical improvement does not occur in the same measure, even with a successful bony fusion. What may be assumed to be certain is that the instability in the motion segment caused by the vertebral disc height loss is a trigger for the frequency of reoccurring lumbago. Non-physiologic movements that are possible only due to vertebral disc height loss lead to a shift of the nucleus pulposus within the vertebral disc and a subsequent ingrowth of pain-conducting nerve ends.[5] This increased innervation of the degenerative vertebral disc is also responsible for the so-called memory pain in discography.[6]

The term instability used in this context has been better defined by Panjabi as a "clinical instability" that leads to a pathologic movement and pain, deformities, and neurologic failures.[7] The operative treatment of the symptomatic lumbar vertebral column degeneration has so far consisted of stabilizing the diseased segment or segments and correcting and adequately decompressing these segments, always in connection with fusion. In recent years, the various different forms of fusion (anterior lumbar interbody fusion [ALIF], posterior lumbar interbody fusion [PLIF], transforaminal lumbar interbody fusion [TLIF], posterior lateral fusion [PLF]) have been discussed very intensively, as one believed to be able to increase the clinical success rate above all by means of a 360 degree fusion.

This could be rejected in a prospective randomized double blind study. The clinical results were independent of the selected fusion form. Complications naturally increased in line with the increased surgical work effort (360 degree fusion). In this study, pseudoarthrosis did not have any influence on the clinical results.[8]

Following a spondylodesis, 16.5% of symptomatic vertebral disc degenerations were expected in the neighboring segment after 5 years, and 36.1% after 10 years.[9] Obviously, there is a lower risk for a posterior lateral spondylodesis without the use of pedicle screw systems.[10] It must be questioned whether the risk for the adjacent segment increases with the rigidity of the fusion construct, which would concern the currently favored 360° fusions with cage in combination with a pedicle screw system.[11–13] Interestingly, the incidence of adjacent-level disease appears to be less in fusion constructs that were carried out for the correction of extended deformities. After 20 years or more following a Harrington fusion, low back pain was found in only 13% of cases.[14]

## WHEN IS A CORRECTION NECESSARY?

In contrast to the treatment of adolescent scoliosis, in which the correction of the deformity is also the objective of the treatment, there are not many indications for the correction of the degenerative lumbar vertebral column that actually serve the direct objective of the operation with subsequent pain release and restoration of neurologic function.

Positional deformities in the sagittal and frontal planes that do not lead to a loss of the body vertical plumb line need not be corrected. This concerns most lateral deviations. Therefore, the correction of a degenerative lumbar scoliosis is necessary only in exceptional cases. The reduction of the vertebral disc always leads also to a flattening of the lumbar vertebral column, which also does not need to be corrected as long as the patient assumes an upright well-balanced posture. True and degenerative olisthesis vera in an adult are not usually progressive. Stabilization and decompression without correction lead to the objective of the treatment. Therefore, it is not meaningful to transfer the principles of surgery of scoliosis in adolescents noncritically to the surgery of the degenerative lumbar vertebral column.

### Indications for Dynamic Stabilization with Cosmic

1. Symptomatic lumbar stenosis (neurogenic claudication): A stand-alone decompression of the spinal canal carries the risk of a recurrence of spinal stenosis because the instability that led to the hypertrophy of the yellow ligament and the facet joints is not taken into consideration. In addition, back pain and deformities may increase as an expression of the increased clinical instability. For this reason, we perform stabilization with Cosmic (Ulrich AG, Germany) (Fig. 64–1A to C).
2. Chronically recurring low back pain in the case of discogenic pain and facet syndrome: Degenerative disc disease is present if vertebral disc dehydration with height loss and positive Modic signs are detected. In the presence of additional vertebral discs (black disc), we carry out an additional discography. The presence of memory pain confirms the suspicion of a symptomatic vertebral disc degeneration.[15] In the case of a facet syndrome, we carry out diagnostic local anesthesia under x-ray control, using 2 mL local anesthetic respectively. If the pain subsides for several hours, the suspected diagnosis is confirmed. In such cases, we carry out the Cosmic stabilization using a paraspinous transmuscular approach according to Wiltse (Fig. 64–2A and B).
3. Recurrent disc herniation: In the case of a second recurrence of a disc herniation, we carry out a stabilization with Cosmic in addition to the nerve root decompression.
4. In combination with an arthrodesis: Cosmic can also be used if, in addition to the nonfusion stabilization, there is an indication of an arthrodesis in one or two segments; for example, if there is a spondylolisthesis with a clear shift in the function radiographs and there is symptomatic vertebral disc degeneration in another segment. In addition to the Cosmic stabilization in situ, a posterolateral fusion is set up within the area of the spondylolisthesis. A laminectomy or facetectomy is carried out if there is an indication for this purpose (Fig. 64–3).
5. Extension of an existing arthrodesis in the case of a painful adjacent-level degeneration: Typically, in the case of a rigid 360 degree fusion with cage and pedicle screw rod or pedicle screw plate fixation, there is the risk of developing a painful connection instability. In these cases, we remove the pedicle screw rod or plate system and stabilize the adjacent segment with Cosmic together with a decompression, if indicated. We fill up the existing pedicle drill holes with bone chips and use a 7-mm revision screw for this purpose. (Fig. 64–4).

## CONTRAINDICATIONS

### Correction

If corrections are necessary to relieve the patient's symptoms (as stated above, in almost all cases of a degenerative deformity this is not indicated), a spondylodesis must be provided in addition to the Cosmic instrumentation.

### Stabilizations Extending Beyond Three Segments

Cosmic may be used beyond three segments only in combination with a posterolateral fusion. If there is a degenerative kyphoscoliosis with a loss of balance in the sagittal plane, in which there is a necessity to correct the kyphosis, longer extended instrumentations are required as a rule. Here, in the area to be corrected, Cosmic can be used with a posterolateral fusion and in the other cranial segments with the nonfusion technology.

### Severe Osteoporosis in Combination with Obesity

In obese patients with osteoporosis, there exists a higher risk of screw breakage or loosening when drilling or screwing. In this case, posterolateral spondylodesis should be added.

## DESCRIPTION OF THE DEVICE

A posterior nonfusion implant system should have minimal rigid characteristics. However, in order to be able to control instabilities effectively the system must also feature some stable characteristics. The Cosmic system is a stable nonrigid implant. Stability is ensured by the 6.25-mm rod, and nonrigidity is ensured by the hinged screw head. The screws have an outer diameter of 6 or 7 mm and a length of 35 to 55 mm. The screw features a hinged joint between its head and the threaded section, which causes the load to be shared between implant system and anterior vertebral column (Fig. 64–5).

Cosmic, a form of endoprosthesis, requires optimal healing of the bone-screw interface. For this reason, the threaded part of the screw is coated with Bonit. Bonit is the second generation of bioactive calcium phosphate coatings on implants. In 1995, it was originally used for the first time in oral surgery for dental implants.[16] In the area of vertebral column surgery, there exists a study on the use of a first generation of bioactive calcium phosphate coating on Schanz screws. It was found that there was a significantly improved fixation of the coated screws in comparison to the uncoated screws.[17] In order to achieve a sufficient press-fit behavior, the pedicle is widened by drilling to a 3.2 mm maximum

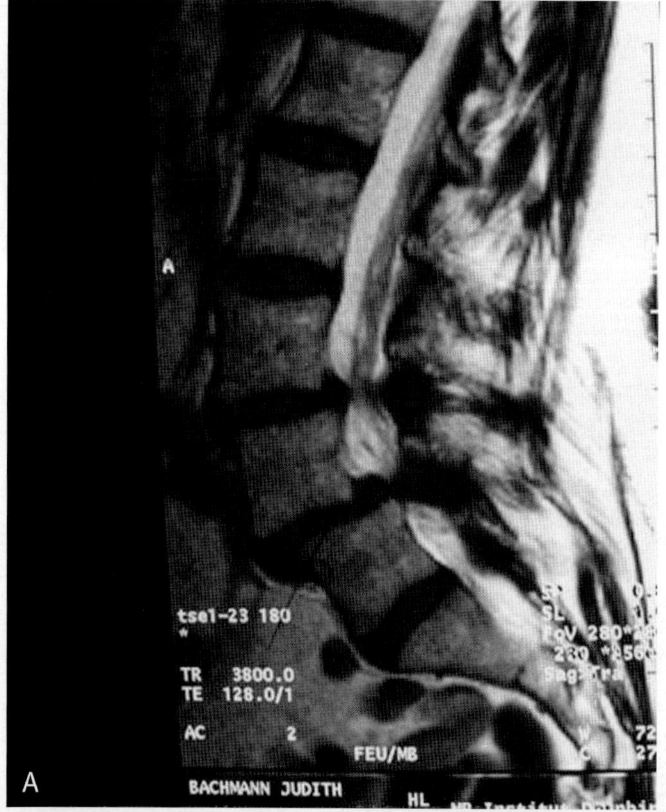


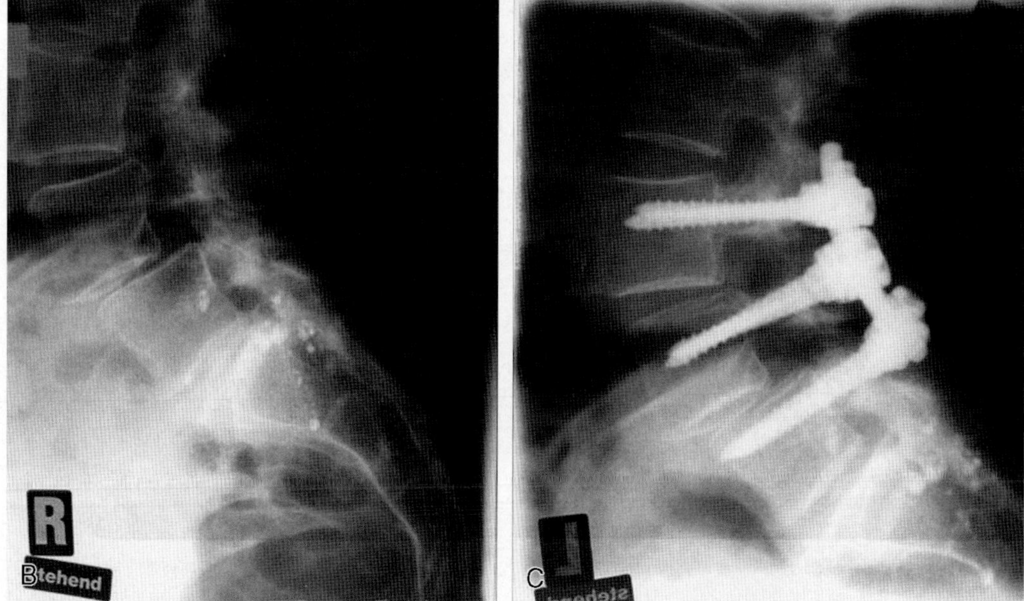


■ **FIGURE 64–1.** **A** to **C,** Spinal stenosis, pseudospondylolisthesis, decompression, and stabilization with Cosmic.

but only along approximately 50% of the screw. The screw has a self-tapping thread so that the tapping instrument needs to be used only in cases of extremely hard spongiosa. In order to prevent any early loosening of the screw, the screw must not be manipulated in any major way. Before the rods are implanted, these must be pre-bent so that they can be connected without any problems to the screw heads.

After the screw heads have been connected to the longitudinal rods, there remains only micromobility in the hinges which, without rod connections, are caudally and cranially mobile by approximately 20 degrees (Fig. 64–6). Owing to rotational stability, Cosmic can be used not only for purely discogenic pain conditions but also in pathologies that require conventional laminectomy or even a facetectomy. A transverse stabilizer is used only for a monosegmental

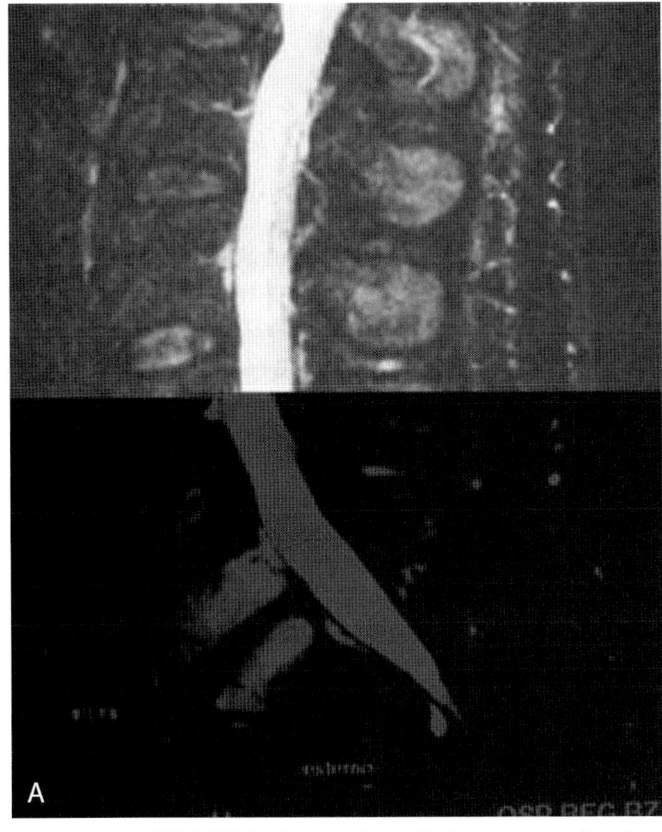


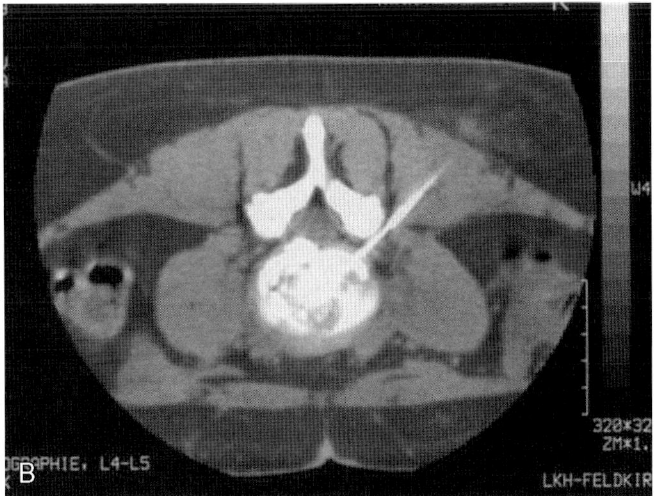


■ **FIGURE 64–2.** **A** and **B,** Degenerative disc disease, positive Modic sign, contrast computed tomography.

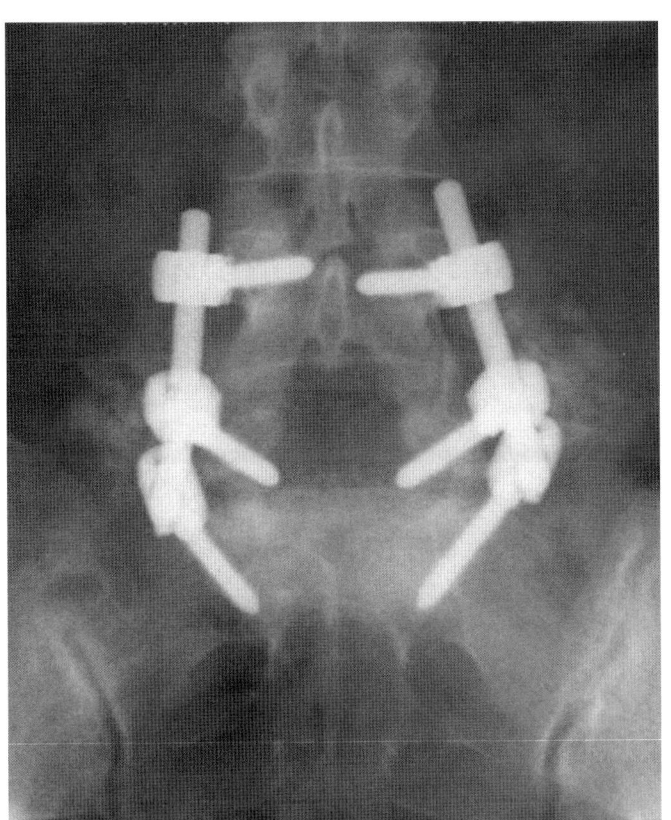

■ **FIGURE 64–3.** Unstable spondylolisthesis vera, stenosis, L5-S1; degenerative disc disease, L4-L5; Cosmic, L4-S1; laminectomy, L5; PLF L5-S1.

application in combination with a laminectomy. For two- or three-segmental applications, no transverse stabilizer is used.

Surgical implantation of the device can be performed through a conventional midline approach, with a point of entry lateral to the facet joint and an angle of approximately 15 degrees horizontal to the sagittal plane, or by means of the more laterally situated Wiltse approach, with a somewhat more ventrally located point of entry close to the base of the transverse continuations and an angle of 20 to 25 degrees horizontal to the sagittal plane [Fig. 64–7]. A purely sagittal implantation direction is not recommended because this will lead to a parallel positioning of the hinges and thus to an increased mobility in the sagittal plane. Before the rod is implanted, the correct positioning of the patient will be checked again by means of a lordosis, that is, as physiologic as possible. In order to avoid any early loosening, correction forces must not be applied to the screw.

## BACKGROUND OF SCIENTIFIC TESTING/CLINICAL OUTCOMES

Compared with a rigid system, the hinged-screw device permits greater load through the disc and allows for greater axial displacement without any decrease of rotational instability.[18] Load sharing and axial displacement are important factors for a long-term survival of the implant and for the preservation of the pump function (shock-absorbing function) of the disc. Because of this dynamic stabilization, we expect a better protection of adjacent segments from increased degeneration. It was possible to show by means of laboratory tests that Cosmic allows the same rotation stability

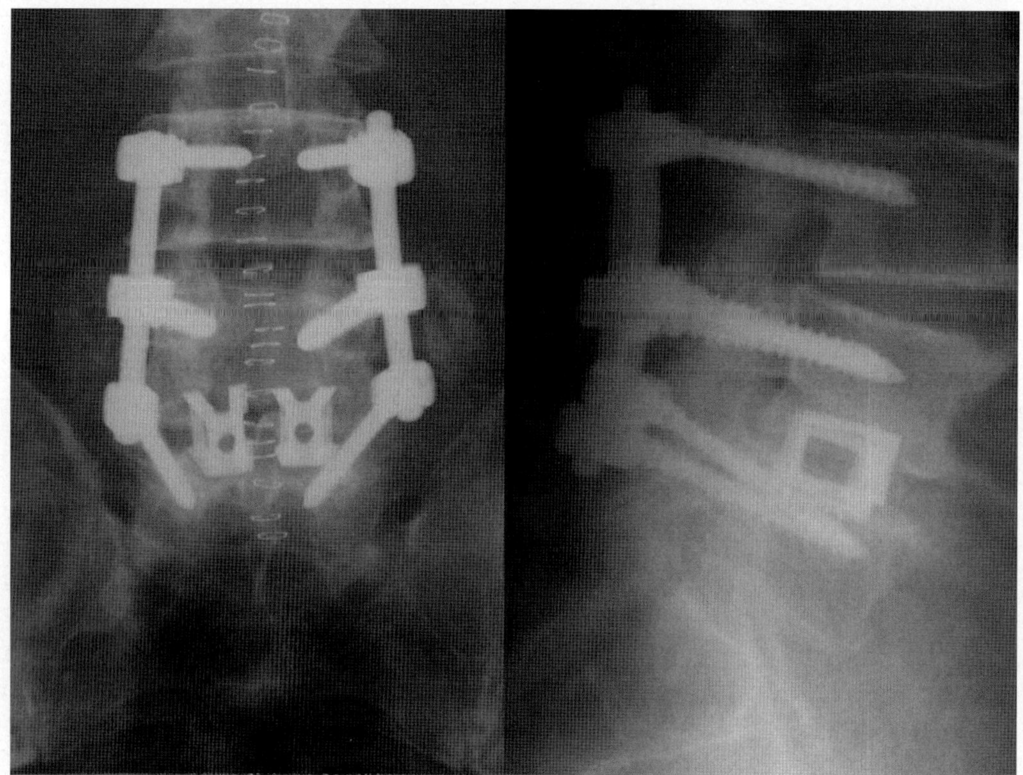

■ **FIGURE 64–4.** Cosmic, L3-L5; laminectomy, L3; pre-existing fusion, L4-L5.

as a healthy motion segment.[19] In a cyclic loading test with 0.3 to 3.0 KN/1 Hz, we did not find an implant breakage or any debris after 10 million cycles.[20]

## In Vivo Clinical Data

From January 2002 to June 2006, 253 patients underwent surgery in Feldkirch, Austria.

The clinical results of 75 patients with a follow-up of 24 months were compared with those from 75 patients with a follow-up of 24 months that, for the same indications, had been treated with Segmental Spinal Correction System (SSCS) (Osteotech, Eatontown, NJ), which also contains a jointed head pedicle screw but without coating, and with a conventional posterolateral fusion. The SSCS had been used since 1989.

In both groups, the indications were comparable: symptomatic lumbar stenosis, painful olistheses, painful osteochondroses, painful spondyloarthroses, recurring vertebral disc prolapse, and discogenic pain.

The average age in the nonfusion group was 67.2 years, and in the fusion group, it was 55.9 years. The reason for the increased age of the group without fusion is that, during the first year, we predominantly used the nonfusion technique for the treatment of older patients in order to keep the surgery trauma as low as possible. With increasing experience, we then used the nonfusion technique also in the case of middle-aged patients.

In the nonfusion group, the pain ratings on the Visual Analog Scale (VAS) were 5.7 preoperatively and 2.9 postoperatively, and in the fusion group, the pain ratings were 5.8 preoperatively and 3.4 postoperatively.

The Oswestry Disability Index (ODI) in the nonfusion group was 25.4 points or 50.8% preoperatively and 17.0 points or 34,0% postoperatively. In the fusion group, the ODI was 23.7 points or 47.4% preoperatively and 14.7 points or 29.4% postoperatively.

The hospital stay in the nonfusion group was 7.4 days (6 to 18 days) and, in the fusion group, 16.9 days (9 to 36 days).

The duration of surgery (skin to skin) in the nonfusion group was 118.8 minutes (62 to 200 minutes), and in the fusion group, it was 172.4 minutes (120 to 215 minutes). Perioperatively, a total of 0.60 units of eryconcentrate were transfused in the non fusion group (0 to 4 units), and in the fusion group, 2.96 units of eryconcentrate (0 to 6 units) were transfused on average.

In the nonfusion group, revisions were carried out in the case of four patients, and in the fusion group, revisions were carried out in the case of six patients. The revisions were caused by wound infections (once in the case of the nonfusion group, as well as three times in the case of the fusion group), twice by symptomatic loosening of a screw in the nonfusion group, once when a screw broke off in the nonfusion group, and a total of three times due to pseudoarthrosis in connection with an implant fracture or implant loosening in the fusion group.

In June 2004, a multicenter study on an Internet platform was started in cooperation with six international spine centers. So far, 301 patients up to June 2006 have been documented. Two hundred and three patients had primary surgery, and 98 patients had secondary surgery. One hundred and sixty were women, and 141 men. The age range was from 24 to 94 years. Sixty-three percent of patients were between 41 and 70 years old. One hundred and seventy-eight patients had a degenerative disc disease, 115 had spinal stenosis, 65 had spondylolisthesis, 9 had fusion before, and 11 underwent fusion

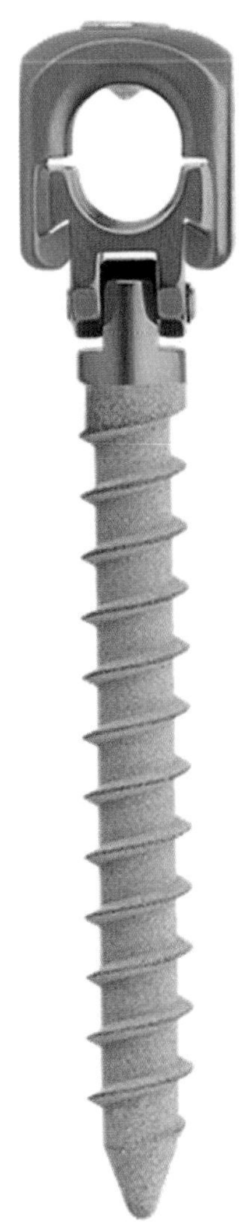

■ **FIGURE 64–5.** Cosmic screw.

together with nonfusion stabilization (more than one diagnosis is possible). One hundred and eighty-three patients received one-level instrumentation, 107 patients received two-level instrumentation, and 11 patients received three-level instrumentation.

One hundred and thirty-one patients out of these 301 had a 12-month follow-up. Preoperatively, the ODI was 50.3%, and after 12 months, it was 28.7%. Preoperatively, the VAS was 7.2, and after 12 months, it was 3.2.

Preoperatively, the lumbar lordosis was 50.3 degrees, and after 12 months, it was 50.5 degrees. The disc height of the adjacent level did not change. Six hundred thirty six screws and 262 rods were implanted. One rod (0.3%) and two screws (0.3%) broke, and seven screws became loose (1.1%) in seven patients (5.3%) who underwent revision. Ten screws (1.5%) showed a halo without clinical symptoms. No screw dislocation was observed. Four revisions were performed for other reasons.

## OPERATIVE TECHNIQUE

While the patient is under general anesthesia, he or she is positioned in the knee-chest position, with hip joints flexed to 90 degrees to avoid any pressure on the abdomen. The lordosis is radiologically controlled and can be increased by lifting the leg section of the operating table. For pure stabilizations, two skin cuts are made paraspinally, each one in position located 4 cm laterally to the processus spinosus vertebrarum. The fascia thoracolumbalis is split, and the finger is used to prepare the muscular system between the multifidus and longissimus, until the transverse processes or the ala of the sacrum can be felt. The screw implantation is performed under lateral imager control (C-arm). In the case of a monosegmental stabilization, only closed screws are used (Fig. 64–8A to C); for a two- or three-segmental stabilization closed screws are used at the caudal end of the instrumentation, and in all other respects, open screws are used (Fig. 64–9). In the sacrum, we recommend bicortical screw implantation, if the screw length is 50 mm or less.

In the case of a monosegmental instrumentation, a straight rod is implanted, and in the case of two- and three-segmental instrumentations, the rod will first be bent, in accordance with the profile. With open screws, the rod is fixed by a clamp to the screw base and the cap is then put on. The rod and screw base feature a thread for guaranteeing a high degree of rotation stability between rod and screw (Fig. 64–10). Fixation is then performed with a small grub screw that is tightened by a force of 6 Nm.

Lateral decompressions can also be carried out from this access point. If a laminectomy is necessary, we carry out a midline incision from which either the muscular system is then prepared beyond the joint continuations in order to carry out screw implantation and decompression from the same access point, or the screws are first set, using the technique described earlier, and followed by the economical preparation of the spinal muscular system from the processus spinosus vertebrarum and the vertebral laminae to a medial position relative to the facet joints to make the decompression. The advantage of this procedure is that damage to the spinal muscles is reduced and that there is less blood loss.

## POSTOPERATIVE CARE

In the case of pure stabilizations, the patient will be mobilized on the first postoperative day. In the case of a conventional midline approach with decompression, such mobilization will be done on the second day. Drains are removed on the first day. For infection prophylaxis, a dose of cephalosporin is given before the skin is incised. The thrombosis prophylaxis is carried out with a low-molecular-weight heparin for 2 weeks postoperatively. External support will not be used. Patients are discharged from the hospital when they are able to climb stairs, after 2 days (stabilization only) to 8 days (stabilization and decompression). We do not recommend physical activities like sports and manual labor for 6 weeks. Follow-up examinations are performed after 6 weeks, 12 weeks, 12 months, 24 months, and 60 months. Anteroposterior and lateral standing radiographs are taken.

## COMPLICATIONS AND AVOIDANCE

Manipulation of the screws should be minimal to avoid primary screw loosening. The pedicle should be entered laterally to the facet joint, close to the base of the transverse process to position the screw head anteriorly as much as possible. This method

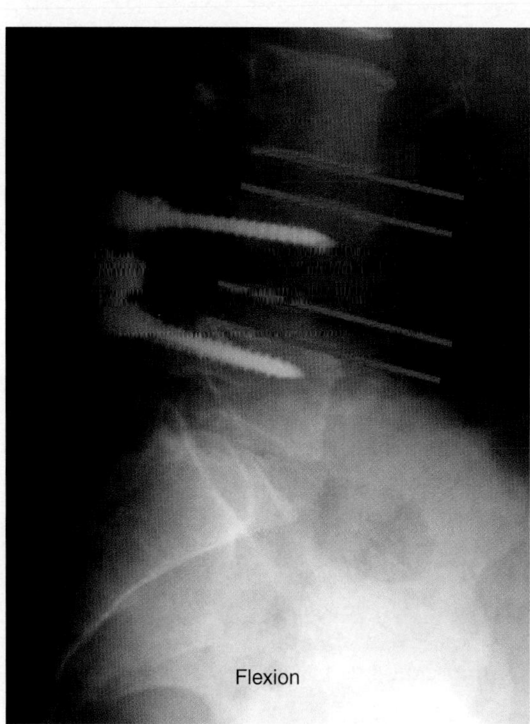


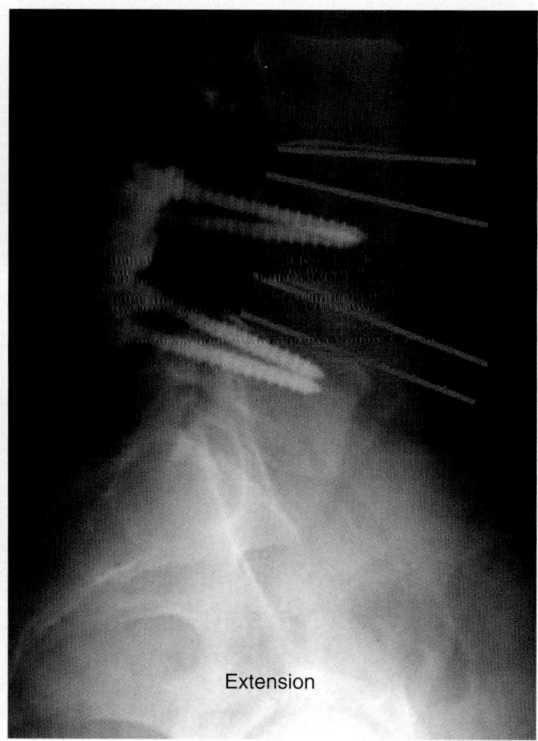


■ **FIGURE 64–6.** Flexion-extension view after 1 year.

reduces the shear forces on the implants and the risk of screw breakage. In a small sacrum, the screws should be implanted bicortically, with the perforation in the anterior middle third of the promontorium. This avoids sacral screw loosening.

Patients who are overweight or who have concurrent severe osteopenia or osteoporosis are considered to be high risk for complications. A posterolateral fusion can prevent screw loosening. Patients who have normal weight and good bone quality are considered to be at low risk for complications.

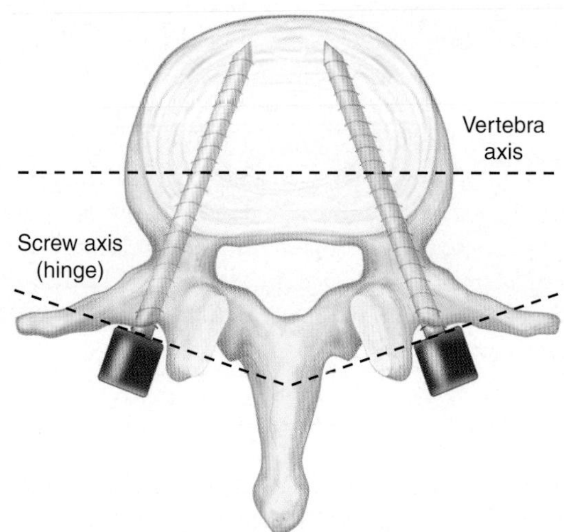


■ **FIGURE 64–7.** Angle of screw direction in the horizontal plan is 15 to 25 degrees.

**ADVANTAGES/DISADVANTAGES: COSMIC**

- Cosmic does not destroy important structures of the vertebrae, and it retains the disk. It is an alternative for fusion or disc replacement in many indications.
- Cosmic is not indicated if correction is necessary. Fusion must be used as well.

## CONCLUSIONS AND DISCUSSION

Degenerative diseases of the lumbar vertebral column represent their own nosologic entity. So far, they have been treated primarily in accordance with the principles of deformity and traumatic surgery. In the past, the goal of surgery has been to correct existing deformities as completely as possible; and in order to ensure this result, rigid implants were used that were able to provide for three-dimensional correction, if at all possible. The fact that fusion of individual segments of the degenerative lumbar vertebral column may cause painful connection instabilities—and this applies obviously in particular to the rigid 360 degree fusions—increasingly calls into question the use of these techniques for the treatment of degenerative diseases.[21–33] The postoperative sagittal profile of the lumbar spine did not have any influence on the development of adjacent instabilities.[34]

In addition, in older patients the quality of the bone frequently does not allow for any secure fixation of rigid implants nor for any corrections. Some elderly patients also show additional secondary diseases that cause an increased perioperative complication rate in the case of more invasive operations on the vertebral column. The idea that fusion is the gold standard for the treatment of

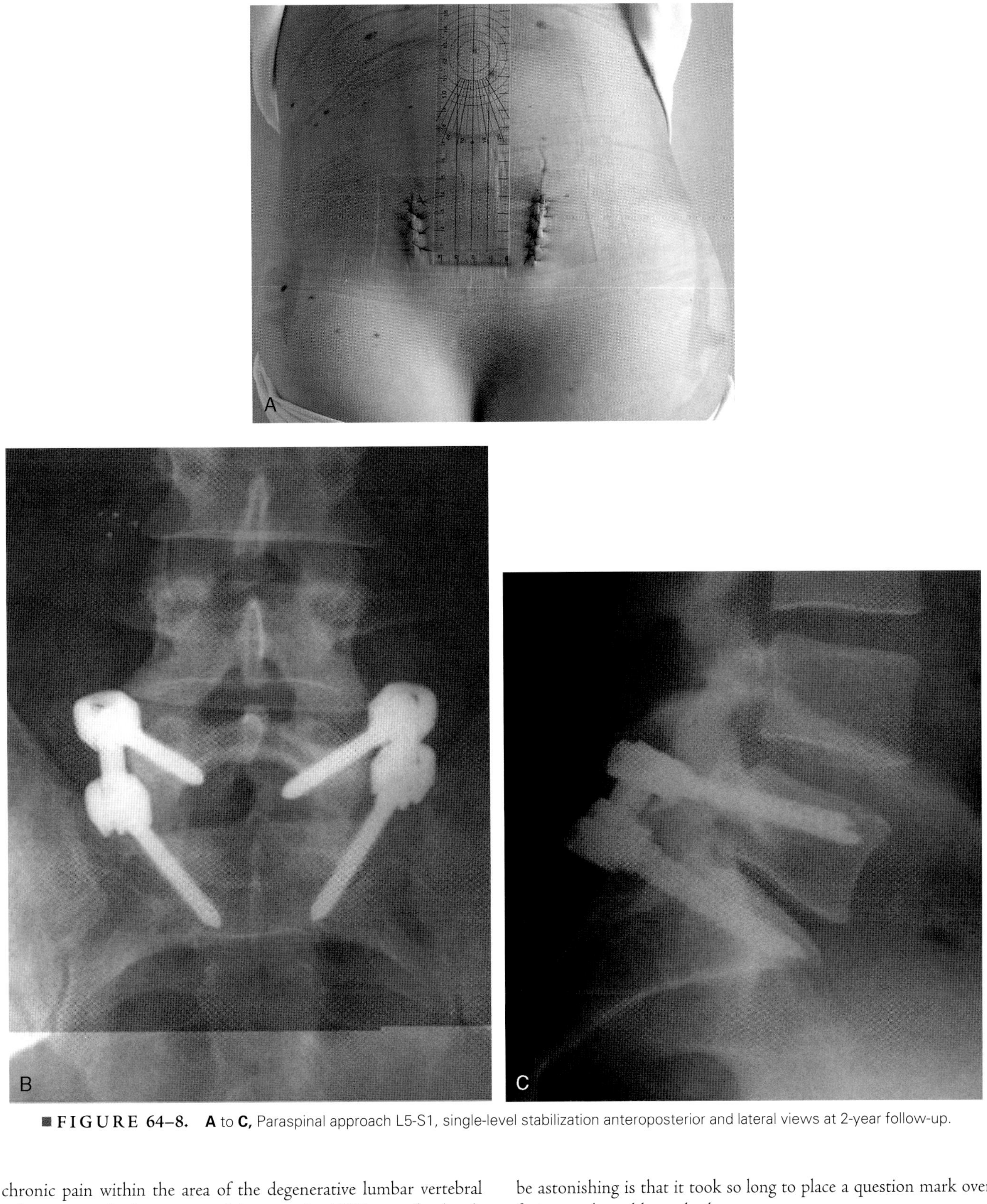

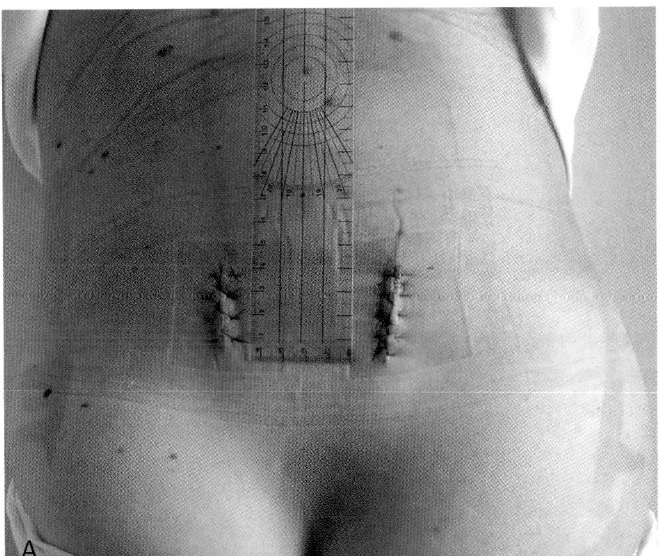

■ **FIGURE 64–8.** **A** to **C,** Paraspinal approach L5-S1, single-level stabilization anteroposterior and lateral views at 2-year follow-up.

chronic pain within the area of the degenerative lumbar vertebral column must also be questioned, because the 100% rate of arthrodeses is not the equivalent to a 100% clinical success rate.[35,36] The significance of patient selection is justifiably regarded as a decisive criterion for achieving a good clinic result.[37] For this reason it is not astonishing that there is a search for different alternative operative techniques that prevent any fusion.[38] But what may possibly be astonishing is that it took so long to place a question mark over fusion as the gold standard.

There have been individual efforts to develop alternative solutions other than fusion. The Graf band is possibly the first pedicle screw-supported nonfusion system used in the treatment of painful degenerative instabilities in the lumbar vertebral column. Biomechanically, it increases the use of dorsal tension chords and reduces painful

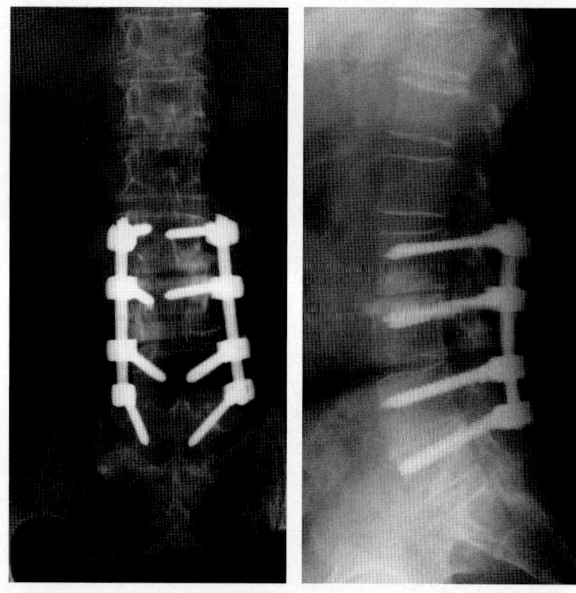

■ **FIGURE 64–9.** Three levels of stabilization at 2-year follow-up.

movements in the facet joints and also in the disc. Clinical success has been reported with the use of this technique.[39–43]

The disadvantages of the Graf system are the missing rotational stability and the risk of early failure of the cable. The Dynesys (Zimmer Spine, Inc., Warsaw, IN) system represents further development of the Graf system. The band is provided with a plastic sleeve, and the band is tensioned against this sleeve. This causes the stability to be increased, but it also produces an increase in the load on the interface between vertebral bone and screw, which may cause loosening to occur.[44] In relation to the rotational forces, the Dynesys system does not show any stability comparable to that of an intact vertebral column.[45] The clinical reports that have so far been published on the Dynesys system are mostly positive.[46,47] In combination with decompressions, these two systems are used somewhat more rarely because even partial removal of the facet increases rotational instability.[48]

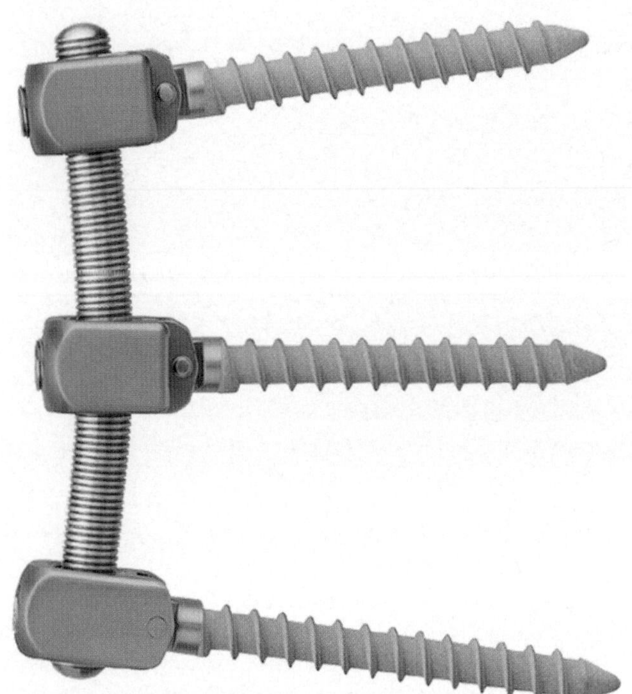

■ **FIGURE 64–10.** Cosmic screws and rod.

Other nonfusion techniques that are not based on pedicle screws stabilize the motion segment by spreading the processus spinosus vertebrarum and thereby also expand the spinal canal. The indications are limited to minimal spinal stenosis. Interspinous spreaders can be implanted with minimal invasion.

## SUMMARY

In contrast to the above-mentioned posterior nonfusion systems, Cosmic is used for symptomatic spinal stenosis, in combination with decompressions, as well as in the case of purely discogenic or facet joint-related pain. The hinged screw provides for a sufficient degree of dynamization and load sharing between the implant and the vertebral column and minimizes any rotation and translation instability. The rotation stability corresponds to that shown by an intact lumbar vertebral column.[19]

Because nonfusion implants act like stability prostheses and must last permanently without the protection of a fusion, the Cosmic screw was additionally coated with Bonit in order to ensure a better anchoring in the vertebral bone.[17] When compared with conventional fusions, the clinical results found so far are equally good. Careful tiner-muscular (between musculus multifidus and musculus longissimus) access to the pedicles may further decrease the operation trauma.

Even when using Cosmic, a careful selection of patients is necessary for clinical success.

The radiologic implant-related complications are in the lower range of those specified in the literature with regard to rigid implants in combination with a fusion. Here, between 2.5% and 15% screw fractures were reported.[49,50]

In those cases in which a patient again develops pain after experiencing a temporary relief from symptoms and in which an implant-related complication can be radiologically detected, the revision is recommended in all cases. In principle, when using a nonfusion implant system, there is the option to carry out a conventional fusion in addition to the replacement of implants. The results found so far with the Cosmic system are very encouraging. However, additional long-term observations are necessary. For this reason, we will continue our international multicenter study, which began in June, 2004.

## REFERENCES


1. Fujiwara A, Tamai K, Yamato M, et al: The relationship between facet joint osteoarthritis and disc degeneration of the lumbar spine: An MRI study. Eur Spine J 8:396–401, 1999.
2. Fujiwara A, Lim T-H, An HS, et al: The effect of disc degeneration and facet joint osteoarthritis on the segmental flexibility of the lumbar spine. Spine 25:3036–3044, 2000.
3. Krismer M, Haid C, Behensky H, et al: Motion in lumbar functional spine units during side bending and axial rotation moments depending on the degree of degeneration. Spine 25:2020–2027, 2000.
4. Tanaka N, An HS, Lim TH, et al: The relationship between disc degeneration and flexibility of the lumbar spine. Spine J 1:47–56, 2001.
5. Rauschning W: Pathoanatomy of lumbar disc degeneration and stenosis. Acta Orthop Scand Suppl 251:3–12, 1993.

6. Peng B, Wu W, Hou S, et al: The pathogenesis of discogenic low back pain. J Bone Joint Surg Br 87:62–67, 2005.
7. Panjabi MM: Clinical spinal instability and low back pain. J Electromyogr Kinesiol 13:371–379, 2003.
8. Fritzell P, Hagg O, Nordwall A: Complications in lumbar fusion surgery for chronic low back pain: Comparison of three surgical techniques used in a prospective randomized study: A report from the Swedish Lumbar Spine Study Group. Eur Spine J 12:178–189, 2003.
9. Ghiselli G, Wang JC, Bhatia NN, et al: Adjacent segment degeneration in the lumbar spine. J Bone Joint Surg Am 86-A:1497–1503, 2004.
10. Park P, Garton HJ, Gala VC, et al: Adjacent segment disease after lumbar or lumbosacral fusion: Review of the literature. Spine 29:1938–1944, 2004.
11. Chosa E, Goto K, Totoribe K, Tajima N: Analysis of the effect of lumbar spine fusion on the superior adjacent intervertebral disk in the presence of disk degeneration, using the three-dimensional finite element method. J Spinal Disord Tech 17:134–139, 2004.
12. Brantigan JW, Neidre A, Toohey JS: The lumbar I/F cage for posterior lumbar interbody fusion with the variable screw placement system: 10-year results of a Food and Drug Administration clinical trial. Spine J 4:681–688, 2004.
13. Rahm MD, Hall BB: Adjacent-segment degeneration after lumbar fusion with instrumentation: A retrospective study. J Spinal Disord 9:392–400, 1996.
14. Helenius I, Remes V, Yrjonen T, et al: Comparison of long-term functional and radiologic outcomes after Harrington instrumentation and spondylodesis in adolescent idiopathic scoliosis: A review of 78 patients. Spine 27:176–180, 2002.
15. Guyer RD, Ohnmeiss DD: Lumbar discography: Position statement from the North American Spine Society Diagnostic and Therapeutic Committee. Spine 20:2048–2059, 1995.
16. Lacefield WR: Current status of ceramic coating for dental implants. Implant Dentistry 7:315–318, 1998.
17. Sanden B, Olerud C, Petren-Mallmin M, Larsson S: Hydroxyapatite coating improves fixation of pedicle screws: A clinical study. J Bone Joint Surg Br 84:387–391, 2002.
18. Goel VK, Konz RJ, Chang HT, et al: Hinged-dynamic posterior device permits greater loads on the graft and similar stability as compared with its equivalent rigid device. JPO 13:17–22, 2001.
19. Scifert JL, Sairyo K, Goel VK, et al: Stability analysis of an enhanced load sharing posterior fixation device and its equivalent conventional device in a calf spine model. Spine 24:2206–2213, 1999.
20. Ettinger C: Test report No. 27.011019.30.95, Endolab Mechanical Engineering. Rosenheim, Germany, 02.15.2002: 1–7.
21. Aota Y, Kumano K, Hirabayashi S: Postfusion instability at the adjacent segments after rigid pedicle screw fixation for degenerative lumbar spinal disorders. J Spinal Disord 8:464–473, 1995.
22. Esses SI, Doherty BJ, Crawford MJ, Dreyzin V: Kinematic evaluation of lumbar fusion techniques. Spine 21:676–684, 1996.
23. Kumar MN, Jacquot F, Hall H: Long-term follow-up of functional outcomes and radiographic changes at adjacent levels following lumbar spine fusion for degenerative disc disease. Eur Spine J 10:309–313, 2001.
24. Gillet P: The fate of the adjacent motion segments after lumbar fusion. J Spinal Disord Tech 16:338–345, 2003.
25. Etebar S, Cahill DW: Risk factors for adjacent-segment failure following lumbar fixation with rigid instrumentation for degenerative instability. J Neurosurg 90:163–169, 1999.
26. Eck JC, Humphreys SC, Hodges SD. Adjacent-segment degeneration after lumbar fusion: A review of clinical, biomechanical, and radiologic studies. Am J Orthop 28:336–340, 1999.
27. Chou WY, Hsu CJ, Chang WN, Wong CY: Adjacent segment degeneration after lumbar spinal posterolateral fusion with instrumentation in elderly patients. Arch Orthop Trauma Surg 122:39–43, 2002.
28. Booth KC, Bridwell KH, Eisenberg BA, et al: Minimum 5-year results of degenerative spondylolisthesis treated with decompression and instrumented posterior fusion. Spine 24:1721–1727, 1999.
29. Axelsson P, Johnsson R, Stromqvist B: The spondylolytic vertebra and its adjacent segment: Mobility measured before and after posterolateral fusion. Spine 22:414–417, 1997.
30. Sudo H, Oda I, Abumi K, et al: In vitro biomechanical effects of reconstruction on adjacent motion segment: Comparison of aligned/kyphotic posterolateral fusion with aligned posterior lumbar interbody fusion/posterolateral fusion. J Neurosurg 99:221–228, 2003.
31. Okuda S, Iwasaki M, Miyauchi A, et al: Risk factors for adjacent segment degeneration after PLIF. Spine 29:1535–1540, 2004.
32. Hilibrand AS, Robbins M: Adjacent segment degeneration and adjacent segment disease: the consequences of spinal fusion? Spine J 4:190S–1904S, 2004.
33. Wenger M, Sapio N, Markwalder TM: Long-term outcome in 132 consecutive patients after posterior internal fixation and fusion for Grade I and II isthmic spondylolisthesis. J Neurosurg Spine 2:289–297, 2005.
34. Lai PL, Chen LH, Niu CC, Chen WJ: Effect of postoperative lumbar sagittal alignment on the development of adjacent instability. J Spinal Disord Tech 17:353–357, 2004.
35. Bohnen IM, Schaafsma J, Tonino AJ: Results and complications after posterior lumbar spondylodesis with the "Variable Screw Placement Spinal Fixation System." Acta Orthop Belg 63:67–73, 1997.
36. Tunturi T, Kataja M, Keski-Nisula L, et al: Posterior fusion of the lumbosacral spine: Evaluation of the operative results and the factors influencing them. Acta Orthop Scand; 50:415–425, 1979.
37. Fritzell P: Fusion as treatment for chronic low back pain—existing evidence, the scientific frontier and research strategies. Eur Spine J 14:519–520, 2005.
38. Huang RC, Wright TM, Panjabi MM, Lipman JD: Biomechanics of nonfusion implants. Orthop Clin North Am 36:271–280, 2005.
39. Sengupta DK, Mulholland RC: Fulcrum assisted soft stabilization system: A new concept in the surgical treatment of degenerative low back pain. Spine 30:1019–1029, 2005.
40. Kanayama M, Hashimoto T, Shigenobu K, et al: Adjacent-segment morbidity after Graf ligamentoplasty compared with posterolateral lumbar fusion. J Neurosurg 95:5–10, 2001.
41. Kanayama M, Hashimoto T, Shigenobu K: Rationale, biomechanics, and surgical indications for graf ligamentoplasty. Orthop Clin North Am 36:373–377, 2005.
42. Kanayama M, Hashimoto T, Shigenobu K, et al: Non-fusion surgery for degenerative spondylolisthesis using artificial ligament stabilization: Surgical indication and clinical results. Spine 30:588–592, 2005.
43. Brechbuhler D, Markwalder TM, Braun M: Surgical results after soft system stabilization of the lumbar spine in degenerative disc disease—long-term results. Acta Neurochir (Wien) 140:521–525, 1998.
44. Schwarzenbach O, Berlemann U, Stoll TM, Dubois G: Posterior Dynamic Stabilization Systems: DYNESYS. Orthop Clin North Am 36:363–372, 2005.
45. Schmoelz W, Huber JF, Nydegger T, et al: Dynamic stabilization of the lumbar spine and its effects on adjacent segments: An in vitro experiment. J Spinal Disord Tech 16:418–423, 2003.
46. Putzier M, Schneider SV, Funk J, Perka C: Application of a dynamic pedicle screw system (DYNESYS) for lumbar segmental degenerations—comparison of clinical and radiological results for different indications. Z Orthop Ihre Grenzgeb 142:166–173, 2004.
47. Stoll TM, Dubois G, Schwarzenbach O: The dynamic neutralization system for the spine: A multi-center study of a novel non-fusion system. Eur Spine J 11(2):S170–S178, 2002.
48. Zander T, Rohlmann A, Klockner C, Bergmann G: Influence of graded facetectomy and laminectomy on spinal biomechanics. Eur Spine J 12:427–434, 2003.
49. McAfee PC, Weiland DJ, Carlow JJ: Survivorship analysis of pedicle spinal instrumentation. Spine 16:S422–S427, 1991.
50. Marchesi DG, Thalgott JS, Aebi M: Application and results of the AO internal fixation system in nontraumatic indications. Spine 16: S162–S169, 1991.

CHAPTER **65**

# Innovative Spinal Technologies Dynamic Stabilization Device

**Dennis Colleran**

## KEY POINTS

- Back pain may be due to irregular load distribution, not to instability alone. Must off-load disc throughout entire range of motion (ROM), not just extension.
- Adjacent-level disease (ALD) may be minimized with proper motion preservation. Pedicle-to-pedicle distance changes are important to normal spinal motion, and optimal dynamic stabilization systems should allow large motions.
- Proper motion is needed for implant longevity. Incorrect or limited motion can lead to early failure, including implant loosening or breakage, subsidence, or failure to maintain mobility.
- Minimally invasive surgery benefits are more important in motion-preserving techniques.
- Dynamic stabilization devices must be dynamic by allowing certain motions and also stabilize by controlling or limiting other motions.

## INTRODUCTION

Many dynamic stabilization devices have been developed or are in the process of being developed with the promise of delivering a better clinical outcome when compared with fusion. The goal of any dynamic stabilization system is to restore normal loading to reduce pain, to allow normal motion, to prevent further degeneration at the adjacent levels, to maintain the function of the surrounding anatomy by minimizing collateral damage to all adjacent tissues, and to provide a simple revision strategy. Early dynamic stabilization devices may have addressed some, but not all, of these goals.

The goals of any back surgery are to relieve pain and restore normal function. Pain may be associated with spondylolisthesis, stenosis, mechanical back pain due to disc degeneration, or facet degeneration, or the pain may originate from ligaments, tendons, or muscles. Complex loading patterns on the degenerated discs are a likely a source of mechanical back pain due to disc focal loading on the sensory nerves of the vertebral end plates, disc shear stress concentrations causing a response by the nociceptors in the annulus, or buckling of the disc annulus causing the lamellae to be torn apart.[1] Alternatively, pain may generate from a narrowing foramen, causing nerve root compression. Posterior stabilization systems may provide benefit by restoring foraminal space or balancing disc loading to reduce pain without the loss of movement by creating a more normal loading pattern.[2]

The surgical technique and spine implant system must be designed to minimize the incidence of recurrence at the operative level and to minimize the acceleration of degeneration at the adjacent levels seen in fusion in order to provide long-term pain relief. It is theorized that reduced motion at the operative level causes increased motion and stress at the adjacent levels, leading to degeneration.[3] Postoperative studies of total disc replacement show no evidence of adjacent-level disease when the operative level has greater than five degrees of motion yet demonstrate a 24% incidence rate of adjacent-level disease in patients who have less than five degrees of motion at the operative level.[4] A dynamic stabilization system should allow for these normal motions ($\geq$5 degrees) at the operative level to minimize the stresses and degeneration at the adjacent levels.

## INDICATIONS/CONTRAINDICATIONS

As with all spinal implant systems, indications for posterior dynamic stabilization devices are based on their design and biomechanical effects. The Innovative Spinal Technologies (IST; Mansfield, MA) Dynamic Stabilization device addresses instabilities of all kinds, including excessive or pathologic motion, and addresses low back pain as well as neurogenic pain. The device can be used as an adjunct to fusion in the treatment of acute and chronic instabilities or deformities of the thoracic, lumbar, and sacral spine. The IST Dynamic Stabilization device will treat grade 0 or 1 degenerative spondylolisthesis with objective evidence of neurologic impairment. The IST Dynamic Stabilization device will treat lateral, central, and midsagittal stenosis as well as discogenic back pain with disc degeneration, facet joint degeneration, and loss of disc height of at least 2 mL. The IST Dynamic Stabilization device can be used at a single level or two contiguous levels.

## DESCRIPTION OF THE DEVICE

Dynamic stabilization solutions can be segmented into three categories: facet replacement, nucleus replacement, and posterior dynamic stabilization. Posterior dynamic stabilization can be further segmented into interspinous process spacers, partial motion, and full motion pedicle screw–based dynamic stabilization systems. Figure 65–1 shows the dynamic stabilization market segmentation.

Each posterior dynamic stabilization subsegment has advantages and disadvantages in terms of procedure, cost, reliability, clinical outcome, and ease of revision. Although interspinous spacers are less complex and can be implanted with a relatively simple surgical technique, they are generally indicated for radicular pain from nerve root compression and neurogenic claudication caused by stenosis. Insertion of an interspinous spacer with or without decompression may provide good results in this limited indication, but these interspinous devices do not offer the more broad functionality of the pedicle screw–based dynamic stabilization systems, which also aim to relieve mechanical back pain.

To relieve mechanical back pain, pedicle screw–based posterior dynamic stabilization devices should provide a more normal load distribution to the disc and through the vertebral end plate. McNally[1] and Sengupta[5] present the theory that nonuniform distribution of load within the degenerated nucleus and annulus causes localized anisotropic concentrations of stress leading to possible pain in the vertebral end plates that contain pain-sensitive nerve endings. Insertion of a posterior load-sharing dynamic stabilization system could supplement this loading on the nucleus, annulus, and vertebral end plates, thus reducing the localized high-contact stresses.

These systems must provide for natural and controlled motion at the operative level to minimize compensatory increased motion and stress at the adjacent levels to prevent accelerated degeneration at those levels. Huang and colleagues[3] show the effect of fusion increasing intradiscal pressures, and end plate and annular stresses at the adjacent levels. Controlled motion allows all biomechanically normal motions, flexion-extension, lateral bend, and axial rotation, while resisting abnormal motions like anteroposterior (AP) shear and overcompression of the disc or facets.

To determine normal extent of motion of a pedicle screw–based system, Cunningham and colleagues[6] studied the range of motion (ROM) between adjacent pedicles of preoperative total disc patients at the operative and adjacent levels, as shown in Figure 65–2. Although the average change in pedicle-to-pedicle distance throughout the ROM was between 2 and 3 mm, many patients realized greater motion and as much as 8 mm to 9 mm change in distance between pedicles during the flexion-extension cycle as shown in Figure 65–3.

To minimize the bone-to-implant interface stresses and the incidence of pedicle screw loosening, any pedicle screw–based dynamic stabilization system must allow the pedicle screws to follow a natural motion about the kinematic center of rotation. The dynamic rod connecting the pedicle screws must allow for both change in length and change in relative angulation between the pedicle screws, as shown in Figure 65–4.

Similarly, this normal motion must also be allowed in lateral bending and axial rotation. It is important for the posterior dynamic stabilization device to allow this motion, not only to minimize implant-bone interface stresses at the operative level but also to minimize increased compensatory motion and elevated stress at the adjacent levels.

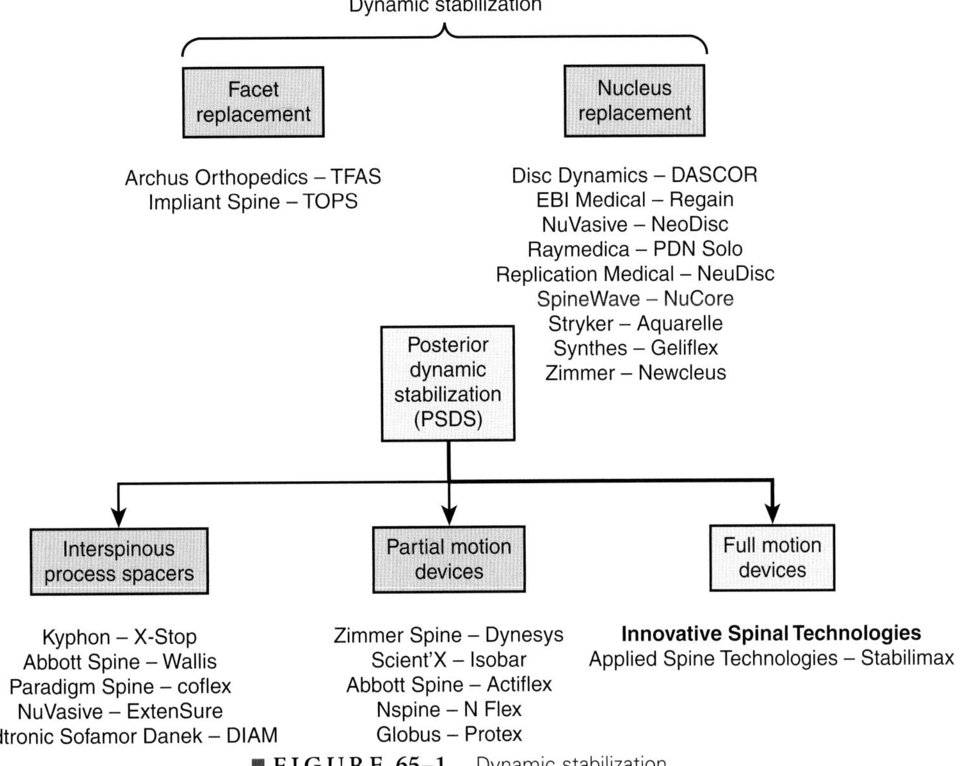


■ **FIGURE 65–1.** Dynamic stabilization.

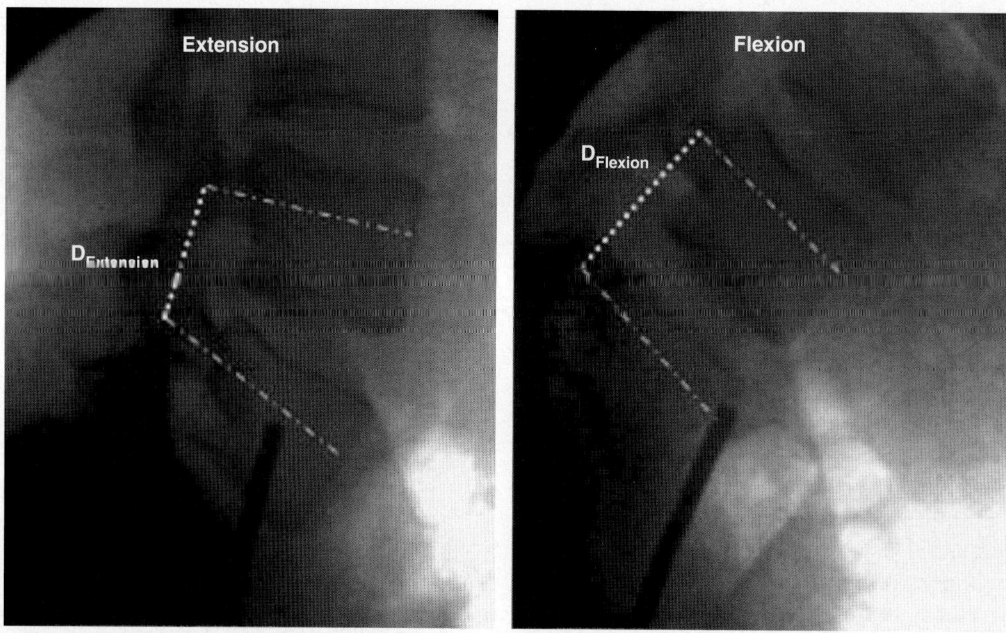


■ **FIGURE 65–2.** Pedicle-to-pedicle measurements in extension and flexion.

Although the Paramount MM DS (Innovative Spinal Technologies, Mansfield, MA) device allows natural motion in flexion-extension, lateral bending and axial rotation, it resists AP translation (shown as the "Z" axis in Fig. 65–5) and also off-loads the compressive loads on the disc (shown as the "Y" axis on Fig. 65–5).

The IST Dynamic Stabilization product line has two levels of implant. The IST Paramount MM (Fig. 65–6) is used for micromotion similar to many of the current pedicle screw–based dynamic stabilization systems. The IST DS FM (Fig. 65–7) is used when greater motions are desired. The IST Dynamic Stabilization device uses curved telescoping cobalt chrome metal-on-metal links on the IST Paramount MM and a pair of spherical cobalt chrome linkages on the IST DS FM Device to allow rotations about a spherical center of rotation while resisting translation. Polymer and elastomeric flexion and extension limiters are used to control the extent of the ROM. These dynamic rods are mounted onto typical titanium pedicle screws similar to a fusion system using a minimally invasive technique. It is well recognized that minimally invasive surgery has many benefits: preserving ligaments, muscle, and bony anatomy; reducing recovery time, and providing less scarring. These benefits may be much more advantageous with motion-sparing devices than with fusion techniques in long-term results.[7]

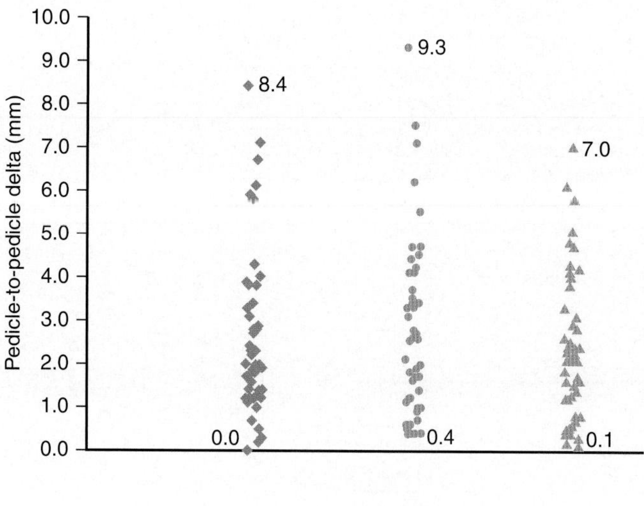


■ **FIGURE 65–3.** Change in pedicle-to-pedicle distance throughout range of motion.

Dynamic stabilization devices may address earlier stage degeneration and a broader patient population, increasing the need for long-term reliability and, in some cases, revisability. These devices may need to be adjusted, revised to a fusion, or possibly removed. The device should maximize future options by minimizing collateral damage to adjacent anatomic structures.

## BACKGROUND OF SCIENTIFIC TESTING/CLINICAL OUTCOMES

Motion-preserving devices may be used in younger patients and thus require a substantial amount of evaluation to ensure that they can both provide the added functionality over fusion devices and also perform long term. Although fusion devices may be loaded for only 6 months, a motion-preserving implant may need to function for 20, 30, or even 40 years. For this reason, there is a significant amount of mechanical testing on any dynamic stabilization device, including strength, wear, kinematic, biocompatibility, and functional nonhuman testing. Although the American Society for Testing and Materials (ASTM) is currently developing methods to test new motion-preserving devices, no standards currently exist for these systems. It should be noted that there is a wide variety of designs under development and that no one test will fit all devices.

The implant mechanical strength was determined using an in vitro static and fatigue corpectomy model per the ASTM standard

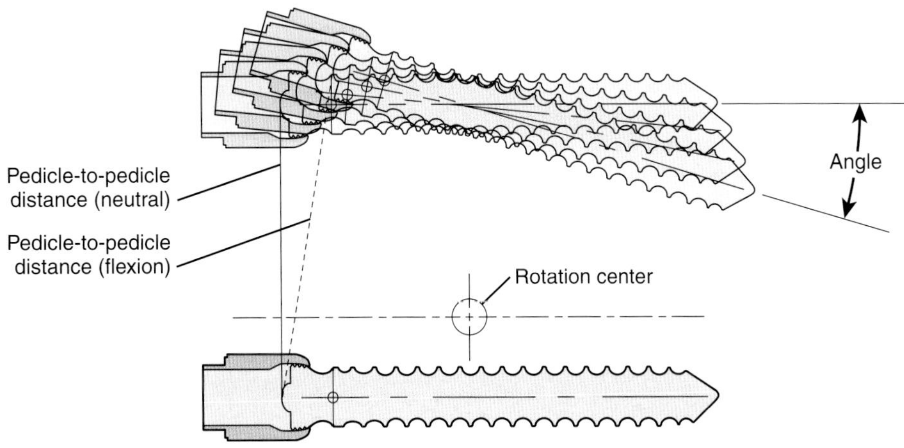


■ **FIGURE 65–4.** Pedicle screw kinematics.

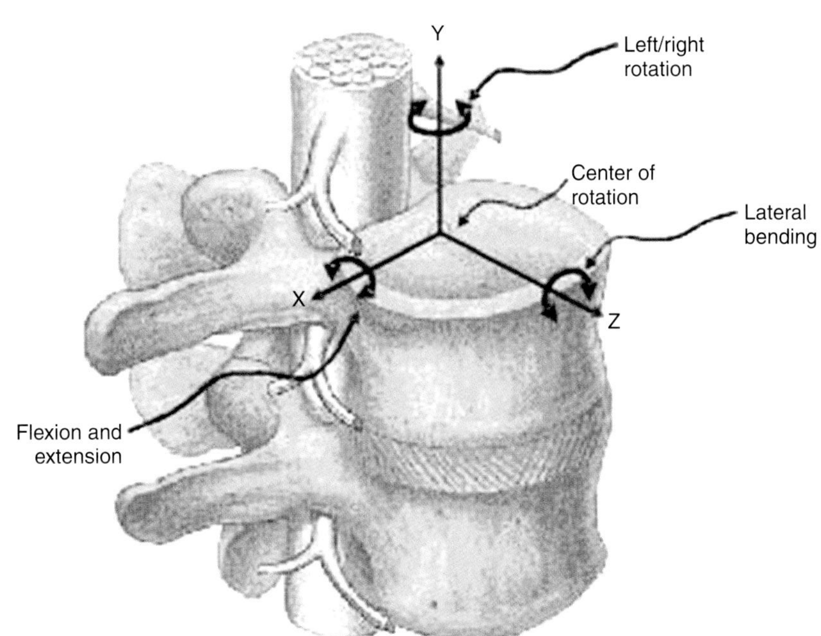


■ **FIGURE 65–5.** Allowed motions in dynamic stabilization.

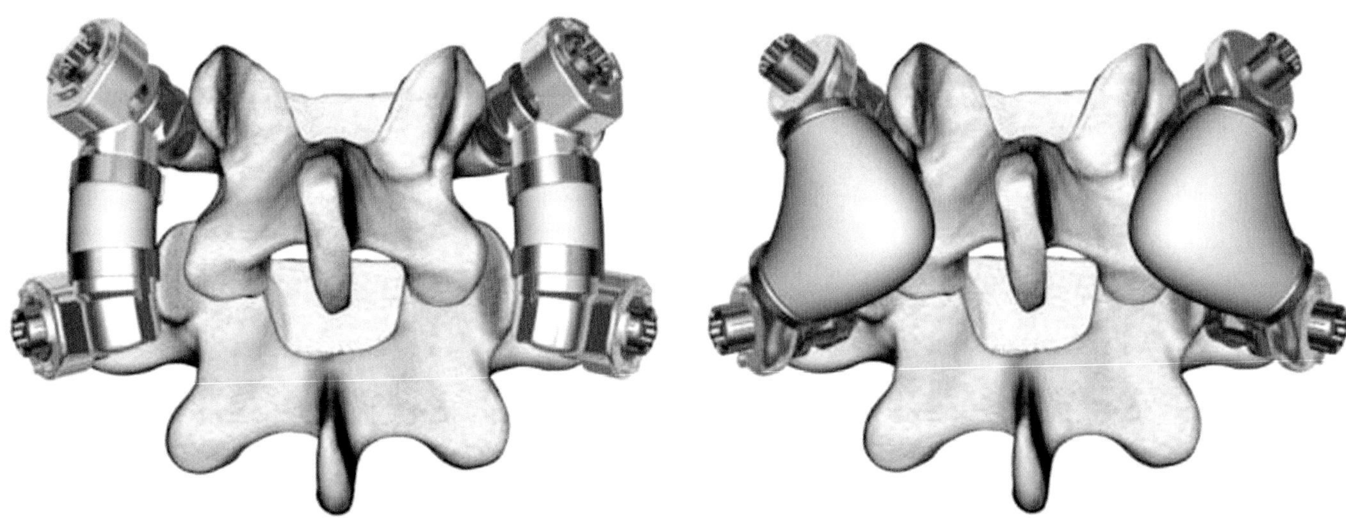

■ **FIGURE 65–6.** IST Paramount MM.

■ **FIGURE 65–7.** IST DS FM.

F1717. This model tested the ability of the implant construct to handle physiologic loads in compression and torsion similar to standard fusion systems. This test will verify the ability of the dynamic stabilization device to off-load the disc. During development, finite element analysis was used to evaluate interim designs and determine optimal component geometry.

Wear characteristics were tested about multiple axes of motion, including flexion-extension, lateral bending, and rotation, out to 10 million cycles per the ASTM Draft for Extradiscal Nonfusion devices.

Kinematics were tested using an in vitro human cadaveric model. Multidirectional flexibility properties were quantified for flexion-extension, lateral bending, and rotation at both operative and adjacent levels. This kinematic testing determined the ability of the dynamic stabilization system to attain normal motions under physiologic loading conditions. Adjacent-level kinematics were also studied to ensure that stresses due to the implant design were minimized.

Nonhuman primate (baboon) and nonprimate (sheep) models may be used to evaluate the effects of tissue ingrowth histologically and the mechanical effect of any ingrowth, to study the effects of axial loading in vivo and ROM after implantation, to look at regional disc effects, and to assess for in-growth.

Other mechanical tests are needed based on specific materials and designs. When polymers and elastomers are used for load-bearing components, a creep study should be completed to analyze the long-term effects of loading. Other additional functionalities should be examined to ensure that the device functions as intended.

Dynamic stabilization device failure can include implant failure, implant loosening, or a failure of the implant to maintain mobility or proper motion. Improper motion due to implant design or surgical placement can either cause loss in optimal ROM or create high implant-bone interface stresses, leading to screw loosening. DS devices will need to function for many years, and the implants will need to withstand long-term cyclic loading without failure of the individual implant components.

## OPERATIVE TECHNIQUE

The patient is placed in a neutral prone position under general anesthesia. The IST dynamic stabilization systems use a minimally invasive technique under fluoroscopic guidance for pedicle targeting using a bone biopsy needle and guide wire placement. The guide wire is then used to tap and insert the pedicle screw. After screw placement is completed, a precise pedicle-to-pedicle distance will be measured in the neutral flexion-extension position. Dynamic rods are then inserted into position attached to the pedicle screw heads; left and right dynamic rods are aligned to each other using a floating alignment jig. Then the alignment jig and both left and right constructs are aligned to the anatomic center of rotation on the posterior aspect of the upper end plate of the lower vertebral body. Once alignment is complete, the orientation is locked down.

### ADVANTAGES/DISADVANTAGES

The IST DS FM device has several potential advantages over current dynamic stabilization devices, including a greater ROM to minimize stress at the adjacent levels, a more natural motion about an anatomic center of rotation to minimize bone-implant interface stresses, ability to off-load the disc uniformly, and easy revision technique. The device will require alignment to the center of rotation.

## CONCLUSIONS/DISCUSSION

There are many varied approaches under development to create the optimal motion-preserving implant. The main goal of these devices should be to relieve pain, restore or maintain motion at the operative level, minimize degeneration at the adjacent levels, and use a surgical technique that minimizes damage to collateral structures to improve outcomes and allow for easy revisions. Also, whereas many of the new motion-preserving designs seem reasonable from a theoretical standpoint, all need to be proven in randomized, controlled studies and long-term follow-up.

## REFERENCES

1. McNally DS, Shackleford IM, Goodship AE, Mulholland RC: In vivo stress measurement can predict pain on discography. Spine 21:2580–2587, 1996.
2. Nockels RP: Dynamic stabilization in the surgical management of painful lumbar spinal disorders. Spine 30:S68–S72, 2005.
3. Huang RC, Wright TM, Panjabi MM, Lipman JD: Biomechanics of nonfusion implants. Orthop Clin North Am 36:271–280, 2005.
4. Huang RC, Girardi FP, Cammisa Jr. FP, et al: Correlation between range of motion and outcome after lumbar total disc replacement 8.6-year follow-up. Spine 30:1407–1411, 2005.
5. Sengupta DK, Herkowitz HN: Nonfusion: The physiologic solution. Nonfusion Techniques for the Spine 28–37, 2006.
6. Cunningham B, Colleran D, et al: Lumbar Spine Kinematics—a Radiographic Assessment of the Change in Interpedicular Distance Throughout the Range of Motion. SAS, 2006.
7. Sengupta DK, Herkowitz HN: Degenerative spondylolisthesis: Review of current trends and controversies. Spine 30:S71–S81, 2005.

CHAPTER 66

# NFlex

**Corey J. Wallach, Andelle L. Teng,** and **Jeffrey C. Wang**

## KEY POINTS

- The NFlex Dynamic Stabilization System allows elongation of the stabilizing construct through flexion while still allowing compression during extension.
- The NFix II Pedicle Screw System exhibited greater static and fatigue strength in compression bending tests than several commercially available rigid pedicle screw systems.
- Cadaveric studies in a bovine model with three-dimensional motion analysis revealed that after decompression, specimens instrumented with NFlex provided motion similar to that of the intact spine.

## INTRODUCTION

NFlex (N Spine Inc., San Diego, CA), a dynamic stabilization device, has been designed in response to several of the concerns with earlier motion preservation devices and aims to more closely emulate the physiologic range of motion of the lumbar spine. The following is a brief review of the proposed design advantages the system incorporates, biomechanical studies of the device, and its early clinical use.

Several "lumbar stabilization" devices are now available and attempt to control or limit specific aspects of lumbar motion. Static lumbar stabilization devices are implants that limit range of motion but are not intrinsically dynamic themselves, such as interspinous spacers and facet screws. Dynamic lumbar stabilization devices aim to mimic desired physiologic movements and load transfers while limiting unwanted motion, specifically shear, within the lumbar spine. Several such devices are currently under investigation and target different regions of the lumbar spine, such as total disc arthroplasty, nucleus replacements, and those that provide stabilization in concert with the posterior spinal structures. It is hoped that these posterior dynamic stabilization systems support the physiologically desired range of motion and load sharing while still limiting pathologic motion within the lumbar motion segment. Several theoretical benefits exist for an implant capable of providing adequate stability and permitting range of motion while still decreasing the load to the facet and intervertebral disc. Relieving pressure at the facet may allow for normalized mobility, as well as mitigating facet-triggered pain. At the intervertebral disc, the reduced load may allow for decreased intradiscal pressure, normalization of disc metabolism, and a decrease in its rate of degeneration. Perhaps most important are the potential benefits to the adjacent levels, in which physiologic load transfer from one motion segment to the next may minimize the accelerated adjacent segment disease frequently seen following arthrodesis.[1]

Although early clinical results from other motion-preserving dynamic stabilization systems[2] have yet to show any clear advantage to traditional decompression and arthrodesis,[3,4] this may reflect certain design flaws in these previously studied systems that may potentially be improved upon. Certainly, the current enthusiasm for motion preserving spinal procedures is widespread, with many new devices being designed in response to the marginal success of earlier dynamic stabilization systems. These new designs attempt to more accurately mimic lumbar range of motion, and it is hoped that these advances will result in improved clinical outcomes.

## DESCRIPTION OF THE DEVICE

Although several devices adequately restrict lumbar extension, reproduction of normal spinal flexion has proved more difficult to emulate. In the unaltered lumbar spine, flexion is necessarily coupled with elongation of the posterior segments; therefore, any device hoping to provide support through physiologic flexion would be required to elongate as well. The NFlex system attempts to incorporate this capacity and allow elongation through its connecting rod during flexion as well as allow compression during extension (Fig. 66–1).

The NFlex system is a semirigid rod composed of titanium, 6.0 mm in diameter, with one end containing a composite titanium and polycarbonate urethane sleeve. The sleeve is positioned over a 3.25-mm titanium core, which contains the spacer by connecting a titanium end cap to the 6-mm titanium rod. The rod may be attached to pedicle screws in the standard fashion, with one pedicle screw attached to the titanium ring of the sleeve and one or more pedicle screws attached to the titanium rod (Fig. 66–2).

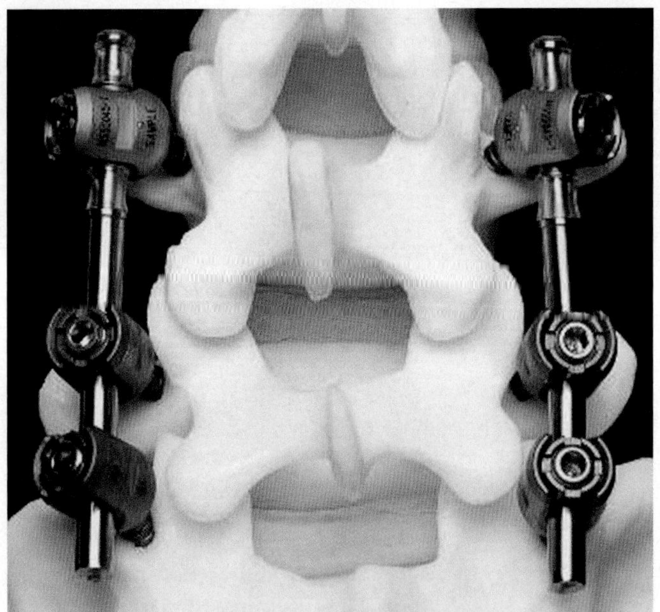

■ **FIGURE 66–1.** The NFlex Dynamic Stabilization System.

As shown in Figure 66–3, the composite sleeve is not bonded to the titanium components of the rod, and compressive loads are borne primarily by this dynamic structure as opposed to the titanium core. Additionally, the titanium core of the NFlex rod provides resistance to translation of one vertebra relative to the adjacent vertebra.

The NFlex is produced in a single configuration (i.e., single elongation and compression stiffness). However, the connecting rod's resistance to compression is decoupled from the resistance to extension because these features are controlled by separate polymer elements on either side of the pedicle screw. The resistance to translation is controlled by the thickness of the polymer between the titanium sleeve and titanium core, which is also independent of the flexion and extension stiffness. Clinically, it may be necessary to bias the stiffness of the device in the direction of one or more motions to treat various indications and pathologies. The independence of resistance in each direction in NFlex will allow for NFlex devices in the future to achieve a more physiologic balance of flexion, extension, and translation motion, once appropriate clinical evidence is available to substantiate a stiffness bias.

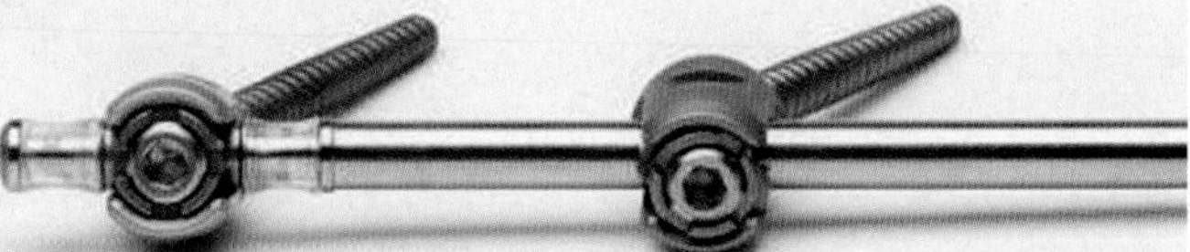

■ **FIGURE 66–2.** The rod may be attached to pedicle screws in the standard fashion, with one pedicle screw attached to the titanium ring of the sleeve and one or more pedicle screws attached to the titanium rod.

## BACKGROUND OF SCIENTIFIC TESTING/CLINICAL OUTCOMES

The NFix II Pedicle Screw System has been tested for static and fatigue durability in three primary modes, compression bending (to simulate bending motion in vivo), axial tension and compression (to simulate worst-case compression of the polymer), and torsion (to simulate axial rotation in vivo). These tests were performed according to the American Society for Testing Materials (ASTM) specification number F1717. In compression

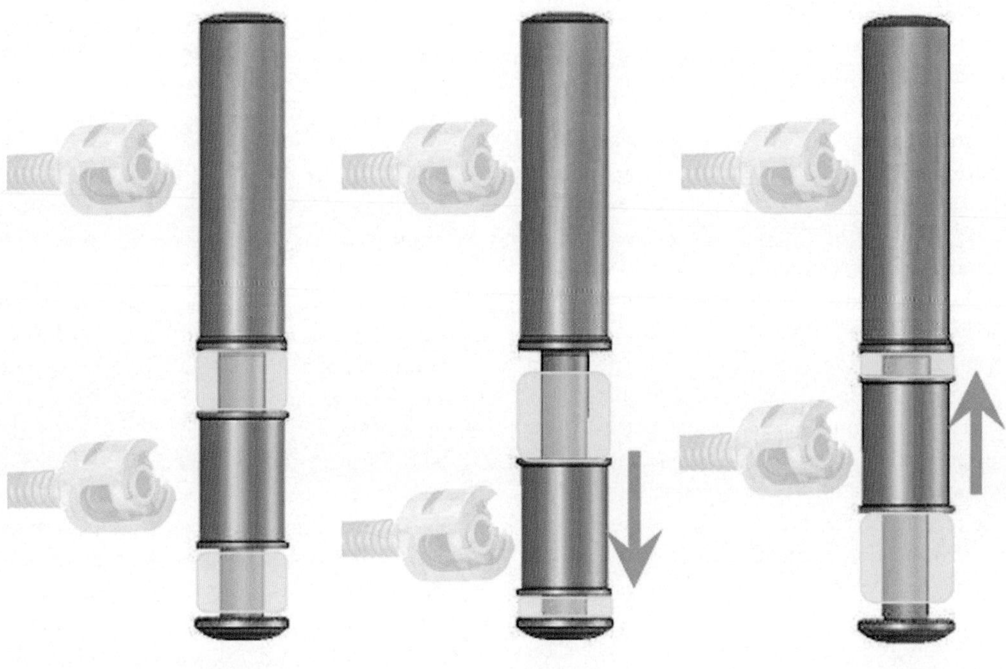


■ **FIGURE 66–3.** The composite titanium and polycarbonate urethane sleeve, which allows compressive loads to be borne primarily by this dynamic structure as opposed to the titanium core.

TABLE 66–1. NFlex ASTM F1717 Static Compression Bending Test Results

| Specimen | 2% Yield Displacement (mm) | Elastic Displacement (mm) | 2% Yield Load (N) | Compressive Stiffness (N/mm) |
|---|---|---|---|---|
| 232804-N-AC1 | 10.58 | 9.41 | 194.50 | 20.67 |
| 232804-N-AC2 | 10.06 | 8.89 | 185.19 | 20.83 |
| 232804-N-AC3 | 10.36 | 9.19 | 192.24 | 20.91 |
| 232804-N-AC4 | 10.73 | 9.56 | 197.94 | 20.70 |
| 232804-N-AC5 | 10.54 | 9.37 | 195.85 | 20.90 |
| 232804-N-AC6 | 10.72 | 9.55 | 200.38 | 20.98 |
| Mean | 10.50 | 9.33 | 194.35 | 20.83 |
| Std. Dev. | 0.254 | 0.254 | 5.290 | 0.125 |

bending, the NFix II Pedicle Screw System was tested for both static and fatigue strength. The data for each test are presented in Tables 66–1 and 66–2. The NFix II Pedicle Screw System exhibited greater static and fatigue strength in compression bending tests than several commercially available rigid pedicle screw systems.

The NFix II Pedicle Screw System was also tested for durability under static and repeated torsional loads. This test employs the same bilateral construct as the ASTM compression bending test but is subjected to a direct torsion load through the cross-pins. The static torsion test results are presented in Table 66–3.

The NFix II Pedicle Screw System allows for axial elongation and compression of the NFix II rod between the pedicle screws. This axial elongation and compression occur in both rods during flexion and extension respectively, as well as alternately in each rod from side to side during lateral bending. The maximum static elongation and compression were tested on individual NFix II rods, and the results are shown in Table 66–4. The NFlex device was also successfully tested 10 million cycles in axial tension and compression of +/−1 mm under physiologic conditions of 37 °C in saline solution. During the first 200,000 cycles of axial fatigue testing, the composite sleeve exhibits approximately 25% stress relaxation before reaching a steady-state level of resistance. This behavior, shown graphically in Figure 66–4, is similar to stress relaxation observed in other devices fabricated from polycarbonate urethane.[5]

Although no results from clinical trials are available for analysis, in vitro studies have been performed to characterize the stability provided by this system. Cadaveric studies in a bovine model with three-dimensional motion analysis revealed that after decompression, specimens instrumented with NFlex provided motion similar to that of the intact spine (Table 66–5). Rigid fixation, however, significantly limited motion.[6]

TABLE 66–2. NFlex ASTM F1717 Compression Bending Fatigue Test Results

| Specimen ID | Max. Compressive Load (N) | Nf Cycles | Remarks |
|---|---|---|---|
| Compression-A-FO6 | 160 | 5,000,000 | Run out |
| Compression-A-FO3 | 130 | 10,000,000 | Run out |
| Compression-A-FO7 | 130 | 10,000,000 | Run out |
| Compression-A-FO1 | 110 | 6,398,747 | Run out |
| Compression-A-FO2 | 110 | 5,000,000 | Run out |

## CLINICAL PRESENTATION AND EVALUATION

The NFlex device has been in use clinically since the fall of 2006. No clinical data are yet available for this device; however, several applications of the device are being evaluated. The images in Figures 66–5 to 66–8 illustrate various ways in which the NFlex device may be applied clinically. Figure 66–5 is a single-level application of the device for discogenic back pain. Figure 66–6 is a two-level application of the device for grade 1 degenerative spondylolisthesis in which L4-L5 has been fused and L5-S1 has been treated with the dynamic portion of the device. In Figure 66–7, a patient with degenerative spondylolisthesis has been fused at L4-L5 and treated dynamically at L3-L4. Last, Figure 66–8 shows a two-level application of NFlex in revision of a previous three-level fusion that was operated on for pain due to adjacent level degeneration.

TABLE 66–3. NFlex ASTM F1717 Static Torsional Test Results

| Specimen | 2% Yield Angle Displacement (degrees) | Elastic Angle Displacement (degrees) | 2% Yield Torque (N-m) | Torsional Stiffness (n-m/degrees) |
|---|---|---|---|---|
| 232804-N-TR1 | 5.50 | 4.00 | 12.79 | 3.20 |
| 232804-N-TR2 | 6.85 | 5.35 | 11.86 | 2.22 |
| 232804-N-TR3 | 5.94 | 4.44 | 11.04 | 2.48 |
| 232804-N-TR4 | 5.71 | 4.21 | 12.25 | 2.91 |
| 232804-N-TR5 | 7.13 | 5.64 | 12.88 | 2.29 |
| 232804-N-TR6 | 6.49 | 4.99 | 12.19 | 2.44 |
| Mean | 6.27 | 4.77 | 12.17 | 2.59 |
| Std. Dev. | 0.655 | 0.655 | 0.674 | 0.383 |

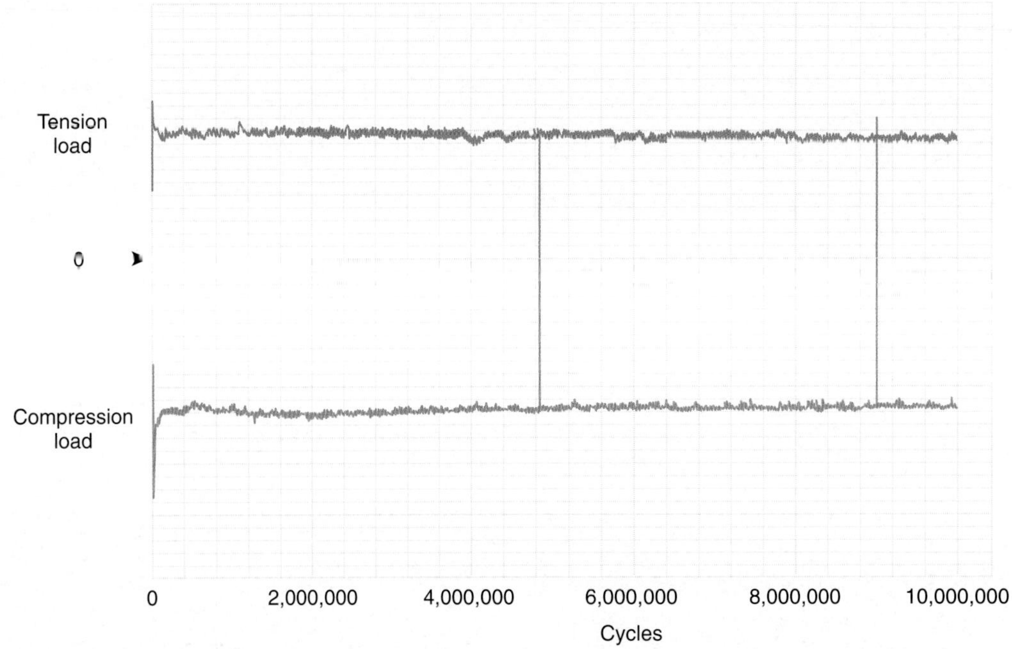


■ **FIGURE 66–4.** NFlex modified ASTM F1717 tension and compression fatigue results.

**ADVANTAGES/DISADVANTAGES: NFLEX**

**Advantages**

- The device was designed to emulate physiologic range of motion, with elongation of construct through flexion and compression during extension.

**Disadvantages**

- At present, there is no clinical outcome data to assess benefits of this system.

**TABLE 66–4. NFlex Modified ASTM F1717 Static Tension and Compression Test Results**

| Specimen | Peak Load (N) | Disp at Peak Load (mm) |
|---|---|---|
| 266609-AC2 | 908.19 | 5.52 |
| 266609-AC3 | 807.38 | 5.58 |
| 266609-AC4 | 910.51 | 5 |
| Mean | 875.36 | 5.37 |
| Std Dev. | 58.881 | 0.317 |

## CONCLUSIONS/DISCUSSION

Clearly, prospective randomized clinical trials need to be undertaken to objectively identify any sustained benefit from dynamic stabilization and to clarify its role in the treatment of patients with various degenerative lumbar conditions. Despite the success of traditional decompression and arthrodesis,[3,4,7] the morbidity associated with iliac crest graft harvesting,[8] the variable potency of demineralized bone graft products,[9] and the legitimate concerns of adjacent-segment disease,[10,11] make the theoretical benefits of dynamic stabilization appealing. If these dynamic systems can in fact reliably improve patient outcomes, prevent progressive instability, and minimize adjacent-segment disease, the current enthusiasm for these technologies will be more than warranted.

**TABLE 66–5. NFlex Bovine Cadaver Range-of-Motion Test Results**

| | | Intact | Decompression | NFlex | Inverted | Solid Rod |
|---|---|---|---|---|---|---|
| FXL | Average | 3.3 | 5.14 | 2.71 | 2.63 | 1.26 |
| | Std. Dev. | 1.05 | 1.29 | 1.01 | 1.04 | 0.16 |
| EXT | Average | 3.45 | 4.37 | 1.88 | 1.68 | 1.14 |
| | Std. Dev. | 0.88 | 1.16 | 0.53 | 0.45 | 0.28 |
| LB | Average | 6.22 | 5.99 | 4.82 | 4.31 | 2.56 |
| | Std. Dev. | 2.54 | 2.24 | 1.4 | 1.23 | 0.55 |
| AR | Average | 1.91 | 1.93 | 1.19 | 1.55 | 1.15 |
| | Std. Dev. | 1.62 | 0.62 | 0.24 | 0.83 | 0.31 |

AR, axial rotation; EXT, extension; FXL, flexion; LB, lateral bend.

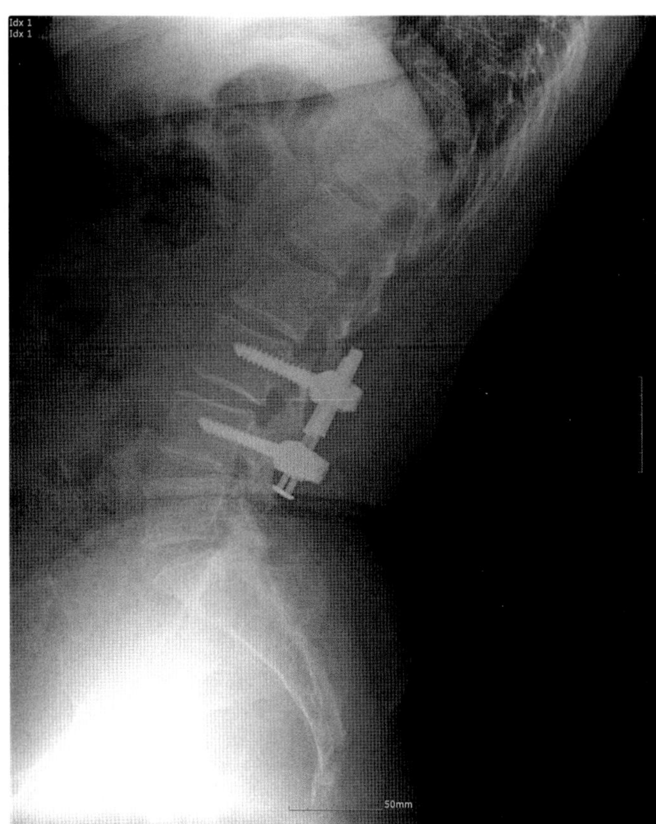


■ **FIGURE 66–5.** Single-level NFlex device at L3-L4. *(Courtesy of Tae-Ahn Jahng, MD, Seoul, Korea.)*

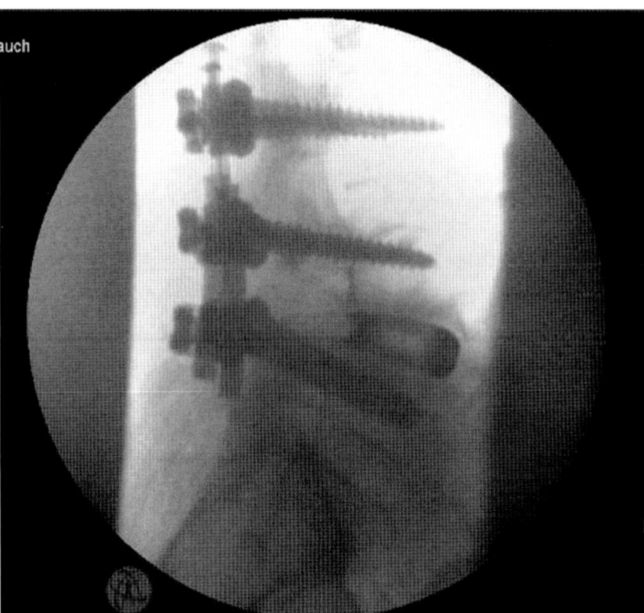

■ **FIGURE 66–7.** NFlex two-level device with dynamic section cephalad to L4-L5 fusion. *(Courtesy of H. Jörg Meisel, MD, and Mark Schnöring, MD, Halle, Germany.)*

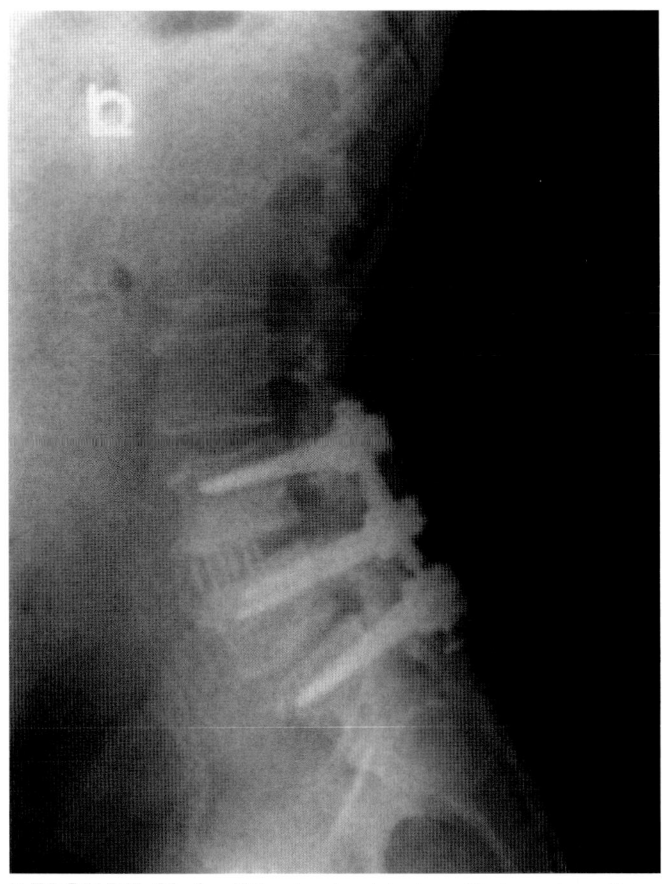

■ **FIGURE 66–6.** NFlex two-level device with dynamic section caudal to L4-L5 fusion. *(Courtesy of Jeffrey D. Coe, MD, Los Gatos, CA.)*

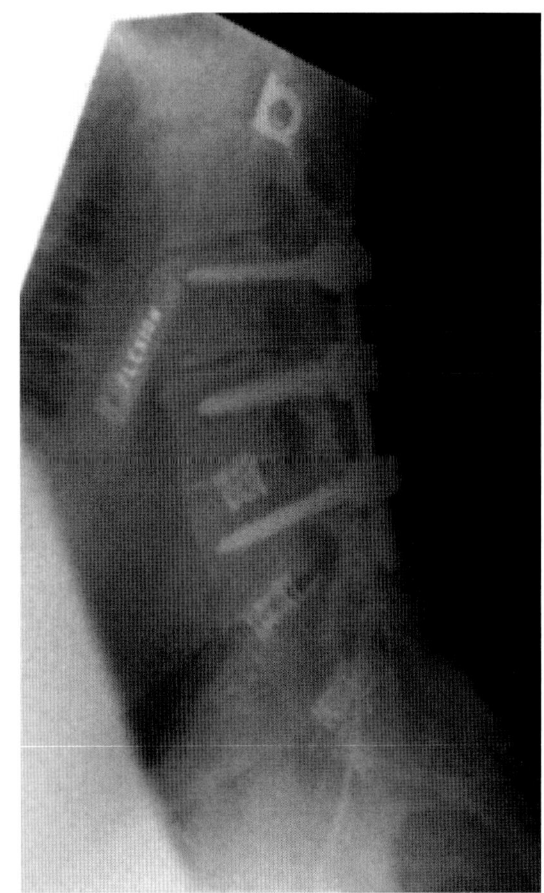

■ **FIGURE 66–8.** NFlex two-level device adjacent to a previous fusion. *(Courtesy of Jeffrey D. Coe, MD, Los Gatos, CA.)*

## REFERENCES


1. Aota Y, Kumano K, Hirabayashi S: Postfusion instability at the adjacent segments after rigid pedicle screw fixation for degenerative lumbar spinal disorders. J Spinal Disord 8:464–473, 1995.
2. Grob D, Benini A, Junge A, Mannion AF: Clinical experience with the Dynesys semirigid fixation system for the lumbar spine: Surgical and patient-oriented outcome in 50 cases after an average of 2 years. Spine 30:324–331, 2005.
3. Herkowitz HN, Kurz LT: Degenerative lumbar spondylolisthesis with spinal stenosis: A prospective study comparing decompression with decompression and intertransverse process arthrodesis. J Bone Joint Surg Am 73:802–808, 1991.
4. Kornblum MB, Fischgrund JS, Herkowitz HN, et al: Degenerative lumbar spondylolisthesis with spinal stenosis: A prospective long-term study comparing fusion and pseudarthrosis. Spine 29:726–733; discussion 733–734, 2004.
5. Maxwell JH, Griffith SL, Welch WC: *In* Welch WC (ed): Nonfusion Techniques for the Spine: Motion Preservation and Balance. St. Louis, Quality Medical Publishers, 2006.
6. Lim TH, HKS, Keller L, et al: Biomechanical Evaluation of Dynamic Fixation Device: NFlex. Spine Arthroplasty Society Annual Meeting, Montreal, Canada, 2006.
7. Zdeblick TA: A prospective, randomized study of lumbar fusion: Preliminary results. Spine 18:983–991, 1993.
8. Younger EM, Chapman MW: Morbidity at bone graft donor sites. J Orthop Trauma 3:192–195, 1989.
9. Bae HW, Zhao L, Kanim LE, et al: Intervariability and intravariability of bone morphogenetic proteins in commercially available demineralized bone matrix products. Spine 31:1299–1306; discussion 1307–1308, 2006.
10. Lee CK, Langrana NA: Lumbosacral spinal fusion: A biomechanical study. Spine 9:574–581, 1984.
11. Lee CK: Accelerated degeneration of the segment adjacent to a lumbar fusion. Spine 13:375–377, 1988.

CHAPTER 67

# The PercuDyn System

**Juan M. Dipp, Ricardo Flores,** and **German Rodríguez**

**KEY POINTS**

- Posterior extension-limiting device that is pedicle screw–based; facet-blocking mechanism is employed.
- At present, the device is being evaluated for the treatment of low back pain secondary to lumbar degenerative disc disease.
- The device can be used from L1 to S1.
- Percutaneous or open implantation is possible.

## INTRODUCTION

Low back pain (LBP) is an ever-present problem that affects more than 60% of the general population at least once in a lifetime, with a lower percentage evolving into chronicity.[1] This problem has a significant social and economic impact due to incapacitating pain and sometimes long treatment periods, as well as extended absence from work.[2,3]

A high percentage of LBP is due to degenerative disc disease (DDD), which causes fluctuation in disc pressure, thus producing disc dehydration with consequent loss of height, loss of resistance, disc prolapse, and instability.[4,5]

There are multiple treatment options, from conservative to surgical, all of which have the common goal of alleviating LBP. Surgical procedures vary from neurologic decompression to stabilization, or a combination of both procedures. Through the 1990s, the gold standard for treatment of LBP due to DDD was surgical decompression and fusion. With the advent of modern hardware and biologic materials, these procedures have obtained 100% fusion rates in some series. However, other series question the efficacy of fusion due to DDD because of residual pain in fusion patients. In these patients, the clinical outcome was comparable to those patients with good response to aggressive physical therapy. Moreover, there is significant concern for the incidence of adjacent-level disc disease in patients who have undergone fusion surgery.

In the last decade, the demand and use of nonfusion devices, ranging from artificial discs to dynamic stabilization devices, have multiplied. These devices are designed to alleviate LBP without the need to fuse segments.[6]

The definition of dynamic stabilization is a system that can favorably modify movement and load transmission through a mobile, functional vertebral unit, without the need to fuse the segment.[7–9]

The PercuDyn is a facet-allocated dynamic stabilization device for the lumbar spine. It works as an extension-limiting for load sharing. It unloads the degenerated disc, thus reducing load transmission and abnormal movement through the disc, maintaining segment mobility while controlling abnormal movement, thus alleviating LBP.

## INDICATIONS

The PercuDyn posterior dynamic stabilization implant (Interventional Spine, Irvine, CA) is indicated for treatment of patients with chronic LBP due to DDD for whom conservative treatment has failed. These patients also have loss of disc height of up to 50% shown on plain films. Also, the presence of a dehydrated "black" disc at one or more levels of the lumbar spine is noted on magnetic resonance imaging (MRI), with a minimal Oswestry Disability Index score of 30%.[10]

## CONTRAINDICATIONS

Insertion of the device is contraindicated in patients with good clinical outcome after aggressive physical therapy, patients with radicular pain without LBP, previous surgery at the affected level, local or systemic infection, osteoporosis, known allergy to titanium or polycarbonate-urethane (PCU), extreme obesity, spondylolisis or spondylolisthesis, Paget's disease, or osteomalacia or other metabolic disease.[11]

## DESCRIPTION OF THE DEVICE

The PercuDyn device is composed of two pieces: 1) a titanium alloy cannulated 4.5-mm anchor with a 16-mm double helix thread and a total length of 38 mm, and 2) a 12-mm long, cannulated, 10-mm-diameter PCU stabilizer. The two pieces come together intraoperatively by means of a compression locking anchor with secondary purchase (CLASP) technology (Fig. 67–1).

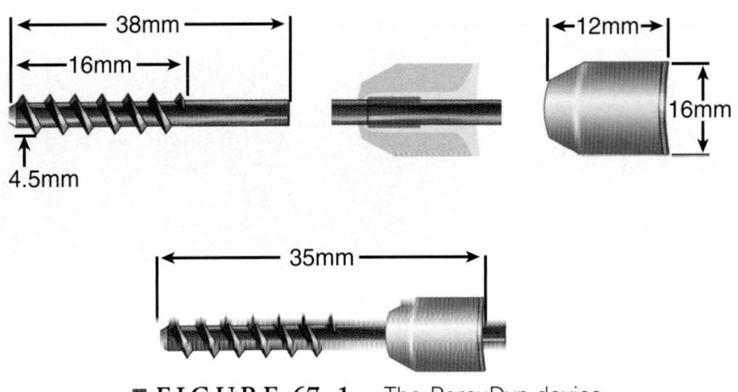


■ FIGURE 67–1. The PercuDyn device.

TABLE 67–1. Treated Levels

| Level Treated | Number of Patients Treated | Number of Levels Treated |
|---|---|---|
| L2/L3 | 1 | 1 |
| L2/L3/L4 | 1 | 2 |
| L3/L4/L5/S1 | 1 | 3 |
| L4/L5 | 12 | 12 |
| L4/L5/S1 | 11 | 22 |
| L5/S1 | 9 | 9 |
| Total | 35 | 49 |

## BACKGROUND OF SCIENTIFIC TESTING

Scientific and biomechanical testing was performed at the Orthopedic Biomechanics Research Center, Children's Hospital, San Diego, CA.

Six human cadaveric spines were dissected from L2 to L5, leaving all ligamentous structures intact. The intact spines were first tested in flexion and extension, lateral bending, and axial rotation at ± 7.5 Nm. The PercuDyn devices were inserted at L3-L4, and testing was repeated. Fluorosocopic analysis of posterior disc height and foraminal area of the intact and instrumented spines while loading was performed. All test data were compared using a one-way analysis of variance (statistical significance was set at $P<0.05$).

Instrumented spines had 62% less motion during flexion and 49% less motion during extension compared with the intact spines. Neuroimaging analysis showed 84% less compression of the posterior disc of the instrumented spines during extension and no difference during flexion compared with intact spines. After the instrumentation was inserted, the foraminal area was 36% larger than in intact spine during extension, and 9% larger during flexion. During axial loading, compression of the posterior disc was decreased by 70%, and analysis showed 10% decompression before loading just from implanting the devices.

## CLINICAL STUDIES

A prospective nonrandomized clinical study was performed to evaluate a posterior facet-based extension-limiting device that has been developed to support and cushion the facet complex. It is a titanium-based anchor with a PCU stabilizer that lies against the inferior articular process and is anchored into the pedicle for posterior dynamic stabilization.

Thirty-five patients were included in the study. All of the patients suffered from LBP due to DDD, and in all of them, conservative treatment consisting of aggressive physical therapy and, in some instances, treatment in a pain clinic failed to relieve the pain. The study included 22 male and 13 female patients, with a total of 49 treated segments from February 2006 to March 2007. The age of the patients ranged from 21 to 67 years, with a median of 37.9 years. The patients underwent evaluation at baseline before surgery, and at 2 weeks, 6 weeks, 3 months, 6 months, and 1 year after surgery depending on the study enrollment date. The patient's pain was evaluated using the Oswestry Disability Index (ODI) and the Visual Analog Scale (VAS) at each visit (ODI scores ranged from 0 to 100%; VAS scores ranged from 1 to 10).[12,13] In addition, lumbar spine MRIs were obtained during the preoperative evaluation and at the 12-month follow-up period. Lumbar spine radiographs were obtained at the preoperative evaluation, immediately after surgery, and 6 and 12 months after surgery.

Thirty-five patients (13 female/22 male) with DDD were enrolled for placement of the PercuDyn device at the affected level. A total of 49 levels were treated (Table 67–1).

Figures 67–2 and 67–3 and Table 67–2 present the ODI and VAS outcomes for the different evaluation periods. It can be seen that after PercuDyn placement, there is a marked improvement in both scores at every evaluation period.

Figure 67–4A and B show a lateral projection of the lower lumbar and sacral segments. Figure 67–4A is part of the preoperative evaluation of a 34-year-old man who was diagnosed with DDD. His baseline VAS and ODI were 8 and 42%. At the 6-month follow-up examination, the VAS score was 0 and ODI score was 1, and at the time of these images (12-month follow-up), he improved to a VAS score of 0 and an ODI score of 0. We can see that there is considerable loss of disc height at the L4-L5 level. The 12-month follow-up image (Fig. 67–4B) shows the PercuDyn implant in the pedicles of L5 with a noticeable improvement in L4-L5 disc height.[14]

## CLINICAL PRESENTATION

Most of the patients in our study group are young, active people with DDD. Owing to the age and high level of activity of these patients, they are not candidates for fusion procedures.[10] So in

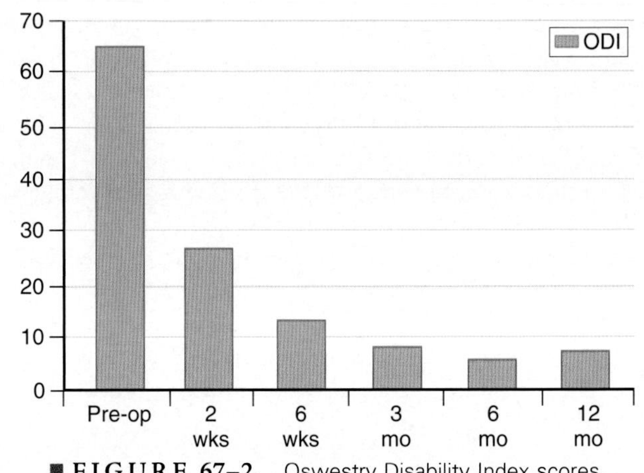


■ FIGURE 67–2. Oswestry Disability Index scores.

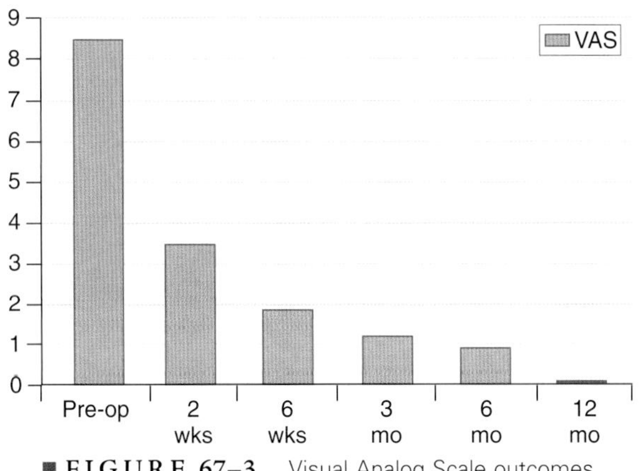


■ **FIGURE 67–3.** Visual Analog Scale outcomes.

the past, physical therapy and the pain clinic were the only two treatment options for these patients. Once these methods failed, the patient had to undergo fusion or learn to live with the pain. Most report chronic lower lumbar back pain that radiated to their lower extremities in some cases. As can be inferred from the preoperative data of the study, most patients had a very low quality of life owing to the severity of the pain. Figure 67–5, an MRI scan of the lumbar spine, represents the usual "black disc" image seen in patients with DDD (L4-L5).[10,16–18]

## OPERATIVE TECHNIQUE

The surgical procedure is performed under intravenous sedation or light anesthesia with local infiltration of lidocaine and epinephrine over the marked surgical area. The patient is positioned prone over a William's frame and the vertebral levels to treat localized with fluoroscopy. The patient is prepped in the typical manner, target pedicles are marked, and a 12-mm incision is made, being careful to incise the muscular fascia. A Jamsheedy needle is placed in the pedicle to treat with care to place the Jamsheedy tip in the middle half of the pedicle image, and placed immediately under the superior facet, the Jamsheedy is then directed 10 degrees medial to lateral and 10 degrees caudal to cephalic, and is then introduced into the pedicle with a mallet, until the tip reaches the posterior third of the vertebral body. The Jamsheedy needle is replaced with a 0.62' Kirschner wire, which is advanced to the second half of the vertebral body. Serial dilation of the musculature is carried out, and after fluoroscopic confirmation of Kirschner wire positioning, the pedicle is drilled by a cannulated 3.2-mm drill bit, tapped with a 4.5-mm bone tap. Care should be taken not to place the drill bit or tap beyond the deepness of Kirschner wire, because this would dislodge the K-wire. After drilling and tapping, the superior facet is decorticated by a 10-mm countersink, which mimics the PCU stabilizer until the depth mark in the countersink is in line with the posterior cortex of the superior facet. The titanium alloy anchor is inserted with a special instrument that will release the anchor once it reaches optimal depth. The PCU stabilizer is then guided over the K-wire. Once it reaches the anchor, the ratcheting mechanism can be felt and heard when the stabilizer is locked into the anchor and then malleted slightly to obtain a press-fit, aligning the posterior mark of the stabilizer with the posterior cortex of the superior facet. After positioning is verified in both lateral and AP views, both the guide wire and muscle dilator are removed and the wound is cleansed. The same procedure is then carried out on the contralateral pedicle; both wounds are cleansed and closed with subcuticular absorbable suture and steri-strips. The bilateral procedure should take approximately 15 to 40 minutes.

**TABLE 67–2. Clinical Outcome Data**

| | Preoperative | 2 wk | 6 wk | 3 mo | 6 mo | 12 mo |
|---|---|---|---|---|---|---|
| VAS | 8.5 | 3.5 | 1.9 | 1.3 | 1.0 | 0.14 |
| ODI | 65.3 | 26.1 | 13.4 | 8.4 | 5.3 | 7 |

ODI, Oswestry Disability Index; VAS, Visual Analog Scale.

## POSTOPERATIVE CARE

After surgery, the patient is moved to recovery and discharged 4 to 6 hours postoperatively. At home, routine care for wounds is indicated and nonsteroidal anti-inflammatory drugs (NSAIDs) are prescribed. Patients who do nonphysical labor are permitted to return to customary work after 3 or 4 days. Those who have physically demanding occupations are permitted to go back to work in 10 to 14 days. The use of back support is not advocated, and there is no need for initial bed rest.

## COMPLICATIONS AND AVOIDANCE

In our series, complications have been minimal and include one implant misplacement, which was corrected intraoperatively; one skin irritation due to aseptic substance reaction; one unilateral muscle herniation; and one incidence of unilateral facet pain, which subsided after use of NSAIDs for 21 days.

### ADVANTAGES/DISADVANTAGES: THE PERCUDYN SYSTEM

**Advantages**
- Non fusion
- Facet augmentation device
- Percutaneous outpatient procedure
- Involves light sedation and local anesthesia
- Preserves posterior ligamentous structures
- Placement inferior to instrumented segment
- Can be used at L5-S1 level
- Neutralizes lateral bending
- Device is closer to rotational axis

**Disadvantages**
- Learning curve involved in correct placement
- Bilateral placement required
- Contraindicated in spondylolysis or spondylolisthesis
- Cannot be placed superior to instrumented segment

Care must be taken during the procedure not to invade the spinal canal, and maintain both Jamsheedy needle and guide wire within the pedicle margin to avoid neurologic damage. Also the anterior cortex of the treated vertebrae should not be breeched to avoid an

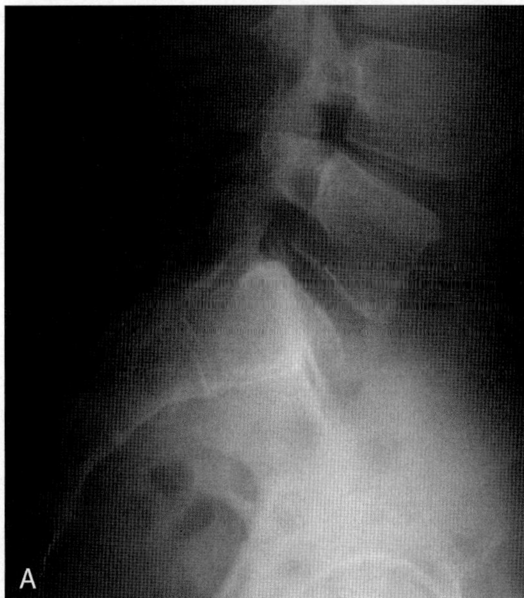


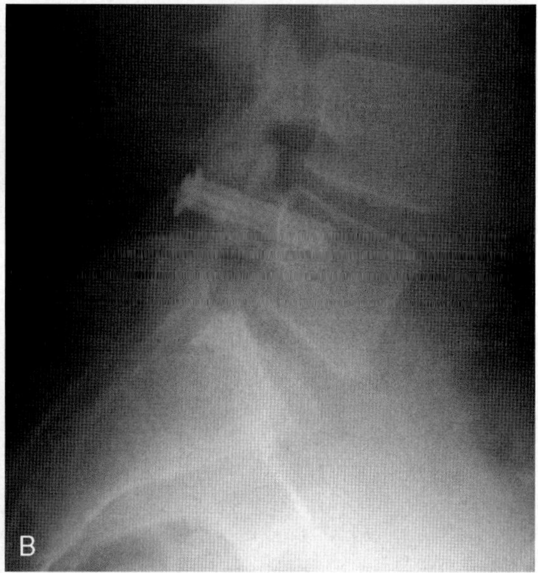


■ **FIGURE 67–4.** Lateral projection of the lower lumbar and sacral segments. **A,** Preoperative evaluation of a 34-year-old man who was diagnosed with degenerative disc disease. **B,** Twelve-month follow-up image shows the PercuDyn implant in the pedicles of L5 with a noticeable improvement in L4-L5 disc height.

intra-abdominal lesion. Also, it is critical to place the PercuDyn device from medial to lateral to ensure correct stabilization. The device should not be placed from lateral to medial because this could produce facet impingement and consequent facet pain.

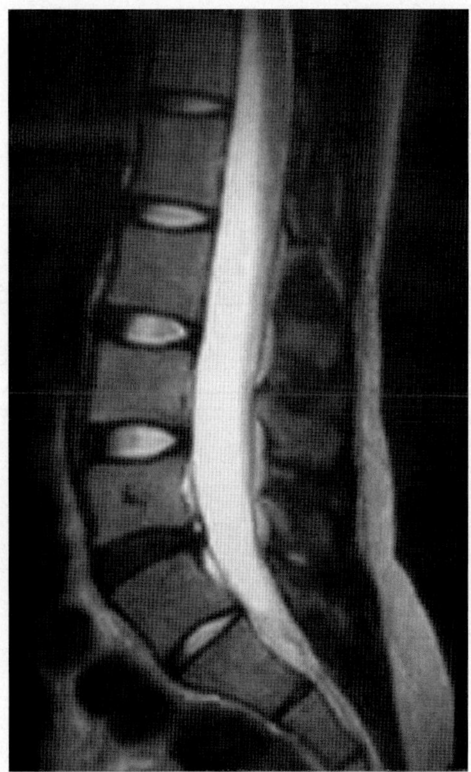

■ **FIGURE 67–5.** Magnetic resonance imaging scan of the lumbar spine represents the usual "black disc" image seen in patients with degenerative disc disease (L4-L5).

## CONCLUSIONS

The degenerating lumbar spine is a source of pain for many individuals. The pain generator can be the disc itself or spondylitic changes in the facet joints. Painful conditions of the aging spine include DDD,[4] facet arthropathy, central and foraminal stenosis, and spondylolisthesis.[3] There is significant clinical interest in developing technologies that would alleviate pain while maintaining the spine's natural biomechanics and not resorting to fusion.[15]

Similar to extension-limiting devices, the PercuDyn System has been designed to treat the pain caused by degenerative conditions like DDD and spondylosis by stabilizing the lumbar spine without fusion. Specifically, the PercuDyn implant has been designed to prevent extension motion by providing support for the articulating facets.[19] The PercuDyn device is implanted as described earlier. The implants are percutaneously placed posteriorly at the base of the superior articular facet, through the pars, and into the pedicles. A countersink is used to remove a small portion of the superior articular facet and the pars interarticularis to obtain an anatomically snug fit for the stabilizer. Once the implants are placed bilaterally, they act as a stop to prevent extension motion of the facets. The elastic modulus of the material used in the stabilizer is less than that of bone and serves to cushion the facets and to relieve stress.[20–23] Pain associated with activities of daily living may also be reduced by limiting potential bulging of the disc or closure of the spinal foramen during extension.

Biomechanical testing showed that the PercuDyn device maintained posterior disc height and foraminal area during extension while also unloading the disc in flexion, without altering axial rotation and lateral bending at the treated segment. At the same time, it does not overload the adjacent levels.[24]

In our series, patient selection included those with chronic LBP secondary to DDD of one or more levels of the lumbar spine, and conservative treatment had failed to relieve the pain.

The patients did not present any neurologic affection. Informed consent was signed by each individual, and the surgical procedure was carried out in typical fashion. ODI and VAS scores were obtained preoperatively and at 2, 6, 12, and 24 weeks postoperatively. Plain radiographs were taken at 3 and 6 months, with a postoperative MRI taken at 1-year follow-up. Initial ODI scores ranged from 36% to 90%, with a median of 64%. VAS scores ranged from 5 to 10, with a median of 8.5. The PercuDyn System is a new concept in implant technology for dynamic stabilization of the lumbar spine in patients with chronic LBP due to DDD at one or more levels of the lumbar spine. The implant is performed as a percutaneous outpatient surgical procedure, which has demonstrated a fast recovery and short-term progressive clinical improvement in ODI and VAS scores.

## REFERENCES


1. Kothari MVL, Lopa Mehta, Natarajan M, Kothari VM: Spine revisited: Principles and parlance redefined. Neurol India 53:397–398, 2005.
2. Gibson JN, Grant IC, Waddell G: The Cochrane review of surgery for lumbar disc prolapse and degenerative lumbar spondylosis. Spine 24:1820–1832, 1999.
3. Kirkaldy-Willis WH, Farfan HF: Instability of lumbar spine. J Clin Orthop 165:110–123, 1982.
4. Adams MA, Roughley PJ: What is intervertebral disc degeneration, and what causes it? Spine 31:2151–2161, 2006.
5. Ariga K, Miyamoto S, Nakase T, et al: The relationship between apoptosis of endplate chondrocytes and aging and degeneration of the intervertebral disc. Spine 26(22):2414–2420, 2001.
6. Freudiger S, Dubois G, Lorrain M: Dynamic neutralisation of the lumbar spine confirmed on a new lumbar spine simulator in vitro. Arch Orthop Trauma Surg 119:127–132, 1999.
7. Cakir B, Richter M, Huch K, et al: Dynamic stabilization of the lumbar spine. Orthopedics 29:716–722, 2006.
8. Dubois G, de Germany B, Schaerer NS, Fennema P: Dynamic neutralization: A new concept for restabilization. *In* Szpalski M, Gunzburg R, Pope MH (eds): Lumbar Segmental Instability. Philadelphia, Lippincott Williams & Wilkins, 1999, pp 233–240.
9. Bordes-Monmeneu M, Bordes-Garcia V, Rodrigo-Baeza F, Saez F: Sistema de neutralizacion dinamica en la columna lumbar: Dynesys system experience of 94 cases. Neurocirugía 16:499–550, 2005.
10. Modic M, Pavlicack W, Weinstein M, et al: Magnetic resonance imaging of intervertebral disk disease. Radiology 152:103–111, 1984.
11. Triage LSPW Data Summary.
12. Fairbank JCT, Cooper J, Davis JB, O'Brien JP: Oswestry Low Back Pain Disability Questionnaire. Physiotherapy 66:271–273, 1980.
13. Fairbank JCT, Pynsent PB: The Oswestry Disability Index. Spine 25:2940–2953, 2000.
14. Kroeber MW, Unglaub F, Wang H, et al: New in vivo animal model to create intervertebral disc degeneration and to investigate the effects of therapeutic strategies to stimulate disc regeneration. Spine 27:2684–2690, 2002.
15. Graf H: Lumbar instability: Surgical treatment without Fusion. Rachis 412:123–137, 1992.
16. Modic M, Ross J: Magnetic resonance in the evaluation of low back pain. Orthop Clin North Am 22:283–301, 1999.
17. Natarjan RN, Williams JR, Andersson GB: Modeling changes in intervertebral disc mechanics with degeneration. J Bone Joint Surg 88(2):36–40, 2006.
18. Ross J, Modic M, Masaryk T: Tears of the annulus fibrosus: Assessment with Gd-DTPA-enhanced MR imaging. AJNR Am J Neuroradiol 10:1251–1254, 1989.
19. Mulholland RC, Sengupta DK: Rationale, principles and experimental evaluation of the concept of soft stabilization. Eur Spine J 11(2): S198–S205, 2002.
20. Rohlmann A, Burra N, Zander T, Bergman G: Comparison of the effects of bilateral posterior dynamic and rigid fixation devices on the loads in the lumbar spine: A finite element análisis. Eur Spine J 16(8):1223–1231, 2007.
21. Sato K, Kikichu S, Yonezawa T: In vivo intradiscal pressure measurement in healthy individuals and in patients with ongoing back problems. Spine 24:2468–2474, 1999.
22. Schmoelz W, Huber JF, Nydegger T, et al: Dynamic stabilization of the lumbar spine and its effects on adjacent segments: An in vitro experiment. J Spinal Disord Tech 16:418–423, 2003.
23. Sengupta DK: Dynamic stabilization devices in the treatment of low back pain. Neurol India 53:466–474, 2005.
24. Swanson KE, Lindsey DP, Hsu KY, et al: The effects of an interspinous implant on intervertebral disc pressures. Spine 28:26–32, 2003.
25. Schnake KJ, Putzier M, Haas NP, Kandziora F: Mechanical concepts for disc regeneration. Eur Spine J Suppl 15:354–360, 2006.

PART

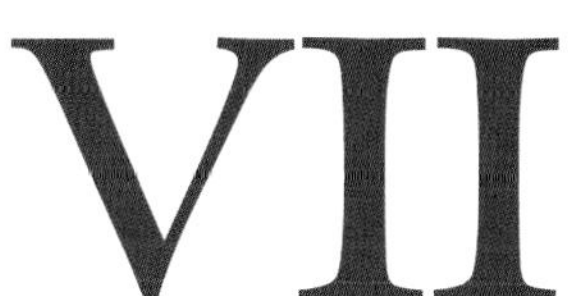

# VII

# Lumbar Posterior Dynamic Stabilization: Interspinous Based

CHAPTER 68

# DIAM Spinal Stabilization System

**Giancarlo Guizzardi** and **Piero Petrini**

## KEY POINTS

- DIAM (Device for Intervertebral Assisted Motion) is a polyethylene terephthalate (polyester)–covered shock-absorbing biomedical silicone device, in the form of an H.
- It is implanted between the spinous process, sacrificing only the interspinous ligament and leaving the fibrous upper spinous complex intact, which is therefore placed under stress.
- Preserving the fibrous upper spinous complex creates a rear stress band that prevents the abnormal kyphosis of the segment.
- Two solid ligaments anchor the device to the two adjacent spinous processes (Fig. 68–1).
- At the present time, DIAM is available in four sizes: 8, 10, 12, and 14 mm.

## INDICATIONS AND CONTRAINDICATIONS

The indications for use of the DIAM device (Medtronic Sofamor Danek, Memphis, TN) are

1. Black disc–facet syndrome
2. Soft or foraminal stenosis
3. Lumbar canal stenosis after decompression (no laminectomy)
4. Large-dimension lumbar disc herniations in young patients[1]
5. Topping off (to prevent the junctional pathology after arthrodesis)

The contraindications are

1. Tumors
2. Infections
3. Fractures
4. Clinically overt osteoporosis
5. Clinically overt instability (spondylolisthesis)
6. Hypoagenesis of the spinous processes
7. Intolerance to the material

## DESCRIPTION OF THE DEVICE

- Rongeur for removal of the interspinous ligament (Fig. 68–2A)
- Distractor of the interspinous area (Fig. 68–2B)
- Phantom for the correct determination of the device size (four measures) (Fig. 68–2C)
- DIAM deformation rongeur (Fig. 68–2D)
- Ligament-anchorage rongeur (Fig. 68–2E)
- Clamp for maintenance of the DIAM deformation (three measures) (Fig. 68–2F)

## BACKGROUND OF THE SCIENTIFIC TESTING/CLINICAL OUTCOMES

### Biocompatibility

The biocompatibility of the material was determined through tests carried out on animals and in vitro. The results are presented in Table 68–1.

Other tests of biocompatibility were recently carried out in the United States, all with excellent success. However, we believe that the best proof of nontoxicity and biocompatibility is the more than 15,000 implants carried out in humans, already with a follow-up of approximately 7 years.

#### Mechanical Tests

Ultimate static strength (with 8-mm DIAM)[2]:

- Compression 2,199 ± 83 N: maximum load determined by 90% compression; no device failure observed.
- Tension 565 ± 84 N: failure mode in cable; no spacer failure noted.

Ten million–cycle fatigue strength (maximum run out of load):

- Compression 480 N peak, 48 N valley.
- Tension 155 N peak, 15.5 N valley.
- Tests conducted in 37 °C saline solution. Minimal wear debris observed and analyzed.

Compression creep:

- Static 450 N: only 1.2 mm (steady-state value, which was determined through regression analysis).
- Dynamic 480:48 N: peak 1.67 mm, valley 1.17 mm.

### Dynamic Interspinous Process Technology

In a recent publication, some American authors carried out a review of the literature[3] to evaluate the mechanisms of action and effectiveness

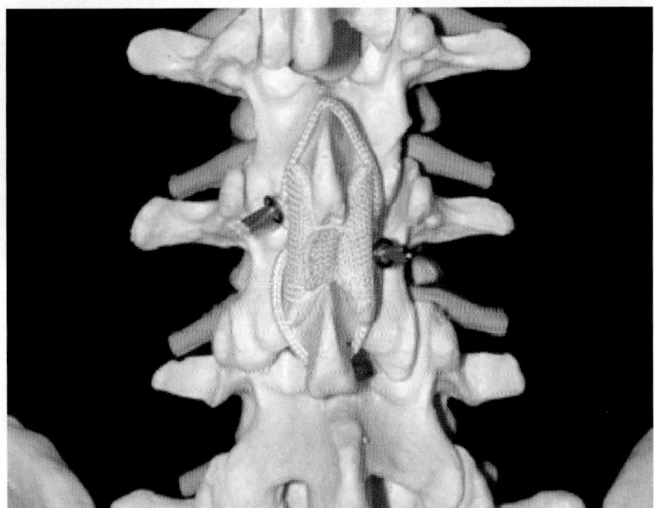

■ **FIGURE 68–1.** DIAM.

of interspinous distraction devices in managing symptomatic lumbar spinal pathology. They concluded that because of the anatomic structure of the S1 spinous process, these implants are not favorable and are not currently recommended for use at L5-S1. The concept of dynamic stabilization, as opposed to fusion, is particularly attractive, especially for young patients who would bear a life-long burden on adjacent segments. In addition, its use does not restrict or eliminate any potential future therapeutic options. Interspinous implants share the mechanism of limiting extension of the lumbar spine and, as result, appear to improve clinical symptoms. The interspinous implants distract the spinous process and restrict extension, thereby reducing the pressure on the posterior annulus and enlarging the neural foramen.

In another recent work conducted by American colleagues,[4] it is furthermore clearly demonstrated how the interspinous implants significantly reduced the mean peak pressure, average pressure, contact area, and force at the implanted level.

### The Crane Principle

According to Harms,[5] we support the Crane principle, in which the posterior elements protect the disc, restricting the range of flexion. As early as 1857, Gordon,[6] engineer in the Royal Aeronautical Society and professor of Materials Technology at Reading University, stated:

> Within the body framework of the vertebral column, nature has employed nicely placed soft elements to limit the loads that are burdened and also helps to protect from the consequences of its fragility.

Certainly, these two old but still very valid concepts are the best justification to explain and understand the use of an elastic interspinous prosthesis.

## CLINICAL PRESENTATION AND EVALUATION

Our clinical experience includes 1,120 patients with a follow-up from 12 to 60 months. The percentage of age groups in which the DIAM device was implanted are as follows:

5% from 15 to 30 years
26% from 31 to 40 years
31% from 41 to 50 years
19% from 51 to 60 years
10% from 61 to 70 years
9% older than 70 years

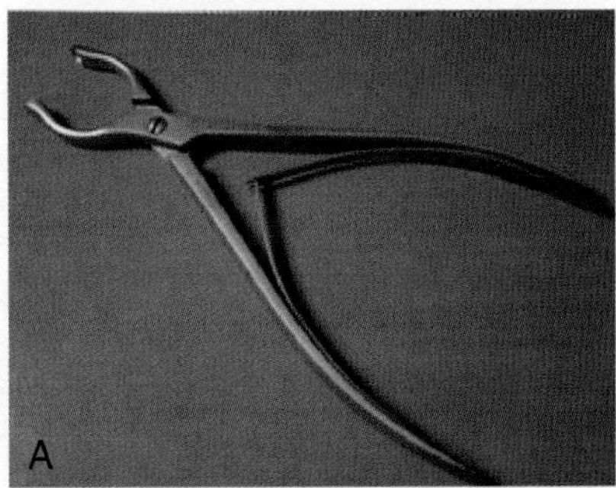


Rongeur for removal of the interspinous ligament

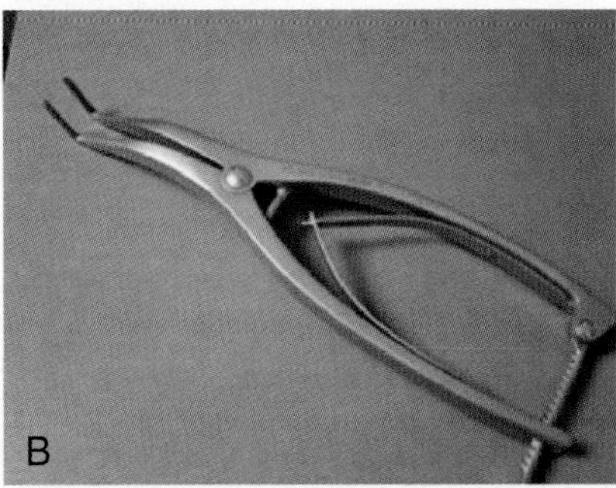


Distractor of the interspinous area

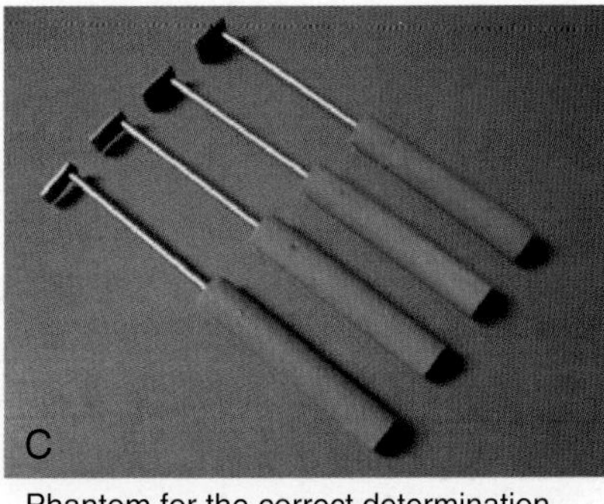


Phantom for the correct determination of the device size (4 measures)

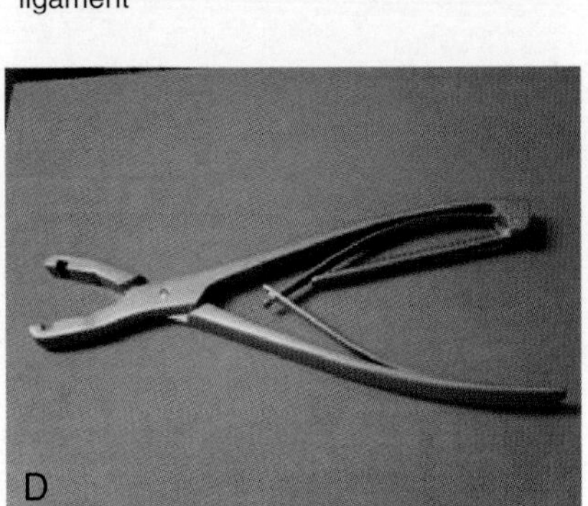


DIAM deformation rongeur

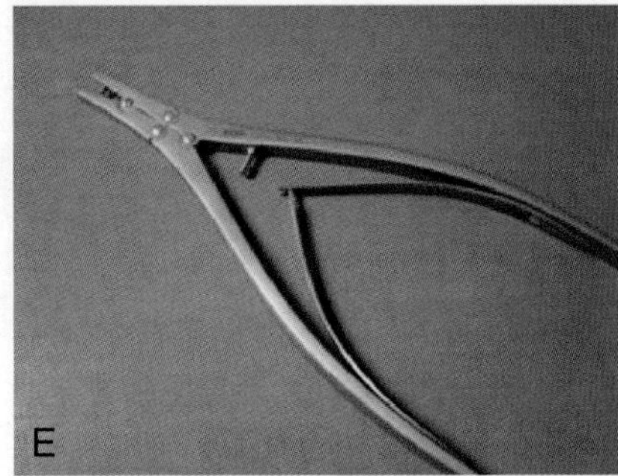


Ligament-anchorage rongeur

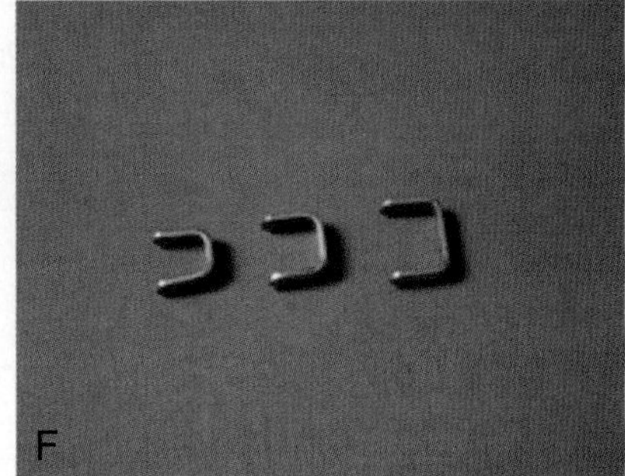


Clamp for maintenance of the DIAM deformation (3 measures)

■ **FIGURE 68–2.** **A** to **F,** Instrumentation.

TABLE 68–1. Results of Biocompatibility Testing

| Study Title | Procedural USP | Compliance ISO | Result |
|---|---|---|---|
| Cytotoxicity Testing using the ISO Elution Method in the L-929 Mouse Fibroblast Cell Line | Yes | Yes | MEM test extracts were not cytotoxic |
| In Vitro Hemolysis Study (extraction method) | Yes | No | Nonhemolytic |
| Rabbit Pyrogen Study—Material mediated | Yes | Yes | Extract is nonpyrogenic; within acceptable USP limits |
| USP Systemic Toxicity in the Mouse (extracts) | Yes | Yes | Extracts not systemically toxic; meets USP requirements |
| Acute Intracutaneous Reactivity Study in the Rabbit (extracts) | Yes | Yes | Extracts showed nonsignificant irritation or toxicity |
| USP Muscle Implantation Study in the Rabbit (with histopathology) (13 weeks) | Yes | No | Macroscopic reaction was not significant as compared to USP negative control; implant material met USP requirements; microscopically classified as slight irritant |
| Delayed Contact Sensitization Study (a maximization method) in the Guinea Pig (saline extract) | Yes | No | No evidence of delayed dermal contact sensitization to guinea pig |
| AMES *Salmonella* Mammalian Microsome Mutagenicity Assay | Yes | Yes | Nonmutagenic to *Salmonella typhimurium* |

ISO, international standards organization; MEM, minimal essential medium—an extract evaluated to assess the biological safety of extracted chemicals from the test articles. The extract is examined using a sensitive in vitro method to determine whether leachables extracted from the material would cause cytotoxicity or cell death. The results thereby give "predictive evidence of material biocompatibility." See ISO 10993-5 for further clarification.; USP, United States Pharmacopeia, a legally recognized compendium of standards for drugs published by the United States Pharmacopeial Convention, Inc., and revised periodically. It includes assays and tests for the determination of strength, quality, and purity.

The DIAM device was used to treat several pathologic conditions, including 374 cases of black disc or facet joint syndrome, 491 cases of mono- or multilevel stenosis, 203 extruded disc herniations (153 in patients younger than 40 years), and 52 cases in topping off. The implants were 65% at one level, 32% at two levels, and 3% at three levels. The treated levels were 0% at L1-L2, 4% at L2-L3, 20% at L3-L4, 61% at L4-L5, and 15% at L5-S1.

### Results

Pre- and postoperative evaluations with the Visual Analog Scale (VAS) relative to low back pain (follow-up 24 to 70 months) showed statistically significant variations of 88% in the extruded lumbar disc herniations, 78% in black disc or facet joint syndrome, 74% in lumbar stenosis. Relative to the topping-off application of this device, we have no evidence of junctional pathology in 98% of the patients controlled at maximum follow-up of 5 years.

Therefore, we can state that 87% of patients experienced between very satisfactory and satisfactory results; in 7% of patients, the condition was unchanged; and in 6% of patients, the results were unsatisfactory.

### Complications

Complications occurred in 3.8% of patients, with 12 cases of infection, nine cases of breakage of a spinous process that required the removal of the DIAM, and 21 cases in which we had to use arthrodesis, always after the removal of the device.

## OPERATIVE TECHNIQUE

Anesthesia can be local. In cases in which it is necessary to bypass the yellow ligament, or for operations of more than one device, general anesthesia is recommended.

Usually the prone position is preferred, with a modest delordosis, but without creating a genu-pectoral position.

The procedure includes a sterile operating area, markers in the area involved using floroscopy, incision of the skin corresponding to the upper and lower spinous of the space involved (in less-invasive techniques no greater than 3 to 4 cm). Isolation of the superspinous fibrous complex and incision of the same bilaterally, amply avoiding the upper spinous ligament. Detaching the paravertebral muscles with bilateral peeling of at least two insertions of the divided muscle and removal with the appropriate rongeur of the interspinous ligament. Application of the interspinous distractor in the situ thus created, attempting to obtain good retention of the upper spinous ligament to recreate its natural "tension band."[9] Measurement with the appropriate fantom of the more correct measurement of the interspinous prosthesis and insertion of the DIAM before its deformation and containment: From an H shape, it passes temporarily to a T obtained with the appropriate callipers and held by an appropriate measurement clamp included in the instruments. Once the DIAM is inserted in the interspinous area, the clamp is removed (from the part opposite to the side of insertion), allowing the prosthesis to recover its original H shape. The retractor is removed and the prosthesis is lodged correctly with the appropriate hitting unit. At this point, two ligaments are passed over and under the contiguous spinous processes, which are fixed with the appropriate rivets. Careful suturing is carried out on the upper spinal fibrous complex and the layers of skin.

There are two fundamental points in the technique that must be respected in order to obtain the desired results:

- The distraction of the interspinous space must retain the supraspinous ligament, otherwise we easily risk using an undersized device.
- The prosthesis must be placed as anteriorly as possible by creating a correct situ for the device; if necessary even with the occasional sacrifice of small amounts of bone (hypertrophy of the articular processes and/or the laminae, osteophytes, and so on) (Fig. 68–3).

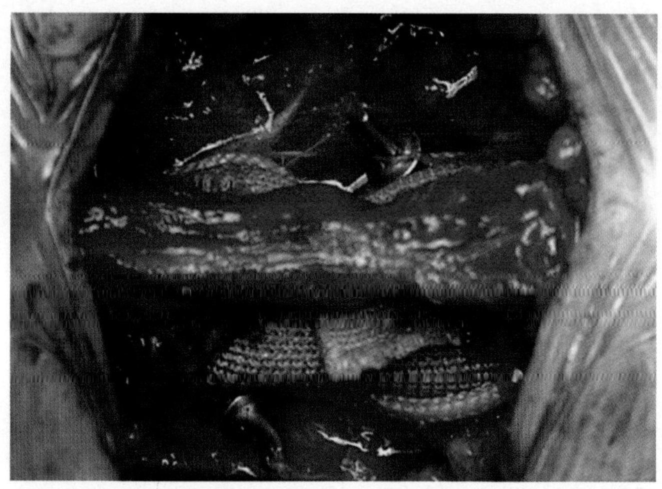

■ **FIGURE 68–3.** Intraoperative view.

## POSTOPERATIVE TREATMENT

The patient gets out of bed on the day of the surgery. He or she is advised to sit in an ergonomic position for at least 3 weeks and to use shoes with a firm sole for at least a month. After this time, it is mandatory to initiate a period of rehabilitative physiokinesitherapy for a time of no less than 4 weeks, using (this is our experience) the GPR (Global Postural Rehabilitation). After this, we recommend the patient maintain constant hygiene of the vertebral column.

> **ADVANTAGES/DISADVANTAGES: DIAM SPINAL STABILIZATION SYSTEM**
>
> **Advantages**
> - Creates a support after the work of the intervertebral disc
> - Simple technique
> - Less invasive than arthrodesis
> - Does not cause irreversible variations to the anatomic structures
> - Absence of complications linked to the material
> - Evident clinical advantages in studies with follow-up beyond 6 years
>
> **Disadvantages**
> - Lodging too far back, and thus far from the center of instant rotation
> - Impedes the recovery of the lumbar curvature and physiology
> - Damage to muscles and soft tissue too significant for a device that must support the function of the mobile segment

## CONCLUSIONS/DISCUSSION

Based on the experience we gained in more than 1,500 implants carried out from December 1998 to the time of this writing and in theoretical and practical comparisons with colleagues with extensive experience in vertebral surgery, we believe that the DIAM is currently the interspinous prosthesis that is closest to the physiologic movement for material, form, and elasticity, determining the tolerability and good clinical results even at a distance.

Our data are confirmed by a recent biomechanical study presented by a German group[7] that states:

> In extension, the defect (bilateral hemifacetectomy with transaction of yellow ligament and transsected supra- and interspinous ligaments) increased the ROM by less than 10%, in flexion it leads to an increase of about 30% above intact values. The interspinous implants with crimped wings restricted flexion by about 20% to 30% (compared to intact). Only the DIAM implant still allowed more motion in extension than the intact specimens. This has to be discussed with care, because the implants lead to different kyphosis of the segments, most with the DIAM. In lateral bending and in axial rotation, the ROM increased with our decompression model by less than 10% and stayed at about these values with all implants.

## FUTURE DEVELOPMENTS

Thanks to this significant experience and the support of new biomechanical studies on cadavers carried out by GISSER (Interdisciplinary Group Development Elastic Systems of the Vertebral Column), we created a new device that maintains the advantages of the DIAM but the same time eliminates the disadvantages. Thus, the new interlaminar device INTRASpine is born.

The INTRASpine has properties and peculiarities (like elasticity, positioning closer to the center of rotation, and monolateral less-invasive approach) allow recovery of the physiologic movement of the mobile lumbar segment.[10]

The first international randomized study of this new device is in the start-up phase, and in the next few months, we will have the first clinical results.

## REFERENCES


1. Guizzardi G, Petrini P, Morichi R, Paoli L: The use of DIAM in the prevention of chronic low back pain in young patients operated on for large dimension lumbar disc herniations. Proceedings 12th European Congress of Neurosurgery, Monduzzi ED, International Proceedings Division, 2003, pp 835–839.
2. Shepherd DET, Lehaj JC, Mathias KJ, et al: Spinous process strength. Spine 25:319–323, 2000.
3. Christie SD, Song JK, Fessler RG: Dynamic interspinous process technology. Spine 30:S73–S78, 2005.
4. Wieseman CM, Lyndsey DP, Fredrick AD, Yerby SA: The effect of Interspinous process implants on facet loading during extension. Spine 30:903–907, 2005.
5. Matthies A: Medieval treadwheels. Artist's views of building construction. Technology and Culture 33(3):510–547, 1992.
6. Gordon JE: Structures under stress or why things don't fall down, Mondadori ED, 1st edition, September 1979.
7. Wilke HJ, Drumm J, Haussler K, Claes L: Biomechanical comparison of the segmental stability and intradiscal pressure achieved with different interspinous implants: Abstracts Proceedings, SAS, 2006, pp 54–55.
8. Caserta S, The Maida GA, Misaggi B: Elastic stabilization alone or combined with rigid fusion in spinal surgery: A biomechanical study and clinical experience based on 82 cases. Eur Spine J 11(suppl 2): S192–S197, 2002.
9. Senegas J: La ligamentoplastie intervertebrale, alternative à l'artrodese dans le traitement des instabilitè degeneratives. Acta Orthop Belg 57 (suppl 1):221–226, 1991.
10. Mimura M, Panjabi MM, Oxland TR: Disc degeneration affects the multidirectional flexibility of the lumbar spine. Spine 19:1371–1380, 1994.

CHAPTER 69

# Wallis Dynamic Stabilization

**Nicholas R. Boeree**

## KEY POINTS

- Off-loads the disc and facet joints and restores normal biomechanics in the moderately degenerative motion segment.
- Simple, minimally invasive, nondestructive, and low-risk surgical technique.
- Indicated in a range of conditions associated with mild to moderate degenerative disease.
- Preserves all important anatomic structures so retains surgical options, including reversal.
- Outcomes compare favorably with spinal fusion and disc replacement.

## INTRODUCTION

Our aim in treating symptomatic lumbar degenerative disease is, of course, the relief of the patient's symptoms while maintaining functional capacity. We hope to achieve these objectives with the minimum of risk and potential comorbidity for the patient. As such, we must consider the potential impact of our intervention, bearing in mind the overriding principal in surgery: "First, do no harm." This philosophy inherently drives us toward more minimally invasive techniques that respect and, where possible, conserve the patient's anatomy and that do not compromise the normal biomechanics of the spine.

For very advanced degenerative disease at a particular level, there may be little alternative to a spinal fusion. Some would argue that even in this situation, prosthetic replacement surgery may offer a viable alternative. However, total disc replacement (TDR) has several significant risks and long-term uncertainties. The procedure is irreversible, and salvage techniques, in the event of a complication or failure, are technically extremely challenging with somewhat uncertain outcomes. In this context, particularly for mild to moderate degenerative disease, less destructive and less invasive dynamic stabilization procedures that aim to preserve the existing motion segment by providing support and protection offer a number of advantages. These procedures fall into two broad categories: (1) those relying on pedicle screw fixation (for example, the Dynesys device [Zimmer Spine Inc., Warsaw, IN]), and (2) interspinous process devices (such as the Wallis Stabilization System [Abbott Spine Inc., Austin, TX]). This chapter discusses the Wallis stabilization procedure.

## DESCRIPTION OF THE DEVICE

The Wallis implant is in fact the second generation of a device developed by Professor Sénégas in the 1980s. His first-generation implant comprised a titanium interspinous process spacer, to accommodate load sharing and to limit extension, combined with two Dacron bands, which controlled flexion movements. This design required no direct fixation to bone, thus eliminating the risks of screw loosening or failure. This alternative approach to degenerative problems in the lumbar spine was supported by good long-term results concerning the implant's efficacy.[1] The survivorship of these first-generation implants has also been impressive at 84.1% at 10 years.[2] In contrast to the usual survivorship behavior, the rate of failure actually decreased very notably with the passage of time.

Although these first-generation implants fared well, conceptually it was considered that certain design changes might be advantageous. Alternative materials and changes in implant design offered an elastic modulus closer to that of bone, providing better stress shielding of the spinous processes. A flatter band distributed loads more effectively and could be combined with a controlled means of band tightening. These changes led to the second-generation implant, the Wallis Stabilization System (Fig. 69–1). The new interspinous spacer is made from polyetheretherketone (PEEK), which has an elastic modulus close to that of bone, a feature further enhanced by compressible spaces in the implant itself. The implant shape fits securely between the spinous processes. The flat bands are woven polyester and are anchored at opposing corners of the implant, from which they can be passed around the corresponding spinous process. To secure and tension the bands, each is looped through a PEEK strap fastener, which snap-fixes to the implant. A range of sizes is available, from 8 mm to 16 mm. The implant is radiolucent, and tantalum markers allow radiographic assessment of implant positioning.

## BACKGROUND OF SCIENTIFIC TESTING

Why certain degenerative motion segments cause mechanical back pain is not, of course, fully understood. However, the abnormal

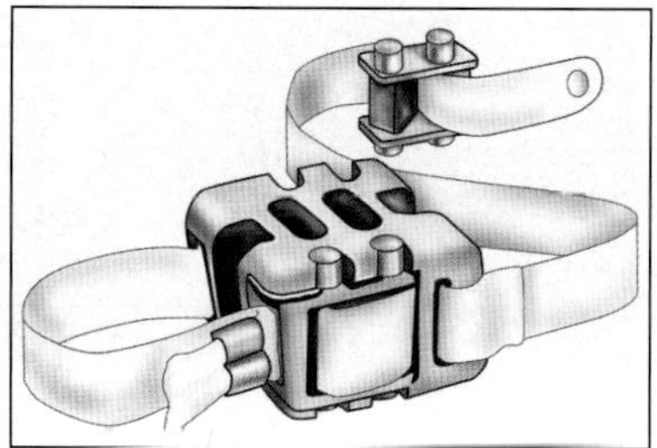
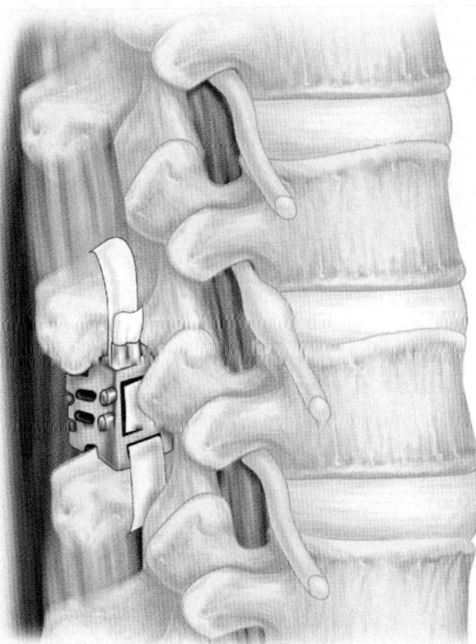

■ **FIGURE 69–1.** The Wallis Stabilization System. The polyetheretherketone (PEEK) interspinous device is shown with the bands *(left)* and in place *(right)*. These bands pass around the adjacent spinous processes and then back to the implant, where they can be tightened and secured with the PEEK clips. After tightening, the excess band is cut off after crimping to prevent fraying.

biomechanics of the degenerative motion segment have been well described in detail in various texts. The contrasting kinematic behavior of the normal and moderately degenerative motion segment can be seen in Figure 69–2. With the motion segment in the neutral position, little force is required to cause significant displacement, and the relationship between load and displacement is fairly linear. This is the central portion of the graph and is defined as the neutral zone. The slope of this central portion of the graph defines the stiffness of the motion segment. Figure 69–2 shows that in the degenerative motion segment the range of movement increases, the initial stiffness is reduced, and the neutral zone is broadened. This results in excessive translation and greater displacement in response to physiologic loading. This behavior effectively falls within the definition of instability (abnormal displacement in response to physiologic loads). For the patient, excessive translation and instability equate to painful episodes with trivial movements in a very unpredictable fashion.

The degenerative disc also loses the capacity to distribute loads evenly. Abnormal peak loads are seen particularly in the posterior annulus.[3] This results in progressive pathologic changes with fissuring and tearing of the annulus, loss of nuclear matrix, reduction in disc height, and facet joint changes. The spectrum of degenerative pathology and the range of clinical problems that can ensue are well recognized.

Cadaveric testing and finite element analysis allow an assessment of the Wallis Stabilization System upon the pattern of loading through the degenerative disc and degenerative kinematic behavior. The findings from six cadaveric specimens[4] are summarized in schematic form in Figure 69–3. The Wallis stabilization technique virtually restores normal kinematic behavior to the

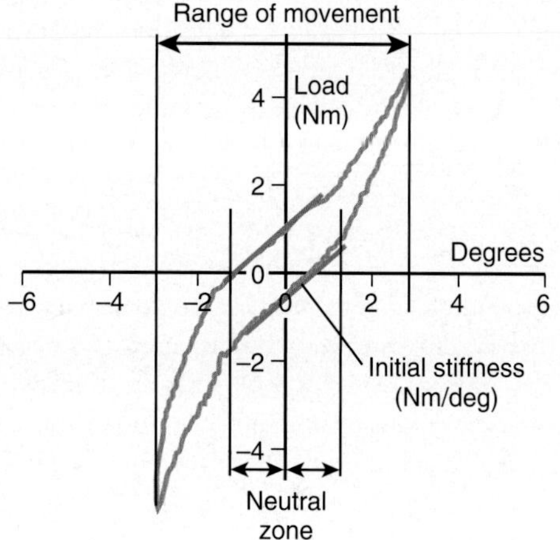


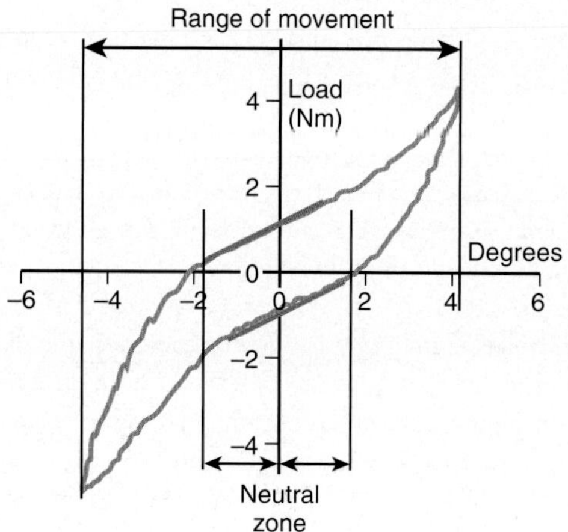


■ **FIGURE 69–2.** The load-displacement curves obtained from cadaveric testing of normal *(left)* and moderately degenerative *(right)* motion segments. In the degenerative segment, the neutral zone is broadened and the slope of the graph in this section is reduced, indicating lower stiffness. In this region, small loads will cause a significant displacement. There is excessive translation, and the overall range of movement is increased.

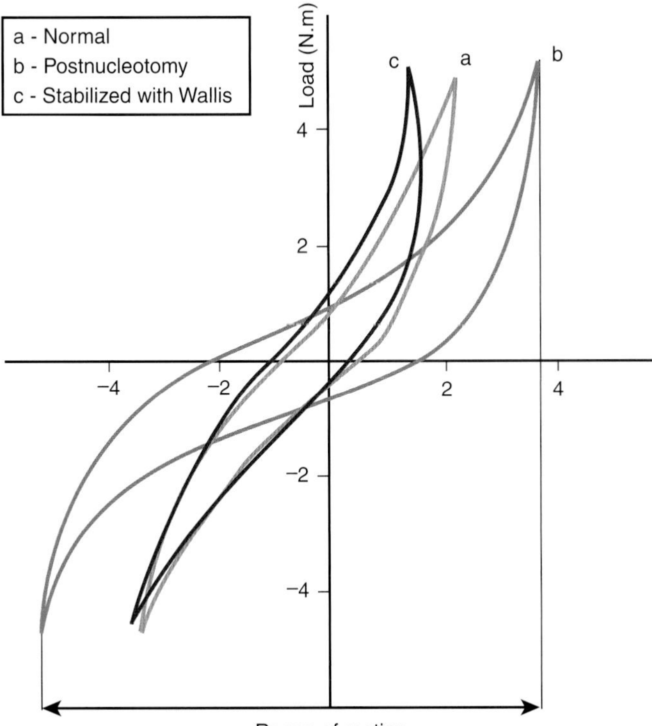


■ **FIGURE 69–3.** Six cadaveric motion segment studies. The normal motion segments give rise to the load-displacement curve shown by (a) when subjected to physiologic flexion and extension loading moments. After controlled nucleotomy, the segment shows the curve in (b), which is typical of a degenerative motion segment with features of instability (see body of text). However, after instrumentation with the Wallis Stabilization System, the kinematic behavior returns virtually to normal, as shown by the curve shown in (c).

motion segment. Stiffness is restored, the neutral zone is reduced, and with it, excessive translation is abolished. The range of movement is almost restored to normal. Finite element analysis shows that the peak loads through the annulus are reduced to less than in the normal disc[4] and, furthermore, demonstrates that there is no stress transfer to adjacent levels with this technique. Pressure transducer studies confirm the off-loading of the motion segment with interspinous process devices. There is a 63% reduction in the loading of the annulus.[5] Facet joint loads are also relieved, with a 39% reduction in mean loads and a 55% reduction of peak loads.[6] Thus, the Wallis device stabilizes the motion segment while at the same time supporting and off-loading the degenerative structures, such as the intervertebral disc and the facet joints.

## CLINICAL OUTCOMES

With any new surgical technique, the first priority must be to confirm its safety, ensuring that the technique does not adversely influence clinical outcomes in those indications for which it seems to be suited. This was the objective in the ongoing multicentered prospective safety and efficacy study that commenced in 2002 involving eight centers in six countries.

The clinical outcome measures included the Visual Analog Scale (VAS) for overall pain, the SF-36, the Japanese Orthopaedic Association score (JOA), and the Oswestry Disability Index (ODI). Radiologic data included interval static and dynamic radiographs and magnetic resonance imaging (MRI) preoperatively and yearly postoperatively. Levels instrumented were restricted to L4-L5 and above, the L5-S1 level being excluded because it is particularly lordotic and has unsuitable spinous processes for interspinous process devices.

The clinical indications were restricted to those in which the Wallis Stabilization System was considered by the investigators as a group to represent either a potentially beneficial supplement or an alternative to traditional surgical techniques. For example, those with discogenic low back pain being considered for other forms of surgical intervention, such as fusion or TDR, were included provided the degenerative changes were not too advanced (Pfirrmann grade IV or less). Patients who had developed a very large or massive disc protrusion, in whom subsequent progressive degenerative changes and problems with low back pain were considered more likely to occur, were also included. The same future risk applies to those who develop a disc protrusion at a level above a transitional anomaly (a partially sacralized L5, for example) or who present with a recurrent disc protrusion. For these cases, protection with Wallis stabilization in addition to excising the extruded disc fragment offered potential benefit with minimal additional risk. Also included in the study were those with stenosis in whom disc height at the affected level was still reasonably preserved. Decompression was performed, but the Wallis Stabilization System was then used to provide stability and help improve the dimensions of the canal and foramina.

The clinical results over the first 2 years are summarized in Figures 69–4 to 69–12. It will be seen that the low back pain VAS (see Fig. 69–4), the JOA (see Fig. 69–7), and the ODI (see Fig. 69–8) show a very clear and statistically significant improvement at 3 months that continues subsequently with further significant improvement between 3 months and 1 year. The mean VAS pain score improved from 77 preoperatively to 12 at 1 year. Figure 69–5 shows the VAS scores at the different review intervals for the principal surgical indications. There were no significant differences in the outcomes for these groups. The VAS change for individual patients at 1 year is illustrated in Figure 69–6. Ninety-three percent of patients reported an improvement in VAS scores of at least 50%. The change in ODI scores at 1 year

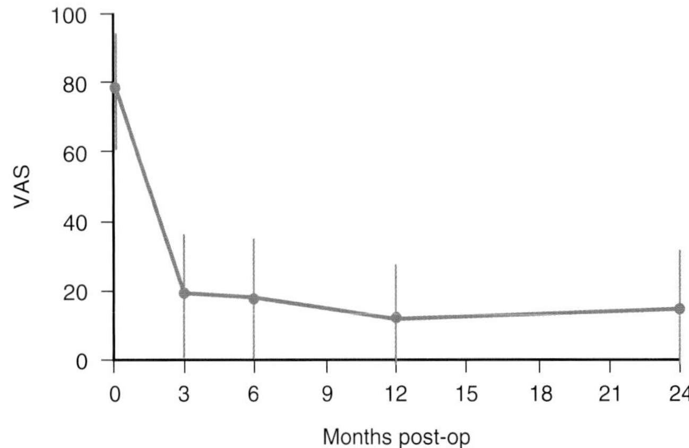


■ **FIGURE 69–4.** Back pain Visual Analog Scale scores for the multicenter study patients.

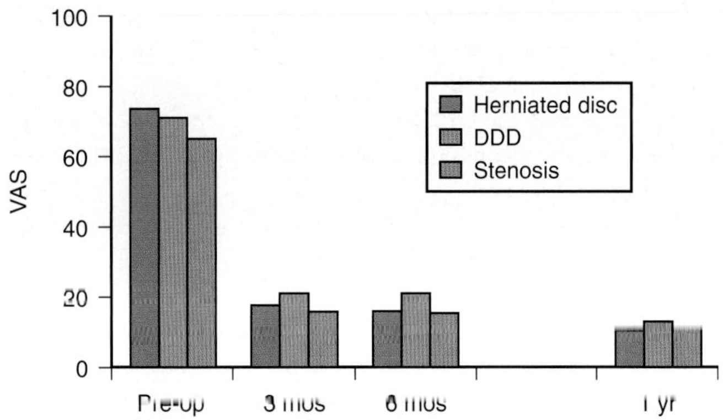


■ **FIGURE 69–5.** Course of Visual Analog Scale (VAS) for the three principal surgical indications. There is no significant difference between the various groups in terms of improvement in VAS. DDD, degenerative disc disease.

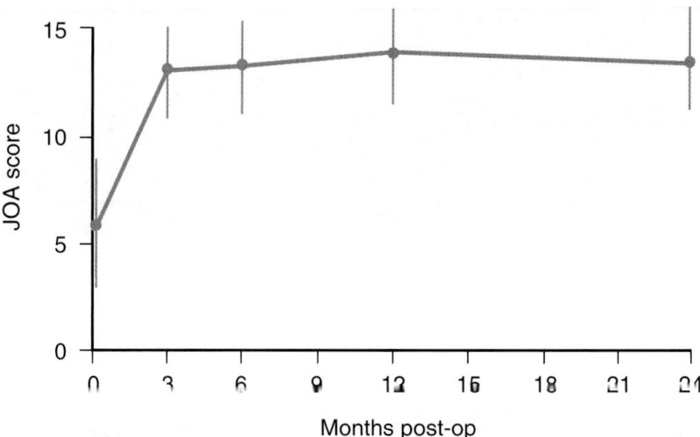


■ **FIGURE 69–7.** The progression of the Japanese Orthopaedic Association (JOA) scores for the multicenter study patients.

as a function of individual preoperative ODI scores is shown in Figure 69–9. Overall, 82% of patients achieved an improvement of more than 50% in their preoperative ODI score, and 60% of patients improved their scores by over 75%. There was a marked reduction in analgesic use (see Fig. 69–10). The SF-36 scores also showed a marked improvement (see Fig. 69–11). Although the SF-36 scores at 2 years are not perfect, they have been compared with a similar age- and sex-matched control population, with no difference being found (see Fig. 69–12). This simply reflects the fact that we all have our aches and pains, and this is revealed in the SF-36 scores. However, those symptoms are no worse in the study group 2 years following surgery than they are in a similar normal population.

## INDICATIONS

The relative merits of the Wallis stabilization technique in different spinal pathologies will require clarification from prospective comparative clinical studies. Until such studies are available, guidance concerning appropriate indications must rely upon our understanding of what the implant can do biomechanically and experience in clinical use. The broad clinical indications are discussed here and illustrated by some cases.

### Disc Support—Discogenic Back Pain

The aim here is to provide support and protection to the degenerative disc and facet joints also. Abnormally high loads through the disc and facet joints, and altered biomechanics seem to be implicated in pain generation. The Wallis Stabilization System reduces the loads through both of these structures and also restores more normal biomechanics, as noted earlier. However, for the Wallis system to be effective, the motion segment must be capable, with appropriate support, of reasonably normal biomechanical function. Severely degenerative discs (Pfirrmann grade V) do not have this capacity. There is little point in trying to support a disc that is very narrow and extensively disrupted. The first illustrative case provides a good example of disc support and shows how Wallis stabilization can provide a treatment option in which alternatives such as fusion or TDR might be regarded as inappropriate.

The patient was a 24-year-old student who had 4 years of severe and very restricting back pain that had not responded

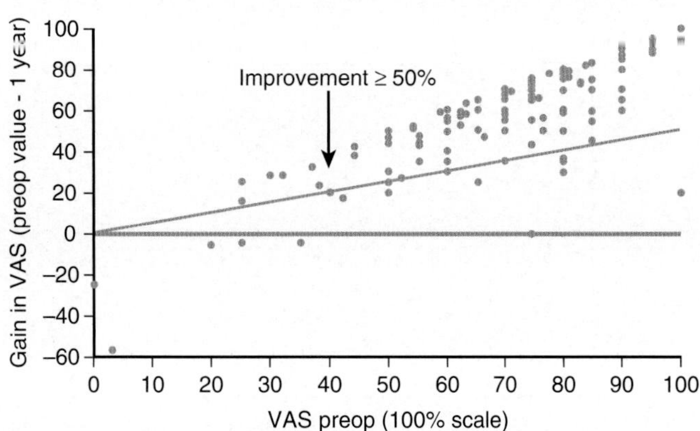


■ **FIGURE 69–6.** Change in Visual Analog Scale (VAS) score at 1 year. Note that 92.7% of the patients reported an improvement in VAS of at least 50% and that the three patients with initial VAS scores lower than 20 were the only ones whose pain worsened.

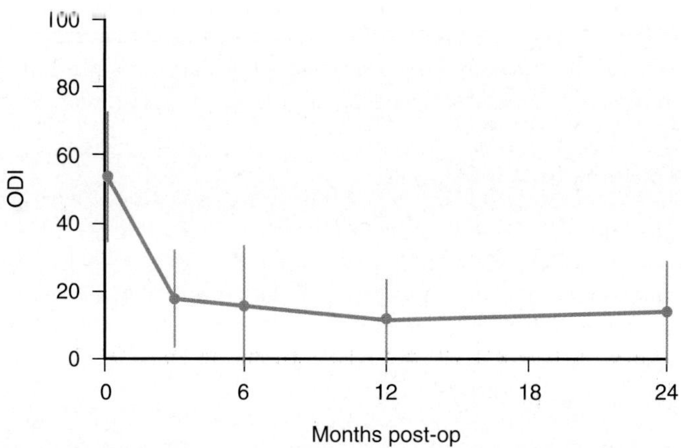


■ **FIGURE 69–8.** The improvement seen in the Oswestry Disability Index (ODI) for the study group.

■ **FIGURE 69–9.** Oswestry Disability Index (ODI) values at 1 year as a function of the preoperative ODI values for individual patients.

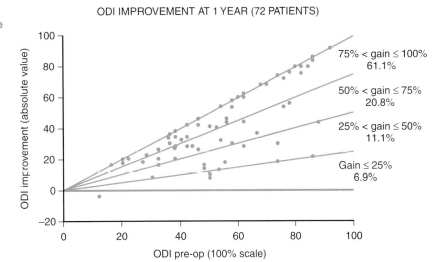

ODI IMPROVEMENT AT 1 YEAR (72 PATIENTS)

ODI improvement (absolute value)

ODI pre-op (100% scale)

75% < gain ≤ 100% 61.1%

50% < gain ≤ 75% 20.8%

25% < gain ≤ 50% 11.1%

Gain ≤ 25% 6.9%

to extensive conservative treatment. Her MRI is shown in Figure 69–13. Fusion and TDR were considered, but in a woman of this age, there were concerns about possible long-term complications such as adjacent-level disease in the case of fusion and uncertainties about very long-term viability in the case of TDR. Wallis stabilization, in contrast, offered the opportunity to support the disc while at the same time presenting no significant long-term risks. At worst, the implant could be removed and the motion segment would not have been compromised in any way. Alternative surgical procedures were still retained as an option for the future.

Flexion and extension radiographs at 1 year (Fig. 69–14) confirm that movement is maintained. It is clear that the Wallis system does not kyphose the motion segment. The MRIs at this stage (Fig. 69–15) are very encouraging, showing that disc height has been maintained and revealing some improvement in the T2 signal return from the instrumented disc. The patient had an excellent clinical outcome (no back pain at all and full return to normal function, including sports), which has been sustained at 3 years.

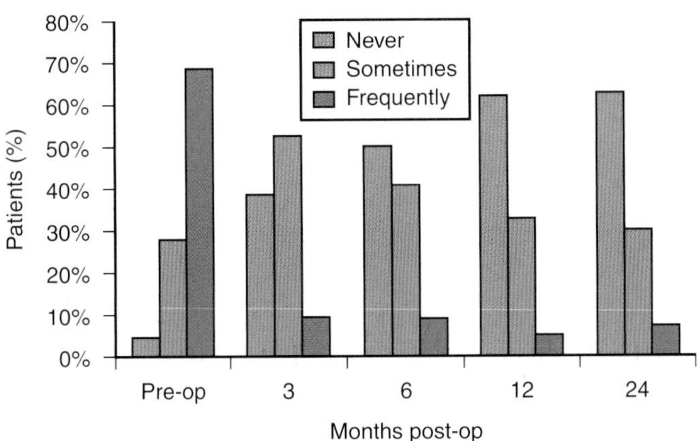


■ **FIGURE 69–10.** The change over time in analgesic use for the study group patients.

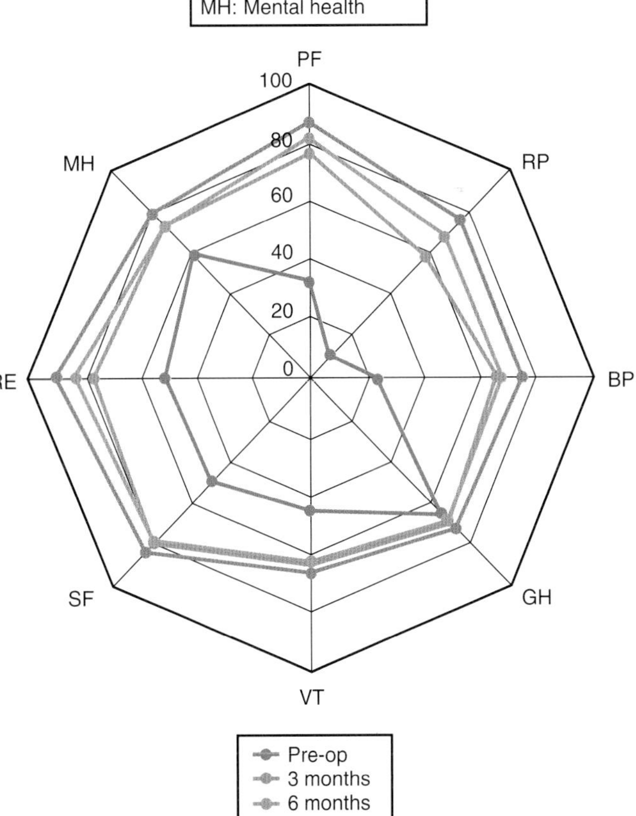


■ **FIGURE 69–11.** The progressive improvement seen in global Short-Form 36 (SF-36) scores for the study group (the results at 2 years are shown in Fig. 69–12).

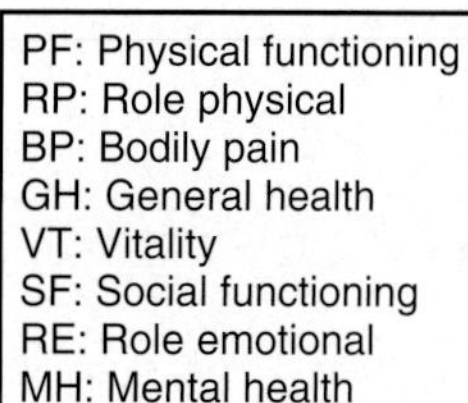
PF: Physical functioning
RP: Role physical
BP: Bodily pain
GH: General health
VT: Vitality
SF: Social functioning
RE: Role emotional
MH: Mental health

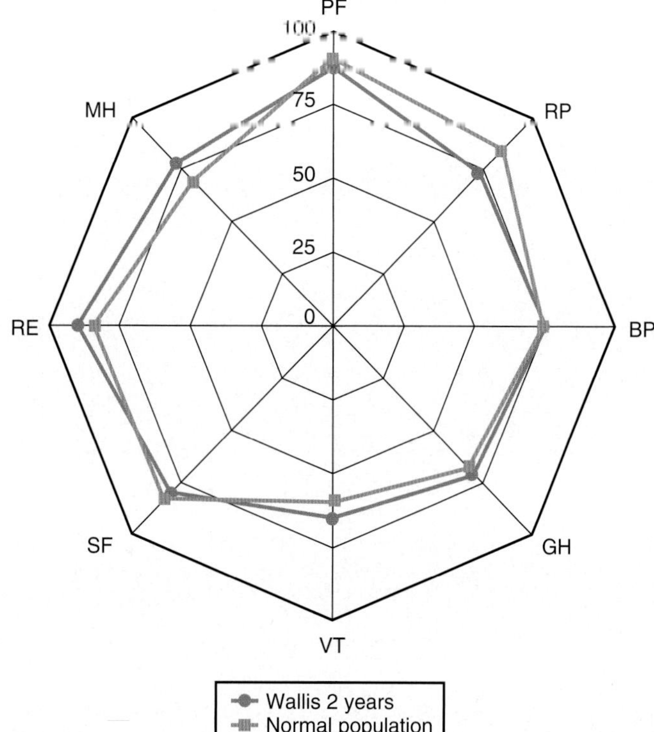


■ **FIGURE 69–12.** The 2-year Short-Form 36 results for the study group when compared with an age- and sex-matched normal population. There was no significant difference between the two groups.

## Disc at Risk—Large or Recurrent Disc Prolapse or Prolapse at Transitional Levels

The principal indication for surgery in this somewhat diverse group of patients will, of course, be sciatica. If the problem is purely one of radicular leg pain, the option of limiting surgery to a simple discectomy is reasonable. However, these patients are at risk of going on to develop problems of back pain in future years. The disc at a transitional level is exposed to greater stresses than normal and therefore will be vulnerable to accelerated degenerative changes and thus to problems of back pain. Similarly, the sudden loss of a considerable volume of nuclear material in very large protrusions, or the additional loss in recurrent protrusions, predisposes the disc to biomechanical dysfunction and thus to problems of back pain.

It is doubtful that the risk of future back pain in these cases would justify the risks and morbidity of more major surgical procedures such as fusion, but Wallis stabilization provides protection to these discs at risk, with minimal additional operating time (mean implantation time 18 minutes), no increased morbidity, and very little additional risk. Clearly, the decision is even more straightforward if, as is often the case, the patient has had back pain in addition to more recent sciatica.

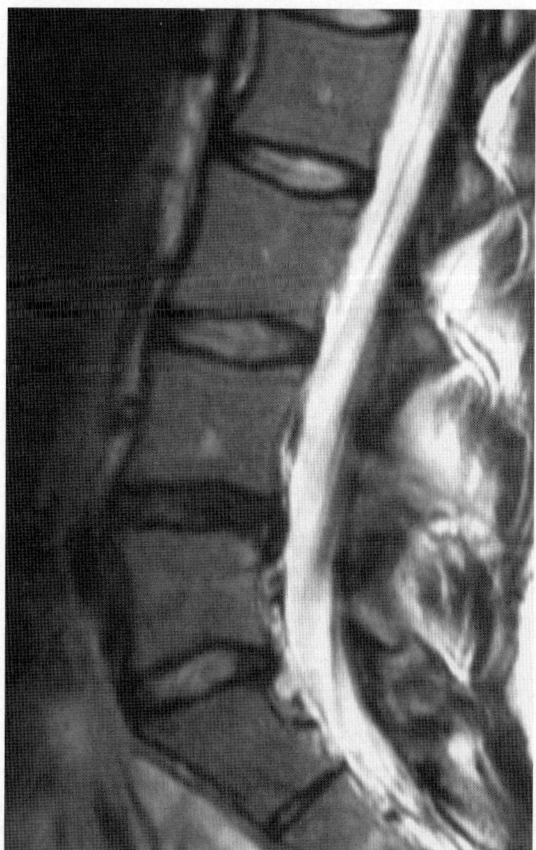

■ **FIGURE 69–13.** The preoperative magnetic resonance imaging scan of the 24-year-old woman with a 4-year history of low back pain (case 1). There are focal degenerative changes seen at L4-L5, but disc height and architecture remain well preserved.

The MRI in Figure 69–16 illustrates the treatment dilemma often encountered in this situation. The patient was a 43-year-old light manual worker with 3 years of intermittent but quite troublesome low back pain. He then developed severe right-sided sciatica. He estimated that 60% of his problem was leg pain and

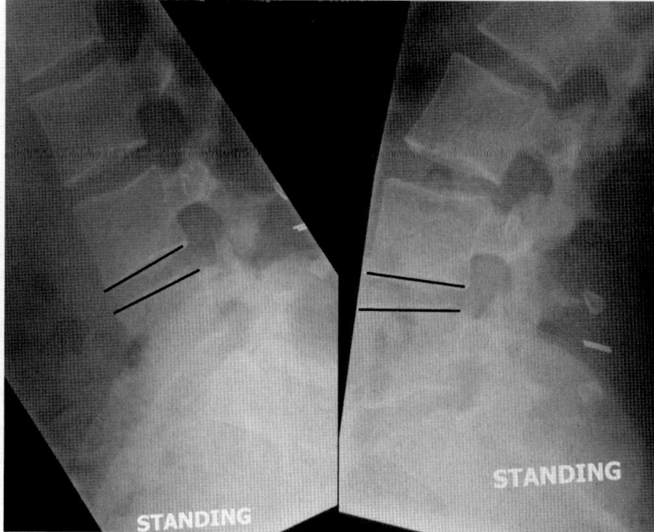


■ **FIGURE 69–14.** The flexion and extension radiographs from case 1 at 1 year following Wallis stabilization. Good movement is retained.

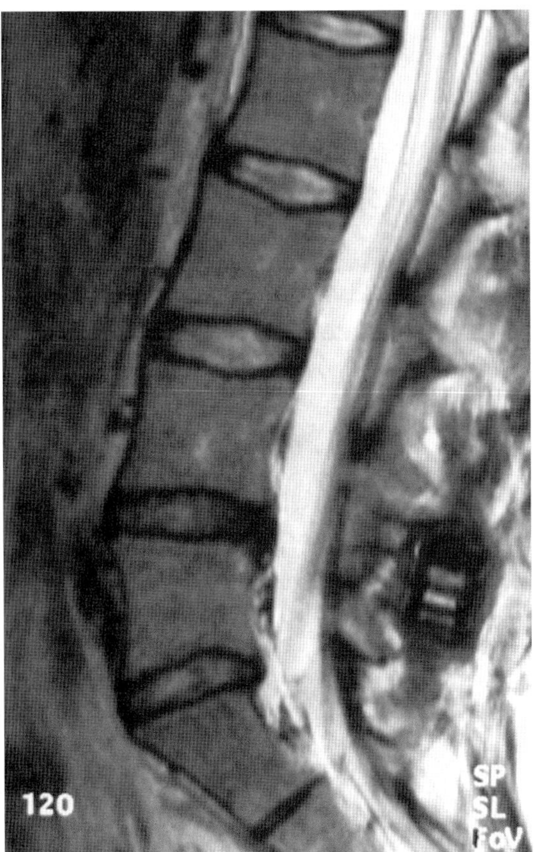


■ **FIGURE 69–15.** The 1-year postoperative magnetic resonance imaging scan for case 1. The disc height remains well preserved, and there has been some improvement in T2 signal return from the disc nucleus.

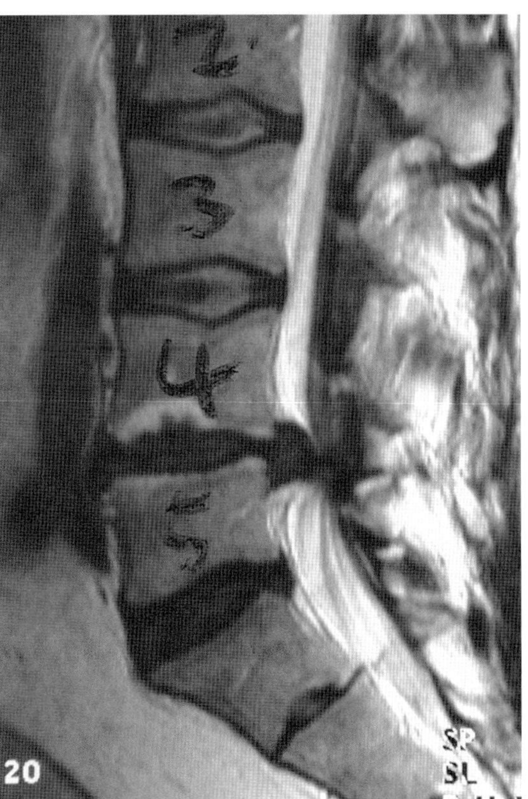


■ **FIGURE 69–16.** The preoperative magnetic resonance imaging scan for case 2, a 43-year-old man with a combination of sciatica and back pain.

40% was back pain. Discectomy alone would undoubtedly have helped with his sciatica, but what should be done to alleviate his back pain and the risk that this would deteriorate further? A fusion procedure, given the changes at L5-S1, would probably have had to extend over two levels. Much less invasive, the Wallis procedure allowed support and stability to be provided to the more damaged L4-L5 level. Because movement is retained, no additional stress is transferred to the adjacent L5-S1 level. The patient returned to light work at 4 weeks and normal duties at 8 weeks. His leg pain resolved. At 3 months, his back pain VAS had improved from 50 to 15, and he stopped all analgesia. His preoperative and 3-month postoperative radiographs are shown for comparison in Figure 69–17. Note the improvement in posterior disc height, illustrating how the implant off-loads the disc, and the lack of any kyphosis. Over the subsequent months the patient's improvement continued and was sustained at his most recent 2-year review.

## Top-Off—Support and Protection for Levels Adjacent to a Fusion

Fusion is still the mainstay of treatment for severe intractable back pain resulting from more advanced degenerative disease. However, the surgeon is frequently presented with a quandary following detailed investigation of the lumbar spine. The patient may have one level of advanced degenerative disease that is confirmed as the principal pain source on provocative discography, but with moderate and perhaps minimally symptomatic changes (on MRI and provocative discography) present at an adjacent level. Should the patient be denied surgery in view of the risk of accelerated adjacent-level disease? Or should the fusion be extended to include the additional level, with the increased risks and additional morbidity that this implies? Wallis stabilization offers a viable alternative, protecting the motion segment from the additional stresses adjacent to a fused segment.

The MRI shown on the left in Figure 69–18 is from a 55-year-old light manual worker who had 2 years of significant back pain, representing about 70% of his overall problem; the remaining 30% was left-sided sciatica.

The author considered that fusion was required at L5-S1. The disc protrusion at L4-L5 was responsible for his sciatica, but there was concern about undertaking discectomy alone at L4-L5 and leaving the level exposed above a fusion. To avoid extending the fusion to L4-L5, Wallis stabilization was undertaken at this level at the same time as a posterior lumbar interbody fusion (PLIF) at L5-S1. The patient made a good recovery, returning to light duties after 4 months. At 1 year, he reported mild intermittent low back pain. His VAS improved from 75 to 10 and his ODI from 54 to 15. At 2 years, he felt that his back was "no longer a problem." His radiographs and MRIs at that stage are shown in the center and on the right in Figure 69–18.

The Wallis Stabilization System also provides a simple and minimally invasive method of addressing symptomatic adjacent-

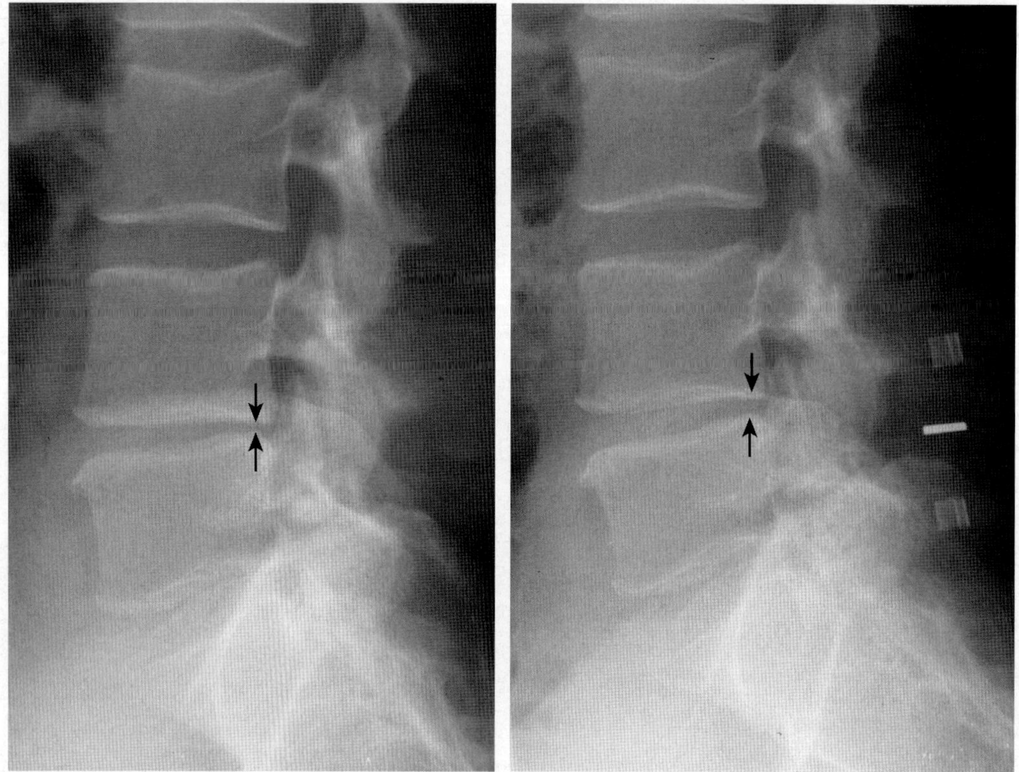

■ **FIGURE 69–17.** The preoperative and 3-month postoperative lateral radiographs for case 2. Following Wallis stabilization, the posterior disc height has been improved, suggesting that the disc has been off-loaded. Note also that the implant does not induce kyphosis at the instrumented level.

level disease that develops following a previous fusion but should not be used if there are advanced changes, marked disc narrowing or more than a minor degenerative spondylolisthesis (≤3 mm). However, in more moderate but nonetheless significantly symptomatic adjacent-level disease, the Wallis Stabilization System provides a minimally invasive means of addressing the condition without recourse to the much more destructive alternative of explanting the prior instrumentation and extending the fusion to an additional level, an option that inevitably risks yet further problems at the next level up in future years.

## Distraction Decompression—Central, Lateral Recess, and Foraminal Stenosis

The role of interspinous process spacers in improving the capacity of the spinal canal has been shown in several studies, achieving an

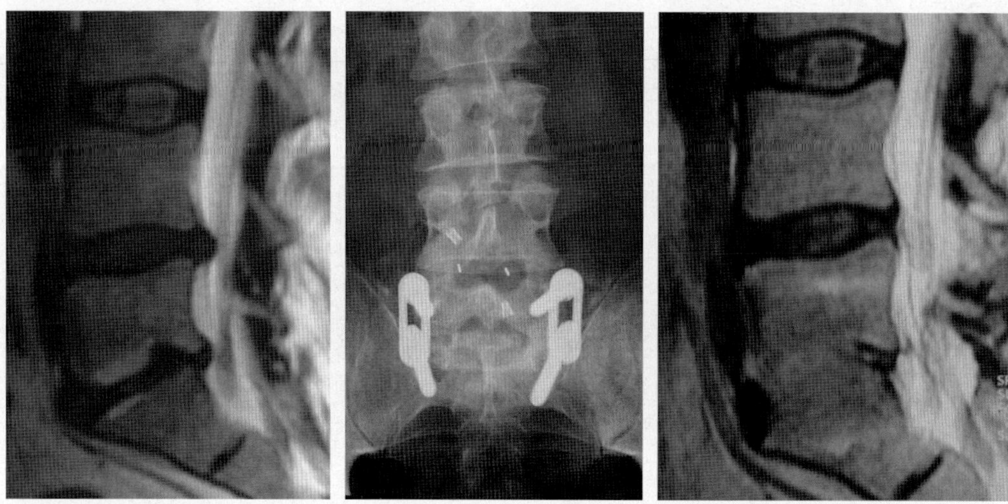

■ **FIGURE 69–18.** On the left are the preoperative magnetic resonance imaging (MRI) scans of a 55-year-old light manual worker (case 3) with a combination of low back pain and left sciatica. PLIF at L5-S1 was undertaken, together with discectomy and Wallis stabilization at L4-L5. His radiographs and MRI scans at 2-year review are shown (*center* and *right*).

increase in the cross-sectional area and diameter of the spinal canal and the width and area of the neural foramina.[7,8] Interspinous process devices may be used alone to achieve a distraction decompression in the lumbar spine, at least in certain cases, without recourse to surgical intrusion into the spinal canal. However, where there is a hard stenosis with facet hypertrophy and osteophyte contributing to neurologic compromise, surgical decompression may still be required. However, even then interspinous process distraction can be used to enhance surgical decompression, particularly in areas where access may be more restricted.

Surgical decompression is perhaps most reliably and safely performed after division and reflection (for later repair) of the supraspinous ligament and clearance of the interspinous ligament and the central ligamentum flavum. The spinous processes can then be spread apart, allowing access to the lateral recess and neural foramina. This technique precludes the use of unconstrained floating devices such as X-Stop (Kyphon, Inc., Sunnyvale, CA), which rely on the integrity of the supraspinous ligament but is an integral part of the procedure of Wallis Stabilization System, which does not depend on constraint by the supraspinous ligament. The stability provided by the Wallis Stabilization System is likely to confer additional benefits because stenosis is, in many cases, an adaptive response to instability in the motion segment.

## DISCUSSION

### Safety

The Wallis Stabilization System exposes the patient to very little additional risk or operative morbidity compared with procedures such as discectomy or decompression. Also, the implant is certainly far less destructive and invasive than alternative procedures such as fusion or TDR. The system does away with the need for pedicle screw fixation, reducing both the risk and seriousness of any complications. Pedicle screws are a significant cause of complications in posterior fusion procedures.[9,10] Dynamic stabilization systems that rely on pedicle screws, such as Graf ligamentoplasty and Dynesys, have significant rates of screw loosening and screw breakage,[11] as well as other screw-related complications. This is not surprising because in such systems, the screws will continue to be subjected to repetitive loading over many years. Dynesys may overcome some of the problems seen with Graf ligamentoplasty, but the Dynesys interpedicular blockers may be insufficiently flexible to prevent adjacent-level degeneration.[12,13] Revision of pedicle screw–based dynamic stabilization systems can be very challenging when there is screw loosening or breakage. In contrast, it will be appreciated that with the Wallis Stabilization System, even were structural failure of the implant to occur (which in fact is almost unknown), the failure mode is safe and does not compromise any options, including a revision Wallis procedure or some alternative surgery.

### Clinical Benefit

Clinical success in any surgical technique for low back pain is determined primarily by patient selection and accurate identification of a focal and treatable pain source. In comparison, the selection of a specific form of surgical technology is probably of much less importance. However, the Wallis technique appears to be very effective in providing clinical benefit, as shown by the significant improvement in VAS pain scores in the multicenter study patients and by the marked reduction in analgesic use. An improvement in the VAS score of at least 50% was seen in 93% of patients and overall the VAS scores improved from 77 preoperatively to 12 at 1 year.

It is interesting to compare these results with those achieved with other treatment options. The gold standard is often regarded as fusion (although many now would question this rather lofty status). In the landmark study by Fritzell et al[14] comparing lumbar fusion to conservative treatment for chronic low back pain, the VAS values for those undergoing fusion operations dropped from a preoperative value of 64 to 30 at 1 year. In the conservative treatment arm, the VAS was reduced from 63 to 55 at 1 year. Different fusion techniques were compared by Kim et al.[15] In the different groups, the VAS pain scores decreased from 75 preoperatively to between 17 and 20 at 1 year. As an alternative to fusion, TDR is increasingly popular, providing outcomes that appear to be at least as good but at an earlier stage and with quicker functional recovery. Blumenthal et al[16] compared TDR and anterior lumbar interbody fusion in symptomatic degenerative disc disease. The mean preoperative VAS pain score was 72 in both groups and this improved to 33 at 1 year in the TDR group and to 40 in the anterior lumber interbody fusion (ALIF) group. In this study, among those considered to have been successfully treated, 64% of the TDR patients and 80% the fusion patients described their analgesic use at 1 year as "frequent" or "sometimes." Only 38% of the patients who received the Wallis Stabilization System had the same level of analgesic use at 1 year. Facet joint arthrosis may compromise the results with TDR and was an exclusion criteria for TDR investigational studies.[16] Some TDR designs may contribute to facet joint changes. In contrast, interspinous stabilization systems such as the Wallis Stabilization System may relieve facet joint pain.[6] Results for VAS pain scores are also available for Dynesys stabilization. Stoll et al[13] reported that pain scores improved from 74 at baseline to 31 after an average 38 months. In a separate series, low back pain VAS improved from 70 preoperatively to 47 at 2 years.[17]

Clinical benefit in terms of improvement in quality of life is best reflected by the SF-36 scores. The Wallis device's therapeutic success in this area was once again seen to be very good in the multicenter study. The postoperative values at 2 years were no different to a comparable normal population. Again, this can be compared with a further study of patients undergoing one of four different fusion techniques.[18] Their preoperative physical component scores (PCS) were 25 (possible score of 100), similar to the Wallis preoperative PCS (28/100). At 1 year, improvement in the PCS ranged from 8.4 to 12.6 points. In comparison, the PCS of the patients with the Wallis Stabilization System improved by more than 19 points at 1 year.

The most commonly used and best-validated measure of functional disability is, of course, the ODI. In recent investigational studies of total TDR, one criterion for clinical success has been an improvement in ODI scores of 25%.[16] By this standard, the Wallis stabilization technique achieved clinical success in 93% of patients. Once again, the Wallis technique may be compared with other techniques. In the study of four fusion techniques cited earlier,[18] the preoperative ODI scores of between 46 and 56 improved at 1 year by between 16 and 23 points. The Wallis study patients had similar preoperative ODI scores, but at 1 year, their average improvement was more than 40 points. This apparently better functional outcome is likely to be related to the less invasive nature of the surgery, the preservation of the posterior paravertebral musculature, and, most particularly, the maintenance of motion at the instrumented level.

Caution must clearly be exercised in drawing conclusions from comparison of such diverse studies in which many factors are uncontrolled. Nonetheless, Wallis stabilization clearly stands up well to comparison with alternative techniques and can be achieved with simpler surgical techniques and far less risk to the patient.

### Adjacent-Segment Preservation

The finite element model predicts that the Wallis system should not affect the mechanical loading of adjacent segments. Therefore, there should be a much lower risk of symptomatic adjacent-level disease compared with the rate seen in fusion procedures. The evidence available thus far confirms this to be the case. In a series of lumbar fusion patients with more than 5 years' follow-up, Gillet[19] reported a 20% rate of revision surgery to extend the arthrodesis to adjacent segments. At levels adjacent to fusion, Ghiselli et al[20] reported a reoperation rate of 16.5% at 5 years and 36.1% at 10 years in 215 patients who had undergone posterior lumbar arthrodesis. The latter figure is almost double the rate of all revisions for all causes combined in the long-term retrospective Wallis study, at a follow-up interval of between 10 and 18 years. This clearly suggests a much lower rate of adjacent-level degeneration.

### Potential Disc Restoration

In discussing the first illustrative case, it was noted that 1 year following Wallis stabilization, there had been a notable improvement in the T2 signal return from the disc compared with the preoperative scans. This was not an isolated observation and has been seen in a significant proportion of paired MRIs. This change is likely to reflect the off-loading of the disc, perhaps allowing some rehydration of the nuclear matrix. It is hoped that by restoring more favorable physiologic conditions within the disc, there may be an improvement in cellular function, potentially allowing for some regeneration and repair of the extracellular matrix.

## CONCLUSION

In the treatment of degenerative conditions of the lumbar spine, there has been a palpable void between conservative treatment and the surgical option of spinal fusion. Fusion has been perceived as very invasive and destructive, associated with significant risks, and often rather mediocre outcomes.

There is good evidence now that TDR, in suitable cases, probably represents a better alternative to fusion. However, there remain uncertainties about the long-term viability of this procedure. Although less destructive than fusion, TDR nonetheless has major surgical risks. When complications or failures occur, their management can be very challenging. Both fusion and TDR represent steps that, once taken, cannot be retraced. As such, the void between conservative treatment and surgical intervention has remained wide, with a large number of patients finding neither option very satisfactory.

Wallis dynamic stabilization offers a real alternative for at least a portion of these patients. The results appear to compare favorably with other more radical procedures but can be achieved with minimally invasive surgery. This itself carries major advantages such as quicker recuperation and shorter hospital stay, but there are further important benefits. The risks of the procedure are few and none are very serious. Furthermore, unlike fusion or TDR, the procedure is not an irrevocable step but can be reversed, thus preserving other surgical options should they become necessary.

The Wallis Stabilization System is clearly a valuable addition to the range of surgical techniques available in the treatment of degenerative disorders of the lumbar spine.

## REFERENCES

1. Sénégas J: La ligamentoplastie intervertébrale, alternative à l'arthrodèse dans le traitement des instabilités dégénératives. Acta Orthop Belg 57(suppl I):221–226, 1991.
2. Sénégas J, Vital JM, Pointillart V, Mangione P: Long-term actuarial survivorship analysis of an interspinous stabilization system. Eur Spine J 16(8):1279–1287, 2007.
3. Adams MA, McNally DS, Dolan P: Stress distributions inside intervertebral discs: The effects of age and degeneration. J Bone Joint Surg Br 78:965–972, 1996.
4. Lafage V, Gangnet N, Sénégas J, et al: New interspinous implant evaluation using an in vitro biomechanical study combined with finite element analysis. Spine 32(16):1706–1713, 2007.
5. Swanson KE, Lindsey DP, Hsu KY, et al: The effects of an interspinous implant on intervertebral disc pressures. Spine 28:26–32, 2003.
6. Wiseman CM, Lindsey DP, Fredrick AD, Yerby SA: The effect of an interspinous implant on facet load during extension. Spine 30:903–907, 2005.
7. Richards JC, Majumdar S, Lindsey DP, et al: The treatment mechanism of an interspinous process implant for lumbar neurogenic intermittent claudication. Spine 30:744–749, 2005.
8. Siddiqui M, Nicol M, Karadimas E, et al: The positional magnetic resonance imaging changes in the lumbar spine following insertion of a novel interspinous process distraction device. Spine 30:2677–2682, 2005.
9. Katonis P, Christoforakis J, Kontakis G, et al: Complications and problems related to pedicle screw fixation of the spine. Clin Orthop 41:86–94, 2003.
10. Lonstein JE, Denis F, Perra JH, et al: Complications associated with pedicle screws. J Bone Joint Surg Am 81:1519–1528, 1999.
11. Nockels RP: Dynamic stabilization in the surgical management of painful lumbar spinal disorders. Spine 15(16):S68–S72, 2005.
12. Schnake KJ, Schaeren S, Jeanneret B: Dynamic stabilization in addition to decompression for lumbar spinal stenosis with degenerative spondylolisthesis. Spine 31:442–449, 2006.
13. Stoll TM, Dubois G, Schwarzenbach O: The dynamic neutralization system for the spine: A multi-center study of a novel non-fusion system. Eur Spine J 11(2):S170–S178, 2002.
14. Fritzell P, Hagg O, Wessberg P, Nordwall A: Lumbar fusion versus nonsurgical treatment for chronic low back pain. Spine 26:2521–2532; discussion 2532–2534, 2001.
15. Kim KT, Lee SH, Lee YH, et al: Clinical outcomes of three fusion methods through the posterior approach in the lumbar spine. Spine 31:1351–1357, 2006.

16. Blumenthal S, McAfee PC, Guyer RD, et al: A prospective, randomized, multicenter Food and Drug Administration investigational device exemptions study of lumbar total disc replacement with the CHARITÉ artificial disc versus lumbar fusion, part I: Evaluation of clinical outcomes. Spine 30:1565–1575; discussion E387–E391, 2005.
17. Grob D, Benini A, Junge A, Mannion AF: Clinical experience with the Dynesys semi-rigid fixation system for the lumbar spine: Surgical and patient-oriented outcome in 50 cases after an average of 2 years. Spine 30:324–331, 2005.
18. Glassman S, Gornet MF, Branch C, et al: MOS Short Form 36 and Oswestry Disability Index outcomes in lumbar fusion: A multicenter experience. Spine J 6:21–26, 2006.
19. Gillet P: The fate of the adjacent motion segments after lumbar fusion. J Spinal Disord Tech 16:338–345, 2003.
20. Ghiselli G, Wang JC, Bhatia NN, et al: The fate of the adjacent motion segments after lumbar fusion. J Bone Joint Surg Am 86A:1497–1503, 2004.

CHAPTER 70

# coflex Interspinous Implant for Stabilization of the Lumbar Spine

**Gary L. Lowery, Rudolf Bertagnoli,** and **Robert J. Chomiak**

## KEY POINTS

- The coflex is intended to treat patients suffering from lumbar spinal stenosis.
- The coflex is a nonfusion interspinous process stabilization device.
- The coflex has up to 11 years of clinical history.
- The coflex is functionally dynamic, is compressible in extension, and allows flexion.
- The coflex has been implanted in more than 15,000 patients worldwide.

Spinal stenosis is any type of narrowing of the central spinal canal or intervertebral foramina.[1] Symptoms most often occur in patients 50 to 70 years of age. On initial presentation, patients may complain of low back pain, buttock pain, or trochanteric and posterior thigh pain that may radiate to the knee and occasionally into the feet.[2] These symptoms may be relieved by sitting or lying down in the earlier stages of the disease. Symptoms may be exacerbated by walking, known as neurogenic claudication, especially downhill.[3] Although plain radiographs, computed tomography (CT scan), magnetic resonance imaging (MRI), and other studies are useful in confirming the diagnosis of spinal stenosis, a careful clinical history is most often the means for establishing the diagnosis.[4] Spinal stenosis may be congenital, but it is most often the result of degenerative changes to the spine, typically beginning in the nucleus pulposus. As the disc degenerates and narrows, the vertebrae become more closely positioned to one another, which may result in ligament laxity and lead to intersegmental instability.[5] These changes lead to osteophyte formation as the body attempts to restabilize the unstable spinal segment. These circumferential osteophytes, together with loss of disc space height, contribute to narrowing of the neural foramen. As the degenerative changes progress, the ligamentum flavum shortens and buckles, producing thickening, which may further contribute to central spinal stenosis.[2] Finally, degenerative changes to the facet joints with secondary osteophyte formation may add a component of lateral recess stenosis. This cascade often results in antero- and retrolisthesis (sagittal plane deformity) and degenerative scoliosis (coronal deformity).

## DESCRIPTION OF THE DEVICE

The coflex device was invented by Dr. Jacques Samani in 1994 and has been in continuous use since that time outside the United States. Initially, the product was known as the Interspinous "U" and was marketed in 1995 by Fixano SAS (Péronnas, France), with ownership being transferred to Paradigm Spine, LLC (New York, NY), in 2005. The device was renamed coflex for "cofunctioning of flexion and extension." The design of the product has remained substantially the same during its entire history, except for tightening of tolerances. The design and materials have not changed, although two new sizes have been added.

After an extensive 589-patient international multicenter retrospective study, the coflex device was promoted to address the clinical needs of spinal stenosis patients by providing nonfusion stabilization of the affected level(s) after microsurgical decompression. The coflex is an interspinous functionally dynamic implant, and it consists of a single, U-shaped component fabricated from medical grade titanium alloy ($Ti_6Al_4V$), a material with a long history of safe use in implantable orthopaedic products. In clinical use, this U is positioned horizontally, with its apex oriented anteriorly under the facets; the two long arms of the U portion are parallel to the long axis of the spinal processes, and these bone-facing surfaces are ridged to provide resistance to migration. A photograph of the implant is provided in Figure 70–1.

A set of two wings extends vertically from the superior long arm of the U, with a second set of wings extending below the inferior long arm. Both sets of wings have serrated bone-facing surfaces, which are designed to secure the coflex to the superior and inferior spinous processes through crimping. In addition, the opposing wing surfaces are offset such that they allow two contiguous levels to be stabilized. This design allows for a degree of mobility of the spinous process in flexion while preventing anterior or posterior migration. The device is compressible in extension, and spinal balance becomes normalized in the upright position. Facet pressures are off-loaded at the index level owing to a slight permanent facet distraction resulting from a deeper insertion than for any other interspinous device. This also maintains foraminal

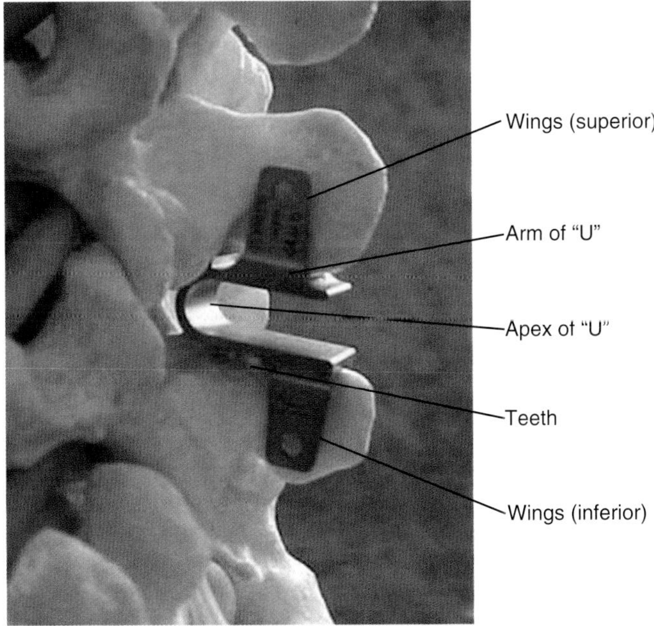


■ **FIGURE 70–1.** coflex interspinous stabilization device.

distraction. As the coflex is functionally dynamic, posterior intradiscal pressures are decreased at the index level. The adjacent levels appear not to be adversely affected in their biomechanical parameters. Rotational mobility may possibly be further constrained initially by crimping the wings.

## INDICATIONS

The following are the currently promoted indications for the coflex, as exemplified in an ongoing U.S. FDA IDE study. The patient may have, but is not required to have, the following for inclusion in clinical use:

1. Spinal deformity (stenosis, listhesis, or scoliosis)
   a. Moderate to severe central spinal stenosis
   b. Facet hypertrophy and subarticular recess stenosis at the affected level(s)
   c. Foraminal stenosis at the affected level(s)
   d. Up to stable Grade I degenerative spondylolisthesis (Meyerding classification) or equivalent retrolisthesis as determined by flexion/extension x-ray study
   e. Mild lumbar scoliosis (Cobb angle up to 25 degrees)
2. Radiographic confirmation of no angular or translatory instability of the spine at index or adjacent levels (instability as defined by White and Panjabi: sagittal plane translation >4.5 mm or 15% or sagittal plane rotation >15 degrees at L1-L2, L2-L3, and L3-L4; >20 degrees at L4-L5 based on standing flexion/extension x-rays)
3. Age between 40 and 80 years
4. At least 6 months of prior conservative care, including at least one epidural injection, without adequate and sustained symptom relief
5. Neurogenic claudication as defined by leg/buttocks or groin pain that can be relieved by flexion such as sitting in a chair
6. Oswestry Low Back Pain Disability Questionnaire score of at least 20/50 (40%)
7. Visual Analog Scale (VAS) back pain score of at least 50 mm on a 100-mm scale
8. Appropriate candidate for treatment using posterior surgical approach

## CONTRAINDICATIONS

1. More than two vertebral levels requiring surgical decompression
2. Prior fusion, implantation of a total disc replacement, complete laminectomy, or implantation of an interspinous process device at any lumbar level
3. Radiographically compromised vertebral bodies at any lumbar level(s) caused by current or past trauma or tumor (e.g., compression fracture)
4. Severe facet hypertrophy that requires extensive bone removal which would cause instability
5. Isthmic spondylolisthesis or spondylolysis (pars fracture)
6. Degenerative lumbar scoliosis (Cobb angle >25 degrees)
7. Disc herniation at any lumbar level requiring surgical intervention
8. Osteopenia: A screening questionnaire for osteopenia (SCORE, Simple Calculated Osteoporosis Risk Estimation) will be used to screen patients who require a dual-emission x-ray absorptiometry (DEXA) bone mineral density measurement. If DEXA is required, exclusion will be defined as a DEXA bone density measured T score at or below −1.0 (The World Health Organization definition of osteopenia).
9. Back or leg pain of unknown etiology
10. Axial back pain only, with no leg, buttock, or groin pain
11. History of significant peripheral neuropathy
12. Significant peripheral vascular disease (e.g., with diminished dorsalis pedis or posterior tibial pulse)
13. Unremitting back pain in *any* position
14. Morbid obesity (defined as a body mass index >40)
15. Pregnant or interested in becoming pregnant in the next 3 years
16. Known allergy to titanium, titanium alloys, or MRI contrast agents
17. Active or chronic infection—systemic or local
18. Chronically taking medications or any drug known to potentially interfere with bone or soft tissue healing (e.g., steroids), not including a medrol dose pack
19. Uncontrolled diabetes
20. Known history of Paget's disease, osteomalacia, or any other metabolic bone disease (excluding osteopenia, which is addressed above)
21. Rheumatoid arthritis or other autoimmune diseases
22. Known or documented history of communicable disease, including AIDS, HIV, active hepatitis
23. Active malignancy: a patient with a history of any invasive malignancy (except nonmelanoma skin cancer), unless he/she has been treated with curative intent and there have been no clinical signs or symptoms of the malignancy for at least 5 years. Patients with a primary bony tumor are excluded as well.

24. Cauda equina syndrome, defined as neural compression causing neurogenic bowel (rectal incontinence) or bladder (bladder retention or incontinence) dysfunction
25. Fixed and complete motor, sensory, or reflex deficit

## SCIENTIFIC TESTING RESULTS AND CLINICAL OUTCOMES

### Mechanical Testing

The preclinical testing of the coflex was designed to evaluate all the relevant loading conditions that may affect the device. The worst-case device size was used in all tests, which is generally the smallest size (8 mm), except as otherwise noted. The key areas of the device with respect to mechanical strength are the interface between the wings and the U-shaped body of the implant, and the apex of the U, as illustrated in Figure 70–1.

With respect to the wing/U interface, there is no difference in dimensions across device sizes that would affect mechanical strength. With respect to the U, all devices have the same radius of curvature. The smallest device size has the minimum thickness at the dorsal aspect and will therefore sustain maximum stresses when loaded in axial compression. It should be noted that the size and geometry of the superior and inferior teeth, as well as the size and geometry of the lateral wings, are the same for all implant sizes.

The design and dimensions of the coflex remained unchanged. The current device is manufactured via a milling process, and the prior version of the device was made via wire-electrical discharge machining (EDM) manufacturing. In addition to ensuring that the coflex provides adequate mechanical strength to withstand worst-case physiologic loading conditions, these tests were designed to verify that the milled coflex was not significantly worse than the wire-EDM coflex with respect to the property being tested.

### Compression Testing

Compression testing of the coflex was performed under both static and dynamic loading conditions. With respect to the dynamic testing, the coflex is not secured to the bone of the spinous process; rather, the bone can move between the crimped wings in general without exerting any significant tensile load on the device when the spine is in flexion. However, in extension, the U-shaped portion of the device imposes a limitation between the spinous processes, and this portion of the device is therefore dynamically compressed. Thus, dynamic compression fatigue of the U-shaped portion of the device was performed to assess cyclic loading in flexion-extension.

It should also be noted that the material ($Ti_6Al_4V$) is relatively insensitive to frequency for purposes of fatigue testing. The cyclic plastic straining of alloys near the fatigue limit or near the threshold of fatigue crack growth is limited. Therefore, plastic strain rates are low, even at high loading frequencies. Thus, it was concluded that cycling $Ti_6Al_4V$ at frequencies less than 15 Hz would not alter the material properties of the metal.

#### Static Compression

The purpose of this test was to measure the static compressive strength of the coflex to ensure that it can withstand the worst-case compressive loads anticipated in clinical use. Only the U portion of the device was tested in static compression to permit direct application of compressive force to the long arms of the U.

The results demonstrated that the mean yield force of the coflex implant was 239 N.

#### Dynamic Compression

The purpose of this test was to determine the maximum load the coflex can withstand for a run-out of 10 million cycles. Only the U portion of the device was tested in cyclic compression to permit direct application of compressive force to the long arms of the U. The coflex devices survived a maximum load of 150 N to run-out.

For comparative analysis, the loading conditions of the spinous process on the coflex device were derived based on an independent digitized radiographic analysis of dynamic flexion-extension x-rays (>200 patients). This analysis indicated that the median load on the spinous process in extension is 45.8 N. Thus, the endurance limit of the coflex demonstrates that it can withstand approximately three times the expected loads exerted on the spinous process in vivo for 10 million cycles.

### Torsional Analysis (Wing Bending)

To assess the mechanical performance of the coflex in torsion, it was determined that the key design feature of the device in torsion is in the wings where they provide resistance to rotation of the spinous processes and are affected by a perpendicular load directed on the wing.

#### Static Torsion Testing

Static torsion testing on the coflex was not performed. Only the wings are expected to bear any load when the spine is in axial rotation. Owing to the low amount of axial rotation in the lumbar spine, it is expected that the amount of loading that will be seen on these wings is also very low. However, two tests were performed: a dynamic test placing a perpendicularly dynamic load on a wing and a biomechanical analysis evaluating the coflex in worst-case bending modes.

#### Torsion Fatigue Testing

The purpose of this test was to determine the maximum torsional load the coflex can withstand for a run-out of 10 million cycles. The coflex device survived a maximum load of 75 N to run-out.

### Finite Element Analysis and Mechanical Evaluation of Physiologic Loading on coflex

When evaluating the loading conditions of the coflex, one must consider the loading of the apex of the U because of its positioning near the physiologic loading of the facets. A finite element analysis (FEA) and a static compression test evaluating the stress on the coflex when a load is placed near the apex of the U were performed.

This FEA model was validated in the load deformation analysis to the static compression testing. The stresses observed increase significantly. In the FEA model, the resultant load observed for the size 8 mm coflex was 717 N. This load is much higher than those seen physiologically (400 N) for the entire posterior column.

The static compression test was performed for comparison by placing a load approximately 8 mm from the apex of the U portion of the coflex. This loading condition was set to mimic the loads placed on the spine by the posterior elements, such as the facets. When a load was placed toward the apex of the U, the yield load was approximately 1,212 N. This load greatly exceeds the loads cited in the literature and is the quoted axial load on the entire spine in the upright position.

### Biomechanical Wing Test

Biomechanical testing was performed to determine the worst-case loads exerted on the wings of the implant. Strain gauges were placed at five locations in the device (one on each side of each wing, and another in the arch of the U), and then the coflex devices were implanted in cadaveric lumbar spines. Each specimen was then articulated in flexion-extension, lateral bending, and rotation to determine the maximum forces exerted on the wings. The tests were designed to produce a 7.5 Nm external moment in each mode, which was based on prior testing in the same laboratory, indicating that this represents a worst-case in vivo moment. The results demonstrated that under these test conditions, the largest forces exerted on the wings were in lateral bending. However, even in lateral bending with an external moment of 7.5 Nm, the maximum wing-bending moment was only 0.42 Nm, and the maximum force on the wing was only 42 N. In axial rotation, the maximum wing-bending moment was only 0.26 Nm, and the maximum force on the wing was 26 N. In flexion-extension, the maximum wing-bending moment was only 0.16 Nm, and the maximum force was 16 N. Thus, the endurance limit of 75 N provides adequate assurance that the coflex can withstand the worst-case moments that may be applied to the device in vivo. When comparing the resulting loads seen in the study, specifically those in axial rotation, an endurance limit of 75 N at 10 million cycles is more than a 2.7 factor of safety.

### Wear Characteristics of the coflex

The coflex device consists of one piece of milled titanium alloy without any articulating surfaces. This design eliminates the possibility of fretting corrosion and the generation of wear debris. Therefore, in vitro wear testing is not warranted for the coflex.

### Biomechanical Evaluation of the Effect of the coflex on Range of Motion

Biomechanical testing was performed in a series of tests on cadaveric specimens to assess the impact of the coflex on spinal segment motion in flexion-extension, lateral bending, axial rotation, and compression.[6] The following testing conditions were evaluated sequentially in each of eight cadaveric spine specimens: (1) the intact spine, (2) the partially destabilized spine (resection of all ligaments, ligamentum flavum, facet capsules, and bilateral 50% resection of inferior facets), (3) the partially destabilized spine then implanted with coflex, then (4) the complete destabilization of the spine via total laminectomy (coflex removal), and finally (5) the completely destabilized spine restabilized with pedicle screw fixation.

In the first test, for purposes of characterizing the effect of the coflex on motion, eight cadaveric specimens (L4-L5) were tested to represent a range of potential anatomic presentations. The center of rotation was established as part of the test set up to minimize off-axis bending, and the specimens were preconditioned via dynamic compressive loading for 1,000 cycles at 500 N. After determining the center of rotation, compression (900 N at 0.25 cm/minute), flexion-extension (±12 Nm), lateral bending (±12 Nm), and axial rotation (±9 Nm) were applied to each cadaveric spine under a 600-N preload. Each specimen and device was then tested in each mode three times, and a load-deformation curve was generated.

The results of this test demonstrated that the coflex principally serves to stabilize motion in flexion-extension and initially in axial rotation. In each mode, the motion permitted by the coflex was normalized to the amount of motion permitted by the intact spine.

Similar results were observed in axial rotation, with a significant increase in the range of motion observed after partial destabilization, but restoration of near-normal rotational motion following implantation of the coflex. Because the coflex device is located centrally between the spinous processes, it is not designed to provide any significant limitation on lateral bending, which was confirmed by the results of the cadaveric testing.

### In Vivo Loading Environment of the coflex

The coflex is intended to be implanted with the superior and inferior wings facing the sides of the cranial and caudal spinous processes, respectively. The apex of the U is inserted in line with the facets and leads to a slight distraction of the facets.

The loads exerted on the coflex in vivo are applied initially at the apex of the U at the level of the facets and to the arms of the U in extension (and the wings at the contacting interfaces with the cranial and caudal spinous processes). Therefore, relatively little load is expected to be exerted on the spinous process, as the majority of the load on the lumbar spine is carried by the intervertebral disc and the facets.

In flexion, the loads on the spinous processes are generally expected to be reduced, as flexion causes the spinous processes to separate further. If bony ingrowth or crimping causes the coflex to become fixed to both the upper and lower spinous processes, the arms of the U could be separated slightly in flexion, placing the device in tension. As each spinous process moves between the wings in flexion, low bending forces are also applied to the wings. However, in extension, the spinous processes move closer together, increasing the compressive load that is exerted on the U. When the coflex is properly inserted, low loads are exerted on the spinous processes generally. This fact is coupled with the limitations on the extent of compression that are imposed anatomically by the facets. The typical compressive loads on the coflex in extension are not expected to exceed approximately 45.8 N as extrapolated from direct in vivo x-ray measurements in more than 200 patients.

In lateral bending, the spinous processes transmit load to the coflex via contact with the wings. Direct measurement of the forces on the device when implanted in cadaveric specimens has been performed using strain gauges. These measurements have demonstrated that even under lateral-bending moments of 7.5 Nm, the degree of force applied to the wings of the coflex is relatively low, averaging approximately 23 N. A maximum bending force on the wing is estimated at 42 N for extreme bending moments of up to 10 Nm and overall very little bending (torsional) load is transmitted to the U. There is no significant "twisting" force at the apex of the U, and instead the wings are designed to bend at the point of attachment to the U arms.

Based on the direct measurement of forces on the device in cadavers, the magnitude of this load under a 7.5-Nm external-bending moment is less than in lateral bending with an average of approximately 16 N (a maximum bending load of 27 N at extreme-bending moments of 10 Nm). The degree of torsional loading transmitted to the U is thus minimal.

Maximum compressive loading of the device is expected to occur when the spine is in full extension, and maximum-bending loads will occur in lateral bending. The mechanical testing, together with the extensive prior clinical experience with the device, demonstrates that it can withstand the worst-case physiologic loads that are expected to occur in vivo without permanent deformation or breakage of the device and without fracture of the spinous processes.

### In Vivo Deflection and Loading Analysis

To assess the maximum load that may be exerted on the device in vivo, a comprehensive review of the degree of implant deflection was performed by an independent Radiographic Analysis Core Laboratory (Medical Metrics, Inc., Houston, TX) using radiographs obtained in the retrospective study. Review of the neutral, extension, and flexion radiographs for the 209 subjects with stenosis, which was the population eligible for participation in the U.S. IDE study, was performed. The collected ranges were then inserted into a validated finite element analysis. Based on this analysis, a load/deformation curve was developed. Medical Metrics, Inc. took the validated FEA and applied the formula to the retrospective data patients. The median load in extension was 45.8 N. This demonstrated that the maximum estimated load exerted on the implant was less than the 150 N endurance limit found for 97.1% of the implants, with only one case (0.5%) in which the calculated load on the coflex device in extension was greater than the reported yield load for the device (239 N). This load deformation analysis demonstrates that the compressive static and fatigue strength of the coflex is adequate to withstand the worst-case dynamic loading conditions that are expected in clinical use.

In addition, Medical Metrics, Inc. conducted an analysis of the range of motion of the coflex and adjacent levels in 180 patients. This number of patients was based on the original cohort of patients (209). The analyses determined that the range of motion for one-level coflex implantations at preoperative time was 4.3 degrees, 2.1 degrees at 1 year, 2.3 degrees at 2 years, and 2.1 degrees beyond the 2-year point. The range of motion (flexion-extension) for the two-level patients was 4.0 degrees at the preoperative time, 2.1 degrees at 1 year, 1.6 degrees at 2 years, and 3.4 degrees beyond the 2-year point.

## CLINICAL PRESENTATION AND EVALUATION

The company has gathered retrospective data on the clinical outcomes of 429 coflex patients, as well as contemporaneous clinical and x-ray data on the same cohort of patients. These patients represent a portion of the 589 patients treated with the coflex at four clinical sites from which data were available. Of these 429 patients, 209 patients were treated for spinal stenosis at a single level or two adjacent levels, a population that is substantially similar to the population for the protocol that is the subject of the IDE study. In this population, the coflex demonstrates a clear record of safety as well as preliminary evidence of efficacy.

Patient data for the retrospective study were gathered via a questionnaire that captured the following information: gender, preoperative diagnosis, preoperative clinical evaluation, previous conservative therapy, previous spinal therapies, concomitant medical conditions, operative data, radiographic and diagnostic tests, postoperative tests, postoperative clinical examination, and qualitative postoperative x-ray analysis. All patients from the four sites who were more than 6 months past operation were given the option of participating in this data collection, which the company believes helped to minimize selection bias. Of the 589 patients identified by the surgeons, 429 (73%) responded and agreed to participate. All patients were asked to return for contemporaneous history, clinical examination, and dynamic x-rays. These results were compared to available patient records and pre-existing x-rays pertaining to their quality of life and implant survivorship.

The patient case report forms and x-rays from 429 patients were reviewed by an independent orthopaedic spine surgeon who identified 209 patients with spinal stenosis. The remaining patients were treated for various indications such as "topping-off" of spinal fusions, use of the device with other spinal implants, disc herniation, and other diagnoses.

Table 70–1 evaluates patients' clinical success outcomes, satisfactions, and adverse events relative to the three time intervals of follow-up. For the follow-up groups of 6 to 12, >12 to 24, and >24

**TABLE 70–1. Composite Pertinent Patient Outcomes Over Time***

| Postoperative Outcomes ($n$ = 209) | Overall | Follow-Up Time Intervals | | |
|---|---|---|---|---|
| | | $n$ = 72<br>6 to 12 mo | $n$ = 69<br>>12 to 24 mo | $n$ = 68<br>>24 mo |
| Improvement in moderate or severe preoperative low back pain | 75% | 73% | 82% | 72% |
| Improvement in preoperative claudication | 87% | 90% | 85% | 87% |
| Improvement in preoperative walking distance | 74% | 83% | 75% | 66% |
| Patient satisfaction | 89% | 90% | 91% | 88% |
| "Would have surgery again" | 92% | 96% | 90% | 91% |
| Adverse events ($n$ = 17) | 8.1% | 8.1% | 0% | 0% |
| "Device-related" issues ($n$ = 7) | 3.3% | 1.9% | 0.5% | 0.5% |

*Percentage calculations relative to total spinal stenosis population per side.

months the mean follow-up times were 8.8 ± 1.5, 18.4 ± 1.7, and 53.7 ± 9.4 months, respectively, with the median follow-up times being 9, 19, and 33 months, respectively. Again, no differences were noted between one- and two-level decompressions relative to clinical outcomes, and the incidence of adverse events was low and not different between these two groups. Therefore, Table 70–1 was constructed to see the composite pertinent patient outcomes overall and their relationship over time. Overall, 75% of the patients had improvement in their moderate or severe preoperative low back pain, and this improvement remained constant over time. Claudicatory symptoms improved overall in 87% of the patients and again remained reasonably constant over time. Postoperative walking distance improved overall in 74% of the patients with a slight tapering effect at the longer term follow-up period (a decrease to 66%). This observation could be related to the increasing age/activity of the patient. Patient satisfaction was positive in 89% of the patients overall, and 92% of the patients stated they "would have surgery again." Both of these results remained constant during all three time intervals. Non-device–related adverse events (8.1%) occurred uniquely in only the short-term follow-up group (6–12 months). "Device-related issues" were low (3.3% overall), and although few, the majority were noted less than 13 months postoperatively (2.4%). Only one patient in the long-term follow-up (>24 months) was noted to need a second operation and removal of the U with subsequent conversion to fusion after a fall (no device fracture or deformation, but a new L4-L5 spondylolisthesis).

The retrospective data demonstrated an extremely low incidence of breakage or deformation of the U component, with the primary mode of mechanical failure at the wing (two cases). Wing breakage was noted intraoperatively secondary to opening and closing of the wings with standard surgical pliers.

## OPERATIVE TECHNIQUE

### Preparation

The patient is placed in a prone position on the surgical frame, avoiding hyperlordosis of the spinal segment(s) to be operated on. A neutral position or a slight kyphosis may be advantageous for surgical decompression as well as for the necessary interspinous distraction.

A routine (midline) skin incision is performed. The muscle is sharply dissected lateral to the supraspinous ligament, preserving the entire thickness of the supraspinous ligament. Resection of the supraspinous ligament should be avoided, if possible. If maintenance of the supraspinous ligament is impossible, however, it may be resected. If resection is needed, it should be reconstructed following insertion of the device.

Paraspinal muscles are then stripped off the laminae while preserving the facet capsules. The supraspinous ligament is dissected subperiosteally and preserved as a thick cuff and retracted laterally. If resection is necessary, a small portion of the bony tip can be resected together with the supraspinous ligament. This method will aid in faster healing after reconstruction of the ligament.

Depending on the pathology, a microsurgical unilateral decompression can then be performed, and the supraspinous ligament together with the fascia and muscle from the opposite side can be mobilized. Completion of the microsurgical decompression can then be performed. The interspinous ligament is sacrificed, and any bony overgrowth of the spinous process that may interfere with insertion is resected.

### Microsurgical Decompression

The ligamentum flavum is resected and microsurgical decompression is performed. This procedure includes bilateral laminotomy or hemilaminectomy with appropriate resection of overgrown facets and foraminotomies as needed in order to relieve all points of neural compression.

### Implant Site Preparation

Trials of the device are utilized to define appropriate implant size. Selection of the appropriate implant size is essential in obtaining proper function of the device and good clinical results.

The trial instrument is placed to evaluate proper contact with spinous process and the amount of interspinous distraction. Some bony resection of the spinous process may be needed to ensure proper contact of the implant.

Distraction is considered to be appropriate to prevent any settling of the interspinous distance after successful decompression of the spinal stenosis. The appropriate sized implant will fit securely on the spinous processes and lead to a 1- to 2-mm slight distraction of the facet joints. To ensure proper depth of implant insertion, a small portion of the laminar surface may need partial resurfacing before implantation of the device (Fig. 70–2).

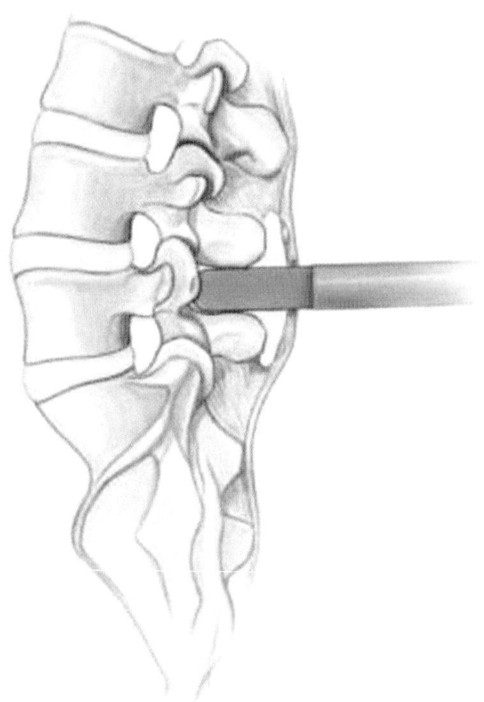

■ **FIGURE 70–2.** Implant site preparation.

### Implant Insertion

First, the surgeon must determine if the wings have to be bent open at all by holding the coflex over the spinous processes and checking the width. The wings do not need to be opened if it is felt that in the process of insertion, they will make good bony contact and be placed deep into the interspinous space, ensuring appropriate distraction.

Bending pliers are available to bend the wings open prior to application while avoiding any damage to the spinous processes during implant insertion. If the spinous processes are felt to be too thick, or will impede safe insertion, special pliers are utilized for controlled bending of the implant wings. Use only the special wing-bending pliers provided. The wings are bent open (or crimped together) until both sets of wings are approximately 2 mm smaller in width than the receiving spinous processes. The bending result should correlate with the actual thickness of the spinous processes and allow easy implantation without any stress on the adjacent spinous processes. The implant is introduced via impaction utilizing a mallet. Proper depth is determined if a beaded tip probe can be passed freely leaving 3 to 4 mm of separation from the dura (Fig. 70–3). If the implant is not seated appropriately, further resurfacing or slightly more impaction force may be utilized. For appropriate bony contact after insertion, additional stability is achieved by crimping the wings, utilizing the coflex crimping pliers. The crimping pliers close the wings in a controlled manner after insertion. It is important to note that crimping has to correlate with the initial bending. After impaction, crimp the implant until the teeth on the contact surface of the wings penetrate into substantia corticalis. Appropriate stability is achieved if surrounding fat tissue starts to squeeze around the wings. In the event that there is wing breakage during the insertion process, the coflex device should be explanted and replaced with a new one. In the event of a spinous process fracture, the coflex should remain explanted.

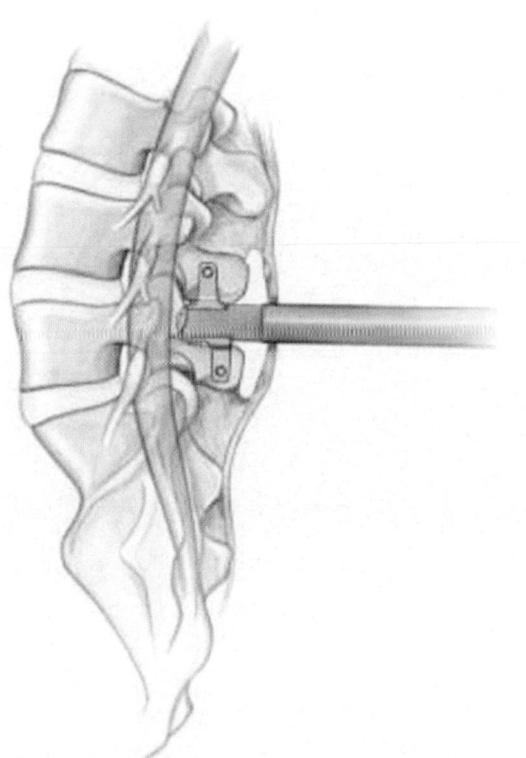

■ **FIGURE 70–3.** Implant insertion.

In the case of ligament reconstruction a figure-of-eight suture can be passed through two bone holes in the superior spinous process and the supraspinous ligament. If, due to Baastrup's disease, the patient has minimal or no supraspinous ligament, tight closure of the muscle and fascia around the spinous processes should be performed. A surgical drain may be placed as per surgeon preference. Paraspinal muscles are reattached to the supraspinous ligament. Skin is closed in the usual manner. Alternatively, the fascia and the supraspinous ligament can be closed in one layer over the spinous processes.

### Double-Level Implantation

If a two-level decompression is mandated, the implants must be sequentially placed to the appropriate depth, avoiding any overlap (contact) of one set of wings on the other. The inferior implant should be inserted first, followed by the superior implant. After appropriate anteroposterior and lateral radiographs are taken intraoperatively, the wings should be crimped.

## POSTOPERATIVE CARE

Compliance with postoperative care is important to the success of the coflex device. A soft corset or brace may be used for patient comfort. The patient should avoid excessive lumbar flexion and extension as well as lifting heavy objects for 6 weeks after surgery. Gradual return to daily living activities and exercise, such as walking, can be initiated as soon as the surgical incision is healed.

## CONCLUSION

The coflex interspinous stabilization device is ideal for spinal stabilization after surgically addressing neural decompression from soft or bony stenosis of the spinal canal. The device is functionally dynamic, is compressible in extension, allows flexion, and increases rotational stability. Insertion is a less invasive, tissue-sparing procedure. The coflex has up to 11 years of clinical history and more than 15,000 implantations worldwide to prove its safety.

## REFERENCES


1. Arnoldi CC, Brodsky AE, Cauchoix J, et al: Lumbar spinal stenosis and nerve root entrapment syndrome: Definition and classification. Clin Orthop 115:4–5, 1976.
2. Yong-Hing K, Kirkaldy-Willis WH: The pathophysiology of degenerative disease of the lumbar spine. Orthop Clin North Am 14:501–503, 1983.
3. Delamarter RB, Howard M: Lumbar spinal stenosis. *In* Hochschular S, Cotler H, Guyer R (eds): Rehabilitation of the Spine, Science and Practice. St. Louis, Mosby, 1993, pp 443–456.
4. Deyo RA, Rainville J, Kent DL: What can the history of physical examination tell us about low back pain? JAMA 268:760–765, 1992.
5. Fast A, Greenbaum M: Degenerative lumbar spinal stenosis. Phys Med Rehabil St Art Rev 9:673–682, 1995.
6. Tsai KJ, Murakami H, Lowery GL, Hutton WC: A biomechanical evaluation of an interspinous device (coflex) used to stabilize the lumbar spine. J Surg Orthop Adv 15(3):167–172, 2006.

CHAPTER 71

# X-STOP Interspinous Process Decompression for Lumbar Spinal Stenosis

**Cary Idler, James F. Zucherman, Kenneth Y. Hsu,** and **Matthew Hannibal**

## KEY POINTS

- The X-STOP, FDA approved November 2005, can be used for neurogenic intermittent claudication at one- or two-level lumbar spinal stenosis.
- The X-STOP preserves the interspinous and supraspinous ligaments.
- The X-STOP preferred approach is performed with local anesthesia as an outpatient procedure.
- The 1-, 2-, and 4-year outcomes are at least as good as those for laminectomy, with lower cost and lower surgical risk.
- The X-STOP can be used in low-grade spondylolisthesis.

The X-STOP (Kyphon, Inc., Sunnyvale, CA), an interspinous process spacer, is a promising surgical treatment alternative for neurogenic intermittent claudication (NIC) caused by lumbar spinal stenosis (LSS). The device provides an unloading distractive force to the stenotic middle column of the motion segment and can relieve claudicatory symptoms of central, lateral, and foraminal stenosis. Other devices currently being tested are suggested for degenerative disc disease, adjacent level syndromes, lumbar spinal stenosis, and herniated disc.[1] Some spacers require either the supraspinous ligament or interspinous ligament to be significantly altered or removed before they can be inserted, and some spacers require the spinous processes themselves to be either modified or shaped. Some spacers are designed to function as stand-alone devices while others incorporate an artificial ligament as an integral part of the design. The artificial ligament helps to limit flexion and it may also decrease the laxity of the motion segment, which could be an important component in treating certain pathologies such as degenerative disc disease. NIC is the most common symptom seen in lumbar spinal stenosis. Patients typically obtain relief with sitting or positions of flexion and are exacerbated with standing or walking. Moreover, elderly patients tend to be osteopenic and at risk for osteoporosis so any shaping or remodeling of the spinous process would reduce bone strength and should be avoided. In fact, care should be taken to avoid decorticating or damaging any bone surrounding the spinous process.

The first interspinous process decompression device approved in the U.S. by the FDA for general use (Nov. 21, 2005) was the X-STOP. It was approved for use in Europe in July 2002. Since then, over 10,000 devices have been implanted. Placement of this device requires preservation of the spinous process and interspinous and supraspinous ligaments. This chapter will describe current treatment options, patient selection, biomechanical studies, the technique for performing interspinous process decompression (IPD) with the X-STOP, as well as outcomes from all clinical, biomechanical, and radiographic studies published to date.

## CURRENT TREATMENT

Treatment for NIC involves conservative and operative measures. Conservative treatment usually begins with activity management as well as non-steroidal anti-inflammatory medications, physical therapy, and a short course of oral steroids. Trunk stabilization and core muscle strengthening is typically the goal in physical therapy. However, bracing and physical therapy alone have little proven efficacy.[2] Hurri and associates showed 44% had some improvement with nonoperative treatment.[3] Atlas and associates found that 45% of patients had improvement in leg pain,[4] and Johnsson and associates reported 32% considered their symptoms improved with conservative treatment.[5]

Epidural steroid injections are often used as an adjunct in patients with severe or unremitting radiculopathy or NIC. In about one third of cases, this treatment can result in enough relief to avoid surgery for a short period of time. However, long-term relief is less likely.[6]

If conservative treatment fails to provide relief or the condition is worsening, operative treatment is indicated. Traditionally, the surgeries include decompressive laminectomy, laminotomy, or foraminotomy, depending on the anatomic region of the stenosis. Moreover, fusion may be indicated where the motion segment is unstable. The success of these surgeries varies with severity, surgical technique, patient selection, and outcomes measures.

A meta-analysis of 74 studies related to surgery for spinal stenosis reveals a rate of good to excellent results of 64% at 1 year.[7] Prospective studies such as the Maine Lumbar Study have shown superior outcomes for operative treatments of symptomatic lumbar stenosis compared to nonoperative treatment.[8]

Surgical decompression, while offering the potential to improve the quality of life for the patients, also has the potential for significant complications, especially when a fusion is performed and in revision surgery. Postoperative complications may include the cardiovascular and pulmonary complications of general anesthesia, infection, iatrogenic instability, pseudarthrosis, hardware failure, and the need for future surgery due to the development of disease at adjacent levels.[9] A meta-analysis of the literature of spinal stenosis surgery by Turner and associates in 1992 showed the following complication rates for lumbar decompressive surgery: perioperative mortality (0.32%), dural tears (5.91%), deep infection (1.08%), superficial infection (2.3%), deep vein thrombosis (2.78%), and any complication (12.64%).[10] In a study by Yuan and co-workers, 2% to 3% of patients undergoing lumbar decompression and arthrodesis, with or without internal fixation, suffered an infection, and the risk of nerve root injury from placement of pedicle screws was 0.4%.[11]

## INDICATIONS AND CONTRAINDICATIONS

Patient selection criteria include leg, buttock, or groin pain with or without back pain which is relieved with sitting or flexion. Once the diagnosis is confirmed with either magnetic resonance imaging (MRI) or computed tomography (CT), at one or two levels, and the patient has undergone a trial of conservative management (typically up to 6 months), placement of the device can be considered. Moreover, patients should be able to sit for at least 50 minutes without pain. Contraindications include cauda equina syndrome, scoliotic Cobb angle greater than 25 degrees, gross instability at the motion segment, fragility compression fracture or severe osteoporosis, Paget's disease, metastasis to the vertebrae, ankylosis at the affected segment, spinal anatomy that would cause the device to become unstable (such as aplastic spinous process or spina bifida occulta), isthmic spondylolisthesis, olisthesis, and degenerative spondylolisthesis greater than Meyerding Grade 1. Spondylolisthesis up to Grade 1 is indicated and described in more detail later. Patients with prior spinal surgery were excluded from the study trials, however, patients who have had prior laminotomy from a microdiscectomy may be considered, assuming the interspinous and supraspinous ligaments are intact. Although, extensive prior laminectomy would be a contraindication. X-STOP may also be indicated for the patients unable to undergo general anesthesia.

Although in the clinical study conducted in the U.S., patients with symptomatic stenosis at L5-S1 were excluded, the X-STOP has been successfully implanted at the L5-S1 level in Europe in patients with sufficiently sized S1 spinous processes. Approximately one third of patients in the United States have received implants at two levels, but three-level procedures were not performed in the U.S. study. As with L5-S1 procedures, triple-level procedures are performed in Europe, but less frequently.

## DESCRIPTION OF THE DEVICE

The X-STOP was developed to provide a safer, less invasive treatment option for those who fail conservative management and those needing the riskier decompression surgery. The X-STOP was designed specifically to reduce extension only at the individual level(s) that provokes symptoms, while allowing unrestricted movement in flexion, axial rotation, and lateral bending of the treated as well as untreated level(s).[12] Because the implant was designed to be placed without removing any bony or soft tissues, the technique is minimally invasive and is usually performed with the patient under local anesthesia.

Thickened lamina, hypertrophied ligamentum flavum, spondylolisthesis, disc bulges, and facet hypertrophy can concomitantly lead to canal, foraminal, and lateral recess stenosis.[13] NIC is often related to position so that symptoms such as pain, numbness, tingling, and weakness are elicited with extension of the lumbar spine and relieved in flexion or sitting.[14,15] The level affected primarily is L4-L5, followed by L3-L4, L5-S1, L2-L3, L1-L2.[16]

Several key design features allow for the straightforward implantation of the X-STOP. The oval spacer separates the spinous processes and limits extension at the implanted level (Fig. 71–1). The oval spacer helps distribute the load along the generally concave shape of the spinous processes and, by eliminating any sharp edges, reduces the likelihood of damaging the cortical bone. The two lateral wings prevent migration laterally, the lamina prevents migration anteriorly, and the supraspinous ligament, as well as the concave space between the spinous processes, prevents the implant from migrating posteriorly. The tapered tissue expander facilitates lateral insertion, from right to left, allowing the supraspinous ligament and its insertions to be preserved (Fig. 71–2).

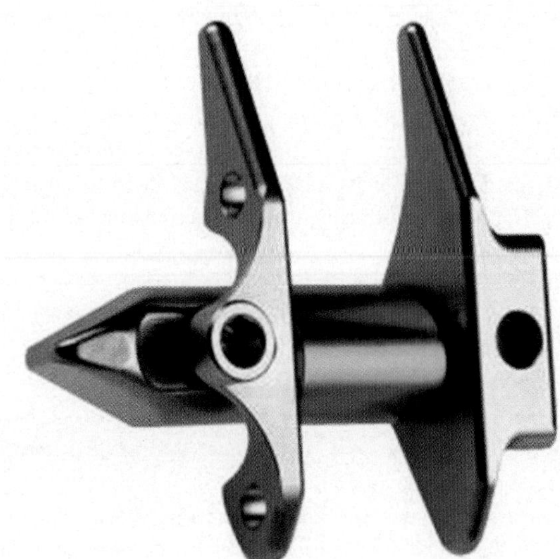

■ **FIGURE 71–1.** An image of the X-STOP depicting the adjustable universal wing, tissue expander, fixed wing, and spacer. The tapered tissue expander allows for easier insertion between the spinous processes. The universal and fixed wings limit anterior and lateral migration. The spacer limits extension of the treated spinous processes.

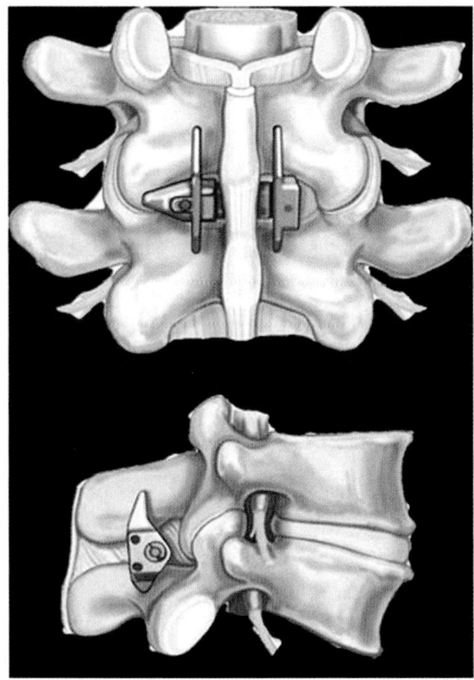

■ **FIGURE 71–2.** Posterior and lateral views of a lumbar motion segment with an implanted X-STOP. The implant is placed posterior to the lamina and away from the nerve roots and spinal cord. The supraspinous ligament is retained to prevent posterior migration. The implant is not fixed to any bony structures.

The L5-S1 level may present a difficult challenge. Most people lack an S1 spinous process large enough to support the device. Those who do have a large S1 spinous process usually are those who have a lumbarized S1 segment. In these cases, the X-STOP can be placed in the same manner as the proximal segments.

## SCIENTIFIC TESTING

Biomechanical studies have shown that the X-STOP significantly prevents narrowing of the spinal canal and neural foramina, limits extension, and reduces intradiscal pressure and facet loading. In an MRI cadaver study, Richards and associates reported that the X-STOP increased the neural foramina area by 26% and the spinal canal area by 18% during extension. In addition, foraminal width was increased by 41% and subarticular diameter by 50% in extension.[17] In a kinematics cadaver study, Lindsey and associates[18] showed terminal extension at the implant level was reduced by 62% following X-STOP placement, although lateral bending and axial rotation range of motion were unchanged. In a cadaveric disc pressure study, Swanson and associates[19] reported that the pressures in the posterior annulus and nucleus pulposus were reduced by 63% and 41%, respectively, during extension and by 38% and 20%, respectively, in the neutral standing position. Rohlmann and associates performed a similar study and found a slight increase in intradiscal pressure, which reduced dramatically with extension at the implanted segment. This finding, however, occurred only when the interspinous space was distracted more than 6 mm.[20] They recommend not placing an implant much larger than the interspinous space. Finally, Wiseman and associates[21] performed a cadaveric facet loading study and reported that the mean facet force during extension decreased by 68%. In each of those studies, the adjacent level measurements were not significantly changed from the intact specimen state. These preclinical studies indicate that the X-STOP increases spinal canal and neural foramina space and produces significant unloading of the disc and facets.

In a 6-month clinical follow-up MRI study, Wardlaw and associates and Siddiqui and associates reported equal results in their clinical studies evaluating positional MRI changes after X-STOP implantation.[22,23] Siddiqui and associates found in 17 levels an increase in the dural sac from 77.8 to 93.4 mm$^2$ ($P = 0.006$). In a later study, Siddiqui and associates found in 26 patients no differences in disc heights, end plate angles, and segmental and lumbar range of movement.[24]

The supraspinous ligament is a substantial structure, and its presence, as well as the preservation of its original osseous insertion, prevents overdistraction of the segment. The ultimate load and tensile strength of the interspinous-supraspinous ligament complex are 203 N and 1.2 Mpa, respectively.[25] In another biomechanical study, the supraspinous-interspinous ligament complex was the largest contributor to resisting applied flexion moments in the porcine lumbar spine.[26]

A relative contraindication for its use is in a patient with severe osteoporosis. Talwar, and associates showed that the spinous process is significantly weaker in those with low bone mineral densities, and therefore, care must be taken when implanting the X-STOP in these patients.[27]

## CLINICAL OUTCOMES

A multicenter prospective, randomized controlled trial was performed in the United States, comparing the outcomes of mild-to-moderate NIC patients treated with the X-STOP interspinous process decompression system to those of patients treated nonsurgically.[28] There were 191 patients treated at nine centers. Inclusion criteria included patients older than 50 years old and patients with leg, buttock, or groin pain with or without back pain while walking, relieved with forward flexion, and able to sit for at least 50 minutes pain free. Exclusion criteria includes a fixed motor deficit, cauda equina syndrome, significant instability, previous lumbar surgery, dense peripheral neuropathy, scoliosis with Cobb angle greater than 25 degrees, spondylolisthesis greater than Grade 1 (25% slip or less), history of pathologic compression fractures including fragility fractures, severe osteoporosis, obesity (BMI >40), and active infection.

Eligible patients were randomized to either the X-STOP group or the conservative care group. Those randomized to the conservative care group received one or more epidural steroid injections and had the option to receive non-steroidal anti-inflammatory drugs (NSAIDs), analgesics, and physical therapy and additional injections as needed. Physical therapy consisted of "back school," which included stabilization exercises, pool therapy, massage, and cold/hot packs.

Assessments were based on baseline (prior to initial treatment) values and findings at 6 weeks, 6 months, 1 year, 2 years, and 4 years. Assessment data were based on outcomes measured specifically for neurogenic claudication, the Zurich Claudication Questionnaire (ZCQ), as well as the SF-36.

One hundred patients received the X-STOP, and 91 patients were treated nonoperatively. A total of 136 levels were implanted in 100 patients: 64 single levels and 36 double levels. One-level procedures took an average of 51 minutes, and two-level procedures took 58 minutes. Blood loss was negligible: 40 mL for one-level procedures and 58 mL for two-level procedures. The most common level implanted was L4-L5 (89/136), and the second most common level was L3-L4 (43/136). The most common implant size was 12 mm. There were five X-STOP sizes available during the trial, ranging from 6 mm to 14 mm. The procedure was performed under local anesthesia in 97 patients and under general anesthesia in 3 patients. The length of stay was, on the average, less than 24 hours.

At 2-year follow-up, data from 93 of the 100 X-STOP patients and 81 of the 91 control patients were available for analysis. The X-STOP group had a significantly greater percentage of patients with an improvement in Symptom Severity Domain of ZCQ than did the control group at each posttreatment visit. At 2-year follow-up, 56/93 (60.2%) of the patients reported a clinically significant reduction in the severity of symptoms compared to the 15/81 (18%) of the control group. The X-STOP group also had a significantly greater percentage of patients with an improvement in Physical Function Domain of ZCQ than did the control group at each posttreatment visit. At the 24-month evaluation, 57% of the X-STOP patients reported a clinically significant improvement in their physical function compared to 15% of the control patients. At 2-year follow-up, 73% of the X-STOP patients were at least "somewhat satisfied" compared to 36% of the control group. Interestingly, patients with two-level X-STOPs had greater symptom relief than those with the single level, although not significantly greater. This is opposite to the trend seen in laminectomy and fusion cases, in which multilevel procedures tend to have less favorable outcomes.

Results of the SF-36 scores showed no significant differences in the pretreatment enrollment scores between the X-STOP and control groups for any SF-36 domain. At all follow-up time points, the X-STOP group scored significantly better than the control group in every physical domain including the mean scores, whereas in the control group, none of the mean scores were better.

More recently, based on the original 18 patient FDA pilot study group who all received X-STOP, Kondrashov and associates showed 78% had successful outcomes at 4-year follow-ups. They had a 15 point improvement in Oswestry Disability Index (ODI) compared with the baseline (Table 71–1).

TABLE 71–1. Zurich Claudication Questionnaire Success Rates at 1 and 2 Years

| Period | Category | X-STOP | Control | *P* Value |
|---|---|---|---|---|
| One year N100/N91 | Symptom Severity | 64% | 21% | 0.001 |
| | Physical Function | 70% | 21% | 0.001 |
| | Patient Satisfaction | 75% | 45% | 0.001 |
| Two years N93/N81 | Symptom Severity | 60% | 19% | 0.001 |
| | Physical Function | 57% | 15% | 0.001 |
| | Patient Satisfaction | 73% | 36% | 0.001 |

## GERMAN REGISTRY

In Germany, a registry is being maintained to gather prospective data on NIC patients who are treated with the X-STOP implant in general practice. Patients are assessed pre- and postoperatively using the validated, condition-specific ZCQ. The ZCQ is the only validated LSS-specific outcome measure. The questionnaire consists of three domains: Symptom Severity (SS), Physical Function (PF), and Patient Satisfaction (PS). To date, 212 patients have been evaluated 1 year after surgery with very good results (Table 71–2). Two patients had a reoperation because of lack of efficacy and one because of dislocation of the implant.

## EUROPEAN CLINICAL EXPERIENCE

A prospective clinical evaluation of 15 patients at 3- and 6-month follow-ups was carried out by Wardlaw and associates in conjunction with pre- and postoperative positional MRI scan measurements. All cases demonstrated clinical improvement, and the X-STOP implant increased the cross-sectional area of the dural sac and exit foramina without affecting overall movement of the lumbar spine.[29]

Heijnen and Kramer reported on the satisfaction of 14 patients with NIC who were treated with the X-STOP implant. One patient died of a non-back-related disorder. Eleven of the other 13 patients expressed great satisfaction. They are free of NIC symptoms, and all but one would undergo the surgery again, if the choice had to be made again.[30]

## PATIENTS WITH DEGENERATIVE SPONDYLOLISTHESIS

Interestingly, 39 patients in the U.S. FDA study with Grade I degenerative spondylolisthesis were treated with the X-STOP and 22 patients were treated nonoperatively. Using 15-point improvement over baseline scores in the ZCQ as the criterion of clinical success, 69% of the 39 X-STOP patients had a successful outcome at 2-year follow-up, compared to 9% of the control patients. The mean improvement score for the 39 X-STOP patients was 26 points. There were no significant differences in the mean percentage of slip between X-STOP and control patients at baseline or at 2-year follow-up. Spondylolisthesis patients are often treated with spinal fusion and decompression.

Moreover, Anderson and associates in a cohort of 75 patients, 42 X-STOP and 33 nonoperative control patients at 2-year follow-up, showed statistically significant clinical success in 63.4% of X-STOP patients and 12.9% of control patients using ZCQ and SF-36 outcome measures. Sagittal balance (listhesis and kyphosis) remained unaltered.[31] The X-STOP represents a

TABLE 71–2. German Registry Success Rates 6 and 12 Months After Surgery

| ZCQ Category | 6 Months | 12 Months |
|---|---|---|
| Symptom Severity | 82% | 82% |
| Physical Function | 81% | 77% |
| Patient Satisfaction | 82% | 82% |

ZCQ, Zurich Claudication Questionnaire.

significantly less invasive alternative therapy for these patients, resulting in very good clinical outcomes and, most importantly, no evidence that the implant results in any instability of the motion segment.

## SAGITTAL BALANCE

The requirement to maintain proper sagittal alignment and balance in patients receiving spinal implants is well understood. Experience with lumbar fusion procedures that cause a flat back has overwhelmingly resulted in unacceptable clinical outcomes. Three different radiologic studies were therefore undertaken to measure any possible effect of the X-STOP on sagittal alignment. In the U.S. study, radiographs were taken at each follow-up visit for both X-STOP and control patients, and measurements were made of the lumbosacral angle (L1 to S1) and the treated intervertebral angle. At 2-year follow-up, there were no significant differences in the mean angles between the two groups of patients. Preoperative x-rays from a subset of X-STOP patients were also compared to standing films taken at 2-year follow-up. In 23 patients with single-level implants, the change in the intervertebral angle was only 0.5 degree, and the change in the lumbosacral angle was 0.1 degree.

A newly published report by Siddiqui and associates using a positional MRI scanner, in addition to confirming in vivo the increases in the area of the foramen and canal that were measured in the preclinical in vitro cadaver study, confirms a minor change in angulation for both the lumbosacral angle and intervertebral angle of approximately 1 degree.[32] These studies confirm that the X-STOP results in only minimal changes to sagittal alignment. This is due to preserving the supraspinous ligament and its original insertions. This ligament is a very robust structure receiving the confluence of the lumbodorsal fascia, and its preservation prevents overdistraction of the segment.

## X-STOP VERSUS DECOMPRESSIVE LAMINECTOMY

It is not easy to interpret X-STOP clinical results in the context of published outcomes of surgical treatment for stenosis. To date, no randomized controlled multicenter study has been performed for X-STOP versus laminectomy. The X-STOP was clearly superior to conservative treatment in the U.S. study, but it does not permit a comprehensive comparison between the X-STOP and laminectomy.

Hannibal compared patients from the U.S. FDA Pivotal X-STOP Trial (June 2000–July 2001) with those who received laminectomy during the same time period at the same institution, using the same criteria used in that trial in a nonrandom manner. At 4 years after surgery and with a 15 point improvement from baseline ODI score as a success criterion, 80% (12/15) of X-STOP patients and 38% (5/13) of laminectomy patients had successful outcomes.[33]

Compared to literature-reported outcomes of decompressive surgery, there are significant differences in operative time, estimated blood loss, length of hospital stay, complication rate, and reoperation rates, favoring the X-STOP.[34,35]

The results of the X-STOP patients showed 59.8% statistically significantly improved in Symptom Severity, 56.5% improved in Physical Function, and 72.8% were satisfied. During the course of the U.S. study, 24 patients in the control group underwent decompressive laminectomy for the relief of their stenosis symptoms, and outcomes are available for 22 patients at a mean follow-up time of 12.8 months. Sixty-four percent had clinically significant improvement in Symptom Severity Domain of ZCQ, 68.2% had clinically significantly improvement in Physical Function Domain of ZCQ, and 59.1% were satisfied with the outcome of their treatment. Furthermore, Katz and associates[36] published a large series of surgically treated spinal stenosis patients also using the ZCQ outcomes tool at 2-year follow-up. In that study, 63% of the patients significantly improved in Symptom Severity, 59% improved in Physical Function, and 72% were satisfied. Fokter and Yerby looked at pre- and post-laminectomy ZCQ scores at 12 to 54 months in 58 patients, and 63.8% of the patients had significant clinical improvement in Symptom Severity, 55.2 had significant clinical improvement in Physical Function, and 58.6% of the patients were at least somewhat satisfied (Table 71–3).[37]

There is striking similarity in outcomes between the X-STOP and laminectomy groups. However, there are some important differences between these procedures. The mean operative time for the X-STOP was less than an hour for two levels, compared with 72 to 278 minutes reported for laminectomies. Mean blood loss of 40.1 to 58 mL during the X-STOP was negligible compared with 115 to 1040 mL reported for decompression.[38] Moreover, the X-STOP procedure can be performed under local anesthesia, thus nearly eliminating the risk associated with general anesthesia. Finally, a comparison of the incidence and severity of complications cited in the laminectomy literature with the X-STOP indicates that the X-STOP is a much safer procedure.

## OPERATIVE TECHNIQUE

The patient is placed in the right lateral decubitus position on a radiolucent table (Fig. 71–3). The level(s) to be treated is identified by fluoroscopy using an 18-guage needle taped to the skin. An indelible ink mark is made at the appropriate level. The site is prepped with usual sterile technique and draped using shower curtain type drape. Two 22-guage spinal needles can be placed at the caudal and cephalad ends of the proposed incision to accurately identify the level(s) and length of the incision. The spinal needles may be used to instill local anesthetic with epinephrine

**TABLE 71–3. ZCQ Scores Comparing X-STOP with Laminectomy**

| | Symptom Severity | Physical Function | Satisfaction |
|---|---|---|---|
| X-STOP, 2-year follow-up | 59.8% | 56.5% | 72.8% |
| Katz laminectomy, 2-year follow-up | 63% | 59% | 72% |
| Laminectomy after failed conservative management | 63.6% | 68.2% | 59.1% |
| Fokter laminectomy | 63.8% | 55.2% | 58.6% |

ZCQ, Zurich Claudication Questionnaire.

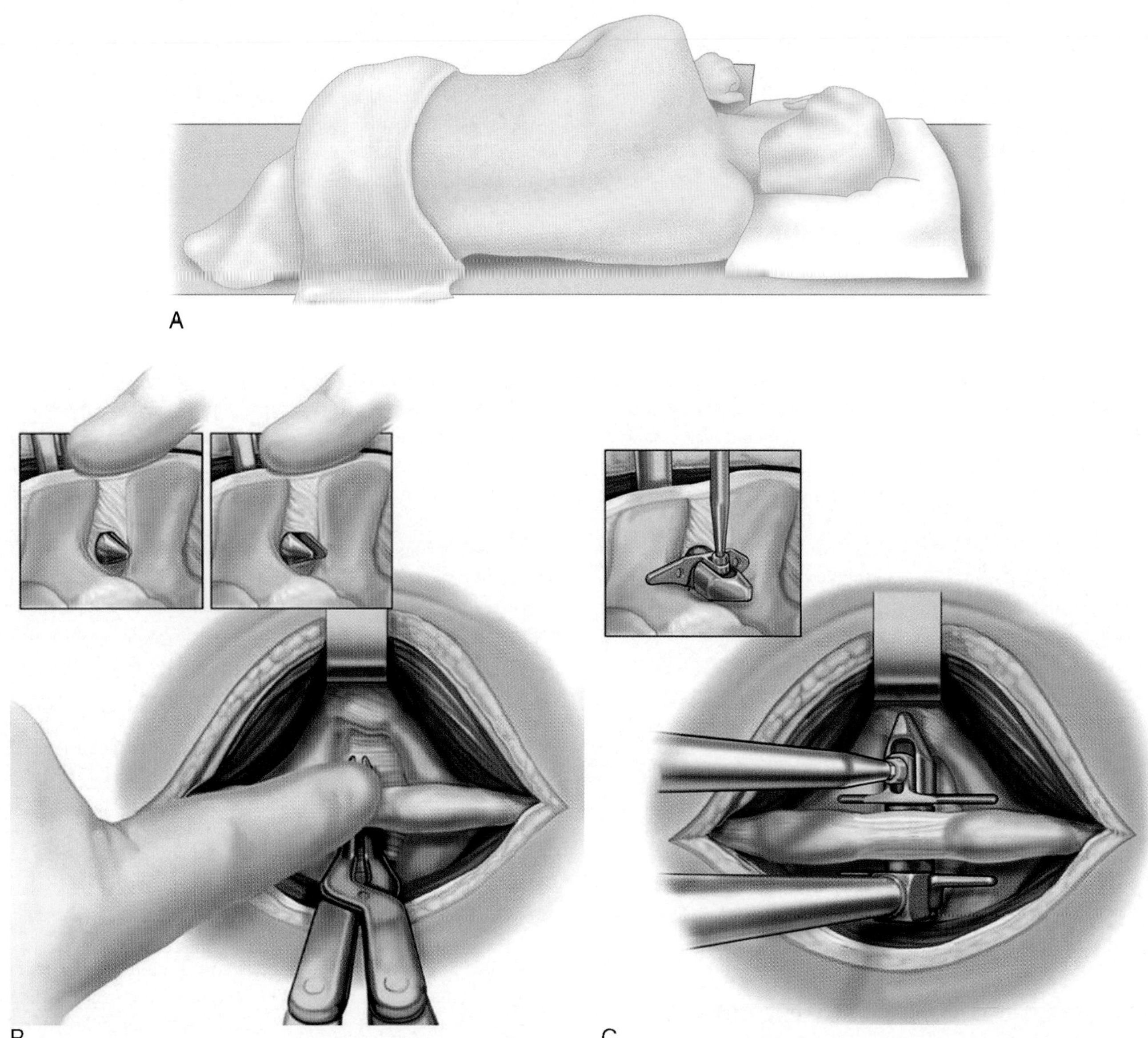


■ **FIGURE 71–3.** Surgical technique. **A,** Patients are placed in a right lateral decubitus position, and a midsagittal incision of approximately 4 cm is made over the spinous processes of the stenotic level(s). **B,** The small curved dilator sizing instrument is then inserted at the most anterior margin of the interspinous space. **C,** The universal wing is attached.

to block the posterior rami bilaterally. A midsagittal incision about 4 cm is made over the spinous process to the dorsal fascia. A Cobb elevator is used to sweep the subcutaneous tissue from the dorsal fascia. After further local anesthesia to the dorsal fascia, two longitudinal incisions are made through both layers of the dorsal fascia about 1 cm from the lateral aspect of the spinous processes. The paraspinal musculature is then subperiosteally elevated from the spinous processes and medial lamina bilaterally using a large Cobb elevator. A large Cobb is appropriate to ensure that the canal is protected, especially in cases with prior laminotomy. The spinal canal should never be violated and neither laminectomy nor laminotomy is performed. Removal of any portion of the ligamentum flavum is unnecessary.

If the facets are hypertrophied, they may block proper insertion of the device, causing them to be positioned too posterior; thus, they may be partially trimmed medially with a rongeur to ensure adequate anterior placement. Fuchs and associates found in a cadaveric biomechanical study that the facets can be safely trimmed without destabilizing the motion segment while using the X-STOP. However, one should avoid aggressive bilateral facetectomies.[39]

Prior to starting the insertion process, the patient is asked to curl up and flex the back by trying to place the chin to the knees. A small curved dialator is inserted across the interspinous space at the most anterior margin of the interspinous space. After the correct level is verified by fluoroscopy, the small dilator is removed and replaced with a larger curved one. A finger is placed on the left side at the point where the small dilator is removed to ensure placement of the large dilator as well as the sizing distractor, which are placed at the same location. The interspinous ligament is dilated, not excised. After the larger dilator is removed, the sizing distractor is inserted. Because the patient is in the flexed, pain-free position, the sizing distractor should be opened until it contacts the spinous process and slightly distracts the interspinous space. If the interspinous space is sized between two available X-STOP sizes, choose the next smallest size. The X-STOP is then implanted from right to left, again with a finger on the left side to help guide the beveled tip of the device through the appropriate point. The right wing should be flush against the side of the spinous process. The screw hole for the universal wing on the left side is directly visualized, and the wing screw is engaged. The two wings are approximated medially, and the universal wing screw is secured using a torque-limiting screwdriver. Anteroposterior and lateral fluoroscopy views are obtained to ensure proper placement. The two fascia incisions are closed separately along with subcutaneous tissue and skin. A drain is rarely indicated. The procedure can typically be performed in less than an hour, and most patients can be released from the hospital within 24 hours.

## POSTOPERATIVE CARE

Patients are encouraged to get up and ambulate as soon as they feel comfortable. They should avoid hyperextension activities for 2 to 6 months.

## COMPLICATIONS

Reported complications related to the X-STOP have been minor and resolved easily without further sequelae. In the U.S. clinical study, there was one wound dehiscence, one seroma that was aspirated, one hematoma, and one report of incisional pain. No spinous process fractures occurred during X-STOP implantation. There have been no reports of either vascular or neurologic complications, an outcome which is anticipated because the laminae are left intact and the spinal canal and neuroforamina are not entered. Device-related complications included one patient who fell, causing the implant to dislodge; it was removed without any sequelae. A review of the patient's radiographs showed a very prominent facet that prevented the implant from being properly positioned anteriorly. One patient reported worsening pain about 1 year after the procedure, which was determined to be possibly related to the implant. One implant was placed too posterior and was considered to be malpositioned. An asymptomatic spinous process fracture was diagnosed in another patient on routine 6-month follow-up radiographs.

Revising the implant is rather uncomplicated. Once the set screw on the wing is removed, the implant can be easily removed or replaced. Should an adjacent level need to be instrumented with the X-STOP, there would be little added difficulty. Placement of the X-STOP adjacent to a prior fusion remains a subject for further testing.

## COST ANALYSIS

Kondrashov and associates recently evaluated the cost-effectiveness of X-STOP patients versus those treated with laminectomy. They found X-STOP to be significantly more cost-effective. There were 18 X-STOP and 11 laminectomy patients. Average hospital costs for one-level X-STOP and one-level laminectomy groups were $17,059 and $45,302, respectively. Average hospital costs for two-level X-STOP and two-level laminectomy groups were $24,353 and $45,739, respectively. The main savings in the X-STOP group (cost drivers) were in operating room costs (shorter operative time), hospital charges (X-STOP is an outpatient procedure), and anesthesia charges (X-STOP is placed under local or MAC anesthesia). The cost of the X-STOP implant and higher radiology charges due to use of fluoroscopy during X-STOP placement were significantly offset by those savings.[40]

### ADVANTAGES/DISADVANTAGES: X-STOP

**Advantages**

Clinically proved to be an effective treatment for symptoms of LSS with or without degenerative spondylolisthesis
Safe
Short surgery time, implanted under local anesthesia
Minimally invasive
An outpatient procedure
Immediate relief of NIC
Cost-effective
Easily be revised to other procedures
No violation of the spinal canal
No tissue removal

**Disadvantages**

Cannot be used with lytic spondylolisthesis
No published prospective controlled studies comparing X-STOP with laminectomy

## CONCLUSION

Decompression of the lumbar spine with the X-STOP offers a well-proved, safe, effective, and cost-effective treatment of patients suffering from NIC secondary to LSS. The X-STOP can be implanted using local anesthetic, and many patients can return home within hours after surgery. The X-STOP implant offers the benefits of decompression, yet with a low-risk profile, for NIC patients. It utilizes ligamentotaxis to indirectly increase the foraminal and canal dimensions by reconstituting tension in the posterior ligamentous structures.

The comparative analyses suggest that the outcomes of the X-STOP decompression may at least be comparable to outcomes reported in the literature for decompressive laminectomy.

The X-STOP interspinous process decompression is indicated for patients 50 years of age or older with one- or two-level mild-to-moderate LSS symptoms and back and lower extremity complaints that are relieved in flexion. X-STOP outcomes have been demonstrated to be vastly superior to nonoperative therapy in the U.S. multicenter prospective randomized trial in LSS patients with mild-to-moderate symptoms. Complications with the X-STOP are relatively minor and uncommon. X-STOP also prevents the risks of pedicle screw placement and pseudarthrosis. Most importantly, being a motion-sparing device, X-STOP does not increase the adjacent segment stresses and probably does not contribute to adjacent segment degeneration and adjacent segment disease.

## REFERENCES


1. Senegas J: Mechanical supplementation by non-rigid fixation in degenerative intervertebral lumbar segments: The Wallis system. Eur Spine J 11(2):S164–S169, 2002. Epub 2002 Jun.
2. Postacchini F: Management of lumbar spinal stenosis. J Bone Joint Surg Br 78(1):154–164, 1996.
3. Hurri H, Slatis P, Soini J, et al: Lumbar spinal stenosis: Assessment of long-term outcome 12 years after operative and conservative treatment. J Spinal Disord 11(2):110–115, 1998.
4. Atlas SJ, Keller RB, Robson D, et al: Surgical and nonsurgical management of lumbar spinal stenosis: Four-year outcomes from the Maine lumbar spine study. Spine 25:556–562, 2000.
5. Johnsson KE, Uden A, Rosen I: The effect of decompression on the natural course of spinal stenosis: A comparison of surgically treated and untreated patients. Spine 16(6):615–619, 1991.
6. Riew KD, Yin Y, Gilula L, et al: The effect of nerve-root injections on the need for operative treatment of lumbar radicular pain: A prospective, randomized, controlled, double-blind study. Bone Joint Surg Am 82-A(11):1589–1593, 2000.
7. Turner JA, Ersek M, Herron L, Deyo R: Surgery for lumbar spinal stenosis: Attempted meta-analysis of the literature. Spine 17:1–8, 1992.
8. Atlas SJ, Keller RB, Robson D, et al: Surgical and nonsurgical management of lumbar spinal stenosis: Four-year outcomes from the Maine lumbar spine study. Spine 25:556–562, 2000.
9. Wang JC, Bohlman HH, Riew KD: Dural tears secondary to operations on the lumbar spine: Management and results after a two-year-minimum follow-up of eighty-eight patients. J Bone Joint Surg Am 80:1728–1732, 1998.
10. Turner JA, Ersek M, Herron L, Deyo R: Surgery for lumbar spinal stenosis: Attempted meta-analysis of the literature. Spine 17:1–8, 1992.
11. Yuan HA, Garfin SR, Dickman CA, Mardjetko SM: A historical cohort study of pedicle screw fixation in thoracic, lumbar, and sacral spinal fusions. Spine 19:2279S–2296S, 1994.
12. Lindsey DP, Swanson KE, Fuchs P, et al: The effects of an interspinous implant on the kinematics of the instrumented and adjacent levels in the lumbar spine. Spine 28(19):2192–2197, 2003.
13. Verbiest H: A radicular syndrome from developmental narrowing of the lumbar vertebral canal. J Bone Joint Surg 36B:230–237, 1954.
14. Porter RW: Spinal stenosis and neurogenic claudication. Spine 21:2046–2052, 1996.
15. Willen J, Danielson B, Gaulitz A, et al: Dynamic effects of the lumbar spinal canal: Axially loaded CT-myelopathy and MRI in patients with sciatica and/or neurogenic claudication. Spine 22:2968–2976, 1997.
16. Jonsson B, Annertz M, Sjoberg C, Strömqvist B: A prospective and consecutive study of surgically treated LSS, Part II: Five-year follow-up by an independent observer. Spine 22:2938–2944, 1997.
17. Richards JC, Majumdar S, Lindsey DP, et al: The treatment mechanism of an interspinous process implant for lumbar neurogenic intermittent claudication. Spine 30:744–749, 2005.
18. Lindsey DP, Swanson KE, Fuchs P, et al: The effects of an interspinous implant on the kinematics of the instrumented and adjacent levels in the lumbar spine. Spine 28(19):2192–2197, 2003.
19. Swanson KE, Lindsey DP, Hsu KY, et al: The effects of an interspinous implant on intervertebral disc pressures. Spine 28:26–32, 2003.
20. Rohlmann A, Zander T, Burra NK, Bergmann G: Effect of an interspinous implant on loads in the lumbar spine. Biomed Tech (Berl) 50(10):343–347, 2005.
21. Wiseman CM, Lindsey DP, Fredrick AD, Yerby SA: The effect of an interspinous process implant on facet loading during extension. Spine 30:903–907, 2005.
22. Wardlaw D, Smith F, Pope M, et al: Change in spinal canal and nerve root foraminal measurements before and six months following insertion of the X-STOP Interspinous Process Distraction Device in relation to early clinical outcome. Presented at Trans ISMISS Zurich, Switzerland, 2004.
23. Siddiqui M, Nicol M, Karadimas E, et al: The positional magnetic resonance imaging changes in the lumbar spine following insertion of a novel interspinous process distraction device. Spine 30(23):2677–2682, 2005.
24. Siddiqui M, Karadimas E, Nicol M, et al: Effects of X-STOP devices on sagittal spine kinematics in spinal stenosis. J Spinal Disord Tech 19(5):328–333, 2006.
25. Iida T, Abumi K, Kotani Y, et al: Effects of aging and spinal degeneration on mechanical properties of lumbar supraspinous and interspinous ligaments. Spine J 2(2):95–100, 2002.
26. Gillespie KA, Dickey JP: Biomechanical role of lumbar spine ligaments in flexion and extension: Determination using a parallel linkage robot and a porcine model. Spine 1;29(11):1208–1216, 2004.
27. Talwar V, Lindsey DP, Fredrick A, et al: Insertion loads of the X-STOP interspinous process distraction system designed to treat neurogenic intermittent claudication. Eur Spine J 15(6):908–912, 2006. Epub 2005 May 31.
28. Zucherman JF, Hsu KY, et al: A prospective randomized multi-center study for the treatment of lumbar spinal stenosis with the X-STOP interspinous implant: 1-year results. Eur Spine J 13 (1):22–31, 2004.
29. Wardlaw D, Smith F, Pope M, et al: Change in spinal canal and nerve root foraminal measurements before and six months following insertion of the X-STOP Interspinous Process Distraction Device in relation to early clinical outcome. Presented at Trans ISMISS Zurich, Switzerland, 2004.
30. Heijnen SAF, Kramer FJK: Spinale distractie als therapie bij lumbale wervelkanaalstenose—De eerste resultaten. Ned Tijdschr Orthop 11(4):199–203, 2004.
31. Anderson PA, Tribus CB, Kitchel SH: Treatment of neurogenic claudication by interspinous decompression: Application of the X-STOP device in patients with lumbar degenerative spondylolisthesis. J Neurosurg Spine 4(6):463–471, 2006.
32. Siddiqui M, Karadimas E, Nicol M, et al: Effects of X-STOP devices on sagittal spine kinematics in spinal stenosis. J Spinal Disord Tech 19(5):328–333, 2006.
33. Hannibal M: Interspinous process decompression with the XSTOP device for lumbar spinal stenosis: a 4-year follow-up study. Journal of Spinal Disorder Technology 19, 2006.
34. Benz RJ, Ibrahim ZG, Afshar P, Garfin SR: Predicting complications in elderly patients undergoing lumbar decompression. Clin Orthop 384:116–121, 2001.
35. Timothy J, Pal D, Ross S, Marks P: Early experience with the X-STOP a lumbar spinous process distractor for the treatment of lumbar canal stenosis. Abstract Br J Neurosurg 2005. (in press).
36. Katz JN, Stucki G, Lipson SJ, et al: Predictors of surgical outcome in degenerative lumbar spinal stenosis. Spine 24:2229–2233, 1999.
37. Fokter SK, Yerby SA: Patient-based outcomes for the operative treatment of degenerative lumbar spinal stenosis. Eur Spine J 21:1–9, 2005.
38. Reindl R, Steffen T, Cohen L, Aebi M: Elective lumbar spinal decompression in the elderly: Is it a high-risk operation? Can J Surg 46:43–46, 2003.
39. Fuchs PD, Lindsey DP, Hsu KY, et al: The use of an interspinous implant in conjunction with a graded facetectomy procedure. Spine 30(11):1266–1272; discussion 1273–1274, 2005.
40. Kondrashov DG, Hannibal M, Hsu KY, Zucherman JF: XSTOP versus decompression for neurogenic claudication: economic and clinical analysis. The Internet Journal of Minimally Invasive Spinal Technology 1(2), 2007.

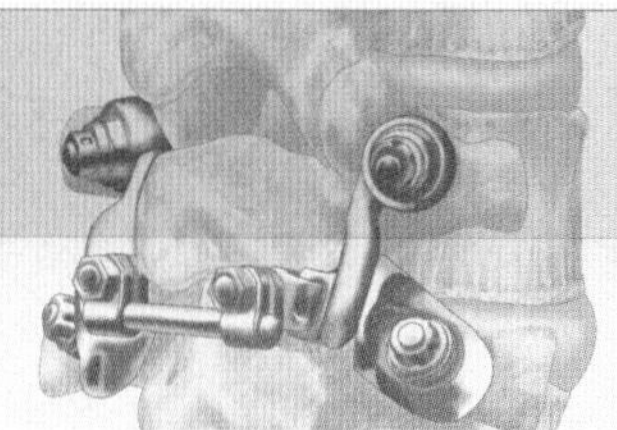

PART

# VIII

# LUMBAR FACET REPLACEMENT

CHAPTER 72

# TOPS: Total Posterior Facet Replacement and Dynamic Motion Segment Stabilization System

**Larry T. Khoo, Luiz Pimenta,** and **Roberto Díaz**

## KEY POINTS

- The TOPS device is a total posterior spinal arthroplasty system for the treatment of moderate-to-severe lumbar spinal stenosis.
- The TOPS device replaces not only the facets but also the soft tissue as well as bony elements that are removed at the time of decompression.
- The TOPS device permits complete decompression of the central and lateral zones of the spine, thereby permitting excellent direct decompression of compressed neural elements.
- The TOPS device can be used in conjunction with an adjacent level fusion.
- Adequate bone density should be preoperatively evaluated as in any motion-sparing device.

The pathophysiologic mechanisms of low back pain continue to be poorly elucidated and to be difficult to effectively study. Whereas pain resulting from neurologic compression has been traditionally treated with great success via decompressive procedures, treatment of mechanical or discogenic lumbar pain has proved far more problematic. For many patients who remain refractory to conservative or less aggressive modalities, spinal fusion continues to be the mainstay of surgical treatment for the relief of axial back pain.[1–7] Unfortunately, clinical outcomes have been variable and inconsistent with regard to the efficacy of spinal fusion in relieving lumbago as measured by standardized measures such as the Oswestry Disability Index (ODI), Visual Analog Scales (VAS) for pain, and SF-36.[1] To compound the problem, accelerated degeneration of the adjacent segment has also been observed in biomechanical laboratory investigations, on long-term radiologic studies, and in numerous retrospective clinical surgical series.[8–15] Although the exact incidence of this "adjacent segment disease" (ASD) remains poorly defined, it is clear that ASD is one of the most dreaded long-term clinical sequelae after successful fusion. From biomechanical investigations and clinical radiographic studies, it appears that there is an alteration of load sharing with an increase in mobility, shear, strain, and pressure at the invertebral disc, uncovertebral joints, and facet joints of the adjacent segment(s) after rigid spinal fusion.[13,15] With this in mind, many postulate that preservation of motion and load sharing at the index pathologic level would help to mitigate or reduce the overall incidence of ASD.

## RATIONALE FOR POSTERIOR FACET REPLACEMENT AND ARTHROPLASTY

In the hope of decreasing adjacent segment forces, total anterior disc replacement (TDR) devices such as the CHARITÉ III (DePuy Spine, Raynham, MA) and the ProDisc II (Synthes, Paoli, PA) were developed in an attempt to preserve motion at the etiologic intervertebral disc. From the clinical federal Food and Drug Administration (FDA) Investigational Device Exemption (IDE) study, the CHARITÉ III was able to provide equivalent relief of low back pain as compared to the randomized control arm of anterior fusion.[2,16] However, numerous authors have cited that severe facet arthropathy, spinal stenosis, neurogenic claudication, significant canal disease, spondylolisthesis, and translational instability are all relative or absolute contraindications to placement of an anterior total disc replacement.[11,17] In a study by Huang and Camissa examining the typical makeup of patients seen in a tertiary spinal clinic, there was a majority preponderance of such patients with dorsal disease, spinal stenosis, spondylolisthesis, and spinal instability. These patients were ideally suited for classical spinal decompression and, in many cases, posterior spinal fusion and not candidates for TDR.[9] As such, it is clear that motion-preserving devices that can be used for patients requiring dorsal surgical treatment are needed.

When we examine the issue of posterior spinal disease and spinal stenosis, it is clear that we face not only the natural history of the disease process but also the iatrogenic instability that results from surgical decompression of these patients. As a large majority of these patients are symptomatic from radicular or central canal compression, they require decompression of the paramedian lamina and at least the medial third or medial half of the facet complex. As a result, progressive resection for neural decompression can lead to progressive spinal instability when the facet orientation is more sagittal than coronal.[1] In many patients with spinal stenosis who require aggressive decompression for extensive neural foraminal narrowing, spinal fusion is often necessitated after facet resection.[5,18] In Fischgrund's analysis, patients with spondylolisthesis and stenosis overall did better with regard to their low back pain scores when they had a primary fusion in addition to decompression as opposed to those who had decompression alone.[6,7] However, it is also clear that many patients with stenosis or stenosis with spondylolisthesis do well without fusion and do not go on to have gross or glacial spinal instability after decompressive surgery. As such, a motion-preserving technology that can be placed via a standard posterior approach can help to avoid fusion in the many stenotic patients who are either preoperatively only mildly unstable or made unstable after surgical decompressive destabilization of the facet complex.

With this in mind, questions remain as to the ideal nature of such a posterior motion-preserving stabilizer of the spine. Whereas numerous theories regarding the etiology of low back pain exist, perhaps the most developed of these is the concept of the biomechanical neutral zone as postulated by Panjabi.[19,20] In this useful heuristic system, a motion segment functions to share load, move, and impinge within a given set of mechanical parameters. During biomechanical testing, any given spinal motion segment will thus move a given amount per quantum of applied load as determined by the viscoelastic properties of the surrounding structures that bind the two verterbrae such as the intervertebral nucleus and annulus, facet joint and capsule, interspinous ligaments, spinal longitudinal ligaments, attached paraspinal muscles, and truncal musculature. Plotted in any of three dimensions, this leads to a classical load-displacement plot of the "neutral zone" (Fig. 72–1). Degeneration, acute injury, or other pathology alters the biomechanical limiters of the system, leading to laxity, altered load sharing, and a widening of the load-displacement curves, thereby altering the neutral zone itself. As movement of the spinal segment begins to exceed its intial set points, joint, nociceptive, and stretch receptors begin to activate and signal pain and injury in the area, which may lead to progressive pain and inflammation in that area. As such, induced injury of the ligaments, facets, or disc complex will lead to a widened neutral zone as seen on load-displacement curves during biomechanical cadaveric testing (Fig. 72–1). This model thus provides a useful point of reference for the cause of mechanical back pain in patients.

Whereas decompression will help to relieve radicular pain, surgical restoration of proper load-sharing and normalization of the "neutral zone" may help to decrease pain and inflammatory stimuli in the treated spinal segment(s). Thus, the efficacy of rigid spinal fusion may ultimately result from its ability to radically correct the load displacement characteristics of the motion segment to near-zero movement for any applied load after rigid fusion and instrumentation. With this in mind, a proper motion-preserving stabilizing device must also be able to correct the load-displacement curves back to an anatomically natural neutral zone and still preserves some degree of native spinal mobility above that of rigid fusion. Additionally, by preserving load-sharing of the treated segment, it must also decrease the "stress-riser" effect on adjacent untreated levels to potentially minimize the incidence of ASD. Finally, the motion-preserving dorsal device must also be secured to the spine in such a way that the device-bone interface remains stable over several million cycles. For example, devices that are to be implanted through the vertebral pedicles must thereby minimize the stress at the screw-bone interface to prevent screw pullout. The motion-preserving device must be able to not only provide motion but must also do so in a way that does not significantly load the screws.

## DESCRIPTION OF THE DEVICE

### Design Parameters

The TOPS system (Impliant Spine, Princeton, NJ) is a unitary device (Fig. 72–2) composed of a titanium "sandwich" with an interlocking polycarbonate urethane (PcU) articulating construct.

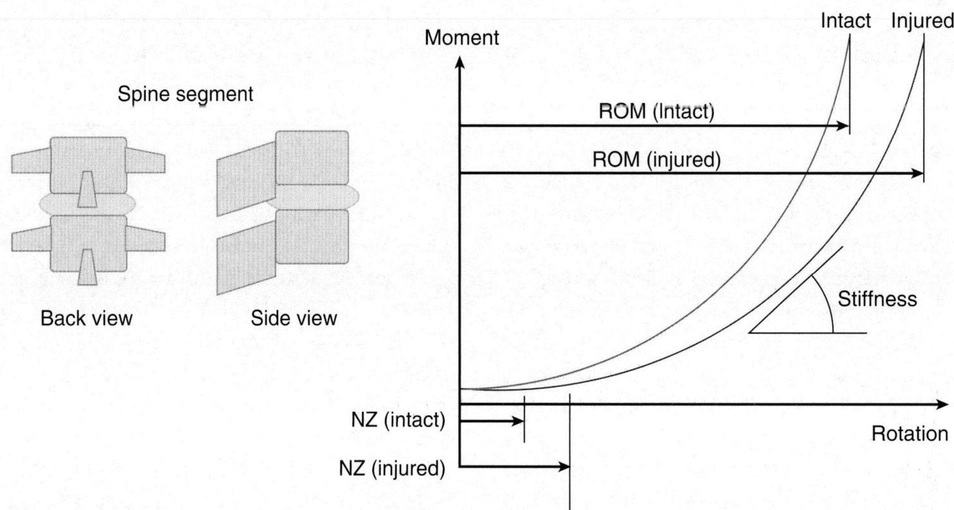


■ **FIGURE 72–1.** Mechanical properties of intact and injured spine. NZ, neutral zone; ROM, range of motion.

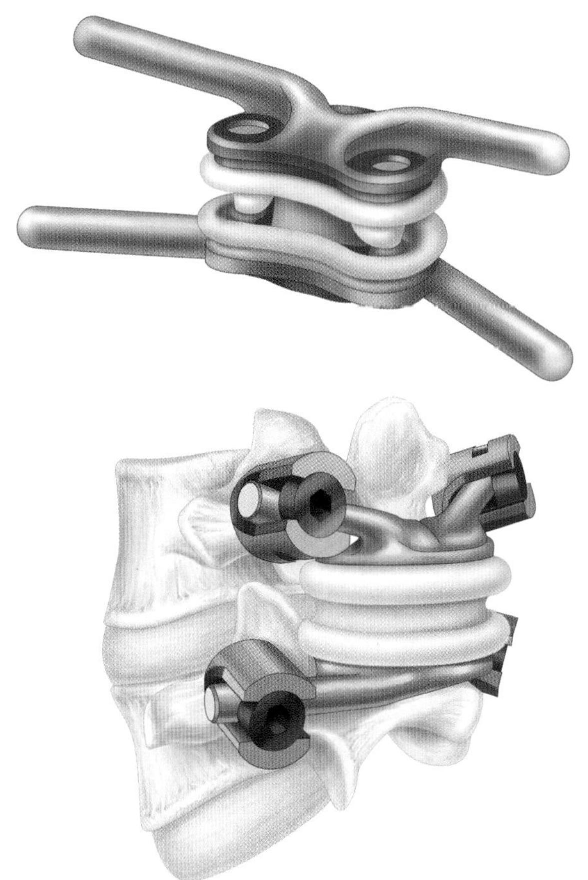

■ FIGURE 72–2. Artificial facet joint capsule. Polyurethane capsule enhances stability and internal bumpers.

The flexible PcU elements within the construct allow relative movement between the titanium plates so as to create axial rotation, lateral bending, extension, and flexion. The internal construct mechanically restricts motion to ±1.5 degrees of axial rotation, ±5 degrees of lateral bending, 2 degrees of extension, and 8 degrees of flexion. The implant also blocks excessive posterior and anterior sagittal translation. The TOPS system uses four standard hydroxyapatite-coated (HA-coated) polyaxial pedicle screws for fixation to the vertebrae (Fig. 72–3). As the internal configuration of the PcU bumpers ultimately acts as the limiter of motion, the TOPS device has an inherent dampening property that serves to dissipate energy that is passed through it during standard load-sharing of the moving spinal motion segment. Furthermore, as the PcU elements also have some "shock-absorption" properties in the vertical axis, vertical load transmitted through the cross-bars through the centroid of the device is somewhat dampened as well. These features serve not only to allow nearly full spinal motion but also to decrease stresses at the adjacent levels and at the screw-bone interface.

The TOPS system provides patients suffering from degeneration or hypertrophy of the facet joint, Grade I degenerative spondylolisthesis, and spinal stenosis with three major advantages. The surgeon can perform a wide decompression to eliminate the pain generators. The procedure stabilizes the posterior spine. The procedure allows a controlled range of motion. The implanted device, made of flexible materials and titanium, allows for constrained bending, straightening, and twisting movements in the affected segment after surgery. As such, the TOPS system serves to achieve the goals detailed earlier of restoring the physiologic neutral zone, maintaining a degree of spinal motion over rigid fusion, decreasing abnormal load-sharing at the adjacent levels, and minimizing screw-bone interface stresses, through the dampeners of the PcU elements contained therein.

## SCIENTIFIC TESTING RESULTS

### Finite Element Analysis

As part of the overall development program on early designs of the TOPS device, a finite element analysis (FEA) was performed on the implant using ANSYS computational software. The original model developed for this theoretical stress analysis was a half section representation of the device. The model was chosen because the device itself and the loading conditions on it were found to be symmetric about the central plane. This hemi-model analysis allowed for faster computation without loss of precision. The results of this assessment show the principal stresses acting on the model as a result of the applied loading. The principal stress generated in the device during maximum anticipated loading is well below the yield stress for the titanium alloy from which it is fabricated[21] (Fig. 72–4).

### Biomechanical in Vitro Motion Segment Analysis

The TOPS system was tested on six frozen cadaver specimens to (1) evaluate the capability of restoring motion to the intact spinal segment and (2) evaluate the effects on motion to the adjacent spinal segment after stabilization.

The test showed that the TOPS system almost ideally restores the motion behavior of a segment in left and right lateral bending (Fig. 72–5A) and left and right axial rotation (Fig. 72–5B) after facet removal compared to the intact segment. In flexion and extension (Fig. 72–5C), the range of motion was 55% of that of an intact segment. By way of comparison, these results are significantly better than the Dynesys system (Zimmer Spine, Inc., Warsaw, IN).[21] There was no effect shown on the adjacent segments. This finding, however, has to be interpreted carefully, as it might be due to the loading condition with pure moments.

The intradiscal pressure data showed that the implant allows the disc to take part of the load, which is consistent with the natural biomechanics of the disc. However, the absolute values cannot be compared directly to the in vivo conditions because no preload could be simulated. Additionally, the hydrostatic pressure can be determined accurately only in a nondegenerated disc.

### Load on the Pedicle Screws

To evaluate the efficacy of the polyaxial pedicle screws and the ability to fixate the TOPS device to the lumbar spinal vertebrae, a comparative test was performed. The examination was performed on a cadaveric spine with the same polyaxial screws. Strain gauges were applied to the same four screws so that the mechanical stress and resulting strains transferred to them from the leading

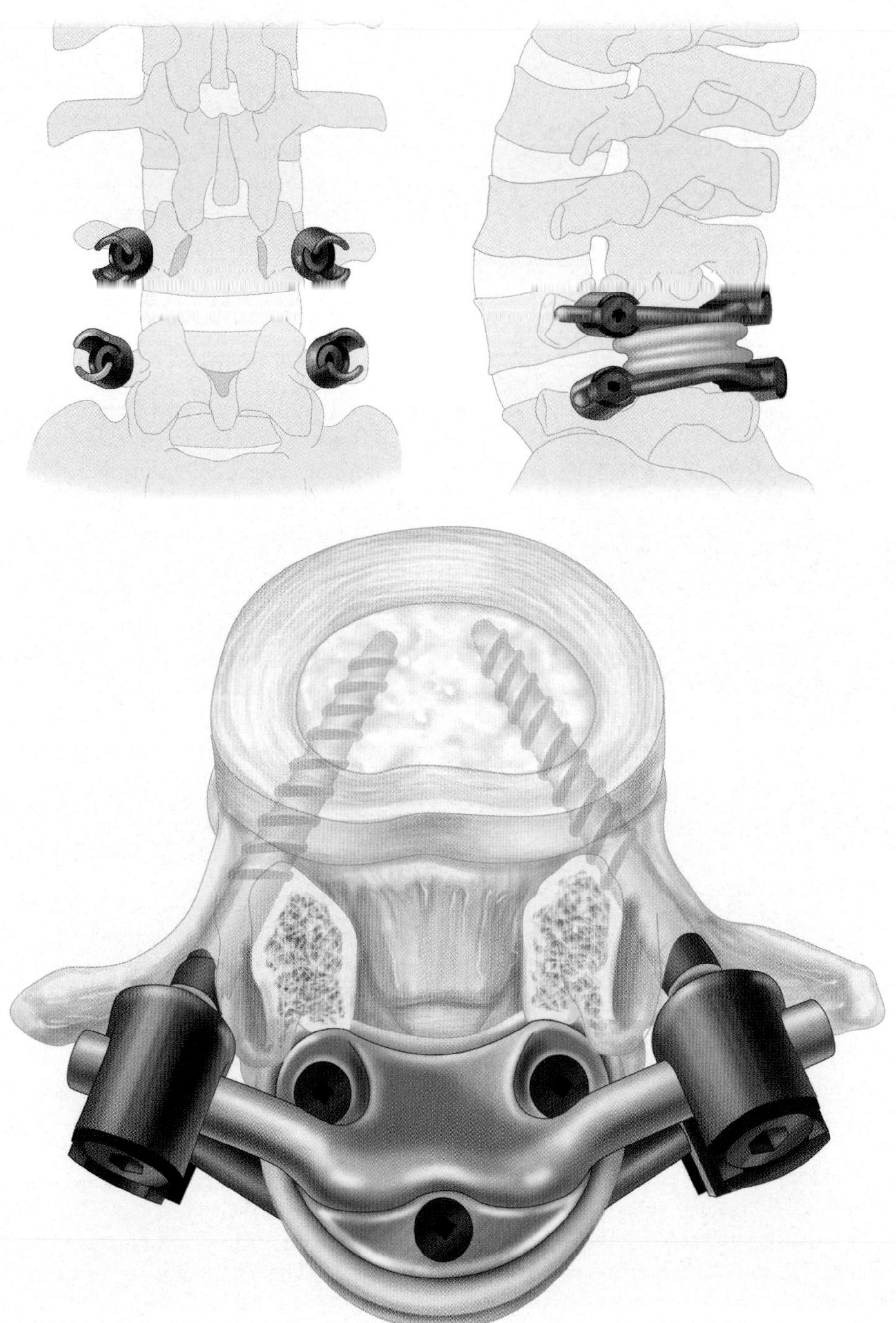

■ **FIGURE 72–3.** The TOPS system uses four standard hydroxyapatite-coated (HA-coated) polyaxial pedicle screws for fixation to the vertebrae.

competitor (Dynesys) and TOPS devices could be monitored while the spine simulator manipulated the spine segments (Fig. 72–6). Results of this study indicate that the load transmission to the pedicle screws is significantly less with the TOPS system than the leading competitor.[21] As clinical results of the Dynesys device have indicated a 6% to 8% screw loosening rate at 2- to 3-year clinical follow-ups, it would be expected that the TOPS device will fare as well if not better after long-term clinical implantation.[8,22]

## OPERATIVE TECHNIQUE

The patient is positioned prone on the operative frame with either a four-poster or double-roll type configuration to simultaneously recreate the lumbar lordosis as well as to ensure that the abdomen is free and uncompressed. Preoperative biplanar fluoroscopic confirmation of the spinal alignment and the target level incision is obtained. Preinjection of the skin, fascia, and musculature with 0.25% lidocaine with 1:200,000 epinephrine is useful to decrease

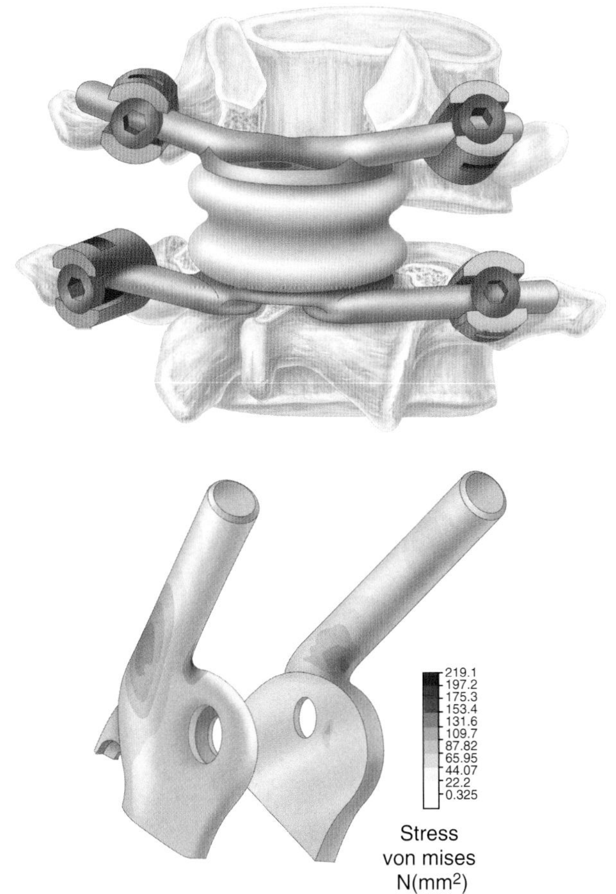


■ **FIGURE 72–4.** The principal stress generated in the device during maximum anticipated loading is well below the yield stress for the titanium alloy from which it is fabricated.

postoperative pain as well as to decrease intraoperative bleeding. The surgical field is then prepped and draped in the usual sterile fashion.

Using a No. 10 scalpel blade, a vertical incision is made down to the level of the lumbodorsal fascia. Subperiosteal dissection is then continued with the use of bovie cautery in combination with periosteal elevators to elevate the dorsal musculoligamentous complex off the spinous processes, laminae, and facets of the vertebrae above and below the target motion segment. As compared to classical spinal arthrodesis, in which exposure of the transverse processes is needed for future bone graft placement, exposure and retraction of the musculature for TOPS placement need only be carried to the lateral aspect of the facet complex. Additionally, particular care should be taken to preserve the capsule and muscular attachments surrounding the superior facet complex above the target level. The surgical exposure is then secured using a self-retaining retractor system.

Standard decompression of the index level is then completed via laminectomy and facetectomy techniques. Classically, spinal stenosis occurs at the central canal, lateral recess, and lateral neural foramen from a combination of disc herniation, dorsal uncovertebral joint spurring and lipping, facet osteophytes, and facet subluxation. Depending on the exact pathology of the individual case, the degree of bony, synovium, ligamentum flavum, and disc resection may thus vary accordingly (Fig. 72–7). With specific regard to the TOPS implant, there are three unique points that should be taken into account. First, it is recommended that aggressive resection of the intervertebral disc be avoided and that only herniated or bulging material be removed as needed to decompress the neural elements. Thermal annuloplasty with the bipolar forceps may be desired to stiffen and reinforce the annulus at the point of bulge or herniation.

Due to the specific design of the TOPS implant, total or near-total resection of the spinous process at the lower vertebrae of the index segment is needed to properly seat the four arms and centroid of the device. An implant trial is provided in the system and can be used to estimate the degree of laminar and spinous process removal that will be required (Fig. 72–8). Finally, as the TOPS implant serves to functionally replace the motion restraint of the native facet complex, it is recommended that the facet joint be effectively decoupled. This can be achieved by aggressive resection through the joint itself or by removing the superior articulating processes from the inferior vertebrae. This maneuver is often readily achieved by creating two surgical osteotomies at the level of the pars interarticularis with either an osteotome or powered drill-bit. Once the necessary degree of bony resection has been achieved, adequate neural decompression is confirmed with a Woodson elevator bilaterally over the thecal sac, exiting and traversing nerve roots. Meticulous hemostasis should be obtained at this point with a combination of bipolar cautery, bone wax, Gelfoam with thrombin, and Surgicel as needed. Some of the authors also advocate placement of a collagen-barrier type material (e.g., Duragen, Helostat) above the exposed neural elements to decrease the incidence of scarring and to create a readily accessible surgical plane in case of revision or implant removal.

The pedicle screw entry points are then identified at the superior and inferior vertebral levels. Particular attention should be paid to obtain a more lateral-to-medial vector of pedicle cannulation such that more triangulation of the final screws can be achieved. Careful preservation of the superior facet complex is again desired. A cannulated system is provided with the TOPS implant for use via a semipercutaneous technique if desired. In this fashion, a Jamshidi needle can be used to cannulate the pedicles, and then is exchanged for a Kirshner wire once confirmation of the needle trajectory has been obtained on biplanar fluoroscopic guidance. A unique pendulum type guide is provided in the TOPS system that will ensure that the angle of pedicle cannulation will remain within the acceptable range of angles that can be tolerated by the four-arm extensions of the implant (Fig. 72–9). Then, using the provided serial tissue dilator tubes, a working corridor is obtained through the lateral musculoligametous complex. In this fashion, excessive initial stripping and lateral exposure of the muscles can be minimized. A cannulated awl and tap can then be used to prepare the pedicle for instrumentation. It is recommended that a bicortical or near-bicortical triangulating passage be obtained as to massive the pull-out strength of the individual pedicle screw. Further, utilization of the largest diameter screw that can be accepted by the anatomy of the pedicle is recommended for similar reasons. Last, undertapping by 0.5 to 1 mm will also serve to increase the ultimate strength of the screw threads' purchase.

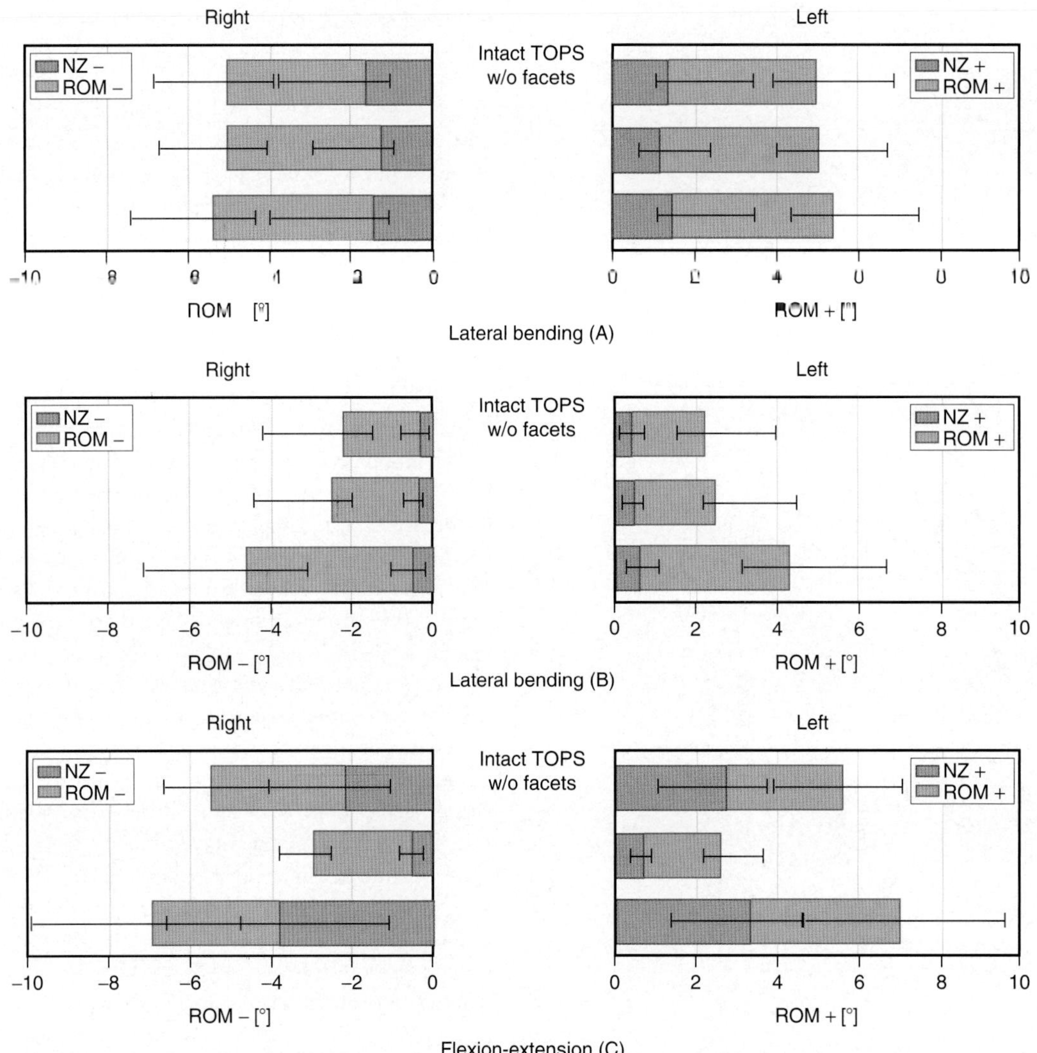


■ **FIGURE 72–5.** **A,** TOPS system almost ideally restores the motion behavior of a segment in left and right lateral bending. **B,** Left and right axial rotation after facet removal compared to the intact segment. **C,** In flexion and extension, the range of motion was 55% of that of an intact segment. NZ, neutral zone; ROM, range of motion.

Once the desired length of screw has been determined, the pedicles are then instrumented with the standard cannulated tulip-head polyaxial screws that are provided in the TOPS system. Snap-on slotted extension sleeves are available to facilitate final implantation of the TOPS device (Fig. 72–10). The pedicle screws can be placed with or without the sleeves attached according to the surgeon's preference. Whereas the top two screws should be advanced to the end of their passage as low as desired, it is recommended that the bottom two screws be kept slightly more prominent initially. Using a separate four-armed targeting jig (Fig. 72–11), the crossbars are first placed into the tulip heads of the superior screws. Then, using the adjustable sliding inferior arms of the targeting jig, the inferior screws can be advanced to the appropriate depth to ensure that it will readily accept the four-arm geometry of the TOPS implant. It is recommended by the authors that the screws not be "backed-up" if possible to again maximize their purchase and pull-out strength.

At this point, the TOPS device is prepared for implantation. Earlier in the process, the exact profile (regular or low-profile) has been determined using the sizing jigs already described. A small amount of sterile saline is injected through a small port in the gasketed portion of the centroid of the implant to serve as a nonhydraulic lubricant. The device is then loaded on a specialized claw-armed holder (Fig. 72–12). The four arms of the TOPS implant are then passed into the tulip heads of the polyaxial screws. If the screw-extension sleeves were utilized, these can help to facilitate the passage of the arms at this point. Once in place, each of the four crossbar arms are secured using a standard locking nut and then countertorqued to their final tightness (Fig. 72–13). Careful inspection of the implant should confirm that all crossbars are well seated with no evidence of cross-threading or inadequate surface area of the bars within the tulip-head channels. If present, the extension sleeves are then unclipped from the tulip heads to complete the TOPS device implantation

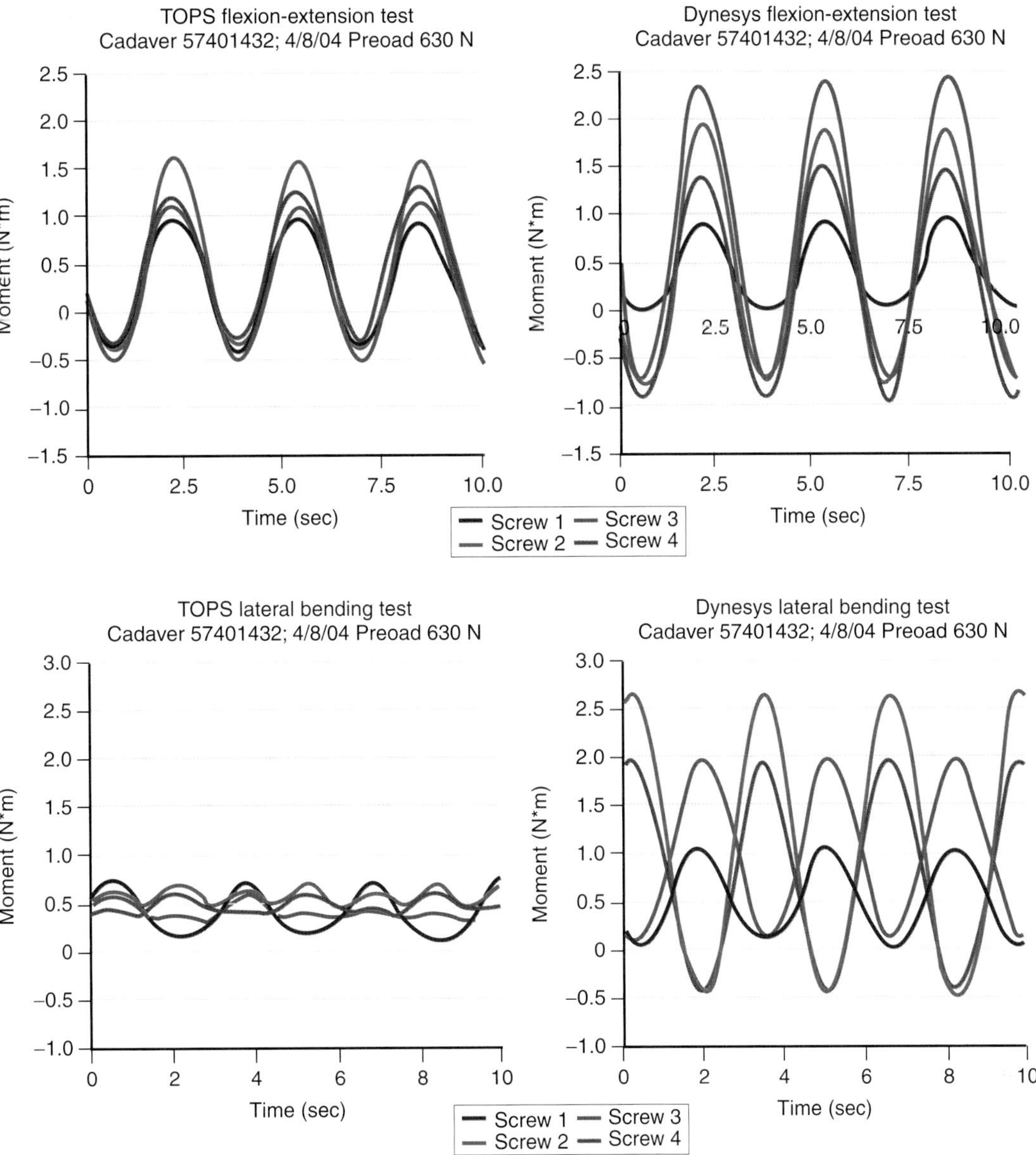


■ **FIGURE 72–6.** Spine simulator manipulating the spine segments.

procedure. Biplanar fluoroscopic confirmation of the device and screw positions should be obtained prior to final closure to ensure good alignment and angle of the overall segment and construct (Fig. 72–14).

Copious antibiotic-impregnated irrigation of the entire wound and implants is completed. A Davol or Jackson-Pratt wound drain should be placed at this time if there are concerns regarding hemostasis or seroma accumulation in the potential surgical dead space. Interrupted O-Vicryl sutures are then used to appose and close the lumbodorsal fascia in a near-watertight fashion. Inverted 2–0 or 3–0 absorbable sutures are then used to appose the subcutaneous layer of the skin. Skin closure can proceed according to the preference of the surgeon.

Postoperatively, a rigid clamshell lumbosacral orthosis is generally not recommended due to the motion-preserving nature of the TOPS implant. However, a lumbar corset or semirigid brace is often useful in the early perioperative period for support and the comfort of the patient. In comparison to spinal fusion patients, patients after TOPS implantation are encouraged to mobilize and ambulate early in their recovery process.

## CLINICAL OUTCOMES

### Patients and Methods

A total of 29 patients with the diagnosis of moderate-to-severe lumbar spinal stenosis were enrolled in a prospective clinical trial using the TOPS system (Class II). The sites included in this study are São Paulo, Brazil; Istanbul, Turkey; Zreifin, Israel; and Antwerp, Belgium. The average age of the enrolled patients was 64.2 years (range, 52–72 years) (Table 72–1). Inclusion

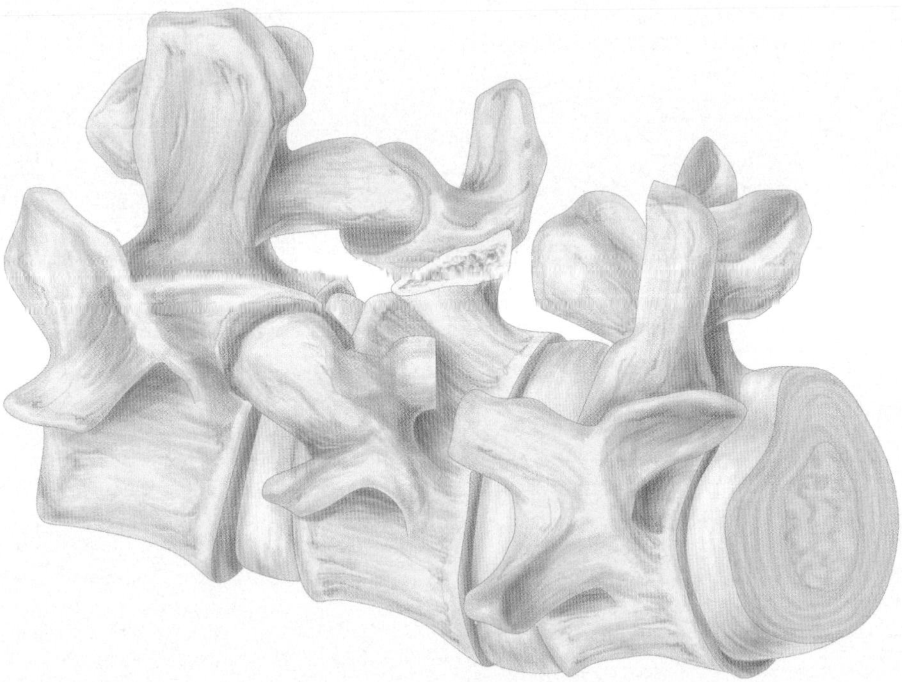

■ **FIGURE 72–7.** Depending on the exact pathology of the individual case, the degree of bony, synovium, ligamentum flavum, and disc resection may thus vary accordingly.

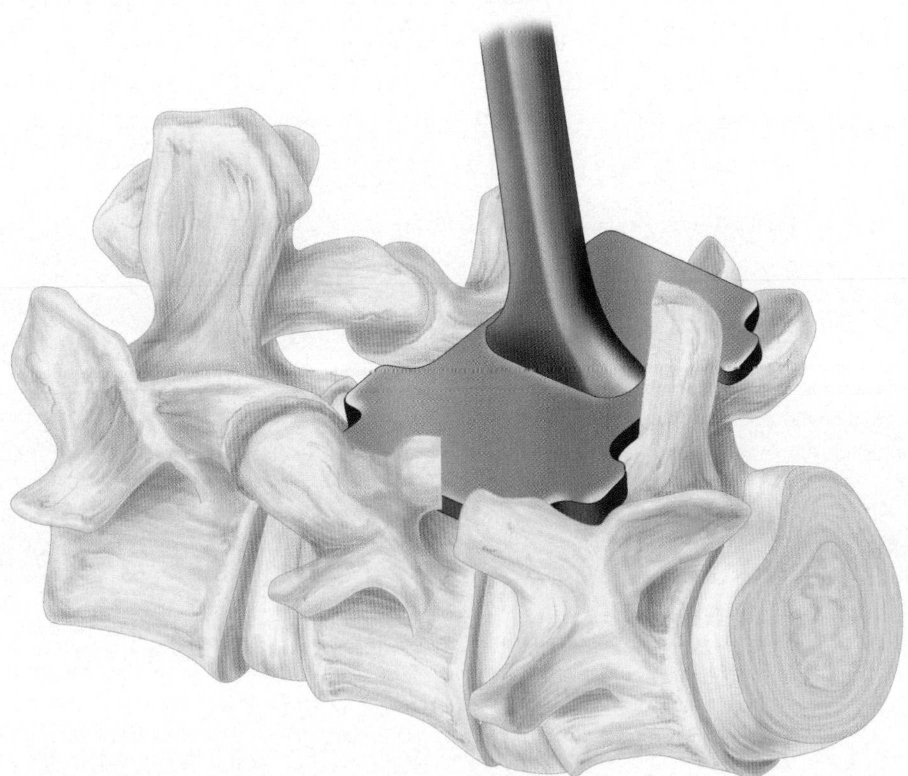

■ **FIGURE 72–8.** An implant trial used to estimate the degree of laminar and spinous process removal that will be required.

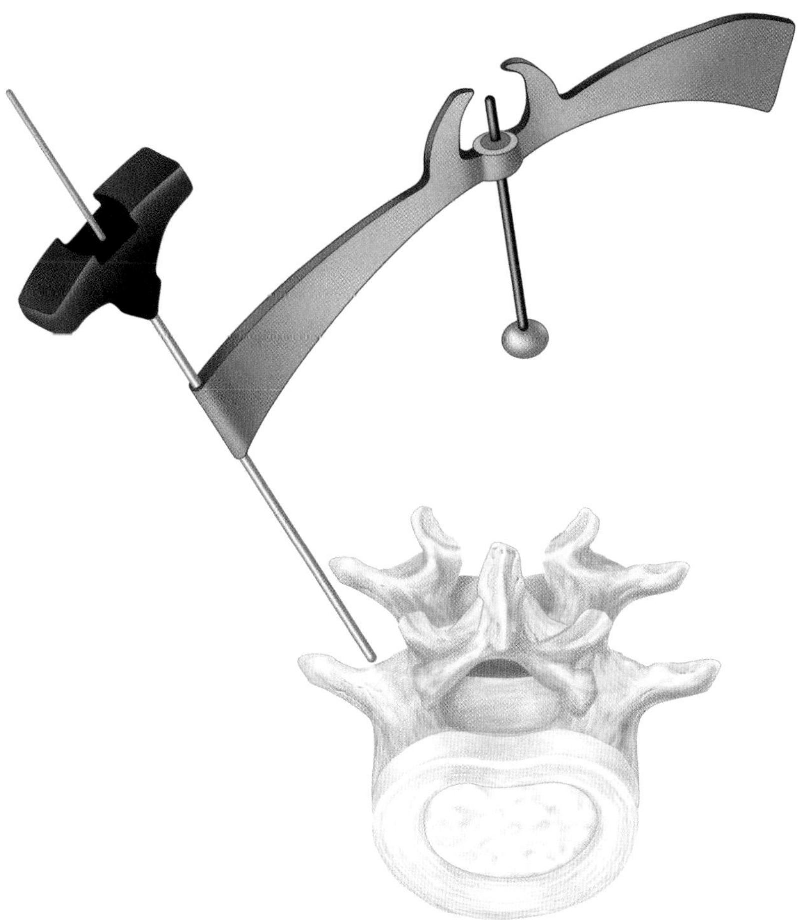

■ **FIGURE 72–9.** The pendulum guide provided in the TOPS system will ensure that the angle of pedicle cannulation will remain within the acceptable range of angles that can be tolerated by the four-arm extensions of the implant.

criteria for this population included patients requiring single-level spinal decompression and fusion surgery between L2 and L5. Radiographic analysis using computed tomography (CT), magnetic resonance imaging (MRI), myelography, or plain x-ray was performed to diagnose and better characterize the exact location of lumbar spinal stenosis. Specifically, these studies were used to confirm the presence of any of the following: thecal sac or cauda equina compression, nerve root impingement by either osseous or nonosseous elements, or hypertrophic facets with canal encroachment. All patients displayed both low back and sciatic pain, with or without claudication. Secondary inclusion criteria for this study included, but did not require, degenerative spondylolisthesis up to Grade 2, advanced facet arthrosis, and radiologic segmental instability (based on dynamic flexion-extension radiographic analysis).

Standard anteroposterior, lateral, flexion, and extension radiographs were obtained preoperatively and at 3 weeks, 6 weeks, and 6 months. Sagittal angulation was measured on the lateral radiographs from L1 to S1 using the Cobb method. Flexion, extension, and total range of motion were measured. The radiographs were examined by two independent observers for evidence of hardware failure, loosening, or signs of spinal instability. Clinical outcomes were assessed using Visual Analog Score (VAS), Oswestry Disability Index (ODI), and Zurich Claudication Questionnaire (ZCQ) questionnaires administered preoperatively and at 6 weeks, 3 months, 6 months, and 1 year following surgery.

## Results

To date, the patients enrolled are at various stages of follow-up ranging from 6 weeks to 1 year (Table 72–2). Of the 29 patients enrolled, 28 study patients were treated at L4-L5 and one patient was treated at L3-L4. Fifteen of the 29 patients had degenerative spondylolisthesis of Grade 1 or 2 (see Table 72–1). The mean surgical duration was 3.1 hours, with a standard deviation of 0.89 hour. The mean blood loss was approximately 200 mL. The average preoperative ODI score was 57%. The ODI scores were 20% and 16% at the 6-month and 1-year time points, respectively (Fig. 72–15). The mean VAS leg score was 88 at baseline, 21 at 6 weeks, 19 at 3 months, 18 at 6 months, and 12 at 1 year (Fig. 72–16). The mean ZCQ score was 57% initially and 26% at 1 year (Fig. 72–17).

The radiographic findings were reviewed by an independent panel of radiographic specialists at 6 weeks, 3 months, 6 months, and 1 year after the procedure. These studies revealed that all the motion segments instrumented with the TOPS device were stable and that no device migrations or malfunctions occurred. The preoperative disc heights at the treatment level and adjacent

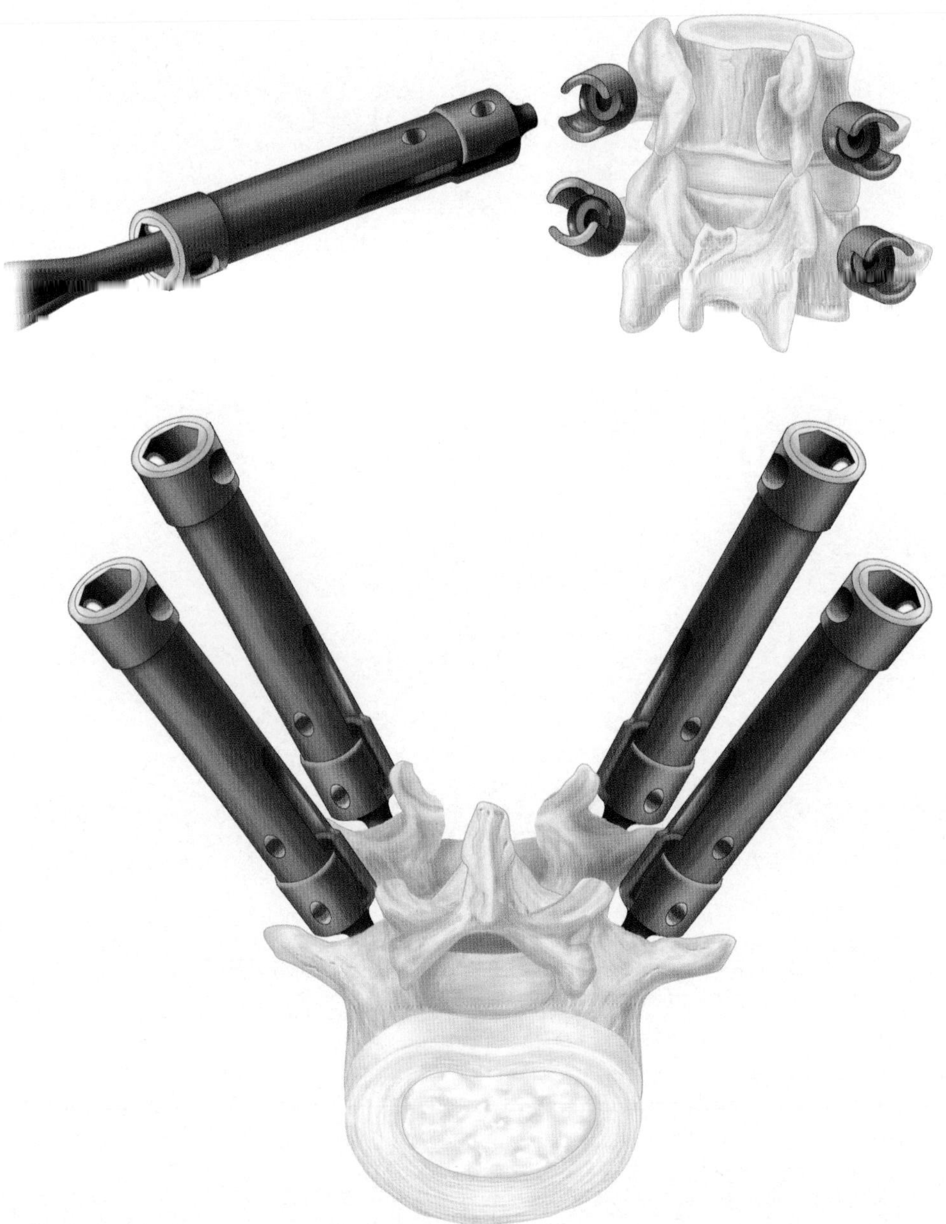

■ **FIGURE 72–10.** Snap-on slotted extension sleeves facilitate final implantation of the TOPS device.

levels were measured and recorded using plain x-rays and confirmed with sagittal CT scans. This was reevaluated at 3 months and 1 year and no subsequent disc height loss was observed. The degree of spondylolisthesis was recorded at all time points and no cases of slip progression were observed. The screw-bone interface was analyzed with thin-slice CT scans. In this independent analysis, none of the 29 patients exhibited any signs of screw loosening at any time point. Global spinal motion was also evaluated using flexion-extension films taken at 3 months and 12 months (Fig. 72–18). This evaluation confirmed that global motion was preserved in all patients ($n = 11$) through the 1-year time point.

Safety analysis revealed no device-related adverse events (AEs) during this study. Non-device–related AEs included three dural tears, four postoperative seromas, and one neurologic deficit. The non-device–related AEs occurred during the normal course of decompression and were not due to implant insertion. None of the dural tears or seromas developed long-term sequelae. None of the non-device–related AEs required additional surgery. During the study, one patient developed a transient neurologic deficit 1 day following surgery. CT evaluation showed that the position of the TOPS device and pedicle screws were normal. However, it also revealed the presence of a postoperative hematoma that was causing central canal compression. Although the patient's preoperative blood coagulation parameters were normal, the patient reported similar postoperative bleeding complications following previous knee surgery, with a late hemorrhage that required surgical intervention. The patient has been treated conservatively and demonstrated rapid improvement in neurologic function.

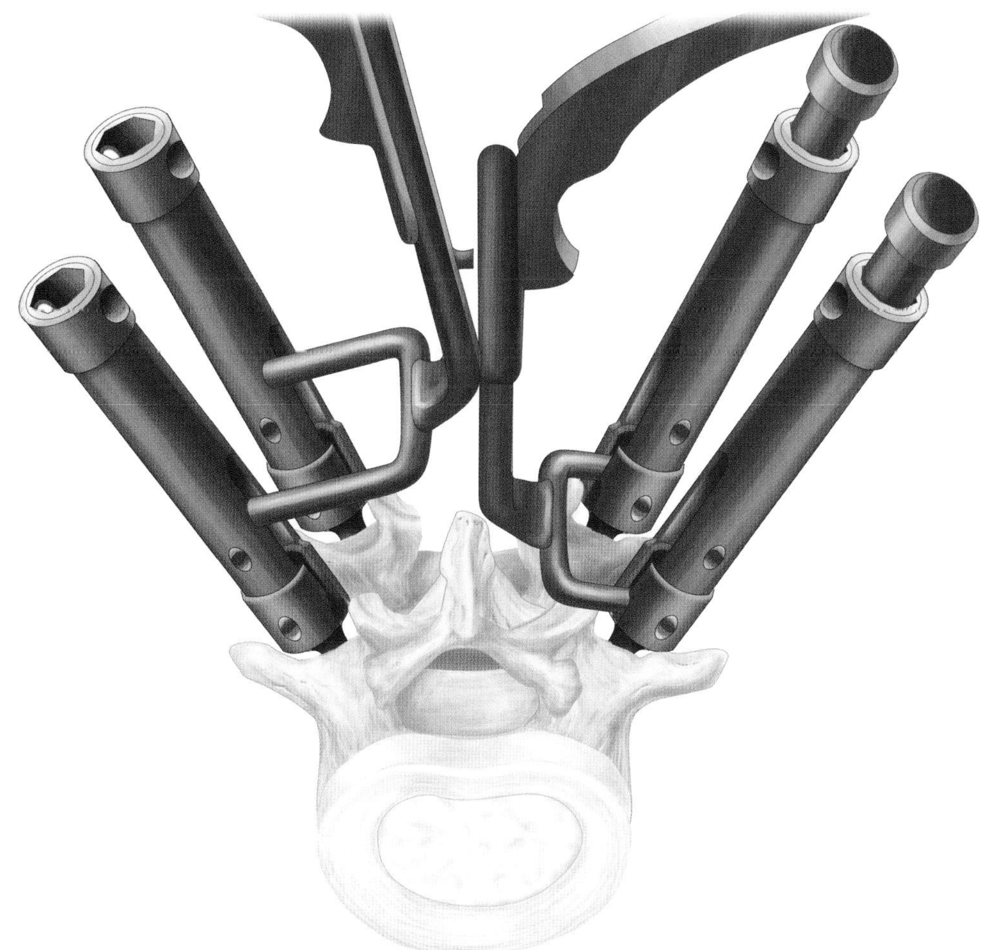

■ **FIGURE 72–11.** Four-armed targeting jig.

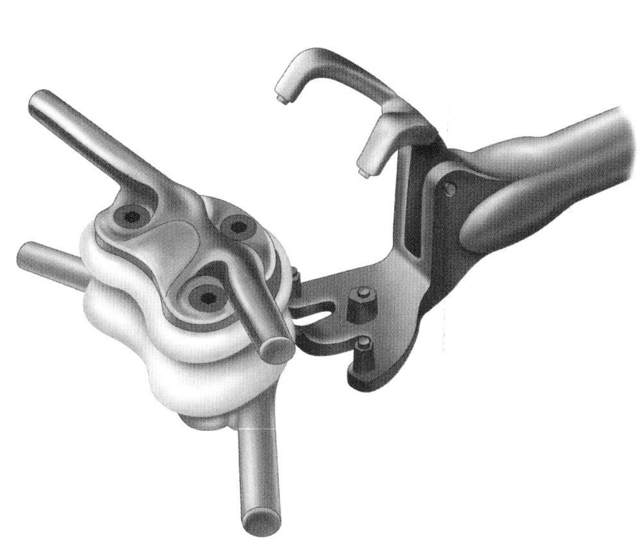

■ **FIGURE 72–12.** Claw-armed holder.

## CONCLUSION

The TOPS total facet replacement system is a novel posterior stabilizing device able to preserve motion, restore the biomechanical neutral zone, and prevent abnormal load-sharing at the treated and adjacent spinal motion segments. Within the limited clinical study, it appears that decompression combined with implantation of the TOPS device is able to achieve functional outcomes as favorable as historical control arms for fusion for stenosis and spondylolisthesis. ODI and VAS scores indicate that the device is effective in treating the back pain component of these patients as well as rigid spinal fusion in prior studies. Although the device itself has been tested for over 10 million cycles with no functional failures and minimal wear debris, questions concerning screw purchase and pullout will require far more extensive follow-up and study. As the device appears to have less screw-bone interface stresses than other predicate devices, it would be reasonable to expect a failure rate less than or equivalent to previously published predicate screw pullout rates of 6% to 8%.[8, 22] Additional long-term studies will also be required to examine the effect this device has on the incidence of ASD as well. Overall, the TOPS device represents a novel means of treating back pain while still preserving the native motion of the pathologic spinal segment.

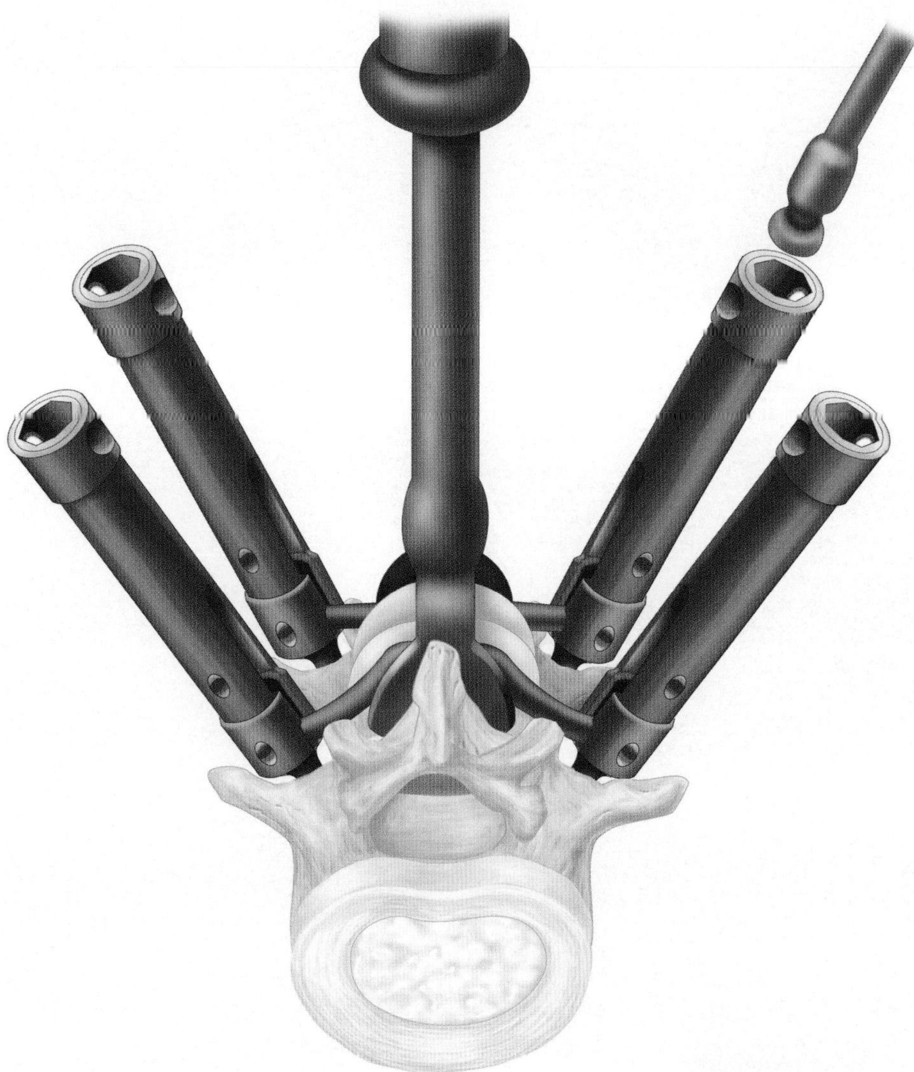

■ **FIGURE 72–13.** Once in place, each of the four cross-bar arms are secured using a standard locking nut and countertorqued to their final tightness.

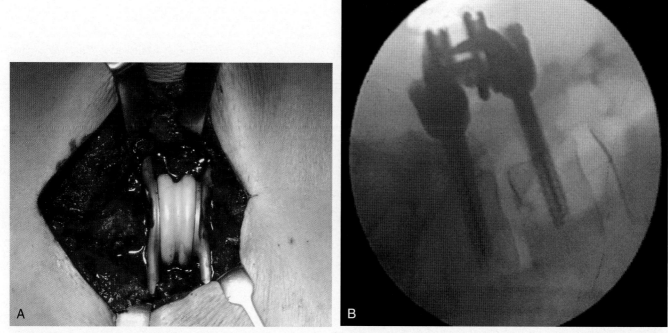

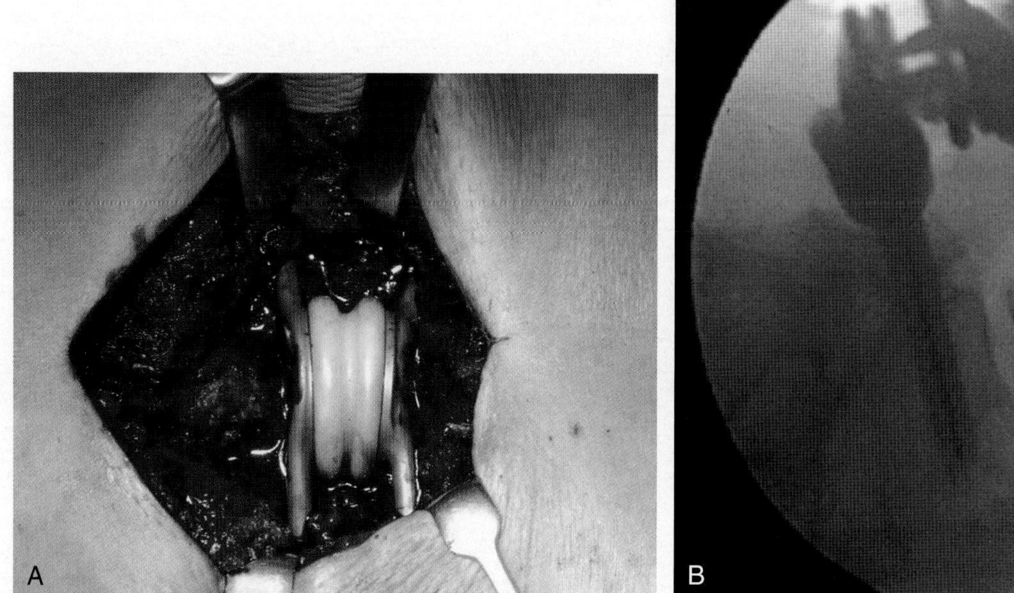

■ **FIGURE 72–14.** Biplanar fluoroscopic confirmation of the device and screw positions should be obtained prior to final closure to ensure good alignment and angle of the overall segment and construct.

TABLE 72–1. Patient Demographics in TOPS Clinical Trial

| Category | Data |
|---|---|
| Gender | |
| Male | 12 (41.4%) |
| Female | 17 (58.6%) |
| Age | |
| Mean (SD) | 64.2 (6.10) |
| Min, max | 52.0, 72.0 |
| Body mass index | |
| Mean (SD) | 28.8 (4.94) |
| Min, max | 18.1, 39.2 |
| Spondylolisthesis | |
| Grade 0 | 48.3% |
| Grade I | 44.8% |
| Grade II | 6.9% |

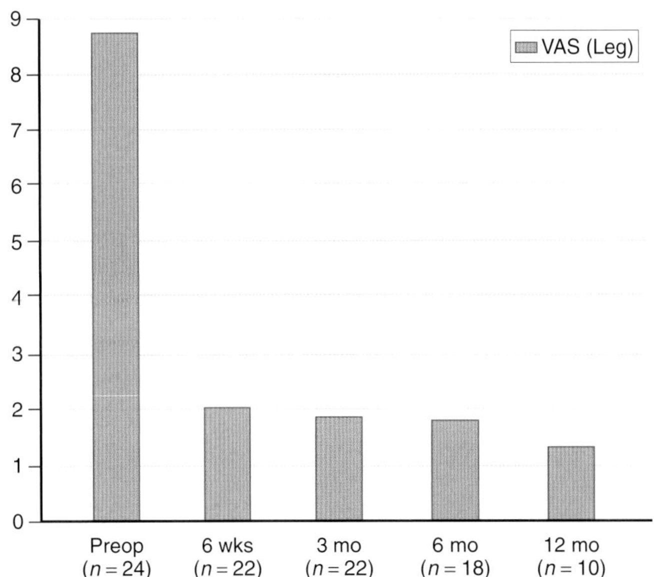


■ FIGURE 72–16. Visual Analog Score (VAS) for the leg at baseline (preop) and at 6 weeks, 3 months, 6 months, and 1 year after surgery.

TABLE 72–2. Patient Follow-Up Distribution per Study Site

| | Baseline | Patient Follow-Up Distribution | | | |
|---|---|---|---|---|---|
| | | 6 wks | 3 mo | 6 mo | 12 mo |
| Theoretical | 29 | 29 | 29 | 25 | 17 |
| Expected | 29 | 29 | 28 | 20 | 12 |
| Actual | 29 | 25 | 18 | 18 | 11 |
| Follow-up (%) | | 86 | 79 | 90 | 92 |

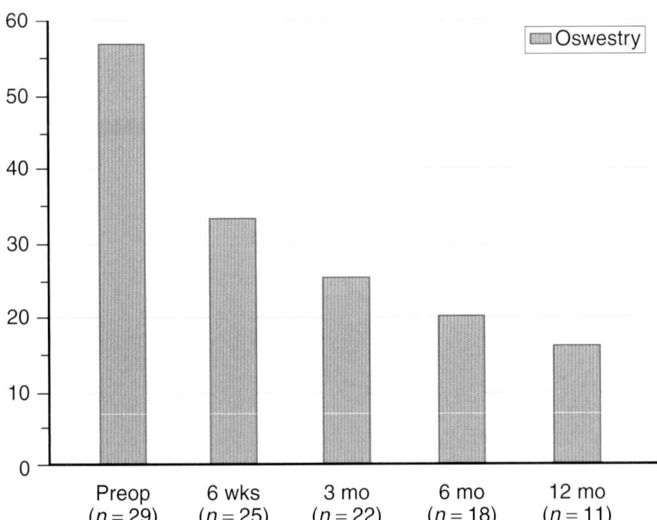


■ FIGURE 72–15. Oswestry Disability Index (ODI) scores before surgery (preop) and at 6 weeks, 3 months, 6 months, and 1 year.

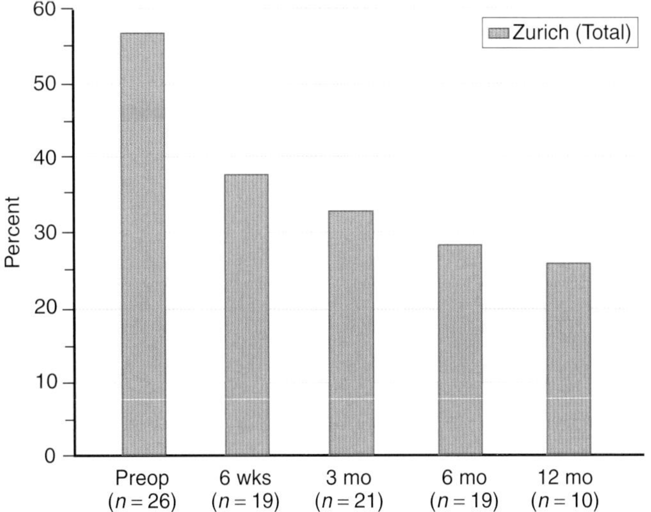


■ FIGURE 72–17. Mean Zurich Claudication Questionnaire (ZCQ) score before and after surgery up to 1 year.

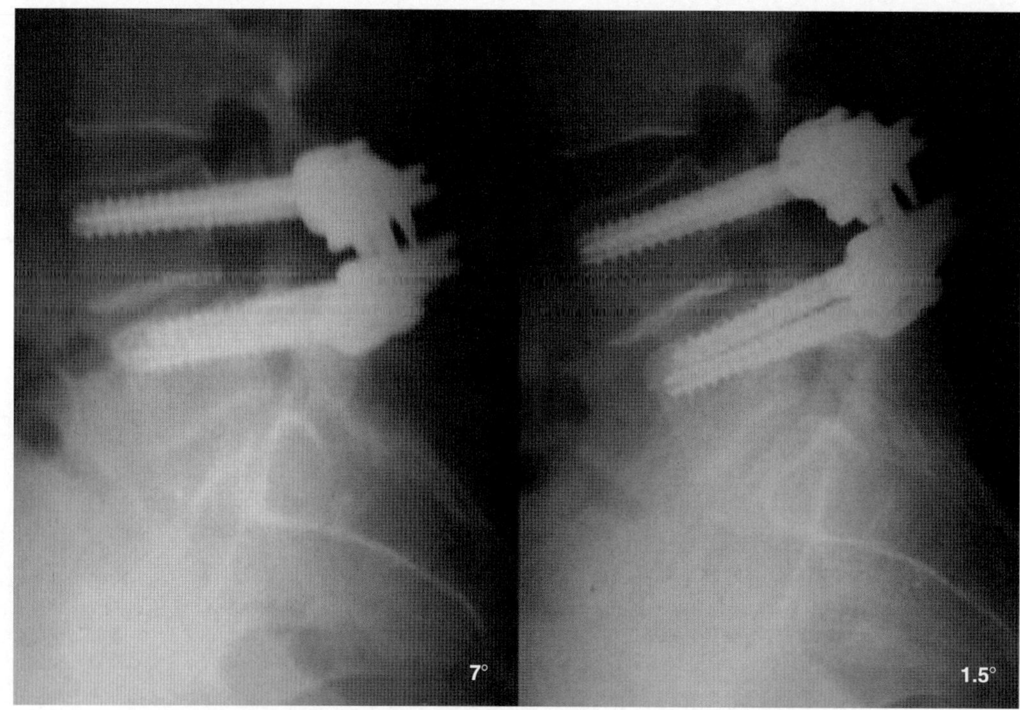


■ **FIGURE 72–18.** Flexion-extension films taken at 3 months and 12 months.

## REFERENCES


1. Abumi K, Panjabi MM, Kramer HM, et al: Biomechanical evaluation of lumbar spinal stability after graded facetectomies. Spine 15 (11):1142–1147, 1990.
2. Blumenthal S, McAfee PC, Guyer RD, et al: A prospective, randomized, multicenter Food and Drug Administration investigational device exemptions study of lumbar total disc replacement with the CHARITE artificial disc versus lumbar fusion, Part I: Evaluation of clinical outcomes. Spine 30(14):1565–1575; discussion E387–E391, 2005.
3. Resnick DK, Chourdhri TF, Dailey AT, et al: Guidelines for the performance of fusion procedures for degenerative disease of the lumbar spine, Part 5: Correlation between radiographic and functional outcome. J Neurosurg Spine 2(6):658–661, 2005.
4. Resnick DK, Chourdhri TF, Dailey AT, et al: Guidelines for the performance of fusion procedures for degenerative disease of the lumbar spine, Part 7: Intractable low-back pain without stenosis or spondylolisthesis. J Neurosurg Spine 2(6):670–672, 2005.
5. Resnick DK, Chourdhri TF, Dailey AT, et al: Guidelines for the performance of fusion procedures for degenerative disease of the lumbar spine, Part 9: Fusion for patients with stenosis and associated spondylolisthesis. J Neurosurg Spine 2(6):679–685, 2005.
6. Resnick DK, Chourdhri TF, Dailey AT, et al: Guidelines for the performance of fusion procedures for degenerative disease of the lumbar spine, Part 10: Fusion following decompression in patients with stenosis without spondylolisthesis. J Neurosurg Spine 2(6):686–691, 2005.
7. Fischgrund JS, Mackay M, Herkowitz HN, et al: 1997 Volvo Award winner in clinical studies: Degenerative lumbar spondylolisthesis with spinal stenosis: A prospective, randomized study comparing decompressive laminectomy and arthrodesis with and without spinal instrumentation. Spine 22:2807–2812, 1997.
8. Grob D, Benini A, Junge A, Mannion AF: Clinical experience with the Dynesys Semirigid Fixation System for the lumbar spine: Surgical outcome and patient oriented outcome in 50 cases after an average of 2 years. Spine 30(3):324–331, 2005.
9. Huang J, Girardi F, Camissa F: The prevalence of contraindications to total disc replacement in a cohort of lumbar surgical patients. Spine 29(22):2538–2541, 2004.
10. Hunter LY, Braunstein EM, Bailey RW: Radiographic changes following anterior cervical spine fusions. Spine 5:399–401, 1980.
11. Kostuik JP: Complications and surgical revision for failed disc arthroplasty. Spine J 4:289S–291S, 2004.
12. Lee CK: Accelerated degeneration of the segment adjacent to a fusion. Spine 13:375–377, 1988.
13. Lee CK, Langrana NA: Lumbosacral spinal fusion: A biomechanical study. Spine 9:574–581, 1984.
14. Lu WW, Luk KD, Holmes A: Pure shear properties of lumbar spinal joints and the effect of tissue sectioning on load-sharing. Spine 30 (8):E204–E209, 2005.
15. Olsewski JM, Garvey TA, Schendel MJ: Biomechanical analysis of facet and graft loading in a Smith-Robinson type cervical spine model. Spine 19:2540–2544, 1994.
16. Geisler FH: Surgical technique of lumbar artificial disc replacement with the Charite Artificial Disc. Neurosurgery 56(1):46–57; discussion 46–57, 2005.
17. Gamradt SC, Wang JC: Lumbar disc arthroplasty. Spine J 5:95–103, 2005.
18. Yone K, Sahou T, Kawauchi Y, et al: Indication of fusion for lumbar spinal stenosis in elderly patients and its significance. Spine 21:242–248, 1996.
19. Panjabi MM: Clinical spinal instability and low back pain. J Electromyogr Kinesiol 13(4):371–379, 2003.
20. Panjabi MM: The stabilizing system of the spine, Part II: Neutral zone and instability hypothesis. J Spinal Disord 5(4):390–396; discussion 397, 1992.
21. McAfee P: Biomechanics and results of implant testing of the TOPS Facet Replacement Device (Luncheon Symposium presentation—TOPS Device). Presented at the 5th Annual Spine Arthroplasty Society Meeting, New York, New York, May 9, 2005.
22. Stoll TM, Dubois G, Schwarzenbach O: The dynamic neutralization system for the spine: A multi-center study of a novel non-fusion system. Eur Spine J 11(2):170–178, 2002.

CHAPTER 73

# Total Facet Arthroplasty System (TFAS)

**Scott A. Webb** and **Gordon Neil Holen**

## KEY POINTS

- Total Facet Arthroplasty System (TFAS) is a nonfusion spinal implant developed for the treatment of patients with moderate-to-severe lumbar spinal stenosis.
- TFAS allows for the replacement of the diseased facets and laminae and is an alternative to traditional spinal fusion.
- The potential benefits for posterior motion devices include stabilization with controlled kinematics, excision of pain generators, allowance of a more complete lateral recess decompression compared to standard laminectomy, and avoidance of increasing loads at and accelerating degeneration of adjacent levels.

Total Facet Arthroplasty System (TFAS) (Archus Orthopedics Inc., Redmond, WA) is a nonfusion spinal implant developed for the treatment of patients with moderate-to-severe lumbar spinal stenosis. TFAS allows for the replacement of the diseased facets and laminae and is an alternative to traditional spinal fusion. This procedure allows for a wide decompression and maintains, and often restores, intervertebral motion, stability, and sagittal balance in the replaced spinal segment. In contrast to spinal fusion, TFAS also eliminates the need for autologous bone grafting and its well-known associated comorbidities. Currently, TFAS is limited to investigational use only within the U.S. The current clinical trial is a multicenter prospective randomized controlled study comparing the safety and effectiveness of TFAS to spinal fusion for patients with moderate-to-severe lumbar spinal stenosis.

A great deal of time and interest has been focused on the development of motion-preserving technology and artificial disc replacement, with little attention paid to the posterior structures. Huang and associates showed that the majority of contraindications for total disc replacement candidates (89%) involve stenosis and facet arthritis.[1] The potential benefits for posterior motion devices include stabilization with controlled kinematics, excision of pain generators, allowance of a more complete lateral recess decompression compared to standard laminectomy, and avoidance of increasing loads at and accelerating degeneration of adjacent levels.

## BIOMECHANICS

The functional spine unit (FSU) comprises the five-joint complex of the intervertebral disc, corresponding facet joints, and ligaments. The FSU has three main roles: (1) to stabilize the vertebrae in relation to each other and protect the nerves through a range of motion and under various loads; (2) to provide proper motion of each segment and of the spine as a whole; and (3) to transfer and share loads within the spinal column. The balance of these three biomechanical elements can be disrupted by disease as well as surgical procedures.

The primary role of the facet joints is to both allow and limit motion, thus acting as spinal segment stabilizers. Facet joints also act to protect the lumbar disc from excessive stress. They are complex synovial joints which bear loads in both compression and shear (Fig. 73–1A and B). Facet joint load depends on location and can be increased by degeneration of the intervertebral disc.

Facet joint capsules are innervated by Type I, II, and III mechanoreceptors. It is thought that their proprioceptive role can be compensated for by the balance of non-removed capsules in the spine. Work done by Jiang and associates in 1995 showed that the supraspinous and interspinous ligaments were innervated by bundles of Type III receptors suggesting that spinal ligaments are indeed active in monitoring the loading of spinal joints.[2] This provides at least static positional awareness for postural control. This offers additional support to the concept that ligaments act as part of the neurologic feedback mechanism for protection and stability of the spine. Thus, the neural input from the facets may indeed be important for proprioception and may modulate muscular action that could control joint stability.

Damage to and pain from the facet joints and corresponding capsular ligaments can be independent of surgical intervention and result from trauma, disease, and degeneration. Extensive work has been published on facet joints as pain generators. Ghormley first described this as *Facet syndrome* in 1933.[3] The facet synovial linings and capsules are highly innervated and have free nerve endings within their tissues. Cartilage breakdown can lead to progressive joint

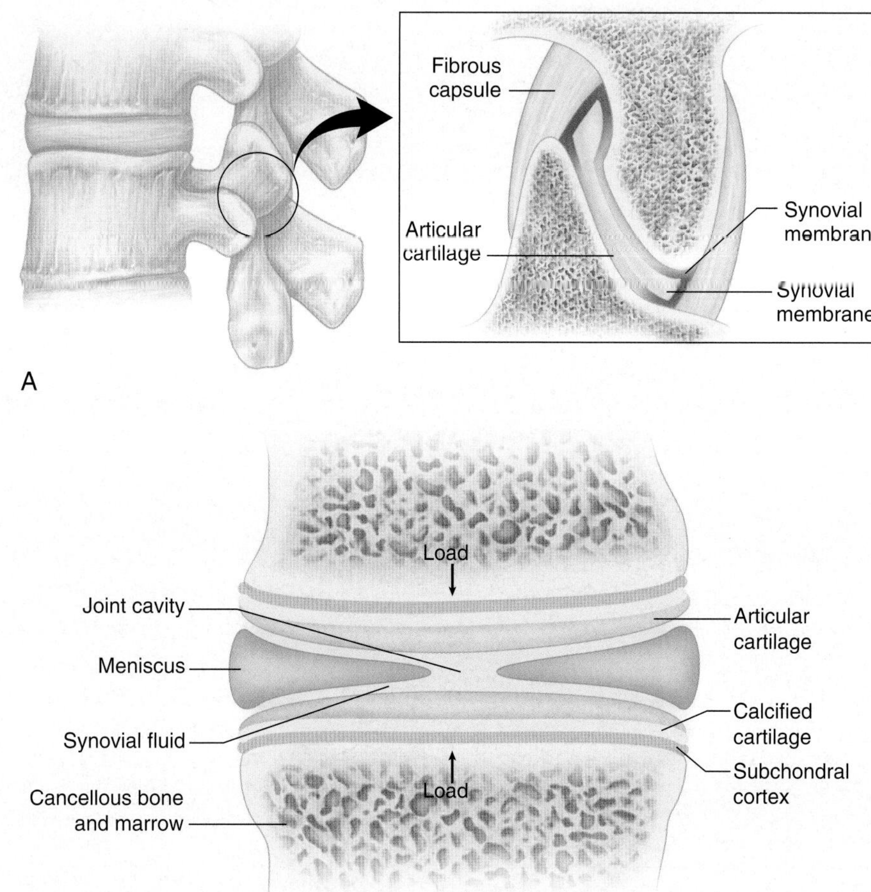


■ **FIGURE 73–1.** **A,** Schematic drawing of an apophyseal joint. (Adapted from Adams MA, Hutton WC: The mechanical function of the lumbar apophyseal joints. Spine 8(3):327–330, 1983.) **B,** Generic drawing of a diarthrodial (synovial) joint. (Adapted from Mow VC, Hayes WC (eds): Basic Orthopaedic Biomechanics, 2nd ed. Philadelphia, Lippincott-Raven, 1997.)

degeneration, inflammation, spur formation, and possible synovial cyst formation. Cyst formation may also lead to stenosis and radiculopathy. A grading system was proposed for facet degeneration by Fujiwara[4] (Figs. 73–2 and 73–3).

The function of the facet joints is determined by their shape, size, orientation, and location (Fig. 73–4). In the cervical spine the facets are located laterally and are tilted in abduction in the coronal plane. This allows significant freedom in lateral bending, extension, and axial torsion. Cervical facets are subjected to the lowest effective transmitted loads in the spine.

Lumbar facets, in contrast, are larger, more centrally located, and oriented in a more sagittal or adducted position. This orientation allows for the main motion of the lumbar segments, which is flexion and extension. Axial rotation and lateral flexion are limited. The joints act as cam-like stops, preventing hyperextension and axial torsion. Lumbar facets are also subjected to the highest magnitude load in the spine.

## INDICATIONS AND CONTRAINDICATIONS

TFAS is currently indicated for use as an adjunct to decompressive procedures in place of traditional fusion. It can be used in degenerative diseases of the facets, central or lateral recess stenosis with claudication, and in cases with Grade I degenerative spondylolisthesis. It is currently allowed for single-level implantation at L3-L4 and L4-L5. A U.S. Investigational Device Exemption (IDE) study allows for decompression of up to three levels but limits implantation of the device to a single level. The first TFAS within the U. S. was performed on August 26, 2005, under the FDA IDE study, and TFAS is not yet available outside study centers within the U. S. The European Commission, however, approved the general use of TFAS within the European Union on March 2, 2005.

Contraindications in the current U.S. IDE study include a dual-emission x-ray absorptiometry (DEXA) scan with a T score below −2.5, immunosuppressive disorder, metal implant sensitivities, BMI greater than 35, scoliosis with a Cobb angle greater than 25 degrees, and endocrine or metabolic disorders that may affect osteogenesis.

## DESCRIPTION OF DEVICE

The Total Facet Arthroplasty System is a modular implant with a metal-on-metal articulation. The present device is fixated to the

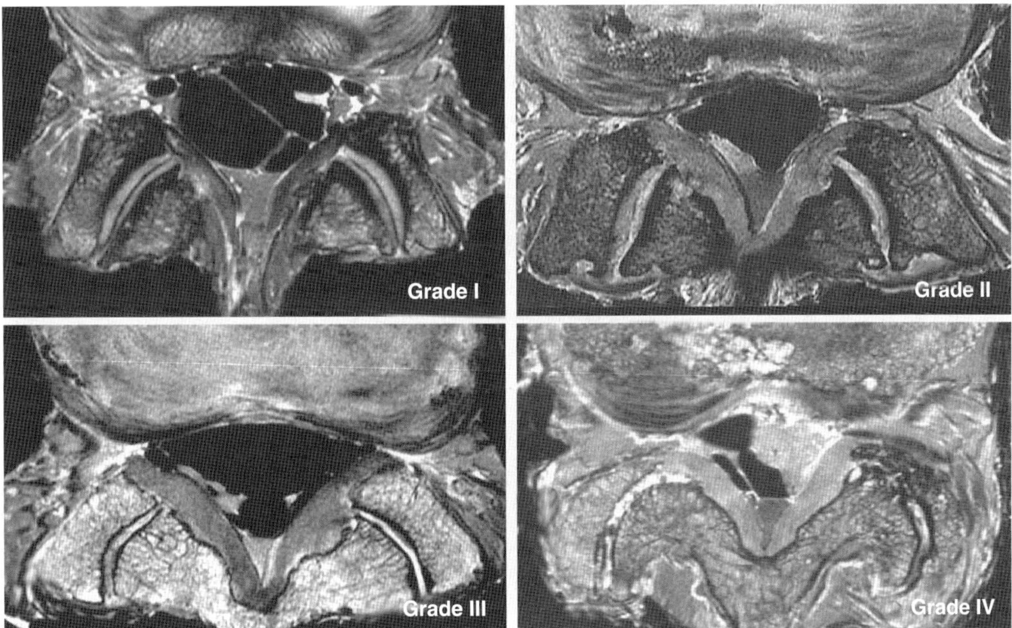


■ **FIGURE 73–2.** Facet cartilage degeneration MRI scale proposed by Grogan. Grade I: Uniformly thick cartilage covers the articular surfaces completely. Grade II: Cartilage covers the entire surface of the articular processes but with erosion of the irregular region evident. Grade III: Cartilage incompletely covers the articular surfaces, with regions of the underlying bone exposed to the joint. Grade IV: Cartilage is absent except for traces on the articular surfaces. (From Fujiwara A, Lim T, An H, et al: The effect of disc degeneration and facet joint arthritis on the segmental flexibility of the lumbar spine. Spine 25(23):3036–3044, 2000.)

pedicles with standard polymethyl-methacrylate (PMMA) cement, although a cementless implant is under development. It comprises two cephalad bearings and two caudal housings or cups, which articulate via a cross-arm assembly (Figs. 73–5 and 73–6).

TFAS allows flexion of 13 degrees and extension of 2 degrees. Lateral bending is allowed up to 7.5 degrees and axial rotation up to 2 degrees. The instant axis of rotation is in the posterior third of the vertebral body.

Kinematic testing has demonstrated that the TFAS implant restores motion of an unstable FSU to that of an intact FSU. Motion was stabilized in flexion and lateral bending and restored in extension. Motion was limited in axial rotation.

In vivo loading has been performed comparing TFAS to a pedicle screw fusion system. With similar loads applied to both systems, the strains in the actual metal surfaces are lower than the rigidly connected pedicle screw system because of the motion capability of the system. This implies that TFAS will transmit lower loads to the implant-bone interface.

Strength testing demonstrates that the construct strength, utilizing cement, is two to three times greater than maximum static in vivo loads that the device will experience (Fig. 73–7). The strength of the fixation in vertebral bone is two times stronger than that of pedicle screws. The integrity of the construct and interconnection mechanisms were tested in vitro to 10 million

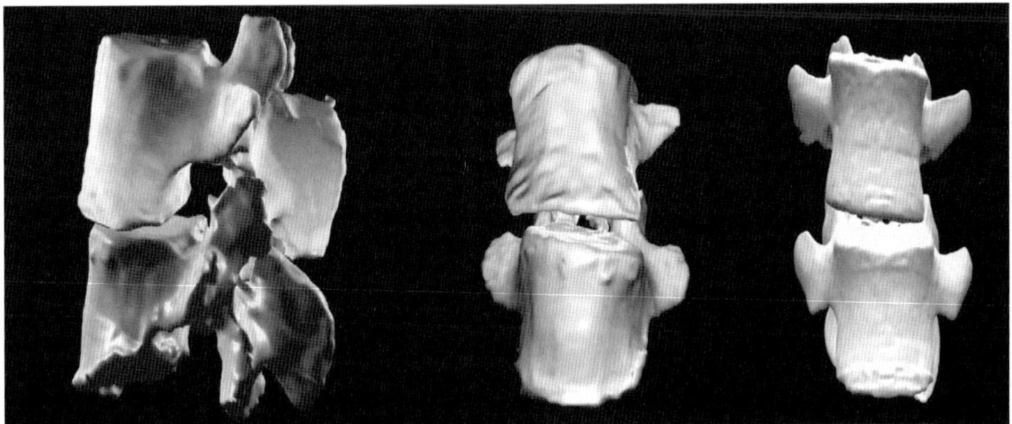

■ **FIGURE 73–3.** Examples of lumbar vertebrae from highly degenerative *(left)* to normal *(right)* patients contrasting the large variability in geometry which affects load-bearing and motion.

■ **FIGURE 73–4.** The three-dimensional morphology of the facets is complex but can be well characterized through computed anthropometric analysis of CT-scan reconstructions. Accurate characterization of facet morphology is necessary because curvature, pose, and location of vertebral facet joints play an important role in their load-bearing characteristics.

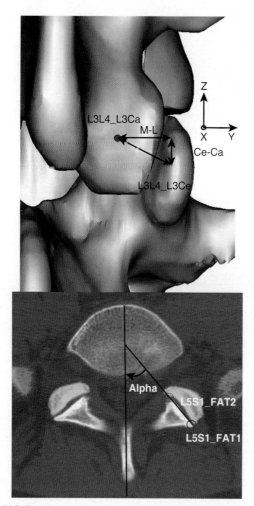

cycles and there were no implant connection failures or dissociations of the device and PMMA under maximum static loading. The strength of the system is key, and TFAS sets the standard for bone-implant interface strength.

Implant wear was assessed through 10 million cycles of testing in a custom-designed wear simulator that allows variable and cross-coupled motion and load application to replicate the activity of daily living conditions of the intact spine. The structural members of the implant are titanium-aluminum-vanadium alloy ($Ti_6Al_4V$) while the articulating surfaces are cobalt-chromium (CoCr). The amount of debris generated is similar to that generated by other orthopaedic implant-bearing surfaces under physiologic testing conditions. Particle size and distribution also were comparable to current metal-on-metal hips. In animal studies there was no neurotoxic response noted locally or systemically.

Load-sharing has been shown to be more physiologic with TFAS when compared to a pedicle fusion construct as demonstrated in tests using strain gauges. Testing was performed with strain gauges placed in the disc space. The disc loads were measured and the TFAS-treated disc segment acted similar to an intact FSU, while the pedicle screw system demonstrated significantly lower non-physiologic loads at the disc space.

TFAS has been studied in complete laminectomy-facetectomy models. Studies have shown that TFAS is able to restore segmental stability to that of an intact functional spine unit (Fig. 73–8).

Because TFAS is designed to be a total joint replacement, it not only restores the physiologic range or limits of motion but also the quality of motion of the operated segment to that of an intact spinal segment. Quality of motion can be defined as the ability of a device (e.g., posterior stabilizing or spinal arthroplasty) to replicate the characteristic kinematic signature of the intact spine in both its limits as well as profile.

The highly nonlinear nature of lumbar spine kinematics, especially in flexion-extension and lateral bending, is a result of the interaction of all the multiple nonlinear subsystems of the spine, such as ligaments, discs, nucleus, muscles, and cartilaginous facet contact. Therefore, the TFAS implants have been designed to physiologically reproduce the biomechanics of the spine after implantation. A design objective of reproducing only the limits of motion rather than the whole motion path during activities of

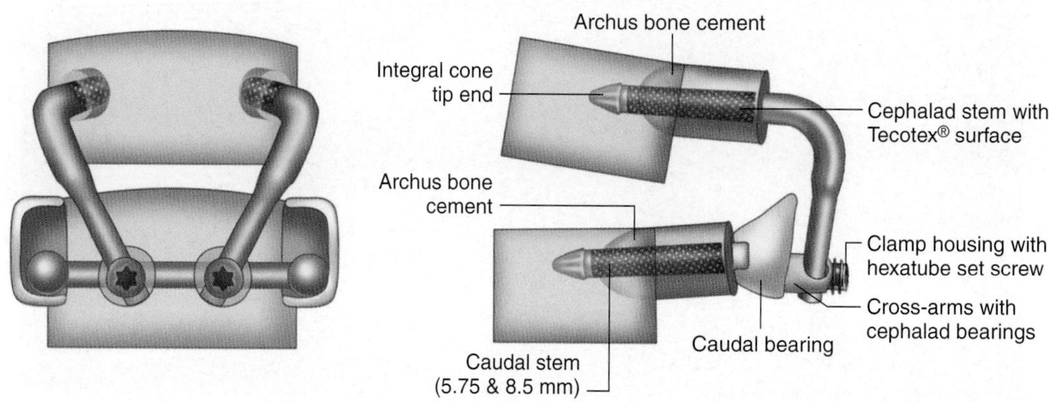


■ **FIGURE 73–5.** The TFAS construct in relation to the vertebral bodies with individual component labels.

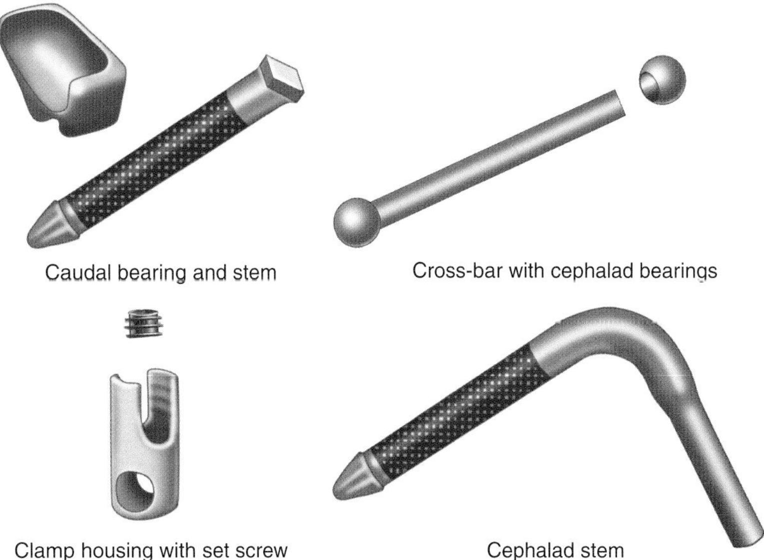


■ **FIGURE 73–6.** Schematic of the TFAS components that are assembled in order to custom-fit the highly variable patient anatomy.

daily living could result in a non-physiologic loading of the tissues and implants and lead to morphologic changes in the tissues due to disuse or overload during the duty cycle of the device after implantation. Other devices that are meant to dynamically stabilize and preserve motion rather than restore physiologic motion may only grossly reproduce the kinematic behavior of the lumbar spine and not truly reproduce the physiologic motion profile of the spine but rather allow only for similar motion ranges or limits (Fig. 73–9).

## SCIENTIFIC TESTING RESULTS

Our initial experience with TFAS was in Romania. We prospectively evaluated 13 consecutive patients who underwent total facet arthroplasty. Our first operation was on May 13, 2005. Our initial series involved eight male and five female patients with an average age of 60.7 years and average BMI of 28.9. Four operations were at L3-L4 and nine at L4-L5. Results were quantified using the Zurich Claudication Questionnaire (ZCQ) for both symptom and function as well as Visual Analog Scale (VAS) measurements.

The mean percentage of improvement in ZCQ Symptom Raw Score was 50.2%, ZCQ Function Raw Score was 46%, VAS Leg improvement was 78.2%, and VAS Back was 63.7%.

## CLINICAL PRESENTATION

Standard preoperative planning, as with any surgical spine procedure, begins with a systematic history and physical examination. Radiographs should include a minimum of anteroposterior, lateral, and flexion-extension radiographs. Magnetic resonance imaging (MRI) or myelography is performed to document underlying stenosis. An attempt should be made to verify that the diameter of the involved pedicles will allow creation of a 6.5-mm diameter drill channel. Otherwise, no special testing is required preoperatively for total facet arthroplasty.

## OPERATIVE TECHNIQUES

### Positioning

The patient is positioned on a Jackson table in the prone position after general endotracheal intubation. This position allows the chest to be supported, legs extended, and the abdomen free from external compression and will place the patient in good lordotic alignment and allow C-arm visualization. Lordotic positioning is important so that when the implant is inserted, the cephalad bearing is bottomed out on the caudal bearing. This will allow full range of motion postoperatively. If the patient is positioned in a nonlordotic or flexed position and the implant is bottomed

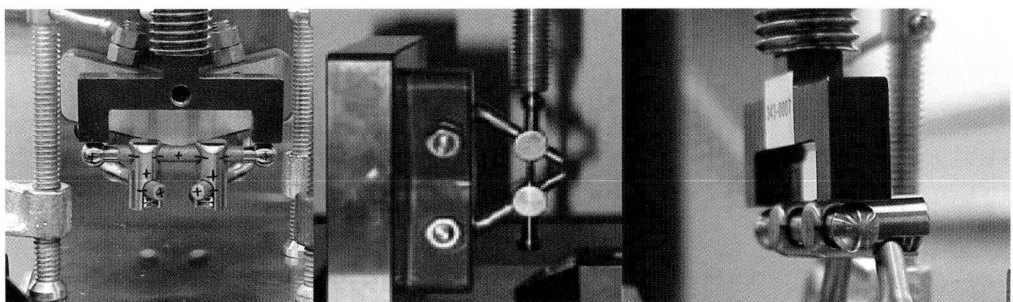

■ **FIGURE 73–7.** Examples of test apparatus utilized for static and fatigue strength testing of the TFAS constructs.

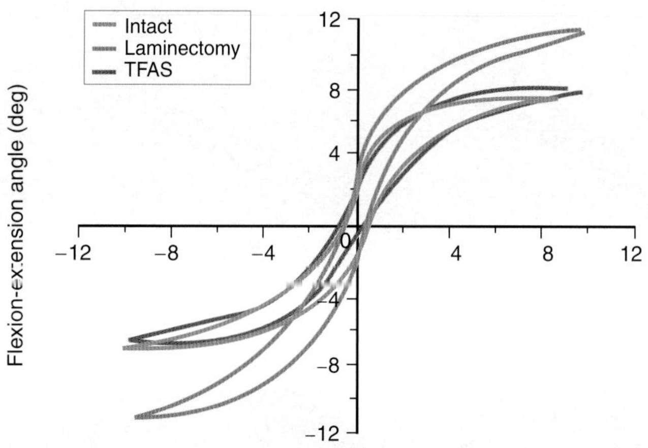


■ FIGURE 73–8. Kinematic signature in flexion-extension from a spine simulator of a cadaveric spine tested intact, surgically destabilized, and then implanted with TFAS. Note that TFAS restored quality of motion to an otherwise unstable FSU (no facets or posterior ligaments) by completely re-establishing the characteristic kinematic signature of the intact spine in both its limits as well as profile. This was accomplished for motion in all planes.

out when implanted, extension and potentially flexion may be restricted by the implant.

## Exposure

After verification of the appropriate level, the spine is exposed in standard fashion. Decompression is performed and associated bone is removed as needed. Care should be taken not to destabilize levels undergoing decompression adjacent to the TFAS level.

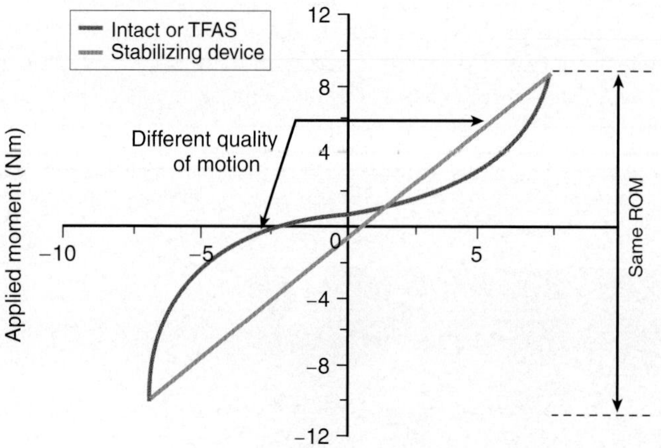


■ FIGURE 73–9. Utilizing range of motion (ROM) can be deceiving when evaluating the ability of a motion-restoring spinal implant, because two devices having identical ranges of motion can have drastically different kinematic signatures and thus may not be attaining total proper motion quality.

## Facet Removal

The articulating facets for the desired instrumented level are excised. Because TFAS restores stability to the operative level, a full laminectomy may be performed. The facet capsules at adjacent levels should be preserved.

The inferior articulating surfaces should be resected at their intersection with the pedicle. A portion of the facet may be left to help in identifying the appropriate entry point of the pedicle stem. This portion of the facet is then subsequently removed. The superior articulating surface should be resected to the level of the lamina. In cases of wide decompressive laminectomy, the entire spinous process and lamina will be removed.

## Pedicle Preparation

The entry point of each involved pedicle is used by identifying the intersection of the midline of the transverse process and the lateral border of the superior facet. A burr or awl is utilized to access the pedicle. Although the pedicle dictates the angulation of the probe, the ideal trajectory is 20 degrees lateral from the sagittal plane.

The 4.0 drill bit is then used to create a channel to within 10 mm from the anterior cortex of the vertebral body or the 55 mm marking is reached on the drill bit. Utilize fluoroscopy to verify that the drill bit is centered in the pedicle. Measure the distance from the end of the channel to the exit point of the pedicle to confirm appropriate drill depth and corresponding stem size.

Repeat the steps above for the remaining pedicles. Note and record the depth measurement for all four holes (left and right caudal, left and right cephalad). These lengths will be needed in order to select the appropriate stem implants later in the surgical technique.

A pedicle probe should be used to verify that there is no breach in the pedicle. If a significant breach is detected, the TFAS should not be implanted in order to avoid cement extravasation and a standard pedicle screw fusion system should be implanted. Smaller breaches can be managed by the insertion of bone graft prior to cement insertion under fluoroscopic visualization.

## Caudal Stem Selection

After obtaining an accurate anteroposterior (AP) C-arm image, the appropriate caudal selector (left or right) is placed into the 4-mm caudal hole. The trial does not need to be fully seated in order for the correct measurement to be obtained, but it should be stable (Fig. 73–10). The lateral edge of the trial should be visually aligned with the spinous processes.

An AP C-arm image is taken of the target level with the trial in place. The image displayed on the C-arm screen will show three indicator lines and a ball. The surgeon should determine which line is closest to the ball. Intermediate markings are provided for guidance when the ball is in the middle. The line chosen provides the correct angulation for the caudal stem. When combined with the previously measured length of the pedicle hole, the caudal stem may be selected for both the left and right sides (Fig. 73–11).

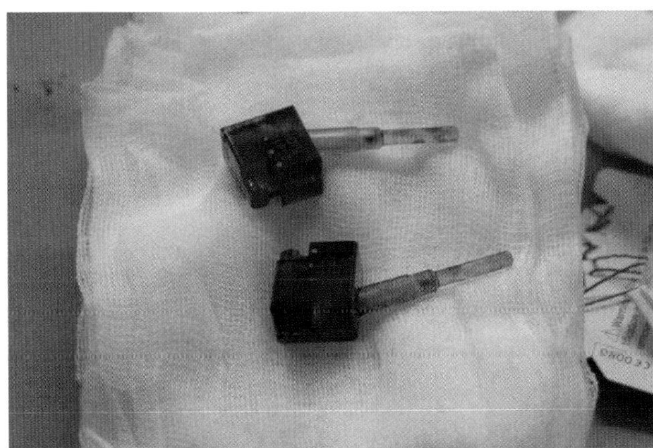
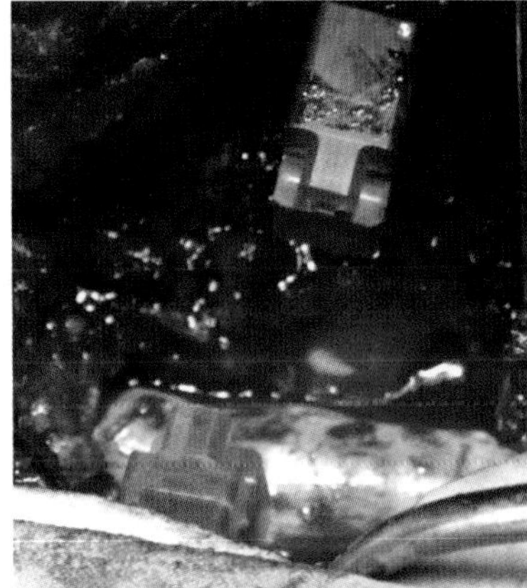

■ FIGURE 73–10. Caudal alignment trials on the back table *(left)* and in situ *(right)* during surgery.

## Caudal Cup Selection

A direct lateral image should then be taken. The C-arm is positioned such that the cephalad end plate of the inferior vertebral body is visible. With the same caudal selector instrument in place, an image is taken. Three short lines on the implant, which are divergent, appear on the C-arm image. The ridged marker lines correspond to the right side and the smooth lines to the left. Outside the sterile field, the caudal selector template is applied over the image on the C-arm screen, and the lines of the template are laid over the ridged and smooth lines on the C-arm image. The superior end plate of the templated vertebral body is now aligned with the appropriate lines on the template. The line that appears most parallel to the cephalad end plate will be the correct angulation of the cup (−9, −4, 1, 6, or 11 degrees) (Fig. 73–12).

Using this angle, the correct (left or right) caudal cup is selected, and the same procedure is performed on the contralateral side. Care should be taken to avoid scratching or marring the highly polished cup surfaces.

## Cephalad Arm Selection

Caudal trials corresponding to the correct angulation are placed into the pedicles. Verify that the caudal trial is fully seated, and if necessary, bone should be removed until the caudal trial sits on the bone. The narrow body housing trial is placed into the caudal trials. If the narrow housing trial does not span the distance between the cup trials, the wide housing trial should be used.

The 85-degree cephalad trial is placed into the pedicle and the housing trial. The necessary final position is completely seated in

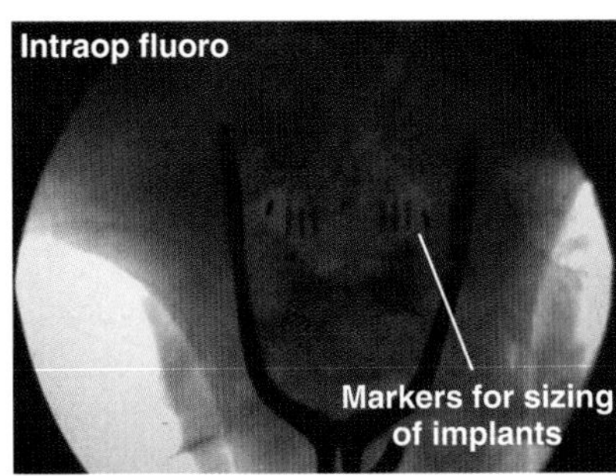


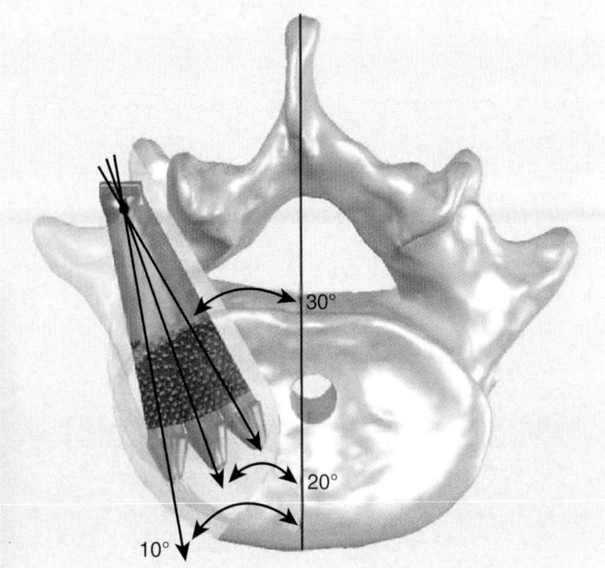


■ FIGURE 73–11. Caudal trial fluoroscopic image indicating radiopaque features clearly visible . When the indicator (ball) is closest to the most lateral line, a 10-degree caudal stem is selected. When the indicator is closest to the middle line, a 20-degree caudal stem is selected, and when the ball is closest to the most medial line, a 30-degree caudal stem is indicated.

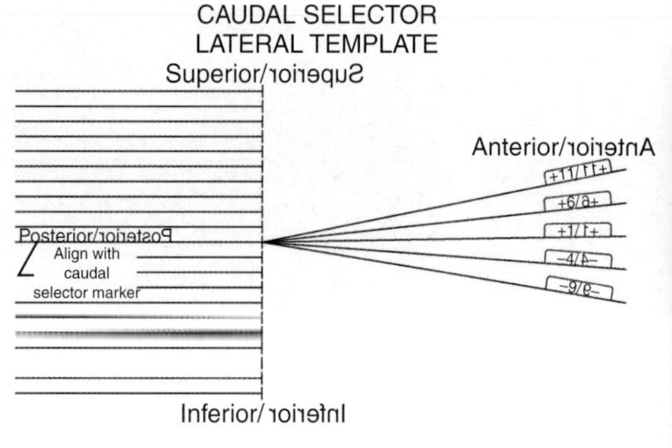


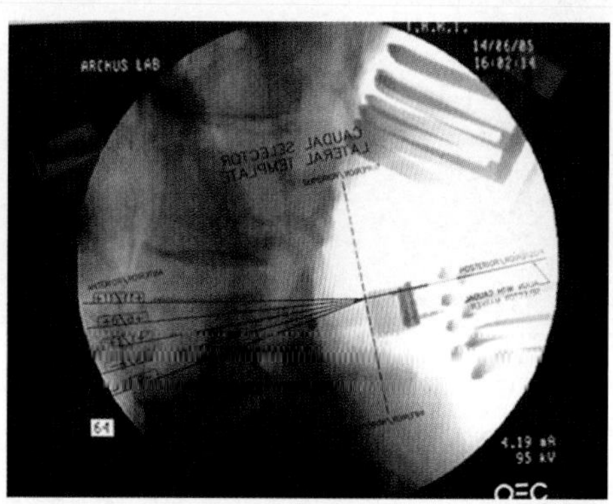

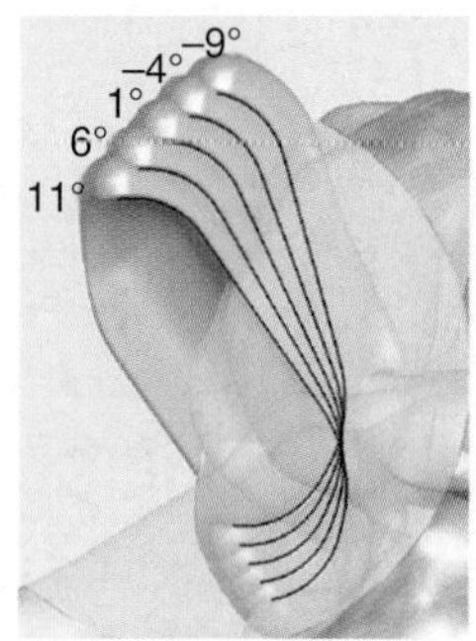


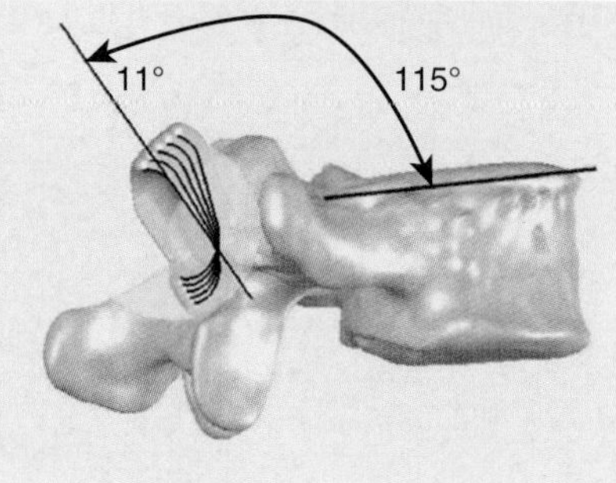


■ **FIGURE 73–12.** Caudal trial fluoroscopic image indicating radiopaque features clearly visible. When the alignment lines on the template are parallel with the alignment lines on the trial, the indicator (angled) line on the template, which is parallel to the superior end plate of the inferior vertebral body of the treated FSU, is used to select the proper caudal cup angulation. *(From Archus Orthopedics, Inc., Redmond, WA.)*

the pedicle, while also being flush with the bottom of the housing, and the cephalad trial must extend at least even with the far edge of the housing. If the medium cephalad trial is too short, the long cephalad trial should be used. If the medium cephalad trial extends significantly outside the housing trial, potentially causing impingement on the level below, the short cephalad trial should be used (Fig. 73–13).

If the 85-degree cephalad trial of the correct length (short, medium, long) impinges on the caudal trial housing or otherwise cannot be fully seated, a 75-degree cephalad trial of the same length should be evaluated.

With both cephalad trials in the trial housings, the arms should be placed so they are as symmetric as possible. Both trial arms should sit flush on the bottom slots of the housings.

Using the lengths previously noted, the appropriate small, medium, or large cephalad arm implants are selected.

### Housing Implant Selection

With the cephalad trials seated in the housing trial, look at the markings on the inside of the trial housing. If the line is in the shaded portion of the trial housing, the 15-degree housing implant is selected. If the line is in the unshaded part of the housing, the 35-degree housing implant should be selected. Selection is completed for both housing implants, and the selected implants are set aside (Fig. 73–14).

Upon completion of the housing selection, remove all trials from the implant site. All appropriate implant components except for the cross-arm and bearings should now have been selected and placed in the selection tray.

### Final Preparation of the Pedicle Channels

Based on dimensions of the isthmus of the pedicle, the appropriate 5.75-mm or 6.5-mm drill bit is chosen and attached to the T-handle. Observe the drill bit depth markings (35–55 mm in 5-mm increments) for the previously measured pedicle depth.

Maintaining good alignment with the previously drilled hole to avoid breaching the pedicle, the pedicle is drilled to the appropriate depth. A ball-tipped probe is used to verify the integrity of the pedicle.

The drill bit stop is adjusted for the measured depth for each pedicle and drilled in a similar fashion. A 5.75- or 6.5-mm blunt-tipped reamer is also available and, though less aggressive, is less likely to penetrate the pedicle wall or anterior vertebral body.

The reamer and drill allow for a 1-mm nominal cement mantle surrounding the implant within the pedicle.

## CAUDAL IMPLANT ASSEMBLY

The appropriate caudal implants are prepared for assembly. Verify that both the caudal stem and cup are for the same side, and slide the cup onto the caudal stem via the dovetail connection. The cup will slide onto the stem only in one direction, from medial to lateral.

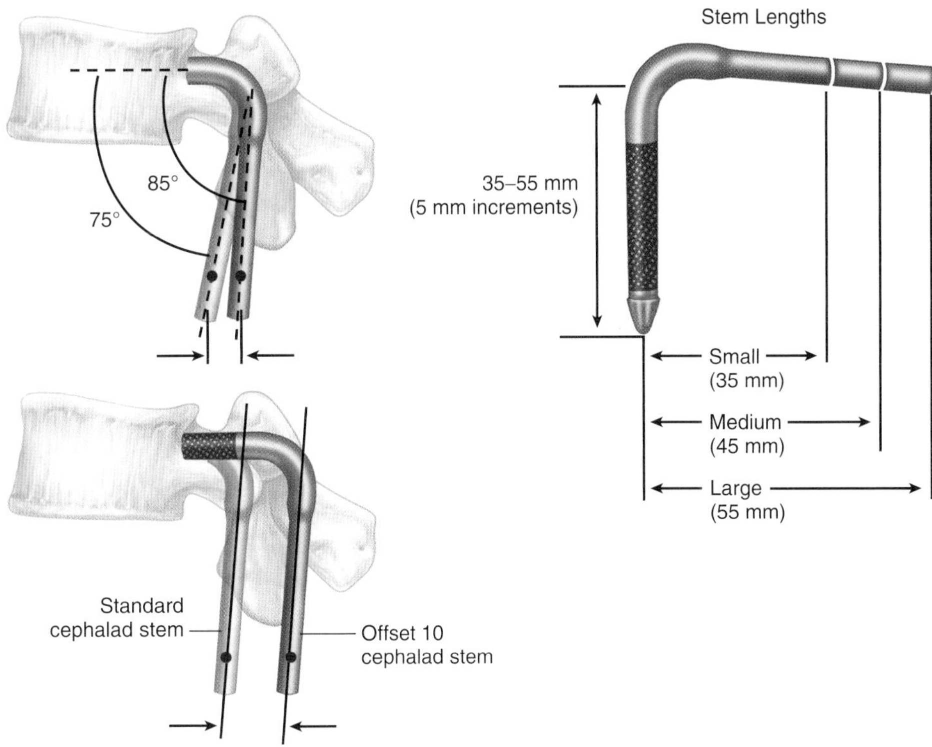


■ **FIGURE 73–13.** Superimposed schematic representations of the size and angular permutations of the TFAS cephalad stems.

The ratcheting quick-release T-handle is attached to the caudal assembly instrument. The cup and caudal stem are placed into the caudal assembly instrument, and the retention lever is turned flush with the instrument. The screw mechanism is advanced completely to the visual stop, locking the cup and stem together. Assembly is completed in the same fashion for the opposite side. Once fully locked, cup and stem components cannot be disassembled.

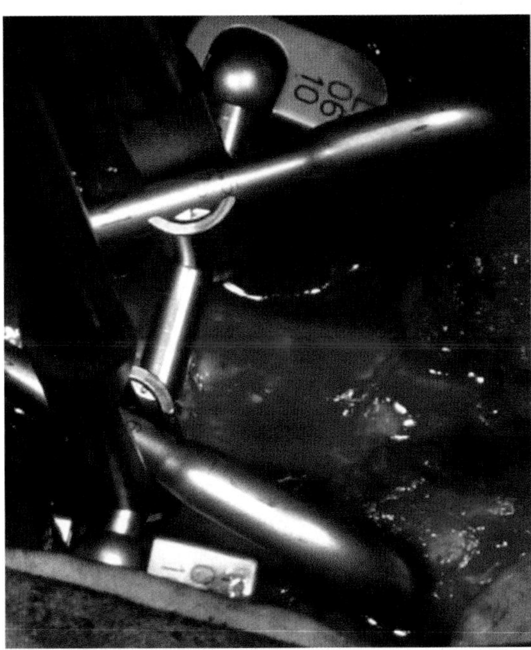

■ **FIGURE 73–14.** Cephalad trials sitting with housing trials. The upper trial housing line is outside the shaded area so a 35-degree final housing should be used. The lower trial housing line is inside the shaded area, so a 15-degree final housing should be used. A universal design housing has been created that accommodates all variation in angulation so this measurement is no longer required.

## Cement Mixing and Preparation

The cement is then mixed in the provided container. Mixing is continued for 30 to 60 seconds or until the cement appears to be smooth and consistent; 10-mL syringes are then filled by drawing the cement from the cement mixing bowl or vial. The cement cannula is then screwed onto the front of the syringe. Once it reaches a "doughy" state, the cement is ready for delivery (Fig. 73–15).

## Cementing the Caudal Stem/Cup Assembly

The cement cannula is inserted into the bottom of the pedicle channel. Using fluoroscopy, dispense cement slowly into the bottom of the drill channel, verifying penetration into the surrounding cancellous bone. After verifying a bolus of cement has been delivered into the surrounding cancellous bone, begin backfilling the pedicle drill channel in retrograde fashion by slowly withdrawing the cement cannula. Imaging should be used to check carefully for any extravertebral or extrapedicular extrusion of cement or any venous uptake of cement. Extrusion or venous uptake during delivery should be monitored. Excess cement should be removed from around the opening of the pedicle drill hole.

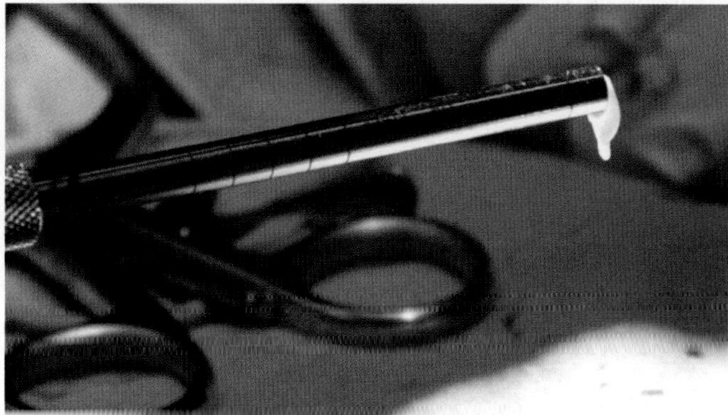

■ **FIGURE 73–15.** PMMA (polymethyl-methacrylate) bone cement extruding from the delivery gun. When ready, the cement will flow, will have a dull sheen, and will not drip freely when expressed from the syringe.

The caudal holder (left or right) is attached to the corresponding left or right caudal assembly. A small amount of cement is applied to the distal portion of the stem and around the cone tip. The medial (open side) face of the cup is aligned so that it is parallel to the spinous process, and the caudal stem is inserted slowly until the cup is fully seated. Cement that extrudes from the pedicle should be removed. No cement should be allowed around the dovetail connection of the stem and cup or any part of the articulating surface.

A final visual check is again made to ensure that the pedicle has not been breached. If a breach is noticed, the surgeon should remove all cement from the exterior of the breach and verify, after the cement has fully hardened, that no additional cement removal is needed. The contralateral caudal assembly implant is implanted in similar fashion. Remove the caudal holders.

### Cross-Arm Assembly

The cross-arm selector is placed into the caudal cups, and a corresponding cross-arm size is read directly from the size indicator on the instrument dial. Using the bearing cross-arm assembly chart, select the correct bearings and cross-arm combination from the implant tray to achieve the measured dimension.

The cross-arm selector is placed with smooth spheres to articulate with the caudal cups. Once it is locked in place, a measurement can be made to determine cross-arm length (Fig. 73–16).

The cross-arm and bearings are assembled by manually pressing one bearing onto the end of the cross-arm. Then, sequentially transfer the already selected housings, verify one left and one right, and slide them onto the cross-arm. Manually press the second bearing onto the cross-arm.

Place the assembled cross-arm housing assembly into the cross-arm assembly instrument and attach the T-handle. Turn the T-handle assembly until the handle has been advanced completely to the visual stop. Once fully locked, the cross-arm, housing, and bearing components cannot be disassembled or reused. If the incorrect components are assembled, they must be discarded.

### Cross-Arm Assembly Insertion and Cementing of Cephalad Arms

Attach the cross-arm holder onto the cross-arm assembly and place the assembly into the caudal cups. Cement should be mixed as previously described.

Dispense cement slowly into the bottom of the pedicle channel, again verifying penetration into the surrounding cancellous bone using fluoroscopic imaging. After verifying a bolus of cement has been delivered into the surrounding cancellous bone, begin backfilling the pedicle drill channel in retrograde fashion while slowly

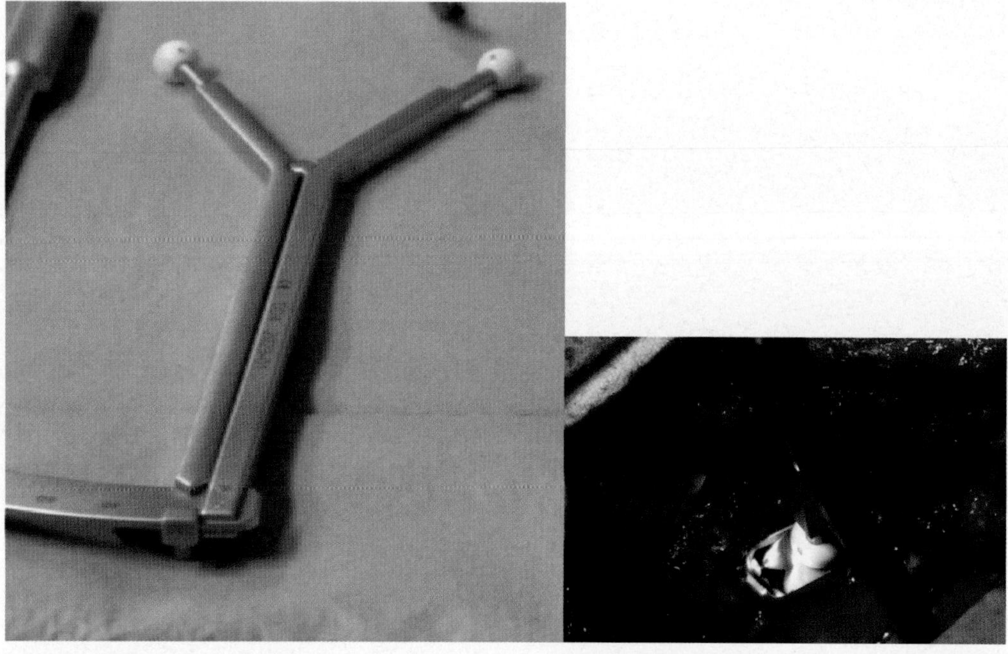

■ **FIGURE 73–16.** The cross-arm selector *(left)* is put in place and engaged with the final caudal implants *(right)* to determine cross-arm size.

withdrawing the cement delivery nozzle. Imaging should be used to check for cement extrusion and excess cement should be removed.

The appropriate cephalad arm implant is attached to the cephalad stem holder. A small amount of cement is applied to the distal portion of the stem and around the cone tip.

The cephalad stem implant is inserted in line with the appropriate housing and slowly pushed into the pedicle until it rests flush against the bottom of the housing. Excess cement is again removed (Fig. 73–17). The same technique is used on the contralateral side to cement the other arm.

### Alignment Verification and Locking of Cephalad Arms

Place the bearing positioner instrument onto the bearings and into the caudal cups to center the bearings in the caudal cups. Apply a set screw to each housing using the initial set screwdriver and provisionally tighten each set screw so that the arm is flush against the bottom of the housing.

Slide the countertorque wrench over the housing and engage the arm. Attach the torque adapter to the T-handle and final set screwdriver and tighten the set screws until the torque wrench reaches its slip limit, signifying that the set screws have been tightened to the required torque. Perform the same technique to the other housing and set screw. This completes the assembly of the structure (Fig. 73–18).

Allow the cemented components to fully cure and remove all implant holders. Verify that all excess cement has been removed. Irrigate and close in a standard fashion (Fig. 73–19).

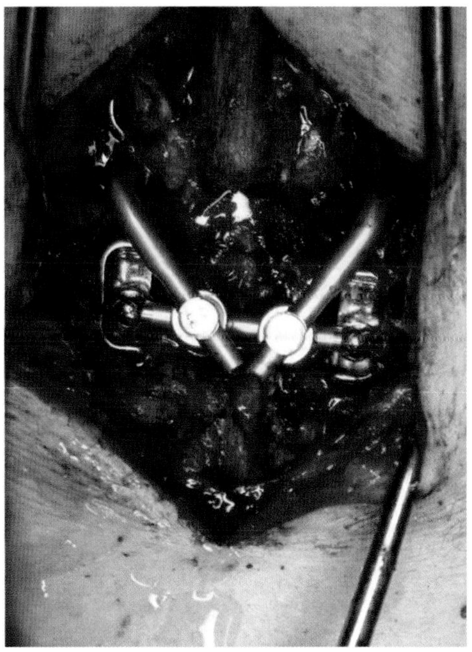

■ **FIGURE 73–18.** Final TFAS construct.

## POSTOPERATIVE CARE

Postoperative antibiotics are continued for 24 hours. A lumbosacral orthotic brace is worn for 6 weeks while out of bed. Patients are instructed to discontinue smoking and avoid using NSAIDs (non-steroidal anti-inflammatory drugs). Bending, lifting, twisting, and particularly hyperextension are to be avoided initially. At 3 months patients can resume light activities. At 4 months a progressive trunk strengthening and stabilization program is initiated.

## COMPLICATIONS

In our initial European experience, we had no operative complications. There was one death in the follow-up period unrelated to the surgery or device. In our U.S. IDE experience, we have had one device-related complication. This involved a patient who presented for his first postoperative visit on which radiographs revealed a unilateral dislocation of the cup and ball assembly. The patient was asymptomatic with this, but was taken back to surgery and successfully revised.

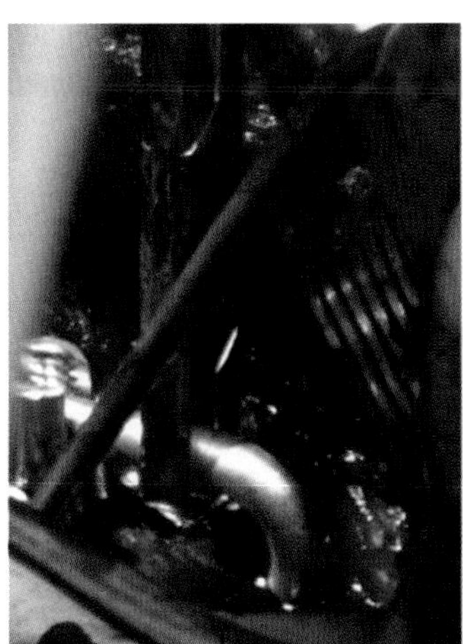

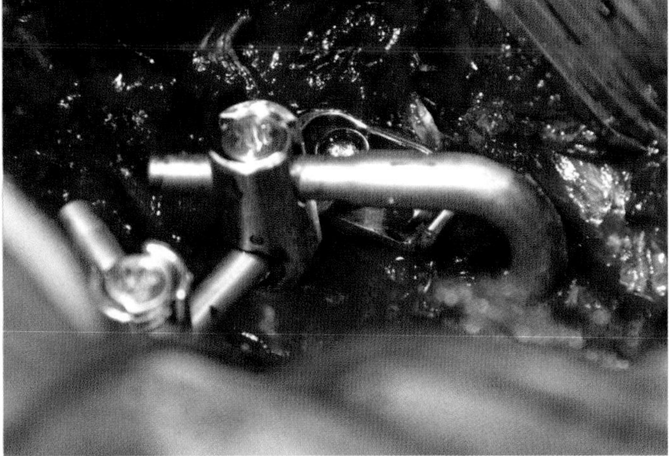

■ **FIGURE 73–17.** Cephalad stem being inserted into pedicle and housing *(left)* and after set screw is used to fix construct.

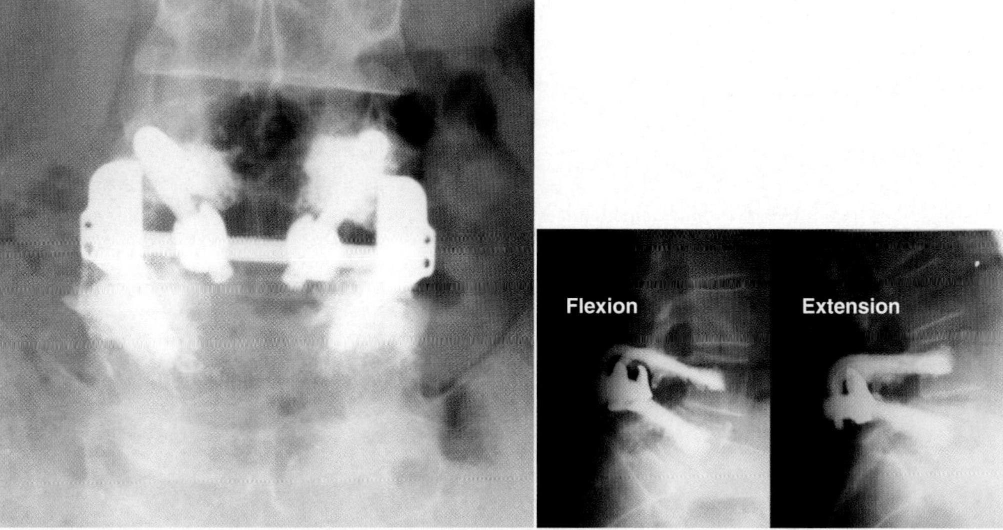


■ **FIGURE 73–19.** Typical TFAS postoperative anteroposterior radiograph *(left)* along with flexion-extension radiographs *(right)* indicating the full range of motion attained.

## CONCLUSION

Our initial clinical experience is promising. It demonstrates that posterior element replacement can be successfully used as an adjunct treatment for adult patients in the treatment of lumbar spinal stenosis. The device can restore functional spine unit biomechanics without off-loading the disc and increasing stress at adjacent segments. Long-term outcome studies will be the only way to determine its final efficacy as a stand-alone device and in the future may play a potential role in the development of 360-degree spinal arthroplasty.

## REFERENCES

1. Huang RC, Lim MR, Girardi FP, et al: the prevalence of contraindications to total disc replacement in a cohort of lumbar surgical patients. Spine 29:2538–2541, 2004.
2. Huang RC, Lim MR, Girardi FP, Cammisa FP: The prevalence of contraindications to total disc replacement in a cohort of lumbar surgical patients. Spine 29(22):2538–2541, 2004.
3. Ghormley RK: Low back pain, with special references to articular facet, with presentation of an operative procedure. JAMA 101:1773–1777, 1933.
4. Fujiwara A, Lim T, An H, et al: The effect of disc degeneration and facet joint arthritis on the segmental flexibility of the lumbar spine. Spine 25(23):3036–3044, 2000.

## BIBLIOGRAPHY

Bowden AE, Villarraga ML, et al: In Situ Biomechanics of Total Facet Replacement Using Finite Element Analysis. Presented at NASS, Sept. 2006.

Larson CR, Qingan Z, et al: Tissue Loading of the Total Facet Arthroplasty System (TFAS®). Presented at SAS, May 6, 2005.

Mow VC, Lai WM, Hou JS: A triphasic theory for the swelling and deformation behaviors of articular cartilage. J Biomech Eng 113 (3):245–258, 1991.

Sjovold SG, Zhe Q, et al: Loading of the Total Facet Arthroplasty System (TFAS®) Compared to a Rigid Posterior Instrumentation System. Presented at SAS, May 2005.

Webb SA, Presbeana R, Branea R: Preliminary Experience with Total Facet Arthroplasty (TFAS®). Presented at SAS, May 2006.

Zhu Q, Larson CR, et al: Biomechanical Evaluation of the Total Facet Arthroplasty System (TFAS®) Kinematics. Presented at SAS, May 2005.

CHAPTER 74

# Anatomic Facet Replacement System (AFRS)

**Allen Carl, Carlos E. Oliveira, Robert W. Hoy, William Lavelle, Vijay K. Goel,** and **Bryan W. Cunningham**

## KEY POINTS

- Fusion and dynamic stabilization may lead to accelerated adjacent level disease due to the reduction or elimination of segmental motion.
- There is a clinical need for motion preservation devices that address the posterior spine.
- Anatomically based long bone joint replacement designs have historically resulted in clinical success.
- Successful arthroplasty systems have utilized precision instrumentation to place implants accurately and repeatably.
- Building on the clinical success achieved by total hip and total knee arthroplasty systems, the Facet Solutions AFRS uses the general principles of anatomic design and reproducible instrumentation to provide pain relief, normal motion with stability, and optimal implant survival.

The recognition of adjacent level disease as a condition linked to spinal arthrodesis[1] has led to the emergence of spinal motion preservation devices as alternatives to fusion. Initially, the focus was on developing disc replacement devices to treat patients with anterior column pathologies. However, more recently, posterior devices have been developed as well. Lumbar spinal stenosis cases in which posterior element neural decompressions lead to instability and thus require fusion[2,3] have spawned an interest in motion preservation devices that attempt to replace and mimic the function of the facet joints. In addition, these devices may provide a treatment option for patients with low-grade spondylolisthesis or isolated posterior pain and total disc replacement patients with postoperative facet-related pain.

Arthroplasty procedures for many other articulating synovial joints have used implant systems designed to mimic normal healthy anatomy with excellent clinical results for decades.[4,5] The Facet Solutions Anatomic Facet Replacement System (AFRS) (Facet Solutions, Inc., Logan, UT) has evolved adhering to the basic concepts that brought success to total hip and knee prostheses. Although their development arose during different eras, their success is due to the same fundamental understanding of materials and biomechanics. Long-term cyclic loading success in long bone joint replacements is felt to be due to meticulous operative intervention while mimicking the normal anatomy with implant design. Preservation of surrounding soft tissues, ligaments, and proper tissue balancing allows for structural conformity, retained stability, and a uniform distribution of forces leading to optimal implant life.

The objective for the Facet Solutions AFRS was to address posterior lumbar spinal pathologies while preserving natural lumbar biomechanics (stability with natural motion), thereby mitigating the adjacent level effects resulting from the reduction or elimination of motion as seen in dynamic stabilization and fusion devices.[6] To this end, the development of a facet arthroplasty system comprising anatomic facet implants and precision instrumentation providing for reproducible implant placement was undertaken.

## INDICATIONS AND CONTRAINDICATIONS

The Facet Solutions AFRS implant is intended for use in the treatment of patients with osteoarthritis of the facet joints resulting in subarticular, lateral, or central canal stenosis. In addition, patients with stenosis caused by low-grade spondylolisthesis (Grade I or less) may benefit from this procedure. The implant is specifically designed to preserve motion for patients who are susceptible to adjacent level disorder, commonly caused by spinal arthrodesis. While not included in the clinical trial indications, patients with isolated facet joint pain and no stenosis or nondegenerative patients with recent traumatic facet fractures would also be considered candidates for this surgery.

This procedure is contraindicated for patients with the following conditions. (*Note*: This list is not complete and only includes contraindications that may be of interest to the reader.)

1. Previous fusion attempt(s) with pedicle instrumentation at the operative or adjacent levels
2. Osteoporosis
3. Greater than a Grade I spondylolisthesis at the operative level
4. A recent traumatic pars fracture at the operative level or either adjacent level
5. Trauma to the lumbar spine
6. Metabolic bone disease (osteomalacia, osteogenisis imperfecta)
7. Spondylolisthesis at levels other than the operative level
8. Scoliosis of the lumbar spine (defined as more than 11 degrees of sagittal deformity), as indicated by plain x-ray films, magnetic resonance imaging (MRI), or discography

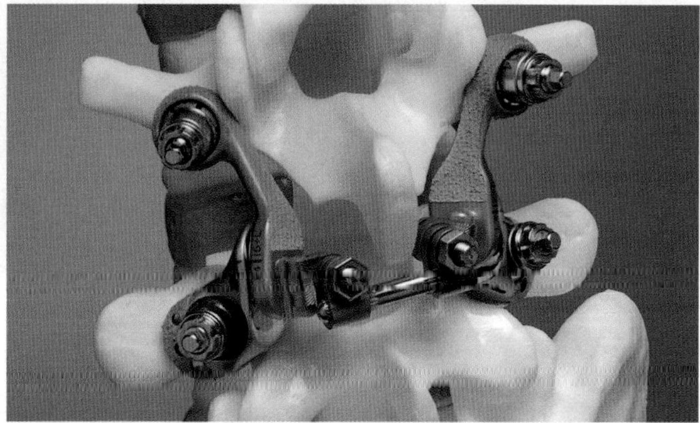

■ **FIGURE 74–1.** Anatomic Facet Replacement System (AFRS).

9. Medically significant obesity as defined by a body mass index (BMI*) greater than 40 kg/m$^2$
10. Known allergy to cobalt-chromium-molybdenum

## DESCRIPTION OF THE DEVICE

The Facet Solutions AFRS is composed of superior and inferior facet implants and utilizes conventional pedicle screw fixation (Fig. 74–1). A crossbar links the left and right inferior facet implants, providing additional construct stability. The conforming articulating surfaces of the facet implants are manufactured from cobalt-chromium-molybdenum, a highly polished, superhard, wear-resistant alloy. This material has a long and successful history of clinical use in total joint replacement systems.[7,8]

■ **FIGURE 74–2.** Kinematics test setup. (Courtesy of Vijay Goel, University of Toledo, Spine Research Center.)

## SCIENTIFIC TESTING OUTCOMES

Preclinical testing consisted of a series of implant static strength, fatigue strength, and fixation strength evaluations. This testing demonstrated that the construct's strength far exceeded physiologic loads. Additionally, a cadaveric kinematics study was performed in which the intact, destabilized, and implanted conditions were evaluated for each specimen (Fig. 74–2). This test established that the AFRS restored intact kinematics (Fig. 74–3).

A coupled-motion 20 million cycle wear debris biocompatibility assessment was performed in which no adverse histopathologic response was observed (Fig. 74–4).

The Investigational Device Exemption (IDE) study submission for this device was approved by the FDA on the first attempt, illustrating the rigorous and thorough nature of the bench-top testing regimen.

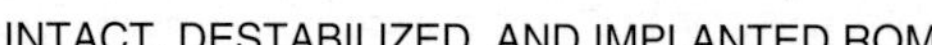


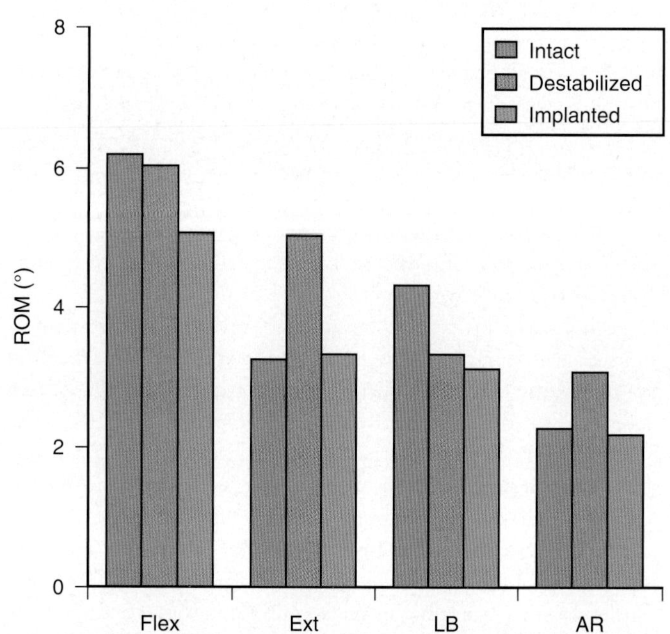


■ **FIGURE 74–3.** Kinematics test results. (Courtesy of Vijay Goel, University of Toledo, Spine Research Center.)

## CLINICAL PRESENTATION AND EVALUATION

The clinical evaluation of the Facet Solutions AFRS began in São Paulo, Brazil in 2005 where the first implantations were performed by Dr. Carlos Oliveira and Dr. Allen Carl. In 2006 Facet

*BMI = weight(kg) ÷ (height [m])$^2$

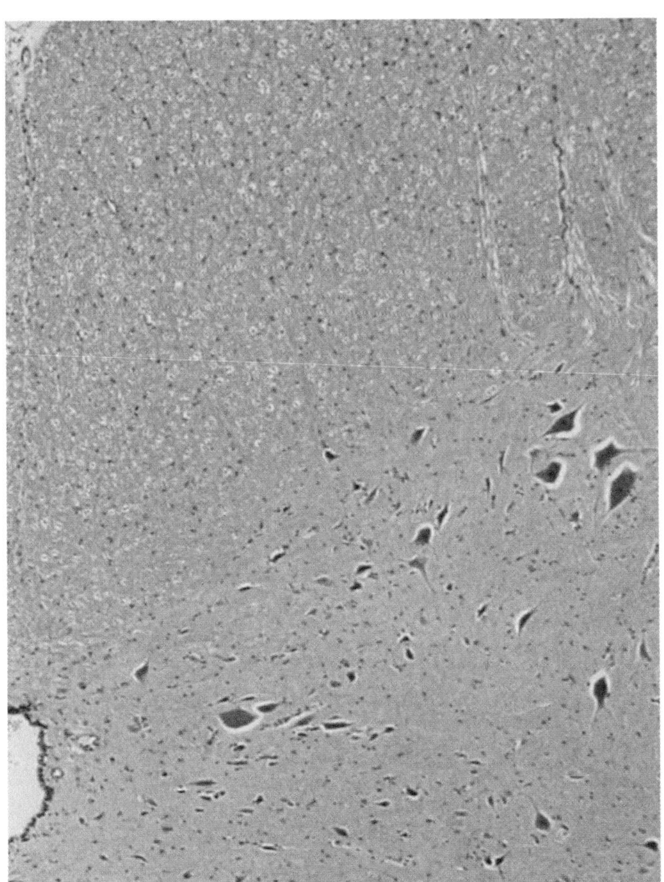

■ **FIGURE 74–4.** There was no adverse histopathologic response to an implantation of wear debris representing 20 million coupled motion cycles. (Courtesy of Bryan Cunningham, Orthopedic Biomechanics Laboratory, Union Memorial Hospital.)

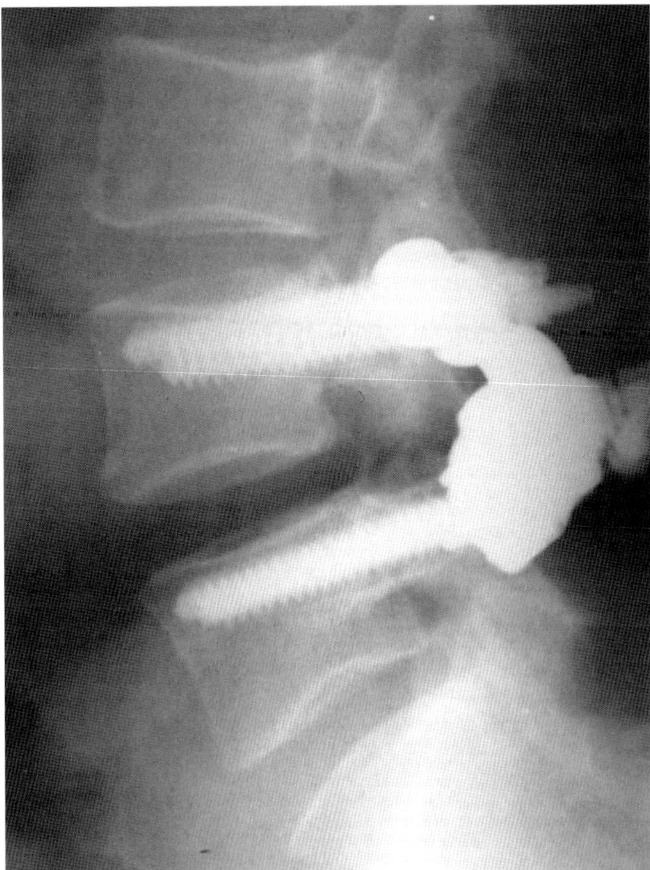

■ **FIGURE 74–5.** AFRS lateral standing radiograph.

Solutions was granted CE mark approval and FDA IDE study approval for the AFRS. The company is currently in the patient enrollment phase for their U.S. study.

Although the 1-year follow-up results from the OUS clinical study are encouraging, the small number of patients that have reached that time point limits the data's statistical power. All of the patients will continue to be followed and outcome measures will be recorded per protocol. When more OUS patients reach the later follow-up periods, statistically meaningful results will be reported (Fig. 74–5).

## OPERATIVE TECHNIQUE

The patient will be placed in a prone position with padded prominences and no pressure on the abdominal contents. General anesthetic typical for any posterior spine procedure will be administered. The procedure calls for a standard midline approach with an incision length comparable to a posterior instrumented lumbar fusion. However, the instrumentation also lends itself to a minimally invasive double Wiltse approach. A decompression is performed to relieve any subarticular, lateral, or central canal stenosis. A set of precision instrumentation then allows for repeatable bony preparation and implant trials. Finally, the pedicle screws and facet implants are installed and secured much like a screw and rod system. This technique was designed to build upon what spine surgeons are comfortable with today. The "look and feel" of the procedure is not all that different from a posterior instrumented fusion. As the general population of spine surgeons migrates toward more minimally invasive muscle-splitting approaches, micro-decompressions, and image or computer guidance systems, the Facet Solutions AFRS technique will easily accommodate those advances.

## POSTOPERATIVE CARE

The hospital stay and postoperative care will be similar to what is expected for a posterior lumbar instrumented fusion. The patient requires 6 weeks of soft corset bracing and curtailing of aggressive activity, but walking activity is permissible.

## COMPLICATIONS AND AVOIDANCE

Adhering to the indications for use as defined in the IDE clinical study protocol is the best way to avoid complications and steer clear of high-risk patients. Like any new procedure, there is an absence of long-term clinical data to support broadly defined indications. For the sake of study clarity and safety, the FDA and sponsors tend to err on the conservative side when establishing study indications. As the base of clinical knowledge grows, the indications can be refined to include all the patients who will benefit from this procedure.

**ADVANTAGES/DISADVANTAGES: AFRS**

**Advantages**
Anatomic by design
Easy-to-use and reproducible instrumentation
Provides stability with natural motion
Conventional pedicle screw fixation

**Disadvantages**
Investigational use only

## CONCLUSION

As improvements in diagnostic capabilities and a more complete understanding of pain generators are achieved, the degeneration of the three-joint complex can be broken down into more discrete stages. Filling the surgeon's armamentarium with technologies that specifically address each stage of the degenerative process is where the future of spinal motion preservation will take us. These therapies will range from nonoperative care to procedures that address multilevel anterior and posterior disorders simultaneously with minimal invasion. The Facet Solutions Anatomic Facet Replacement System has a unique place in this continuum for patients suffering from facet-related, subarticular, lateral, and central stenosis. Building from the clinical success achieved by total hip and total knee arthroplasty systems, the Facet Solutions AFRS uses the general principles of anatomic design and reproducible instrumentation to provide for pain relief, normal motion with stability, and optimal implant survival.

*Caution*: The Facet Solutions AFRS is an investigational device and is limited by U.S. law to investigational use.

## REFERENCES

1. Shono Y, Kanada K, Abumi K, et al: Stability of posterior spinal instrumentation and its effects on adjacent motion segments in the lumbosacral spine. Spine 23(14):1550–1558, 1998.
2. Knaub MA, et al: Lumbar spinal stenosis: Indications for arthrodesis and spinal instrumentation. Instr Course Lect 54:313–319, 2005.
3. Yuan PS, Booth RE Jr, Albert TJ: Nonsurgical and surgical management of lumbar spinal stenosis. Instr Course Lect 54:303–312, 2005.
4. Ramaniraka NA, Rakotomanana LR, Rubin PJ, Leyvraz P, et al: Noncemented total hip arthroplasty: Influence of extramedullary parameters on initial implant stability and on bone-implant interface stresses. Rev Chir Orthop Reparatrice Appar Mot 86(6):590–597, 2000.
5. Kelley MA: Patellofemoral complications following total knee arthroplasty. Instr Course Lect 50:403–407, 2001.
6. Schmoelz W, Huber JF, Nydegger T, et al: Dynamic stabilization of the lumbar spine and its effects on adjacent segments an in vitro experiment. J Spinal Disord Tech 16(4):418–423, 2003.
7. Howie DW, McCalden RW, Nawana NS, et al: The long-term wear of retrieved McKee-Farrar metal-on-metal total hip prostheses. J Arthroplasty 20(3):350–357, 2005.
8. Rieker CB, Schon R, Kottig P, et al: Development and validation of a second-generation metal-on-metal bearing: Laboratory studies and analysis of retrievals. J Arthroplasty 19(8 suppl 3):5–11, 2004.

CHAPTER 75

# The Zyre Facet Replacement Device

**Carl Lauryssen, Scott H. Kitchel,** and **Jason D. Blain**

## KEY POINTS

- The Zyre device is used to perform lumbar facet spacer arthroplasty.
- Implantation of the device is a minimally invasive procedure.
- The procedure can be performed with or without decompression procedures.

A proliferation of motion preservation technologies has surfaced in recent years with the bulk of the development being focused on devices intended to relieve or supplement the forces seen by the anterior column of the spine. These developments follow the relative successes of the ProDisc (Synthes, West Chester, PA) and CHARITÉ (DePuy Spine, Raynham, MA) intervertebral total disc arthroplasty devices. These devices along with other total disc arthroplasty, nucleus replacement, and dynamic stabilization devices are well covered in other chapters of this book.

Relatively few new technologies have focused exclusively on the two posterior elements of the three-joint complex that comprises a spinal functional unit. Although this area of development is still emerging, there appear to be two basic disciplines of thought with respect to addressing the facts with implantable device technology.

The predominate focus thus far appears to be on technologies that require the resection of substantial amounts of the facet joint or the entire facet joint in conjunction with a midline incision approach. The facet joints are then replaced with a mechanical functioning means.

The Zyre Facet Replacement Device from Spinal Elements, Inc. (Carlsbad, CA), differs from this approach. The Zyre device is an interpositional arthroplasty device that requires no bony resection and can be implanted using less disruptive techniques with small bilateral incisions directly over the facets.

The primary functions of the facets are to absorb loads transmitted through the spine and to restrict motion. The facets may be a source of pain generation themselves. Their composition of a synovial-bathed articulation of hyaline cartilage over subchondral bone leaves them susceptible to the same degenerative osteoarthritis mechanism that affects other joints.

Degeneration of the facet joints alters normal spinal kinematics. Without the healthy functioning of this motion component, other motion preservation devices are in jeopardy of failure. Radiographic facet degeneration following CHARITÉ lumbar disc replacement has already been shown.[1]

The technology behind the Zyre device, interpositional arthroplasty, has been applied in both large and small joints of the appendicular skeleton. As of this writing, the clinical efficacy of the device has yet to be proved; however, the design, mechanical testing, and background technology provide strong evidence that this implant will be capable of providing a solution to maintaining motion in the posterior elements in a simple, elegant manner that makes it attractive as a stand-alone device or as an adjunct to the implantation of other motion preservation technologies.

## INDICATIONS AND CONTRAINDICATIONS

As previously stated, the clinical efficacy of the Zyre device has yet to be proven. Therefore, the indications and contraindications presented represent the authors' best estimate of application of the device based on preclinical testing that has been performed to date.

The indications for use of this device are similar to those for other synovial joints: painful degeneration in the appendicular skeletal system that is unresponsive to conservative treatment. Additionally, we are exploring the device and its use to address neurologic claudication.

Any diagnosis must involve a survey of the topography of the facets through computed tomography (CT) scans. Magnetic resonance imaging (MRI) will provide an evaluation of the fluid content within the joint as well as an assessment of the articular cartilage and the joint capsule. A bone scan will also be a key diagnostic tool, demonstrating evidence of uptake in a painful facet joint. Anesthetic blocks of the facet joint may offer the best method of isolating back pain to the facets.[2]

The use of the Zyre device to address isolated degeneration of the facet joint is an enticing possibility, as the degeneration of each aspect of the three-joint complex of the spine concordantly is a well-documented phenomenon.[3]

Additionally, this device may be best used as an adjunct to the implantation of other motion preservation devices that address the anterior column. This combined usage would give the practitioner the tools to address each segment of the spinal joint.

Contraindications to the implantation of the Zyre device are similar to those for posterior spinal surgery and those of other motion preservation devices. They include systemic diseases; infection; failed previous procedures at the operative level, including hemilaminectomy and facetectomy; previous fusion at the operative level; ankylosed discs or facets; pars fracture; and other factors that may prevent a positive surgical outcome (obesity, neurologic disorder, chemical abuse, etc.).

## DESCRIPTION OF THE DEVICE

The Zyre Facet Replacement Device is an interpositional spacer that consists of three basic components—a dish-shaped spacer, a polymer cord, and retainers. The spacer is manufactured from cobalt-chromium and is designed to reside within the joint space. Multiple sizes of the spacer are available, varying in diameter and thickness to fit the individual anatomy and pathology. The spacer has a central hole that allows passage of the polymer cord. The cord is made from polyester (PET) fiber and is threaded across the facet joint and through the spacer. The retainers are also made from cobalt-chromium. They slide over the cord on either side of the facet joint and secure to the cord by means of a set screw. A picture of the individual components can be seen in Figure 75–1, and a picture of the device implanted in a spine model is provided in Figure 75–2.

## SCIENTIFIC TESTING AND CLINICAL OUTCOMES

Biomechanical testing was performed on the Zyre Facet Replacement Device with the goal of determining several factors related to the device's performance. The device was implanted in excised cadaveric functional spinal units (FSUs) and loaded both statically and dynamically to determine the range of motion, stability, and endurance of the device. After mechanical testing was completed, the Zyre devices were removed and examined for histologic evidence of wear.

Four adult cadaveric excised spines with adequate bone quality and adequate intervertebral discs were obtained for the testing. DEXA (dual-emission x-ray absorptiometry) scans were performed on all specimens as part of the pretest evaluation. The spines were then sectioned into L2-L3 and L4-L5 FSUs, and all nonfunctional soft tissue was removed. This provided eight FSUs for testing.

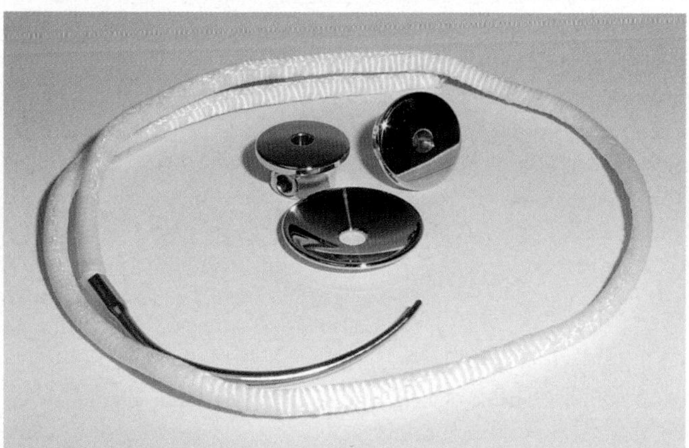

■ **FIGURE 75–1.** Components of the Zyre Facet Replacement Device.

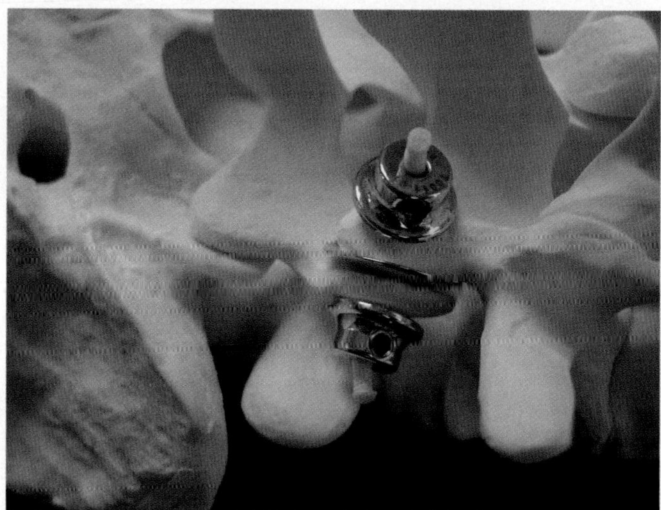

■ **FIGURE 75–2.** Construct in spine model.

The FSUs were potted in fixtures with the aid of bone cement, and each unit was tested prior to implantation by the application of a 500-N load placed 15 mm anterior to the neutral loading axis to cause the FSU to go into flexion. The units were loaded a total of 20 times each and data related to flexion angle and stiffness were recorded.

Following the short-run testing of the undisturbed FSUs, six of the units were implanted with the Zyre Facet Replacement Device, and the short-run testing described above was repeated for an additional 20 cycles. All constructs and controls were then cycled in a similar fashion to 1 million cycles. The FSUs were kept in a saline solution bath that was temperature regulated to 37 °C.

After the completion of the dynamic cycling, all FSUs were again subjected to the short-cycle loading to get final values for range of motion and construct stiffness. A chart indicating the initial and final data is illustrated in Figure 75–3.

The Zyre implants were then removed from the FSU constructs, and the facets and posterior vertebral bodies and discs were sectioned from the FSU, dehydrated, and infiltrated with methyl/methacrylate reagent grade polymer. Once the polymer cured, the specimens were cut into 2-mm sections using a diamond blade saw. Sagittal section cuts were taken across the right side of the specimens, and transverse cuts were made across the left side of the specimens. An image of a typical section can be seen in Figure 75–4. No evidence of wear was seen in any of the sections taken.

The interpositional spacer was not able to be removed from one specimen. A picture of this specimen is depicted in Figure 75–5. This image depicts the conformance of the interpositional spacer to the surrounding anatomy.

The static and dynamic tests indicated that the Zyre Facet Replacement Device is capable of withstanding cyclic loading in a cadaveric model, and the histologic examination after the testing indicates that wear is not evident.

SUMMARY OF STATIC FLEXION TEST, ($n=3$)

Relevant unit

16.0
14.0
12.0
10.0
8.0
6.0
4.0
2.0
0.0

Without
With
With post
Control ($n=1$)
Control post ($n=1$)

EBS (Nm/Deg) NZ (Deg) ROM (Deg) EBS (Nm/Deg) NZ (Deg) ROM (Deg)

L2-L3 L4-L5

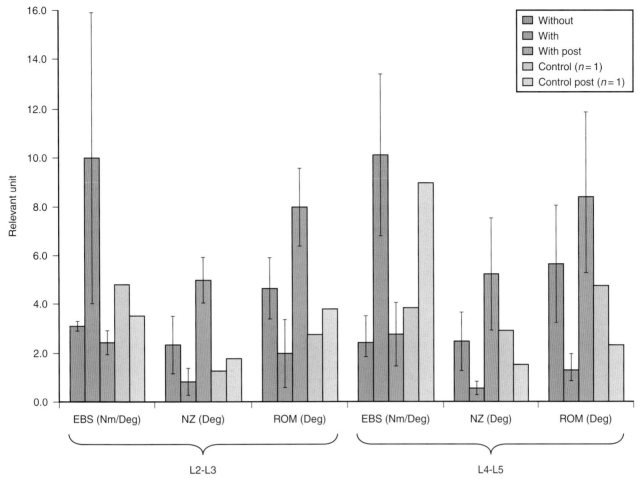

■ **FIGURE 75–3.** Chart of test data.

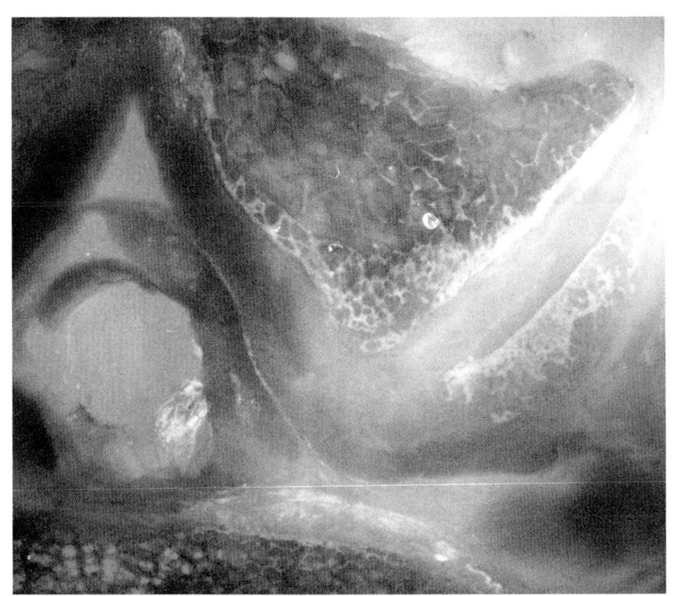

■ **FIGURE 75–4.** Histologic section of normal non-operated facet complex.

## OPERATIVE TECHNIQUES

The implantation of the Zyre facet system may be performed in line with a minimally invasive technique that involves very little muscle disruption. Each joint of the affected level is addressed with its own incision and exposure. The first incision of about 25 mm may be made over the first facet to be implanted. Soft tissues are then retracted to expose the facet capsule.

Care should be taken to maintain as much of the facet capsule as possible. An incision can then be made at the joint line of the capsule. The incision should be long enough to fit the interpositional component of the implant system into the joint space.

By placing a trial into the joint space, the facet can be sized for the appropriate corresponding implant. Fluoroscopic verification will reveal if the trial is the appropriate size by comparison to the overall joint space and position relative to the neural foramen. The trial and subsequent implant should cover the articular surfaces without interfering with surrounding structures.

The appropriately sized interpositional implant may be place in the articular space. Some forming may be necessary to get the implant to better match the native anatomy. This is accomplished with specialized instruments. If distraction is needed during the implantation of the interpositional spacer, the joint space may be opened by

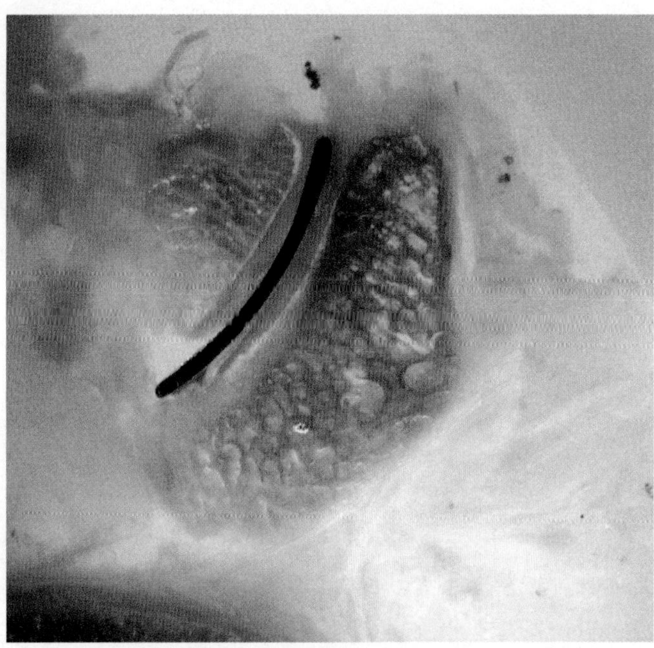

■ **FIGURE 75–5.** Histologic section of device with spacer.

distracting on the spinous processes. The spinous processes may be accessed through the incision made over the contralateral facet.

Once the interpositional component is placed, a hole is drilled across the facet joint and through the spacer. The polymer cable may then be threaded through the hole in a suture-like fashion. Retainers are placed on the medial and lateral aspect of the joint and secured by a set screw that bears against the cable.

The contralateral facet may be addressed in a similar fashion. Radiographic assessment is performed with anteroposterior and lateral fluoroscopic imaging to assure appropriate placement.

## COMPLICATIONS

As with any implant, the complications for this device will fall into one of two categories—device-related and non-device–related. Non-device–related complications will be similar to those for any posterior lumbar spine procedure and will be related to anesthesia, infection, and underlying medical conditions of the patient.

Additional experience with the Zyre device will reveal what, if any, device-related complications will arise. As with any motion preservation device, whether for the spine or extremities, wear, implant migration, and failure of adequate pain relief will be the complications to monitor.

## CONCLUSION

There are many exciting new developments in the area of motion preservation for the spine. Many of the technologies remain to be proved, and finding a position in the continuum of spine care may take years of exposure to these devices.

The Zyre Facet Replacement Device is a new technology that appears capable of providing a solution to motion preservation in the posterior elements. Its capacity to be a stand-alone device or used in concert with other motion preservation technologies, in addition to its ease of implantation, makes the device seem like a promising innovation for the future of spine surgery.

## REFERENCES

1. Phillips FM, Piment LF: Facet degeneration after CHARITÉ Disc replacement. Orthop Today 25:45, 2005.
2. Lewinnek GE, Warfield CA: Facet joint degeneration as a cause of low back pain. Clin Orthop Rel Res 213:216–222, 1986.
3. Kirkaldy-Willis WH: Managing Low Back Pain. New York, Churchill Livingstone, 1983.

CHAPTER 76

# FENIX Facet Resurfacing Implant

**Teddy Fagerstrom** and **Horace Hale**

## KEY POINTS

- Concept of facet joint resurfacing versus replacement
- Preserves supportive structures of the spine
- Mimics normal motion of the intact spine
- Eliminates origin of pain
- Compatible with any disc replacement techniques

Spinal degeneration and arthritis are well-known causes of several conditions of the spine leading to surgical intervention. The origin of pain in the degenerated lumbar spine is diagnostically a challenge, sometimes making the choice of surgical technique difficult.[1,2] Resurfacing techniques have effectively been used in other areas of the body as an alternative to more extensive joint replacement techniques.[3] The FENIX Facet Resurfacing Implant (Gerraspine, St. Gallen, Switzerland) is the first resurfacing system for use in the lumbar spine.

Osteoarthritis of the spine appears much like osteoarthritis elsewhere in the body. Affecting the synovial facet joint, it can result in osteophytosis, joint space narrowing, subchondral sclerosis, and subchondral cyst formation.[4] The prevalence of facet joint pain is considered common and estimated at 15% in younger, injured workers with chronic low back pain and about 40% in older, noninjured, rheumatology patients.[5] Several clinical studies have shown that back pain and referred pain in patients can be relieved by anesthetizing one or more of the facet joints. Other studies have shown that facet joint injections and facet nerve blocks may be of equal value as diagnostic tests.[2]

Total disc replacement has become a popular technique over the last several years. This technique does not address the potential pain arising from the facet joints. Actually, Philips and associates showed in a recent study that 44% of the patients undergoing total disc replacement developed symptomatic pain from the facets and increased facet degeneration. Facet joint arthritis is considered a contraindication to total disc replacement.[6,7]

Besides being a potential source of low back pain, facet joint osteoarthritis, with osteophytosis, may cause nerve root impingement or compression when extending into the lateral recess of the spinal canal (Fig 76–1).

Facet joints are the only true articulation in the lumbar and lumbosacral spine. In conjunction with the soft tissue supporting structures, they provide axial, rotational, and shear load support to the spine as well as sliding articulation, thus being an important component of the spinal motion segment. Therefore, if normal function of the spine is to be restored and subsequently maintained, the facet joints must be addressed, while taking care to preserve the natural supporting structures, during surgical treatment of debilitating low back pain.

The FENIX Facet Resurfacing Implant is manufactured from cobalt-chromium alloy. It is designed to resurface—not replace—the degenerated or otherwise diseased articulating surfaces of the human facet joint and restore its function in subjects with low back pain derived from degenerated facets of the lumbar spine (from L1 to S1), while preserving the supporting soft tissue structures. The cause of the degeneration may be primary or secondary.

These implants are designed for single-use only and are fixed by means of the following:

1. A translaminar screw for immediate fixation of the *inferior* facet component
2. Crossed fins for immediate fixation of the *superior* facet component
3. Titanium-plasma sprayed contact surfaces for *osseous ingrowth* and to facilitate and ensure long-term fixation of both the inferior and superior components of the implant

## INDICATIONS AND CONTRAINDICATIONS

### Indications

1. Significant facet disease, including facet arthrosis, clinically restricted or painful extension range of motion (ROM), or facet blocks
2. Single- or multilevel symptomatic lumbar facet syndrome from L1-L2 to L5-S1 confirmed by subject history, physical examination, diagnostic facet injections, and radiographic studies

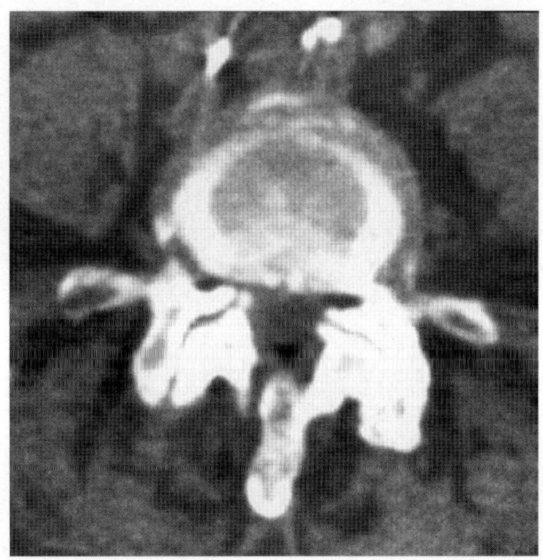

■ **FIGURE 76–1.** Radiographic image showing marked osteophytosis in the spine of a patient with osteoarthritis of the lumbar facet joints.

3. Radicular symptoms caused by lateral canal stenosis
4. Chronic low back pain with a pain intensity of a minimum of 4 on a scale of 10 on the Visual Analog Scale (VAS) lasting for more than 6 months
5. Age between 18 and 85 years old; males and females
6. Intact posterior elements of the involved segment
7. Failed at least 6 months of nonoperative care

### Contraindications

1. Age is greater than 85 or less than 18 years
2. Osteoporosis or osteomalacia
3. Isthmic spondylolisthesis
4. Prior spine surgery at the involved segment (other than nucleotomy, total disc replacement, or decompression of the medial spinal canal)
5. Congenital conditions altering the posterior anatomy
6. Medication that may reduce bone metabolism
7. Facet joints that are absent or fractured
8. Morbid obesity, having a body mass index (BMI) of 40 or greater*
9. Active infection at the operative site or other systemic site

## DESCRIPTION OF THE DEVICE

The FENIX Facet Resurfacing Implant consists of three primary components: the FENIX superior facet resurfacing component, FENIX inferior facet resurfacing component, and the FENIX locking screw (Fig. 76–2).

## SCIENTIFIC TESTING RESULTS

### Three-Dimensional Flexibility Testing L2-S1

In flexion-extension, the total range of motion (from 8 Nm extension to 8 Nm flexion) of the spine specimen was slightly increased following implantation of the Gerraspine device (34.3 degrees vs. 30.9 degrees). The neutral zone was also slightly increased (≈6 degrees vs. 4 degrees) (Fig. 76–3A).

In lateral bending, the total range of motion (from 8 Nm right to 8 Nm left) of the spine specimen was slightly increased following implantation of the Gerraspine device (31.2 degrees vs. 29.6 degrees). The neutral zone was similar (Fig. 76–3B).

In torsion, the total range of motion (from 8 Nm right to 8 Nm left) of the spine specimen was *unchanged* following implantation of the Gerraspine device (18.5 degrees vs. 18.4 degrees) (Fig. 76–3C). *The neutral zone was unchanged.*

1. The L4-L5 segmental range of motion is not affected by the device.
2. The centers of rotation lie in the same range for the intact spine and for the spine after implantation. The progression of centers of rotation through the entire flexion-extension, lateral bending, or rotation motions seems "smoother" with the implant compared to the intact spine.
3. The coupled motions (i.e., lateral bending or torsion in response to a principal motion of flexion-extension) are much cleaner with the implant. With the intact spine,

*BMI = weight (in kg) ÷ [height (in meters)]$^2$.

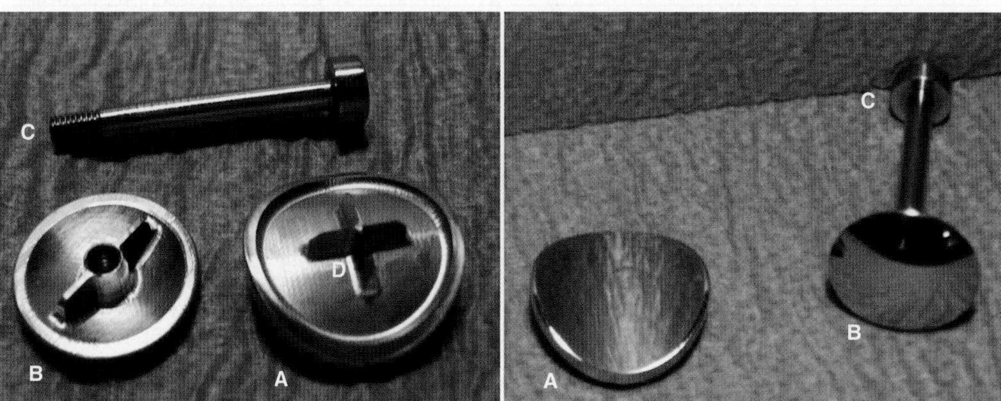


■ **FIGURE 76–2.** FENIX implant parts from above *(left)* and below *(right)*. **A,** superior component; **B,** inferior component; **C,** locking screw; **D,** crossed fins.

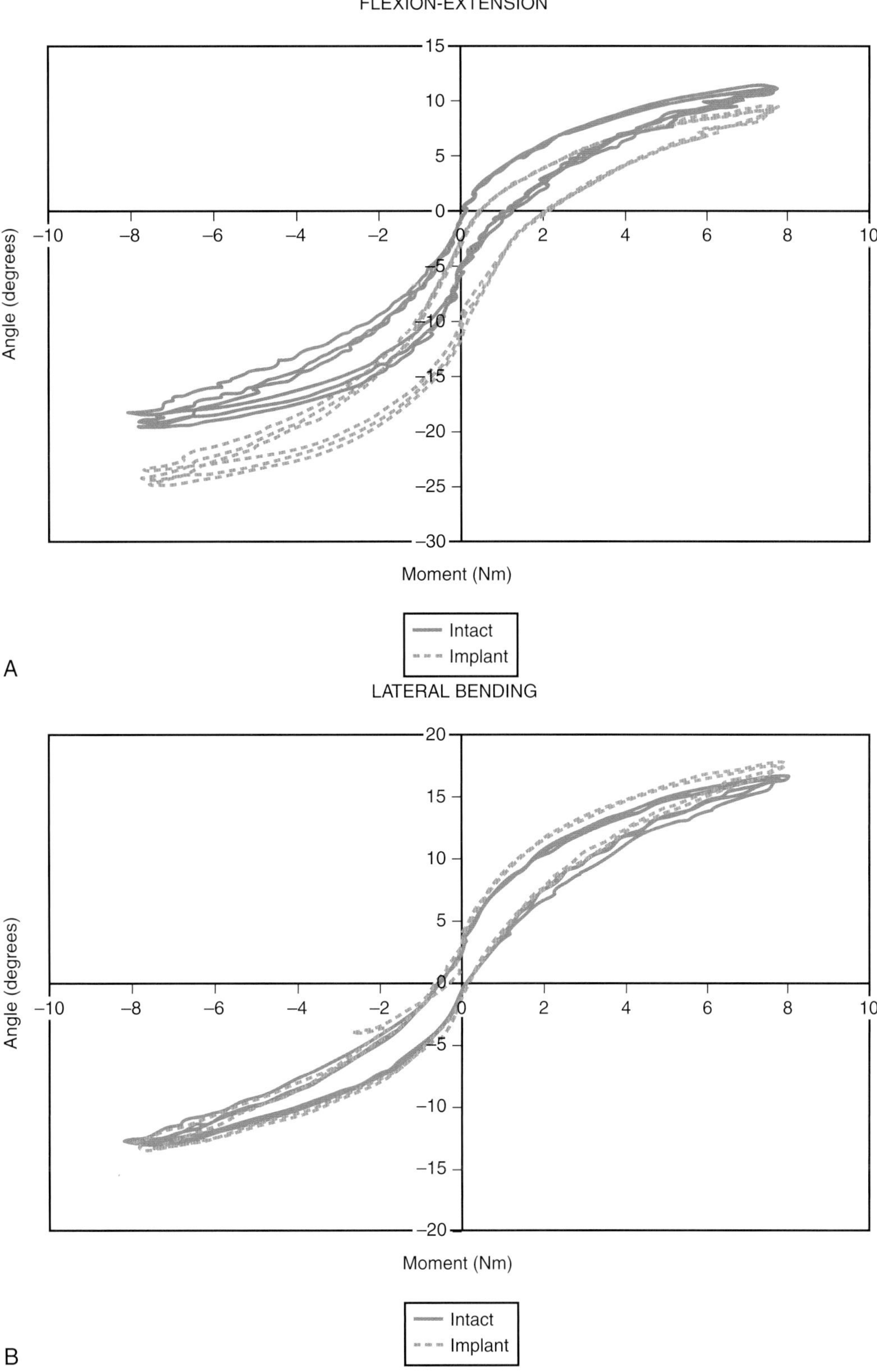


■ **FIGURE 76–3.** Results of three-dimensional flexibility testing.

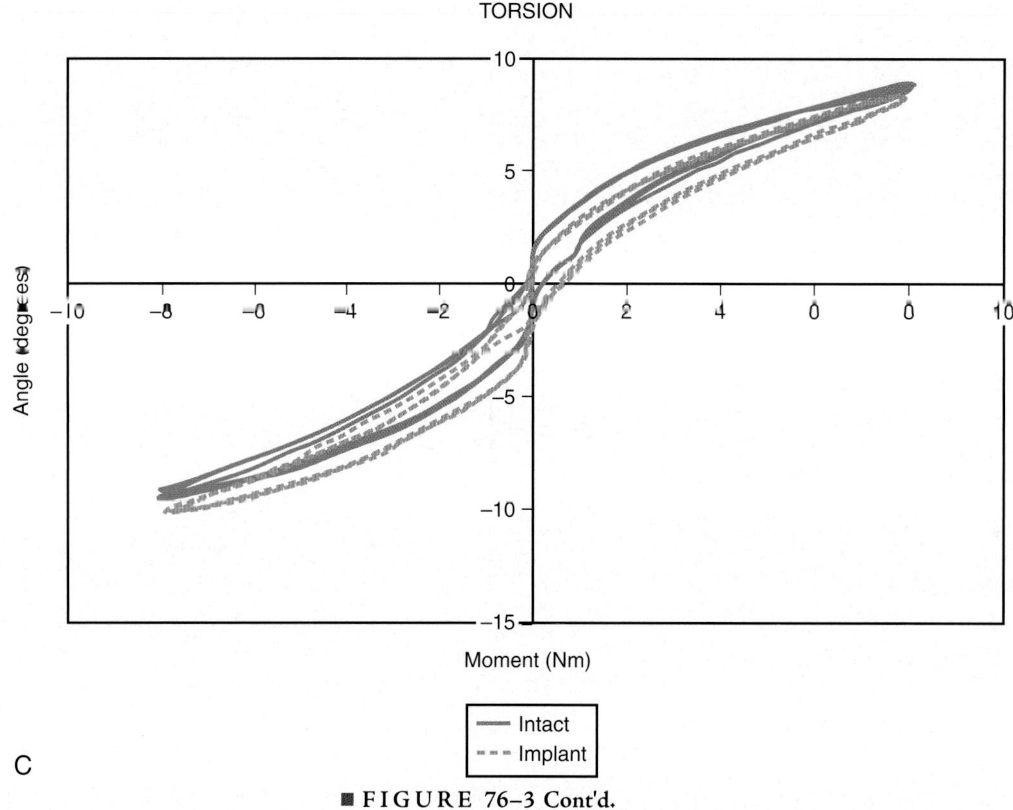


■ **FIGURE 76–3 Cont'd.**

coupled motions in torsion are quite erratic and do not follow the timing or magnitude of the principal motion. With the implant in place, the coupled motions follow the timing of the principal motions and are the same for each successive load application. In general, it seems that the implant cleans up the motion of the segment without having a negative influence on range of motion[8] (Fig. 76–4A and B; Table 76–1).

## OPERATIVE TECHNIQUE

The surgical procedure can be performed by traditional open exposure or by minimally invasive techniques and requires the following steps:

**Step 1: Preoperative.** Preoperatively, the surgeon must decide which intervertebral levels to treat. This may be done using a variety of diagnostic techniques such as diagnostic facet injections, radiographs, magnetic resonance imaging (MRI), discography, patient history, and physical examination.

**Step 2: Patient Positioning.** The patient is positioned in the prone or kneeling position. A table should be used that accommodates both lateral and anteroposterior radiographs.

**Step 3: Exposure.** Exposure of the facet joints at the affected level can be effected through a classical midline approach or a paramedian approach modified according to Wiltse to reduce surgical trauma to the erector trunci muscles.

The surgeon should use the approach that he is trained in and that is appropriate for the patient being treated.

Commercially available surgical instruments are used to perform the exposure down to the level(s) to be treated. They are also used to maintain the exposure via the appropriate retractors.

The exposure is complete when the facets of the appropriate level are exposed and sufficient retraction has been done to permit access.

**Step 4: Identify Location and Orientation.** The identification of the target facet is done by imaging control or based on the local anatomy.

Beginning on the side of your choosing, remove the capsule. Moving the spinous processes with towel clamps of the involved vertebrae may help to identify the joint space and the orientation of the facet.

The yellow ligament is detached by inserting a blunt dissector along the ventral side of the cranial lamina and the medial border of the facet is identified. A simultaneous decompression with removal of the medial border of the facet can be performed to decompress the lateral part of the spinal canal and the entry to the foramen.

**Step 5: Joint Preparation.** With a small curette and rongeur, create a 3- to 4-mm intraarticular space by removing the cartilaginous surfaces of the facet joint. The removal of cartilage should be complete, and the subchondral bone has to be carefully decorticated without weakening the bone. If the narrowness of the joint requires removal of bone, this should be done on the side of the *inferior* facet and *not* of the superior facet.

With the specially designed *inferior facet burr*, prepare the *inferior facet* for placement of the inferior facet implant. Be

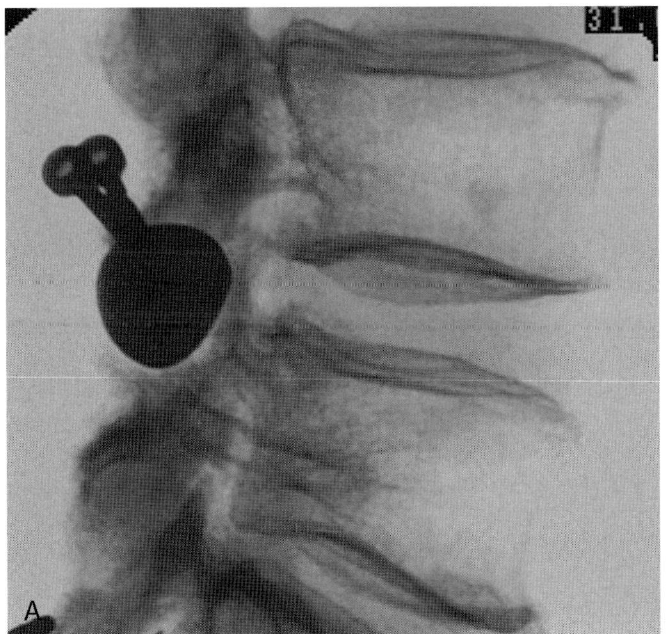

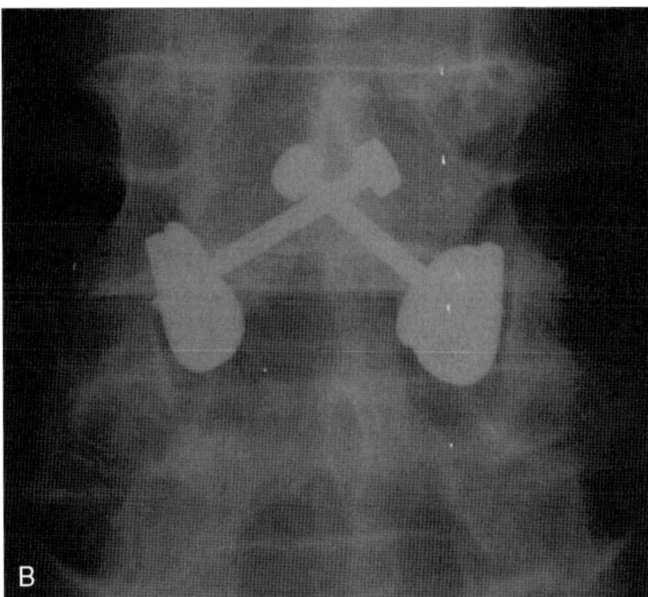

■ **FIGURE 76–4.** Radiographic imaging; anteroposterior **(A)** and lateral **(B)** images of specimen.

careful to "lateralize" the apex of the curve of the preparation tool. The resection plane should be chosen in a way that the plane is parallel to the original plane of the facet.

The power burr is moved in a caudal to cephalad direction achieving a clean bony surface to receive the prosthesis. The penetration of the canal is avoided by the normal curve of the facet in the ventral part and should be controlled by insertion of the dissector along the medial border of the facet (Fig. 76–5A and B).

With the specially designed *superior facet burr,* prepare the *superior facet.* Ensure that the flat superior end of the rasp is in contact and in alignment with the previously prepared inferior facet. The rasp is then moved in a cephalad to caudal direction with the power on. This motion effects a clean and uniform resection of the joint space in the shape and dimension of the superior implant. This cephalad to caudal motion is continued until a bleeding bone bed is achieved.

*CAUTION: Do not remove more than 2 mm of the medial aspect of the superior facet.*

**STEP 6: LAMINAR PREPARATION.** With the specially designed aiming device, drill a 3.2-mm hole for the placement of the translaminar screw.

The spacer is mounted on the aiming device and is placed centrally in the prepared space of the facet and in contact with the resected inferior facet.

Through the drill guide, the hole for the translaminar fixation screw is made. The drill hole exits ideally in the center of the previously prepared inferior facet surface.

With the specially designed fin-cutting instrument, prepare the lamina for acceptance of the fins of both the *superior* and the *inferior* implants.

By *hammering upward,* this instrument will create a space at the location of the drill hole, in the center of the prepared

**TABLE 76–1. Values of Motion-Testing Results Compared to Control Levels**

| L4-L5 Instrumented Level | | | | | | | | | | | |
|---|---|---|---|---|---|---|---|---|---|---|---|
| Frame | Disc Angle (deg) | Disc Angle C | Ant Disc Hgt | Pst Disc Hgt | Ant Disc Disp | Pst Disc Disp | Avg Disc Hgt | Avg Disc Disp | Translation (p) | COR X (pix) | COR Y (pix) |
| 0 | 8.02 | 0 | 64.08 | 38.94 | 0 | 0 | 51.51 | 0 | 0 | 0 | 0 |
| 1 | 6.18 | −1.84 | 60.78 | 41.38 | −3.29 | 2.44 | 51.08 | −0.43 | −2.21 | −16.22 | −34.94 |
| 2 | 10.84 | 2.82 | 70.2 | 36.32 | 6.12 | −2.63 | 53.26 | 1.75 | 2.82 | −31.39 | −40.73 |

| L5-S1 Intact Level | | | | | | | | | | | |
|---|---|---|---|---|---|---|---|---|---|---|---|
| Frame | Disc Angle (deg) | Disc Angle C | Ant Disc Hgt | Pst Disc Hgt | Ant Disc Disp | Pst Disc Disp | Avg Disc Hgt | Avg Disc Disp | Translation (p) | COR X (pix) | COR Y (pix) |
| 0 | 19.52 | 0 | 72.65 | 16.89 | 0 | 0 | 44.77 | 0 | 0 | 0 | 0 |
| 1 | 17.11 | −2.41 | 69.79 | 20.68 | −2.86 | 3.79 | 45.24 | 0.47 | 0.17 | 12.71 | −78.52 |
| 2 | 21.69 | 2.17 | 75.11 | 13.42 | 2.46 | −3.47 | 44.27 | −0.5 | 1.49 | 12.45 | −56.3 |

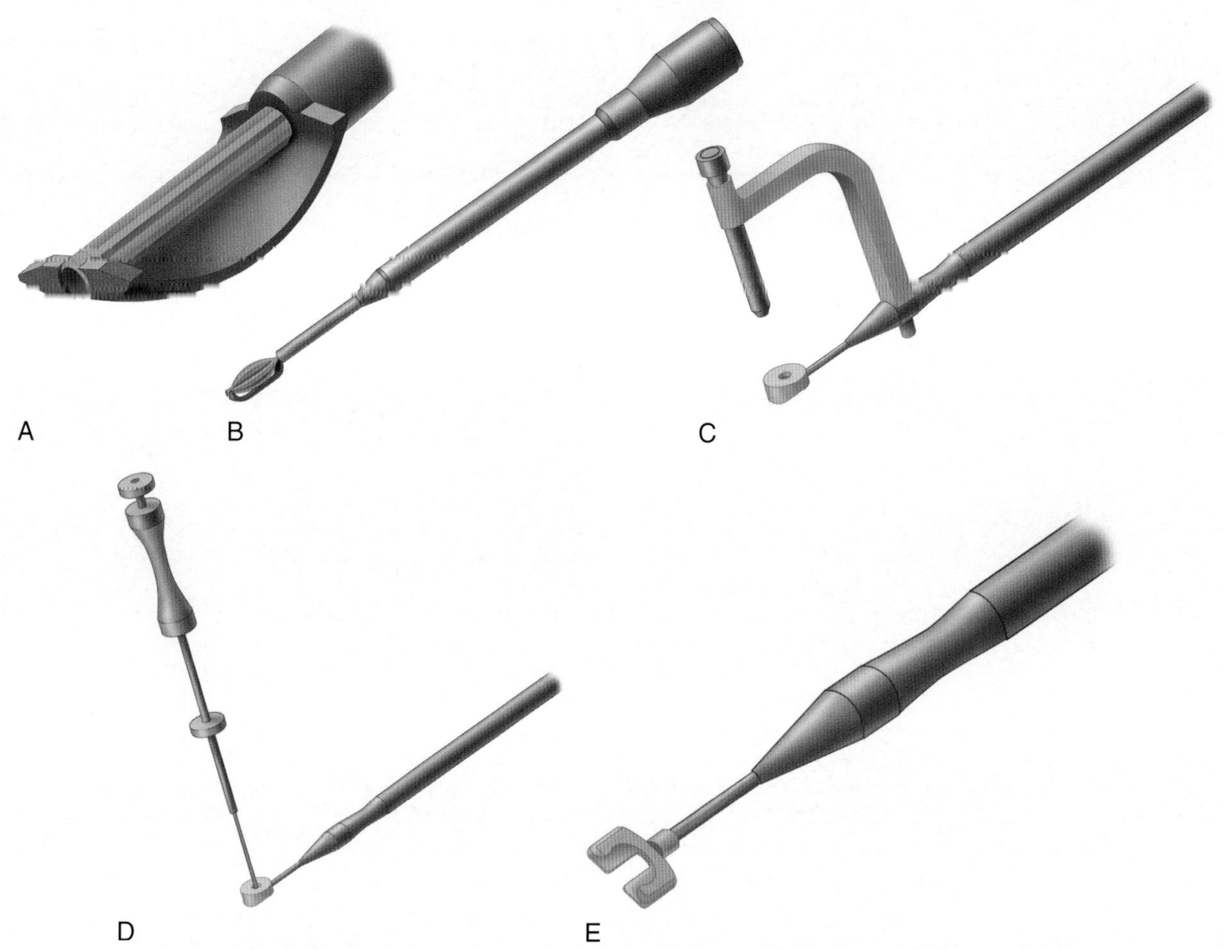


■ **FIGURE 76–5.** Instrumentation for facet surface preparation and implant introduction.

inferior facet, in order to receive the small tower and the fins of the *inferior* implant.

By *hammering downward*, the trench on the *superior* facet is made in appropriate size, depth, and position to receive the fins of the *superior* prosthesis (Fig. 76–5C and D).

**STEP 7:** Repeat steps 3 to 6 on the contralateral side.

**STEP 8: INFERIOR IMPLANT INSERTION.** With the screw measurement gauge, determine the correct length of translaminar fixation screw required.

Place the *inferior facet component* in the prepared bed, using the specially designed implant introducer. Distraction of the segment by interspinous spreading facilitates the introduction of the components.

By placing the tower of the prosthesis into the bony excavation, the prosthesis is placed automatically in the correct position.

*Insert the translaminar screw.* Tightening the screw will "lag" the inferior facet implant to the lamina thereby ensuring tight contact between the prosthesis and the bony surface.

Repeat on the contralateral side (Fig. 76–5E).

**STEP 9: SUPERIOR IMPLANT INSERTION.** Place the superior facet component in the prepared bed, using the specially designed implant introducer. Distraction of the segment by interspinous spreading facilitates the introduction of the components.

The *superior facet component* must be introduced from *caudal to cranial.* Avoid unnecessary and gross movement of the implant before final positioning in order to maintain the integrity of the cross-fin trenches, which were cut earlier. The prosthesis is pressed against the bony surface by relieving segmental distraction and is held in place by the fins.

Repeat on the contralateral side.

Following final implant insertion, lateral and anteroposterior radiographs may be taken to assure proper implant placement.

**STEP 10: CLOSURE.** The muscle and skin are closed in the usual fashion (Fig. 76–6A and B).

## POSTOPERATIVE CARE

The recommended postoperative regimen for surgeons and their patients is as follows:

1. Mobilization is begun on the first or second postoperative day.
2. A soft brace is worn during daily activities for 3 months to restrict gross motions.
3. The patient is encouraged to walk but instructed to limit activity until advised by the surgeon. Specifically, heavy lifting, repetitive bending, and extension of the spine should be avoided. No physical therapy is performed during the first 2 months.
4. Avoid steroidal drugs for at least 60 days postoperatively.

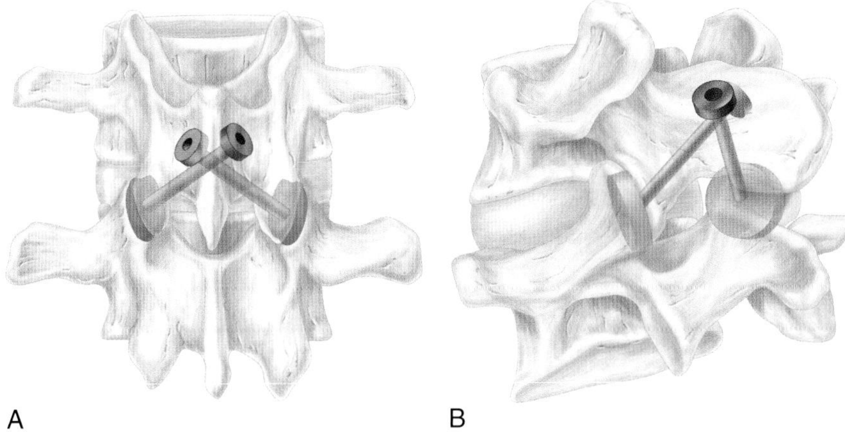


■ **FIGURE 76–6.** **A,** FENIX implant in place, posterior view. **B,** FENIX implant in place, posterolateral view, with transparent vertebrae to show positioning of and the translaminar fixation of the superior part of the implant, which is attached to the inferior facet of L4.

## COMPLICATIONS

This implant relies on the support of the posterior elements of the vertebrae for immediate and long-term fixation. Therefore, based on this requirement, there will be some complications and contraindications for its use.

- Severe osteopenia or systemic bone disease may cause implant loosening through the absence of bony ingrowth into the porous surfaces of the implant.
- The posterior elements should be able to receive a 3-mm screw.
- For anatomic reasons, isthmic spondylolysis patients should be avoided.
- Degenerative and mild (Grades 1–2) dysplastic sponylolisthesis patients should be considered because the joints, interarticular surfaces, and the laminae are usually intact, even when altered. However, great care should be taken in the preparation of the joint surfaces and when preparing the path for the translaminar screw.
- MRI diagnostic techniques can be difficult with cobalt-chromium alloys. However, we are hopeful that the new generation of low-carbon, cobalt-chromium alloys will be better suited to these diagnostic techniques.
- In the event that the implant should be explanted (loosening, infection, etc.), implant removal should be simple, and all salvage options (e.g., for fusion) will still be open to the surgeon.

### ADVANTAGES/DISADVANTAGES: FENIX

**Advantages**

Unique, innovative, simple concept
Mimics normal motion
Resurfacing procedure—minor osseous and no ligamentous resection required
Eliminates pain source
Stand-alone implant
Works with any presently available disc opportunity for complete motion segment repair
Adds additional stability and longevity to the diseased spine when used alone or in conjunction with an anteriorly placed implant
Easy, straightforward implant insertion
Broadens the treatment modalities for spine disease
Gives spine surgeons a viable alternative to fusion or a more traumatic procedure
A complementary anterior device is easily added
A true multilevel device; able to implant from L1 to S1 in the same patient

**Disadvantages**

Patient selection sometimes difficult
Addresses only pain originating from the facet joints
Limited experience with use of resurfacing techniques in the spine

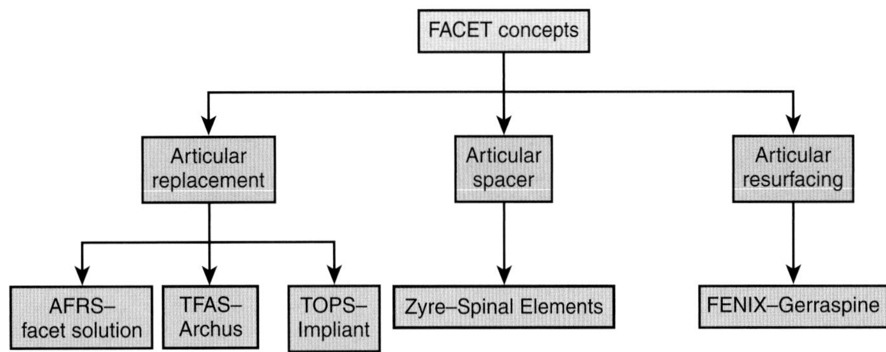


■ **FIGURE 76–7.** Chart depicting the different surgical approaches to the facet arthroplasty.

## CONCLUSION

Ongoing questions center on the following issues:

- Indications
- Pain source
- Actual efficacy of and need for a facet implant

Even the best proven prophylactic, diagnostic, and therapeutic methods must continuously be challenged through research for their effectiveness, efficiency, accessibility, and quality (Fig. 76–7).

Our in vitro investigations show the FENIX Facet Resurfacing Implant to be a safe and effective implant that improves the function of an arthritic facet joint without destroying surrounding and needed supporting structures, mimicking the function and motion of a normal facet joint.

Such an implant has the potential to enhance the quality of life of patients suffering from debilitating low back pain due to degenerative osteoarthritis.

Further work is needed to gather experience and results from clinical use of the FENIX, our intention being to develop a safe and effective implant which in the future can be expanded for use in all areas of the human spine.

## REFERENCES


1. Bogduk N, Long DM: The anatomy of the so-called "articular nerves" and their relationship to facet denervation in the treatment of low-back pain. J Neurosurg 51(2):172–177, 1979.
2. Marks RC, Houston T, Thulbourne T: Facet joint injection and facet nerve block: A randomised comparison in 86 patients with chronic low back pain. Pain 49(3):325–328, 1992.
3. Roberts P, Grigoris P: Removal of acetabular bone in resurfacing arthroplasty of the hip. J Bone Joint Surg Br 88(6):839, 2006.
4. Richardson ML: Approaches to differential diagnosis in musculoskeletal imaging. University of Washington Medical School, version 2.0. October 2001 web posting.
5. Schwarzer AC, Aprill CN, Derby R, et al: Clinical features of patients with pain stemming from the lumbar zygapophysial joints: Is the lumbar facet syndrome a clinical entity? Spine 19(10):1132–1137, 1994.
6. Cammisa FP: The prevalence of contraindications in a cohort of lumbar surgical patients. Spine 29(22):2538–2541, 2004.
7. Philips FM, Diaz R, Pimenta L: The fate of the facet joints after lumbar total disc replacement: A two-year clinical and MRI study. Global Symposium on Intervertebral Disc Replacement and Non Fusion Technology. New York, New York, 2005.
8. Ferguson S: Summary of results of flexibility with the FENIX facet implant: Report from biomechanical testing. MEM Research Center: 2004.

PART

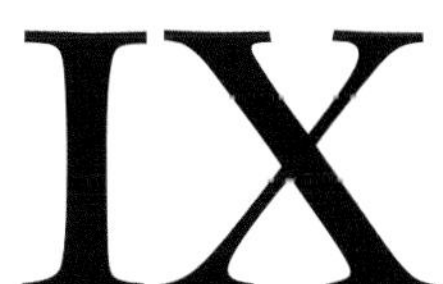


# Hybrid Nonfusion Techniques

CHAPTER 77

# Cervical Disc Replacement Combined with Cervical Laminoplasty

**Seok Woo Kim*** and **Paul C. McAfee**

## KEY POINTS

- Cervical laminoplasty techniques were developed in Japan, and they are a time-honored method of increasing the cross-sectional area of the spinal canal without requiring spinal fusion. They are the original motion preservation method for the cervical spine.
- Cervical spinal radiculopathy can be treated either anteriorly or posteriorly, whereas multilevel cervical spinal stenosis is preferred to be treated by posterior decompressive techniques.
- Cervical disk replacement can be combined with multilevel cervical laminoplasty in myeloradiculopathy patients with multilevel stenosis and one- or two-level herniated discs. Posterior laminoplasty is performed first to relieve myelopathy, and if the patient has persistent or recurrent symptoms of radiculopathy, anterior cervical disk replacement could be added.
- Of the several methods of expanding the spinal canal with laminoplasty, the two methods that are most widely used are (1) the hinge door from the junction of the lamina and facet and (2) the midline French door, splitting the spinous processes in the midline. Both types are meticulous surgical techniques that decompress the spinal cord and roots and frequently require spacers or plates to keep the neural arch open.

Recently, cervical laminoplasty has received increased attention for the treatment of multilevel cervical compressive myelopathy. Laminoplasty was developed to widen the spinal canal dimensions without permanently removing the dorsal elements of the cervical spine. The retained dorsal elements should prevent scar formation on the dura and potentially reduce the incidence of postoperative instability.

Cervical motion is theoretically preserved. Although the clinical relevance of the range of motion (ROM) after laminoplasty is controversial, several authors have noted the benefit of maintaining the cervical ROM. This improved ROM has the potential to decrease axial neck pain and prevent adjacent segment cervical disease.

Although most cervical myelopathy can be addressed surgically with an isolated anterior or posterior approach, some patients present with more complex cervical spine disease, such as myelopathy with superimposed radiculopathy. The problem with anterior cervical decompression and fusion (ACDF) for the treatment of acute disc herniation could be that there is reduction of motion and there could be significant morbidity if autologous bone graft harvesting is done. Consequently, there has been more recent emphasis on cervical disc arthroplasty to maintain motion, reduce adjacent segment deterioration, allow for an adequate decompression, and avoid the use of iliac bone grafts.

Cervical disc replacement combined with laminoplasty could be successful. Anterior total disc replacement (TDR) combined with posterior multilevel laminoplasty could preserve ROM after laminoplasty for multilevel cervical compressive myelopathy in addition to correcting radiculopathy in patients presenting with myeloradiculopathy due to multilevel stenosis and a herniated disc at one or two levels.

This chapter will focus on the possible merits of the cervical disc replacement combined with laminoplasty, especially from the perspective of the maintenance of ROM, by first reviewing classical laminoplasty methods used to treat complex compressive myelopathy and radiculopathy in the cervical spine.

## DEVELOPMENT OF LAMINOPLASTY—HISTORICAL BACKGROUND OF OPERATIVE TREATMENT IN CERVICAL SPONDYLOTIC MYELOPATHY

Degenerative cervical spondylosis and ossification of the posterior longitudinal ligament (OPLL), rheumatoid arthritis, and trauma remain common causes of compression of the spinal cord that can result in cervical spondylotic myelopathy (CSM). Patients suffer from clumsiness of the hands, difficulty walking, impaired balance and coordination, and sensory complaints of numbness or tingling in the hands and feet. Cervical spondylosis, which most commonly occurs after age 50, is the most common cause of cervical myelopathy. It evolves from degeneration of the disc that leads to reduced disc height and bulging of the disc posteriorly into the spinal canal. The bulging disc may then calcify. This calcified disc, along with marginal osteophyte formation and uncovertebral spurring, plays an important role for narrowing the spinal canal. The resultant foraminal and spinal canal stenoses produce radiculopathy and myelopathy, respectively.

*Seok Woo Kim should be credited as the first spinal surgeon in the world to innovate and to combine cervical disc replacement and cervical laminoplasty in the successful treatment of patients.

Operative treatment is usually required to decompress the neural elements, restore lordosis, and stabilize the spine to prevent additional degeneration at the affected level.

Surgery for cervical myelopathy has been performed by both posterior (laminectomy with or without fusion, laminoplasty) and anterior (corpectomy, multilevel discectomy) approaches.

The decision to use either an anterior or posterior approach depends on many factors, including the number of vertebral segments involved in the disease process, cervical alignment, the source of spinal cord compression, presence of instability on dynamic radiographs, and surgeon's preference for the various surgical techniques. Other clinical factors to consider include axial neck symptoms, presence of congenital spinal stenosis, medical comorbidities, previous surgery, and the presence of radiculopathy.

Anterior decompression with stabilization obtained by anterior arthrodesis allows direct removal of the compressive sources. The procedure is accomplished through multilevel discectomies and fusions with segmental instrumentation or through cervical corpectomy with vertebral reconstruction using autograft, allograft, or titanium mesh cages with plate fixation. The disadvantages include the risks of an extensive anterior cervical approach, the need for graft healing, and the potential problems at adjacent levels. Emery and associates reviewed 108 cases of cervical spondylotic myelopathy which had been managed with anterior decompression and arthrodesis via partial or subtotal corpectomy.[1] In their report, 46% of patients with preoperative gait abnormality had a normal gait at follow-up, and 62% presenting with a preoperative motor deficit had full recovery. However, 15% of the patients developed pseudarthrosis after surgery. It has been well documented that the rate of pseudarthrosis increases with each segmental level added to an anterior decompression and fusion.[2] Additional complications of anterior cervical decompression and fusion surgery include graft fracture, dislodgement or settling, and surgery-related complications including dysphagia, recurrent laryngeal nerve dysfunction, esophageal injury, carotid vessel injury, and late adjacent segment degeneration.

Historically, laminectomy has been regarded as the standard procedure to decompress the spinal cord for cervical myelopathy secondary to multisegmental spondylosis, ossification of the posterior longitudinal ligament (OPLL), with or without developmental spinal canal stenosis. However, segmental instability, kyphosis, perineural adhesions, and late neurologic deterioration occurred and became well-known complications after laminectomy. Pal and Cooper tested load transmission in the anterior (vertebral bodies) and posterior (facet joints and articular processes) cervical columns in cadavers.[3] They demonstrated that 36% of load transmission was through the anterior columns, whereas 64% was through the posterior columns. Therefore, the posterior neural arch is responsible for most of the load transmission in the cervical spine, and significant loss of integrity of these posterior columns can result in instability, causing the weight-bearing axis to shift anteriorly. Kyphosis progresses subsequent to this loss of sagittal balance and places the cervical musculature at a mechanical disadvantage, requiring constant contractions to maintain upright head posture. This progression causes most of the weight to be borne by the discs and anterior vertebral bodies, which leads to further degeneration and spondylosis. Some authors advocate to augment with fusion after laminectomy because of the frequency of instability and loss of normal cervical lordosis.

To avoid these problems, surgeons developed a different strategy in which decompression of the spinal cord could be achieved while preserving posterior arch, which was thought to contribute to postoperative cervical alignment and stability.

Oyama and associates introduced the expansive Z-shaped laminoplasty in which the posterior wall of the spinal canal was preserved by Z-plasty of the thinned laminae.[4] Hirabayashi developed "expansive open door laminoplasty" in 1978.[5] Since then, many modifications of the procedure have been reported, such as "double-door laminoplasty," which was introduced by Kurokawa and co-workers in 1982.[6] In this procedure, spinal canal enlargement is achieved by splitting the spinous process, and graft bones are inserted between the split spinous process. This procedure has shown several new features, including symmetric configuration of reconstructed posterior elements that theoretically allow symmetric expansion of the spinal cord, closed-ring configuration of the neural arch for each segment through insertion of bone graft, and wide access to the spinal canal to perform additional procedures. Because of these advantages, this procedure is widely accepted and a variety of modifications have been developed. In 1992, Nakano and associates developed a hydroxyapatite (HA) spacer instead of an autogenous bone graft to decrease the operation time, decrease blood loss, and avoid postoperative pain around the donor site.[7] Over time various modifications and supplementary procedures were devised for posterior decompression of the spinal canal while preserving stability and mobility of the cervical spine: reattachment of the spinous process and extensor musculature, dome-like decompression on the C2 lamina, use of thread wire saw (T-saw) to minimize the bony loss at the time of sagittal cutting of laminae, and modification of the spinous process spacer.

With refinements of the surgical technique and the development of more stable fixation devices, the reproducibility of the procedure has been improved. All of the laminoplasty variants effectively expand the cross-sectional area of the spinal canal while preserving alignment, stability, and motion. Surgeons have demonstrated equivalent neurologic outcomes utilizing the various laminoplasty methods.

Many authors have shown that laminoplasty can be effectively utilized in a patient to multilevel cervical spondylotic myelopathy with similar or superior clinical outcomes as compared to multilevel anterior surgery or laminectomy combined with fusion.[8] In addition, laminoplasty can be combined with posterior foraminotomies to relieve compression of the nerve roots and with fusion at one or two levels if instability such as spondylolisthesis is present.

## TECHNIQUES OF LAMINOPLASTY

Nearly all of the laminoplasty variants effectively expand the cross-sectional area of the spinal canal while preserving alignment, stability, and motion. The following techniques are most commonly used:

- Z-plasty
- Hirabayashi laminoplasty (open-door laminoplasty)
- French door laminoplasty (double-door laminoplasty)
- Kurokawa modification
- Tomita modification

Novel techniques designed to reposition the laminae and open the spinal canal continue to evolve. There are two basic types of procedures. The first is the "open-door laminoplasty," whereby one side of the lamina is hinged open, along with the ligamentum flavum on the same side. The other procedures involve creating a midline opening with the left and right hemilaminae hinging on both sides.

Newer techniques, such as the use of hydroxyapatite (HA) or ceramic spacers and titanium miniplates, have been proposed to decrease the surgical time and improve the safety of the procedure.

## Z-Plasty

This technique was first described by Oyama and associates.[4] In the Z-plasty, troughs are first drilled into the laminae at the junction of the lateral mass. Then the laminae are thinned. After this, a Z-shaped cut in the laminae is done with a high-speed drill. After the Z cut, the thinned sections of laminae may then be separated and the canal opened or expanded. The laminae may then be secured or wired to maintain the expanded canal. Naito and associates reported Z-plasty had longer operation time and more blood loss, and it has subsequently disappeared.[9]

## Hirabayashi Laminoplasty

Hirabayashi and collegues described the expansive open-door laminoplasty.[5, 10–12] In this technique, a trough is first drilled in the laminae at the junction of the lateral mass. The cut is taken down to dura. The ligament and any remaining thinned bone should be removed with a Kerrison rongeur. After drilling the complete trough on the open-door side, a second trough is drilled on the closed side. After the troughs have been cut, the ligamentum flavum between ventral and caudal vertebrae and remaining structures should be removed with a Kerrison rongeur. After cutting on the open side, the block of laminae is rotated toward the closed (hinged) side This effectively opens and expands the spinal canal. The laminae may be held open with sutures passing around or through the spinous processes and the facet capsule on the hinged side or held open with titanium miniplates. Hirabayashi advocated stay sutures within the spinous process and paraspinal muscles to avoid closure of the opened laminae. Even with the added sutures, there were several cases of a spring-back phenomenon (i.e., the door closed), in which patients showed both progressive neurologic and radiologic deterioration. Since then, in order to prevent the spring-back phenomenon, many techniques were developed to maintain canal patency. Recently, a novel technique augmented by titanium miniplates to maintain patency of the open-door laminoplasty was introduced by O'Brien and associates[13] (Figs. 77–1, 77–2). They reported a significant improvement in sagittal canal diameter and canal area with no hardware failure during their follow-up.

## French Door Laminoplasty (Double-Door Laminoplasty, Midline Opening Laminoplasty)

In this type of laminoplasty, the spinous processes are split in the midline; therefore, the door is opened in the midline and creates a symmetric opening in the canal, unlike Hirabayashi type open-door laminoplasty in which the canal is opened on one side and hinged on the other and thus creates an asymmetric expansion of the canal. Troughs are then cut into the laminae at the junction of the lateral masses. The laminae are only thinned and are not cut completely through. After the completion of the trough cuts, the spinous processes are split in the midline. Then the spinous processes are spread in the midline and held open, just like French doors. They may be held open with small bone grafts or other grafts. Ceramic or hydroxyapatite (HA) spacers have also been reported as a substitute for autogenous bone graft (Figs. 77–3, 77–4).

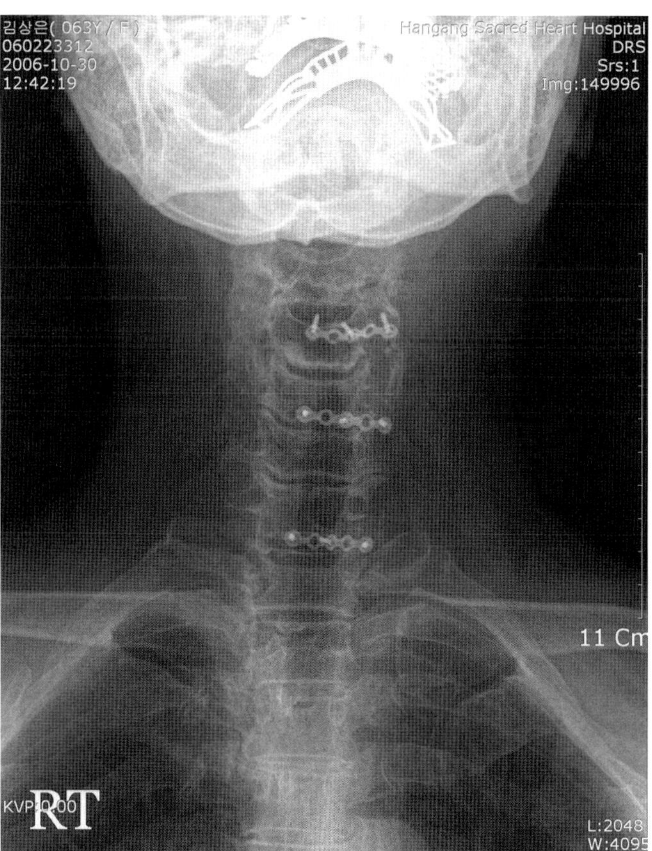


■ **FIGURE 77–1.** Anteroposterior radiograph of a 63-year-old female patient after Hirabayashi open-door laminoplasty augmented by titanium miniplates.

The Kurokawa modification means that the dorsal aspect of the spinous processes is removed and used as grafts.[6] The spinous processes are cut in the midline. The spinous processes are split in the midline and held open with bone grafts that are wired in place. The main disadvantages of this procedure are the technical difficulty and high risk of the procedure associated with sagittal splitting of the spinous processes with a burr in such close proximity to the spinal cord.

In the Tomita modification, the spinous processes are split with a wire saw (threadwire saw; T-saw) to avoid the use of a burr while splitting the midline. The polyethylene sleeve enclosing the T-saw is passed cranially along the epidural space, and then the sleeve is withdrawn over the saw. The saw is pulled tight to cut the midline of the inner wall of the lamina arch by using a reciprocating saw motion (Figs. 77–5 to 77–7). An important safety consideration is that cervical kyphosis places the cord at risk during the splitting of the spinous processes.

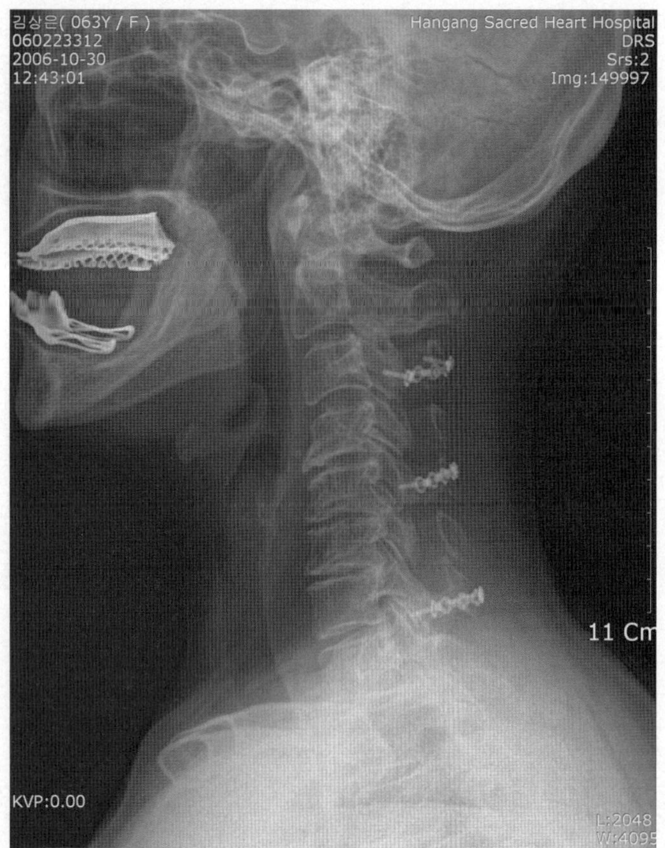

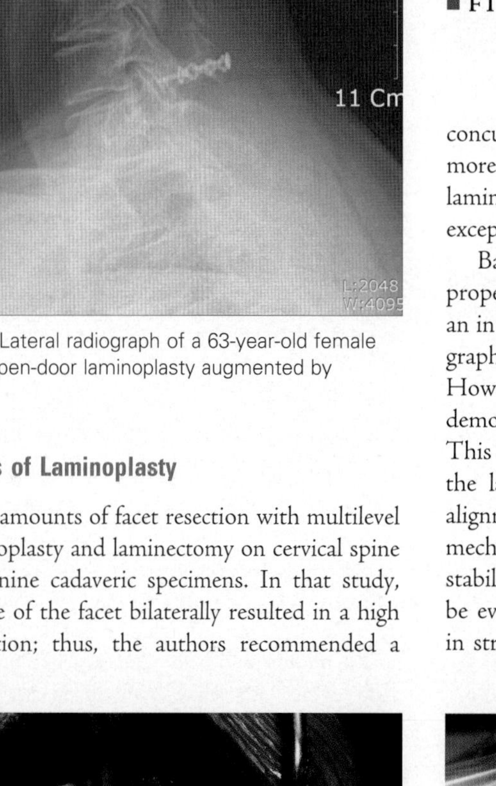

■ **FIGURE 77–2.** Lateral radiograph of a 63-year-old female patient after Hirabayashi open-door laminoplasty augmented by titanium miniplates.

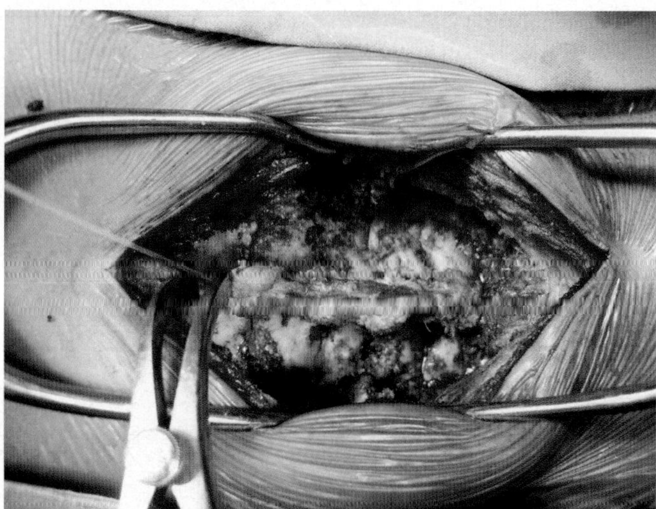

■ **FIGURE 77–4.** Polyethylene sleeve enclosing the T-saw.

## Biomechanical Studies of Laminoplasty

The effects of increasing amounts of facet resection with multilevel cervical open-door laminoplasty and laminectomy on cervical spine stability were tested in nine cadaveric specimens. In that study, resection of 25% or more of the facet bilaterally resulted in a high increase in cervical motion; thus, the authors recommended a concurrent arthrodesis should accompany a laminectomy with more than 25% bilateral facectectomy. On the other hand, cervical laminoplasty was not significantly different from the intact control except for a marginal increase in axial torsion.

Baisden and associates[14] observed the effects on structural properties between multilevel laminectomy and laminoplasty using an in vivo goat model over a 6-month period. No significant radiographic differences in cervical alignment were observed initially. However, at 16 weeks after surgery, the laminectomy group demonstrated a significant decrease in normal cervical lordosis. This decrease progressed throughout the 6-month period, whereas the laminoplasty group did not significantly change its cervical alignment during the study period. Unfortunately, few in vitro biomechanical studies evaluate the ability of laminoplasty to maintain stability of the cervical spine. More biomechanical studies need to be evaluated on a long-term basis analyzing stability and changes in structural alignment parameters.

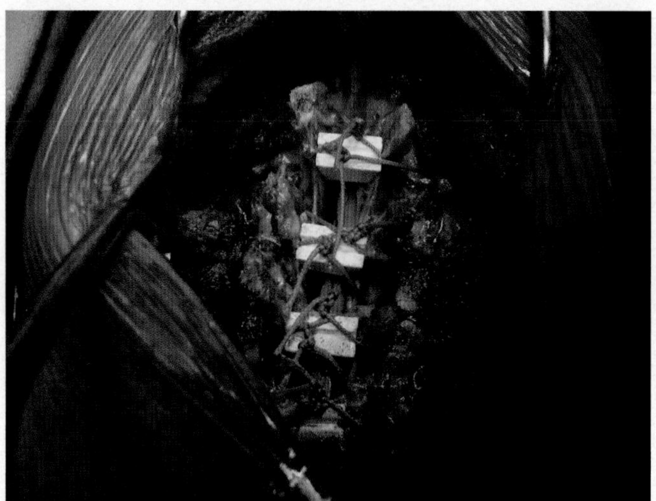

■ **FIGURE 77–3.** Hydroxyapatite (HA) spacer as a substitute for autogenous bone graft.

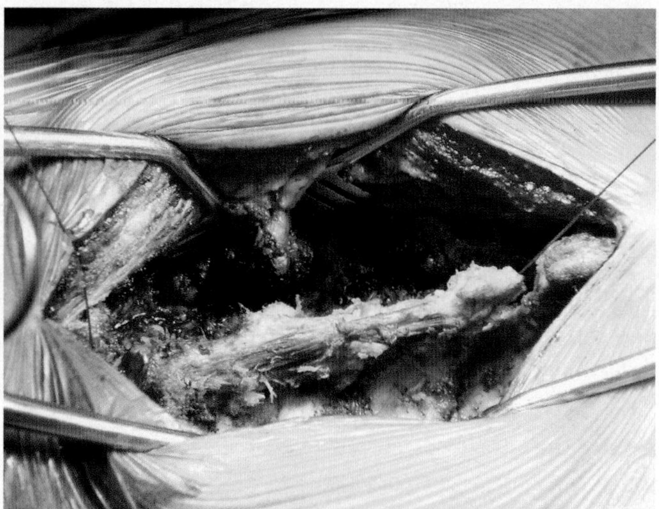

■ **FIGURE 77–5.** Threadwire saw (T-saw) used to split the spinous process.

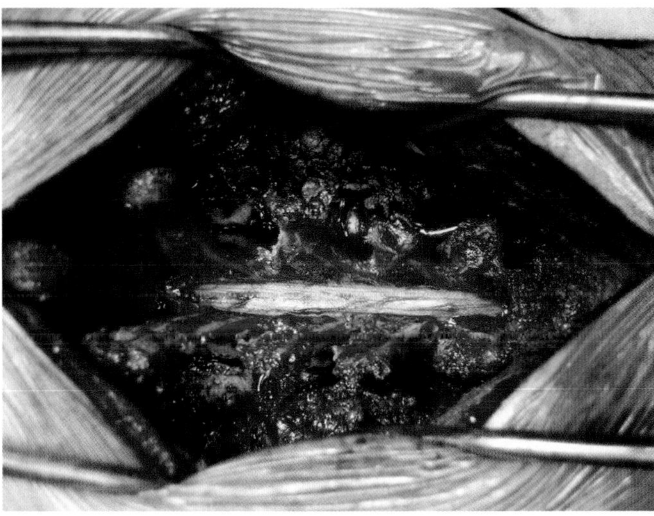

■ FIGURE 77–6. Exposed dura after splitting the spinous processes with T-saw (modified French door laminoplasty).

## CLINICAL OUTCOMES

Many studies have evaluated the clinical outcomes after various laminoplasty procedures. Most studies report clinical outcomes based on JOA (Japanese Orthopaedic Association) scores to demonstrate some improvement in preoperative neurologic deficits.

### Hirabayashi Open-Door Laminoplasty

The mean recovery rate after Hirabayashi expansive laminoplasty is approximately 50% to 60%.[5,10–12,15,16] Hirabayashi and Satomi reported a 54% neurologic improvement rate over an average 3-year follow-up.[12] Satomi and associates[17] found recovery rates of 56% for OPLL and 61% for cervical spondylotic myelopathy over an average 8-year follow-up for 33 patients with OPLL and 18 patients with cervical spondylotic myelopathy. Herkowitz[18] reported a 90% neurologic recovery rate after Hirabayashi laminoplasty with unilateral foraminotomy on the open-door side. Overall, the majority of studies reported some neurologic improvement.

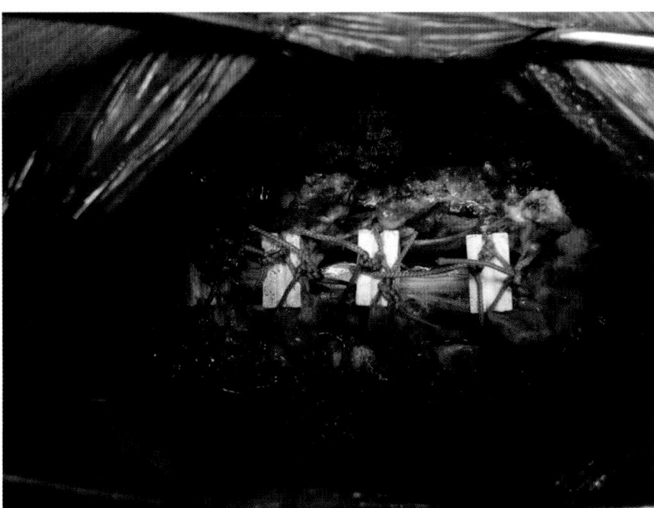

■ FIGURE 77–7. Postoperative photograph showing modified French door laminoplasty using hydroxyapatite (HA) spacers.

### French Door Laminoplasty and Its Modifications

The mean recovery rate after French door laminoplasty is approximately 50% to 70%.[19] The recovery rate is not likely related to the specific surgical procedure. Clinical outcome is more likely related to preoperative neurologic status.

### Short-Term Results

Almost all of the studies based on short-term follow-up have shown satisfactory results after any types of laminoplasty.

### Long-Term Results

A few studies have evaluated the long-term clinical outcome after laminoplasty. Miyazaki and associates[20] reported that improved neurologic status was maintained at a mean of 12 years after surgery.

Kawaguchi and associates[21] observed the long-term outcome over 10 years of 126 patients after en bloc laminoplasty. They found that neurologic recovery rates were maintained to 55.1% at the last follow-up. Most of the patients improved their JOA scores after surgery and maintained them at the final follow-up, although 20 patients has a worsened JOA score during follow-up. Postoperative ROM decreased to 25.1% of preoperative motion, with 61% of patients showing some reduction in ROM. Kyphotic changes were noted in eight patients, who showed poor neurologic recovery rates.

Seichi and associates[22] also examined the average 12-year follow-up of 25 patients who underwent a double-door laminoplasty. They observed that the average preoperative JOA score was improved after surgery, and the average score increased by 5-year follow-up. However, 10 years after surgery, the average score had decreased slightly until the final follow-up. Late neurologic deterioration was noted in four patients at an average of 8 years.

Another long-term study by Chiba and associates[23,24] examined the average 14-year follow-up of 80 patients who underwent expansive open-door laminoplasty. They reported that the average JOA score and recovery rate improved significantly until 3 years after surgery and remained at an acceptable level in both cervical spondylosis and OPLL patients with slight deterioration after 5 years. Segmental motor palsy developed in 8 patients. Late neurologic deterioration, mainly lower extremity motor score decline, was noted in 8 CSM and 16 OPLL patients. Overall, cervical range of motion decreased by 36%. Cervical lordosis decreased gradually in both patient groups. Such changes in alignments did not affect surgical results in CSM patients, and OPLL patients with preoperative kyphosis had lower recovery rates than those with straight and lordotic alignments. OPLL progression was detected in 66% of patients but did not affect clinical results.

## POSTOPERATIVE COMPLICATIONS

Most studies report similar problems after laminoplasty, which include postoperative axial neck pain, reduced range of motion, motor nerve root palsy (canal stenosis), and the loss of cervical lordosis (development of some degree of kyphosis). In addition to these complications, the issue of range of motion will be discussed later at the end of this chapter.

### Axial Neck Pain

Sani and associates[25] reported that the overall incidence of neck pain ranged from 6% to 60% without apparent dependence on the specific variation of laminoplasty using meta-analysis in 71 retrospective studies. Hosono and associates[26] also reported that the prevalence of postoperative axial symptoms was significantly higher (60%) after laminoplasty than after anterior fusion (19%). In a study by Wada and associates[27] comparing subtotal corpectomy and laminoplasty, axial pain was observed in 15% of the corpectomy group and in 40% of the laminoplasty group. The etiology of axial neck pain remains unclear, but it might be related to posterior soft tissue and muscle dissection or facet joint disruption.

### Motor Nerve Root Palsy

Segmental motor nerve paralysis is common after laminoplasty. Motor paralysis most commonly involves the C5 nerve root, possibly caused by the result of a tethering effect on the nerve root at or near the apex of lordosis induced by excessive posterior cord migration after decompression. Sani and associates[25] reported the incidence of C5 root palsy as 8%, and most cases resolved spontaneously. The motor palsy usually recovers to normal or near normal within 12 months after surgery.

### Loss of Cervical Lordosis (Development of Kyphosis)

The range of worsening spinal alignment, not necessarily kyphosis, has been reported to range from 22% to 53%.[27,30] However, with the use of modern instrumentation techniques, the incidence of development of kyphosis has been reported to range from 2% to 4%, with 0% in the hardware augmentation group.[13]

Although many studies have evaluated the preoperative and postoperative cervical alignment using various methods, there are few reports on the correlation between loss of normal lordosis and potential long-term neurologic deterioration.

## DISCUSSION

### Laminoplasty versus Laminectomy and Fusion

In a retrospective matched cohort analysis of cervical laminoplasty versus cervical laminectomy with fusion for the treatment of multilevel cervical myelopathy, laminoplasty was associated with a higher improvement in function and a lower frequency of complications.

Although most studies that used laminectomy and fusion for the treatment of multilevel cervical myelopathy have reported favorable neurologic outcomes, complications seem to occur in 12% to 40% of patients. These complications include screw loosening, broken hardware, pseudarthrosis, adjacent segment degeneration, progression of myelopathy, development of cervical kyphosis, deep wound infection, epidural hematoma, seroma, and donor site discomfort.

Importantly, no laminoplasty technique is effective for the restoration of lordosis in an already kyphotic spine, because the first goal of laminoplasty is maintaining the expanded spinal canal and cervical alignment. On the other hand, laminectomy should decompress the cervical canal; therefore, any type of fusion must be followed until bony fusion has been documented radiographically. In addition, the fusion procedure is likely to have a higher rate of adjacent segment degeneration due to the lost motion through several spinal motion segments.

### Laminoplasty versus Multilevel Anterior Corpectomy and Discectomy

In a retrospective matched cohort analysis of multilevel cervical corpectomy and fusion versus laminoplasty for the treatment of multilevel cervical myelopathy, the percentage of patients with subjective improvement in symptoms was similar between the two groups; however, complications in the corpectomy group were more frequent than in the laminoplasty group.[29] Complications were progression of myelopathy, nonunion, screw malposition, persistent dysphagia, and persistent dysphonia. Yonenobu and associates[24] also reported similar clinical results (neurologic outcomes) after multilevel anterior decompression and fusion compared with laminoplasty; however, complications were more frequent in the subtotal corpectomy and strut graft group than in the laminoplasty group. Overall, multilevel anterior cervical discectomies and corpectomies have been shown to have more frequent complications. To reduce these complications, combined anterior and posterior surgery might be an alternative treatment to address the nonunion and instrumentation-related problems, but greater surgical risk could arise.

### Range of Motion in Laminoplasty

In almost all the reviewed studies, cervical ROM has been reported to decrease 17% to 50%, with an average of approximately 50% after the Hirabayashi laminoplasty. Cervical ROM was decreased greatly (70% to 80%) when laminoplasty was augmented with fusion. The clinical relevance of this decreased ROM is controversial. Some authors emphasized the importance of limiting cervical ROM after laminoplasty. Kimura and associates[31] reported that the 40% reduction in cervical ROM after laminoplasty and this decreased ROM were thought to contribute to limiting dynamic factors, which are some of the possible reasons for the development of myelopathy. Yoshida and associates[32] documented that the decreased ROM may prevent late deterioration caused by progression of OPLL.

In contrast, other authors emphasized the importance of preservation of cervical ROM after laminoplasty. They thought that axial neck pain was decreased and adjacent segment degeneration was prevented by preserving cervical ROM. Morimoto and associates[28] reported that 83% of "normal range of cervical motion" was preserved at 3-year follow-up using their modification of the Kurokawa laminoplasty and noted the importance of preserving cervical ROM.

Hirabayashi and Bohlman[10] proposed that the restrictive effects of cervical laminoplasty produce spinal stability without the complete restriction of motion that is obtained by fusion techniques.

In long-term follow-up studies, there is a trend to loss of cervical ROM after laminoplasty. Seichi and co-workers[22] observed that a significant rate of spontaneous facet fusion occurred in patients followed for at least 10 years after a Kurokawa laminoplasty. They therefore recommended use of hydroxyapatite spacers instead of autogenous bone graft and reduced postoperative neck immobilization to prevent these effects.

One of the most confusing aspects of the laminoplasty might be related to the cervical ROM. The gain from this changed ROM after laminoplasty appears to lie between solid fusion with elimination of cervical motion and laminectomy alone with complete preservation of normal cervical range of motion. And it is clear that this wide range of cervical motion was retained after surgery while maintaining cervical stability regardless of the type of laminoplasty, patient age, and postoperative immobilization, although there has been inconsistent emphasis in the literature regarding maintenance of preoperative ROM and its effect on progressive myelopathy. Also, the range of remaining ROM must lie between the ROM from solid fusion and the ROM from laminectomy alone. Therefore, if the patient is doing well without any loss of cervical stability and any undesirable complications after laminoplasty, it is not necessary to try to reduce the remaining motion from the surgery, because nobody knows whether this motion could be of a beneficial nature, such as decreasing neck pain and preventing adjacent segment level disease.

## Range of Motion in Cervical Arthroplasty

There have been more recent interests on new emerging technologies, such as cervical disc arthroplasty, to maintain motion, avoid deformity, reduce adjacent segment deterioration, and allow for an adequate decompression without having to use bone graft.

Although there are no long-term data available yet, most of cervical arthroplasty prostheses available on the market have shown satisfactory clinical and radiographic outcomes, including maintaining ROM at the treated level and overall cervical spine (C2-C7; to check the global cervical motion) without any remarkable device-related complications.

Goffin and associates[33]observed that motion was maintained at the treated segment, and this motion was similar to preoperative motion in almost 90% of the group at the 2-year follow-up after implantation of the Bryan cervical disc (Medtronic Sofamor Danek, Memphis, TN). Duggal and associates[34] demonstrated quantitatively the functional motion-preserving capabilities of cervical arthroplasty (Bryan device). They found that the mean sagittal ROM at the treated disc space was 7.8 degrees on follow-up assessments, and this did not differ significantly from the 10.1 degrees measured before surgery. Moreover, no significant changes in ROM were noted at individual segments either adjacent to or distant from the operative site, and global cervical sagittal motion distributed across all levels (C2-C7) increased moderately in the late follow-up evaluations. Bertagnoli and associates[35]reported that ROM at level of implants was 12 degrees after implantation of ProDisc-C cervical artificial disc. McAfee and associates[36] demonstrated that ROM was maintained at the treated level in their biomechanical study using the porous-coated motion (PCM) device (Cervitech, Inc., Rockaway, NJ) and reported that ROM was corroborated with dynamic fluoroscopy in 23 patients (32 implants) who underwent PCM cervical artificial disc replacement surgery.

## Cervical Disc Replacement Combined with Cervical Laminoplasty

Recently, the capability of maintaining motion of the treated level makes it possible to extend the indications of cervical artificial disc. Sekhon[37] reported the use of an artificial disc at one or two levels in the management of cervical spondylotic myelopathy. In his study, a total of seven patients who underwent Bryan artificial disc prosthesis preserved motion at the final follow-up, and improvement in lordosis was achieved in 29% of cases. McAfee also reported the use of PCM cervical arthroplasties in the management of radiculopathy, myelopathy, and especially Klippel-Feil syndrome to preserve the motion. It is known that cervical motion is important to assist in chewing in this class of Klippel-Feil patients.

Therefore, the proven advantages of the foregoing procedures, which can preserve and maintain ROM at the treated level, might have a major impact on the primary indications for cervical arthroplasty and more widespread use of implantations.

## Case Report

A herniated nucleus pulposus occurred in a 51-year-old male patient with classic symptoms of cervical spondylotic myelopathy due to cervical stenosis, and the patient underwent posterior cervical laminoplasty (Figs. 77–8 and 77–9). He was suffering from hand clumsiness (both hands), gait disturbance, and difficulty in fine finger movement bilaterally. The senior author (SWK) performed a posterior cervical modified French door midline splitting laminoplasty using a T-saw and hydroxyapatite spacers to preserve the motion. After surgery, the patient was dramatically improved neurologically. He could walk independently without aids and moved all his extremities unassisted. However, several months later, he was starting to complain of a tingling sensation and pain in his right hand; herniated nucleus pulposus was noted at the C5-C6 level on a new MRI. As he was completely happy from the previous laminoplasty surgery, especially in terms of preservation of motion, even after such a major surgery like multilevel laminoplasty, he wanted to have a surgery which afforded him the opportunity to maintain the motion at the herniated disc level. Therefore, an anterior decompression and PCM artificial disc implantation were performed at C5-C6. He was completely satisfied with the results after cervical artificial disc replacement. At 1-year follow-up, he has returned to work and is unrestricted in performance of the activities of daily living without any limitation of neck motion (Figs. 77–10 and 77–11). Although there has been much debate on the beneficial or harmful effects of the motion after laminoplasty, we have realized how motion is important for the patient's life quality (satisfaction).

It is hoped that by combining posterior cervical laminoplasty with anterior cervical artificial disc replacement surgery, the

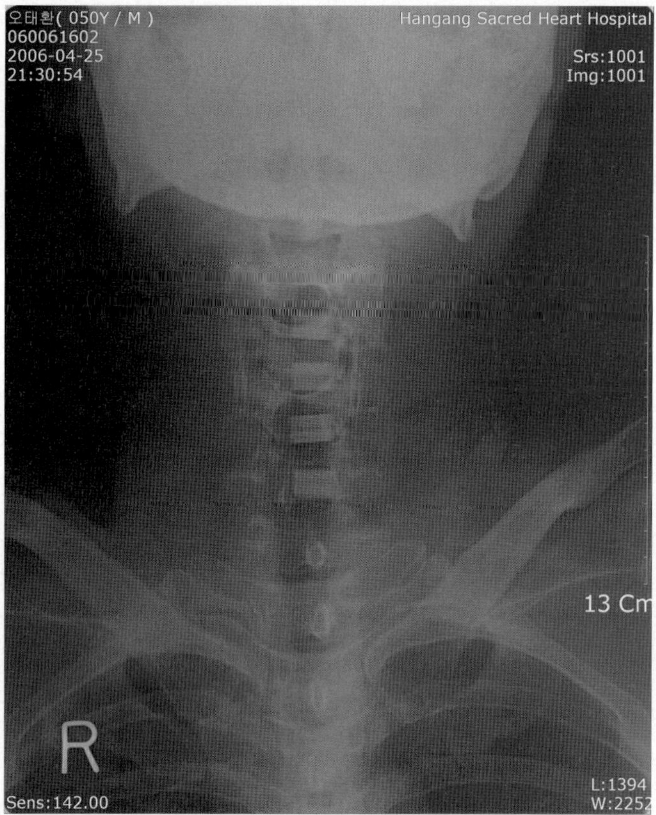


■ **FIGURE 77–8.** Anteroposterior view of a 51-year-old male patient after posterior laminoplasty (modified French door laminoplasty using hydroxyapatite spacers).

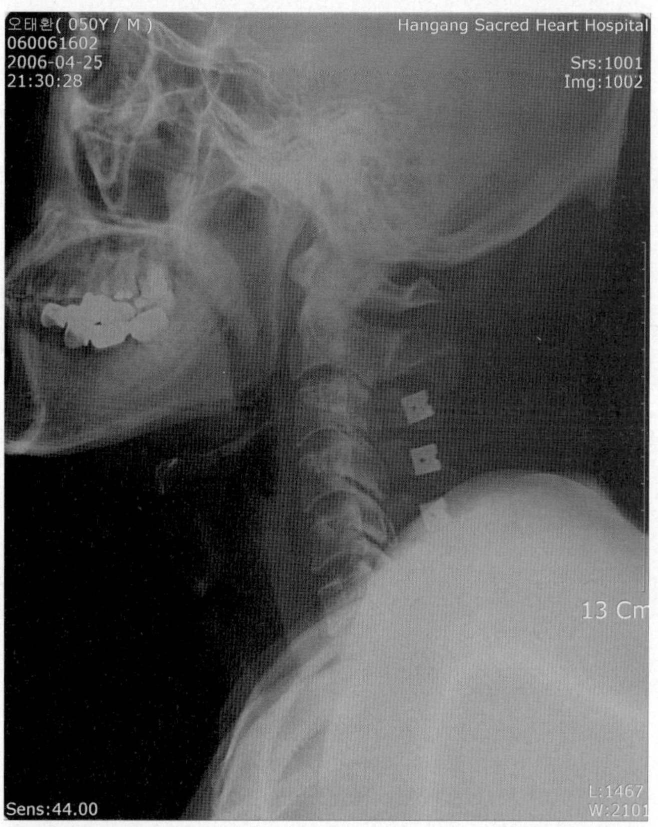


■ **FIGURE 77–9.** Lateral radiographs of a 51-year-old male patient after posterior laminoplasty (modified French door laminoplasty using hydroxyapatite spacers).

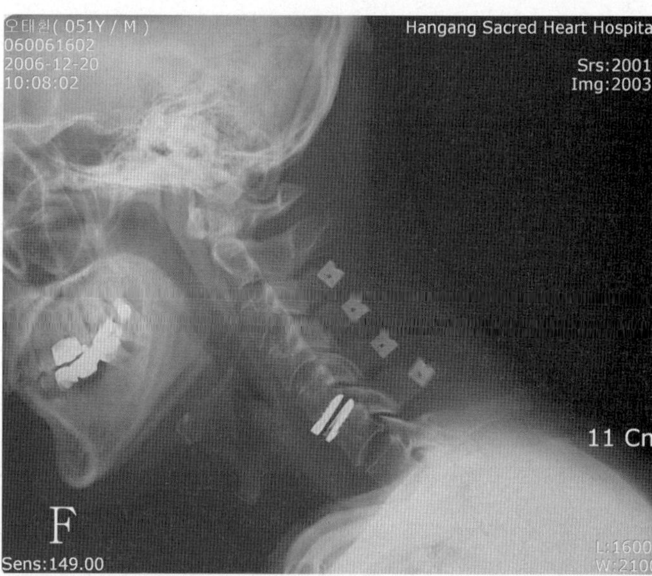


■ **FIGURE 77–10.** PCM artificial disc implantation in a patient who underwent previous multilevel posterior laminoplasty (flexion-lateral radiograph).

historically successful outcomes attained by posterior laminoplasty can be married to the known advantages of maintenance of normal motion attained by cervical artificial disc replacement.

Currently, there is a tremendous interest in the maintenance of the biomechanical properties of the cervical spine that focus on the preservation of the motion segment.

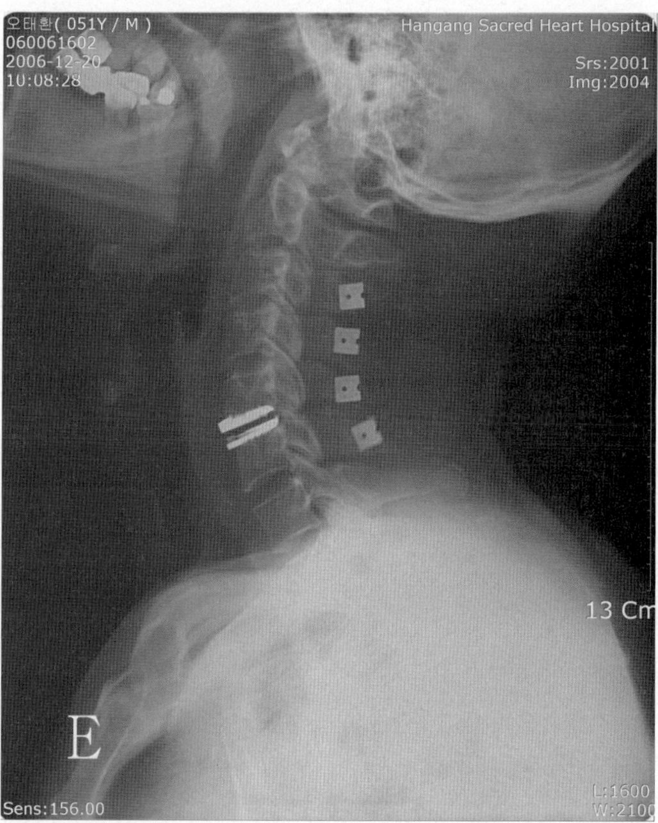


■ **FIGURE 77–11.** PCM artificial disc implantation in a patient who underwent previous posterior laminoplasty (extension-lateral radiograph).

The patient's anticipation for a better postoperative outcome and avoidance of the known problems associated with fusion suggest that the new procedures such as cervical artificial disc replacement and laminoplasty may play an important role in the management of cervical spondylotic myelopathy combined with radiculopathy. A larger series of patients with long-term follow-up data is needed before recommending this technique routinely.

## REFERENCES


1. Emery SE, Bohlman HH, Bolesta MJ, Jones PK: Anterior cervical decompression and arthrodesis for the treatment of cervical myelopathy:two to seven-year follow-up. J Bone Joint Surg Am 80:941–951, 1998.
2. Farey ID, McAfee PC, Davis RF, Long DM: Pseudoarthrosis of the cervical spine after anterior arthrodesis: treatment by posterior nerve-root decompression, stabilization, and arthrodesis. J Bone Joint Surg Am 72:1171–1177, 1990.
3. Pal PP, Cooper HH: The vertical stability of the cervical spine. Spine 13:447–449, 1988.
4. Oyama M, Hattori S, Moriwaki N: A new method of posterior decompression(in Japanese). Centr Jpn J Orthop Traumatol Surg 16:792–794, 1973.
5. Hirabayashi K: Expansive open-door laminoplasty for cervical spondylotic myelopathy(in Japanese). Operation 32:1159–1163, 1978.
6. Kurokawa T, Tsuyama N, Tanaka H: Enlargement of spinal canal by the sagittal splitting of the spinous process. Bessatsu Seikeigeka 2:234–240, 1982.
7. Nakano K, Harata S, Suetsuna F, et al: Spinous process-splitting laminoplasty using hydroxyapatite spinous process spacer. Spine 17:41–43, 1992.
8. Heller JG, Edwards CC, Murakami H, et al: Laminoplasty versus laminectomy and fusion for multilevel cervical myelopathy: an independent matched cohort analysis. Spine 26:1330–1336, 2001.
9. Natio M, Ogata K, Kurose S, Oyama M: Canal-expansive laminoplasty in 83 patients with cervical spondylotic myelopathy. Int Orthop 18:347–351, 1994.
10. Hirabayashi K, Bohlman KH: Controversy: multilevel cervical spondylosis. Spine 20:1732–1734, 1995.
11. Hirabayashi S, Kumano K: Contact of hydroxyapatite spacers with split spinous processes in double-door laminoplasty for cervical myelopathy. J Orthop Sci 4:264–268, 1999.
12. Hirabayashi K, Satomi K: Operative procedure and results of expansive open-door laminoplasty. Spine 13:870–876, 1988.
13. O'Brien MF, Peterson D, Casey AT, et al: A novel technique for laminoplasty augmentation of spinal canal area using titanium miniplate stabilization. A computerized morphometric analysis. Spine 21:474–483, 1996.
14. Baisden J, Voo LM, Cusick JF, Pintar FA, Yoganandan N: Evaluation of cervical laminectomy and laminoplasty: a longitudinal study in the goat model. Spine 24:1283–1289, 1999.
15. Kawaguchi Y, Matsui H, Ishihara H: Surgical outcomes of cervical expansive laminoplasty in patients with diabetes mellitus. Spine 25:551–555, 2000.
16. Kimura K, Oh-Hama M, Shingu H: Cervical myelopathy treated by canal-expansive laminoplasty: computed tomographic and myelographic findings. J Bone Joint Surg Am 66:914–920, 1995.
17. Satomi K, Nishu Y, Kohno T, Hirabayashi K: Long-term follow-up studies of open-door expansive laminoplasty for cervical stenotic myelopathy. Spine 19:507–510, 1994.
18. Herkowitz H: A comparison of anterior cervical fusion, cervical laminectomy, and cervical laminoplasty for the surgical management of multiple level spondylotic radiculopathy. Spine 13:774–780, 1988.
19. Takayasu M, Takagi T, Nishizawa T, et al: Bilateral open-door cervical expansive laminoplasty with hydroxyapatite spacers and titanium screws. J Neurosurg(Spine 1) 96:22–28, 2001.
20. Miyazaki K, Korohuji E, Ono S: Extensive simultaneous multisegmental laminectomy and posterior decompression with posterolateral fusion. J Jpn Spine Res Soc 5:167, 1994.
21. Kawaguchi Y, Knamori M, Ishihara H, et al: Minimum 10-year follow-up after en bloc cervical laminoplasty. Clin Orthop 411:129–139, 2003.
22. Seichi A, Takeshita K, Ohishi I, et al: Long-term results of double-door laminoplasty for cervical stenotic myelopathy. Spine 479–487, 2001.
23. Chiba K, Ogawa Y, Ishii K, et al: Long-term results of expansive open-door laminoplasty for cervical myelopathy-average 14-year follow-up study. Spine 31(26):2998–3005, 2006.
24. Chiba K, Toyama Y, Watanabe M, et al: Impact of longitudinal distance of the cervical spine on the results of expansive open-door laminoplasty. Spine 25:2893–2898, 2000.
25. Sani S, Ratliff JK, Cooper PR: A critical review of cervical laminoplasty. Neurosurg Ouart 14:5–16, 2004.
26. Hosono N, Yonenobu K, Ono K: Neck and shoulder pain after laminoplasty: a noticeable complication. Spine 21:1969–1973, 1996.
27. Wada E, Suzuki S, Kanazawa A, et al: Subtotal corpectomy versus laminoplasty for multilevel cervical spondylotic myelopathy: a long-term follow-up study over 10 years. Spine 26:1443–1448, 2001.
28. Morimoto T, Matsuyama T, Hirabayashi H, Sakaki T, Yabuno T: Expansive laminoplasty for multilevel cervical OPLL. J Spinal Disord 10:296–298, 1997.
29. Edwards CC, Heller JG, Murakami H: Corpectomy versus laminoplasty for multilevel cervical myelopathy: an independent matched cohort analysis. Spine 27:1168–1175, 2002.
30. Yonenobu K, Hosono N, Iwasaki M, Asano M, Ono K: Laminoplasty versus subtotal corpectomy: a comparative study of results in multisegmental cervical spondylotic myelopathy. Spine 17:1281–1284, 1992.
31. Kimura I, Shingu H, Nasu Y: Long-term follow-up of cervical spondylotic myelopathy treated by canal-expansive laminoplasty. J Bone Joint Surg Br 77:956–961, 1995.
32. Yoshida M, Otani K, Shibasaki K, et al: Expansive laminoplasty with reattachment of spinous process and extensor musculature for cervical myelopathy. Spine 17:491–497, 1992.
33. Goffin J, Van Calenberg F, Van Loon J, et al: Intermediate follow-up after treatment of degenerative disc disease with the Bryan cervical disc prosthesis: single-level and bi-level. Spine 28:2673–2678, 2003.
34. Duggal N, Pickett GE, Mitsis DK, et al: Early clinical and biomechanical results following cervical arthroplasty. Neurosurg Focus 17:62–68, 2004.
35. Bertagnoli R, Yue JJ, Pfeiffer F, et al: Early results after ProDisc-C cervical disc replacement. J Neurosurg Spine 2:403–410, 2005.
36. McAfee PC: The indications for lumbar and cervical disc replacement. Spine J 4:177s–181s, 2006.
37. Sekhon LH: Cervical arthroplasty in the management of spondylotic myelopathy: 18-month results. Neurosurg Focus 17:55–62, 2004.

CHAPTER 78

# Hybrid Nonfusion Techniques

**Rudolf Bertagnoli**

## KEY POINTS

- The use of motion sparing and/or fusion technologies should be assigned based on the specific pathology or pathologies in a patient.
- Patients may require a combinaton of motion sparing or fusion technologies concurrently or during different temporal surgical times.
- The anterior and posterior spinal compartments should be carefully and individually evaluated.
- Select patients with prior fusions may be candidates for motion sparing surgery.
- Contraindications to motion sparing technology should be reviewed prior to any hybrid surgery technique.

Classical fusion technologies display a wide range of disadvantages such as obliteration of normal anatomy, elimination of mobility, and increased stiffness. Each consequence can increase the possibility of other long-term complications ("fusion diseases"), such as facet hypertrophy, facet arthritis, spinal stenosis, osteophyte formation, posterior muscular debilitation, and adjacent-level disc degeneration.[1–6] In order to avoid (circumvent) these problems, nonfusion motion-preserving techniques (disc arthroplasty and posterior dynamic stabilization) have been developed that offer the possibility of achieving intersegmental stabilization while preserving/restoring physiologic mobility.

In cases in which total disc replacement (TDR) technologies fail to produce the expected result, cannot address the complete disease process, or are contraindicated, hybrid techniques may be the resultant method of choice.

## CLASSIFICATION OF HYBRID CONSTRUCTS

In principle, hybrid constructs can be subgrouped into two categories: single-level hybrid constructs and multilevel hybrid constructs (Tables 78–1, 78–2), which may be single-stage and multistage. Multilevel hybrids can be subgrouped into pure motion-sparing technologies and a mixture of fusion and motion-sparing technologies.

### Single-Level Hybrid Constructs

#### Single-Stage Motion-Preserving Hybrids: Types 1, 2a, 2b (see Table 78–1)

Because the motion segments consist of three moving areas, disc arthroplasty technologies (partial and total disc arthroplasty) may need to be combined with elements that achieve posterior stabilization, such as dynamic pedicle screw devices, interspinous devices, or facet replacements.

#### Multistage Motion-Preserving Hybrids (Types 2a, 2b)

Patients who had a prior surgery in which a motion-preserving device was implanted can also receive an additional implantation at a later date. This is defined as "multistage" (Table 78–1, types 2a, 2b) and allows the combination of primary anterior or primary posterior technologies with secondary posterior or secondary anterior technologies.

### Multilevel Hybrids: Types 3, 4, 5a to 5c (see Table 78–2)

The combination of anterior motion-preserving technologies (nucleus arthroplasty, total disc arthroplasty) with posterior motion-preserving technologies (interspinous devices, pedicle screw systems, facet replacement) at more than one level is termed a *multilevel hybrid*. With these combinations, a three-dimensional, motion-preserving, and biomechanically stable reconstruction of the affected motion segments can be achieved, and a physiologic range of motion can be reestablished. These multilevel motion-preserving hybrids can be classified in three subgroups: single stage type 3; fusion (single stage type 4); and previous fusion (multistage type 5a to c).

#### Motion-Preserving Hybrid: Single Stage Type 3

Anterior (nucleus arthroplasty, total disc arthroplasty) and posterior (interspinous devices, pedicle screw systems, facet replacement) technologies can be implanted in different levels and can be combined in a single stage. The dynamic treatment of all affected segments with motion-preserving technologies can be achieved with this type of hybrid.

TABLE 78–1. Single-Level Hybrid Constructs

| Type | Timing of Surgical Procedures | Anterior | Posterior |
|---|---|---|---|
| 1 | Single stage | Yes | Yes |
| 2a | Multistage | Previous surgery | Yes |
| 2b | Multistage | Yes | Previous surgery |

### Motion-Preserving Hybrid: Fusion (Single Stage Type 4)

In some cases, it makes sense to apply a hybrid construct in which a motion-preserving device and a fusion technique are combined. If different pathologies are found within multiple motion segments, it is not advantageous to reconstruct only the most affected segment with motion-preserving technologies. This is the case if, for example, one segment shows severe spondyloarthritis, spondylolysis, and/or spondylolisthesis, the second segment has a reduced disc height of at least 50%, and the third segment shows a large central disc herniation (in conditions with no severe posterior element disease at all levels). With the application of a fusion device in the lower or middle area, a mechanically stable construct can be achieved and should be taken into consideration. In these cases, single-stage surgery is preferred.

TABLE 78–2. Multilevel Hybrid Constructs

| Type | Timing of Surgical Procedures | Type of procedure: Level X to Z | Type of procedure: Level Y to Z |
|---|---|---|---|
| 3 | Single stage | Motion-preserving technology (anterior, posterior, or combinations) | Motion-preserving technology (anterior, posterior, or combinations) |
| 4 | Single stage | Fusion procedure (any kind) | Motion-preserving technology (anterior, posterior, or combinations) |
| 5a | Multistage | Previous surgery: fusion procedure (any kind) | Motion-preserving technology (anterior, posterior, or combinations) |
| 5b | Multistage | Previous surgery: motion preservation (any kind) | Fusion procedure (any kind) |
| 5c | Multistage | Previous surgery: motion preservation (any kind) | Motion preservation (any kind) |

### Motion-Preserving Hybrid: Previous Fusion (Multistage Type 5a to c)

For symptomatic adjacent level instability, a surgery with implantation of a motion-preserving technology subsequent to a prior fusion surgery may be beneficial to the patient. The hybrid is then a combination of a fusion device with a motion-preserving technology implanted in different, consecutive sessions. Anterior and posterior technologies or combinations of single-level hybrids can be used in these cases.

## INDICATIONS AND CONTRAINDICATIONS

### Indications

Indications for hybrid constructs are similar to those for the anterior or posterior motion-sparing technologies. The reconstruction of a motion segment should be analyzed on a three-dimensional basis, taking biomechanical and morphologic changes into consideration. Therefore, the degree of degeneration and the degree of mechanical insufficiency must be considered by the surgeon before deciding which combinations of technologies to use. The scenarios in which hybrid constructs might be beneficial for the patient typically involve multilevel-diseased spines in which all affected levels are symptomatic. Thus, multilevel degenerative disc disease (DDD) with or without degenerative spondylolisthesis, degenerative scoliosis, combinations of isthmic or hyperplastic spondylolisthesis with DDD-affected adjacent levels, and progressively degenerated motion segments above or below a fusion (TZS, transitional zone syndrome) are typical indications for hybrid constructs.

### Contraindications

In general, the same contraindications that are valid for fusion and nonfusion technologies can be considered for hybrid constructs as well. Major contraindications are osteopenia (T-score $< -1.5$), osteoporosis, and other severe bone pathologies; infectious diseases; and severe psychosocial factors. These disorders significantly reduce the load-bearing capacities of the ventral bodies and their end plates. In fusion-only reconstructions, however, this is of less concern. Additionally, acute spinal fractures, spine tumor, and discitis should be excluded as well.

## CASE STUDIES

**Posterior Dynamic Stabilization and Lumbar TDR**

***Hybrid Construct Type 1: Dynesys System plus ProDisc-L Prosthesis***

A 68-year-old male patient underwent a previous fusion surgery at level L4-L5 (posterior lumbar interbody fusion) with two titanium cages (Fig. 78–1A, B). At 6 months after the surgery he developed continuous low back pain due to a failure of bony ingrowth. In a revision surgery with anterior explantation of the cages, a ProDisc-L prosthesis (Synthes, Inc., Paoli, PA) was implanted (Fig. 78–1C, D). In the same session, a posterior stabilization procedure with a modified Wiltse approach was used to implant a dynamic instrumentation system (Dynesys; Zimmer Spine, Inc., Warsaw, IN). The patient reported significant pain reduction a few days after the surgery with maintainance of relief at the 1-year follow-up.

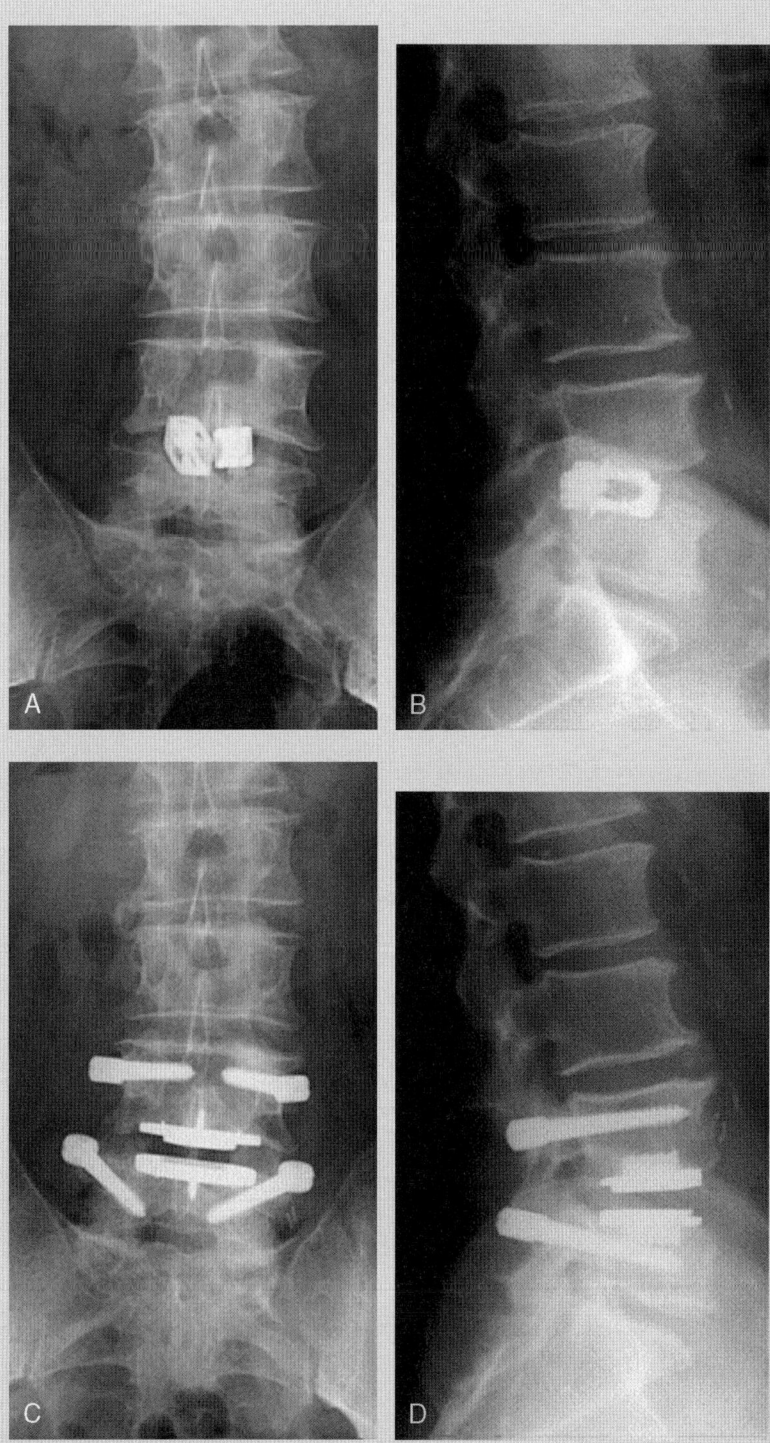


■ **FIGURE 78–1.** Preoperative radiographs: anteroposterior **(A)**, lateral **(B)**. Postoperative radiographs: anteroposterior **(C)**, lateral **(D)**.

***Hybrid Construct Type 2a: ProDisc-L Prosthesis plus Coflex System***

A 44-year-old female patient underwent ProDisc-L surgery in level L4-L5. The prosthesis was placed too far posterior, impinging the existing nerve root and creating a segmental scoliosis with facet compression pain (Fig. 78–2A, B). Posterior repositioning of the ProDisc and implantation of a coflex (Paradigm Spine, LLC, New York, NY) interspinous implant were performed at level L4-L5 (Fig. 78–2C, D) to unload the facets. Patient reported improvement after surgery.

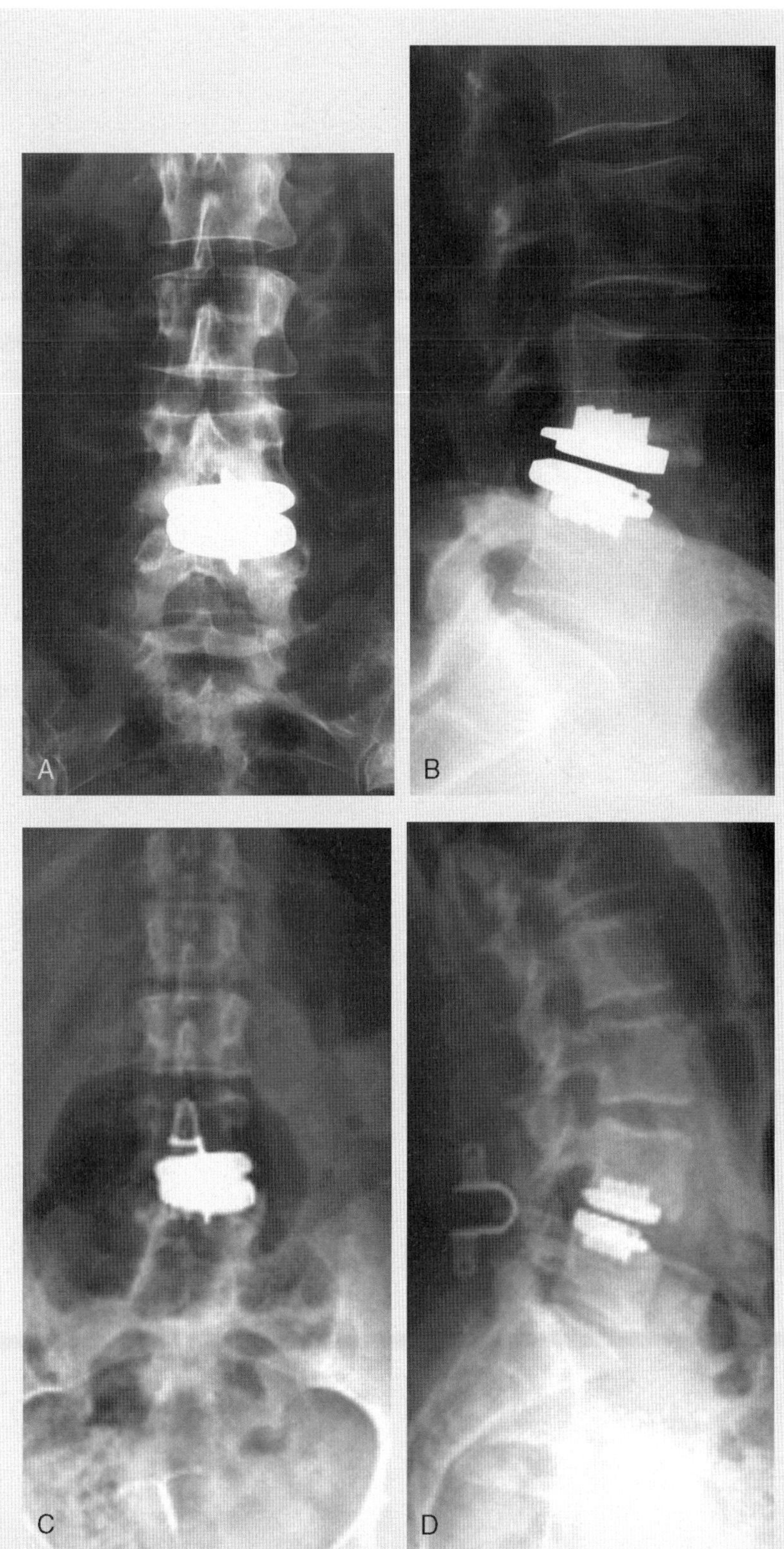


■ FIGURE 78–2. Preoperative radiographs: anteroposterior **(A)**, lateral **(B)**. Postoperative radiographs: anteroposterior **(C)**, lateral **(D)**.

***Hybrid Construct Type 3: Dynesys System plus ProDisc-L Prosthesis (Three-Level Procedure)***

A 42-year-old male patient underwent laminectomy at L2-L3 and L4-L5 and a disectomy at L3-L4 with progressive low back pain (Fig. 78–3A, B).

Discographically, L2-L3 and L4-L5 disc levels have been negative, and the L3-L4 disc was highly positive.

In a single-stage procedure, first implantation of ProDisc-L prosthesis was done at level L3-L4, and then Dynesys was implanted at levels L2-L3 and L4-L5 (Fig. 78–3C, D).

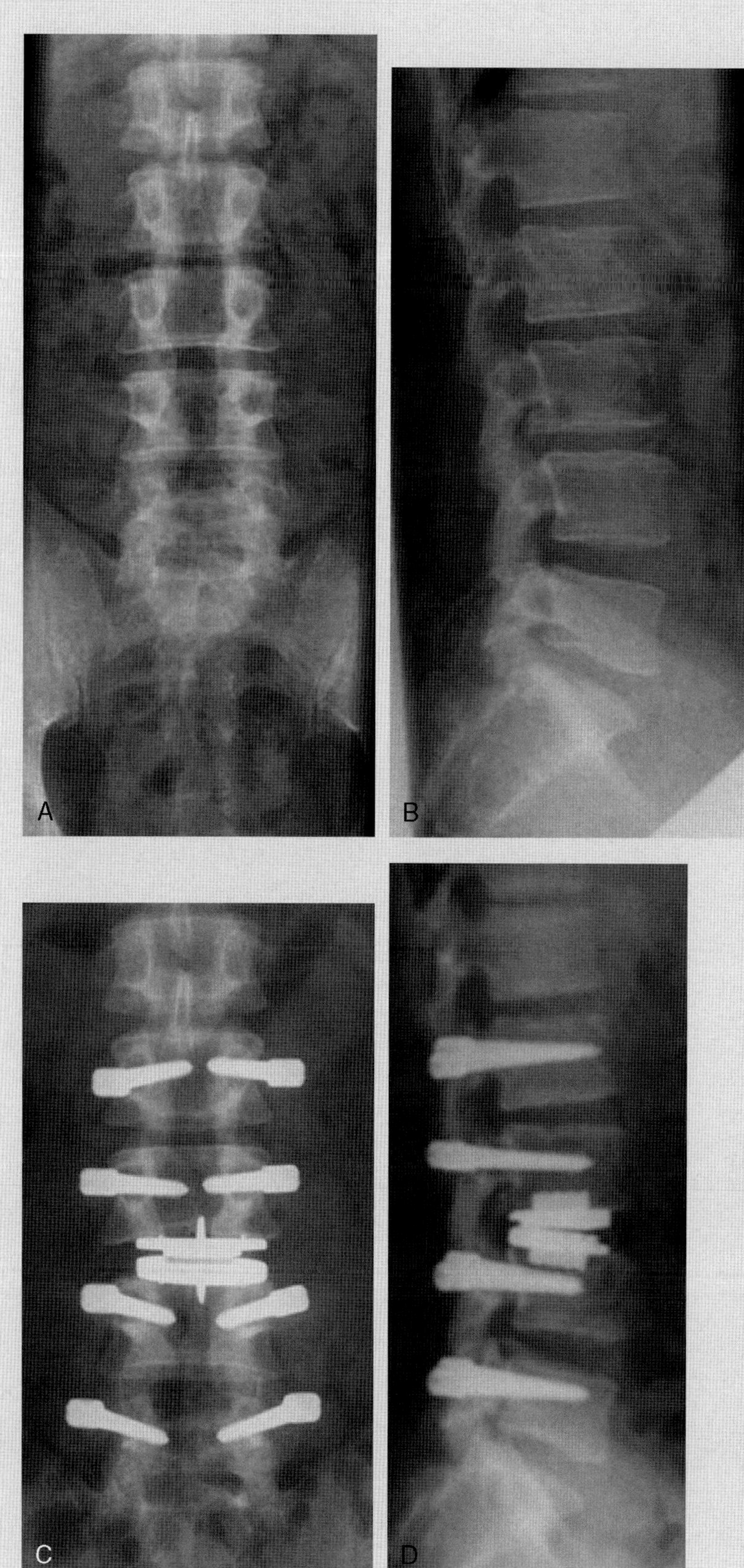


■ **FIGURE 78–3.** Preoperative radiographs: anteroposterior **(A)**, lateral **(B)**. Postoperative radiographs: anteroposterior **(C)**, lateral **(D)**.

***Hybrid Construct Type 5c***

A 46-old-female patient received a ProDisc-L at L5-S1 to relieve her low back pain (Fig. 78–4A, B). Three years later she developed a relevant vertical segmental instability at L4-L5 with back and leg pain. Our treatment choice was to perform a posterior dynamic stabilization with the DSS system (Abbott Spine PLC, Austin, TX) (Fig. 78–4C, D), because a posterior procedure is less risky than an anterior one.

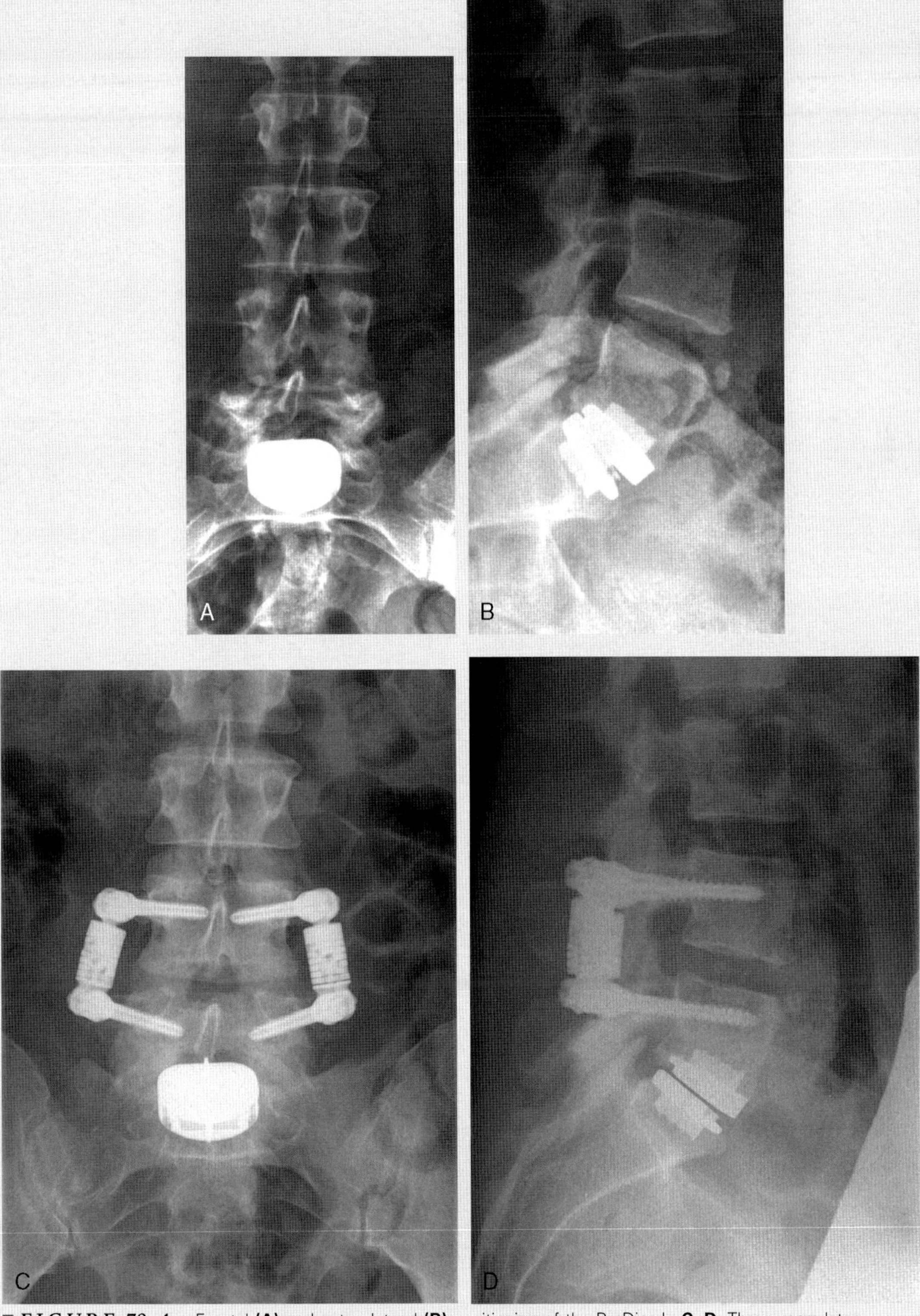


■ **FIGURE 78–4.** Frontal **(A)** and anterolateral **(B)** positioning of the ProDisc-L. **C, D,** Three years later, implantation of DSS.

**Interspinous Implants with Nucleus Replacement**

***Hybrid Construct Type 2a: Nucleus Replacement with NeuDisc plus coflex System***

A 44-year-old female patient underwent nucleus replacement surgery with NeuDisc (Replication Medical, Inc., Cranbury, NJ) at level L4-L5 (Fig. 78–5A). Two years after the surgery, the patient developed a facet hypercompression pain syndrome at the same level that could be confirmed with fluoroscopically guided facet injections (Fig. 78–5B, C). Implantation of a coflex interspinous device (Paradigm Spine, LLC, New York, NY) decompressed the facet joint by maintenance of mobility for dynamic stabilization at level L4-L5 was carried out (Fig. 78–5D, E). Significant pain reduction was reported by the patient.

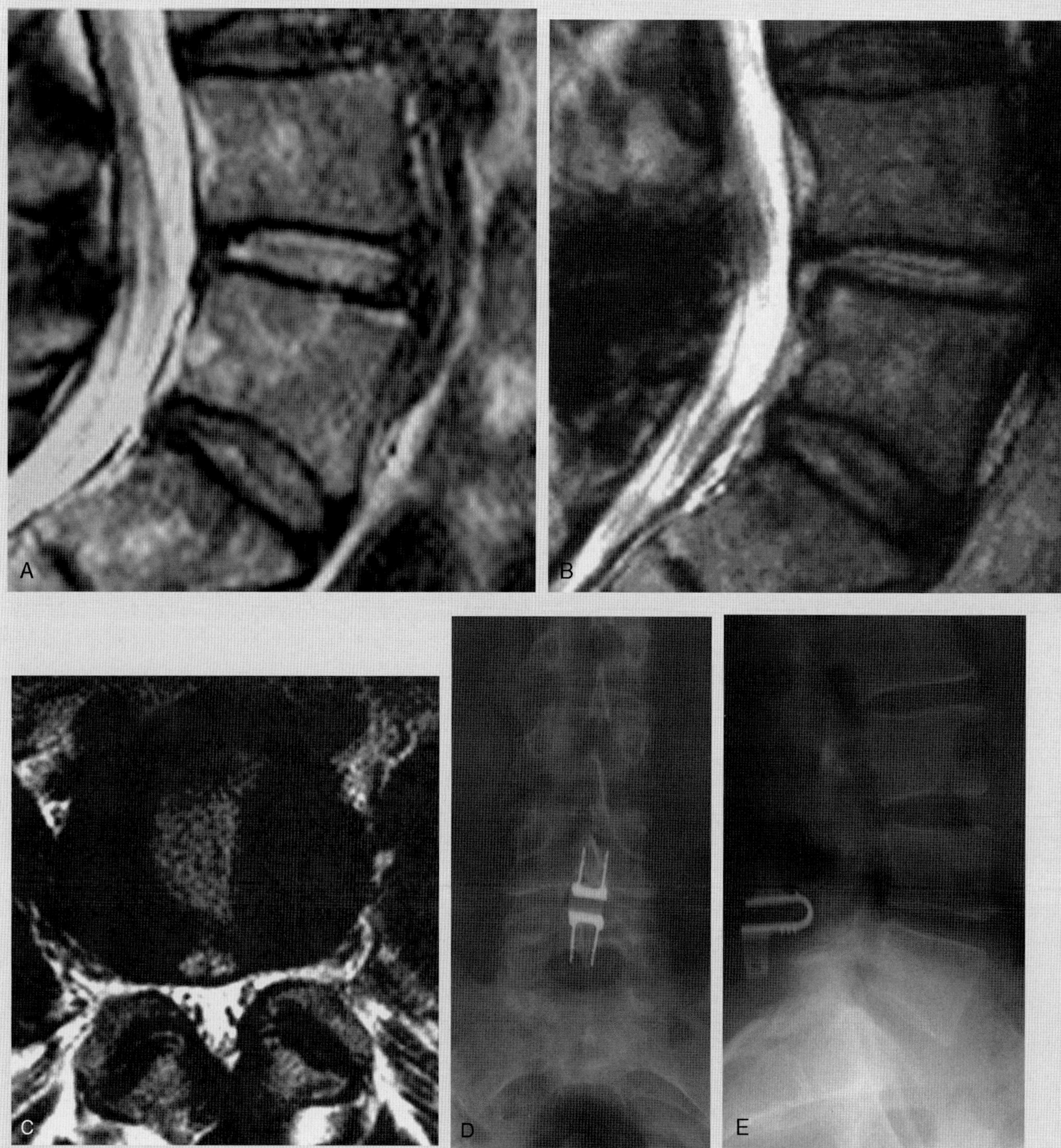


■ **FIGURE 78–5.** **A,** Magnetic resonance images after NeuDisc implantation. **B, C,** Magnetic resonance images after 2 years with facet hypercompression pain. Anteroposterior **(D)** and lateral **(E)** radiographs after coflex implantation.

As a general rule for any surgical procedure, proper adherence to accepted indications and contraindications is crucial for achieving maximum success of the surgery and good postoperative results.

## CONCLUSION

Treatment of only one moving zone of the three-column segment might be in some situations an insufficient solution. In these situations, the use of motion-sparing technologies in all three moving parts could be beneficial in complete reconstruction of the segment by maintaining motion. Especially in multilevel degenerative disc disease in which not all the segments have degenerated to the same degree or in which the pain generators are located in the front and back, very individualized selections of treatment options might be the best solution (multilevel motion-sparing hybrid). In contrast to these cases, highly degenerated or affected areas might need a fusion procedure that can now be combined with motion-sparing technology at another level.

Based on these facts, there has been a dramatic expansion of indications toward patients with multilevel or multicolumn degenerative disease. Early experience with the expansion of indications by using combinations of motion-preserving technologies also revealed promising results. It is very important, however, to verify the results scientifically while performing very stringent patient selection for application of these hybrid combinations. This level of concern is a basic necessity as there are only limited nonrandomized data available for some of these new techniques, and therefore the likelihood for complications can increase drastically when combining them in one patient. Short-, intermediate-, and long-term complications of these combinations are yet unknown, and therefore a careful follow-up of patients is also necessary. In the future, controlled single- and multicenter studies are required to confirm the first promising results from the use of hybrid constructs. It is important that the casual use of these constructs is strictly avoided.

## REFERENCES


1. Bertagnoli R: Disc surgery in motion. SpineLine 6:23–28, 2004.
2. Bertagnoli R, Kumar S: Indications for full prosthetic disc arthroplasty: A correlation of clinical outcome against a variety of indications. Eur Spine J 11(2):S131–136, 2002.
3. Hilibrand AS, Robbins M: Adjacent segement degeneration and adjacent segment disease: The consequences of spinal fusion? Spine J 4 (6):190S–194S, 2004.
4. Malter AD, McNeney B, Loeser JD, Deyo RA: 5-year reoperation rates after different types of lumbar spine surgery. Spine 23(7):814–820, 1998.
5. Bono CM, Lee CK: The influence of subdiagnosis on radiographic and clinical outcomes after lumbar fusion for degenerative disc disorders: An analysis of the literature from two decades. Spine 30(2):227–234, 2005.
6. Bertagnoli R: Review of modern treatment options for degenerative disc disease. *In* Kaech DL, Jinkins JR (ed): Spinal Restabilization Procedures: Diagnostic and Therapeutic Aspects of Intervertebral Fusion Cages, Artificial Discs and Mobile Implants. Amsterdam, Elsevier, 2002, pp 365–375.
7. Bertagnoli R, Tropiano P, Zigler J, et al: Hybrid constructs. Orthop Clin North Am 36:379–388, 2005.

CHAPTER 79

# Dynamic Pedicle-Screw Stabilization with Nucleus Replacement

**Rolando García** and **Brett A. Osborn**

**KEY POINTS**

- The primary function of a nuclear replacement is to help resist axial compressive forces working in conjunction with the annulus.
- The application of hybrid technologies to the lumbar spine theoretically serves to counteract the destabilizing consequences of degeneration, trauma, and standard lumbar procedures.
- While there may be theoretical advantages, surgeons must resist the temptation to combine these technologies purely based on intuition.

The ideal spinal arthroplasty procedure aims to restore normal prepathology anatomy and biomechanics. Although certain individuals are appropriately treated with individual systems, other situations may require more than one technology to achieve this goal. The combined application of these technologies, however, may carry a potentially amplified risk of complication. An unanswered challenge, therefore, is defining the indications for hybrid technologies in the context of the associated risks.

With thousands of nuclear replacement devices and posterior dynamic stabilization devices having been implanted, the major technical complications of these systems individually are now well established.[1–5] A major concern with the utilization of nuclear replacement devices is the potential for migration and subsidence,[6] but the concern of posterior dynamic stabilization is loosening of instrumentation and subsequent need for decompression or fusion.[4] The application of hybrid technologies may theoretically reduce the incidence of complications of motion preservation technologies applied in isolation and potentially extend their inherent limitations.

In a medical environment increasingly scrutinized for cost efficiency, it will be particularly challenging to implement hybrid protocols that will no doubt substantially increase cost.[7] It will be particularly interesting to observe the coverage policies that will be established regarding the combination of implant technologies. Of course, there is precedent for optimism; currently, although the value of bone morphogenetic protein as an adjunct to posterior instrumentation in place of iliac crest bone is not firmly established, their combined use is gaining widespread popularity.[8,9] One can see why when considering that the surgeon's first responsibility is to offer and do what is best for a patient, regardless of effort or cost. In the same vein, it will be interesting to watch how different arthroplasty technologies will be combined at least in part as a result of the surgeon's preference for certain manufacturers.

Utilizing the metaphor that we must learn how to walk before we can run, most surgeons will likely develop considerable experience with individual systems before venturing into hybrid applications. The goal of this chapter is not to propose a manner in which to treat certain disorders with combined arthroplasty techniques but rather to help the reader question and then evaluate the merit and limitations of hybrid techniques.

## ANATOMIC, BIOMECHANICAL, AND PATHOLOGIC CONSIDERATIONS

The intervertebral motion segment includes not only the disc and the facet joints but also a number of secondary structures such as the supraspinous ligament, interspinous ligament, as well as the origin and insertion of a variety of paraspinal muscles. Considering the complexity of this motion model, it should be no surprise that treating global segment instability with either an anterior or posterior approach can sometimes lead to failure. Furthermore, the effect of degeneration on the function of these anatomic structures must be understood in order to apply the proper corrective measures.

In Newtonian terms, in order to properly stabilize a motion segment we must accurately define the instability forces and then apply equal but opposing forces. Failure to properly counteract the destabilizing forces may actually accentuate instability rather than reduce it. A spinal segment lacking axial stability, as is often seen following discectomy, will not be properly served by a system that applies compressive forces, such as a posterior dynamic stabilization. Similarly, a segment lacking posterior flexural control, as can be seen after laminectomy, would not be properly corrected simply by insertion of a nuclear replacement.

The primary function of a nuclear replacement is to help resist axial compressive forces working in conjunction with the annulus. Biomechanical studies have shown that the axial forces on the disc are substantial. Wilke and associates reported that intradiscal pressure can be as high as 2,300 kPa with heavy lifting.[10] In addition, studies have shown that the degree of load shared by the nucleus is proportional to its cross-sectional area.[11]

Although the disc's primary role is that of shock absorption, the facet's primary function is that of rotational control. Furthermore, the function of the facets is influenced by their position and degree of segmental degeneration. Early biomechanical testing by Adams and Hutton has shown that 15% of the total axial compression load is carried by the facets when the segment is in the neutral position and that this load can increase to as much as 40% when the segment is in extension.[12]

Destabilizing or instability forces can take many forms including traumatic, developmental, degenerative, and iatrogenic. Furthermore, destabilizing forces can be subclassified as either anterior or posterior.

Prior to applying hybrid technologies of any sort, one must possess a sound knowledge of the anatomic and biomechanical properties of the spine and familiarity with the application of motion-preservation technologies in isolation. Specifically the facet joint orientation and its favored ranges of motion are crucial. The lumbar facet joints, for example, allow for flexion and extension and resist rotation. The intervertebral discs allow for polyaxial movement but primarily serve to resist compressive forces (axial loading).

The facet joint architecture often is altered during posterior decompressive procedures. Similarly, during discectomies, the intervertebral disc (both annulus and nucleus) is violated. Partial removal of the posterior elements while gaining access to the spinal canal potentially destabilizes the vertebral unit. The altered motion dynamics may, via accelerated facet degeneration, lead to the development of refractory back pain in the postoperative period. Also, the ipsilateral discectomy potentially destabilizes the vertebral unit. The combined motion alterations, albeit subtle, may contribute to the high rate of recurrent disc herniation and refractory low back pain. Alluding to this is Barr's published conclusion that "the thesis that every patient should have a spine fusion done at the time of laminectomy is tenable."[13]

The application of hybrid technologies to the lumbar spine theoretically serves to counteract the destabilizing consequences of degeneration, trauma, and standard lumbar procedures. In order to select the proper combination of spinal arthroplasty systems, we must understand the limitations of each of the individual arthroplasty systems.

In a recently published (2006) study by McAfee and co-workers, the authors concluded that implantation of a total disc replacement (TDR) does not restore rotational stability. Rotational motion is 120% to 140% after one-level TDR and 240% after two-level TDR.[14] By not significantly disrupting the annular architecture, nuclear replacement following microdiscectomy should not alter rotational stability to the same degree as TDR, especially when supplemented by posterior dynamic systems. In fact, nuclear replacement may work in concert with the existing annulus and longitudinal ligmanents to restore segmental stability and motion.[15]

Although rotational instability is a major concern following TDR, sagittal motion behavior or misbehavior is not.[16] In contrast, vertical translation is disproportionately magnified following discectomy and fenestrations, but axial hypermobility is not.[17]

The degree of disc and facet degeneration will play an increasingly important role in the selection process of the surgical approach. In a biomechanical and imaging study, Fujiwara and associates evaluated the effect of disc and facet degeneration on lumbar segmental motion.[18] The authors found that while facet degeneration leads to increased axial motion, axial motion is *most* affected by disc degeneration. Tanaka and colleagues have reported that moderate disc degeneration is associated with greater segmental motion, and severe disc degeneration is associated with reduced segmental motion or stiffening. This is likely secondary to the interference between adjacent osseous structures.[19]

## RATIONALE FOR HYBRID STABILIZATION

In simple terms, the goal of hybrid stabilization is to reduce the limitations of the individual systems while broadening the indications or applications.

In order for arthroplasty techniques to be successful, their relationship must be symbiotic and not parasitic. For example, the combination of interspinous stabilization with posterior pedicle-based dynamic stabilization would be counterproductive because most interspinous devices work as flexion spacers, which would often limit the motion and function in the case of posterior dynamic stabilization.

There are two basic questions that must be addressed before we can support the combination of nuclear replacement and posterior dynamic stabilization:

1. Can posterior dynamic stabilization decrease the rate of migration of nuclear replacement while augmenting stability?
2. Can nuclear replacement decrease the rate of screw loosening while providing anterior column support?

Clinical trials addressing hybrid technologies have yet to be published. The aforementioned questions accordingly remain unanswered but essential to paradigm development as it applies to utilization of motion preservation technologies.

## REVIEW OF THE LITERATURE

The history of spinal arthroplasty is the topic of another chapter in this book. From Fernstrom's original work in the 1960s to Graf's work on ligamentoplasty, there is extensive literature on the individual use of nuclear replacement (NR) and posterior dynamic stabilization (PDS).[20,21] However, there are little data available on the application of hybrid arthroplasty techniques. Although there have been anecdotal reports of the combined use of nuclear replacement with posterior dynamic stabilization, the authors were unable to find any peer-reviewed publications on this topic.

There are no Class I or Class II studies on the use of nuclear replacement with concomitant posterior dynamic stabilization. Furthermore, it will prove particularly challenging to prove the value of such combination techniques for two primary reasons:

First, defining control group criteria will be difficult. Secondary is the foreseen difficulty of two competing instrumentation manufacturers combining their products (and efforts) in an Investigational Device Exemption (IDE) study. The authors believe that the hybrid use of NR and PDS would be best compared with a posterolateral fusion with pedicle screw instrumentation, utilizing newer less invasive techniques and bone morphogenetic protein. A comparison of a NR device in combination with a PDS system with a traditional and open ALIF (anterior lumbar interbody fusion) and PLIF (posterior lumbar interbody fusion) with pedicle screw instrumentation and iliac crest bone graft would hardly seem fair or appropriate.

A major point that can be drawn from publications on the individual use of NR and PDS is the most common limitations and complications of these devices.[1–5] In general, the major complications with nuclear replacement are device migration and subsidence.[1,2] On the other hand, the major complications with posterior dynamic stabilization are screw loosening and persistent back pain.[3–5]

The major complication reported with the use of the PDN (prosthetic disc nucleus) has been device migration.

Shim and associates reported on 46 patients followed for a minimum of 6 months. The authors reported four cases of device migration and one case of infection.[22]

In a prospective multicenter study by Stoll and associates, the authors reported on 83 consecutive patients who underwent flexible stabilization with the Dynesys system (Zimmer Spine, Inc., Warsaw, IN). Although the authors reported favorable clinical results, the authors reported a high rate of additional surgery: three required implant removal and conversion to fusion for persistent pain, seven required additional surgery for transitional level degeneration, one required a laminectomy at the operated level, and one required screw removal because of loosening. In addition, seven patients demonstrated signs of screw loosening.[3]

In a retrospective study by Grob and associates, the authors reported on 31 patients after an average of 2 years following Dynesys stabilization. The authors reported that during the follow-up period 42% of the patients underwent additional decompression. The authors also reported that 67% of the patients reported improvement in back pain, but 33% of the patients reported either no improvement or worsening of their back symptoms at follow-up. Similarly, 35% of the patients reported either no improvement or worsening of their leg symptoms.[4]

In a study by Schnake and associates, the authors reported on 26 patients with a minimum follow-up of 2 years who underwent Dynesys stabilization for degenerative spondylolisthesis. Again, although the authors reported good clinical results, they also reported an implant failure rate of 17%.[23]

## INDICATIONS

Once we have established the intellectual and clinical merit of combining nuclear replacement and posterior dynamic stabilization, we must define the procedure's indications. It would seem logical to look at the indications for nuclear replacement and posterior dynamic stabilization and combine these. However, the combined use may limit some indications while expanding other applications. Furthermore, this chapter deals with the primary and initial combined application of these two techniques. An additional set of indications would be the use of one of the two technologies to "salvage" the motion segment after the failure of one of the individual systems.

Indications for this hybrid procedure in the treatment of herniated nucleus pulposus (HNP) can be classified into two categories: primary and revision (secondary).

### Primary Indications

#### Foraminal HNP Necessitating Vigorous Unilateral Medial Facetectomy

Treatment options for patients with a large foraminal HNP are many. However, most would agree that a discectomy would be the preferred procedure if the patient did not report significant back pain. However, most clinicians would be troubled by the need of some facet resection as well as by the removal of a substantial amount of disc material. In this circumstance, a TLIF (transforaminal lumbar interbody fusion), PLIF, or XLIF (extreme lumbar interbody fusion) would be strong considerations but all at the expense of motion. The isolated application of either NR or PDS in this clinical scenario would be technically feasible but not recommended. On the other hand, the combined application of NR and PDS is particularly appealing because the NR would help to restore disc biomechanics, and the PDS would help to counteract the destabilizing forces from the partial facet violation.

#### HNP with Spondylolysis without Listhesis

The treatment options of a patient with a HNP at the level of a spondylolysis without spondylolisthesis include (1) limited discectomy either endoscopic or open, (2) discectomy and pars repair, and (3) and perhaps the most common, discectomy and fusion. Although all three of these options would address the problem, they all suffer from significant limitations. Discectomy alone may lead to progressive disc collapse and listhesis may ultimately lead to arthrodesis and segmental motion loss. Discectomy and pars repair may lead to bony nonunion or progressive disc collapse and spondylolisthesis. Fusion would, of course, address the problem but at substantial collateral sacrifice. The combined application of NR and PDS would be theoretically attractive because the NR would help to restore anterior column kinematics, and the PDS would help to augment posterior instability, decreasing the potential for progressive spondylolisthesis.

#### HNP at the Apex of a Scoliotic Curve

Most surgeons would address this clinical scenario with either a limited decompression or with a decompression and fusion of the curve. Certainly the extent of the decompression and the magnitude of the deformity would be major determinants of the treatment choice. Nevertheless, a decompression at the apex of the curve, particularly in the presence of any rotatory listhesis, would likely lead to deformity progression and instability. The drawbacks of a multilevel fusion for a moderate deformity otherwise asymptomatic except for the stenotic level are obvious. In this particular presentation, the hybrid use of NR and PDS would work synergistically by restoring disc height and behavior, while the PDS could be used to help correct asymmetric disc height loss and provide supplemental rotational control.

#### HNP and Contralateral Facet (Synovial) Cyst

Two major options are currently used to address this situation: (1) a discectomy and decompression with excision of the facet cyst; (2) a decompression and fusion. The major determinants for the addition of the fusion to the decompression would be the presence of significant disc degeneration and back pain. In this case, the isolated use of NR would be at risk of failure given the need for bilateral decompression and some facet resection. The isolated use of PDS in this case would fail to address the anterior column destabilizing forces potentially leading to persistent mechanical back pain and screw loosening. The joined use of NR and PDS would potentially recalibrate the motion segment after discectomy and facet cyst excision by addressing both anterior column insufficiency as well as by augmenting the loss of posterior motion control.

#### Large Central HNP

The treatment of a young patient with a large central disc herniation is particularly controversial. Although most patients do well with minimally invasive discectomy, surgeons grow particularly wary of removing substantial amounts of disc material.

Although TDR is an attractive alternative to fusion in this patient subgroup, it suffers from two major disadvantages: (1) the risks associated with anterior surgery and (2) the limited ability to decompress the canal in a patient with a migrated, extruded, and potentially sequestered fragment. In this patient population, the application of a NR by itself would be of concern if the posterior longitudinal ligament is deficient and there is a large annular defect. The use of PDS in this application would not serve to properly address the anterior column insufficiency. In this application, the combined use of NR and PDS would allow for restoration of anterior column support with the NR while the PDS would help motion, which would in turn reduce the likelihood of device migration.

### Revision (Secondary)

#### Recurrent HNP

Currently the two main choices in patients with recurrent disc herniation are either a revision discectomy or a discectomy and fusion. Once again, these ends of the treatment spectrum seem sometimes to be either insufficient or overtreatment. The obvious concern with a revision discectomy is the potential for mechanical insufficiency and debilitating discogenic pain. On the other hand, a discectomy and fusion, particularly in a patient without significant back pain, seems overly aggressive. Although some would opt for a nuclear replacement device, the risk of device migration or failure would seem significant given the substantial annular defect and the violation of posterior bony structures usually necessary for safe removal of a recurrent HNP. The combination of NR and PDS would seem to address both the need for anterior column reconstitution as well as the posterior column deficiency while allowing for posterior motion. As alluded to above, however, this option should only be considered in patients with a relative paucity of low back pain (relative to radicular pain).

#### HNP Adjacent to a Fusion

Most surgeons would consider an HNP adjacent to a fusion an indication for extending the fusion. However, others may argue that a minimally disruptive decompression carries little risk of subsequent instability and dysfunction. Newer technologies such as TDR or PDS are attractive choices for this application but experience in this application is limited. In this particular scenario, few, if any, would advocate the use of NR alone, but the combination of NR and PDS would offer substantial biomechanical advantages over PDS alone.

#### "Salvage" Procedures

As stated above, NR and PDS systems may be hybridized (during revision surgery) when the individual systems, implanted in isolation, have failed. For example, in the event that a nuclear replacement migrates from the disc space, the surgeon may consider supplementation with a posterior dynamic stabilization system during reoperation. Similarly, NR systems may be implanted during a reoperative procedure targeting an extruded disc in a level previously stabilized by a PDS system.

## CONTRAINDICATIONS

Contraindications can also be subclassified into two categories: relative and absolute.

### Absolute Contraindications

- Bilateral laminectomies with medial facetectomy
- Markedly collapsed/attenuated disc space
- Total or subtotal facetectomy
- Segmental instability on dynamic x-rays
- Grade II or greater spondylolisthesis
- Infection
- Osteoporosis
- Rheumatoid or inflammatory arthritis

### Relative Contraindication

- Bilateral laminectomies (without significant facet disruption)

## HYBRID PERMUTATIONS

There are myriad nuclear replacement and posterior dynamic stabilization systems. Nuclear replacement options are listed in Table 79–1. Posterior dynamic stabilization systems are given in Table 79–2.

## CONCLUSION

The field of spine arthroplasty is no longer in its infancy but rather in its adolescence, a time of rapid and rebellious growth. The early

**TABLE 79–1. Nuclear Replacement Options**

| Implant Name | Manufacturer |
|---|---|
| Biomet | Regain |
| DASCOR | Disc Dynamics |
| NeuDisc | Replication Medical |
| NUBAC | Pioneer Surgical Technology |
| PDN | Raymedica |
| Nucore | Protein Polymer Technologies |
| SINUX | Sinitec |

**TABLE 79–2. Posterior Dynamic Stabilization Systems**

| Implant Name | Manufacturer |
|---|---|
| Dynesys | Zimmer Spine |
| Graf ligament | SEM Sarl |
| SoftFlex | Globus Medical |
| Cosmic | Ulrich GmbH |
| TFAS | Arcus Othopedics |

promising experience with application of arthroplasty techniques such as nuclear replacement and posterior dynamic stabilization in isolation will undoubtedly lead to the combination of such technologies.

Although there may be theoretical advantages, surgeons must resist the temptation to combine these technologies purely based on intuition. As the art and science of arthroplasty evolve and a myriad of motion preservation options becomes available, it will become increasingly challenging for surgeons to tailor the treatment to each patient. Interestingly, the future will likely show an increase in fusion of arthroplasty techniques in an effort to avoid fusion.

## REFERENCES


1. Ray CD: The PDN prosthetic disc nucleus device. Eur Spine J 11(2): S137–S142, 2002.
2. Bertagnoli R, Karg A, Voigt S: Lumbar partial disc replacement. Orthop Clin North Am 36(3):341–347, 2005.
3. Stoll TM, Dubois G, Schwarzenbach O: The dynamic neutralization system for the spine: A multi-center study of a novel non-fusion system. Eur Spine J 11(2):S170–S178, 2002.
4. Grob D, Benini A, Junge A, Mannion A: Clinical experience with the Dynesys semi-rigid fixation for the lumbar spine. Spine 30:324–331, 2005.
5. Gardner A, Pande KC: Graf ligamentoplasty: A 7 year follow up. Eur Spine J 11(2):S157–S163, 2002.
6. Bertagnoli R, Schonmayr R: Surgical and clinical results with the PDN prosthetic disc nucleus device. Eur Spine J 11(2): S143–S148, 2002.
7. Ray CD: The artificial disc: Introduction, history, and socioeconomics. *In* Weinstein JN (ed): Clinical Efficacy and Outcome in the Diagnosis and Treatment of Low Back Pain. New York, Raven, 1992, pp 205–225.
8. Vaccaro AR, Patel T, Fischgrund J, et al: A pilot study evaluating the safety and efficacy of OP-1 Putty (rhBMP-7) as a replacement of iliac crest bone autograft in posterolateral lumbar arthrodesis for degenerative spondylolisthesis. Spine 29(17):1885–1892, 2004.
9. Boden SD, Kang J, Sandhu H, Heller JG: Use of human bone morphogenetic protein-2 to achieve posterolateral lumbar spine fusion in humans: A prospective, randomized clinical pilot trial: 2002 Volvo Award in Clinical Studies. Spine 27(23):2662–2673, 2002.
10. Wilke HJ, Neel P, Caimi M, et al: New in vivo measurements of pressures in the intervertebral disc in daily life. Spine 24:755–762, 1999.
11. Nachemson A: Lumbar intradiscal pressure. *In* Jayson MIV (ed): The Lumbar Spine and Back Pain. London, Churchill Livingstone, 1987, p 191.
12. Adams MA, Hutton WC: The mechanical function of the lumbar apophyseal joints. Spine 8:327–330, 1983.
13. Barr JS: Ruptured intervertebral disc and sciatic pain. J Bone Joint Surg 29:210–214, 1947.
14. McAfee PC, Cunningham PW, Hayes V, et al: Biomechanical analysis of rotational motions after disc arthroplasty: Implications for patients with adult deformities. Spine 31(19):S152–160, 2006.
15. Ray CD, Hale JE, Norton BK: Prosthetic disk nucleus partial disk replacement: Pathobiological and biomechanical rationale for design and function. *In* Kim DH, Cammisa FP, Fessler RG (eds): Dynamic Reconstruction of the Spine. Thieme, 2006.
16. Cunningham BW, Gordon JD, Dmitriev EV, et al: Biomechanical evaluation of total disc arthroplasty: An in vitro human cadaveric model. Spine 28(20):S110–117, 2003.
17. Lu WW, Luk KD, Ruan DK, et al: Stability of the whole lumbar spine after multi-level fenestration and discectomy. Spine 24(13): 1277–1282, 1999.
18. Fujiwara A, Lim TH, An HS, et al: The effect of disc degeneration and facet joint osteoarthritis on the segmental flexibility of the lumbar spine. Spine 25(23):3036–3044, 2000.
19. Tanaka N, An HS, Lim TH, et al: The relationship between disc degeneration and the flexibility of the lumbar spine. Spine J 1(1): 47–56, 2001.
20. Fernstrom U: Arthroplasty with intercorporeal endoprosthesis in herniated disc and painful disc. Acta Chir Scan Suppl 357:154–159, 1966.
21. Graf H: Lumbar instability: Surgical treatment without fusion. Rachis 412:123–137, 1992.
22. Shim CS, Lee SH, Park CW, et al: Partial disc replacement with the PDN prosthetic disc nucleus device: Early clinical results. J Spinal Disord Tech 16(4):324–330, 2003.
23. Schnake KJ, Schaeren S, Jeanneret B: Dynamic stabilization in addition to decompression for lumbar spinal stenosis with degenerative spondylolisthesis. Spine 31(4):442–449, 2006.

CHAPTER 80

# Simultaneous Lumbar Fusion and Total Disc Replacement

Scott L. Blumenthal, Fred H. Geisler, Thomas F. Roush, and Donna D. Ohnmeiss

## KEY POINTS

- In patients with two-level symptomatic disc degeneration, total disc replacement (TDR) may not be indicated at both levels.
- Combining total disc replacement at one level with fusion at another level may be a viable treatment alternative for two-level painful disc degeneration.
- Biomechanical studies lend support that combined TDR and fusion functions similar to a single-level fusion.
- There is relatively little data available on the use of hybrids at this time, but preliminary results are promising and suggest that if there is no contraindication for TDR at one level, this procedure yields acceptable results.
- The combination of TDR with fusion at separate levels may have a protective effect on the adjacent segment compared to a two-level fusion.

Total disc replacement (TDR) has yielded favorable results in patients with disc degeneration.[1] One of the keys to successful outcome, however, is careful patient selection. This becomes more critical in patients with two-level degeneration. Even though one of the levels may be appropriate for TDR, the other may not be. Theoretically, the potential benefit for TDR may be greater in patients with two-level degeneration because a fusion (which accelerates degeneration at the adjacent segment) may compound the already present degeneration process. In a common case such as this, TDR may play a more important role. However, the enthusiasm to allow motion should not obviate strict adherence to selection criteria. In this chapter, we will review the biomechanical and clinical use of the "hybrid" spine procedure in which TDR is performed at one level and fusion at the adjacent segment during one operative setting (Fig. 80–1). Additionally, a brief review of the clinical experience of performing TDR adjacent to a previously fused segment will be provided.

## RATIONALE

There are many patients with two-level symptomatic disc degeneration who have failed nonoperative management and are considered surgical candidates. Although one may be tempted to perform two-level TDR for potential motion preservation at both painful levels, one must rigorously adhere to the appropriate disc arthroplasty screening regimen. In some of these patients with two-level problems, one level may be suitable for TDR, but the other level may not be. There may be osteophytes or significant facet joint changes, or the disc space may be too collapsed for the prosthesis. In addition, the anatomic environment during a revision operation in the case of prior fusion may be such that accurate placement of the prosthesis may be difficult or improbable and would otherwise compromise the prosthesis' functionality. In such cases, TDR may be undertaken at the level appropriate for it and fusion at the level not appropriate for TDR. The options for fusion are the same as for any patient with respect to graft type, instrumentation, and the combination of a posterior fusion procedure.

Huang and associates reported a relationship between the amount of motion at the level implanted with TDR and degeneration of the adjacent segment.[2] In that study, they found that the segment above a TDR allowing greater motion was less likely to be degenerated than a disc above a TDR that allowed less motion. Similarly, in a study of dynamic posterior stabilization, it was reported that fewer segments adjacent to those treated with Graf ligamentoplasty were degenerated as compared to segments above a fusion at a minimum of 5-year follow-up.[3] These studies lend clinical support for the concept that using dynamic stabilization at a lumbar level reduces the incidence of adjacent segment degeneration compared to the changes seen above immobile or fused segments.

## BIOMECHANICS

The biomechanical concept for the potential benefit of combining TDR with fusion rather than performing a two-level fusion is that the TDR in at least one level will reduce stress on the adjacent segment. Previous biomechanical studies have shown that fusion increases the intradiscal pressure at levels adjacent to a simulated fusion.[4–6] The pressure increased further when an additional

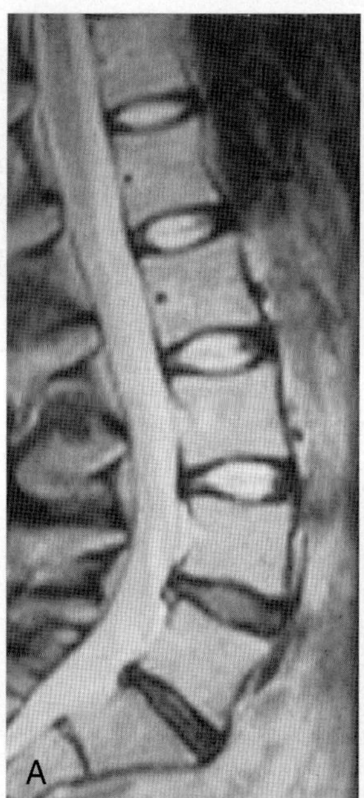


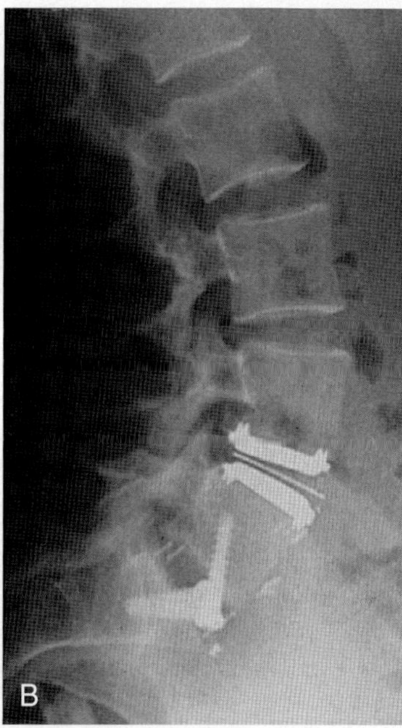


■ **FIGURE 80–1.** **A,** Preoperative MRI showing disc degeneration at the L4-L5 and L5-S1 levels. **B,** Postoperative radiograph showing a CHARITÉ at L4-L5 and a STALIF at the L5-S1 level.

segment was added to the simulated fusion.[6] This finding may be suggestive that multilevel fusions have a greater potential for accelerated deterioration of adjacent segments.

There has been little investigation on the effect of fusion on bone mineral density (BMD). In an early study using canines, it was suggested that the stress shielding caused by posterior instrumentation was related to reduced BMD.[7] In a clinical study of patients undergoing combined anterior/posterior instrumented lumbar fusion at two levels, it was found that the BMD of the vertebral body above fusion decreased significantly as early as 3 months and remained so at 6 months.[8] The authors contributed the decreased BMD to altered biomechanics caused by the two-level combined instrumented fusion. Another study reported that BMD increased during long-term follow-up in patients undergoing single-level posterior fusion; however, their study involved only seven patients.[9] The combined TDR and fusion may help prevent the potential for reduced BMD following fusion procedures.

Serhan and associates performed simulated testing with various combinations of one- and two-level CHARITÉ (DePuy Spine Inc., Raynham, MA) and fusions to investigate the motion patterns of the operated and adjacent segments.[10] They found that single-level TDR preserved physiologic motion, and with two-level TDR, the motion was altered only at the L4-L5 level. With fusion, the motion was significantly altered with one- or two-level surgery. When testing combined TDR and fusion, they found that fusion at L5-S1 combined with TDR at L4-L5 produced results similar to those for a single-level L5-S1 fusion. This is supportive of the use of hybrid surgery, that is, combining fusion at the lower level with TDR at the upper level, in patients with two-level symptomatic disc degeneration.

In a cadaveric model simulating the treatment of two-level disc degeneration, Rivera and associates found that two-level TDR produced motion similar to the intact specimen.[11] However, when the L5-S1 level was replaced with a simulated fusion, the total range of motion was decreased. Additionally, they reported that the L4-L5 level with the TDR did not increase motion to compensate for the reduction of motion at L5-S1.

Grauer and associates used a finite element model to evaluate the effect of two-level TDR to a hybrid TDR and fusion combination on the implanted and adjacent segment.[12] They found that the two-level TDR produced motion and facet loading values very different from those predicted from a combined fusion and TDR hybrid model. For the motion, the magnitude of change from the intact model was the same, but the pattern of change at the various segments were opposites. The potential clinical implication of the changes in motion patterns has yet to be established.

## CLINICAL EXPERIENCE

There are a few reports of the use of TDR combined with fusion at different lumbar levels. Some of these reports deal with procedures performed at the same operative setting, and others are on the results of TDR when performed at the level adjacent to a previous fusion. The second group is primarily using TDR to treat adjacent-segment deterioration following an earlier fusion.

In the area of "true hybrids," that is, combining fusion with TDR at different levels, the indications for such may be a patient with two-level symptomatic disc degeneration, but in whom TDR is not indicated at one of the discs. Rather than fusing both levels, TDR may be used at the level appropriate for this procedure. Possible reasons for not doing TDR at one level are significant facet changes or severely collapsed disc spaces. There have been few reports on this application. In a preliminary report of our own experience with 17 patients,[13] there was approximately a 50% reduction in Oswestry Disability Index (ODI) and VAS pain scores following the combined fusion-TDR procedure (Fig. 80–2). These results were very similar to those from the multicenter Investigational Device Exemption (IDE) trial involving only single-level TDR. Geisler and associates also reported favorable outcomes for this hybrid procedure in a series of 36 patients from

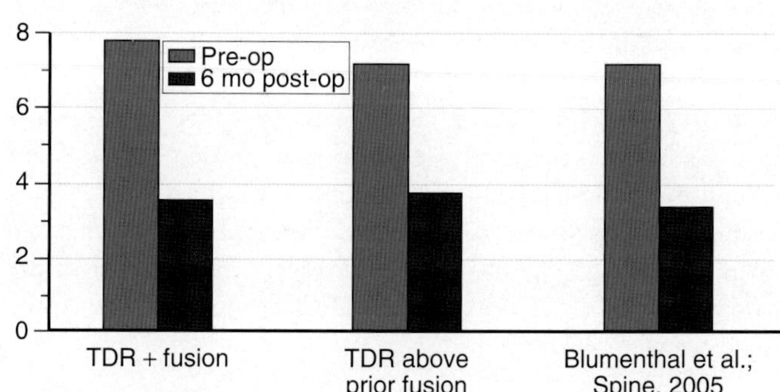


■ **FIGURE 80–2.** VAS (visual analog scale assessing pain) data from our own experience with hybrid TDR and fusion.[13] In both the TDR + fusion group (performed at the same operative setting) and in the TDR above a previous fusion, the preoperative and 6-month postoperative VAS scores were very similar to the values reported from the FDA IDE trial.[1]

10 centers.[14] Aunoble and associates reported on a series of 45 patients undergoing fusion at L5-S1 and TDR with CHARITÉ at L4-L5 with a mean follow-up of 16 months.[15] They noted no pseudarthrosis at L5-S1. The motion at L4-L5 was 8.4 degrees. ODI scores improved 29.6%. The VAS pain scores improved 39.1%, and SF-36 mental and physical components improved significantly.

There have been two reports published dealing with the use of TDR next to a previously fused segment for the treatment of adjacent-segment deterioration. Bertagnoli and associates prospectively assessed the efficacy of treating a degenerated level adjacent to remote prior fusion with ProDisc (Synthes, West Chester, PA) arthroplasty in 20 patients with 2-year follow-up.[16] The authors noted statistical improvements in VAS pain scores and ODI scores both at 3 and 24 months after arthroplasty. The patient satisfaction rate was 86% at 24 months. The authors suggested that patients should be screened carefully for evidence of facet joint impingement/degeneration, hardware-induced pain, and nonunion at prior fusion levels before undergoing disc replacement surgery, but that performing a disc arthroplasty adjacent to prior fusion was both safe and efficacious.

Kim and co-workers also reported their experience with TDR at a level adjacent to a previous fusion.[17] This was a series of five patients with at least 6-month follow-up. They found a decrease in ODI scores from 64 to 24. The authors were encouraged by these early results.

In our clinic's experience with TDR at the level next to a previous fusion, despite heterogeneity in fusion constructs, there was an improvement in the VAS pain score of approximately 50%, which is similar to that reported for single-level TDR in patients with no previous fusion (see Fig. 80–2).[13] In addition, the range of motion was similar to that for single-level TDR.

## SUMMARY

Combining TDR with fusion, either concurrent or remote, appears to be a viable treatment option. The impending research in this area will undoubtedly play a critical role in the routine application of such hybrid technologies. Of particular interest will be the longevity of the prostheses, on which more demand may be placed from the adjacent-segment immobility. Many years must pass before such changes, if present, become evident. In the meantime, theoretical benefits based on current knowledge must be relied upon. At this time, it seems plausible that the incorporation of TDR may help avoid accelerated adjacent disc degeneration in patients with multilevel disc disease.

Although the current clinical experience with hybrid TDR and fusion procedures is relatively limited, the results appear promising. The range of motion and clinical outcomes are comparable to those reported for single-level TDR in patients with no previous fusion.

## REFERENCES


1. Blumenthal S, McAfee PC, Guyer RD, et al: A prospective, randomized, multicenter Food and Drug Administration investigational device exemptions study of lumbar total disc replacement with the CHARITÉ artificial disc versus lumbar fusion, Part I: Evaluation of clinical outcomes. Spine 30:1565–1575, 2005.
2. Huang RC, Girardi FP, Cammisa FP Jr, et al: Long-term flexion-extension range of motion of the Prodisc total disc replacement. J Spinal Disord Tech 16:435–440, 2003.
3. Kanayama M, Hashimoto T, Shigenobu K, et al: Adjacent-segment morbidity after Graf ligamentoplasty compared with posterolateral lumbar fusion. J Neurosurg 95:5–10, 2001.
4. Cunningham BW, Kotani Y, McNulty PS, et al: The effect of spinal destabilization and instrumentation on lumbar intradiscal pressure: an in vitro biomechanical analysis. Spine 22:2655–2663, 1997.
5. Rao RD, David KS, Wang M: Biomechanical changes at adjacent segments following anterior lumbar interbody fusion using tapered cages. Spine 30:2772–2776, 2005.
6. Weinhoffer SL, Guyer RD, Herbert M, et al: Intradiscal pressure measurements above an instrumented fusion: A cadaveric study. Spine 20:526–531, 1995.
7. McAfee PC, Farey ID, Sutterlin CE, et al: The effect of spinal implant rigidity on vertebral bone density: A canine model. Spine 16:S190–197, 1991.
8. Bogdanffy GM, Ohnmeiss DD, Guyer RD: Early changes in bone mineral density above a combined anteroposterior L4-S1 lumbar spinal fusion: A clinical investigation. Spine 20:1674–1678, 1995.
9. Singh K, An HS, Samartzis D, et al: A prospective cohort analysis of adjacent vertebral body bone mineral density in lumbar surgery patients with or without instrumented posterolateral fusion: A 9- to 12-year follow-up. Spine 30:1750–1755, 2005.
10. Serhan H, Malcolmson G, Teng E, et al: Hybrid Testing for Adjacent- and Other-Level Effects Following Arthroplasty with the CHARITÉ Artificial Disc vs. Simulated Fusion. International Meeting on Advanced Spine Technologies. Athens, Greece, 2006.
11. Rivera Y, Mehbod A, Garvey T, et al: Two level disc disease: Two level disc arthroplasty versus a hybrid model. International Meeting on Advanced Spine Technologies. Athens, Greece, 2006.
12. Grauer JN, Biyani A, Faizan A, et al: Biomechanics of two-level CHARITÉ artificial disc placement in comparison to fusion plus single-level disc placement combination. Spine J 6:659–666, 2006.
13. Lhamby J, Guyer R, Zigler J, et al: Patients Undergoing Total Disc Replacement with Spinal Fusion at Different Lumbar Levels. International Society for the Study of the Lumbar Spine. Bergen, Norway, 2006.
14. Geisler F, Banco R, Cappuccino A, et al: Lumbar Total Disc Replacement Combined with Fusion at an Adjacent Level: Early Results from a Multi-Center Retrospective Review of a Hybrid Procedure for Multi-Level Degenerative Disease. International Meeting on Advanced Spine Technologies. Athens, Greece, 2006.
15. Aunoble S, Huec J-CL, Gornet M, et al: Hybrid surgery for DDD: Fusion L5-S1 and disc prosthesis L4-L5. Meeting, Spine Arthroplasty Society. Montreal, Canada, 2006.
16. Bertagnoli R, Yue JJ, Fenk-Mayer A, et al: Treatment of symptomatic adjacent-segment degeneration after lumbar fusion with total disc arthroplasty by using the ProDisc prosthesis: A prospective study with 2-year minimum follow-up. J Neurosurg Spine 4:91–97, 2006.
17. Kim WJ, Lee SH, Kim SS, et al: Treatment of juxtafusional degeneration with artificial disc replacement (ADR): Preliminary results of an ongoing prospective study. J Spinal Disord Tech 16:390–397, 2003.

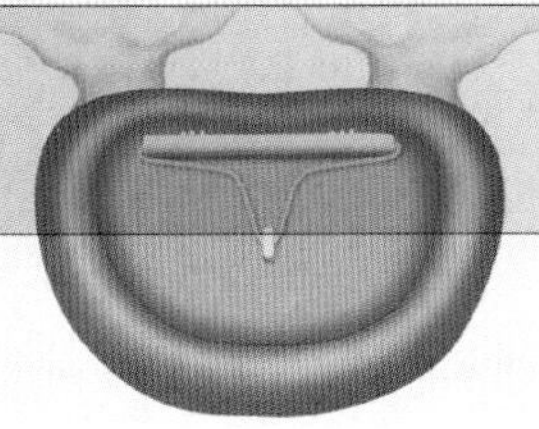

PART

# X

# Annular Repair

CHAPTER 81

# Repair and Reconstruction of the Annulus Fibrosus with the Inclose Surgical Mesh System

Joseph C. Cauthen and Steven L. Griffith

## KEY POINTS

- Reconstruction of the annulus fibrosus after lumbar discectomy is an important consideration, because current procedures without reconstruction might have unsatisfactory clinical outcomes requiring repeat surgery.
- Repair of the annulus fibrosus may reduce subsequent postoperative disc herniation and other secondary operations.
- Nucleus fragment removal with subsequent annular repair, rather than a more extensive nucleus removal without repair, is projected to reduce postoperative back pain that ultimately requires arthrodesis due to instability.
- Biomechanical, animal, and early human clinical studies of a surgical mesh implant (Inclose Surgical Mesh System) are favorable.
- Repair and reconstruction of the annulus with a surgical mesh system, such as Inclose, appears to be a fast, simple, and safe method to close a portal of re-herniation.

There is increasing awareness that postoperative clinical outcomes are less than satisfactory in many cases after discectomy surgery using current standard procedures that do not specifically address the opening in the annulus fibrosus.[1,2] Recurrent disc herniation requiring additional surgery remains a common problem.[3] Further, expulsion of prosthetic nucleus replacement devices has been a perceived negative factor in their development. Recent interest in improving these technical and clinical outcomes has focused on reconstruction and repair of the lumbar disc annulus. In this chapter, preliminary results describing the use of a surgical mesh placed below the aperture in the tissue surface will be presented and include animal and biomechanical studies. Preliminary human trial results will be described.

The Inclose Surgical Mesh System (Fig. 81–1; Anulex Technologies Inc., Minnetonka, MN) is a mesh that supports soft tissue and can be used after disc decompression surgery. It can be inserted into the disc through a tear or incision in the annulus fibrosus. After appropriate positioning inside the intervertebral disc, it is deployed into its final configuration, expanding the implant to act as a barrier and eventually a tissue scaffold, thus containing intradiscal contents that remain after disc decompression.

## INDICATIONS AND CONTRAINDICATIONS

The Inclose Surgical Mesh System in the U.S. has a general indication "...to support soft tissue where weakness exists, or for the repair of hernias requiring the addition of a reinforcing, or bridging material, such as the repair of groin hernias." In the European Union, the device's CE registration includes the repair of "the annulus fibrosus of the intervertebral disc." The mesh is contraindicated where tissue may be contaminated or infected. And the mesh should not be used in infants or children in whom future growth may be compromised by its use. For complete indications, contraindications, potential adverse events, warnings and precautions, the product's Instruction for Use should be consulted.

This chapter addresses a specific use for this system for repair of the annulus fibrosus. Additional information is being assembled to establish long-term outcomes.

## DESCRIPTION OF THE DEVICE

The Inclose Surgical Mesh System is composed of a braided mesh cylinder that is biocompatible and expandable. The basic material is polyethylene-terephthalate (PET). The nonexpanded 3.5-mm cylindrical implant is placed in the recipient's disc site beneath the surface of the annulus by means of a disposable delivery tool. Once in place, the delivery tool is used to expand the implant, which conforms to the available evacuated nucleus cavity. In the cephalad-caudal direction, the disc space is defined by the end plates. It is recommended that at least 6 mm of disc height be available for adequate mesh deployment to avoid overconstraining mesh deployment and expansion. An integral latching mechanism holds the two ends of the cylinder together, forming an implant that acts as a barrier that is larger than the opening in the annulus. In a typical application, the existing pathologic annular tear or fissure is used as the point of insertion for the mesh implant. Alternatively, an incision into the annulus overlying a contained subannular nuclear fragment can be used. The expansion of the mesh into its configuration and latching of the cylinder constitutes

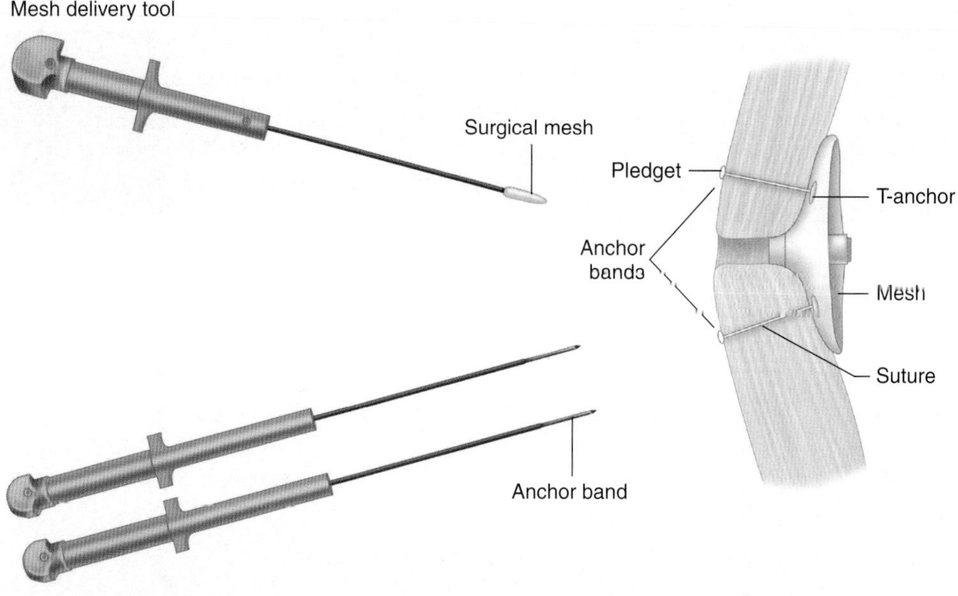


■ **FIGURE 81–1.** The Inclose Surgical Mesh System. The mesh is supplied sterile and premounted on a disposable delivery tool. Anchor bands are used to secure the expanded mesh to available surrounding tissue and below the aperture in the annulus.

a barrier to further displacement of intradiscal tissue or material. After satisfactory nuclear fragment removal and nerve root decompression, the mesh implant is further stabilized by tethering it to the surrounding tissue with suture anchor bands.

## SCIENTIFIC TESTING OUTCOMES

A biomechanical study was conducted by Cunningham and associates using the device.[4] This study evaluated segmental spinal mechanics after placement of Inclose surgical mesh and after cyclic loading. In this acute in vitro study, there was no measurable effect on the spinal mechanics compared to nonrepaired discs (i.e., stiffness, range of motion, or neutral zone) as a result of the placement of the device. This finding is meaningful because the reconstruction and repair of the annulus, in contrast to other intradiscal reparative technologies such as nucleus pulposus replacements or total artificial disc prostheses, should ultimately not affect normal physiology. This study further demonstrated that the device remained in position below the annulus tissue surface after complex cyclic loading. No evidence of mechanical failure (fraying, unraveling, etc.) of the mesh was seen, and no significant particulate debris was noted.

The device was further evaluated in a chronic animal model. The lumbar discs of Nubian cross-bred goats were implanted with smaller prototype mesh implants via a lateral retroperitoneal approach.[5] This study demonstrated that the mesh barrier could be safely placed in proximity to the disc annulus. And when the mesh is properly positioned and affixed, radiographic evidence suggested the device remained in position during a 12-week observation period. Incorporation of the device into the annulus tissue was noted without deleterious effects on the surrounding tissues (Fig. 81–2).

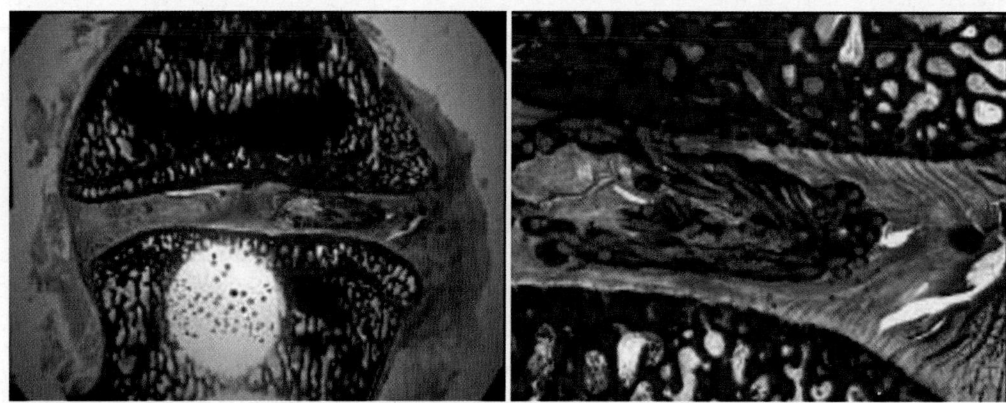

■ **FIGURE 81–2.** Histologic appearance of Inclose mesh. In an undecalcified histologic section from a goat model, the mesh can be seen adjacent to the inner annulus with extracellular matrix in and around the mesh fibers. No adverse tissue reactions were noted.

## CLINICAL PRESENTATION AND EVALUATION

Indications for the use of this device include signs and symptoms of displacement of the intervertebral disc (specifically nucleus pulposus tissue) corroborated by definitive radiographic images. In the ideal candidate, radicular symptoms are predominant and can include gluteal or leg pain, leg weakness or numbness, diminished reflexes, and positive straight-leg raising test. Leg pain should be qualitatively greater than the patient's back pain complaint, thus suggesting nerve root compression or irritation. The pain level is typically intractable and must be concordant with the suspected site of nerve involvement. Additionally, failure of nonoperative measures, including strengthening exercise, epidural steroid injections, and avoidance of lumbar exertional stress, is a prerequisite before surgical intervention. Radiographic correlation to the symptom complex should be confirmed by magnetic resonance imaging (MRI), myelogram, or computed tomography (CT) (Fig. 81–3).

Application of this particular device should be approached cautiously in patients who do not meet the above-mentioned criteria and in those patients who have normal neurologic findings, nonlocalizing pain, infection, significant comorbidities, or a target disc space that will not anatomically accommodate the surgical mesh as discussed next.

## OPERATIVE TECHNIQUES

The use of this mesh implant is adjunctive to standard discectomy or microdiscectomy procedures, and, therefore, no special surgical techniques are needed. The implant has reportedly[6] been used in more than 47 patients in both standard loupe-assisted and microscope-assisted discectomy as well as through endoscopic portal systems such as METRx (Medtronic Sofamor Danek, Memphis, TN).

Under general anesthesia with the patient in the prone position with abdominal compressive forces minimized, the incision is limited to that required to accommodate the preferred open approach, microscopic approach, or minimal access endoscopic approach through a tubular retractor. The surgeon's preferred technique for posterior lumbar laminotomy and nerve decompression can be used. The ligamentum flavum is excised. Closure of epidural veins is achieved using microbipolar forceps allowing isolation and retraction of the dura and exposure of the disc annulus. With the nerve root retracted, a tear or fissure in the annulus fibrosus and herniated disc material is identified. Extradural and intradiscal fragments are removed with exploration of four quadrants of the epidural space. In the case of contained herniations, the annulus fibrosus is opened equidistant between the end plates using a vertical slit followed by evacuation of loose

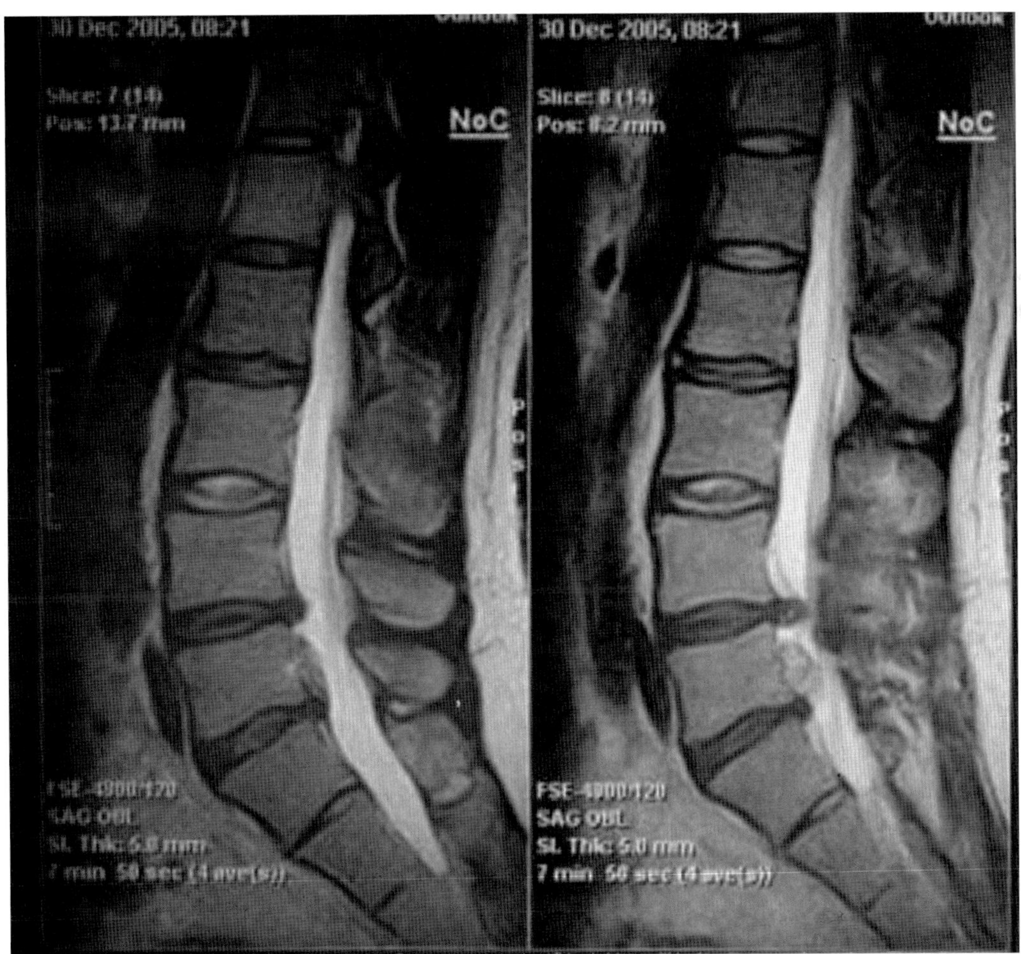


■ **FIGURE 81–3.** Exemplary magnetic resonance image of two-level disc herniation appropriate for Inclose mesh repair. In this clinical example, two lumbar disc herniations are seen at L4-L5 (a contained herniation) and L5-S1 (a sequestration). Adequate disc space for mesh deployment can also be appreciated.

nuclear fragments in the intradiscal space. After satisfactory disc removal and nerve root decompression has been completed, attention can turn to repairing the defect in the annulus fibrosus through which the herniation occurred.

Proof of sufficient disc space height to accommodate the expanded mesh implant can be confirmed by probing the disc with an instrument of known dimensions. A minimum 3-mm opening in the annulus fibrosus is required for insertion of the unexpanded mesh implant. A minimum of 6 mm between the end plates is recommended to allow the mesh to expand and act as a flexible barrier (rather than a load-bearing implant); a tissue space constrained less than 6 mm does not allow the mesh to take the most appropriate shape or to retain its flexibility (tight space constraint, Fig. 81–4). Further qualitative assessment of the integrity of annulus fibrosus should be made to determine whether the annulus is sufficiently competent for annular reconstruction (i.e., the mesh will be attached to a firm tissue base) or if there might be attachment of the mesh to a patulent annulus. In the latter case or in the case of very narrow disc spaces, consideration should be given to an alternative annular repair technique. Tightening of a patulous annulus may best be achieved by reapproximation of the tissue layers with other reparative techniques.

The Inclose surgical mesh is inserted through the fissure in the annulus. Visual depth confirmation is achieved by means of a yellow marker band on the shaft of the instrument. Maintaining the position of this yellow marker band at or near the tissue surface ensures anticipated placement of the deployed mesh below the surface. Deployment is best accomplished by both pulling the finger tabs on the delivery tool and readjusting the position of this yellow indicator band. An audible click is heard when the mesh is fully deployed and it has been latched. Upward pressure on the delivery tool is recommended to further seat the mesh on the inner annular wall.

After the Inclose mesh is deployed below the tissue surface, the delivery tool is held firmly to assure close proximity to the annulus while medial and lateral suture anchor bands are used to tether the implant to the remaining firm annulus fibrosus. Suture anchor bands preloaded in disposable delivery needles are inserted into surrounding annulus tissue and ultimately through the mesh deployed below this tissue surface. A tissue depth indicator located on the shaft of the insertion needle tool protects overpenetration of the distal needle tip. While holding the tissue depth indicator on the tissue surface, the suture anchors are deployed by pulling the finger tabs up. This causes an anchor that is attached to a suture to be placed on the underside of the mesh; simultaneously a circular pledget located on the outer tissue surface and attached to the anchoring suture is cinched down, securing the tissue and the mesh implant.

## POSTOPERATIVE CARE

There is no special perioperative or postoperative care required as a result of the use of this implant. After routine closure, the patient is discharged on the same day as surgery with no modification to standard postoperative precautions. Avoidance of lifting, stretching, or combining compression and twisting are recommended for a period of 12 weeks to allow for tissue healing in and around the implant.

## COMPLICATIONS AND AVOIDANCE

Potential technical or perioperative complications as a result of the use of this mesh device can result if the anteroposterior dimensions of the disc are smaller than the length of the tools. For adequate placement of this device, a minimum depth of 34 mm from the tissue surface is required. Visual marks on the mesh's delivery

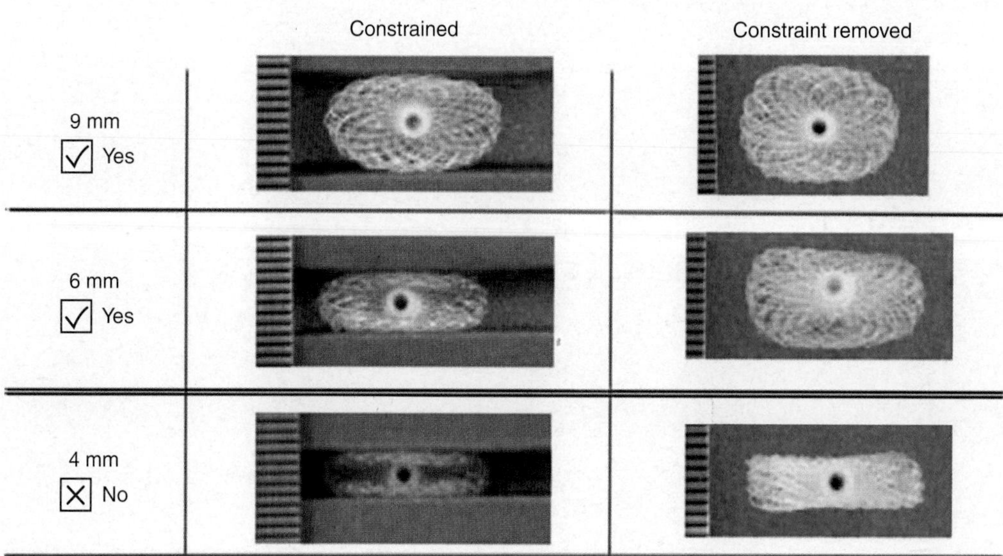


■ **FIGURE 81–4.** Inclose deployed shape comparison. On the left, Inclose mesh was deployed with the noted constraints, and on the right, the same implant is seen after removal of the constraints. With constraints 6 mm or greater, the mesh is adequately deployed in its intended shape and retains its flexibility. As noted in the 4-mm constraint, the mesh becomes overly compressed and can lose its flexibility.

tool and a circular tissue stop on the anchor band delivery tools aid in avoiding overpenetration through the anterior side of the disc. Furthermore, probing the disc after decompression prior to mesh insertion with an instrument of known dimensions also can be used.

Analysis of poor clinical outcomes and complications following laminotomy and partial discectomy is multifactorial. Because this device is adjunctive to the discectomy performed rather than an entirely new procedure, it is difficult to distinguish specific complications of the implant. When using the implant, careful patient selection and meticulous discectomy techniques are critical to prevent untoward or unsatisfactory outcomes. Patients whose symptoms are complex and cannot be corroborated with preoperative or intraoperative imaging studies should be considered a high risk for poor outcomes.

In spite of the intended goal of avoiding repeat surgery, there is certainly the potential for complications requiring additional treatment in cases in which the patient's pain is unresolved or returns. Because this implant is obviously a local barrier, if the implant is not properly placed spanning the opening in the annulus or the herniation, then the implant may not function as intended. The placement of this implant is through an in-line approach, and for instance, a far lateral herniation may not be adequately approached from a standard paramedial, interlaminar approach. As previously described, a patient whose disc space has narrowed below 6 mm should be approached cautiously. In its current configuration, Inclose may not expand effectively into the subannular space because of the constraints of the end plates. Furthermore, intraoperative assessment of the integrity of the annulus is warranted to achieve the best possible technical outcomes for maintaining the position of the mesh. Effective fixation and ultimately the positional stability of the implant may be compromised if these anatomic limitations are not appreciated.

As with any other application of a surgical mesh that supports soft tissue, there is the potential for inadequate attachment or fixation of the implant because of lack of overlying tissue (<2mm) or generalized tissue incompetency.[7] It should come as no surprise that the environment of the soft tissue of the intervertebral disc annulus is not substantially different from other soft tissues in the body. If the annulus soft tissue cannot support fixation of the mesh or the opening is too large relative to the dimensions of the mesh, then there is the potential for re-extrusion of the implant, particularly in light of intradiscal pressures.

In cases in which a secondary surgery is required, the device can be removed if needed. Furthermore, should additional intradiscal decompression be required, the implant would have to be retrieved prior to disc excision. Depending on the timing of any repeat surgery, re-exploration would not be unlike other repeat discectomies in which the surgeon would have to contend with fibrotic scar.

### ADVANTAGES/DISADVANTAGES: INCLOSE SURGICAL MESH SYSTEM

**Advantages**

Rather than leave tears, holes, or fissures in the annulus fibrosus unclosed after discectomy, the Inclose Surgical Mesh System can be used to support the soft tissue of the annulus.

Placement of the Inclose mesh implant does not add significant surgical time and can be performed quicker than manually suturing the tissue.

Placement of the Inclose mesh below the tissue surface and expansion of the mesh greater than the annular tear, fissure, or incision facilitate positional stability.

**Disadvantages**

An incompetent, patulent annulus fibrosus or a degenerative, narrowed disc space is not adequate for this type of annular repair using a flexible barrier implant.

## CONCLUSION

Lumbar discectomy or microdiscectomy is considered to be a successful operation both in terms of technical ease and clinical outcomes. But the wide variety of approaches and techniques used can be debated with respect to their advantages and disadvantages. Simply removing the offending nucleus pulposus fragment without an extensive intradiscal decompression is favored by many surgeons in attempts to maintain disc height. Other surgeons rely on a more aggressive, yet subtotal, disc decompression in attempts to decrease the likelihood that reherniation might occur. Carragee and associates[8] studied this technical aspect prospectively in 86 patients. Two-year follow-up suggested that a "limited discectomy" may result in better patient outcomes, but the reherniation rate in his study was twice as high as in those patients who had subtotal discectomy. These authors ultimately suggested that an effective barrier may be clinically useful.

Description of advantages and disadvantages of a particular device or technique implies comparisons. In the case of annular repair with a barrier, the Inclose Surgical Mesh System is one of the first implants to be used clinically for repairing the soft tissue of the intervertebral disc. Therefore, benefits of this implant are most appreciated in comparison to the current surgical technique of leaving the annulus fibrosus unclosed at the conclusion of the discectomy procedure. The potential advantages of repairing the annulus following discectomy have been suggested previously[9,10] and most extensively studied by Cauthen.[11] In his study of 254 patients with tedious manual suture closure of the annular fissure with or without a fascial autograft patch, he showed a greater than 50% reduction in disc reherniation rates over a 2-year period. In contrast, Ahlgren and associates[12] used studies in animal models to suggest that the healing response of the annulus is not influenced by directly repairing the fissure with sutures or with a muscle-fascial overlay graft.

The ability to achieve closure of the annulus fibrosus with Inclose mesh is a significant advance over the previously described suture methods. Because of the engineering in the delivery instruments, the implant does not add significant time to the procedure. The device can typically be delivered and secured in place in 5 minutes or less. Expansion of the mesh device larger than the opening in the annulus and below the tissue surface further facilitates its function as an effective barrier.

Data from biomechanical testing,[1] laboratory testing in animal implantation trials,[2] and initial clinical experience[13] suggest that a surgical mesh barrier such as Inclose placed into the intervertebral disc affixed with suture anchor bands has a reasonable chance of providing a safe, simple, and fast solution to the problem of recurrent disc herniation in the human spine. As in any pioneering effort, long-term conclusions are not yet possible due to the limited length of follow-up, but early indications strongly suggest that this device is stable and may provide a mechanical barrier to secondary disc herniation. Additional potential benefits of annular repair techniques such as this include the reduction of chemical pain mediators escaping through the open annulus following conventional discectomy, thus reducing secondary effects of irritation of the nerve root ganglion, epidural fibrosis, or the potential for ingrowth of nerve fibers that are mediators of postoperative discogenic pain.[14–16]

## REFERENCES


1. Asch HL, Lewis PF, Moreland DB, et al: Prospective multiple outcomes study of outpatient lumbar microdiscectomy: Should 75 to 80% success rates be the norm? J Neurosurg 96(1):34–44, 2002.
2. Fritsch W, et al: The failed back surgery syndrome—Reasons, intraoperative findings, and long-term results: A report of 182 operative treatments. Spine 21:626–633, 1996.
3. Atlas S, et al: Long-term outcomes of surgical and nonsurgical management of sciatica to a lumbar herniation: 10 year results from the Maine Lumbar Spine Study. Spine 30:927–935, 2005.
4. Cunningham BC, Hu N, Beatson H, McAfee P: Acute in vitro stability of an annular repair device after multi-directional cyclic fatigue evaluated in human specimens. Presented at the Global Symposium on Motion Preservation Technology (SAS), New York, NY, 2005.
5. Peppelman W, Davis R, Sherman J, et al: Feasibility results of a novel anular repair device in a goat model. Presented at the World Spine III—An Interdisciplinary Congress on Spine Care, Rio de Janeiro, Brazil, 2005.
6. Sherman J, Bajares G, Cauthen J, et al: Evaluation of a mesh device to repair the anulus fibrosus. Presented at the 13th Annual International Meeting of Advanced Spinal Techniques (IMAST), Athens, Greece, 2006.
7. Luijendijk RW, Hop WCJ, van den Tol P, et al: A comparison of suture repair with mesh repair for incisional hernia. N Engl J Med 343(6):392–398, 2000.
8. Carragee EJ, Spinnickie AO, Alamin TF, et al: A prospective controlled study of limited versus subtotal posterior discectomy: Short-term outcomes in patients with herniated lumbar intervertebral discs and larger posterior anular defect. Spine 31(6):653–657, 2006.
9. Yasargil MG: Microsurgical operation of herniated lumbar disc. Adv Neurosurg 4:81, 1977.
10. Lehmann T, Titus MK: Refinements in technique for open lumbar discectomy. Proceedings of the International Society for the Study of the Lumbar Spine (ISSLS), June 1997.
11. Cauthen JC: Microsurgical annular reconstruction (annuloplasty) following lumbar microdiscectomy. *In* Guyer RD (ed): Spinal Arthroplasty: A New Era in Spine Care. St. Louis, Quality Medical Publishing, 2005, pp 156–177.
12. Ahlgren BD, Lui W, Herkowitz, HN: Effect of annular repair on the healing strength of the intervertebral disc—A sheep model. Spine 25 (17):2165–2170, 2000.
13. Bajares G, Perz-Oliva A: A pilot study evaluating a novel device for annular repair following spinal discectomy. Presented at the Global Symposium on Motion Preservation Technology (SAS), New York, NY, 2005.
14. Olmarker K: Neovascularization and neoinnervation of subcutaneously placed nucleus pulposus and the inhibitory effects of certain drugs. Spine 30(13):1501–1504, 2005.
15. Nygaard OP, Mellgren SI, Osterud B: The inflammatory properties of contained and noncontained lumbar disc herniations. Spine 22:2484–2488, 1997.
16. Coppes MH, Marani E, Thomeer RT, et al: Innervation of "painful" lumbar discs. Spine 22:2342–2349, 1999.

CHAPTER 82

# The Intrinsic Therapeutics Barricaid Device

**Jacob Einhorn, Oscar Yeh,** and **Greg Lambrecht**

**KEY POINTS**

- Annular repair with the Barricaid may reduce reherniation risk.
- Disc height has been better maintained in prospective, controlled clinical trials.
- The Barricaid covers the entire posterior annulus.
- The Barricaid requires limited removal of nucleus.
- Prospective clinical trials are currently under way.

## THE CLINICAL PROBLEM

Over 275,000 lumbar discectomy procedures were performed in the United States in 2005,[1] with an additional 260,000 projected outside the United States.[2] These patients generally present with radicular symptoms or low back pain that is unresponsive to conservative therapy and magnetic resonance imaging (MRI) or computed tomography (CT) confirmation of a nuclear herniation or extrusion as the immediate cause of their symptoms. Although lumbar discectomy is frequently successful in immediately reducing symptoms of sciatica and radiculopathy, over time many patients suffer a relapse in symptoms, requiring reoperation. One prospective, multicenter study of lumbar discectomy patients reported a 20% rate of reoperation within the first 5 years,[3] and another reported a 13% rate within the first 2 years.[4]

The discectomy procedure itself, despite its short-term efficacy, is not benign to the disc—it is an ablative, not a restorative procedure. Additional nucleus from within the disc space is frequently removed, and the weakness or defect in the annulus, through which the nucleus bulged, protruded, or extruded, remains, or is even enlarged, following discectomy. Both create very real risks for the patient:

- *Reherniation*: Rogers[5] reported a 21% reherniation rate with a fragmentectomy. Carragee and associates[6] reported a 9% reherniation rate in a study of 187 patients done with limited nuclear removal. Asch and colleagues[4] report a 13% reoperation rate for recurrence of herniations in a study of 212 patients in a multicenter study.
- *Loss of disc height*: Almost all discectomy patients lose disc height after surgery,[7] a finding that is not surprising given that material has been removed from their disc, and the hole in the annulus has remained or has been enlarged. Laboratory studies have shown that disc height loss leads to overstressing and degeneration of the annulus,[8,9] while clinical studies have shown that disc height loss of greater than 25% after discectomy is correlated with poor clinical outcomes.[10,11]
- *Increased back pain*: As described earlier, most discectomy patients lose disc height, and those with the most disc height loss have significantly worse clinical outcomes. A large component of this degradation of outcomes is due to increased back pain, which has been reported in greater than 12% of discectomy patients.[10,12]
- *Recurrence of symptoms*: Although discectomy is quite effective in the short term, only about 70% of primary discectomy patients report improvement in their predominant symptoms several years following surgery.[4,10]

## ANNULAR REPAIR

### Patient Characteristics and Surgical Technique

Several prospectively enrolled studies have correlated patient- as well as technique-related risk factors with poor outcomes following discectomy:

- *Size of defect*: Not surprisingly, the size of the defect found at the time of primary discectomy has a huge effect on the reherniation rate. Carragee and associates reported an overall reherniation rate of 9% in 187 patients. However, in patients with massive annular defects (defined as larger than a Penfield-1 probe [~6.5 mm]), the reherniation rate was 27%, but in patients with slit defects the reherniation rate was only 1%. This would indicate that if larger defects could be effectively reduced in size, reherniation rates could fall dramatically in this at-risk group.
- *Amount of nucleus removed*: Aggressive nuclear removal can also impact the risk of reherniation. In a follow-up study, Carragee and associates compared a group of patients in whom nucleus was aggressively removed with an historical cohort from their previous study in whom only the offending

fragments of nucleus were removed.[13] They found that more limited nucleus removal resulted in a doubled risk of reherniation (18% vs. 9% within the first 2 years), while aggressive nucleus removal resulted in significantly higher levels of back pain, worse clinical outcomes (per Oswestry Disability Index), prolonged delay of return to work, and higher levels of required pain medication at 1 year. These data highlight the dilemma a surgeon faces when performing a discectomy: On the one hand, aggressive nuclear removal can reduce reherniations but has been correlated with worse clinical outcomes and increased disc height loss. On the other hand, limited nuclear removal, which results in greater maintenance of disc height and better clinical outcomes, leads to a significantly higher risk of symptomatic reherniation.

In short, for a given herniation type, making the annular defect smaller could reduce reherniation rates. A device that closed and reinforced the annular defect could allow the surgeon to retain as much native nucleus as possible without an increased risk of reherniation. Such a device would provide surgeons and patients with a new option that results in both the best long-term clinical outcome and a reduced risk of reherniation.

### Challenges

The goal of achieving a lasting repair or closure of defects in the annulus is not an easy one. This is in large part due to constraints imposed by the harsh intradiscal environment. These constraints include high pressures, large ranges of motion, lack of natural healing, a wide variety of defect sizes and location, and the risk of weakness on the contralateral side not visible at the time of surgery.

- *High intradiscal pressures*: The highest pressures in the human body have been measured in the lower lumbar discs, with pressures as high as 2.3 MPa (334 psi) having been recorded in vivo during activities of daily living.[14] These high pressures can cause intradiscal devices to be expulsed from the disc space at reported frequencies up to 38% in some studies.[15] Any device intended to close defects in the annulus must remain in place when challenged with these high intradiscal pressures.
- *High ranges of motion*: Even though axial rotation and lateral bending in the lumbar discs are relatively limited, the range of motion of the disc in flexion-extension can be as high as 24 degrees.[8] Because the center of rotation of the disc is typically anterior of the posterior annulus, the strain range of the posterior annulus during these high ranges of motion can often be on the order of 100% (e.g., for a posterior disc height of 4 mm, during flexion-extension this height may go down to 2.5 mm and up to 6.5 mm, for a total strain range of 4 mm). Designing a device that can maintain its integrity while sealing defects that also go through this strain range is extremely challenging.
- *Poor primary annular healing*: Because of the extremely high intradiscal pressures, the high range of motion, and the avascular nature of the disc, the annulus does not heal well. Heggeness and associates[16] reported that posterior extravasation of discography dye is significantly more likely ($P = 0.025$) in a postdiscectomy disc than in an unoperated disc. Ahlgren and associates[17] reported that attempts at direct repair of annular incisions (slit, cruciate, or box) did not significantly affect the strength of the annulus after discectomy as judged by the disc's ability to maintain intradiscal pressure. A successful annular repair device will likely not be able to rely on primary healing of the annulus itself.
- *Variety of defect locations*: The location of the naturally occurring annular defect may range from perfectly central to far lateral. Ninomiya and Muro demonstrated that over 80% of defects are primarily or entirely between the facets.[18] As surgical exposure is limited, the ideal annular repair device would protect aspects of the annulus that are not immediately in front of the surgeon's field of view.
- *Risk of contralateral herniations*: The main goal of annular repair is to contain nuclear material within the disc space following a primary discectomy. As discussed previously, a recurrent herniation occurs in a significant number of these patients. However, this recurrence is not always through the same annular defect, or even on the same side of the disc. Contralateral herniations have been reported in prospective studies to account for up to 37% of recurrent herniations that occur at the operated level.[19] An annular repair device that can protect the contralateral side of the disc, and not just the side of primary access, from recurrence would be ideal.

### Product Requirements

Based on the clinical problems and challenges described here, as well as the ever-present clinical desire to maintain function and reduce operative trauma, the ideal annular repair device would have the following characteristics:

- Prevent reherniation
- Preserve disc height and function
- Cover defects of a variety of sizes and locations
- Protect as much of the posterior annulus as possible
- Require minimal or no removal of nucleus
- Easily used with current surgical approach and techniques
- Have minimal impact on operative time
- Endure the high ranges of motion and pressure without failure or migration

## DESCRIPTION OF THE DEVICE

The Intrinsic Therapeutics (Woburn, MA) Barricaid annular repair device (Fig. 82–1) is designed for use as an adjunct to lumbar discectomy and is intended to close annular defects and support the weakened annular soft tissue. The Barricaid implant serves as an internal patch that is positioned between the annulus and the nucleus and covers substantially all of the posterior annulus (Fig. 82–2). Figure 82–3 shows a herniated disc with nucleus material extruding out of the disc (*left*), and the defect repaired with the Barricaid device (*right*).

The Barricaid consists of a flexible nitinol support frame surrounded by an e-PTFE sleeve, which rests along the posterior

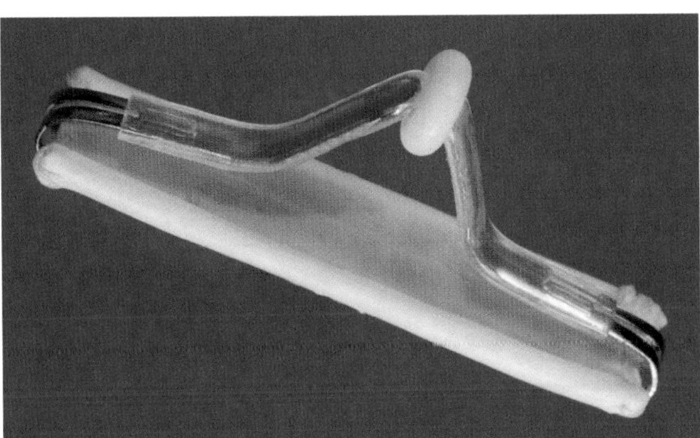

■ FIGURE 82–1. Intrinsic Therapeutics Barricaid annular repair device.

annulus after insertion into the disc. The frame has anterior projections that aid with insertion and serve to stabilize the device in its final position. These projections are connected by a PTFE link and stabilizing ring.

The materials used in the Barricaid were chosen for their unique mechanical properties, excellent biocompatibility, and long clinical implant history. Nitinol is a nickel-titanium alloy known mainly for its shape-memory and superelasticity, and is widely used in implantable medical devices such as stents and bone anchors. Nitinol provides the Barricaid with the strength to resist the extreme pressures within the disc and the flexibility to respond to motions of the treated level. PTFE (also known commonly by the trade names Teflon and Gore-Tex) is an inert polymer that is widely used in implantable medical devices such as abdominal hernia meshes, stent grafts, and dural substitutes. PTFE augments the Barricaid's ability to seal against extrusion of nucleus and increases compliance to the surrounding tissues.

## OPERATIVE TECHNIQUE

The Barricaid annular repair device is implanted via a standard open posterior discectomy approach, with or without the assistance of a microscope. The Barricaid can be implanted through a defect as small as a 5 mm × 5 mm cruciate cut, and can be used to repair defects that are up to 6 mm high and 10 mm wide. As part of a limited discectomy, the offending fragment of nucleus is removed prior to implantation. No additional intradiscal nucleus removal is required to place the Barricaid. Indeed, one of the benefits of the Barricaid is that it enables the retention of intradiscal nucleus without an elevated risk of recurrent herniation.

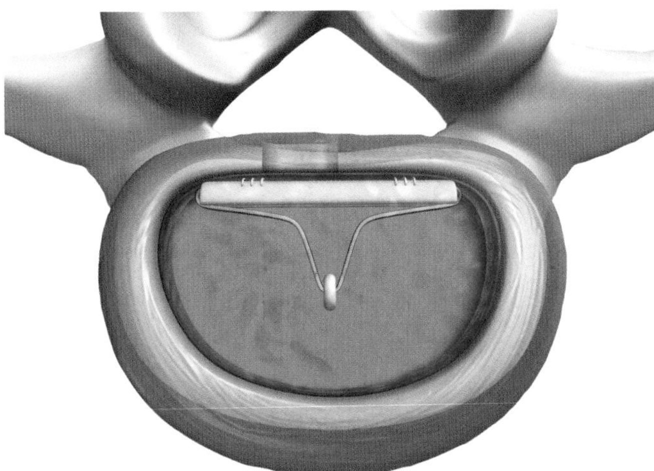

■ FIGURE 82–2. Rendering of the Barricaid in its implanted position between the annulus and nucleus, spanning the defect, and covering substantially all of the posterior annulus.

Following removal of the nuclear fragment and prior to insertion of the implant, two measurements are made using custom tools supplied by Intrinsic Therapeutics. The first is the thickness of the posterior annulus, to ensure that the implant is placed along the border between the annulus and the nucleus; the second is the internal width of the disc, to ensure that the appropriate size Barricaid is implanted to maximize the coverage and protection of the posterior annulus. Once these measurements are made, the implant is folded into the delivery instrument and implanted in the appropriate location. The entire process of measuring the annular thickness and disc width and implanting the device takes approximately 5 to 10 minutes. No changes to postoperative care are required and the patient can return to normal activities per the advice of the treating physician.

## PRECLINICAL TESTING

### Expulsion from the Disc Space

An extremely aggressive mechanical environment exists in the lumbar intervertebral disc. In vivo intradiscal pressures have been reported to be as high as 23 atm (338 psi).[14] The Barricaid serves as a patch that is positioned along the inside of the posterior of the damaged or weakened annulus. The pressure of the nucleus acts to push the Barricaid against the posterior annulus and hold it in place. This intradiscal pressure may also act to expel the Barricaid from the disc space, which represents the device's primary mode of failure in terms of safety.

We test the device's resistance to this failure mode in two ways: (1) on the benchtop in a simulated disc model and (2) in a challenging fresh-frozen human cadaver model, which tests for expulsion resistance following a series of loaded and unloaded motions designed to challenge the stability of the implant. All cadaver and benchtop expulsion testing is done with an annular defect that is 6 mm tall by 10 mm wide, and all testing is conducted at 37°C. Intradiscal pressure is monitored throughout all testing, which is performed to 23 atm (338 psi). When testing intradiscal implants for resistance to expulsion, no test should be considered a "success" unless the appropriate amount of pressure is achieved, and this pressure is accomplished in a disc oriented such that the pressure is acting to expel the implant.

The efficacy of the device in preventing extrusions of nuclear material has also been assessed by performing cadaveric expulsion testing in self-matched specimens. Each specimen was tested in two rounds—first with the device implanted and then with the device removed. A measure of efficacy is obtained by comparing the pressures at which nuclear extrusions occurred in these two scenarios.

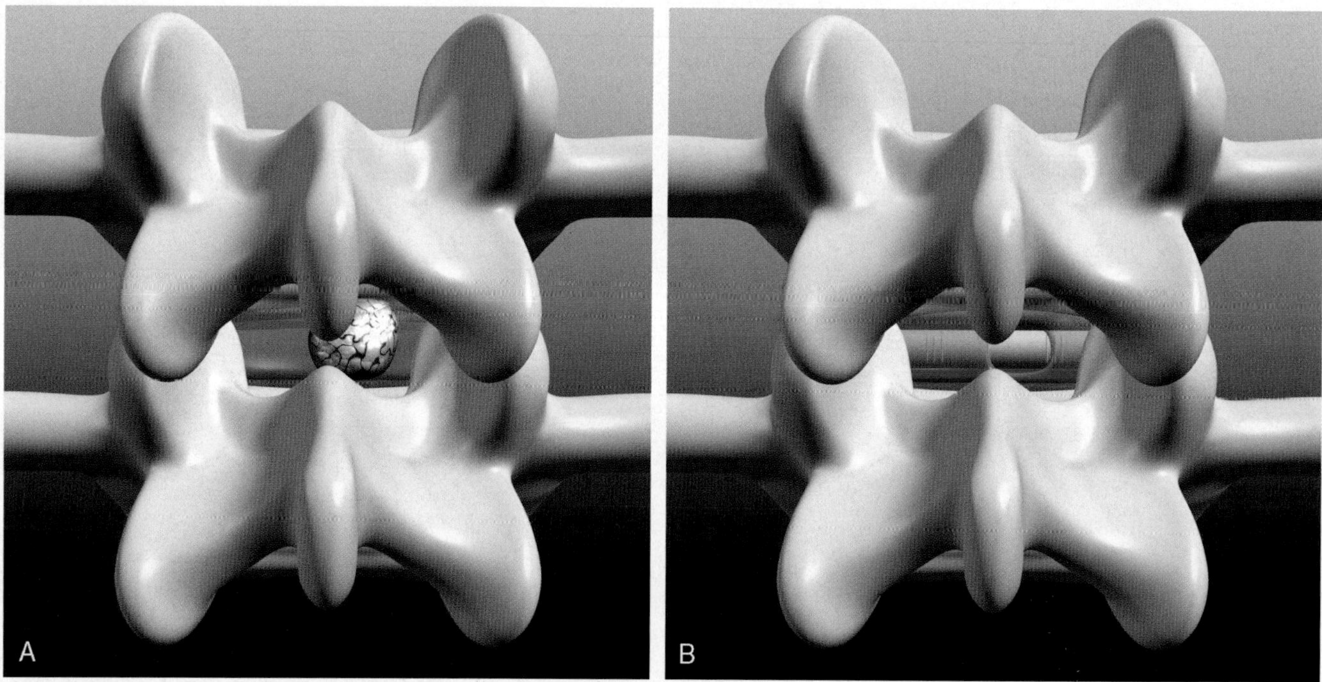


■ **FIGURE 82–3.** Posterior view of a herniated disc **(A)** and a disc whose annulus has been repaired with the Barricaid device **(B)**.

### Cadaver Testing

Loads and moments on the spine have largely been inferred, and no specific combination of loads and specimen orientation reliably produce nuclear extrusions in an in vitro biomechanics model. We have gone to great lengths to develop a cadaver model that can reliably be used to create nuclear extrusions,[20] and we use this model while continuously monitoring intradiscal pressure to challenge the resistance of the Barricaid device against expulsion from the disc.

The Barricaid implant has been implanted in over 150 fresh-frozen cadaver specimens. Over 60 of these have been dynamically tested, with an axial preload of 500 N (to simulate body weight) and unconstrained applied moments of 10 Nm. These motions and loads are applied for several hundred cycles in various orientations—flexion-extension, lateral bending, and flexion combined with each of right and left lateral bending. After this motion testing, the disc is flexed such that the intradiscal pressure is pushing the nucleus and Barricaid posteriorly, and the particular combination of flexion angle and load vector is identified such that intradiscal pressure is maximized. This worst-case orientation is then used to compress the disc until at least 23 atm (338 psi) of pressure is reached, typically around 3 to 5 kN (675 to 1125 lbf). For a test to be considered a success, this pressure must be reached, and the Barricaid implant must remain in position. If a specimen cannot generate this high pressure, or if the specimen fails prior to reaching this pressure (e.g., through an end plate fracture), the device has not been appropriately challenged, and this data point cannot be counted as a success. All the Barricaid implants survived this aggressive testing without incidence of expulsion from the disc space.

To perform efficacy testing, nuclear fragments from an adjacent level were inserted into the disc space from an anterior approach.[21] Use of these fragments increases intradiscal pressure, and the mobility of the fragments fully challenges the device. The fragments were placed anterior to the device after being stained to differentiate the fragments from native nucleus and soaked in radiopaque dye for visualization under fluoroscopy. Expulsion testing, as described earlier, was performed, and the pressure at which extrusion of nuclear material occurred was recorded. After this initial round of testing, the implant was carefully removed. If nuclear material had extruded, an equivalent volume of nuclear material was then inserted back into the disc space. Expulsion testing was then repeated and acted as a control for the first round of testing. In a group of eight specimens, the Barricaid device increased extrusion pressure by at least three times ($P < 0.0001$; Fig. 82–4). During the initial round of testing (i.e., with the Barricaid implanted), extrusions did not occur in all specimens. Testing was stopped at 25 atm of intradiscal pressure in order to preserve the specimens for further testing, so actual extrusion pressures for the implant group were even higher.

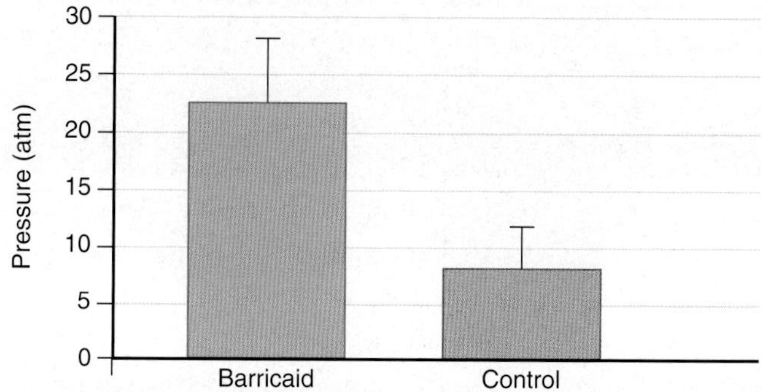


■ **FIGURE 82–4.** Intradiscal pressure at which herniation occurred with and without the Barricaid.

### Benchtop Testing

The benchtop expulsion testing is done following fatigue testing of the Barricaid implant, under the assumption that devices that are challenged by fatigue testing would be theoretically weaker than a virgin device would be against expulsion. All devices are first implanted into a plastic disc model. There are two types of fatigue testing to which implants are subjected in vivo: pressure- (or load-) driven fatigue due to cyclic changes in intradiscal pressure, and displacement-driven fatigue due to cyclic motions of the vertebral bodies.

## Testing Implant Fatigue

### Intradiscal Pressure Changes

As the intradiscal pressure increases and decreases as a result of various activities of daily living, the Barricaid implant may be cyclically deformed and could fatigue as a result. Such fatigue could theoretically result in fragmentation of the Barricaid or decreased resistance to expulsion from the disc space, both of which would constitute device failures. Resistance of the Barricaid implant against fatigue due to this cyclic pressurization is tested as part of our "Cyclic Pressure Fatigue Test."

Intradiscal pressures recorded in living humans in vivo have been reported for a number of different activities of daily life.[14,22] These activities include four general categories: sitting/standing, walking/jogging, climbing stairs, and lifting objects with various techniques. We tested the Barricaid implant in cyclic pressure fatigue in the greatest pressure ranges in each of these four categories, with the following exception: lifting 20 kg with good technique was substituted for climbing stairs to yield an even more rigorous loading protocol.

A loading protocol totaling 10 million cycles was formulated based on the activity frequency estimates provided in other published references, representing the upper end of the range of expected annual cycles for these normal and extreme activities. All tested devices passed this test; no devices fragmented, and all devices survived benchtop expulsion testing, as described earlier, following fatigue testing without extrusion from the disc model.

## Vertebral Body Movement

The Barricaid implant is not intended to support the adjacent vertebrae, or keep them separated from each other in any way. That is, the Barricaid is not intended to support load along the axis of the spine or to support the vertebral bodies in any other way. On the contrary, it is designed to be quite flexible and to move in concert with the surrounding soft tissue and accommodate the natural range of motion of the bony anatomy. As the vertebral bodies move during activities of daily living, the Barricaid implant may be cyclically deformed and could fatigue as a result. Such fatigue could result in fragmentation of the Barricaid or decreased resistance to expulsion from the disc space, both of which would constitute device failures. Resistance of the Barricaid against fatigue due to this cyclic deformation is tested as part of our "Motion Fatigue Test."

Intrinsic Therapeutics has adopted the philosophy of developing benchtop tests from observations of the implant's deformations and motions during aggressive cadaveric testing, and confirming (or modifying) these deformations based on clinical observations when possible. For this benchtop test, Barricaid implants were observed fluoroscopically in fresh-frozen human cadaver specimens while undergoing motions intended to simulate the extreme ranges of motion during daily living activities. The greatest range of implant deformation was seen in lateral bending. This implant deformation was used to simulate a range of activities that occur a combined 400 times per day as estimated from various literature sources.[23,24] These extreme ranges of motion are run for 10 million cycles, or nearly 70 years of simulated activities.

The cadaver specimen group consisted of a population of 23 specimens tested with unconstrained flexion-extension and lateral bending moments of 10 Nm and an axial preload of 500 N simulating the static load of the upper body. Fluorographs were taken at the extreme of each motion, as well as in the neutral position, and analyzed digitally to determine the maximum and minimum implant height (the difference between these being referred to as "implant compression"). These implant compression levels were then compared to implant compression seen in the functional x-rays (i.e., flexion-extension and lateral bending to the patient's limit) of 14 clinical patients implanted with the Barricaid device.

Analysis was also performed to investigate the difference in implant compression between standing and lying down. We did this by testing cadaver specimens with and without the compressive preload, which was meant to simulate the weight of the upper body, in the neutral configuration.

The mean of the maximum mesh compression from all of these cycles was used as the basis for this displacement-controlled test. Testing to these compression levels was accomplished to 10 million cycles without failure; no devices fragmented, and all devices survived benchtop expulsion testing as described earlier for fatigue testing.

## Summary

In summary, mechanical resilience of the Barricaid implant was determined using benchtop and cadaver testing to simulate the following scenarios:

1. Fatigue of the implant due to end plate motion (displacement-controlled, 10 million cycles)
2. Fatigue of the implant due to intradiscal pressure changes of the nucleus pulposus (pressure-controlled, 10 million cycles)
3. Resistance to expulsion from intradiscal pressure of the simulated nucleus in a benchtop model (pressure-controlled "expulsion testing," 338 psi) *after* completion of implant fatigue (motion or pressure)
4. Stability and expulsion resistance in a cadaver model with worst-case disc motion, orientation, intradiscal pressure, and annulus defect size (i.e., physiologic motion simulation, followed by >338 psi of intradiscal pressure with a 10-mm defect in the annulus)

Further, the biocompatibility of the Barricaid was assessed per the requirements of EN/ISO 10993 standards. The results indicate that the Barricaid is biocompatible.

## CLINICAL DATA

### Initial Postmarketing Study

The patients reported here were treated in five European centers and were divided into two cohorts. One group ("treatment") consists of 39 primary discectomy patients treated since March 2006 who were implanted with the Barricaid. The second group ("control") consists of 108 primary discectomy patients treated since January 2003 who were not implanted with the device. All patients were enrolled prospectively, and enrollment in both cohorts is currently ongoing. Exclusion criteria for this initial postmarketing study include prior spine surgery and multilevel herniations. Inclusion criteria include severe sciatica or sciatica unresponsive to conservative therapy for 6 weeks, and MRI or CT confirmation of lumbar herniation as the cause.

Follow-ups occur at 6 weeks, 3 months, 6 months, 12 months, and then annually through 5 years after surgery. Data gathered at each follow-up include Visual Analog Scale (VAS) (back and both legs), Oswestry Disability Index (ODI), and a custom clinical function score. Functional (standing) x-rays and CT scans are taken at each follow-up to assess stability of the implant over time, as well as disc height maintenance. Recurrent herniations (as evidenced by a confirmatory MR image) and reoperations are tracked throughout the follow-up period. Symptomatic reherniations were diagnosed first clinically, through a recurrence of leg pain and neurologic symptoms, and then confirmed by MRI.

Both defect size and amount of disc material removed were measured at the time of surgery. To account for patient variability, the amount of disc material removed was normalized against the total volume of the intervertebral space using a previously reported CT algorithm.[25] See Figure 82–5 for a representation of a CT-based model of the disc space.

Mean follow-up on the control group has been 2.2 years, and on the implanted group 8.0 months. The volume of nucleus removed ranged from 0.4 to 7.0 $cm^3$ (3.6 to 95.9% when normalized for disc volume), and the defect area ranged from 20 to 84 $mm^2$. No patients have been lost to follow-up in the implanted group, and only one patient has been lost to follow-up in the control group at 1 year.

### Symptomatic Recurrent Herniation

There have been no recurrent herniations in any of the 39 treatment group patients. The symptomatic reherniation rate in the control group has been 4% (4 of 108 patients) within the first 3 months and 9% (10 of 108 patients) by the 1-year follow-up (Fig. 82–6). Reherniation rate among the control patients (based on survivorship analysis) was positively correlated on a univariate basis with defect height ($P = 0.0024$) and defect width ($P = 0.0104$), and negatively correlated with nuclear volume removed ($P = 0.0466$). That is, the greater the defect width or defect height created or found at the time of primary discectomy, the greater the risk of reherniation at a given time point. Further follow-up on the treatment group is required to see if the decrease in rate of reherniation remains over time.

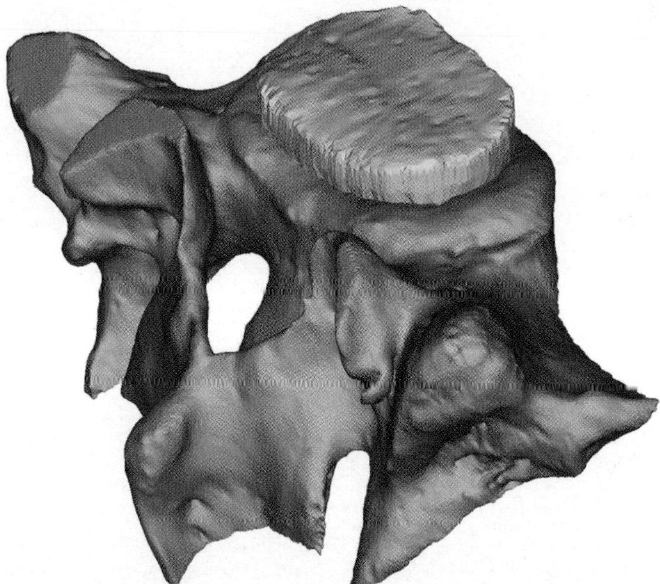

■ **FIGURE 82–5.** This CT-based model of the disc space is used to normalize the volume of nucleus removed during surgery.

### Disc Height Maintenance

Control patients lost an average of 21% of their disc height by 6 months following the surgery and maintained that level at 1 year. Percent disc height loss at 1 year was positively correlated with both preoperative disc height and normalized nuclear volume removed when regressed with defect size (both $P < 0.001$). That is, for a given disc height, the more nucleus removed at the time of primary discectomy, the greater the disc height loss at 1 year following the operation.

At 6 months, Barricaid patients lost only 7.5% of their preoperative disc height versus 21% in nonimplanted patients ($P < 0.0002$, Fig. 82–7). While less nucleus was removed from Barricaid patients ($P < 0.000001$), a multivariate analysis of disc

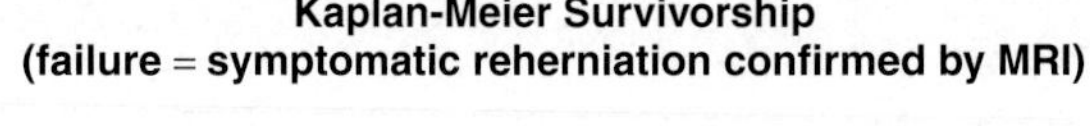


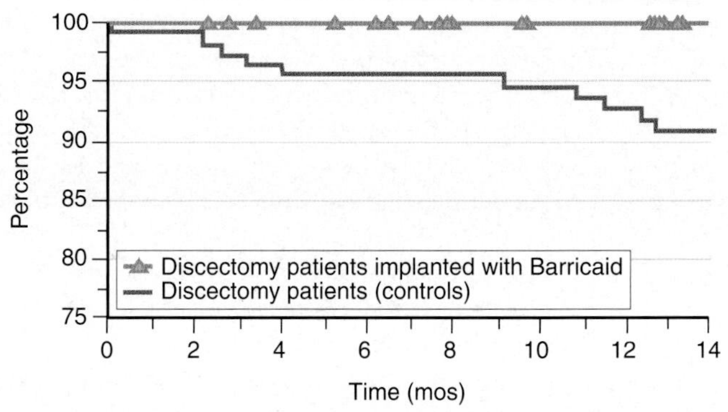


■ **FIGURE 82–6.** Kaplan-Meier survivorship curve comparing Barricaid patients to control discectomy patients (failure defined as symptomatic reherniation confirmed by MRI).

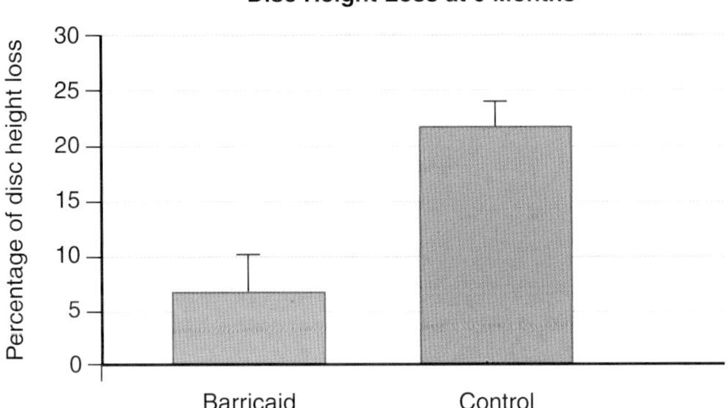


■ **FIGURE 82–7.** Comparison of disc height loss between Barricaid patients and control discectomy patients at 6 months.

height loss as a function of various parameters that may affect it (e.g., gender, body mass index, age, defect size, nuclear volume removed, implantation of Barricaid) demonstrated that Barricaid implantation alone accounts for 13% greater maintenance of disc height at 6 months. As an anecdotal check of this analysis, a subset of the 108 total patients in this abstract was selected with comparable amounts of normalized nucleus removed ($P = 0.97$). At 6 months, Barricaid patients lost significantly less disc height (7.5% compared to 21% in the control group). Further follow-up on the treatment group is required to see if the greater disc height maintenance is retained over time.

### Summary

After a successful initial pilot study, 39 patients have been implanted with the Barricaid annular repair device as part of this ongoing follow-up clinical study. Implantation has been shown to be safe and easy. The device is performing its function of retaining nuclear material within the disc as evidenced both by reherniation rate and disc height maintenance.

Recurrent herniation following primary discectomy is a well-documented clinical problem, reported in up to 21% of the general primary discectomy patient population. To date, there have been no recurrent herniations among patients implanted with the Barricaid at the time of a primary discectomy procedure. This is in contrast to recurrent herniation rates of 4% at 3 months and 16% at 1 year in an equivalent patient population not treated with the Barricaid.

Loss of disc height has been correlated with disc degeneration in both the clinic and the laboratory. Early data indicate that the Barricaid may be effective in maintaining preoperative disc height. In our prospective clinical study, the patients treated with the Barricaid have lost just 7.5% of their preoperative disc height at 6 months, compared to 21% for the control patients. These early data provide a strong indication that an annular closure device may be effective in delaying disc degeneration and improving pain outcomes for discectomy patients.

Further follow-up is ongoing to determine if the decrease in recurrent herniation rate and improvement in disc height maintenance provided by the Barricaid annular repair device remain over time.

## INDICATIONS AND CONTRAINDICATIONS

The indications for the postmarketing study were narrower than clinically necessary in order to have as clean a data set as possible. Many of the contraindications for the postmarketing study (e.g., single level affected, prior spine surgery) will likely go away as further data are gathered. Indications and contraindications for the Barricaid annular repair device are generally in line with those for a standard discectomy procedure. Contraindications specific to the Barricaid include annular defects wider than 10 mm; annular defects taller than 6 mm; foraminal, extraforaminal, or anterior herniations; and disc height in the target level less than 5 mm.

## SUMMARY

The need for annular repair is clear. The annular weakness or defect that is present in every discectomy patient presents a very real dilemma to the surgeons performing the more than 500,000 discectomies that are done each year: remove only the nuclear fragment causing the patient's immediate symptoms and run a high risk of a recurrent herniation, or remove as much nuclear material as possible at the time of the primary discectomy and risk disc collapse and significantly worse clinical outcomes in general.

The Barricaid annular repair device has been designed to meet the product requirements outlined here:

- *Prevent reherniation*: In a prospective clinical study, no reherniations have occurred among patients implanted with the Barricaid.
- *Preserve disc function*: In a prospective controlled clinical study, patients implanted with the Barricaid preserved significantly more disc height at 6 months than the unimplanted control group.
- *Cover defects of a variety of sizes and locations*: The Barricaid can cover defects as tall as 6 mm and as wide as 10 mm and can be inserted through a defect as small as a 5 mm × 5 mm cruciate cut.
- *Protect as much of the posterior annulus as possible*: The Barricaid is sized intraoperatively to cover substantially all of the posterior annulus.
- *Require minimal or no removal of nucleus*: With the Barricaid device, only the fragment of nucleus that is causing the patient's immediate symptoms needs to be removed.
- *Easily used with current surgical approach and techniques*: The Barricaid is implanted through a standard posterior discectomy access.
- *Minimal impact on operative time*: Use of the Barricaid device adds roughly 5 to 10 minutes to the overall operative time.
- *Endure the high ranges of motion and pressure without failure or migration*: Rigorous cadaver and benchtop testing has demonstrated the robustness of the Barricaid design under the aggressive loading environment of the lumbar disc.

The early clinical results described here have shown the Barricaid annular repair device to be an extremely promising solution to the problems associated with the annular defects with which discectomy patients currently leave the operating room.

## REFERENCES


1. Thompson Healthcare, Solucient InpatientView: 2005 estimated data for ICD-9 80.51, 2007.
2. Viscogliosi AG, Viscogliosi MR, Viscogliosi JJ: Spine Arthroplasty: Market Potential and Technology Update. Viscogliosi Bros, LLC. p. 89, 2001.
3. Atlas SJ, Keller RB, Chang Y, et al: Surgical and nonsurgical management of sciatica secondary to a lumbar disc herniation: Five-year outcomes from the Maine lumbar spine study. Spine 26(10): 1179–1187, 2001.
4. Asch HL, Lewis PJ, Moreland DB, et al: Prospective multiple outcomes study of outpatient lumbar microdiscectomy: Should 75 to 80% success rates be the norm? J Neurosurg: Spine 96:34–44, 2002.
5. Rogers, LA: Experience with limited versus extensive disc removal in patients undergoing microsurgical operations for ruptured lumbar discs. Neurosurgery 22(1):82–85, 1988.
6. Carragee EJ, Han MY, Suen PW, Kim D: Clinical outcomes after lumbar discectomy for sciatica: The effects of fragment type and anular competence. J Bone Joint Surg Am, 85-A(1):102–108, 2003.
7. Hanley EN Jr., Shapiro DE: The development of low-back pain after excision of a lumbar disc. J Bone Joint Surg Am, 71-A(5):719–721, 1989.
8. White AA, Panjabi MM: Clinical Biomechanics of the Spine. 2nd edition, Philadelphia, Lippincott Williams & Wilkins, 1990.
9. McMillan DW, McNally DS, Garbutt G, Adams MA: Stress distributions inside intervertebral discs. J Bone Joint Surg Am, 78-B(6): 81–87, 1996.
10. Yorimitsu E, Chiba K, Toyama Y, Hirabayashi K: Long-term outcomes of standard discectomy for lumbar disc herniation: A follow-up study of more than 10 years. Spine 26(6):652–657, 2001.
11. Mochida J, Toh E, Nomura T, Nishimura K: The risks and benefits of percutaneous nucleotomy for lumbar disc herniation: A 10-year longitudinal study. J Bone Joint Surg Am 83-B(4):501–505, 2001.
12. Hanley EN Jr., Shapiro DE: The development of low-back pain after excision of a lumbar disc. J Bone Joint Surg Am, 71-A(5):719–721, 1989.
13. Carragee EJ, Spinnickie AO, Alamin TF, Paragioudakis S: A prospective controlled study of limited versus subtotal posterior discectomy: Short-term outcomes in patients with herniated lumbar intervertebral discs and large posterior anular defect. Spine 31(6): 653–657, 2006.
14. Wilke HJ, Neef P, Caimi M, et al: New in vivo measurements of pressures in the intervertebral disc of daily life. Spine 24(8): 755–762, 1999.
15. Klara PM, Ray CD: Artificial nucleus replacement: Clinical experience. Spine 27(12):1374–1377, 2002.
16. Heggeness MH, Watters WC 3rd, Gray PM Jr: Discography of lumbar discs after surgical treatment for disc herniation. Spine 22: 1606–1609, 1997.
17. Ahlgren BD, Lui W, Herkowitz HN, et al: Effect of anular repair on the healing strength of the intervertebral disc. Spine 25(17): 2165–2170, 2000.
18. Ninomiya M, Muro T: Pathoanatomy of lumbar disc herniation as demonstrated by computed tomography/discography. Spine 17(11): 1316–1322, 1992.
19. Cinotti G, Gumina S, Giannicola G, Postacchini F: Contralateral recurrent lumbar disc herniation: Results of discectomy compared with those in primary herniation. Spine 24(8):800–806, 1999.
20. Yeh O, Chow S, Small M, et al: Novel approach to closing anular defects: a biomechanics study. Poster presented at North American Spine Society, Philadelphia. September 2005.
21. Brinckmann P, Porter RW: A laboratory model of lumbar disc protrusion. Fissure and fragment. Spine 19(2):228–235, 1994.
22. Sato K, Kikuchi S, Yonezawa T: In vivo intradiscal pressure measurement in healthy individuals and in patients with ongoing back problems. Spine 24(23):2468–2474, 1999.
23. Morlock M, Schneider E, Bluhm A, et al: Duration and frequency of everyday activities in total hip patients. J Biomech 34:873–881, 2001.
24. Kaynak H, Kaynak D, Oztura I: Does frequency of nocturnal urination reflect the severity of sleep-disordered breathing? J Sleep Res 13(2):173–176, 2004.
25. Kamaric E, Yeh O, Velagic A, et al: Disc Collapse Following Discectomy: A Novel Approach to Measuring Disc Height. Poster presented at Spine Arthroplasty Society, New York. May 2005.

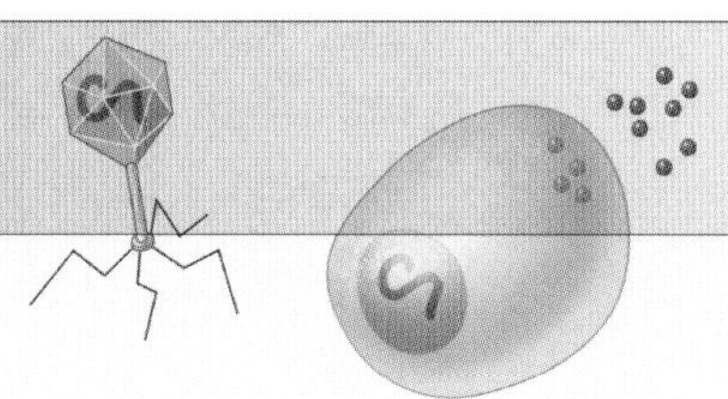

PART

# XI

# Cell-Based Biologic Scientific Methods and Future Clinical Applications

CHAPTER 83

# Animal Models for Human Disc Degeneration

**Kern Singh, Koichi Masuda,** and **Howard S. An**

## KEY POINTS

- The availability of an experimental animal model that consistently reproduces intervertebral disc degeneration would facilitate the investigations of the disease.
- Animal models of human disc degeneration can be subdivided into two main categories: naturally occurring and experimentally induced.
- Naturally occurring animal models have the drawback of the basis for the high rate of disc degeneration not being known.
- Although the interventions in artificial animal models are known, the true relationship between these interventions and the actual events leading to disc degeneration in humans is not.

Intervertebral disc degeneration is a major cause of functional disability in humans.[1] The macroscopic features characterizing disc degeneration include the formation of tears within the annulus substance and progressive fraying and dehydration of the nucleus pulposus (NP).[2–4] Despite the significant impairment associated with this disease, a clear understanding of the basic mechanisms of disease pathogenesis and specific therapeutic agents is still lacking. Unquestionably, disc degeneration is a multifactorial process influenced by genetics, lifestyle conditions (including obesity, occupation, smoking, and alcohol consumption),[1–6] biomechanical loading and activities, and other health factors (diabetes and aging). The availability of an experimental animal model that consistently reproduces the disease would facilitate the investigations of intervertebral disc degeneration. This chapter provides an overview of the reported animal models that have been used to evaluate human disc degeneration.

## INTERVERTEBRAL DISC ANATOMY

The intervertebral disc acts as a load-bearing structure with two distinct components: the NP and the annulus fibrosus (AF). Each component has very distinct biomechanical properties. The NP, rich in proteoglycan, acts as an internal semifluid mass, whereas the AF, rich in collagen, acts as a laminar fibrous container.[5] The hydrostatic properties of the disc arise from its high water content. The NP, when palpated in a young adult, acts as a viscid fluid under applied pressure, but also exhibits considerable elastic rebound, assuming its original physical state upon release.[3] Histologic analysis has shown that the NP is derived from embryonic notochordal tissue. The NP from young individuals is composed of loose, delicate fibrous strands embedded in a gelatinous matrix.[7] The transition from notochordal to chondrocytic cells in NP varies among species, and therefore, the investigator should factor the age of the animals into consideration when performing experiments.[8] This process of transition from notochordal cells to chondrocytic NP cells involves mitochondrial capase,[9] apoptosis of notochordal cells, and migration of chondrocytes from the cartilaginous end plate toward the NP.[9–11] The major function of the NP is to resist and redistribute compressive forces within the spine; the major function of the AF is to withstand tension. The unique combination of biochemical and biomechanical properties of the AF and NP allows the intervertebral disc to absorb and disperse the normal loading forces experienced by the spine.[3,6] The presumption is that when one of these two units, either the AF or the NP, is structurally compromised, degenerative changes will ensue because of the alteration in mechanical force distribution across the functional spinal unit.

## ANIMAL MODELS—REQUIREMENTS AND SELECTION

Animal models are essential in making the transition from scientific concepts to clinical applications. Ethical issues are always of concern. The Animal Welfare Act and the Public Health Service Animal Welfare Policy require that an Institutional Animal Care and Use Committee review and approve each protocol. The use of appropriate technologies to eliminate or reduce pain and euthanize is required. The usage of the minimum number of animals from which significant conclusions can be inferred is not only ethically necessary but also cost-effective. In addition, the species selected should be carefully chosen with serious consideration given to all applicable federal regulations, public health service policy, and institutional policies.

The degree of disc degeneration in an animal model should be controllable and selectable to aid the researcher in proving the hypothesis. The validation of the reproducibility of an animal model allows results from different scientific researchers to be compared. Furthermore, for validation, the interobserver variability of outcome measures should be fully studied. If a surgical technique or other environmental change is used, the procedure should be standardized in detail to increase the transferability of models to other groups.

## CATEGORIES OF ANIMAL MODELS FOR DISC DEGENERATION

Animal models of human disc degeneration (Table 83–1) can be subdivided into two main categories: naturally occurring and experimentally induced.

### Naturally Occurring Disc Changes

#### Sand Rat

The sand rat *(Psammomys obesus)* is indigenous to eastern Mediterranean deserts. Silberberg[12] and Adler[13] first described the spontaneous appearance of disc changes in the rat as similar to those that occur in humans. Cysts, tears, and occasionally bony bars were seen more frequently in the AF of 18- to 30-month-old animals. According to Silberberg, the low water and high salt diet of the sand rat may somehow be related to an altered metabolism potentially leading to the internal derangement of the NP.

Moskowitz and associates[14] further studied the sand rat by analyzing the lumbar as well as the thoracic spine. The authors fed a group of sand rats a normal diet and included radiographic and histologic assessment of the intervertebral disc as well as measurements of serum glucose and insulin. Roentgenographically observed disc degeneration increased with age, leading to 50% of the animals being affected by 18 months of age. The authors believed that the observation of degeneration occurring earlier than 3 months lent support to causative factors other than aging.

Ziv[15] and associates compared hydration, fixed charge density (FCD), and varying osmotic pressures in young, old, and diabetic sand rats. The discs of the young diabetic sand rats demonstrated decreased hydration, FCD, and ability to resist compression under osmotic pressures (assessed by hydration after equilibration in vitro with either 15 or 25 g/dL polyethylene glycol) when compared to young healthy sand rats. The authors noted that the diabetic intervertebral disc was more similar in nature to the older sand rat intervertebral disc.

Gruber and associates[16] recently published a large cross-sectional and prospective analysis of *Psammomys obesus.* They analyzed 158 animals in a cross-sectional study and 22 animals in a longitudinal study (12 months of age). The authors noted that naturally occurring radiographic signs of degeneration were evident by 2 months; wedging, narrowing, irregular disc margins, and end plate calcification were the most common degenerative changes in older animals.

The sand rat was also recently used as a small animal model for autologous disc cell implantation by Gruber and associates.[17] Cells were harvested from a lumbar intervertebral disc, expanded in monolayer tissue culture, labeled with agents that allow subsequent immunolocalization of these cells, and implanted in a second disc site of the donor animal. The cells were either engrafted in a bioresorbable carrier tested for compatibility or injected into the recipient disc. Data from 15 animals were obtained up to 33 weeks. Immunocytologic identification of engrafted cells showed integration into the disc with normal matrix surrounding the cells 8 months after engraftment. Engrafted cells exhibited either a spindle-shaped morphology in the AF or a rounded chondrocyte-like morphology in the NP.

#### Pintail Mouse

Other animal models have also been developed with characteristics that resemble the spontaneous onset of disc degeneration observed in humans. Berry[18] noted that in the pintail mouse (*Anas acuta*), the NP in the subcervical discs underwent changes similar in appearance to those in humans (loss of mucopolysaccharides). This change was much more dramatic in mutant homozygotes (pBr strain mutated by exposure to methylcholanthrene), leading the authors to conclude that disc degeneration in humans may be genetically linked.

#### Chinese Hamster

The Chinese hamster (*Cricetulus griseus*) was used by Silberberg and Gerritsen[19] because of its tendency to develop diabetes. The hamster was evaluated in order to determine a correlation between hyperostotic spondylosis and diabetes. Histologic evaluations revealed a higher incidence of spondylosis (60% versus 39%), but a lower incidence of disc herniations (9% versus 30%) in animals with diabetes. Both spondylosis and disc degeneration increased with age.

#### Rabbit

Kim and associates conducted a biochemical and radiologic comparison of four disc injury models to produce disc degeneration in rabbits.[20] In the first experiment, seven New Zealand white rabbits (1 year old, 3.5–4.5 kg body weight) were used to test four different disc injury models: intradiscal injection of camptothecin (an apoptotic agent) using a 23-gauge needle at L2-L3, nucleus aspiration using a 21-gauge needle at L3-L4, three annulus punctures using a 21-gauge needle at L4-L5, and one annulus puncture using an 18-gauge needle at L5-L6. Lumbar spinal magnetic resonance images were assessed using four grades of disc degeneration. In the second experiment, the 21-gauge three-puncture and the 18-gauge one-puncture models, thought most effective in producing disc degeneration in the first experiment, were again used in a second study. Six rabbits were killed 8 weeks later, the water and sulfated glycosaminoglycan contents being measured as in the first experiment. The authors found that in the first experiment, the 21-gauge three-puncture and the 18-gauge one-puncture models produced the most consistent disc degeneration in the rabbit lumbar spine. When these two models were again studied in the second experiment, the 21-gauge three-puncture technique was superior in producing disc degeneration over a shorter period of time.

#### Dog

Canine models, including those using basset hounds, beagles, and dachshunds, have been extensively described in the literature.[21–24] Several authors have noted that the disc degeneration

TABLE 83–1. Summary of the Animal Models of Disc Degeneration

| Animal Model | Method of Analysis | Onset of Degeneration | Author | Year |
|---|---|---|---|---|
| **Naturally Occurring** | | | | |
| Sand rat (*Psammomys obesus*) | Observation on natural diet—high salt, low water | 6 months | Silberberg[12] | 1979 |
| | Observation on natural diet—high salt, low water | 1.5–2.5 years | Adler[13] | 1983 |
| | Histologic analysis of IVD, measurements of serum glucose/insulin | 3–30 months | Moskovitz[14] | 1990 |
| | Varied hydration, fixed charge density and osmotic pressures (hydration after equilibration in vitro with either 15 or 25 g/dL polyethylene glycol) | 6 weeks | Ziv[15] | 1992 |
| | Biomechanical pressure evaluation of the IVD; peak force and force decay (1 versus 500 s) were measured in response to a flexion-producing step displacement | 3–18 months | Ziran[80] | 1994 |
| | Observational prospective study of natural IVD degeneration | 2–12 months | Gruber[16] | 2002 |
| | Autologous disc cell transplantation; cells were harvested from a lumbar IVD, expanded in monolayer tissue culture, and labeled with agents to allow immunolocalization | 33 weeks | Gruber[17] | 2002 |
| Pin tail mouse | pBr strain mutated by exposure to methylcholanthrene | 2–4 months | Berry[18] | 1961 |
| Chinese hamster (*Cricetulus griseus*) | Comparison of hyperostotic spondylosis and diabetes | 1–3 months | Silberberg[19] | 1976 |
| Beagle/greyhound | Comparison of collagen content | 0–3 months | Goggin[22] | 1970 |
| Multiple canine breeds | Characterization of degenerated disc disease in multiple breeds | 0–124 months | Ghosh[23] | 1976 |
| Beagle | Evaluation of PG content in lumbar IVD | 2 months | Cole[21] | 1986 |
| Baboon (*Papio cynocephalus anubis*) | Roentgenographic evaluation | 0–15.7 years | Lauerman[25] | 1992 |
| **Experimentally Induced** | **Method of Injury** | | | |
| **Surgically/Physically Induced** | | | | |
| | **Posture Change** | | | |
| Wistar rat | Forelimb amputation—midhumeral | 0–6 months | Goff[26] | 1957 |
| Mouse | Midhumeral amputations—effects of experimental posture | 1–6 months | Yamada[27] | 1962 |
| | Light/electron microscopic evaluation of NP in bipedal rats | 3–12 months | Higuchi[28] | 1983 |
| Wistar rat | Observation of lumbosacral herniations in bipedal rats | 1–3 months | Cassidy[29] | 1988 |
| | **Tail suspension** | | | |
| Sprague-Dawley rat | Tail suspension (simulated weightlessness) | 0–4 weeks | Hutton[30] | 1999 |
| | **Axial Loading** | | | |
| Mouse | Mouse tail exposed to external compression | 7–28 days | Lotz[31] | 1998 |
| Sprague-Dawley rat | Rat tail compression using an Ilizarov-type apparatus | 0–56 days | Iatridis[32] | 1999 |
| | Compressive stress via pins inserted in the 6th and 7th caudal vertebrae; cyclic loading of 0.5, 1.5, or 2.5 Hz was applied for 1 hour each day from the 3rd to 17th day; angular compliance, angular laxity, and inter-pin distance were measured | 0–2 wk | Ching[33] | 2002 |
| New Zealand white rabbit | Axial dynamic compression loading | 1–28 days | Kroeber[34] | 2002 |
| | **Torsional Injury** | | | |
| New Zealand white rabbit | Facetectomy and 30-degree lumbar torsion | 60–90 days | Hadjipavlou[35,36] | 1998 |
| | **Resection of Spinal Process or Facet Joint** | | | |
| Mouse | Removal of cervical spinous process and paravertebral muscles | 6–12 months | Miyamoto[37] | 1991 |
| New Zealand white rabbit | Resection of the inferior articular process at one level<br>Resection of the contralateral inferior articular process at an adjacent level | 3–6 months | Sullivan[38] | 1971 |
| | **Adjacent Level Fusion** | | | |
| New Zealand white rabbit | Lumbar fusion L5-L6 | 3–9 months | Phillips[39] | 2002 |
| | **Annulotomy** | | | |
| New Zealand white rabbit | Anterior annulotomy using a scalpel | 0–3 months | Keyes[40] | 1932 |
| | Ventral annulotomy (transverse, mid-disc, 4 mm long and through the AF into the NP) | 0–3 months | Smith[41] | 1951 |
| | Ventral annulotomy similar to Smith and intramuscular ACTH injection every other day | 0–3 months | Haimovichi[42] | 1970 |

(Continued)

**TABLE 83–1. Summary of the Animal Models of Disc Degeneration—Cont'd**

| Animal Model | Method of Analysis | Onset of Degeneration | Author | Year |
|---|---|---|---|---|
| | Full-thickness stab through the anterior part of the AF into the NP (2 mm in length); the NP and anterior AF of the intact IVD and the central region of the lesioned IVD were removed and analyzed; biochemical measures included analysis of PG, water and hyaluronic acid concentration as well as PG monomer size and total PG content | 1–200 days | Lipson[43] | 1981 |
| | Topographic analysis of anterior full-thickness annulotomies | 0–3 months | Urayama[44] | 1986 |
| | Puncture with 16G–21G needle | 12 weeks | Aota[45] | 2002–2004 |
| | Slow degeneration compared to stab model; disc height, MRI and histologic analysis | | Muehleman,[46] Masuda[47] | |
| | Puncture with 16G needle, MRI analysis | 12 weeks | Kompel[48] | 2003 |
| Merino sheep | Left anterolateral annulotomy parallel and adjacent to the inferior end plate with a controlled depth of 5 mm; the inner third of the AF and the NP were left intact closely reproducing the rim Lear lesion | 4–12 months | Osti[49] | 1990 |
| Domestic pig (*Sus scrofa*) | Stab lesion with a No. 11 scalpel midline anteriorly (depth 13 mm) | 0–2 weeks | Kaapa[50–52] | 1994 |
| Gottingen pig | Analyzed lumbar IVDs after a more extensive annulotomy, by a window in the AF anterolaterally, which was then plugged by fibrin glue followed by injection of chymopapain | 0–12 months | Pfeiffer[53] | 1994 |
| | **End Plate Injury** | | | |
| Domestic pig | Analyzed lumbar IVDs after perforation of end plate into the NP | 3 months | Holm[54] | 2004 |
| | **Muscle Stimulation** | | | |
| Rabbit | Repetitive flexion-extension of the C-spine (trapezius stimulation, 200k cycles) | 200k cycles | Wada[55] | 1992 |
| **Chemically/ Genetically Induced** | **Chemonucleolysis** | | | |
| Canine | Injection of chymopapain | 2–26 weeks | Bradford[81,82] | 1983, 1984 |
| Canine | Injection of chymopapain | 6–20 weeks | Kahanovitz[69] | 1985 |
| Canine | Injection of collagenase and chymopapain | 2–52 weeks | Spencer[61] | 1985 |
| Canine | Application of chymodiactin to the lumbar spine IVDs of canines and postinjection biomechanical analysis | 8 weeks | Nitobe[65] | 1988 |
| Pig | Injection of collagenase and chymopapain | 4 weeks | Zook[56] | 1986 |
| Rabbit | Injection of collagenase | 2–4 weeks | Olmarker[64] | 1987 |
| Rabbit | Injection of chondroitinase ABC | 1–12 weeks | Kato,[57] Eurell[83] Takahashi,[59] Sumida[60] | 1990–1999 |
| Canine | Injection of chondroitinase ABC | 1–21 days | Takahashi,[58] Ono[63] | 1997–1998 |
| Sheep | Injection of chondroitinase ABC | 1–4 weeks | Sasaki[62] | 2001 |
| Rat | Injection of trypsin, collagenase, chymopapain, and hyaluronidase | 1 week | Takenaka[84] | 1987 |
| Rat | Effects of chondroitinase ABC on rat tail IVDs | 2 weeks | Norcross[74] | 2003 |
| | **Injection of Fibronectin** | | | |
| Rabbit | Injection of fibronectin fragments, radiographically, histologically, and biochemically analyzed | 16 weeks | Anderson[75] | 2003 |
| | **Smoking** | | | |
| Rabbit | Smoke inhalation via control box | 8 weeks | Oda[77] | 2004 |
| Rat | Nicotine-induced (110 ng/mL) | 8 weeks | Iwahashi[76] | 2002 |
| | **Genetic Knockout** | | | |
| COL2a1 knockout mice | Analysis of skeletal tissues from mice with an inactivated allele of the *Col2a1* gene for type II collagen ("heterozygous knockout"); radiographic analysis; conventional, quantitative, and polarized light microscopy; immunohistochemistry for the major extracellular components, and in situ hybridization for procollagens alpha-1 (I) and alpha-1 (II) | 1 month | Sahlman[85] | 2001 |
| GDF-8 knockout mice | Analysis of skeletal tissues from GDF-8 (myostatin) knockout mice | | Hamrick[79] | 2003 |

AF, annulus fibrosus; G, gauge; IVD, intervertebral disc; MRI, magnetic resonance imaging; NP, nucleus pulposus; PG, proteoglycan.

in these models differs from human intervertebral disc degeneration. Typically, by 1 year of age in these canine models, the NP becomes occupied by chondrocytes with a matrix containing an increased collagen content and decreased proteoglycan and water content. Unlike the human disc, this matrix may become calcified after disc herniations.

### Primates

Primate models, including the baboon (*Papio cynocephalus anubis*), have also been used. Lauerman and associates[25] radiographically demonstrated a significant correlation between age and disc degeneration grade (Spearman correlation coefficient of 0.726, $P < 0.0001$) as well as kyphosis angle (coefficient of 0.6333, $P < 0.0001$).

## Experimentally Induced Disc Changes

Experimentally produced disc changes have been extensively described in the literature. These artificially induced degenerative changes are invaluable in creating clinically applicable and reproducible animal models of degeneration.

### Surgically or Physically Induced Animal Models

#### Postural Change

Goff and Landmesser,[26] as well as Yamada,[27] developed a method for studying disorders of posture and changes in bone dimensions, gait, and behavioral characteristics of bipedal animals. The authors performed neonatal midhumeral surgical bilateral amputations in the Wistar rat and DBA strains of mice. Postural changes resulted in the reduction of the usual lumbar kyphosis and gradual degenerative changes in the AF and NP at 3 to 12 months. The authors also noted that disc herniations developed in some of the bipedal rats. Higuchi and associates[28] used electron microscopy to further analyze changes in the NP of bipedal mice. The authors noted that over time the discs in bipedal mice degenerated in a similar but much more rapid fashion than their quadruped counterparts. Cassidy[29] noted similar findings in bipedal Wistar rats with radiographic evidence of anterior vertebral body wedging, degeneration of the intervertebral discs, and lumbosacral herniations of the NP.

#### Tail Suspension

Hutton and co-workers examined the effects of simulated weightlessness on the intervertebral disc by using a rat-tail suspension model.[30] The authors tail-suspended 32 Sprague-Dawley rats for either 2 or 4 weeks and biochemically evaluated the lumbar discs using enzyme-linked immunosorbent assays. At 4 weeks, the authors noted a significant decrease in proteoglycan content (35%). No appreciable difference was found at 2 weeks. There were no statistically significant differences between the two groups in type I or II collagen content at either time point.

#### Axial Loading

In a mouse model, Lotz and associates studied the biomechanical effects of static compressive loading on tail intervertebral discs.[31] Mouse-tail discs were loaded in vivo with an external compression device. The expression of type II collagen was suppressed at all levels of stress, whereas the expression of aggrecan decreased at the highest stress level in proportion to decreased nuclear cellularity. The authors concluded that compressive loading results in a dose-dependent apoptotic response and a downregulation of collagen II and aggrecan gene expression.

Several authors have described rat-tail compression models.[32,33] Iatridis and associates originally described the rat-tail compression model using an Ilizarov-type apparatus to apply chronic compression.[32] The authors noted that chronically applied compression had effects similar to immobilization but induced the changes earlier and in larger magnitudes. In addition to an increase in proteoglycan content of the intervertebral disc, biomechanically, there was an increase in disc thickness, angular laxity, and axial and angular compliance. Ching and associates also studied the effects of cyclical compression on the rat-tail intervertebral disc.[33] Sixty Sprague-Dawley rats were subjected to daily compressive stress via pins inserted in the sixth and seventh caudal vertebrae over a 2-week loading period. Animals were randomly divided into a sham group (pin insertion, no loading), a static loading group, or cyclic loading group (0.5, 1.5, or 2.5 Hz). Loading was applied for 1 hour each day from the third to seventeenth day following pin insertion. The angular compliance, angular laxity, and inter-pin distance were measured in vivo at days 0, 3, 10, and 17. The authors noted that, in general, cyclical loading resulted in less marked changes than static loading, but cyclical loading at certain frequencies (0.5 and 2.5 Hz) produced severe degenerative changes.

More recently, Kroeber and colleagues[34] reported a new rabbit disc degeneration model (New Zealand white), which applies a controlled and quantified axial mechanical loading. After 14 and 28 days of axial loading, the discs demonstrated a significant decrease in disc height. Histologically, disorganization of the AF occurred, and the number of dead cells increased significantly in the AF and cartilage end plate. These changes were not reversible after 28 days of unloading.

#### Torsional Injury Model

Hadjipavlou and associates described a rabbit model involving a torsional injury that leads to accelerated disc degeneration.[35,36] Sixty-five New Zealand rabbits underwent a surgical facetectomy and a 30-degree torsional lumbar injury. The authors noted that within 60 to 90 days the rabbits that received the torsional strain exhibited clear signs of disc changes, including thinning, increased phospholipase $A_2$, and decreased NP volume. The control group (surgical facetectomy without the torsional strain) did not exhibit these findings, which suggests the role of torsional strain as a possible mechanism of disc degeneration.

#### Resection of Spinal Process or Facet Joint

Miyamoto and associates described an easily reproducible cervical spondylosis model in the rat. The authors noted that cervical disc degeneration was accelerated with detachment of the posterior paravertebral muscles from the vertebrae and resection of the spinous processes along with the supraspinous and interspinous ligaments. Pathologic changes that occurred as a result of the instability included proliferation of cartilaginous tissue and fissures in the AF, shrinkage of the NP, disc herniation, and osteophytic formation.[37]

Facetectomy studies have been performed by Sullivan and associates[38] in the lumbar spine of immature white rabbits. The authors resected the inferior articular process on one side at a selected vertebral level and on the opposite side at the adjacent level. The disc height was decreased at the surgical level in 50% of the discs at 6 months and 74% at 12 months. The discs in the transverse plane at 9 to 12 months showed thinning of the posterior AF, circumferential slits in the peripheral AF, and an increased area and decreased organization of the NP. The facet joints opposite the facetectomy began to show degeneration at 6 months. The authors concluded that the posterior facet joint protects the intervertebral disc against rotational stresses.

### Adjacent-Level Lumbar Fusion

Phillips and associates described a noninjury rabbit model of disc degeneration. Disc degeneration was created at levels proximal (L4-L5) and caudal (L7-S1) to a simulated lumbar fusion and was studied for up to 9 months after arthrodesis.[39] Loss of the normal parallel arrangement of collagen bundles within the annular lamellae was observed in intervertebral discs adjacent to the fusion at 3 months. At 9 months of follow-up, the disc had been replaced by disorganized fibrous tissue. An initial cellular proliferative response was subsequently followed by a loss of chondrocytes and notochordal cells in the NP. Degeneration was accompanied by a decrease in the monomer size of proteoglycans.

### Annulotomy

Annulotomies have been performed both anteriorly and posteriorly in a variety of methods. The annular puncture model of the rabbit intervertebral disc has become a popular and easily reproducible model of disc degeneration. Although Lipson was the first to biochemically analyze the effects of annulotomies, the earliest work in this area was performed by Keyes and Compere in 1930.[40] Both authors described artificially induced injuries to the AF (radiographically and visually) that were noted to be similar to human disc degeneration. Smith and Walmsley[41] performed a similar study, prompted by the superficial healing seen after posterior annulotomies in prior studies. Fifty-five immature adult rabbits were grossly and microscopically examined at times ranging from 1 to 25 months after ventral annulotomy. The ventral annulotomy was transverse, mid-disc, 4 mm long, and through the AF into the NP. The authors found that healing occurred in the outermost portion of the lesion and progressive degeneration occurred throughout the disc even though the lesion was only in the anterior part of the AF. In 1970, Haimovici used a similar rabbit annular laceration model to describe the negligible effects of adrenocorticotropic hormone injections repeated every other day.[42]

Lipson and associates were the first to describe the biochemical effects of full-thickness stab injuries to the anterior part of the AF (ventral annulotomy, 2 mm in length, and through the AF into the NP).[43] From each animal, the NP and the anterior AF of the intact disc and the central region of the lesioned disc were removed and analyzed. Biochemical measures included analysis of proteoglycan, water, and hyaluronic acid concentration as well as proteoglycan monomer size and total proteoglycan content. The authors noted that rabbit discs were similar to human discs in some characteristics (water concentration and proteoglycan size) and different in other characteristics (lower hyaluronic acid concentration and percentage of aggregated proteoglycan).

Urayama[44] focused on the topographic distribution of postannulotomy changes within the AF after annulotomies of rabbit discs as described by Lipson,[43] Relative to the control discs, the greatest changes in the AF were in its inner layer; they were more pronounced for light microscopic measures than for electron microscopic measures.

Our research group has recently developed a new rabbit model of mild, reproducible disc degeneration by an annulus needle puncture. The newly developed annulus needle puncture procedure, utilizing 16- to 21-gauge (G) needles with controlled depth, resulted in a slower decrease in disc height than the classical stab procedure. The gauge size significantly affected the degree of disc degeneration by magnetic resonance imaging (MRI) grading and the histologic score of disc degeneration throughout the experimental period. At all three time points, the histologic scores were significantly higher in the 16-G and 18-G groups than in the control group. The radiographic, histologic, and MRI results suggested that the use of 16-G and 18-G needles for puncture produces the most predictable, slowly progressive disc narrowing. This new model may be more useful in studying changes in the biomechanical and biochemical properties of disc degeneration progression and, due to its milder degeneration, is better suited to test biologic therapy.[45–47]

Kompel and associates showed more detailed findings in the MRI using a 16-G needle puncture. The MRI analysis of eight rabbits revealed that 12 weeks after the anterior annular puncture, the mean NP signal intensity ($T_2$-weighted images) of stabbed discs had significantly decreased to approximately 60% of their respective preoperative values ($P < 0.05$). By week 24, the mean NP signal intensity had significantly decreased further to 34% to 54% of the preoperative values.[48]

Annulotomy models have also been extensively evaluated in larger animal models as well. Annulotomy-induced lesions, similar to those discussed previously, were performed in sheep models. Osti and associates[49] studied only partial thickness anterior annulotomies. In 21 adult sheep, a cut was made in the left anterolateral AF of three randomly selected lumbar discs. The cut was parallel and adjacent to the inferior end plate and had a controlled depth of 5 mm. This left the inner third of the AF and the NP intact and closely reproduced the rim Lear lesion. Using 2-year-old merino sheep, the authors noted that, although the outermost AF showed the ability to heal, the defect induced by the cut led initially to deformation and bulging of the collagen bundles and eventually to inner extension of the tear and complete failure. These findings suggested that discrete tears of the outer AF might have a role in the formation of concentric clefts and in accelerating the development of radiating clefts. Peripheral tears of the AF, therefore, may play an important role in the degeneration of the intervertebral joint complex. Overall, the authors concluded that disc degeneration occurred in an outside-in manner with deterioration occurring first in the AF followed by that in the NP.

Porcine annulotomy models have also been reported in the literature. Kaapa and associates[50–52] studied domestic pigs (*Sus scrofa*). Their iatrogenically induced lesion was an anterior midline stab with a No. 11 blade scalpel to a depth of 13 mm. The concentration of total collagen (hydroxyproline [Hyp]), the activities of the two key enzymes in collagen biosynthesis (prolyl-4-hydroxylase [PH] and galactosylhydroxylysyl glucosyltransferase [GGT]) and the concentration of mature collagen cross-links (hydroxypyridinium [HP]) were determined. Considerable morphologic changes were apparent, particularly in the NP, which became small, fibrous, and yellowish. The annular lamellar structure was partially destroyed and had been replaced by granulation tissue in the region of the injury. Pfeiffer and associates[53] analyzed lumbar discs of Gottingen minipigs after more extensive annulotomies, for example, by a window in the AF anterolaterally, which was then plugged by fibrin glue followed by injection of chymopapain. The authors noted intervertebral disc degeneration in all groups by 3 weeks with an associated decrease in intradiscal pressure.

#### End Plate Injury

Holm and associates developed an animal model of disc degeneration induced by an injury to the end plate.[54] The L4 cranial end plate of domestic pigs was perforated into the NP at the center using a 3.5-mm drill bit from the lateral cortex at the midheight of the vertebral body. After 3 months, biochemical analysis of the L3-L4 disc showed a reduction in the water content in the outer AF of the degenerated disc. Morphologically, the loss of the gel-like nature of the NP as well as the delamination of the AF layer was seen. A $T_2$-weighted MR image of the spine showed the loss of MR signal in the NP of the degenerated disc.

#### Muscle Stimulation

Wada and associates evaluated possible overuse injury and its impact on cervical spondylosis. The authors provided a flexion-extension moment to young rabbit spines through electrical stimulation of the trapezius muscle. After 200,000 cycles, the authors noted severe delamination of the AF with an associated osteophyte formation at the same level. No severe degeneration of the NP occurred despite the repetitive loading.[55]

### Chemically or Genetically Induced Animal Models

#### Chemonucleolysis

Various animal models have been evaluated after the application of chemonucleolytic agents.[32,53,56–73] Canine, murine, porcine, and rabbit models have been extensively described in the literature. Kahanovitz and colleagues reported one of the earlier studies regarding the application of chymodiactin to the lumbar spine of canines.[69] Biomechenically, the authors noted a significant decrease in torsional stiffness, as well as loss of anterior and medial-lateral shear stiffness of the L4-L5 interspace. More recently, Norcross described the effects of chondroitinase ABC on the intervertebral disc of the rat tail.[74] The findings were similar to the changes observed in degenerative disc disease: reduced intervertebral disc height, diminished proteoglycan content, loss of NP cells, and increased stiffness of the disc.

#### Fibronectin Fragment Injection

Anderson and associates have shown that an injection of fibronectin fragments induced the degeneration of intervertebral discs in the rabbit.[75] Fibronectin fragments or control substances were injected, and the discs were examined radiographically, histologically, and biochemically, and the gene expression was measured at the 2-, 4-, 8-, 12-, and 16-week time points. A progressive loss of the normal architecture of the NP and AF was observed over the 16-week study period. Similar biochemical results were shown with decreasing proteoglycan content and downregulation of aggrecan mRNA.

#### Smoking

Iwahashi and associates studied the effects of nicotine on vascular buds in rabbits for elucidating the mechanism of nicotine-induced vertebral disc degeneration.[76] The authors used a pump filled with a dilute nicotine solution placed subcutaneously for 8 weeks. The model maintained nicotine blood concentrations at approximately 110 ng/mL. After 8 weeks of nicotine exposure, necrosis and hyalinization of the nucleus pulposus were noted in all the rabbits. The AF demonstrated a pattern of overlapping laminae with clefts and separation. Furthermore, the authors noted necrotic changes in the endothelial cells and narrowing of the vascular lumen. The authors concluded that the reduction in density of the vascular buds and narrowing of the lumen resulted in a decreased oxygen tension, which leads to the decreased synthesis of proteoglycan and collagen, thereby facilitating disc degeneration.

Similar effects of nicotine on rat intervertebral disc degeneration was noted by Oda and associates.[77] The authors exposed 8-week-old rats to indirect tobacco smoke inhalation resulting in blood concentrations twice that of human smokers. After 8 weeks of exposure, the rats were sacrificed and the chondrocytes were noted to have a disordered AF layer that was larger than normal. Furthermore, the interleukin 1(IL-1)β levels were significantly higher than the nonsmoking control group. The authors concluded that nicotine exposure resulted in an increase in local production and release of inflammatory cytokines and resultant decomposition of chondrocyte activity.

#### Knockout Mouse

Human twin studies suggest that particular genes may play a role in disc degeneration.[78] Sahlman and associates evaluated the heterozygous inactivation ("knockout") of the *Col2a1* gene and its role in growth development and disc degeneration.[85] Skeletal tissues of mice with an inactivated allele of the *Col2a1* gene for type II collagen (heterozygous knockout) were studied. The tissues were studied using radiograph analyses; conventional, quantitative, and polarized light microscopy; immunohistochemistry for the major extracellular components; and in situ hybridization for procollagens α1 and α2. The authors found that the gene-deficient mice had shorter limbs, skulls, and spines, as well as thicker and more irregular vertebral end plates. The mice also had a lower concentration of glycosaminoglycans in the AF, in the end plates, and in the vertebral bone than the controls. The authors concluded that gene-deficient mice (heterozygous knockout of *Col2a1*) showed early skeletal manifestations and late degenerative changes resembling human disc degeneration.

Because these mice were deficient in *Col2a1* it is unclear whether the degenerative changes were from improper development during growth or due to *Col2a1* deficiency as an adult. Similar degenerative changes were also observed in the lumbar spine of mice lacking the GDF-8 (myostatin) gene.[79] Hamrick and colleagues noted that there was a loss of proteoglycan staining in the hyaline end plates and inner AF of the knockout mice. Results from this study suggest that increased muscle mass in mice lacking myostatin is associated with increased bone mass as well as degenerative changes in the intervertebral disc.

## CONCLUSION

Many techniques have been applied in order to develop a successful experimental animal model of human disc degeneration. However, no one particular model currently parallels the complex nature of human disc degeneration. Naturally occurring animal models have the drawback that the basis for the high rate of disc degeneration is not known. The availability of animals is based on the rate of occurrence, so a predictable experiment is difficult. Although the interventions in artificial animal models are known, the true relationship of these changes to the actual events leading to disc degeneration in humans is not. The careful comparison of data obtained from an animal model with those from human pathologic specimens will shed light on the detailed mechanisms of disc degeneration. With recent progress in biomechanics, cell biology, and molecular biology, an easily reproducible and valid animal model may help unlock the complex cascade of events surrounding human disc degeneration. Only then might it be possible to offer insight into the prevalent and disabling condition of back pain. Although there is no perfect animal model to study the degeneration and regeneration of the intervertebral disc, when choosing a proper model to prove a therapeutic hypothesis, careful consideration should be given to balancing the humane treatment and judicious use of animals with the potential benefits to humans.

## REFERENCES


1. Ferguson SJ, Steffen T: Biomechanics of the aging spine. Eur Spine J 12(2):S97–S103, 2003.
2. Boos N, Weissbach S, Rohrbach H, et al: Classification of age-related changes in lumbar intervertebral discs: 2002 Volvo Award in basic science. Spine 27(23):2631–2644, 2002.
3. Lotz JC, Hsieh AH, Walsh AL, et al: Mechanobiology of the intervertebral disc. Biochem Soc Trans 30(Pt 6):853–858, 2002.
4. Ariga K, Miyamoto S, Nakase T, et al: The relationship between apoptosis of endplate chondrocytes and aging and degeneration of the intervertebral disc. Spine 26(22):2414–2420, 2001.
5. Gruber HE, Hanley EN Jr: Ultrastructure of the human intervertebral disc during aging and degeneration: comparison of surgical and control specimens. Spine 27(8):798–805, 2002.
6. Roughley PJ, Alini M, Antoniou J: The role of proteoglycans in aging, degeneration and repair of the intervertebral disc. Biochem Soc Trans 30(Pt 6):869–874, 2002.
7. Oegema TR Jr: Biochemistry of the intervertebral disc. Clin Sports Med 12(3):419–439, 1993.
8. Hunter CJ, Matyas JR, Duncan NA: The functional significance of cell clusters in the notochordal nucleus pulposus: Survival and signaling in the canine intervertebral disc. Spine 29(10):1099–1104, 2004.
9. Kim KW, Ha KY, Park JB, et al: Expressions of membrane-type I matrix metalloproteinase, Ki-67 protein, and type II collagen by chondrocytes migrating from cartilage endplate into nucleus pulposus in rat intervertebral discs: A cartilage endplate-fracture model using an intervertebral disc organ culture. Spine 30(12):1373–1378, 2005.
10. Kim KW, Kim YS, Ha KY, et al: An autocrine or paracrine Fas-mediated counterattack: A potential mechanism for apoptosis of notochordal cells in intact rat nucleus pulposus. Spine 30(11):1247–1251, 2005.
11. Kim KW, Lim TH, Kim JG, et al: The origin of chondrocytes in the nucleus pulposus and histologic findings associated with the transition of a notochordal nucleus pulposus to a fibrocartilaginous nucleus pulposus in intact rabbit intervertebral discs. Spine 28(10):982–990, 2003.
12. Silberberg R, Aufdermaur M, Adler JH: Degeneration of the intervertebral disks and spondylosis in aging sand rats. Arch Pathol Lab Med 103(5):231–235, 1979.
13. Adler JH, Schoenbaum M, Silberberg R: Early onset of disk degeneration and spondylosis in sand rats (*Psammomys obesus*). Vet Pathol 20(1):13–22, 1983.
14. Moskowitz RW, Ziv I, Denko CW, et al: Spondylosis in sand rats: A model of intervertebral disc degeneration and hyperostosis. J Orthop Res 8(3):401–411, 1990.
15. Ziv I, Moskowitz RW, Kraise I, et al: Physicochemical properties of the aging and diabetic sand rat intervertebral disc. J Orthop Res 10(2):205–210, 1992.
16. Gruber HE, Johnson T, Norton HJ, Hanley EN Jr: The sand rat model for disc degeneration: Radiologic characterization of age-related changes: Cross-sectional and prospective analyses. Spine 27(3):230–234, 2002.
17. Gruber HE, Johnson TL, Leslie K, et al: Autologous intervertebral disc cell implantation: A model using *Psammomys obesus*, the sand rat. Spine 27(15):1626–1633, 2002.
18. Berry R: Genetically controlled degeneration of the nucleus pulposus in the mouse. J Bone Joint Surg 43B:387–393, 1961.
19. Silberberg R, Gerritsen G: Aging changes in intervertebral discs and spondylosis in Chinese hamsters. Diabetes 25(6):477–483, 1976.
20. Kim KS, Yoon ST, Li J, et al: Disc degeneration in the rabbit: A biochemical and radiological comparison between four disc injury models. Spine 30(1):33–37, 2005.
21. Cole TC, Ghosh P, Taylor TK: Variations of the proteoglycans of the canine intervertebral disc with ageing. Biochim Biophys Acta 880(2–3):209–219, 1986.
22. Goggin JE, Li AS, Franti CE: Canine intervertebral disk disease: Characterization by age, sex, breed, and anatomic site of involvement. Am J Vet Res 31(9):1687–1692, 1970.
23. Ghosh P, Taylor TK, Braund KG, Larsen LH: The collagenous and non-collagenous protein of the canine intervertebral disc and their variation with age, spinal level and breed. Gerontology 22(3):124–134, 1976.
24. Gillett NA, Gerlach R, Cassidy JJ, Brown SA: Age-related changes in the beagle spine. Acta Orthop Scand 59(5):503–507, 1988.
25. Lauerman WC, Platenberg RC, Cain JE, Deeney VF: Age-related disk degeneration: Preliminary report of a naturally occurring baboon model. J Spinal Disord 5(2):170–174, 1992.
26. Goff C, Landmesser W: Bipedal rats and mice: Laboratory animals for orthopaedic research. J Bone Joint Surg 39A:616–622, 1957.
27. Yamada K: The dynamics of experimental posture: Experimental study of intervertebral disk herniation in bipedal animals. Clin Orthop 25:20–31, 1962.
28. Higuchi M, Abe K, Kaneda K: Changes in the nucleus pulposus of the intervertebral disc in bipedal mice. A light and electron microscopic study. Clin Orthop 1983(175):251–257, 1962.
29. Cassidy JD, Yong-Hing K, Kirkaldy-Willis WH, Wilkinson AA: A study of the effects of bipedism and upright posture on the lumbosacral spine and paravertebral muscles of the Wistar rat. Spine 13(3):301–308, 1988.
30. Hutton WC, Yoon ST, Elmer WA, et al: Effect of tail suspension (or simulated weightlessness) on the lumbar intervertebral disc: Study of proteoglycans and collagen. Spine 27(12):1286–1290, 2002.
31. Lotz J, Colliou O, Chin J, et al: Compression-induced degeneration of the intervertebral disc: An in vivo mouse model and finite element study. Spine 23(23):2493–2506, 1998.

32. Iatridis JC, Mente PL, Stokes IA, et al: Compression-induced changes in intervertebral disc properties in a rat tail model. Spine 24(10):996–1002, 1999.
33. Ching CT, Chow DH, Yao FY, Holmes AD: The effect of cyclic compression on the mechanical properties of the inter-vertebral disc: An in vivo study in a rat tail model. Clin Biomech (Bristol, Avon) 18(3):182–189, 2003.
34. Kroeber MW, Unglaub F, Wang H, et al: New in vivo animal model to create intervertebral disc degeneration and to investigate the effects of therapeutic strategies to stimulate disc regeneration. Spine 27(23):2684–2690, 2002.
35. Hadjipavlou AG, Simmons JW, Yang JP, et al: Torsional injury resulting in disc degeneration in the rabbit, II: Associative changes in dorsal root ganglion and spinal cord neurotransmitter production. J Spinal Disord 11(4):318–321, 1998.
36. Hadjipavlou AG, Simmons JW, Yang JP, et al: Torsional injury resulting in disc degeneration, I: An in vivo rabbit model. J Spinal Disord 11(4):312–317, 1998.
37. Miyamoto S, Yonenobu K, Ono K: Experimental cervical spondylosis in the mouse. Spine 16(10):S495–500, 1991.
38. Sullivan J, Farfan H, Kahn D: Pathologic changes with intervertebral joint rotational instability in the rabbit. Can J Surg 14:71–79, 1971.
39. Phillips FM, Reuben J, Wetzel FT: Intervertebral disc degeneration adjacent to a lumbar fusion: An experimental rabbit model. J Bone Joint Surg Br 84(2):289–294, 2002.
40. Keyes D, Compere E: The normal and pathological physiology of the nucleus pulposus of the intervertebral disc: An anatomical, clinical, and experimental study. J Bone Joint Surg 14:897–938, 1932.
41. Smith J, Walmsley R: Experimental incision of the intervertebral disc. J Bone Joint Surg 33B:612–625, 1951.
42. Haimovici EH: Experimental disc lesion in rabbits: The effect of repeated ACTH administration. Acta Orthop Scand 41(5):505–521, 1970.
43. Lipson SJ, Muir H: Experimental intervertebral disc degeneration: Morphologic and proteoglycan changes over time. Arthritis Rheum 24(1):12–21, 1981.
44. Urayama S: Histological and ultrastructural study of degeneration of the lumbar intervertebral disc in the rabbit following nucleotomy, with special reference to the topographical distribution pattern of the degeneration. Nippon Seikeigeka Gakkai Zasshi 60:649–662, 1986.
45. Aota Y, Masuda K, Nguyen C, et al: Radiological and MRI analyses of a novel rabbit model: A mild, progressive disc degeneration. Ortho Res Soc Trans 27:118, 2002.
46. Muehleman C, Masuda K, Imai Y, et al: Histological assessment of a novel needle puncture model: A mild, progressive intervertebral disc degeneration. Ortho Res Soc Trans 28:86, 2003.
47. Masuda K, Aota Y, Muehleman C, et al: A novel rabbit model of mild, reproducible disc degeneration by an annulus needle puncture: Correlation between the degree of disc injury and radiological and histological appearances of disc degeneration. Spine 30(1):5–14, 2005.
48. Kompel J, Sobajima S, Clarke C, et al: MRI and histological analysis of a rabbit model of disc degeneration. Ortho Res Soc Trans 28:253, 2003.
49. Osti OL, Vernon-Roberts B, Fraser RD: 1990 Volvo Award in experimental studies: Anulus tears and intervertebral disc degeneration. An experimental study using an animal model. Spine 15(8):762–767, 1990.
50. Kaapa E, Holm S, Han X, et al: Collagens in the injured porcine intervertebral disc. J Orthop Res 12(1):93–102, 1994.
51. Kaapa E, Zhang LQ, Muona P, et al: Expression of type I, III, and VI collagen mRNAs in experimentally injured porcine intervertebral disc. Connect Tissue Res 30(3):203–214, 1994.
52. Kaapa E, Gronblad M, Holm S, et al: Neural elements in the normal and experimentally injured porcine intervertebral disk. Eur Spine J 3(3):137–142, 1994.
53. Pfeiffer M, Griss P, Franke P: Degeneration model of the porcine lumbar motion segment: Effects of various intradiscal procedures. Eur Spine J 3:8–16, 1994.
54. Holm S, Holm AK, Ekstrom L, et al: Experimental disc degeneration due to endplate injury. J Spinal Disord Tech 17(1):64–71, 2004.
55. Wada E, Ebara S, Saito S, Ono K: Experimental spondylosis in the rabbit spine: Overuse could accelerate the spondylosis. Spine 17(3): S1–S6, 1992.
56. Zook BC, Kobrine AI: Effects of collagenase and chymopapain on spinal nerves and intervertebral discs of cynomolgus monkeys. J Neurosurg 64(3):474–483, 1986.
57. Kato F, Iwata H, Mimatsu K, Miura T: Experimental chemonucleolysis with chondroitinase ABC. Clin Orthop 1990(253):301–308, 1986.
58. Takahashi T, Nakayama M, Chimura S, et al: Treatment of canine intervertebral disc displacement with chondroitinase ABC. Spine 22 (13):1435–1439; discussion 1446–1447, 1997.
59. Takahashi T, Kurihara H, Nakajima S, et al: Chemonucleolytic effects of chondroitinase ABC on normal rabbit intervertebral discs. Course of action up to 10 days postinjection and minimum effective dose. Spine 21(21):2405–2411, 1996.
60. Sumida K, Sato K, Aoki M, et al: Serial changes in the rate of proteoglycan synthesis after chemonucleolysis of rabbit intervertebral discs. Spine 24(11):1066–1070, 1999.
61. Spencer DL, Miller JA, Schultz AB: The effects of chemonucleolysis on the mechanical properties of the canine lumbar disc. Spine 10 (6):555–561, 1985.
62. Sasaki M, Takahashi T, Miyahara K, Hirosea T: Effects of chondroitinase ABC on intradiscal pressure in sheep: An in vivo study. Spine 26(5):463–468, 2001.
63. Ono A, Harata S, Takagaki K, Endo M: Proteoglycans in the nucleus pulposus of canine intervertebral discs after chondroitinase ABC treatment. J Spinal Disord 11(3):253–260, 1998.
64. Olmarker K, Rydevik B, Dahlin LB, et al: Effects of epidural and intrathecal application of collagenase in the lumbar spine: An experimental study in rabbits. Spine 12(5):477–482, 1987.
65. Nitobe T, Harata S, Okamoto Y, et al: Degradation and biosynthesis of proteoglycans in the nucleus pulposus of canine intervertebral disc after chymopapain treatment. Spine 13(11):1332–1339, 1988.
66. Miyabayashi T, Lord PF, Dubielzig RR, et al: Chemonucleolysis with collagenase: A radiographic and pathologic study in dogs. Vet Surg 21(3):189–194, 1992.
67. Lu DS, Shono Y, Oda I, et al: Effects of chondroitinase ABC and chymopapain on spinal motion segment biomechanics: An in vivo biomechanical, radiologic, and histologic canine study. Spine 22(16):1828–1834; discussion 1834–1835, 1997.
68. Kudo T, Sumi A, Hashimoto A: Experimental chemonucleolysis with chymopapain in canine intervertebral disks. J Vet Med Sci 55 (2):211–215, 1993.
69. Kahanovitz N, Arnoczky SP, Kummer F: The comparative biomechanical, histologic, and radiographic analysis of canine lumbar discs treated by surgical excision or chemonucleolysis. Spine 10 (2):178–183, 1985.
70. Ishikawa H, Nohara Y, Miyauti S: Action of chondroitinase ABC on epidurally transplanted nucleus pulposus in the rabbit. Spine 24 (11):1071–1076, 1999.
71. Henderson N, Stanescu V, Cauchoix J: Nucleolysis of the rabbit intervertebral disc using chondroitinase ABC. Spine 16(2):203–208, 1991.
72. Henderson N, Stanescu V, Cauchoix J: [Nucleolytic action of chondroitinase ABC on the lumbar disc of the rabbit]. C R Acad Sci III 307(7):403–406, 1988.
73. Fry TR, Eurell JC, Johnson AL, et al: Radiographic and histologic effects of chondroitinase ABC on normal canine lumbar intervertebral disc. Spine 16(7):816–819, 1991.
74. Norcross JP, Lester GE, Weinhold P, Dahners LE: An in vivo model of degenerative disc disease. J Orthop Res 21(1):183–188, 2003.
75. Anderson GD, Li X, Tannoury T, et al: A fibronectin fragment stimulates intervertebral disc degeneration in vivo. Spine 28(20):2338–2345, 2003.
76. Iwahashi M, Matsuzaki H, Tokuhashi Y, et al: Mechanism of intervertebral disc degeneration caused by nicotine in rabbits to explicate intervertebral disc disorders caused by smoking. Spine 27 (13):1396–1401, 2002.

77. Oda H, Matsuzaki H, Tokuhashi Y, et al: Degeneration of intervertebral discs due to smoking: Experimental assessment in a rat-smoking model. J Orthop Sci 9(2):135–141, 2004.
78. Sambrook PN, MacGregor AJ, Spector TD: Genetic influences on cervical and lumbar disc degeneration: a magnetic resonance imaging study in twins. Arthritis Rheum 42(2):366–372, 1999.
79. Hamrick MW, Pennington C, Byron CD: Bone architecture and disc degeneration in the lumbar spine of mice lacking GDF-8 (myostatin). J Orthop Res 21(6):1025–1032, 2003.
80. Ziran BH, Pineda S, Pokharna H, et al: Biomechanical, radiologic, and histopathologic correlations in the pathogenesis of experimental intervertebral disc disease. Spine 19(19):2159–2163, 1994.
81. Bradford DS, Cooper KM, Oegema TR Jr: Chymopapain, chemonucleolysis, and nucleus pulposus regeneration. J Bone Joint Surg Am 65(9):1220–1231, 1983.
82. Bradford DS, Oegema TR Jr, Cooper KM, et al: Chymopapain, chemonucleolysis, and nucleus pulposus regeneration: A biochemical and biomechanical study. Spine 9(2):135–147, 1984.
83. Eurell JA, Brown MD, Ramos M: The effects of chondroitinase ABC on the rabbit intervertebral disc: A roentgenographic and histologic study. Clin Orthop 256:238–243, 1990.
84. Takenaka Y, Revel M, Kahan A, Amor B: Experimental model of disc herniations in rats for study of nucleolytic drugs. Spine 12 (6):556–560, 1987.
85. Sahlman J, Inkinen R, Hirvonen T, et al: Premature vertebral endplate ossification and mild disc degeneration in mice after inactivation of one allele belonging to the Col2a1 gene for Type II collagen. Spine 26 (23):2558–2565, 2001.

CHAPTER 84

# Growth Factors for Intervertebral Disc Regeneration

Koichi Masuda and Howard S. An

## KEY POINTS

- In vitro, growth factors, such as bone morphogenetic protein-7 and growth and differentiation factor-5, enhanced cell proliferation and the synthesis and accumulation of proteoglycan and collagen by bovine and human nucleus pulposus and annulus fibrosus cells cultured in alginate beads.
- In vivo, a single injection of a growth factor into the nucleus pulposus resulted in improved radiographic findings and MRI and histologic grades of intervertebral discs in the rabbit annular-puncture disc degeneration model.
- The findings of the biomechanical study provided evidence that an injection of a growth factor restored the biomechanical properties of degenerated discs in the rabbit annular-puncture disc degeneration model.
- The biomechanical and biochemical data in these studies suggested that an injection of a growth factor induced biochemical changes by anabolic stimulation, which may have resulted in the biomechanical restoration of the intervertebral disc.
- Although further efficacy studies with larger animals and studies using pain as a primary end point for a therapeutic approach for disc degeneration are needed, the preliminary evidence in these rabbit studies established that an injection of a growth factor may be clinically applicable as a therapeutic approach to repair the degenerated intervertebral disc.

## MAINTENANCE OF MATRIX HOMEOSTASIS IN THE INTERVERTEBRAL DISC: GROWTH FACTORS AND OTHER BIOLOGIC MOLECULES

Biologically, disc cells actively regulate disc tissue homeostasis by maintaining a balance between anabolism and catabolism. The activity of disc cells is modulated by a variety of substances, including cytokines, growth factors, enzymes, and enzyme inhibitors, in a paracrine or autocrine fashion.[1,2] Recent therapeutic strategies for disc degeneration have included attempts to upregulate important extracellular matrix components (i.e., aggrecan)[3,4] or to downregulate proinflammatory cytokines (i.e., interleukin 1 [IL-1] or tumor necrosis factor-α [TNF-α])[5–12] and matrix-degrading enzymes (i.e., matrix metalloproteinases [MMPs] and members of a *d*isintegrin-like and *m*etalloprotease with *t*hrombo*s*pondin motifs (ADAMTS) family (aggrecanases).[13–15] It may be possible that a combination of both strategies could be most efficacious.

As the name implies, growth factors play an important role in the development of the spine. Interestingly, several growth factors have been found in normal and degenerated intervertebral disc (IVD) tissues, suggesting that IVD cells are capable of expressing and producing growth factors. These factors include insulin-like growth factor-1 (IGF-1),[16,17] basic fibroblast growth factor (bFGF),[18–21] bone morphogenetic-2 (BMP-2),[22] BMP-4,[22,23] growth differentiation factor-5 (GDF-5),[23] platelet-derived growth factor (PDGF),[24] and transforming growth factor-β (TGF-β).[17,25–29] Taken together, the autocrine and paracrine production of growth factors is considered to be a major regulatory mechanism in IVD tissues.[16]

For delivering therapeutic biologic agents into IVD tissue, several methods of administration can be considered. The direct injection of a protein is relatively simple and practical; however, the efficiency, duration of action, and possibility of adverse effects are not currently known. To regenerate or repair a degenerated IVD, the injection of protein anabolic factors would be a simple and practical approach. However, several issues, such as half-life, solubility of the protein, a proper carrier, and a presence of inhibitors, etc., need to be taken into consideration. In the past, the half-life of an injected protein was considered to be very short, in the order of minutes.[30] However, recent research by our group, in collaboration with Stryker Biotech (Hopkinton, MA), revealed that the half-life of injected radiolabeled osteogenic protein-1 (OP-1, otherwise known as BMP-7) was greater than the 1 month observation period; this result may support our contention that a simple protein injection may have therapeutic efficacy.

The preclinical development of an injection of an anabolic factor is one of the most advanced in the biologic treatment of disc diseases. In fact, the first investigational new drug study to test the safety and efficacy of OP-1 has been initiated.

## IN VITRO EVIDENCE FOR THE POSSIBLE THERAPEUTIC ROLE OF GROWTH FACTORS IN DEGENERATIVE DISC DISEASE

A disruption of disc tissue homeostasis may be achieved by stimulating matrix synthesis with cytokines or growth factors, resulting in a shift of cellular metabolism to the anabolic state.[1] Others have shown that the rate of proteoglycan (PG) synthesis by IVD cells increases several-fold by the addition of TGF-β and epidermal growth factor (EGF).[31,32] IGF-1 was found to stimulate matrix synthesis and proliferation in vitro.[16] Using human IVD cells in three-dimensional culture, Gruber and associates first demonstrated that, after 4 days' exposure, TGF-β stimulated cell proliferation by annulus fibrosus (AF) cells.[32] These authors also reported that IGF-1 and PDGF significantly reduced the percentage of apoptotic AF cells induced by serum depletion during culture.[33]

More recently, we have shown that OP-1 enhanced the PG metabolism of IVD cells.[34,35] OP-1, a member of the TGF-β superfamily, was initially found to exert potent effects on osteocyte and chondrocyte differentiation and metabolism.[36,37] In chondrocytes, OP-1 stimulated the synthesis of PGs and type II collagen.[38,39] A series of studies by our laboratory has demonstrated that OP-1 strongly stimulated the production and formation of extracellular matrix molecules, including PGs and collagen, by rabbit IVD cells,[34] as well as by human IVD cells in vitro (Fig. 84–1).[35] After depletion of the extracellular matrix following exposure of IVD cells to IL-1, OP-1 was also found to be effective in the replenishment of a matrix rich in PGs and collagens.[40] A similar result with OP-1 was reported when the matrix was first depleted by in vitro chemonucleolysis using chondroitinase ABC.[41]

Another BMP, BMP-2, stimulated matrix production and cell proliferation by rat IVD cells.[42] Using human IVD cells, Kim and associates reported that BMP-2 facilitated the expression of the chondrogenic phenotype, increased PG synthesis, and upregulated the expression of aggrecan, collagen type I, and collagen type II mRNA, compared to untreated control levels.[43]

GDF-5, another member of the BMP family, was originally found to be a factor responsible for skeletal alterations in brachypodism mice.[44] Recently, an analysis of GDF-5-deficient mice revealed the presence of disc degeneration, as well as a loss of PGs from the IVD.[45] GDF-5 was also shown to stimulate PG and type II collagen expression in mouse IVD cells.[45] Furthermore, we have shown that recombinant human GDF-5 (rhGDF-5) enhanced cell proliferation and matrix synthesis and accumulation by both bovine nucleus pulposus (NP) and AF cells. The response to rhGDF-5 was greater by NP cells than by AF cells (Fig. 84–2).[3]

The application of autologous growth factors may be advantageous for the clinical treatment of degenerative disc disease. Wehling and colleagues showed that the combination of autologous IL-1 receptor antagonist (IL-1ra)/IGF-1/PDGF proteins reduced the percentage of apoptosis and the production of IL-1 and IL-6 by IVD cells.[46]

Platelet-rich plasma (PRP), which is a fraction of plasma that can be produced by centrifugal separation of whole blood in the operating room, contains multiple growth factors concentrated at high levels.[47–50] In porcine NP and AF cells cultured in alginate beads, PRP was found to be an effective stimulator of cell proliferation, PG and collagen synthesis, as well as PG accumulation (Fig. 84–3).[51]

## IN VIVO STUDIES FOR THE DEVELOPMENT OF GROWTH FACTOR INJECTION THERAPY IN DEGENERATIVE DISC DISEASE

Walsh and associates have reported the in vivo effects of a single injection of several growth factors, including bFGF, GDF-5,

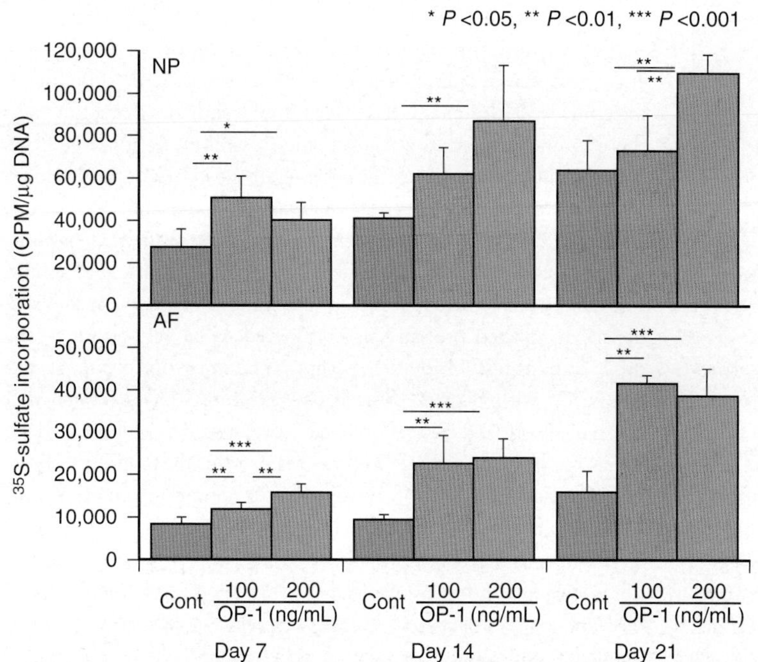


■ **FIGURE 84–1.** The effect of recombinant human osteogenic protein (rhOP-1) on the rate of proteoglycan (PG) synthesis by human nucleus pulposus (NP) and annulus fibrosus (AF) cells cultured in alginate beads. To assess the rate of PG synthesis, the beads were radiolabeled with $^{35}$S-sulfate (20 Ci/mL) for the final 4 hours of culture at each time point. The amount of radiolabeled $^{35}$S-PGs in the cell-associated matrix (CM) and the further removed matrix (FRM) fractions and the media were quantified. The data shown depict the sum of the radiolabeled $^{35}$S-PGs, expressed per μg DNA, found in the CM, FRM, and medium from a representative case (an 84-year-old man). rhOP-1 at 200 ng/mL significantly stimulated PG synthesis by NP and AF cells at all time points. In AF cells, rhOP-1 at 100 ng/mL also significantly stimulated PG synthesis at all time points. *(From Imai Y, Miyamoto K, An H, et al: Recombinant human osteogenic protein-1 upregulates proteoglycan metabolism of human annulus fibrosus and nucleus pulposus cells. Spine 32:1303–1309, 2007.)*

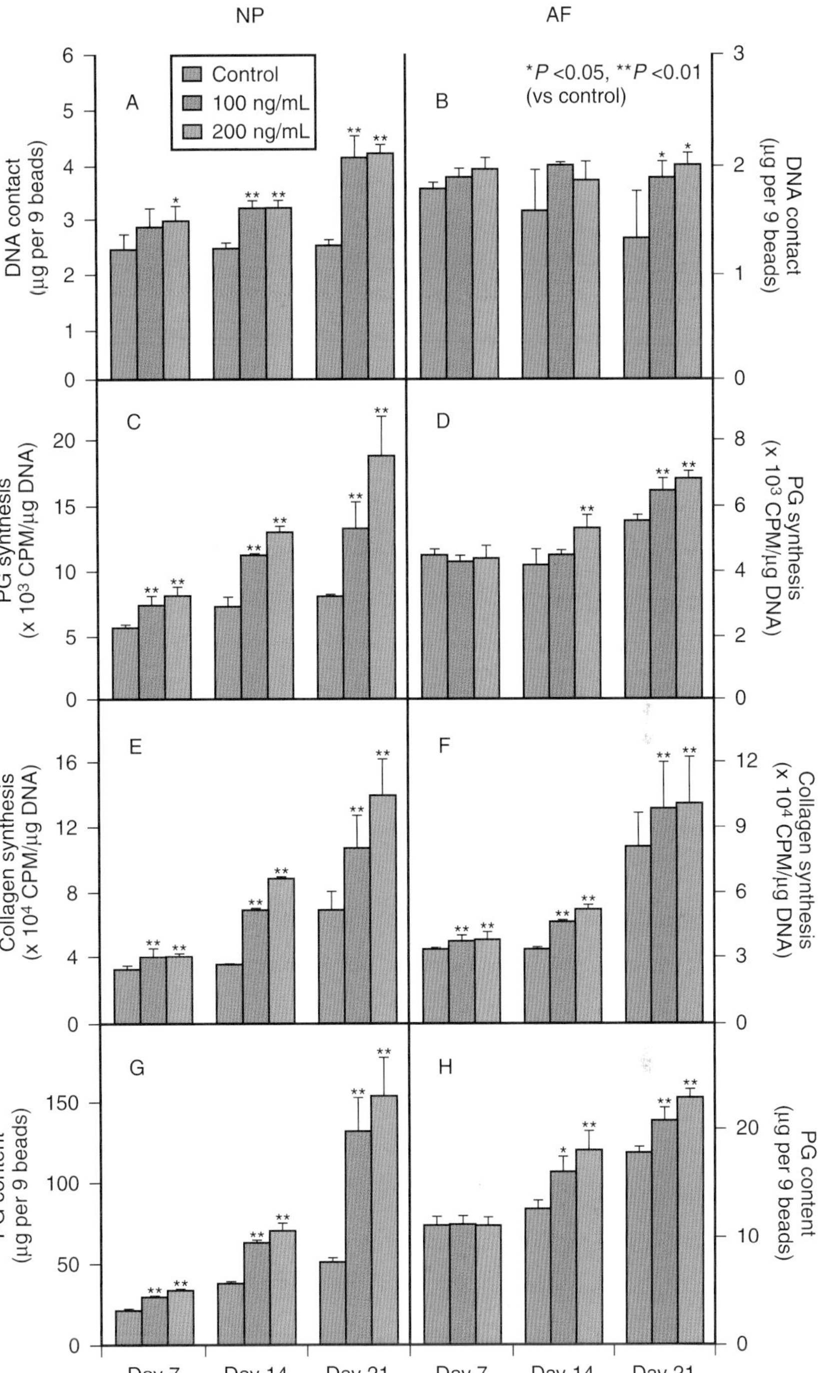


■ **FIGURE 84–2.** The effect of rhGDF-5 on DNA content, proteoglycan (PG) synthesis, collagen synthesis, and PG content by bovine nucleus pulposus (NP) and annulus fibrosus (AF) cells in vitro. **A** and **B,** Cells were cultured in DMEM/F12 + 10% FBS in the presence or absence of 100 and 200 ng/mL of rhGDF-5 for 21 days. The DNA content of alginate beads was significantly higher in the rhGDF-5 group than in the control group at the 14- and 21-day time points with NP cells and only at the 21-day time points with AF cells. **C** and **D,** To assess PG synthesis, beads were radiolabeled with $^{35}$S-sulfate for the final 4 hours of culture at each time point. NP cells treated with rhGDF-5 showed a greater response than AF cells. A dose-dependent effect of rhGDF-5 was observed in NP cells only at day 21. **E** and **F,** Newly synthesized collagens, radiolabeled with $^{3}$H-proline during the final 16 hours of culture, were quantified. The rate of collagen synthesis was significantly higher in the rhGDF-5 groups (100 and 200 ng/mL) than in the control group at all time points in both cell types. **G** and **H,** Cells were cultured in DMEM/F12 +10% FBS in the presence or absence of rhGDF-5 (100 and 200 ng/mL) for up to 21 days. rhGDF-5, at both concentrations, stimulated PG accumulation in beads containing NP cells at all time points and in beads containing AF cells at the 14- and 21-day time points. DMEM, Dulbecco's modified eagle medium; FBS, fetal bovine serum; GDF, growth/differentiation factor 5. *(Used with permission from Chujo T, An HS, Akeda K, et al: Effects of growth differentiation factor-5 on the intervertebral disc—*in vitro *bovine study and* in vivo *rabbit disc degeneration model study. Spine 31(25):2909–2917, 2006.)*

IGF-1, and TGF-β, in the mouse caudal disc with degeneration induced by static compression.[52] An increased cell population was seen only with IGF-1 in the AF. The same group also reported that an injection of GDF-5 was effective in promoting disc regeneration.[53] Multiple injections (four injections, once per week) of TGF-β showed a stimulatory effect on the IVD repair process; the other growth factors studied did not show a significant enhancement of their original effect with multiple injections.[53] The authors suggested that a sustained delivery system or a combined approach with a mechanical or cell-based device was required to achieve a beneficial therapeutic effect with growth factor injection therapy.

## RECOMBINANT HUMAN OSTEOGENIC PROTEIN-1 (rhOP-1)

The results of an in vivo experiment using injections of OP-1 into normal rabbit IVDs also point to the potential therapeutic use of OP-1 in the treatment of degenerative disc disease.[54] In normal rabbits, a single intradiscal injection of OP-1 in vivo has been shown to result in increased disc height and PG content of the NP, neither of which were seen in the saline injection group.[54]

In a rabbit model of disc degeneration, an injection of rhOP-1 into the NP (100 µg/disc) restored the disc height loss and structural changes caused by an annular needle puncture (Fig. 84–4A).[4]

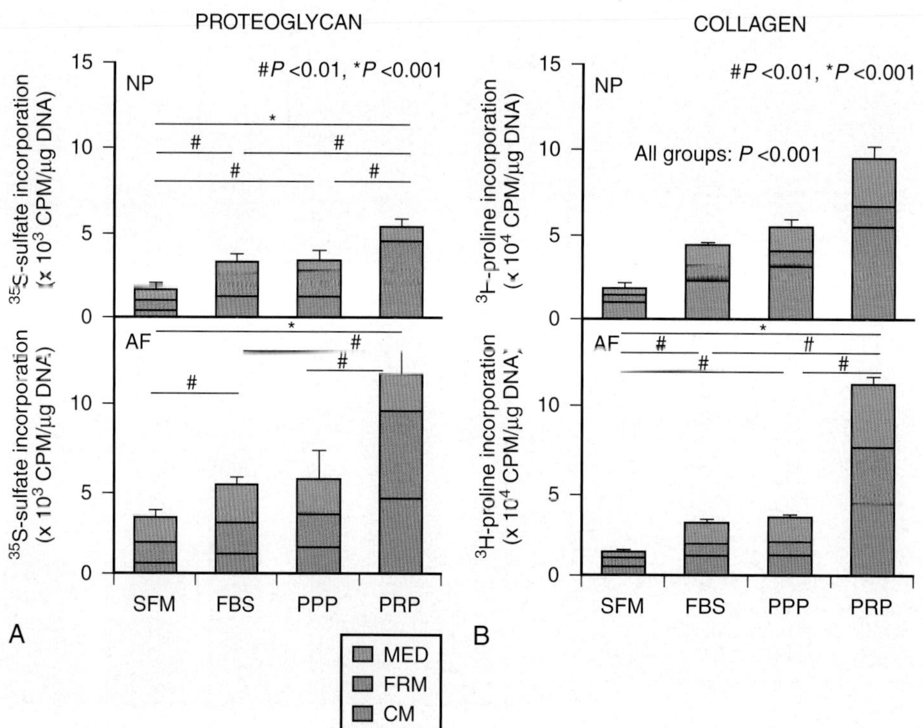


■ **FIGURE 84–3.** Effect of platelet-rich plasma (PRP) on **(A)** proteoglycan (PG) and **(B)** collagen synthesis of porcine intervertebral disc cells. Porcine nucleus pulposus (NP) and annulus fibrosus (AF) cells were cultured in alginate beads. During the last 4 hours of the 72-hour treatment period, the cells were radiolabeled with $^{35}$S-sulfate (20 μCi/mL). The beads were dissolved in sodium citrate buffer, and after mild centrifugation, the cells and their cell-associated matrix (CM) and further removed matrix (FRM) were collected. The amount of radiolabeled $^{35}$S-PGs in the CM, the FRM fraction, and the media were quantified. PG synthesis by the PRP-treated NP and AF cells was significantly higher than that by the platelet-poor plasma (PPP)- or fetal bovine serum (FBS)-treated cells. The incorporation of radiolabeled proline into pepsin-resistant protein was measured as an indicator of collagen synthesis. Porcine NP and AF cells were cultured in alginate beads. During the last 16 hours of the 72-hour treatment period, the cultures were radiolabeled with L-[2,3,4,5-$^{3}$H]-proline (50 μCi/mL). The pepsin-resistant radiolabeled proteins were precipitated with trichloroacetic acid and the radioactivity was measured. The stimulatory effect on the rate of collagen synthesis was greater in the case of PRP-treated cells than in the case of cells treated with PPP or FBS. *(Modified from Akeda K, An HS, Pichika R, et al: Platelet-rich plasma (PRP) stimulates the extracellular matrix metabolism of porcine nucleus pulposus and anulus fibrosus cells cultured in alginate beads. Spine 31(9):959–966, 2006.)*

The annular puncture induced a consistent disc narrowing within 4 weeks. The injection of OP-1, but not lactose, resulted in the restoration of disc height at 6 weeks; this was sustained for the entire experimental period up to 24 weeks after the injection. The MRI grading score showed significant differences between the OP-1-injected and the lactose-injected groups at the 8-, 12- and 24-week time points, suggesting increased water content of the NP in the OP-1 group (Fig. 84–4B). Histologically, the degeneration grades of the punctured discs in the OP-1-injected group were significantly lower than those in the lactose-injected group.

Importantly, the effects of the OP-1 injection on disc height in this study were sustained for up to 6 months after the injection (Fig. 84–4B). The results clearly demonstrated the feasibility of restoring degenerative rabbit discs by a single injection of OP-1 into the NP. The metabolic changes in the cells, following a single injection, might be sustained and thus could induce long-term changes in disc structure.

Using a newly developed dynamic viscoelastic property testing system, we have also demonstrated that an intradiscal injection of OP-1 restored the disc heights (Fig. 84–5) and the biomechanical properties of degenerated IVDs in the rabbit annular puncture model of disc degeneration (Fig. 84–6).[55] The lateral radiographs indicated that the disc space, which showed narrowing 4 weeks after the annular needle puncture, was restored in the OP-1-injected level (Fig. 84–5B). The injection of OP-1 was performed as described previously. The intradiscal injection of OP-1 significantly increased the disc height in the postinjection time course ($P < 0.0001$) (Fig. 84–5B). The viscoelastic properties of the OP-1-injected, the lactose-injected, and the nonpunctured control discs were measured. As a result, the elastic modulus (E′) in the lactose group (triangle) was significantly lower than that in the control group (closed circle) at all loading frequencies (mean: 64% of control, $P < 0.001$). At all loading frequencies, E′ in the OP-1 group was significantly higher than that in the lactose group (mean: +43%, $P < 0.05$) and approached that of the nonpunctured control disc (open circle, OP-1 vs. nonpunctured control, n.s.) (Fig. 84–6A, top panel). The viscous modulus (E″) in the OP-1-injected discs (closed circle) was significantly higher than that in the lactose group (triangle)

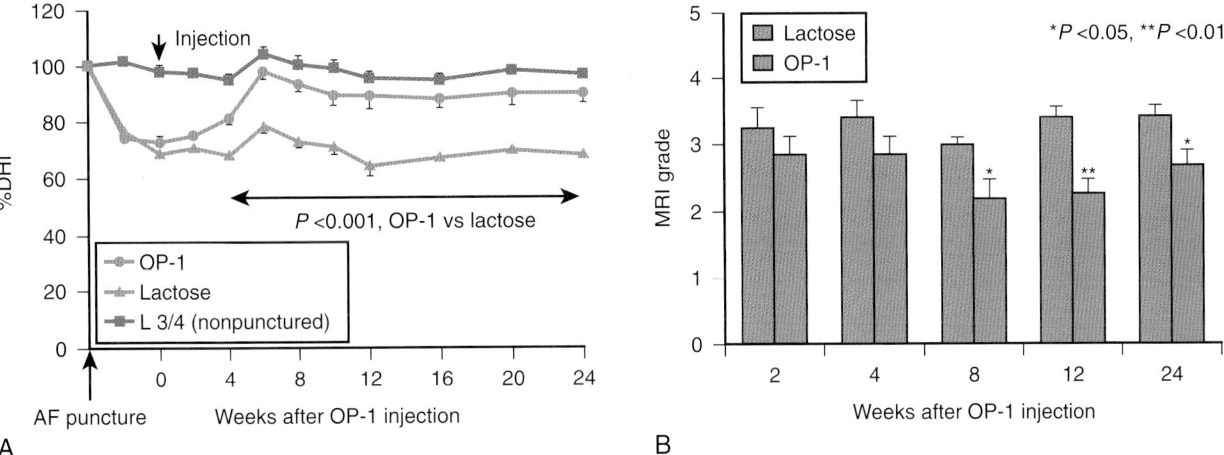


■ **FIGURE 84–4.** Changes in the intervertebral disc height index (DHI, **A)** and magnetic resonance imaging (MRI) grading **(B)** after annular puncture and osteogenic protein-1 (OP-1) injection. Adolescent New Zealand white rabbits (3- to 3.5-kg, 4 to 5 months old) received an annular puncture in two noncontiguous discs with an 18-gauge needle to induce disc degeneration. Four weeks later, either 5% lactose (vehicle control; 10 μL) or osteogenic protein-1 (OP-1; 100 μg in 10 μL 5% lactose) was injected into the center of the nucleus pulposus (NP). The progress of disc degeneration was assessed using the measurement of the percent DHI (%DHI = postoperative DHI/preoperative DHI × 100) radiographically and by MRI scans. By 4 weeks after the OP-1 injection, the mean %DHI of injected discs in the OP-1 group was significantly higher than that in the lactose control group ($P < 0.001$, repeated analysis of variance). This significant difference in mean %DHI was maintained during the follow-up period ($P < 0.001$). MRI examinations were performed on all the spinal columns isolated from the rabbits ex vivo at the time of sacrifice. The magnetic resonance images were evaluated using the modified Thompson classification based on changes in the degree and area of signal intensity from grades 1 to 4. When the degree of disc degeneration by MRI grading was compared between the lactose and OP-1 groups, a significant lower grading of MRI in the OP-1 group was observed ($P < 0.01$, Mann-Whitney U test). *(Modified from Masuda K, Imai Y, Okuma M, et al: Osteogenic protein-1 injection into a degenerated disc induces the restoration of disc height and structural changes in the rabbit annular puncture model. Spine 31(7):742–754, 2006.)*

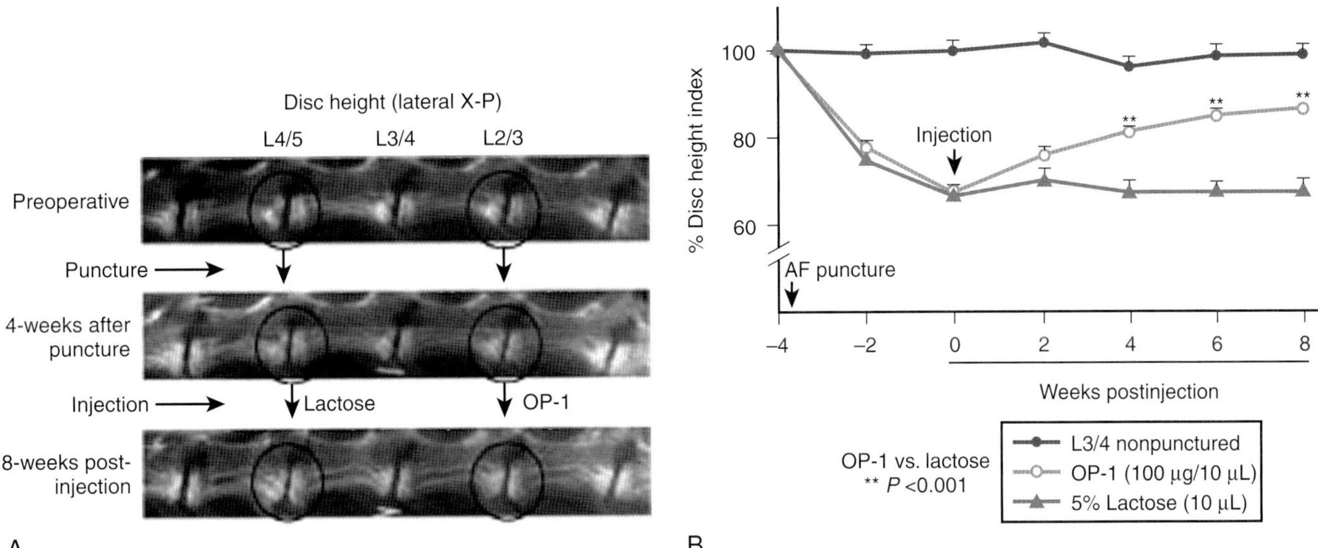


■ **FIGURE 84–5.** Changes in disc height **(A, B)** of intervertebral discs (IVDs) after annular puncture and osteogenic protein-1 (OP-1) injection. New Zealand white rabbits ($n = 16$) underwent annulus fibrosus (AF) puncture, using an 18-gauge needle, at L2-L3 and L4-L5 (L3-L4: nonpunctured control). Four weeks later, the punctured discs received an injection of either 5% lactose (10 μL) or OP-1 (100 μg/10 μL of 5% lactose) into the nucleus pulposus (NP). The progress of disc degeneration was assessed radiographically. The lateral radiographs show that the disc space, which showed narrowing 4 weeks after the annular needle puncture, is restored in the OP-1-injected level, while the narrowing progressed in the lactose-injected level. The graph shows that an annular puncture with an 18-gauge needle decreased the disc height index (DHI) by approximately 32% when compared to the baseline %DHI values before the annular puncture, $P < 0.0001$). The intradiscal injection of OP-1 significantly affected the disc height in the postinjection time course ($P < 0.0001$). *(From Miyamoto K, Masuda K, Kim JG, et al: Intradiscal injections of osteogenic protein-1 restore the viscoelastic properties of degenerated intervertebral discs. Spine J 6(6):692–703, 2006.)*

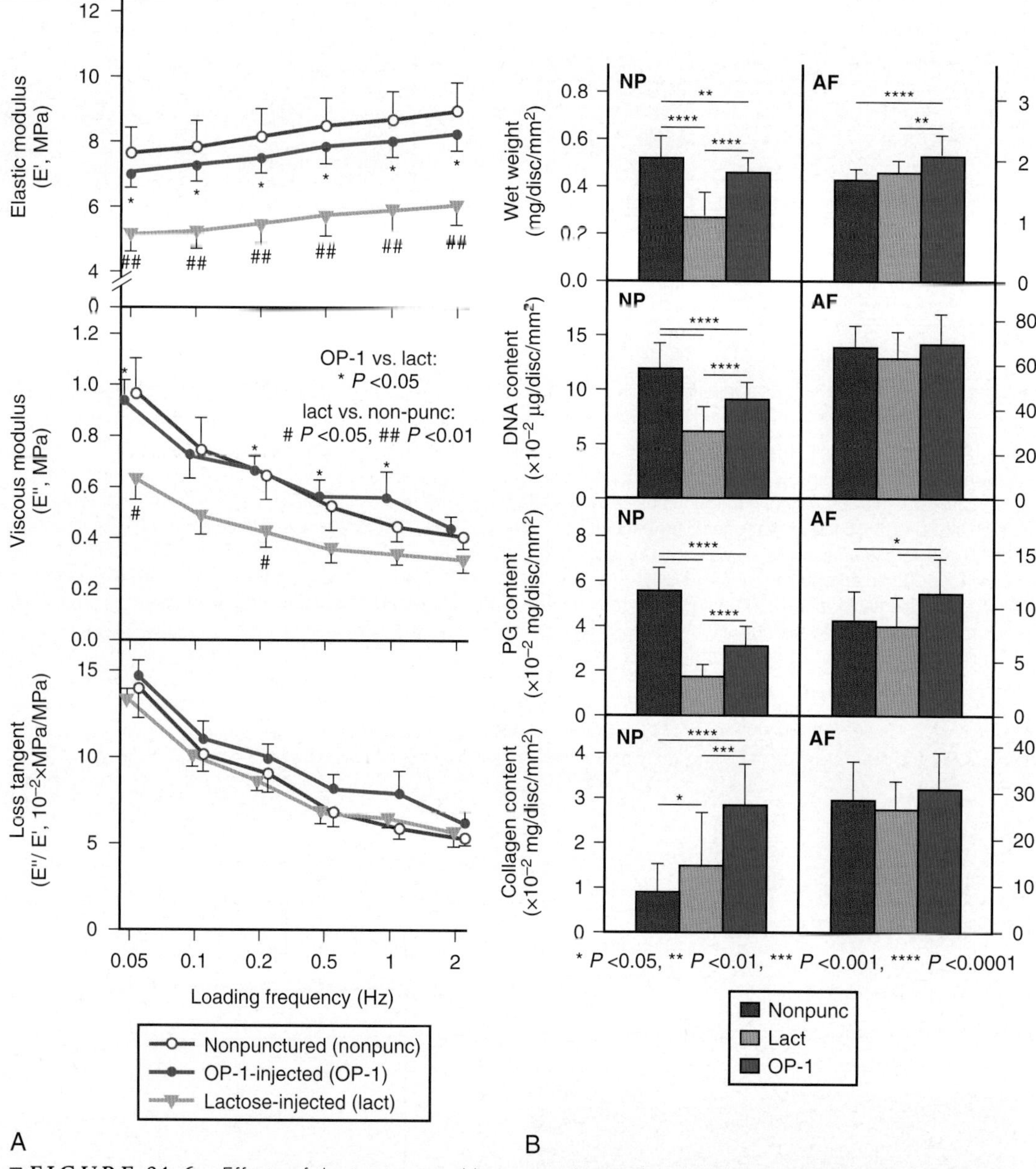


■ **FIGURE 84–6.** Effects of the treatment with osteogenic protein-1 (OP-1) or lactose on the dynamic viscoelastic properties **(A)** and the biochemical properties **(B)** of rabbit intervertebral discs (IVDs). **A,** *Biomechanical properties:* After sacrifice and removal of bone-disc-bone complexes 8 weeks after injection, the dynamic viscoelastic properties of the IVDs were tested by applying a cycle of sinusoidal strain in uniaxial compression at six loading frequencies (0.05 to 2 Hz). Using a custom-made biomechanical testing system, a cycle of sinusoidal strain was applied to each IVD in a uniaxial unconfined compression. After preconditioning by 10 cycles at 1 Hz, six different physiologic loading frequency tests were performed. In the OP-1-injected discs (closed circles), at all loading frequencies, the elastic modulus (E′) was significantly higher than that in the lactose-injected discs (and approached that of the nonpunctured control discs (open circles) (OP-1 vs. nonpunctured control, n.s., upper graph). The viscous modulus (E″) was significantly higher in the OP-1-injected discs (closed circles) than that in the lactose-injected discs (reverse triangles) (middle graph). In both the elastic and the viscous moduli, no significant difference was observed between the OP-1-injected discs and nonpunctured discs at all loading frequencies (upper and middle graphs). No significant difference was observed in the loss tangent (E″/E′) among the nonpunctured control discs and the rhOP-1-injected and lactose-injected discs. **B,** *Biochemical properties:* In the nucleus pulposus, as can be observed in data from the lactose-injected discs, the annular needle puncture induced dramatic decreases in wet weight, DNA content, and proteoglycan (PG) content, while the collagen content was increased (left panel). In the annulus fibrosus, the annular needle puncture did not cause significant changes in any of the four parameters (right panel). The intradiscal injection of OP-1 significantly increased the wet weight and contents of DNA, PG, and collagen in the NP, when compared to the lactose-injected discs. OP-1 also increased the wet weight and PG content of the AF. *(From Miyamoto K, Masuda K, Kim JG, et al: Intradiscal injections of osteogenic protein-1 restore the viscoelastic properties of degenerated intervertebral discs. Spine J 6(6):692–703, 2006.)*

at 0.05, 0.2, and 1 Hz (average: +55%, $P < 0.001$), while showing a strong tendency to be higher at 0.1, 0.5, and 2 Hz ($P = 0.06$–$0.10$) (Fig. 84–6A, middle panel). In both the elastic and the viscous moduli, no significant difference was observed between the OP-1-injected discs and nonpunctured discs at all loading frequencies (Fig. 84–6A, top and middle panels).

PGs and collagen both contribute to the mechanical properties of the NP and AF. PGs endow disc tissues with a fixed negative charge, which results in hydration and swelling of the tissue and the consequent ability to resist compressive loading.[56] To study changes in matrix composition induced by an injection of OP-1, biochemical analyses of the samples used in this biomechanical study were performed. The result revealed that an intradiscal injection of OP-1 resulted in significant increases in wet weight (+57%), DNA content (+48%), PG content (+83%), and collagen content (+76%), compared to the lactose-injected discs, in the NP (Fig. 84–6B, NP, left column). In the AF, significant increases in wet weight (+20%, $P < 0.01$) and PG content (+35%, $P < 0.05$) were also observed (Fig. 84–6B, AF, right column). It is important to note that after the intradiscal injection of OP-1, the PG content in the AF and the collagen content of the NP were significantly higher than those in the nonpunctured control IVDs (PG in the AF: +28%, $P < 0.05$; collagen in the NP: +234%, $P < 0.001$).

When discs from all treatment groups were evaluated together, the elastic modulus (E′) was shown to have a significant positive correlation with the PG content in the NP and the PG and collagen content in the AF (Fig. 84–7, left two panels). Similarly, the viscous modulus was shown to have a significant positive correlation with the PG content in the NP and the PG and collagen content in the AF (Fig. 84–7, right two panels). The positive correlation between the PG content in the NP and the elastic modulus of the IVD suggests that biochemical changes induced by an injection of OP-1 may result in structural and mechanical restoration.

## REGENERATION OF DEGENERATED DISCS AFTER CHEMONUCLEOLYSIS

Intradiscal injections of enzymes (i.e., collagenase[57] or human proteinases[58–62]) have been used to relieve sciatica and low back pain. Recently, chondroitinase ABC (C-ABC), which has a narrow substrate spectrum, and, more importantly, no protease activity, has been studied as an alternative to chymopapain for chemonucleolysis.[63–70] Although matrix regeneration in IVDs treated with C-ABC occurs earlier and to a greater extent than in those treated with chymopapain, disc height and PG content, as well as the biomechanical properties of the disc, do not fully return to normal.[71] In fact, the use of C-ABC was

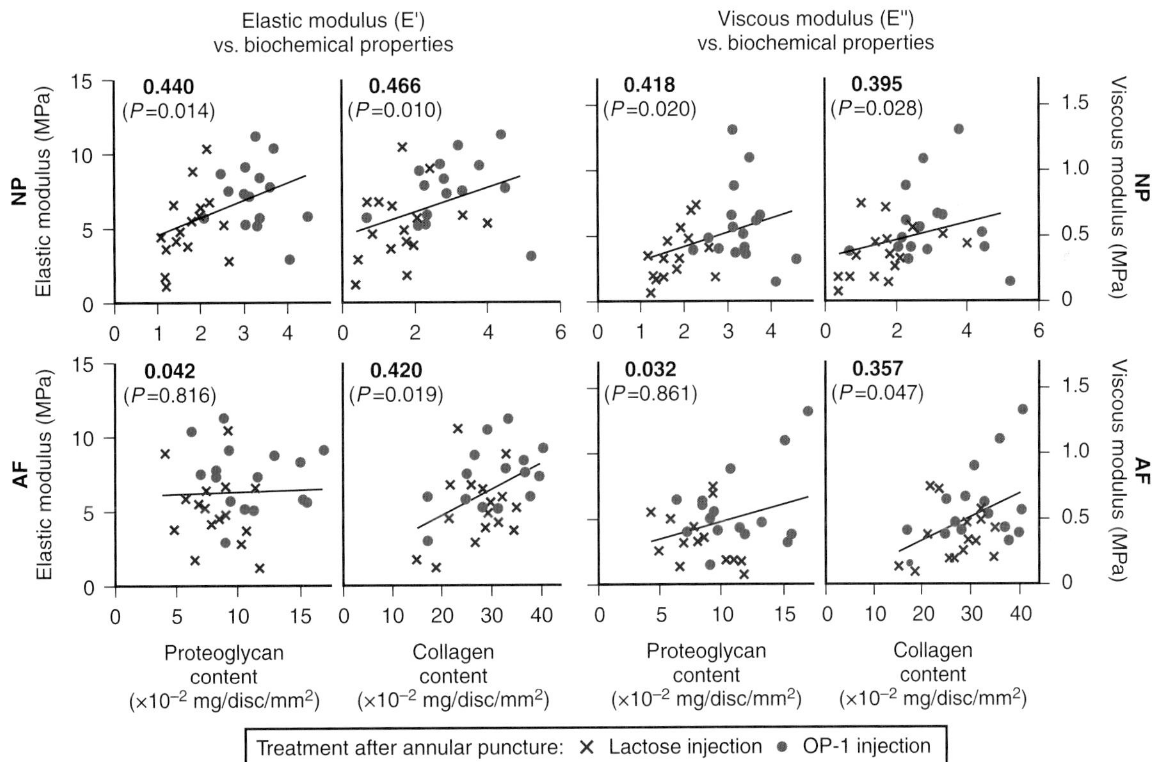


■ **FIGURE 84–7.** Correlations between the biomechanical properties (at 0.5 Hz) and the biochemical properties in lactose-injected and osteogenic protein-1 (OP-1)-injected rabbit intervertebral discs. The elastic modulus (E′) was shown to have a significant positive correlation with the proteoglycan (PG) and collagen contents in the nucleus pulposus (NP) and the collagen content in the annulus fibrosus (AF) tissues when the correlation was assessed using the Spearman signed rank test. Similarly, the viscous modulus was also shown to have a significant correlation with the PG and collagen contents in the NP and the collagen content in the AF. *(From Miyamoto K, Masuda K, Kim JG, et al: Intradiscal injections of osteogenic protein-1 restore the viscoelastic properties of degenerated intervertebral discs. Spine J 6(6):692–703, 2006.)*

proposed as a method to induce disc degeneration in the rat tail as an animal model of disc degeneration.[72]

In consideration of the stimulatory effect on matrix production by OP-1, an injection of rhOP-1 after chemonucleolysis with C-ABC may be useful to counteract the degradative effects of the enzyme and to induce the restoration of IVD structure.[73] In adolescent rabbits, C-ABC (10 mU) was first injected into IVDs to induce chemonucleolytic effects. Four weeks following the injection of C-ABC, OP-1 (100 μg/disc) or vehicle was injected and the disc height was measured for up to 12 weeks after the OP-1 injection. The disc height index (%DHI) of each disc at each time period after the injection of C-ABC was significantly decreased, by approximately 34% (at the 4-week time point), compared to the baseline %DHI values obtained before the C-ABC injection ($P < 0.01$, Fig. 84–8, A, B). In rabbits receiving both C-ABC and rhOP-1, the %DHI began to return toward normal within 4 weeks after the rhOP-1 injection and gradually approached the control level by 6 weeks (Fig. 84–8B). This change was sustained for up to 16 weeks (Fig. 84–8B, DHI, open circle). Biochemically, the PG content of the AF and NP of the C-ABC/rhOP-1 group was higher than that of the C-ABC/lactose group.

The recovery of disc height resulting from an injection of rhOP-1 into enzymatically induced degenerated discs was very similar to that seen in the rabbit annular puncture model.[4] Although the mechanism for the long-lasting effect of rhOP-1 remains to be elucidated, we postulate that this long half-life is due, in part, to the fact that the NP, as an injection site, is a more confined space, being surrounded by the AF, as compared to an articular joint or other locations. Furthermore, rhOP-1 binds to collagen molecules in the NP and AF; this mechanism may be one explanation for its long-acting effects.[74]

The results of our preclinical studies using chemonucleolysis provide further support for the feasibility that a single injection of OP-1 may have the capacity to restore a degenerative IVD.

## Growth and Differentiation Factor-5 (GDF-5)

### Effects of an Intradiscal Injection of rhGDF-5 in Adolescent Rabbits

In the same annular-puncture model of disc degeneration in adolescent rabbits, the therapeutic effectiveness of an injection of rhGDF-5 in the biologic repair of degenerated IVDs was assessed.[3]

The intradiscal injection of rhGDF-5 significantly altered the time course of changes in disc height in degenerated IVDs (Fig. 84–9). At 4 weeks after the injection, the %DHI in the rhGDF-5 group (both 1 μg and 100 μg) began to increase and return toward that of the nonpunctured disc; the PBS control group did not show any recovery of disc height until the end of the observation period. At 12 weeks after injection, the %DHI of rhGDF-5-injected discs remained significantly higher than that of the PBS-injected discs (1 μg and 100 μg) (Fig. 84–9). Although the injection of the lower concentrations of rhGDF-5 (10 ng or 1 μg/disc) did not show any significant effect on the histologic grading score, the total score for the histologic grading scale

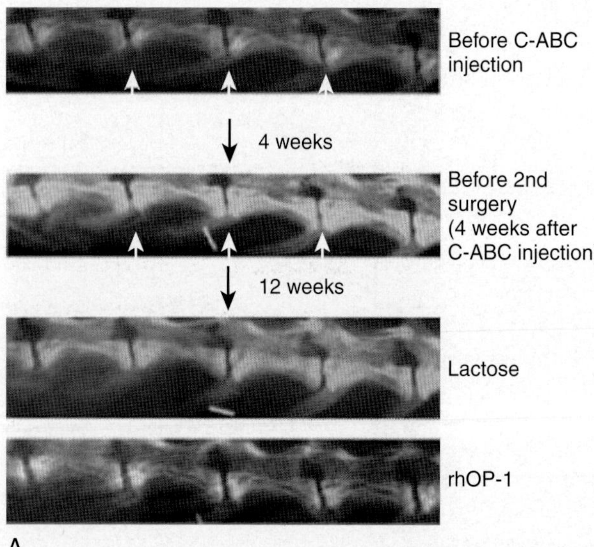


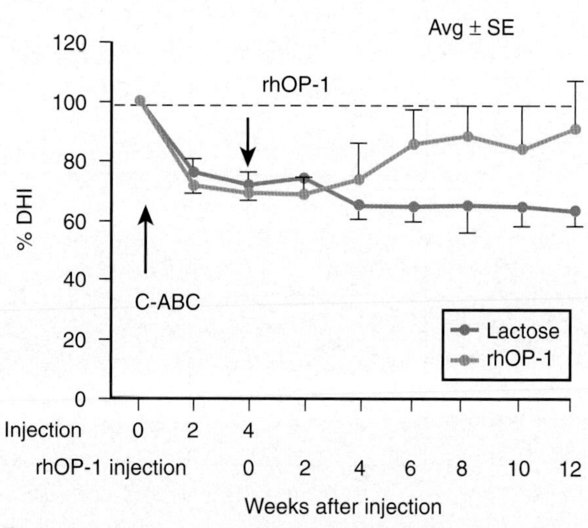


■ **FIGURE 84–8.** Effect of osteogenic protein-1 (OP-1) injection on the disc height after chemonucleolysis by chondroitinase-ABC (C-ABC). **A,** Lateral radiograms of rabbit lumbar spinal segments. Rabbit lumbar intervertebral discs (L2-L5) were exposed through a posterolateral retroperitoneal approach and chondroitinase ABC (C-ABC) at 10 mU in 10 μL of saline was injected into the center of the nucleus pulposus of three consecutive intervertebral discs (L2-L3, L3-L4, L4-L5). A significant decrease of disc height in the lateral radiograph was observed at 4 weeks. Four weeks later after the initial injection of C-ABC, the vehicle (lactose, 10 μL) or rhOP-1 in lactose (100 μg/10μL at each level) was injected. At every second week after the injection, x-rays of the lumbar spine were again taken under general anesthesia. The radiogram of the C-ABC/rhOP-1 group showed a better preservation of disc space after a single injection than the vehicle group. **B,** Changes in the intervertebral disc height index (DHI). The percent DHI (%DHI) was measured, as shown in Figure 84-1, at each time point to quantify changes in disc height. By 6 weeks after the rhOP-1 injection, the mean %DHI of injected discs in the C-ABC/rhOP-1 group was significantly higher than in the C-ABC/lactose group ($P < 0.01$). This significant difference in mean %DHI was maintained during the follow-up period ($P < 0.01$). *(From Imai Y, Okuma M, An H, et al: Restoration of disc height loss by recombinant human osteogenic protein-1 injection into intervertebral discs undergoing degeneration induced by an intradiscal injection of chondroitinase abc. Spine 32(11):1197–1205, 2007.)*

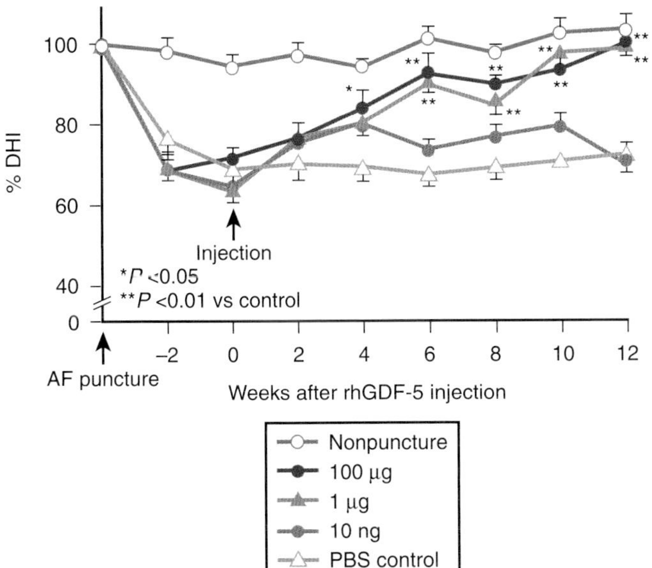


■ **FIGURE 84–9.** Changes in the intervertebral disc (IVD) height index (DHI) after annular puncture and recombinant human growth and differentiation factor-5 (rhGDF-5) injection. Four weeks after inducing disc degeneration by an annular needle puncture in New Zealand white rabbits (weighing 3.5 to 4 kg), the rabbits received an injection of phosphate-buffered saline (PBS) (10 μL) or rhGDF-5 (10 ng, 1 or 100 μg, in 10 μL PBS) and were monitored radiographically for up to 12 weeks after the injections. After sacrifice, the specimens were assessed by magnetic resonance imaging (MRI) and histologic examination. By 4 weeks after the rhGDF-5 injection, the mean %DHI of injected discs in the rhGDF-5 group (100 μg) was significantly higher than in the PBS group ($P < 0.05$). After 12 weeks, the rhGDF-5 groups at two concentrations (1 μg and 100 μg) demonstrated a significantly higher %DHI than the control group ($P < 0.01$). *(From Chujo T, An HS, Akeda K, et al: Effects of growth differentiation factor-5 on the intervertebral disc—in vitro bovine study and in vivo rabbit disc degeneration model study. Spine 31(25):2909–2917, 2006.)*

of the 100 μg rhGDF-5-injected group at the 12-week time point was significantly lower than that of the puncture control group ($P < 0.05$) (Fig. 84–9). The 10 ng group did not show any recovery of disc height (Fig. 84–9).

The MRI of the NP of the rhGDF-5 group showed stronger signal intensity than that in the PBS group (Fig. 84–10A). The MRI grading score was significantly lower in the rhGDF-5 group than in the PBS group (10 ng and 1 μg: $P < 0.05$, 100 μg: $P < 0.01$, Mann-Whitney U test) (Fig. 84–10B). The histologic results showed that the total score for the histologic grading scale of the rhGDF-5 group (100 μg) at the 12-week time point was significantly lower (less degeneration) than that of the puncture control group ($P < 0.05$).

The injection of rhGDF-5 resulted in a restoration of disc height and improvements in MRI and histologic grading scores.[3] The in vitro and in vivo evidence described previously supports the contention that the direct injection of growth factors into the NP or the AF may be clinically feasible as a new therapeutic intervention for treatment of IVD degeneration.

### Effect of an Injection of rhGDF-5 in Mature Rabbits

It is important to recognize that discs from rabbits at the age (3.5- to 4-kg New Zealand white rabbits, 5 months old) used in our previous studies still have a large number of notochordal cells.[75,76] Although most notochordal cells seem to have disappeared after the initial puncture in the needle puncture model, the differences in the cell population remaining in the disc need to be taken into consideration in the interpretation of data.[77] Furthermore, although a longitudinal study has not been performed, it is possible that rabbits develop a spontaneous disc degeneration associated with aging. Yoon and associates have shown an age-related decrease in PG and water content and increased degenerative signs in sagittal MRI scans in their cross-sectional study using 1- to 4-year-old rabbits.[78,79] It has also been reported that aging IVD cells have a lowered matrix metabolic activity.[80,81] Mature rabbits may have less diffusion through the end plate because of decreased vascularity compared to adolescent animals. Therefore, it is possible that the repair of the degenerated disc is age-dependent and that mature rabbits will not restore structure by growth factor injection as seen in the young animals described earlier.

An experiment using older animals that have fewer notochordal cells was conducted to study differences in response to therapeutic treatment. In this study, we tested whether an injection of rhGDF-5 is effective in the repair of the degenerated disc in a mature rabbit annular-puncture disc degeneration model.[82]

The intradiscal injection of rhGDF-5 induced a significant recovery of disc height during the 12-week observation period ($P < 0.001$) (Fig. 84–11A). Two weeks after the injection, the %DHI in the rhGDF-5-injected discs was significantly higher than that in the PBS-injected discs ($P < 0.001$). By 8 weeks after injection, the rhGDF-5-injected discs achieved the %DHI level of the nonpunctured control discs. This recovery continued until the end of the 12-week observation period. Importantly, at sacrifice, the %DHI of the rhGDF-5-injected discs remained significantly higher than that of the PBS-injected discs (PBS vs. rhGDF-5, $P < 0.001$), and had reached the %DHI level of the control discs 8 weeks after the injection. In the MRI analysis, at 12 weeks after the injection, the signal intensity in the NP of the rhGDF-5-injected discs was significantly higher than that of the PBS-injected discs (PBS vs. rhGDF-5, $P < 0.01$) (Fig. 84–8, A, B). The treatment with an intradiscal injection of rhGDF-5 significantly affected both elastic and viscous moduli. The viscous and elastic moduli of the IVDs in the rhGDF-5-injected discs were significantly higher than those in the PBS-injected discs at all loading frequencies (two-way analysis of variance, $P < 0.01$, data not shown).

Although it was of significant concern that age-related changes in cell activity might affect the efficacy of growth factor injection in the rabbit annular-puncture disc degeneration model, discs in mature rabbits responded to rhGDF-5 injection in a similar fashion to that observed in adolescent rabbits.

## POSSIBLE LIMITATIONS OF GROWTH FACTOR INJECTION THERAPY

Although future developments of clinical applications of growth factor injection therapy to treat degenerative disc disease are anticipated, several important limitations arise when the biology of the IVD is taken into account.

It is well known that the cell number is decreased in discs in an advanced stage of degeneration.[83] The lack of viable cells in disc tissues

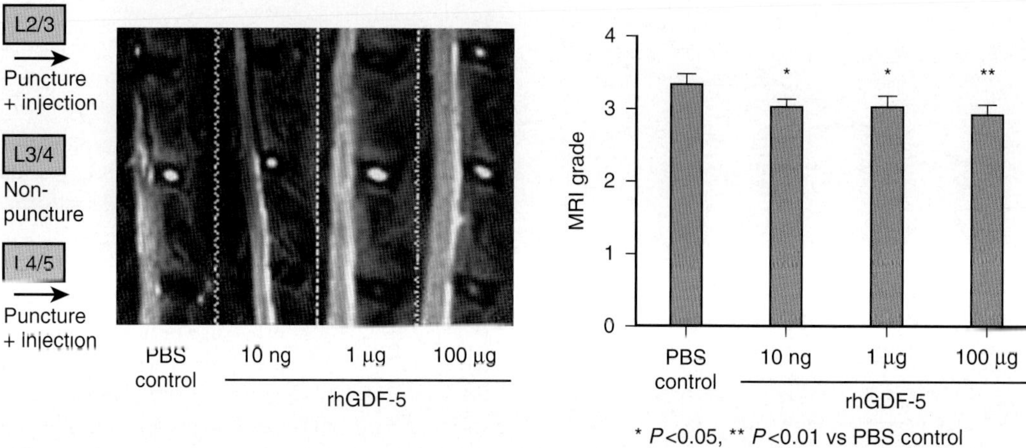


■ **FIGURE 84–10.** Changes in magnetic resonance imaging (MRI) **(A)** and MRI grade scores **(B)** after annular puncture and recombinant human growth and differentiation factor-5 (rhGDF-5) injection. Four weeks after inducing disc degeneration by an annular needle puncture in New Zealand white rabbits (weighing 3.5 to 4 kg), the rabbits received an injection of phosphate-buffered saline (PBS) (10 μL) or rhGDF-5 (10 ng, 1 or 100 μg, in 10 μL PBS) and were monitored radiographically for up to 12 weeks after the injections. After sacrifice, the specimens were assessed by magnetic resonance imaging (MRI) and histologic examination. MRI examinations were performed on all spinal columns isolated from the rabbits ex vivo at the time of sacrifice. At 12 weeks after the rhGDF-5 injection, the MRI of the nucleus pulposus (NP) in the rhGDF-5 group showed stronger signal intensity than that in the PBS group. When the degree of disc degeneration, as assessed by MRI grading (modified Thompson classification from grades 1 to 4), was compared between the PBS and rhGDF-5 groups, significantly lower MRI grades in the rhGDF-5 groups were observed (10 ng and 1 μg: $P < 0.05$, 100 μg: $P < 0.01$, Mann-Whitney U test). *(From Chujo T, An HS, Akeda K, et al: Effects of growth differentiation factor-5 on the intervertebral disc— in vitro bovine study and in vivo rabbit disc degeneration model study. Spine 31(25):2909–2917, 2006.)*

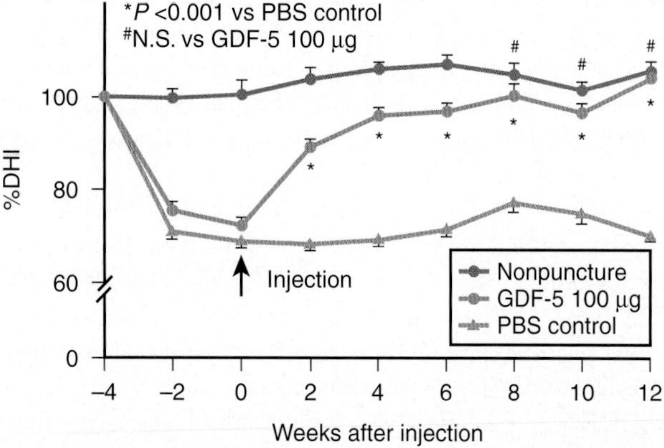


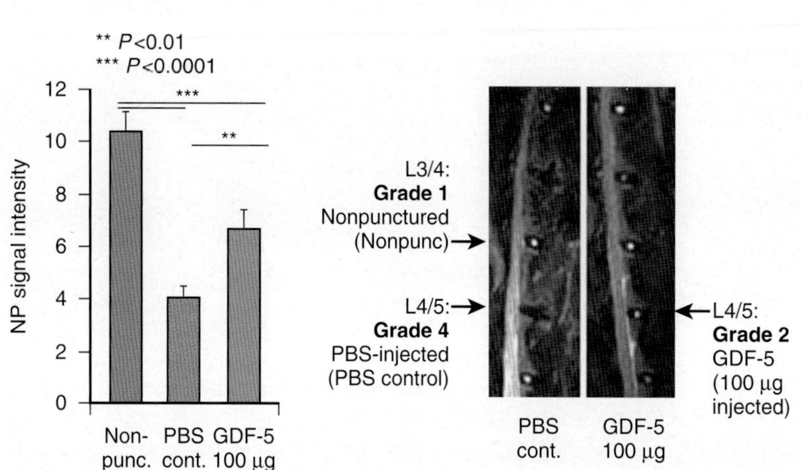


■ **FIGURE 84–11.** Changes in intervertebral disc (IVD) height index (DHI), magnetic resonance imaging (MRI), and MRI grade scores after annular puncture and recombinant human growth and differentiation factor-5 (rhGDF-5) injection in a mature animal model of disc degeneration. New Zealand white rabbits (NZW; $n = 16$; 2 years old) received an annular puncture (18-G) in two noncontiguous discs (L2-L3 and L4-L5) to induce disc degeneration. Four weeks later, either phosphate-buffered saline (PBS) (10 μL) or rhGDF-5 (100 μg, in 10 μL PBS) was injected into the center of the nucleus pulposus (NP) of two previously punctured discs. Disc heights were followed radiographically for up to 12 weeks after the injection. All rabbits were sacrificed 16 weeks after puncture and the spinal columns were removed and subjected to ex vivo MRI analysis. **A,** *Disc height (%DHI):* The intradiscal injection of rhGDF-5 induced significant recovery of disc height during the 12-week observation period ($P < 0.001$). Two weeks after the injection, the %DHI for the rhGDF-5-injected discs was already significantly higher than for the PBS-injected discs ($P < 0.001$); this difference was sustained throughout the 12-week observation period. By 8 weeks after injection, the rhGDF-5-injected discs achieved the DHI level of the nonpunctured control discs. **B,** *MRI analysis:* Twelve weeks after the injection, the signal intensity in the NP of the rhGDF-5-injected discs was significantly higher than in the PBS-injected discs (PBS vs. rhGDF-5, $P < 0.01$). *(Used with permission from Chujo T, An H, Asanuma K, et al: A single injection of recombinant human GDF-5 effectively restores mature rabbit of intervertebral discs degenerated by annular puncture. Trans Orthop Res Soc 32:267, 2007.)*

may lead to the failure of induction of structural restoration by an injected growth factor. To overcome this deficit, the transplantation of healthy functional cells, such as, but not limited to, autologous NP cells, may be required.[84–87] In addition, cells transfected with a therapeutic gene (i.e., those for growth factors and cytokine inhibitors) may be utilized to obtain both a supplementation of cells and the therapeutic effect of the transfected gene.[88]

The importance of nutritional factors in the pathogenesis of disc disease is well recognized.[89] The IVD is the largest avascular tissue in the body and receives its main supply of nutrients by diffusion from the vertebral bodies through the end plates. With the progression of disc disease, end plate sclerosis begins to disrupt the adequate transport of glucose to the cells and appropriate removal of metabolic wastes, such as lactic acid. Importantly, an IVD that lacks proper nutrition or that cannot remove metabolic wastes might experience an adverse environment, such as acidic conditions, and might degenerate significantly because of the loss of steady-state metabolism of its cells. When growth factor injection therapy or cellular therapy is applied under such conditions, the increased demand for energy may negatively affect cell viability. To further develop novel biologic therapies, an improvement in diagnostic methodologies to evaluate the environmental conditions in the IVD is essential.

## GROWTH FACTOR THERAPY AND PAIN

The chief symptom, and complaint, of patients with disc degeneration is pain. Preliminary data from the in vivo rabbit experiments already presented in this chapter have provided evidence that the use of injected growth factors can be effective as a "structural modifying therapy." However, it is not clear whether this approach can be a "symptom-modifying therapy" that is able to resolve the symptoms associated with the pathologic changes. Therefore, further studies are essential to shed light on the mechanism of pain in degenerative disc disease. In order to assess the efficacy of biologic therapies for IVD degeneration, surrogate markers to evaluate pain in animals must be established.

Kawakami and associates evaluated whether intradiscal injections of OP-1 could reverse disc degeneration and reduce hyperalgesia, a pain-related behavior in rats with a compressed NP.[90] In this model, an Ilizarov-type apparatus was applied to the tail to apply the compression load to the disc. Four weeks after surgery, either physiologic saline or OP-1 was injected into the instrumented NP. After an additional 4 weeks, the NP was harvested from the treated disc and applied to the left lumbar nerve roots and hyperalgesia was measured for up to 3 weeks after this surgery. Mechanical hyperalgesia was observed in the sham- and saline-injected groups, but not in the OP-1-treated group. Histologically, the content of the extracellular matrix was markedly increased. The results of the study indicated that OP-1 injection into degenerative intervertebral discs resulted in an increase of the extracellular matrix and the inhibition of pain-related behavior.

Although the rat NP compression model is not a discogenic pain model, but rather a radiculopathy model, the results suggested that changes induced by an injection of OP-1 may influence the biochemical properties of disc tissues and induce some pain relief through the direct effect of OP-1 itself, or through an indirect effect by changing the properties of the restored tissues.

## CONCLUSION

Growth factor injection therapy for treatment of IVD degeneration may have great potential for patients with chronic discogenic low back pain. Currently, the effect of growth factor injection on pain generation is not well known. Although it is difficult to assess back pain in animals, as with any new technology, thorough preclinical studies of growth factor injection therapy should be conducted and followed by well-designed clinical studies to accurately assess safety and efficacy.

## ACKNOWLEDGMENTS

This study was supported by NIH grants P01-AR 48152 and P50-AR39329. The authors would like to thank Ms. Mary Ellen Lenz for her assistance in the preparation of the manuscript.

## REFERENCES

1. Masuda K, Oegema TR Jr, An HS: Growth factors and treatment of intervertebral disc degeneration. Spine 29(23):2757–2769, 2004.
2. Masuda K, An HS: Growth factors and the intervertebral disc. Spine J 4(6):330S–340S, 2004.
3. Chujo T, An HS, Akeda K, et al: Effects of growth differentiation factor-5 on the intervertebral disc—in vitro bovine study and in vivo rabbit disc degeneration model study. Spine 31(25):2909–2917, 2006.
4. Masuda K, Imai Y, Okuma M, et al: Osteogenic protein-1 injection into a degenerated disc induces the restoration of disc height and structural changes in the rabbit anular puncture model. Spine 31(7):742–754, 2006.
5. Ahn SH, Cho YW, Ahn MW, et al: mRNA expression of cytokines and chemokines in herniated lumbar intervertebral discs. Spine 27(9):911–917, 2002.
6. Burke JG, Watson RW, Conhyea D, et al: Human nucleus pulposus can respond to a pro-inflammatory stimulus. Spine 28(24):2685–2693, 2003.
7. Kang JD, Georgescu HI, McIntyre-Larkin L, et al: Herniated lumbar intervertebral discs spontaneously produce matrix metalloproteinases, nitric oxide, interleukin-6, and prostaglandin E2. Spine 21 (3):271–277, 1996.
8. Weiler C, Nerlich AG, Bachmeier BE, Boos N: Expression and distribution of tumor necrosis factor alpha in human lumbar intervertebral discs: A study in surgical specimen and autopsy controls. Spine 30(1):44–53; discussion 54, 2005.
9. Igarashi T, Kikuchi S, Shubayev V, Myers RR: 2000 Volvo Award winner in basic science studies: Exogenous tumor necrosis factor-alpha mimics nucleus pulposus-induced neuropathology: Molecular, histologic, and behavioral comparisons in rats. Spine 25(23):2975–2980, 2000.
10. Olmarker K, Larsson K: Tumor necrosis factor alpha and nucleus-pulposus-induced nerve root injury. Spine 23(23):2538–2544, 1998.
11. Le Maitre CL, Freemont AJ, Hoyland JA: The role of interleukin-1 in the pathogenesis of human intervertebral disc degeneration. Arthritis Res Ther 7(4):R732–745, 2005.
12. Seguin CA, Pilliar RM, Roughley PJ, Kandel RA: Tumor necrosis factor-alpha modulates matrix production and catabolism in nucleus pulposus tissue. Spine 30(17):1940–1948, 2005.
13. Le Maitre CL, Freemont AJ, Hoyland JA: Localization of degradative enzymes and their inhibitors in the degenerate human intervertebral disc. J Pathol 204(1):47–54, 2004.

14. Roberts S, Caterson B, Menage J, et al: Matrix metalloproteinases and aggrecanase: Their role in disorders of the human intervertebral disc. Spine 25(23):3005–3013, 2000.
15. Sztrolovics R, Alini M, Roughley PJ, Mort JS: Aggrecan degradation in human intervertebral disc and articular cartilage. Biochem J 326(Pt 1):235–241, 1997.
16. Osada R, Ohshima H, Ishihara H, et al: Autocrine/paracrine mechanism of insulin-like growth factor-1 secretion, and the effect of insulin-like growth factor-1 on proteoglycan synthesis in bovine intervertebral discs. J Orthop Res 14(5):690–699, 1996.
17. Specchia N, Pagnotta A, Toesca A, Greco F: Cytokines and growth factors in the protruded intervertebral disc of the lumbar spine. Eur Spine J 11(2):145–151, 2002.
18. Tolonen J, Gronblad M, Virri J, et al: Basic fibroblast growth factor immunoreactivity in blood vessels and cells of disc herniations. Spine 20(3):271–276, 1995.
19. Nagano T, Yonenobu K, Miyamoto S, et al: Distribution of the basic fibroblast growth factor and its receptor gene expression in normal and degenerated rat intervertebral discs. Spine 20(18):1972–1978, 1995.
20. Doita M, Kanatani T, Harada T, Mizuno K: Immunohistologic study of the ruptured intervertebral disc of the lumbar spine. Spine 21(2):235–241, 1996.
21. Melrose J, Smith S, Little CB, et al: Spatial and temporal localization of transforming growth factor-beta, fibroblast growth factor-2, and osteonectin, and identification of cells expressing alpha-smooth muscle actin in the injured anulus fibrosus: Implications for extracellular matrix repair. Spine 27(16):1756–1764, 2002.
22. Takae R, Matsunaga S, Origuchi N, et al: Immunolocalization of bone morphogenetic protein and its receptors in degeneration of intervertebral disc. Spine 24(14):1397–1401, 1999.
23. Nakase T, Ariga K, Miyamoto S, et al: Distribution of genes for bone morphogenetic protein-4, -6, growth differentiation factor-5, and bone morphogenetic protein receptors in the process of experimental spondylosis in mice. J Neurosurg 94(1):68–75, 2001.
24. Tolonen J, Gronblad M, Virri J, et al: Platelet-derived growth factor and vascular endothelial growth factor expression in disc herniation tissue: An immunohistochemical study. Eur Spine J 6(1):63–69, 1997.
25. Konttinen YT, Kemppinen P, Li TF, et al: Transforming and epidermal growth factors in degenerated intervertebral discs. J Bone Joint Surg Br 81(6):1058–1063, 1999.
26. Okuda S, Nakase T, Yonenobu K, Ono K: Age-dependent expression of transforming growth factor-beta1 (TGF-beta1) and its receptors and age-related stimulatory effect of TGF-beta1on proteoglycan synthesis in rat intervertebral discs. J Mus Res 4:151–159, 2000.
27. Matsunaga S, Nagano S, Onishi T, et al: Age-related changes in expression of transforming growth factor-beta and receptors in cells of intervertebral discs. J Neurosurg 98(1):63–67, 2003.
28. Tolonen J, Gronblad M, Virri J, et al: Transforming growth factor beta receptor induction in herniated intervertebral disc tissue: An immunohistochemical study. Eur Spine J 10(2):172–176, 2001.
29. Saal JA, Saal JS, Herzog RJ: The natural history of lumbar intervertebral disc extrusions treated nonoperatively. Spine 15(7):683–686, 1990.
30. Larson JW III, Levicoff EA, Gilbertson LG, Kang JD: Biologic modification of animal models of intervertebral disc degeneration. J Bone Joint Surg Am 88(2):83–87, 2006.
31. Thompson JP, Oegema TJ, Bradford DS: Stimulation of mature canine intervertebral disc by growth factors. Spine 16(3):253–260, 1991.
32. Gruber HE, Fisher EC Jr, Desai B, et al: Human intervertebral disc cells from the annulus: Three-dimensional culture in agarose or alginate and responsiveness to TGF-beta1. Exp Cell Res 235(1):13–21, 1997.
33. Gruber HE, Norton HJ, Hanley EN Jr: Anti-apoptotic effects of IGF-1 and PDGF on human intervertebral disc cells in vitro. Spine 25(17):2153–2157, 2000.
34. Masuda K, Takegami K, An H, et al: Recombinant osteogenic protein-1 upregulates extracellular matrix metabolism by rabbit annulus fibrosus and nucleus pulposus cells cultured in alginate beads. J Orthop Res 21(5):922–930, 2003.
35. Imai Y, Miyamoto K, An H, et al: Recombinant human osteogenic protein-1 upregulates proteoglycan metabolism of human anulus fibrosus and nucleus pulposus cells. Spine 32(12):1303–1309, 2007.
36. Asahina I, Sampath TK, Nishimura I, Hauschka PV: Human osteogenic protein-1 induces both chondroblastic and osteoblastic differentiation of osteoprogenitor cells derived from newborn rat calvaria. J Cell Biol 123(4):921–933, 1993.
37. Asahina I, Sampath TK, Hauschka PV: Human osteogenic protein 1 induces chondroblastic, osteoblastic, and/or adipocytic differentiation of clonal murine target cells. Exp Cell Res 222(1):38–47, 1996.
38. Chen P, Vukicevic S, Sampath TK, Luyten FP: Bovine articular chondrocytes do not undergo hypertrophy when cultured in the presence of serum and osteogenic protein-1. Biochem Biophys Res Commun 197(3):1253–1259, 1993.
39. Flechtenmacher J, Huch K, Thonar EJ, et al: Recombinant human osteogenic protein 1 is a potent stimulator of the synthesis of cartilage proteoglycans and collagens by human articular chondrocytes. Arthritis Rheum 39(11):1896–1904, 1996.
40. Takegami K, Thonar EJ, An HS, et al: Osteogenic protein-1 enhances matrix replenishment by intervertebral disc cells previously exposed to interleukin-1. Spine 27(12):1318–1325, 2002.
41. Takegami K, An HS, Kumano F, et al: Osteogenic protein-1 is most effective in stimulating nucleus pulposus and annulus fibrosus cells to repair their matrix after chondroitinase ABC-induced in vitro chemonucleolysis. Spine J 5(3):231–238, 2005.
42. Tim Yoon S, Su Kim K, Li J, et al: The effect of bone morphogenetic protein-2 on rat intervertebral disc cells in vitro. Spine 28 (16):1773–1780, 2003.
43. Kim DJ, Moon SH, Kim H, et al: Bone morphogenetic protein-2 facilitates expression of chondrogenic, not osteogenic, phenotype of human intervertebral disc cells. Spine 28(24):2679–2684, 2003.
44. Storm EE, Huynh TV, Copeland NG, et al: Limb alterations in brachypodism mice due to mutations in a new member of the TGF beta-superfamily. Nature 368(6472):639–643, 1994.
45. Li X, Leo BM, Beck G, et al: Collagen and proteoglycan abnormalities in the GDF-5-deficient mice and molecular changes when treating disk cells with recombinant growth factor. Spine 29 (20):2229–2234, 2004.
46. Wehling P: Antiapoptotic and antidegenerative effect of an autologous IL-1ra/IGF-1/PDGF combination on human intervertebral disc cells in vivo. The International Society for the Study of the Lumbar Spine, 29th Annual Meeting Proceedings, May 14–18, Cleveland, OH, 2002, p 24.
47. Weibrich G, Kleis WK, Hafner G, Hitzler WE: Growth factor levels in platelet-rich plasma and correlations with donor age, sex, and platelet count. J Craniomaxillofac Surg 30(2):97–102, 2002.
48. Okuda K, Kawase T, Momose M, et al: Platelet-rich plasma contains high levels of platelet-derived growth factor and transforming growth factor-beta and modulates the proliferation of periodontally related cells in vitro. J Periodontol 74(6):849–857, 2003.
49. Dugrillon A, Eichler H, Kern S, Kluter H: Autologous concentrated platelet-rich plasma (cPRP) for local application in bone regeneration. Int J Oral Maxillofac Surg 31(6):615–619, 2002.
50. Landesberg R, Roy M, Glickman RS: Quantification of growth factor levels using a simplified method of platelet-rich plasma gel preparation. J Oral Maxillofac Surg 58(3):297–300, 2000.
51. Akeda K, An HS, Pichika R, et al: Platelet-rich plasma (PRP) stimulates the extracellular matrix metabolism of porcine nucleus pulposus and anulus fibrosus cells cultured in alginate beads. Spine 31(9):959–966, 2006.
52. Walsh AL, Kleinstueek F, Lotz J, Bradford D: Growth factor treatment in degenerated intervertebral discs. Trans Ortho Res Soc 26:892, 2001.
53. Walsh AL, Lotz J, Bradford D: Single and multiple injections of GDF-5, IGF-1, or TGF beta into degenerated intervertebral discs. Trans Ortho Res Soc 27:820, 2002.

54. An HS, Takegami K, Kamada H, et al: Intradiscal administration of osteogenic protein-1 increases intervertebral disc height and proteoglycan content in the nucleus pulposus in normal adolescent rabbits. Spine 30(1):25–31, 2005.
55. Miyamoto K, Masuda K, Kim JG, et al: Intradiscal injections of osteogenic protein-1 restore the viscoelastic properties of degenerated intervertebral discs. Spine J 6(6):692–703, 2006.
56. Urban JP, Roberts S: Degeneration of the intervertebral disc. Arthritis Res Ther 5(3):120–130, 2003.
57. Olmarker K, Rydevik B, Dahlin LB, et al: Effects of epidural and intrathecal application of collagenase in the lumbar spine: an experimental study in rabbits. Spine 12(5):477–482, 1987.
58. Dando PM, Morton DB, Buttle DJ, Barrett AJ: Quantitative assessment of human proteinases as agents for chemonucleolysis. Spine 13 (2):188–192, 1988.
59. Grubb A: Safer proteinase treatment of sciatica: A biochemical preview of chymopapain inhibitors. Acta Orthop Scand 59(1):63–65, 1988.
60. Wakita S, Shimizu K, Suzuki K, et al: Chemonucleolysis with calpain I in rabbits. Spine 18(1):159–164, 1993.
61. Kubo S, Tajima N, Katunuma N, et al: A comparative study of chemonucleolysis with recombinant human cathepsin L and chymopapain: A radiologic, histologic, and immunohistochemical assessment. Spine 24(2):120–127, 1999.
62. Shah NH, Dastgir N, Gilmore MF: Medium to long-term functional outcome of patients after chemonucleolysis. Acta Orthop Belg 69(4):346–349, 2003.
63. Eurell JA, Brown MD, Ramos M: The effects of chondroitinase ABC on the rabbit intervertebral disc: A roentgenographic and histologic study. Clin Orthop 256:238–243, 1990.
64. Fry TR, Eurell JC, Johnson AL, et al: Radiographic and histologic effects of chondroitinase ABC on normal canine lumbar intervertebral disc. Spine 16(7):816–819, 1991.
65. Henderson N, Stanescu V, Cauchoix J: Nucleolysis of the rabbit intervertebral disc using chondroitinase ABC. Spine 16(2):203–208, 1991.
66. Kato F, Mimatsu K, Kawakami N, et al: Serial changes observed by magnetic resonance imaging in the intervertebral disc after chemonucleolysis: A consideration of the mechanism of chemonucleolysis. Spine 17(8):934–939, 1992.
67. Ando T, Kato F, Mimatsu K, Iwata H: Effects of chondroitinase ABC on degenerative intervertebral discs. Clin Orthop 318:214–221, 1995.
68. Sugimura T, Kato F, Mimatsu K, et al: Experimental chemonucleolysis with chondroitinase ABC in monkeys. Spine 21(2):161–165, 1996.
69. Takahashi T, Kurihara H, Nakajima S, et al: Chemonucleolytic effects of chondroitinase ABC on normal rabbit intervertebral discs: Course of action up to 10 days postinjection and minimum effective dose. Spine 21(21):2405–2411, 1996.
70. Yamada K, Tanabe S, Ueno H, et al: Investigation of the short-term effect of chemonucleolysis with chondroitinase ABC. J Vet Med Sci 63(5):521–525, 2001.
71. Lu DS, Shono Y, Oda I, et al: Effects of chondroitinase ABC and chymopapain on spinal motion segment biomechanics: An in vivo biomechanical, radiologic, and histologic canine study. Spine 22 (16):1828–1834, 1997.
72. Norcross JP, Lester GE, Weinhold P, Dahners LE: An in vivo model of degenerative disc disease. J Orthop Res 21(1):183–188, 2003.
73. Imai Y, Okuma M, An H, et al: Restoration of disc height loss by recombinant human osteogenic protein-1 injection into intervertebral discs undergoing degeneration induced by an intradiscal injection of chondroitinase ABC. Spine 32(11):1197–1205, 2007.
74. Reddi AH: Morphogenetic messages are in the extracellular matrix: biotechnology from bench to bedside. Biochem Soc Trans 28(4):345–349, 2000.
75. Kim KW, Lim TH, Kim JG, et al: The origin of chondrocytes in the nucleus pulposus and histologic findings associated with the transition of a notochordal nucleus pulposus to a fibrocartilaginous nucleus pulposus in intact rabbit intervertebral discs. Spine 28 (10):982–990, 2003.
76. Scott NA, Harris PF, Bagnall KM: A morphological and histological study of the postnatal development of intervertebral discs in the lumbar spine of the rabbit. J Anat 130(1):75–81, 1980.
77. Masuda K, Aota Y, Muehleman C, et al: A novel rabbit model of mild, reproducible disc degeneration by an anulus needle puncture: Correlation between the degree of disc injury and radiological and histological appearances of disc degeneration. Spine 30(1):5–14, 2005.
78. Yoon S, Li J, Kim K, Boden S: Age related intervertebral disc degeneration in the rabbit. The International Society for the Study of the Lumbar Spine, Porto, Portugal, 2004, p 79.
79. Yoon S, Kim K, Li J, et al: Age related intervertebral disc degeneration in the rabbit. Trans Orthop Res Soc 30:888, 2005.
80. Chiba K, Andersson GBJ, Masuda K, et al: Age-related changes in the metabolism of proteoglycans by intervertebral disc cells cultured *in vitro*. Proceedings of the North American Spine Society Meeting, Vancouver, B.C., Canada, 1996, pp 2–3.
81. Matsumoto T, An H, Thonar E, et al: Effect of osteogenic protein-1 on the metabolism of proteoglycan of intervertebral disc cells in aging. Trans Orthop Res Soc 27:826, 2002.
82. Chujo T, An H, Asanuma K, et al: A single injection of recombinant human GDF-5 effectively restores mature rabbit of intervertebral discs degenerated by anular puncture. Trans Orthop Res Soc 32:267, 2007.
83. Gruber HE, Hanley EN Jr: Analysis of aging and degeneration of the human intervertebral disc: Comparison of surgical specimens with normal controls. Spine 23(7):751–757, 1998.
84. Nishimura K, Mochida J: Percutaneous reinsertion of the nucleus pulposus: An experimental study. Spine 23(14):1531–1538, 1998.
85. Okuma M, Mochida J, Nishimura K, et al: Reinsertion of stimulated nucleus pulposus cells retards intervertebral disc degeneration: An in vitro and in vivo experimental study. J Orthop Res 18(6):988–997, 2000.
86. Gruber HE, Johnson TL, Leslie K, et al: Autologous intervertebral disc cell implantation: A model using *Psammomys obesus*, the sand rat. Spine 27(15):1626–1633, 2002.
87. Ganey T, Libera J, Moos V, et al: Disc chondrocyte transplantation in a canine model: A treatment for degenerated or damaged intervertebral disc. Spine 28(23):2609–2620, 2003.
88. Wehling P, Schulitz KP, Robbins PD, et al: Transfer of genes to chondrocytic cells of the lumbar spine: Proposal for a treatment strategy of spinal disorders by local gene therapy. Spine 22(10):1092–1097, 1997.
89. Urban JP, Smith S, Fairbank JC: Nutrition of the intervertebral disc. Spine 29(23):2700–2709, 2004.
90. Kawakami M, Matsumoto T, Hashizume H, et al: Osteogenic protein-1 (osteogenic protein-1/bone morphogenetic protein-7) inhibits degeneration and pain-related behavior induced by chronically compressed nucleus pulposus in the rat. Spine 30(17):1933–1939, 2005.

CHAPTER 85

# Cell Therapy for Intervertebral Disc Degeneration

**Daisuke Sakai** and **Joji Mochida**

## KEY POINTS

- Among biologic treatments, interest in cell transplantation therapy for disc degeneration has been growing, and various cell types have been examined as possible donor cells.
- Owing to the lack of a definitive cell marker for disc cells, chodrocytes from other sources have been raised as potential donor cells. However, it is not clear if any cells that express a chondrocyte-like phenotype are appropriate.
- Activated nucleus pulposus cells and mesenchymal stem cells have been proved successful as potential donor cell sources for cell transplantation therapy in animal models.
- Mesenchymal stem cells transplanted to degenerative discs in rabbits proliferated and differentiated into cells expressing some of the major phenotypic characteristics of nucleus pulposus cells, suggesting that these stem cells may have undergone site-dependent differentiation.
- Although further research is clearly needed to validate patient selection, method of cell delivery, and safety issues, the use of viable cells in regenerative strategies to treat intervertebral disc degeneration seems promising.

## BIOLOGIC CHANGES DURING DISC DEGENERATION

Low back pain is the second most frequent reason for visits to physicians in modern society.[1] The societal costs, including direct medical costs, insurance, lost production, and disability benefits, are estimated at £12 billion per year in the United Kingdom. In the United States over $50 billion in annual health costs are related directly or indirectly to this disease.[2] Intervertebral disc (IVD) degeneration is responsible for over 20% of low back pain cases and is a leading cause of health care costs, lost wages, and patient morbidity.[3] The causes of IVD degeneration are largely unknown. The disease process is thought to involve sequential events that lead to loss of cells and disc matrix, which is composed of proteoglycans and collagen,[4] and altered biomechanics. As the disc degenerates, the associated loss of functions of the spinal column occurs, with impaired spinal motion and stabilization and protection of the neural elements, possibly ending in symptomatic disc disorders.[5] Surgical procedures, such as discectomy and spinal fusion, are commonly used and generally effective for herniated disc and spondylolisthesis, respectively. These procedures, however, do not preserve the function of the IVD and increase the mechanical load and stresses on adjacent discs.[6] Therefore, development of a treatment that restores biologic function of the IVD and preserves the motion segment is greatly needed. Biologic regeneration of IVD is a major challenge, because of the poor regenerative nature of the IVD cells found in the nucleus pulposus (NP) and annulus fibrosus (AF). Compared with other tissues, the NP, in particular, has a low cell density and is a site where cellular proliferation is difficult. The NP contains different cell types, including notochordal and chondrocyte-like cells, depending on the age of the subject.[7] The microenvironment of NP and AF cells is subjected to high pressure and is characterized by low oxygen tension, low pH, and limited nutrition.[8] Recent studies have shown that NP cells are well adapted to this harsh microenvironment through utilization of lactic acid metabolic cycles and expression of hypoxic-resistible factors. However, it is apparent that the nature of this microenvironment restricts both the timing and procedures for therapeutic intervention.[9,10]

## RECOVERY OF CELL LOSS BY CELL SUPPLEMENTATION

Recent advances in molecular biology and technology have resulted in experimental studies that explored biologic strategies to address disc degeneration. These strategies include the induction of cytokines and growth factors, gene therapy, tissue engineering, and cell supplementation by transplantation therapy.[11–13] Cell transplantation is a new therapy that is based on the supplementation of matrix-producing cells in an attempt to correct the decrease of matrix components, primarily proteoglycan and collagen, a major factor in disc degeneration (Fig. 85–1). In 1996, Mochida and associates demonstrated the importance of preserving NP elements for preventing the acceleration of disc degeneration following discectomy.[14] This clinical study opened a new area of research into replacement of the cells lost by pathologic manifestations or surgical intervention, potentially retarding the progression of disc degeneration. To test this hypothesis, an animal model study, performed by Nishimura and Mochida, demonstrated that reinsertion of autologous fresh or cryopreserved NP cells slowed

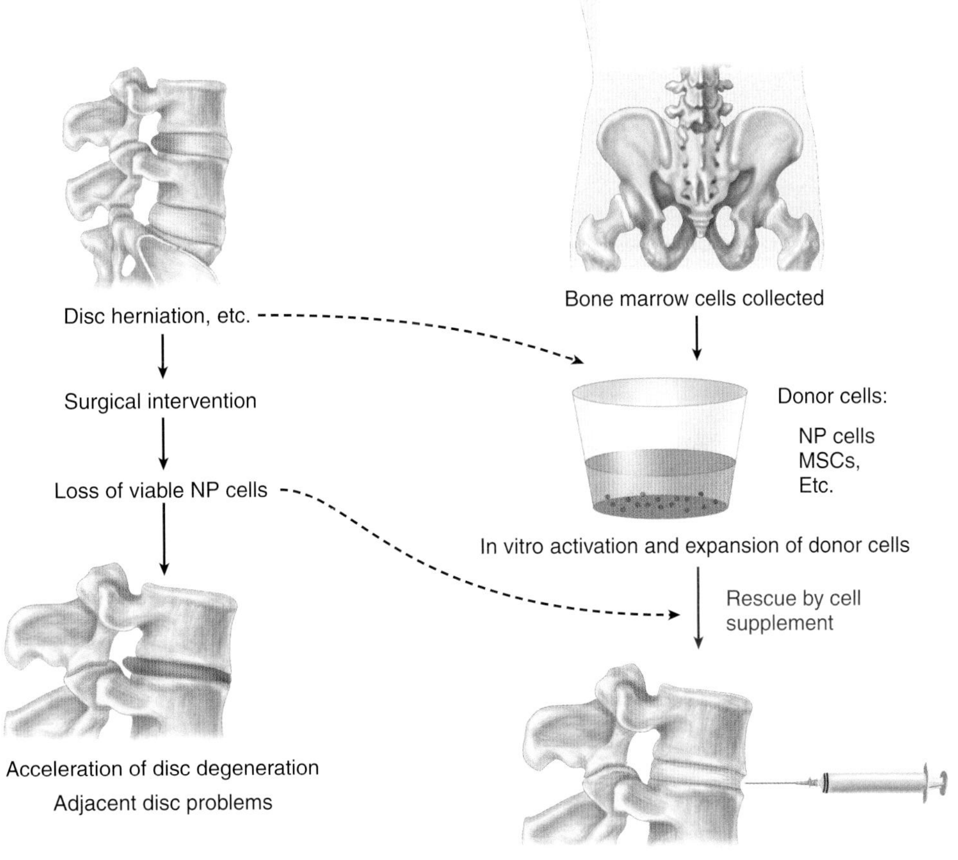


■ **FIGURE 85–1.** Therapeutic scheme for cell therapy in treating disc degeneration. MSCs, mesenchymal stem cells; NP, nucleus pulposus.

degeneration in the rat IVD.[15] Numerous subsequent studies have reported the efficacy of cell transplantation therapy using various animal models and donor cell types. Cell transplantation therapy is facilitated by the unique structure of the IVD: The NP is surrounded by the AF and the end plate, allowing space for donor cells to adapt and preventing cell migration. The contained structure is also thought to play an important role in limiting the immune response following cell transplantation. Cells from the nucleus have been reported to express Fas-ligand (FasL), a specific protein seen in organs that are immune-privileged.[16] Therefore, the NP region may tolerate hosting cells from other areas of the body.

## POTENTIAL CELL SOURCES

A variety of cell types have been proposed or investigated experimentally as candidates for donor cells for IVD cell supplementation. To regenerate normal tissue, it would be most desirable to restore the cellular constituents of the damaged tissues. Therefore, transplanting original NP cells would be most appropriate. A study by Okuma and associates focused on the transplantation of notochordal NP cells in rabbits and demonstrated that notochordal NP cell transplantation activated inner annulus cells, which resulted in the maintenance of the annular structure.[17] However, access to healthy NP cells, especially autologous cells, is difficult in clinical settings. This led to a study by Yamamoto and associates showing that the number of harvested autologous NP cells can be augmented by culture using a direct cell-to-cell contact co-culture system with mesenchymal stem cells (MSCs).[18] Besides differentiating into multiple cell types of mesenchymal origin, MSCs serve as feeder or nursing cells for other cells. This novel coculture system enabled these authors to obtain cell proliferation and proteoglycan synthesis in NP cells three to five times greater than obtained by conventional culture systems. A study by Gruber and associates used sand rats to demonstrate that autologous disc cells harvested from IVDs could be expanded in monolayer culture, labeled, and then implanted into different disc sites. The labeled cells were seen in the discs of the animals as long as 8 months after transplantation, leading to the conclusion that autologous disc cell implantation can result in cell survival and integration into the disc.[19] Ganey and associates studied autologous disc chondrocyte transplantation in a canine disc injury model. The discs in the dogs receiving transplants were significantly better maintained in terms of disc height and structure than in a control group. The effects lasted for about 12 months after transplantation.[20]

These experimental studies confirm that transplantation of cells from an autologous IVD can help prevent disc degeneration in animal models. In a human clinical setting, however, it is almost impossible to obtain donor disc cells from healthy discs. If a suitable cell source is unavailable, the use of alternative donor cells must be explored. Because NP cells, especially in humans, morphologically resemble chondrocytes, Gorensek and associates transplanted chondrocytes from elastic cartilage into rabbit discs. They found that this method also reduces the loss of proteoglycans from injured IVDs when compared to discs not receiving treatment.[21] This raises the question: Can any type of chondrocyte or any other cell that produces proteoglycan and type II collagen be successfully used as an alternative cell source? At present there is no definitive answer for this question because cell markers that clearly distinguish IVD cells from other chondrocytes have not been defined. Studies have shown there are important differences between IVD cells and articular chondrocytes, even between NP and AF cells, notably in the composition and structure of matrix molecules produced. Mwale and associates found the proteoglycan-to-collagen ratio to be distinctly higher in the NP compared to cartilage in same-aged individuals.[22] Such differences result in tissues with quite different mechanical properties. Although cartilage generally exhibits the characteristics of a viscoelastic solid, the NP can behave either as a fluid or as a viscoelastic solid under different loading conditions.[23] Cells from the IVD are therefore commonly referred to as "chondrocyte-like" cells. Recently, several markers have been reported as potential markers for NP cells. Risbud and associates found that NP cells, compared to AF cells or articular chondrocytes, react differently to hypoxia by specifically expressing hypoxia-inducible factor-1 (HIF-1).[24] There have been two separate studies of markers for notochordal NP cells. Fujita and associates reported that CD24 can be used as a NP notochordal cell marker in rodents,[25] and Semba and associates found the sickle tail (*Skt*) gene useful as a NP notochordal cell marker in mice.[26] The heterogeneous cell population found in normal human IVDs differs morphologically and in the production of chondroitin sulfate, keratan sulfate, and collagens. More investigation and discussion of the phenotypic characteristics of human IVD cells are needed.

In addition to autologous disc cells, allografts of NP tissues or cells may be considered. Nomura and associates transplanted allogenic NP cells and tissue in a rabbit disc degeneration model and found that they effectively preserved the disc structure while generating no serious immune reaction. They speculated that the immune privilege of NP cells might be the reason for this result.[27] Although cells from sources other than IVDs may become alternatives, it is doubtful that they would serve better than IVD cells. Because the morphology and function of tissues generated by chondrocytes may differ widely (e.g., NP, AF, articular cartilage, auricular cartilage), the use of differentiated chondrocytes derived from tissues other than the host tissue may not be efficacious.

Emerging techniques of regenerative medicine suggest that progenitor or stem cells may be able to differentiate into IVD cells. There is an increasingly enthusiastic interest in stem cells for use in treating various degenerative diseases and damaged organs.[28] Because the IVD develops from the mesenchyme, the most closely related stem cells for repairing damaged IVDs would be MSCs. MSCs are stem cells found in small numbers in the periosteum, umbilical cord blood, or bone marrow;[29] they possess a unique ability to differentiate into various mesenchymal cell types[30,31] (Fig. 85–2). Experimental MSC transplantation therapies have been effective in a variety of diseases, including disease affecting

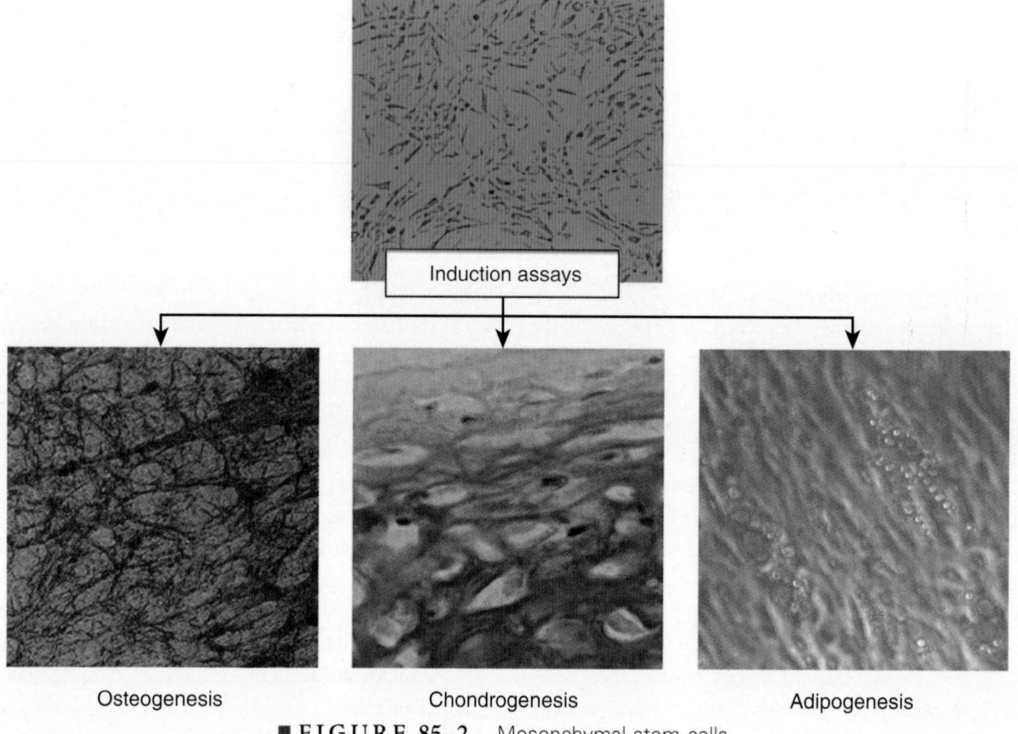


■ **FIGURE 85–2.** Mesenchymal stem cells.

articular cartilage.[32,33] The induction of articular chondrocytes from MSCs in vitro is well established.[34,35] The use of progenitor cells that can differentiate into NP chondrocyte-like cells may be of great value. Autologous MSC transplantation may well become an applicable treatment if MSCs can differentiate into cells expressing the NP cell phenotype. Risbud and associates found that MSCs exposed to hypoxic conditions in vitro, such as those occurring in the NP region of the IVD, differentiate in the direction of NP cells that exhibit an upregulation of hypoxia-responsive genes.[36] Several subsequent studies reported that MSCs can differentiate into cells expressing a phenotype similar to IVD cells in vitro.[37,38] Sakai and associates used autologous MSCs for transplantation in the rabbit disc model and reported that these cells survive, proliferate, and differentiate into cells expressing some of the major phenotype of NP cells.[39–41] This effectiveness of MSC transplantation has been confirmed by several other researchers. Crevensten and associates demonstrated that injected MSCs in a rat disc using hyaluronan as a scaffold maintained viability and proliferated. Viable cells were detected, and disc height was maintained over the 28-day study period.[42] Zhang and associates implanted allogeneic MSCs in rabbits and discovered MSCs survived and increased the proteoglycan content within the disc, supporting their use as a potential treatment for IVD degeneration.[43]

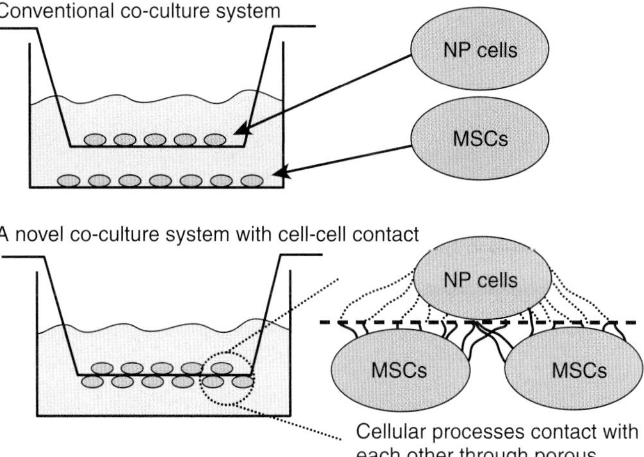


■ **FIGURE 85–3.** Co-culture systems. MSCs, mesenchymal stem cells; NP, nucleus pulposus.

## EXAMPLES OF THERAPEUTIC MODELS

### Development of a Method for Activating NP Cells and Transplantation of Activated NP Cells

Because only a small number of NP cells are obtainable and their biologic activity is low, the development of a new activation method or a new source of cells to replace degenerated NP cells is required.

#### In Vitro Study

Direct cell-to-cell contact is possibly important for the support of hematopoietic stem cells by MSCs in the bone marrow; enhanced signaling between MSCs (feeder cells) and hematopoietic stem cells may result from such contact.[44] Therefore, a new coculture method that allowed intercellular adhesion was developed to facilitate contact between the processes of autologous rabbit MSCs and NP cells. Contact occurred across a membrane with 0.45–μm pores, such that only processes could adhere to each other without more extensive contact between the cultured cells (Figs. 85–3 and 85–4). Activation of NP cells was compared between Group A (NP cells subjected to monolayer culture), Group B (coculture with MSCs performed by the conventional method without intercellular adhesion), and Group C (coculture with MSCs using the new method with intercellular adhesion). Culture was continued for 10 days, at which time confluence had occurred in Group C.

The extent of cell adhesion was determined by scanning electron microscopy, and cell proliferation was evaluated by the WST-8 assay. The syntheses of DNA and proteoglycans were evaluated by the uptakes of $^{3}H$ and $^{35}S$, respectively. The levels of various growth factors and the secretion of cytokines into the culture supernatant were measured by using a cytokine protein array.

Results, confirmed by electron microscopy, demonstrated that MSCs and NP cells adhered to each other by extending processes across the membrane (Fig. 85–5). The number of cells significantly increased in Group C, being approximately fivefold and twofold higher than in Groups A and B, respectively (Fig. 85–6). In addition, DNA synthesis was approximately 22-fold and 15-fold higher in Group C than in Groups A and B, respectively. The synthesis of proteoglycans also showed a significant increase in Group C, approximately 10-fold and 15-fold higher than in Groups A and B, respectively (Fig. 85–7). Thus, these parameters were all significantly higher in Group C. The analysis using the cytokine protein array revealed that the secretion of cytokines known to increase the activity of NP cells was also significantly higher in Group C than in Groups A and B. The secretion of transforming growth factor (TGF-β1) was approximately 3.3-fold and 6.6-fold higher in Group C than in Groups A and B, respectively; the secretion of insulin-like growth factor-1 (IGF-1) was approximately 7.1-fold and 2.1-fold higher; the secretion of platelet-derived growth factor (PDGF) was approximately 7.9-fold and 1.6-fold higher; and the secretion of epidermal growth factor (EGF) was approximately 28.3-fold and 3.0-fold higher. Compared with the conventional NP cell activation method, the co-culture system allowing intercellular adhesion with MSCs led to a marked increase of NP cell proliferation, DNA synthesis, and proteoglycan synthesis. A possible cause for this could be the increased secretion of various cytokines into the culture medium due to the direct contact with MSCs acting as feeder cells.

#### In Vivo Experiment

NP cells activated by coculture with intercellular contact were implanted in a rabbit model of IVD degeneration. The severity of degeneration was determined over time according to Nishimura's histologic classification.[15] The severity of degeneration

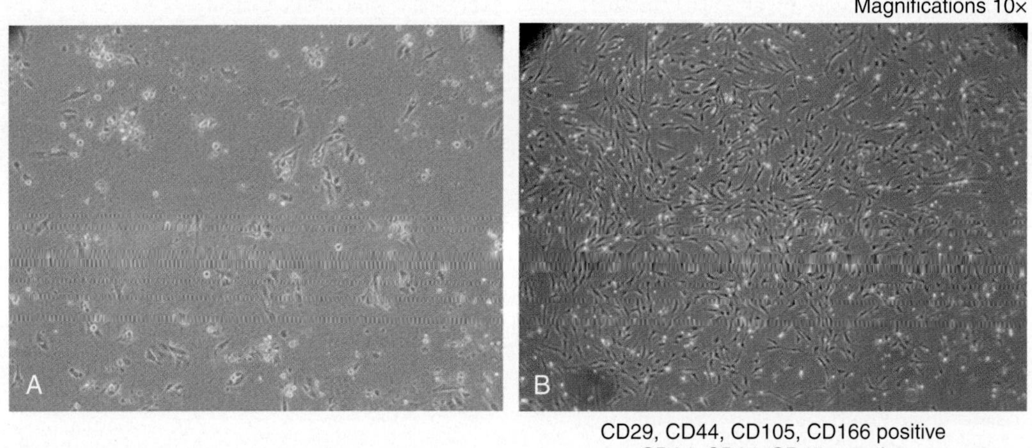


■ **FIGURE 85–4.** Freshy isolated human nucleus pulposus cells **(A)** and mesenchymal stem cells **(B)**.

was compared between cells treated by the new and conventional methods of activation. The Nishimura grade at 24 weeks after transplant was 0 in the normal control group without degeneration induction; 2.8 (the most severe degeneration) in the control group with no treatment; grade 2.1 in the group receiving NP cells

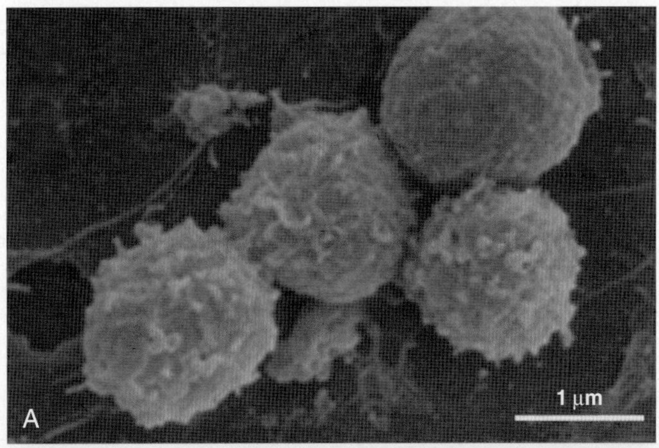


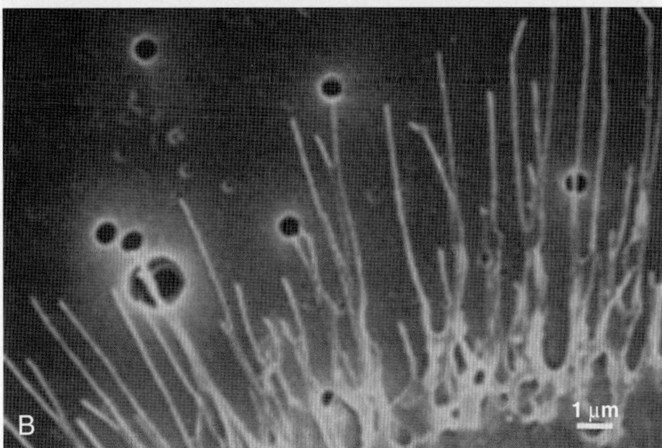


■ **FIGURE 85–5.** Cells in the co-culture system with cell-cell contact photographed by scanning electron microscopy. **A,** Nucleus pulposus cells taken immediately after seeded on a porous membrane. **B,** Mesenchymal stem cells extending their processes toward the membrane pore.

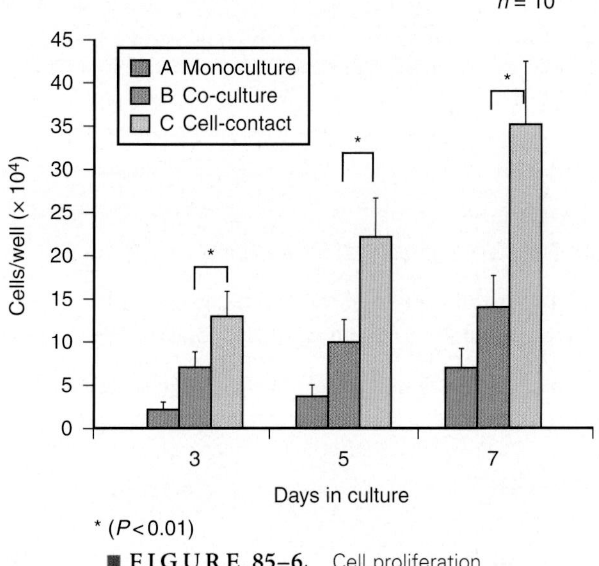


■ **FIGURE 85–6.** Cell proliferation.

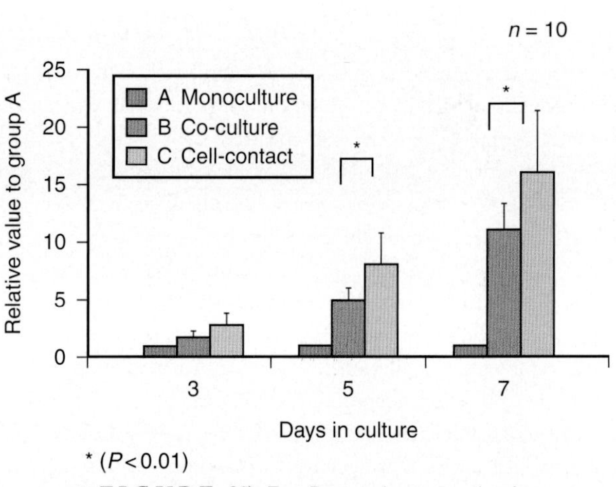


■ **FIGURE 85–7.** Proteoglycan synthesis.

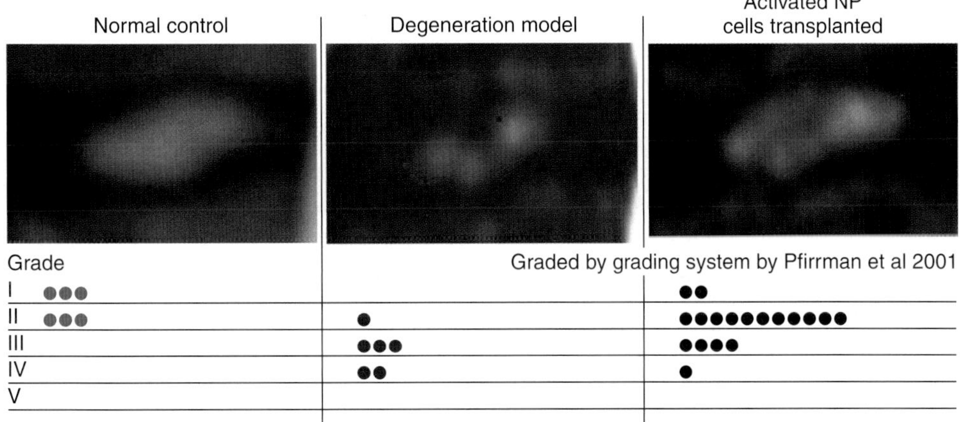


■ **FIGURE 85–8.** Magnetic resonance imaging evaluations of degeneration.

activated by conventional coculture with AF cells; 1.8 in the group receiving NP cells activated by conventional coculture with MSCs; and 1.2, a statistically significant improvement in the degree of degeneration, in the group receiving NP cells activated by co-culture involving contact with MSCs (Figs. 85–8 and 85–9). The positive results of this co-culture system are now being tested by preclinical studies using human cells.

## Mesenchymal Stem Cell Transplantation in a Rabbit Disc Degeneration Model

It has been reported that the inhibition of differentiation of transplanted stem cells is due to the microenvironment at the site of transplantation. In an in vivo experiment, rabbit autologous MSCs transfected with the green fluorescent protein (*GFP*) gene, using a retrovirus vector, were transplanted into a rabbit model of IVD degeneration. The differentiation of transplanted cells within the IVD was assessed for up to 48 weeks after transplantation. Although the transfection efficiency of the viral vector was approximately 35%, purification by cell sorting achieved the level of 98% of the MSCs expressing GFP. Two weeks after transplantation, GFP-positive cells (21 ± 6%) were observed in the NP 2; this increased to 55 ± 8% at 48 weeks after transplantation (Fig. 85–10). GFP-positive cells were also seen around the margin of the AF, and the transplanted MSCs were confirmed to show proliferation. An analysis of MSC differentiation inside the NP demonstrated that GFP-positive cells produced keratan sulfate–containing proteoglycans and type II collagen. Type I collagen was not detected, as is the pattern in native NP cells (Fig. 85–11).

Based on macroscopic and histologic findings, the restoration of NP tissue was markedly better in the transplanted group than in the disc degeneration group at 24 weeks after MSC transplantation (Fig. 85–12). Histologic examinations using Nishimura's classification of IVD degeneration yielded mean scores of 4.8 ± 0.6 in the disc degeneration group and 1.7 ± 0.5 in the MSC transplantation group. The architecture of the AF was significantly more intact in the MSC transplantation group.

When changes in the disc height index (DHI), using plain x-ray films at 24 weeks after transplantation, were compared, the mean index of the untreated control group was set at 100% and

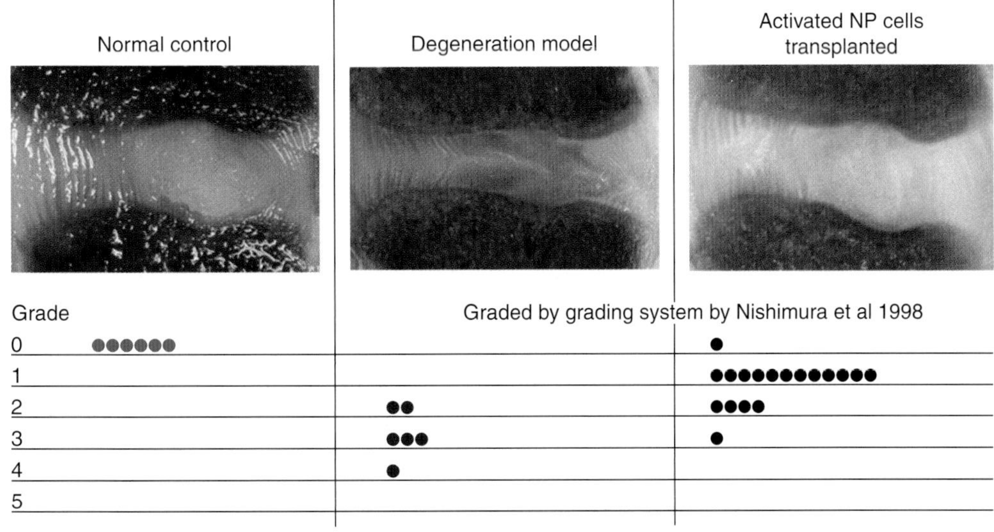


■ **FIGURE 85–9.** Histologic evaluations of degeneration.

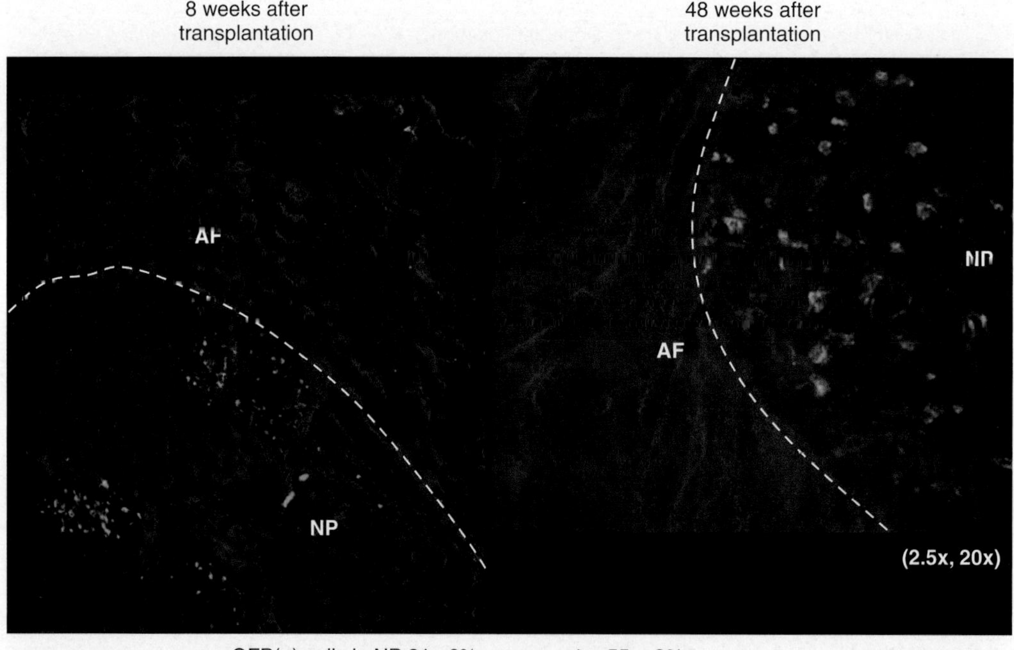


■ **FIGURE 85–10.** Mesenchymal stem cells after transplantation. AF, annulus fibrosis; GFP, green fluorescent protein; NP, nucleus pulposus.

the DHI decreased to 74 ± 8% in the disc degeneration group. This decrease was significantly inhibited in the MSC transplantation group (DHI = 92 ± 4%) at 24 weeks (Fig. 85–13).

Changes in the disc water content were compared using $T_2$-weighted magnetic resonance images. Hydration was 65 ± 2% in the disc degeneration group, and significantly ($P < 0.05$) increased to 80 ± 5% in the MSC transplantation group (Fig. 85–14).

Safranin-0 staining and immunostaining for proteoglycans showed that the intensity of staining markedly decreased in the disc degeneration group; conversely, staining was observably

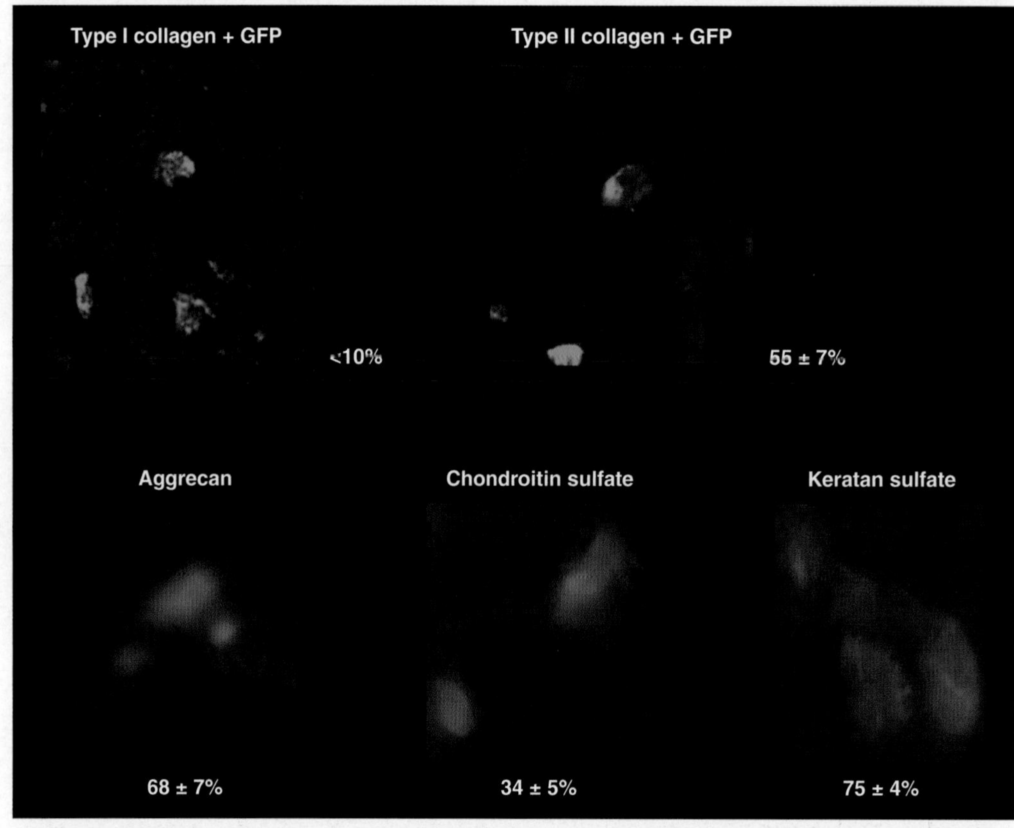


■ **FIGURE 85–11.** Types I and II collagen. GFP, green fluorescent protein.

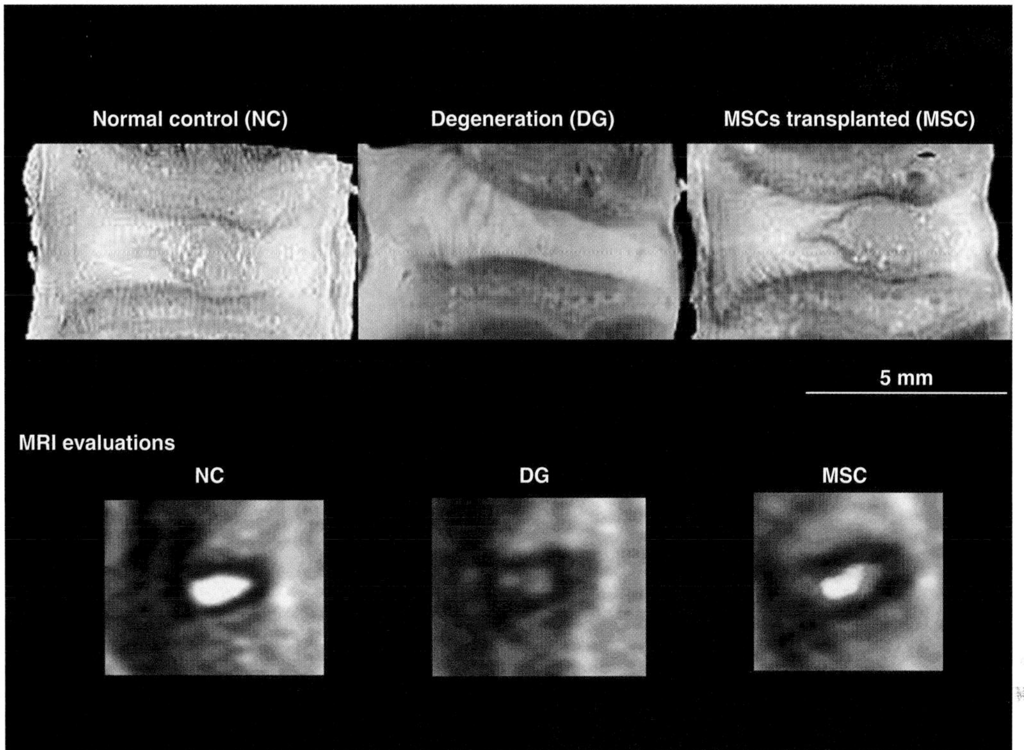


■ **FIGURE 85–12.** Macroscopic evaluations of restoration of nucleus pulposus tissue after mesenchymal stem cell transplantation.

stronger in the MSC transplantation group, indicating restoration of proteoglycan synthesis.

Gene expression in the IVDs was examined by reverse transcriptase-polymerase chain reaction (RT-PCR) at 24 weeks after transplantation. The expression of aggrecan and versican was markedly decreased in the disc degeneration group, but returned toward normal levels in the MSC transplantation group. Collagen gene expression showed no difference between the two groups.

The results of homologous MSC transplantation experiments showed no appreciable differences in the degree of regeneration. Immunostaining for CD4 and CD59 revealed no infiltration of macrophages or lymphocytes, ruling out a rejection reaction. In summary, when bone marrow MSCs were transplanted into experimentally degenerative IVDs, the regenerative effect of these

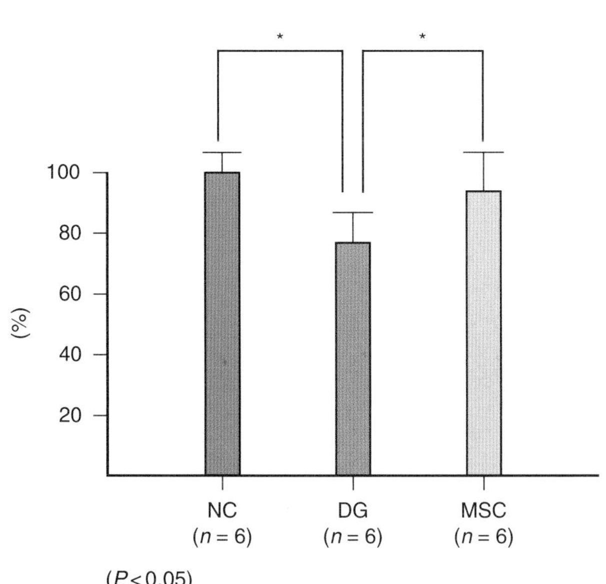


■ **FIGURE 85–13.** Changes in the disc height index seen in radiograph.

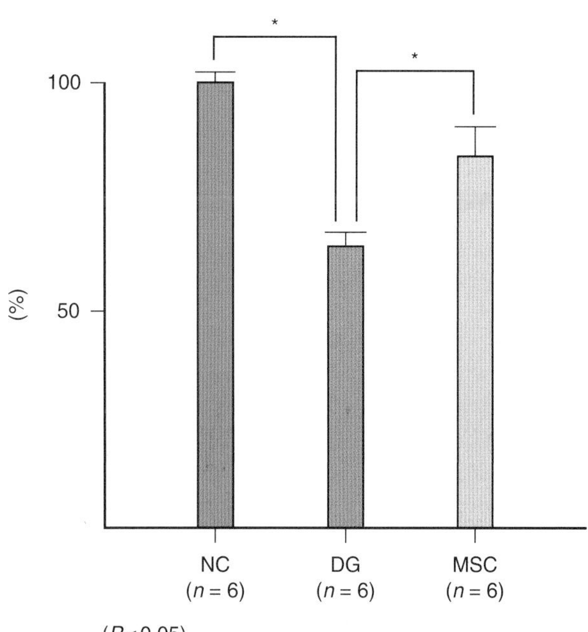


■ **FIGURE 85–14.** High intensity $T_2$-weighted magnetic resonance images showing changes in disc water content.

cells was confirmed by improvements in disc height, water content, and morphologic features. Although the complete inhibition of degeneration or perfect regeneration was not achieved in the MSC transplantation group compared with the normal control group, the antidegenerative and regenerative effects were significantly stronger in the MSC transplantation group than in the disc degeneration group.

Based on these experimental results, three hypotheses may be advanced to elucidate the mechanisms underlying the antidegenerative and regenerative effects of this method: (1) Transplanted MSCs differentiated into NP-like cells and promoted recovery of the disc; (2) residual NP cells and inner layer AF cells were activated by the transplanted MSCs, promoting tissue regeneration; or (3) both of these mechanisms were involved. The relative influence of these mechanisms could not be determined by this experiment. Because both round cells and spindle cells resembling inner layer AF cells were often observed in the NP after MSC transplantation, the possibility exists that transplanted cells differentiated into these cells. In general, transplanted MSCs tend to differentiate into cells that are appropriate for the environment at the site of transplantation.

### Summary of the Therapeutic Models

Through investigation of methods for activation of NP cells, the superiority of co-culture with MSCs and intercellular contact was demonstrated, and progress toward clinical retransplantation of autologous NP cells is expected. Investigating the induction of differentiation of IVD cells from MSCs in vivo confirmed that MSCs could differentiate into cells that synthesized a matrix similar to that produced by native IVD cells. The therapeutic efficacy of intradiscal MSC transplantation was not only confirmed for autotransplantation but also for allotransplantation. This finding is clinically important because it could lead to an increased availability of donor cells for clinical applications. The clinical efficacy of bone marrow MSC transplantation for IVD degeneration may be similar or, taking cell availability into account, superior to NP transplantation. Further assessment of its feasibility is anticipated.

## CONCERNS IN INTERPRETING ANIMAL THERAPEUTIC MODELS

Despite the positive effects of cell transplantation therapy in animal models, many obstacles must be overcome before actual clinical application. A major concern is the different appearance of cells composing the IVD between animal and human species and with age.[44] Histologically, IVD cells in mice, rats, and rabbits have notochord-like cells occurring with large cell size and vacuoles. In larger species, such as pigs, sheep, and cattle, NP cells appear similar to chondrocytes. These cell types are also found in human discs with more notochordal cells dominant in young adolescents and more chondrocyte-like cells in adults.

Environmental nutritional levels are probably changed in actual human disc degeneration; this is not usually the case in animal models of induced disc degeneration. The literature provides a collection of animal models of experimentally induced disc degeneration[45,46]; however, the ideal disc degeneration model that exactly resembles naturally occurring disc degeneration does not exist. Moreover, the multifactorial characteristics of individual variation of disc degeneration in humans make it improbable that a universally applicable animal model can be developed. Absent a universal model, the researcher is challenged to match the model to the objectives of study.

## OBSTACLES TO CLINICAL APPLICATION

### Methods of Cell Delivery

The technique for insertion of transplanted cells also requires more research. The injection technique that is used in the method of discography may be most feasible, but there may be more efficient ways of controlling cell leakage, prevention of injury to the annulus, etc.

### Therapeutic Time Window

The appropriate timing for the application of transplantation therapy to treat disc degeneration has not been thoroughly investigated. It is not realistic to apply this therapy to degenerative IVDs with Thompson Grades 4 to 5 because the discs are essentially biologically inactive.[47] Mild to moderately degenerated IVDs, with Thompson Grades 2 to 3, may prove more appropriate for treatment.

### Restoration of the Annulus Fibrosus and Cartilage End Plate

Attempts to restore the cells and cellular metabolism of the NP have been the subject of research since the late 1990s. The restoration of an injured AF and cartilage end plate has not been focused on. The development of a therapy to accomplish this would be very useful clinically. Cell transplantation would be ineffective if the injury to the AF is severe, or if the cartilage end plate is compromised, leading to malnutrition of the whole IVD.

### Safety Issues

Biologic therapies have focused on cell-based therapies. Researchers should always consider that the introduction of cells may upset the tissue homeostasis, which could produce adverse unintended consequences in the target organ. Phenomena such as tumorigenesis, transformation, or karyotypic abnormalities of cells may be anticipated and need to be closely monitored. The transmission of infectious agents and carcinogenic factors must be guarded against when using exogenous transplants.

## CONCLUSION

Research on cell transplantation for disc disease is in its infancy. Many parameters remain to be defined before clinical efficacy and safety are achieved. However, results from animal therapeutic models are promising for the benefits of cell-based therapy for disc disease.

## REFERENCES


1. Deyo RA, Weinstein JN: Low back pain. N Engl J Med 344:363–370, 2001.
2. Maniadakis N, Gray A: The economic burden of back pain in the UK. Pain 84:95–103, 2000.
3. Frymoyer JW, Cats-Baril WL: An overview of the incidence and costs of low back pain. Orthop Clin North Am 22:263–271, 1991.
4. Buckwalter JA: Aging and degeneration of the human intervertebral disc. Spine 20(11):1307–1314, 1995.
5. Anderson DG, Tannoury C: Molecular pathogenic factors in symptomatic disc degeneration. Spine J 5(suppl):260S–266S, 2005.
6. Phillips FM, Reuben J, Wetzel FT: Intervertebral disc degeneration adjacent to a lumbar fusion: An experimental rabbit model. J Bone Joint Surg Br 84:289–294, 2002.
7. Taylor JR, Twomey LT: The development of the human intervertebral disc. *In* Ghosh P (ed): The Biology of the Intervertebral Disc. Boca Raton, FL, CRC Press, 1988, pp 39–82.
8. Nishida K, Kang JD, Gilbertson LG, et al: 1999 Volvo Award in basic science. Modulation of the biologic activity of the rabbit intervertebral disc by gene therapy: An *in vivo* study of adenovirus-mediated transfer of the human transforming growth factor beta1 encoding gene. Spine 24:2419–2425, 1999.
9. Risbud MV, Guttapalli A, Albert TJ, et al: Hypoxia activates MAPK activity in rat nucleus pulposus cells: Regulation of integrin expression and cell survival. Spine 30:2503–2509, 2005.
10. Risbud MV, Fertala J, Vresilovic EJ, et al: IM. Nucleus pulposus cells upregulate PI3K/AKt and MEK/ERK signaling pathways under hypoxic conditions and resist apoptosis induced by serum withdrawal. Spine 30:882–890, 2005.
11. An HS, Thonar EJ, Masuda K: Biological repair of intervertebral disc. Spine 28:86–92, 2003.
12. Alini M, Roughley PJ, Antoniou J, et al: A biological approach to treating disc degeneration: not for today, but maybe for tomorrow. Eur Spine J 11:215–220, 2002.
13. Nishida K, Kang JD, Suh JK, et al: Adenovirus-mediated gene transfer to nucleus pulposus cells: Implications for the treatment of intervertebral disc degeneration. Spine 23:2437–2442, 1998.
14. Mochida J, Nishimura K, Nomura T, et al: The importance of preserving disc structure in surgical approaches to lumber disc herniation. Spine 21:1556–1563, 1996.
15. Nishimura K, Nochida J: Percutaneous reinsertion of the nucleus pulposus: An experimental study. Spine 23:1531–1539, 1998.
16. Takada T, Nishida K, Doita M, Kurosaka M: Fas ligand exists on intervertebral disc cells: A potential molecular mechanism for immune privilege of the disc. Spine 27:1526–1530, 2002.
17. Okuma M, Mochida J, Nishimura K, et al: Reinsertion of stimulated nucleus pulposus cells retards intervertebral disc degeneration: an *in vitro* and *in vivo* experimental study. J Orthop Res 3:988–997, 2000.
18. Yamamoto Y, Mochida J, Sakai D, et al: Upregulation of the viability of nucleus pulposus cells by bone-marrow-derived stromal cells: Significance of direct cell-to-cell contact in co-culture system. Spine 29:1508–1514, 2004.
19. Gruber HE, Johnson TL, Leslie K, et al: Autologous intervertebral disc cell implantation: A model using *Psammomys obesus*, the sand rat. Spine 27:1626–1633, 2002.
20. Ganey T, Libera J, Moos V, et al: Disc chondrocyte transplantation in a canine model: A treatment for degenerated or damaged intervertebral disc. Spine 28:2609–2620, 2003.
21. Gorensek M, Jaksimovic C, Kregar-Velikonja N, et al: Nucleus pulposus repair with cultured autologous elastic cartilage derived chondrocytes. Cell Mol Biol Lett 9:363–373, 2004.
22. Mwale F, Roughley P, Antoniou J: Distinction between the extracellular matrix of the nucleus pulposus and hyaline cartilage: A requisite for tissue engineering of intervertebral disc. Eur Cell Mater 8:58–63, 2004.
23. Iatridis JC, Weidenbaum, M, Setton LA, et al: Is the nucleus pulposus a solid or a fluid? Mechanical behaviors of the nucleus pulposus of the human intervertebral disc. Spine 21:1174–1184, 1996.
24. Risbud MV, Guttapalli A, Stokes DG, et al: Nucleus pulposus cells express HIF-1alpha under normoxic culture conditions: A metabolic adaptation to the intervertebral disc microenvironment. J Cell Biochem 98(1):152–159, 2006.
25. Fujita N, Miyamoto T, Imai J, et al: CD24 is expressed specifically in the nucleus pulposus of intervertebral discs. Biochem Biophys Res Commun 338(4):1890–1896, 2005.
26. Semba K, Araki K, Li Z, et al: A novel murine gene, Sickle tail, linked to the Danforth's short tail locus, is required for normal development of the intervertebral disc. Genetics 172(1):445–456, 2006.
27. Nomura T, Mochida J, Okuma M, et al: Nucleus pulposus allograft retards intervertebral disc degeneration. Clin Orthop 389:94–101, 2001.
28. Gerson SL: Mesenchymal stem cells: No longer second class marrow citizens. Nat Med 5:262–264, 1999.
29. Horwitz EM, Prockop DJ, Fitzpatrick LA, et al: Transplantability and therapeutic effects of bone marrow-derived mesenchymal cells in children with osteogenesis imperfecta. Nat Med 5:309–313, 1999.
30. Liechty KW, MacKenzie TC, Shaaban AF, et al: Human mesenchymal stem cells engraft and demonstrate site-specific differentiation after in utero transplantation in sheep. Nat Med 6:1282–1286, 2000.
31. Toma C, Pittenger MF, Cahill KS, et al: Human mesenchymal stem cells differentiate to a cardiomyocyte phenotype in the adult murine heart. Circulation 105:93–98, 2002.
32. Caplan AI, Elyaderani M, Mochizuki Y, et al: Principles of cartilage repair and regeneration. Clin Orthop Rel Res 342:254–269, 1997.
33. Wakitani S, Goto T, Pineda SJ, et al: Mesenchymal cell-based repair of large, full-thickness defects of articular cartilage. J Bone Joint Surg 76-A:579–592, 1994.
34. Im GI, Kim DY, Shin JH, et al: Repair of cartilage defect in the rabbit with cultured mesenchymal stem cells from bone marrow. J Bone Joint Surg 83-B:289–294, 2001.
35. Quintavalla J, Uziel-Fusi S, Yin J, et al: Fluorescently labeled mesenchymal stem cells (MSCs) maintain multilineage potential and can be detected following implantation into articular cartilage defects. Biomaterials 23:109–119, 2002.
36. Risbud MV, Albert TJ, Guttapalli A, et al: Differentiation of mesenchymal stem cells towards a nucleus pulposus–like phenotype *in vitro*: Implications for cell-based transplantation therapy. Spine 29:2627–2632, 2004.
37. Steck E, Bertram H, Abel R, et al: Induction of intervertebral disc-like cells from adult mesenchymal stem cells. Stem Cells 23(3):403–411, 2005.
38. Richardson SM, Walker RV, Parker S, et al: Intervertebral disc cell-mediated mesenchymal stem cell differentiation. Stem Cells 24 (3):707–716, 2006.
39. Sakai D, Mochida J, Yamamoto Y, et al: Transplantation of mesenchymal stem cells embedded in atelocollagen gel to the intervertebral disc: A potential therapeutic model for disc degeneration. Biomaterials 24:3531–3541, 2003.
40. Sakai D, Mochida J, Iwashina T, et al: Differentiation of mesenchymal stem cells transplanted to a rabbit degenerative disc model. Spine 30:2379–2387, 2005.
41. Sakai D, Mochida J, Iwashina T, et al: Regenerative effects of transplanting mesenchymal stem cells embedded in atelocollagen to the degenerated intervertebral disc. Biomaterials 27:335–345, 2006.
42. Crevensten G, Walsh AJ, Ananthakrishnan D, et al: Intervertebral disc cell therapy for regeneration: Mesenchymal stem cell implantation in rat intervertebral discs. Ann Biomed Eng 32:430–434, 2004.
43. Zhang YG, Guo X, Xu P, et al: Bone mesenchymal stem cells transplanted into rabbit intervertebral discs can increase proteoglycans. Clin Orthop Relat Res 430:219–226, 2005.

44. Gruber HE, Hanley EN Jr: Ultrastructure of the human intervertebral disc during aging and degeneration: Comparison of surgical and control specimens. Spine 27:798–805, 2002.
45. Singh K, Masuda K, An HS: Animal models for human disc degeneration. Spine J 5:267S–279S, 2005.
46. Masuda K, Aota Y, Muehleman C, et al: A novel rabbit model of mild, reproducible disc degeneration by an annulus needle puncture: Correlation between the degree of disc injury and radiological and histological appearances of disc degeneration. Spine 30:5–14, 2005.
47. Thompson JP, Pearce RH, Schechter MT, et al: Preliminary evaluation of a scheme for grading the gross morphology of the human intervertebral disc. Spine 15:411–415, 1990.

CHAPTER 86

# Gene Therapy for Intervertebral Disc Repair and Regeneration

Corey A. Pacek, Gwendolyn A. Sowa, and James D. Kang

## KEY POINTS

- Intervertebral disc degeneration is a complex biologic and biomechanical process involving multiple pathways that have yet to be completely elucidated.
- Several biologic factors, including TGF-β1, BMP-2, BMP-7 (OP-1), LMP-1, TIMP-1, Sox 9, and IL-1, are involved in the degenerative process.
- Modification of these factors produces effects in vitro and in vivo, and these effects have application to gene therapy.
- Further research is still needed to clarify which of these biologic factors actually has lasting beneficial effects with respect to treating the degenerative process.
- Further research is still needed to refine strategies for safe, efficient, lasting, and controllable gene delivery and expression within the intervertebral disc.

Intervertebral disc degeneration (IVDD) is one of the most common orthopaedic disorders affecting individuals today. It has been identified as an important cause of low back pain, leading to much morbidity and disability. Given the frequency of this condition, multiple treatment modalities have become available, both operative and nonoperative. Nonoperative treatments include nonsteroidal anti-inflammatory drugs, physical therapy, nerve root injections, and chronic pain management. Operative interventions include some of the most common orthopaedic procedures performed today, including, but not limited to, discectomy, laminectomy, fusion, and total disc replacement. Although these therapies do have variable success at treatment, they are all aimed specifically at the endpoint of a chronic degenerative pathway, rather than trying to alter that degenerative pathway.

Although the exact mechanism of IVDD has yet to be elucidated, it is known to involve a complex interaction of biologic and biomechanical factors. The intervertebral disc (IVD) is made up of the outer annulus fibrosus (AF) and the inner nucleus pulposus (NP). The AF is made up primarily of type I collagen, whereas the NP consists primarily of type II collagen, proteoglycans, and water. The proteoglycans, particularly aggrecan, with their multiple negatively charged side chains, are primarily responsible for attracting and maintaining water within the IVD. It has been observed that proteoglycan content decreases with the degenerative process, with a subsequent decrease in water content as well. Multiple biologic mediators are involved in both the synthesis and degradations of proteoglycans. It is believed that this decrease in proteoglycan content is a result of an imbalance in the equilibrium between the anabolism and catabolism of proteoglycans within the IVD (Fig. 86–1).

The goal of gene therapy is to shift the imbalance between the synthesis and breakdown of proteoglycans and thus achieve a net increase of proteoglycans. One strategy is to transduce the cells of the NP using a vector loaded with target genes in order to increase transcription of the target gene with subsequent mRNA translation to protein. This would result finally in a shift in the balance of anabolism and catabolism of proteoglycans, both in the transduced cell and in surrounding cells through a paracrine effect. It is surmised that increasing the proteoglycan content of the IVD will subsequently increase the water content, thereby restoring disc height and the normal physiologic properties of the NP.

## TARGET GENES

Because the end goal of gene therapy is a shift of the balance of anabolism and catabolism of proteoglycans, target genes need to have a relation to the biochemical pathway in either proteoglycan synthesis or degradation. Several groups of such genes are appropriate targets for gene therapy.

One such group includes several growth factors, such as transforming growth factor β-1 (TGF-β1),[1] bone morphogenic protein-2 (BMP-2),[2] and bone morphogenic protein-7 (BMP-7), known also as osteogenic protein-1 (OP-1).[3] These growth factors are important to the production of proteoglycans, the cells of the IVD, specifically the NP cells, and have known chondrogenic and osteogenic effects. Increased levels of these growth factors, both in vitro and in vivo, are known to increase proteoglycan synthesis in the NP.[1–3]

Another category of biologic mediators that has been identified as being involved in the degenerative cascade includes specific

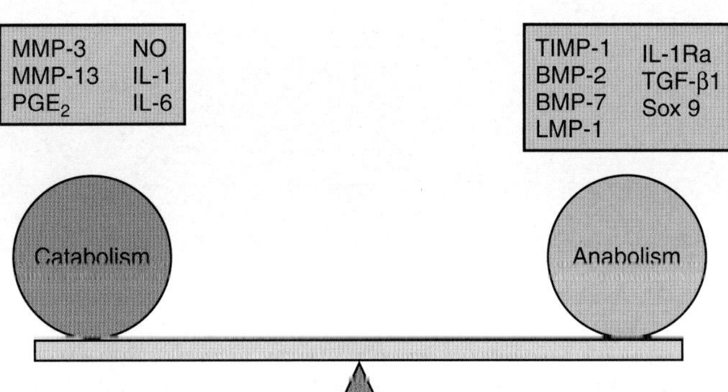


**FIGURE 86–1.** A proposed mechanism of intervertebral disc degeneration (IVDD) is an imbalance of catabolic activity with respect to anabolic activity of proteoglycans within the nucleus pulposus. Factors that modulate each type of activity are listed. BMP, bone morphogenic protein; IL, interleukin; IL-1Ra, interleukin 1 receptor antagonist; LMP, Lim mineralization protein; MMP, matrix metalloproteinase; NO, nitric oxide; $PGE_2$, prostaglandin $E_2$; Sox 9, sex-determining region Y-Box 9; TGF-β1, transforming growth factor β1; TIMP, tissue inhibitor of metalloproteinases.

mediators of degradation and inflammation, such as matrix metalloproteinases (MMPs), prostaglandin $E_2$ ($PGE_2$), nitric oxide (NO), interleukin 1 (IL-1), and interleukin 6 (IL-6). These factors have been reported to be involved in the breakdown or net decrease of the matrix of the NP. Their presence at increased levels is hypothesized to be responsible for increased catabolism of the IVD matrix.[4] Therefore, inhibitors of these catabolic factors would make excellent target genes for gene therapy.

Tissue inhibitors of matrix metalloproteinase (TIMPs) are an example of such a group of proteins that would inhibit mediators of degradation. TIMPs have been identified as natural inhibitors of MMPs, and are found at increased levels in degenerated disc cells along with MMPs. It has been shown that TIMP-1 specifically inhibits MMP-3 and can lead to a net increase of proteoglycan synthesis through this inhibition.[2]

Lim mineralization protein-1 (LMP-1) is another factor that has been identified as having potential for gene therapy. It is a regulatory molecule that can induce the production of other morphogens, including BMP-2 and BMP-7. It has been shown that increased levels of LMP-1 are associated with increases of BMP-2 and BMP-7, which both, in turn, would lead to an increase in proteoglycan synthesis.[5]

Previously mentioned genes have encoded for proteins involved with the regulation of proteoglycan synthesis, which has been the main focus of gene therapy. However, type II collagen has also been shown to be decreased in degenerated IVDs of patients as well.[6] Thus, there is interest in an additional gene, sex-determining region Y-Box 9 (Sox 9), which regulates type II collagen synthesis. An increase in Sox 9 should lead to an increase in type II collagen synthesis, which, it is hoped, could lead to repair of the degenerating IVD.

## GENE DELIVERY SYSTEMS

Identifying target genes that will effectively increase proteoglycan and water content of the NP is only part of the gene therapy equation. In order for the target genes to be transcribed and subsequently translated to protein, they must first enter the cells of the NP. The simplest therapy for the treatment of IVDD would be direct injection of these gene products into the IVD. The half-life of these gene products, which has been reported to be approximately 20 minutes in vivo, makes this strategy unpredictable or short-lasting for the treatment of a chronic condition such as IVDD.[7] In order to apply these products to the cells of the IVD, a stable, continuous supply is needed. This is where the true value of gene therapy can become realized.

A solution to this problem lies in vector-mediated delivery. A vector-mediated delivery system must exist that will provide reliable, efficient transfer of target genes to host cells. Additionally this vector must not have deleterious side effects to the host in which it is being used.

Both viral and nonviral vectors exist for such purposes. Nonviral vectors include liposomes, DNA-ligand complexes, and gene guns. These nonviral vectors are capable of transducing the host cells with the target genes of interest. However, there is some concern with lower efficiencies of transfer of the nonviral vectors as well as limited persistence of gene expression, which has been reported to continue only for days as opposed to the months or years that would be necessary for useful therapy. It is for this reason that the majority of gene therapy for the IVD has focused on viral vectors.[7]

Viral vectors for gene therapy provide reliable, efficient transfer of target genes while providing lasting gene expression. Retroviruses, adenovirus, and adeno-associated virus (AAV) have been investigated as viral vectors for gene transfer. Retroviruses only infect actively dividing cells. However, the IVD undergoes a paucity of cell division, particularly with aging and degeneration, making this a less useful tool when applied to the IVD. Adenovirus has been used extensively for the purpose of gene therapy in the IVD. It has the ability to infect a wide variety of nondividing cells both in vitro and in vivo. Additionally, the transduced cells are able to produce high levels of gene products for long durations, up to 1 year.[7]

One limiting factor for gene expression duration is immunologic activity of the host. Viral infection typically leads to an inflammatory reaction in the host due to the presence of viral proteins, leading to cell-mediated death of those cells producing the inciting protein. This has been associated with the typical decline in gene expression over time. Adenovirus has been used most frequently in recent literature for IVD gene therapy. Specific regions of the viral genome can be removed to continuously decrease the immunogenicity of the viral particle. The newest generation of adenoviral vectors contains no viral genome whatsoever, aside from simple beginning and terminal repeats, and houses only the target gene. These vectors stimulate the least host immune response.

The relatively avascular environment of the IVD appears to vastly decrease the exposure of IVD cells to host immunogenic cells. Nevertheless, in the setting of IVDD, the immune-privileged nature of the IVD may be violated through degenerative injury, leading to neovascularization. This represents a potentially limiting factor of a vector with immunogenic properties. It is for this reason that interest in AAV has also been shown as a potential vector for gene therapy in the IVD. AAV is unable to replicate by itself and requires the molecular machinery of other viruses, such as adenovirus, in order to replicate. It expresses no viral gene products following infection, which leads to little or no immune reaction by the host. This makes AAV an attractive vector as well in terms of both long-term gene expression and host safety.[7]

## GENE THERAPY OF THE INTERVERTEBRAL DISC

The ultimate aim of gene therapy of the IVD entails creating appropriate vectors containing genes of interest that can be transferred in vivo into degenerated IVDs, which in turn will introduce the aforementioned genes of interest into the degenerated NP cells. This will result in overproduction of gene product, causing a signaling cascade that results in a net anabolic or anticatabolic response, leading to repair and regeneration of the IVD.

The first great hurdle of gene therapy is transducing the host cells with the target gene (Fig. 86–2). This was shown to be possible in a very efficient manner by Moon and associates.[8] In their study, the different multiplicities of infectivity (MOI) were tested using adenoviral vectors, *Escherichia coli* β-galactosidase (lacZ), and luciferase as target genes, and human NP tissue as host cells. LacZ and luciferase were chosen as standard markers that transduction has taken place. It was shown that, with appropriate MOI levels, cells could transduce NP cells in vitro with near 100% efficiency with little or no toxic effect on the cells. Additionally, no significant difference was seen in the transducibility between normal and degenerated NP cells. This was a key study in proving the feasibility of gene therapy using adenovirus in not only healthy human IVD cells but degenerated human IVD cells as well.[8]

Studies such as Moon and associates[8] are necessary in order to show in vitro reactions of viral vectors with human cells. However, in vivo experiments with such viral vectors are not yet possible given the lack of sufficient evidence to ethically justify human trials. Fortunately, several animal models of IVDD exist that accurately portray similar pathophysiology of IVDD. The rabbit model, as one example, has been invaluable by giving researchers a valuable tool to continue with in vivo gene therapy studies.

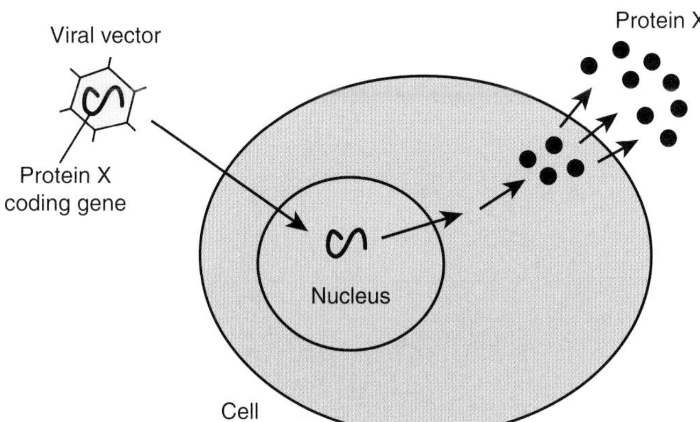


**FIGURE 86–2.** Schematic representation of gene therapy. The target gene encased in a viral vector is transduced into an IVD cell, which in turn produces the gene product of that target gene. *(From Nishida K, et al: Modulation of the biologic activity of the rabbit intervertebral disc by gene therapy: An in vivo study of adenovirus-mediated transfer of the human transforming growth factor beta 1 encoding gene. Spine 24 (23):2419–2425, 1999.)*

This model has been utilized in many key studies that have advanced the fund of knowledge pertaining to gene therapy. The possibility of increasing net proteoglycan synthesis was shown to be possible in vivo utilizing a rabbit model by Nishida and associates.[1] In their study, rabbit IVDs were injected with adenoviral vector containing the gene encoding for TGF-β1. The L2-L3, L3-L4, and L4-L5 disc spaces were injected with either TGF-β1 vectors, luciferase control vectors, or saline (control group). The L1-L2 disc space was used in each rabbit for a control. The experimental group showed a 30-fold increase in TGF-β1 production. No significant increase in TGF-β1 production was seen in the neighboring control disc space of both the saline and TGF-β1 groups, nor was a significant increase in TGF-β1 seen in the cells transduced with the luciferase enzyme (Fig. 86–3). Additionally, by measuring incorporation of radioactively labeled sulfate, newly synthesized proteoglycan was calculated. The discs injected with the *TGF-β1* gene showed a 200% increase in newly synthesized proteoglycan synthesis as compared to both the saline and luciferase groups (Fig. 86–4). This showed that the transduction process in and of itself was not responsible for the increase in proteoglycan production, but that it was a result of the direct action of the TGF-β1 gene inserted into the cells. The rabbits in this study showed no signs of illness following transfection with the viral vectors. This exciting study showed that at least in the healthy rabbit IVD, it was possible to transduce the cells of the IVD and result in both an increase in production of the target gene as well as, and more importantly, the production of newly synthesized proteoglycan.[1]

The bone morphogenic proteins (BMPs) have also shown great promise in terms of gene therapy. BMP-2 has specifically been

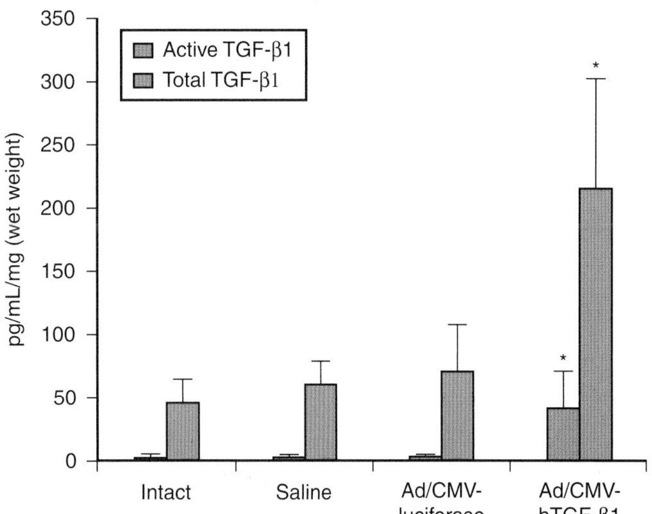


**FIGURE 86–3.** Active and total TGF-β1 synthesis following transduction with the TGF-β1 gene are depicted. Total TGF-β1 = Active TGF-β1 + Latent TGF-β1. Significant values are indicated by an asterisk. Note: CMV indicates that the cytomegalovirus promoter was used in the adenoviral construct. Ad, adenovirus. *(From Nishida K, et al: Modulation of the biologic activity of the rabbit intervertebral disc by gene therapy: An in vivo study of adenovirus-mediated transfer of the human transforming growth factor beta 1 encoding gene. Spine 24(23):2419–2425, 1999.)*

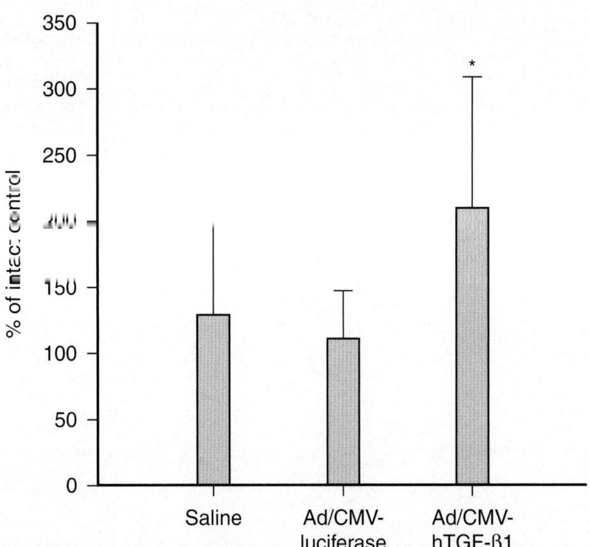


■ **FIGURE 86–4.** Newly synthesized proteoglycans following transduction. Significant values are indicated by an asterisk. Note: CMV indicates that the cytomegalovirus promoter was used in the adenoviral construct. Ad, adenovirus. *(From Nishida K, et al: Modulation of the biologic activity of the rabbit intervertebral disc by gene therapy: An in vivo study of adenovirus-mediated transfer of the human transforming growth factor beta 1 encoding gene. Spine 24(23):2419–2425, 1999.)*

shown in prior studies to lead to an increase in extracellular matrix production, as well as playing a key role in cartilage development as reported by Kim and associates.[9] Given these findings, BMP-2 is another potential choice for gene therapy. There were concerns, however, that BMP-2 could have osteogenic potential within the IVD cells. This question was addressed by Kim and associates[9] in their study using recombinant BMP-2 and human IVD cells suspended in a three-dimensional alginate bead culture. The human IVD cells, when exposed to the recombinant BMP-2, showed an increase in the mRNA of several genes normally produced by the healthy IVD cells, such as aggrecan, type I collagen, and type II collagen. The cells did not, however, show increased mRNA for the osteocalcin gene. Osteocalcin, a marker of bone metabolism, was used as an osteogenic marker for the purposes of this study. Additionally, the IVD cells were shown to positively upregulate the production of proteoglycans when treated with the recombinant form of BMP-2 (Fig. 86–5). This study proved that BMP-2 was another excellent target for gene therapy given its effect on human IVD cells by showing increased production of aggrecan, type II collagen mRNA, and increased net production of proteoglycan, without the increase of markers of bone formation.[9]

Another bone morphogenic protein, BMP-7, also known as OP-1, has shown significant promise as a target gene for gene therapy. An and associates[3] injected OP-1 into the IVD of healthy rabbits and compared subsequent disc height with control rabbits who received injections of saline only. The rabbits injected with OP-1 showed a significantly greater disc height than rabbits injected with saline (Fig. 86–6). The IVD cells of the OP-1–injected rabbits also showed elevated levels of proteoglycan synthesis over the next 2 weeks as compared to a control group

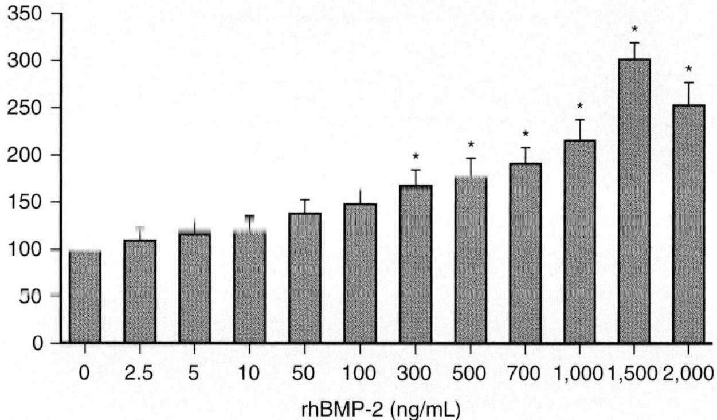


■ **FIGURE 86–5.** Newly synthesized proteoglycan content is significantly increased in cells exposed to recombinant bone morphogenetic protein-2 (rhBMP-2). Significant values are indicated by an asterisk. *(From Kim DJ, et al: Bone morphogenetic protein-2 facilitates expression of chondrogenic, not osteogenic, phenotype of human intervertebral disc cells. Spine 28(24):2679–2684, 2003.)*

(Fig. 86–7). This increased synthesis was not significant past 2 weeks, but again, this study was only showing the effects of OP-1 and did not transduce cells with the *OP-1* gene.[3] This study showed that OP-1 was yet another excellent target for gene therapy in the IVD. Further studies are needed to assess if OP-1 is effective in regenerating degenerated discs over longer periods of time.

Given the positive results seen with the research into BMP-2 and BMP-7 (OP-1), research has continued into an additional growth factor, LMP-1. This growth factor regulates the production of BMP-2, -4, -6, and -7, in that increasing levels of LMP-1 lead to increasing levels of the aforementioned BMPs. Gene therapy

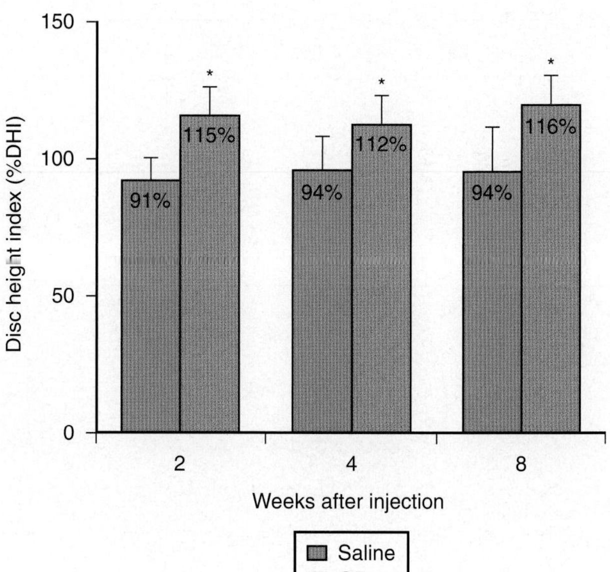


■ **FIGURE 86–6.** Disc height index, a calculated measure of disc height, was significantly increased in OP-1-treated rabbit intervertebral discs. Significant values are indicated by an asterisk. *(From An HS, et al: Intradiscal administration of osteogenic protein-1 increases intervertebral disc height and proteoglycan content in the nucleus pulposus in normal adolescent rabbits. Spine 30(1):25–31; discussion 31–32, 2005.)*

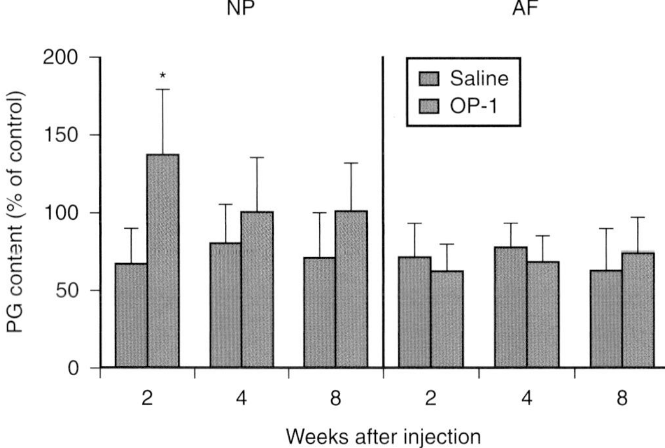


■ **FIGURE 86–7.** Proteoglycan synthesis was found to be significantly increased in OP-1-treated intervertebral disc cells 2 weeks following injection. Significant values are indicated by an asterisk. AF, annulus fibrosus; NP, nucleus pulposus. *(From An HS, et al: Intradiscal administration of osteogenic protein-1 increases intervertebral disc height and proteoglycan content in the nucleus pulposus in normal adolescent rabbits. Spine 30(1):25–31; discussion 31–32, 2005.)*

using this molecule is enticing due to the ability to act on two factors already known to have an effect on the IVD cells by transducing a single gene. Yoon and associates[5] performed studies on both the in vitro and in vivo effects of LMP-1. LMP-1 was shown in vitro with rat lumbar disc cells to lead to both an increase of BMP-2 and BMP-7 mRNA (Fig. 86–8) as well as the actual protein products. There was a net increase in proteoglycan production seen in the transfected cells as well. Additionally, it was also shown that noggin, which is an inhibitor of the BMPs, could completely block the effects of the LMP-1–transfected gene when added to the media in vitro. This result verified that it was the action of the BMPs

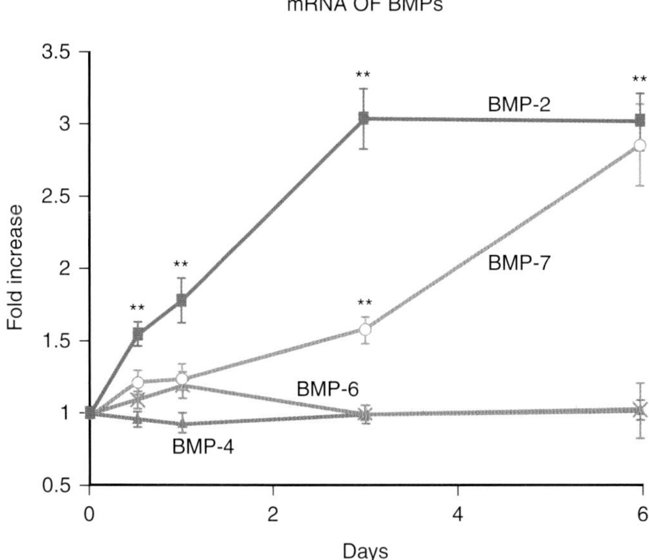


■ **FIGURE 86–8.** Following transduction with LMP-1 (Lim mineralization protein), mRNA of BMP-2 and BMP-7 was significantly increased. Significant values are indicated by double asterisks. BMP, bone morphogenetic protein. *(From Yoon ST, et al: ISSLS prize winner: LMP-1 upregulates intervertebral disc cell production of proteoglycans and BMPs in vitro and in vivo. Spine 29(23):2603–2611, 2004.)*

stimulated by LMP-1 that led to the increase in proteoglycan synthesis in vitro. LMP-1 was shown in vivo in healthy rabbit models to lead to increased production of BMP-2, BMP-7, and aggrecan mRNA without any signs of systemic illness to the rabbits. The data show great promise for yet another target for gene therapy. The ability to act on two growth factors gives a greater effect given one transduction, and it is hoped that this could eventually yield a stronger effect in human IVD cells.[5]

In addition to biologic factors that affect proteoglycan production, there is interest in biologic factors that affect type II collagen synthesis, such as Sox 9. Type II collagen has been shown to represent a high percentage of the NP matrix of healthy adults, and its decrease in synthesis and increased degradation are seen with the aging process. This decrease in type II collagen has therefore been implicated in IVDD, and an increase in its production, much like proteoglycan, has been hypothesized to be beneficial to the IVD. Thus, Sox 9, which leads to increased production of type II collagen, has been studied as a potential target for gene therapy. In a study by Paul and associates,[6] Sox 9 was studied both in vitro and in vivo using human IVD cells and rabbit stab incision models, respectively. Using an in vitro method with human IVD cells, an increased level of *Sox 9* gene product as well as increased type II collagen production was seen in cells transduced with the *Sox 9* gene. The in vivo model involved using a rabbit stab incision model of disc degeneration in which rabbits either received the stab alone, the stab and a marker gene transfer (here, green fluorescent protein), or the stab and the *Sox 9* gene. The rabbit IVD cells that were transfected with adenovirus loaded with the *Sox 9* gene showed preservation of the chondrocytic histologic appearance of the NP compared to control stab models. The rabbit models again showed no signs of systemic illness. Although much of the research into IVD gene therapy has focused on proteoglycan synthesis, type II collagen appears to be an interesting avenue as well given the data that have been revealed.[6]

The growth factors TGF-β1, BMP-2, BMP-7 (OP-1), LMP-1, and Sox 9 have all been shown to have significant promise concerning gene therapy for the IVDD. While these growth factors are anabolic, certain catabolic factors, such as the MMPs, are also important with regard to gene therapy. It has been reported in the literature that degenerated IVD cells contain elevated levels of MMPs, which are associated with increased degradation of the structural matrix of the IVD. The natural inhibitors of MMPs—TIMPs—have also been proposed as effective target genes. Wallach and associates[2] performed an in vitro study that looked at transduction of human IVD cells with TIMP-1 and compared results with that of cells transduced with BMP-2. Both arms of this study produced exciting results. The TIMP-1 group did show significant increase in newly synthesized proteoglycan production. A full fivefold increase in proteoglycan production was seen in the cervical IVD cells treated with a level of 100 MOI of vector. This was shown to be the optimal level, as cervical IVD cells treated with 50 MOI and 150 MOI showed significantly increased levels of proteoglycan as well but were limited to a threefold increase and a fourfold increase, respectively (Fig. 86–9). Lumbar IVD cells showed similar trends. The cells transduced with BMP-2 showed a continued increase in proteoglycan synthesis with increasing MOI, with a significant fourfold increase in newly synthesized

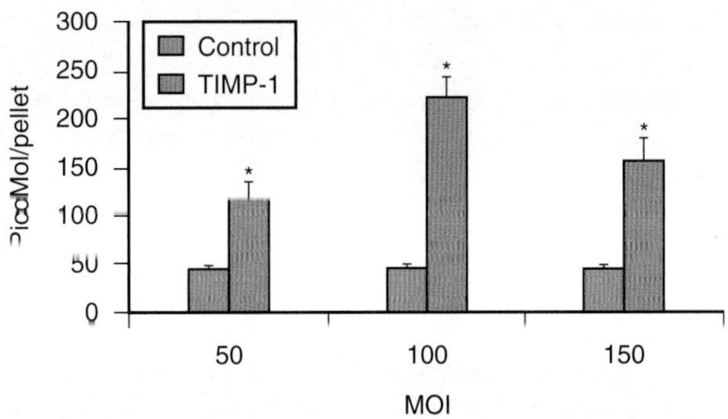


■ **FIGURE 86–9.** Cells transduced with TIMP-1 (tissue inhibitor of metalloproteinases) showed significant increases in proteoglycan synthesis. Significant values are indicated by an asterisk. *(From Wallach CJ, et al: Gene transfer of the catabolic inhibitor TIMP-1 increases measured proteoglycans in cells from degenerated human intervertebral discs. Spine 28(20):2331–2337, 2003.)*

proteoglycans as compared to a control group at 150 MOI. It is unclear, however, as to the exact mechanism of increased proteoglycan synthesis in the face of upregulated TIMP-1 expression. It is possible that the inhibition of MMPs allows the production of proteoglycan that has already taken place to occur in an unopposed fashion or that the appearance of increased levels of TIMP-1 leads to a signaling cascade which results in the increased proteoglycan synthesis. Continued research is needed to delineate the exact biochemical pathways at work, but nonetheless, TIMP-1 has been shown to be another exciting avenue for gene therapy.[2]

IL-1 is another biologic factor that leads to increased catabolism of proteoglycans. As mentioned earlier, this molecule has been found in increased levels in degenerated human IVD cells. IL-1 receptor antagonist (IL-1Ra) is a naturally occurring molecule that, as its name suggests, is able to block the activity of IL-1, and has been identified as a possible target for gene therapy. Preliminary studies of this inhibitor have shown positive results. Human IVD cells were able to be transduced with the *IL-1Ra* gene and produced the protein in significant quantities. The gene expressions of two MMPs, *MMP-3* and *MMP-13* (also known as stromelysin-1 and collagenase 3, respectively), were then measured in response to IL-1 exposure. The cells transduced with IL-1Ra were shown to have significant decrease in *MMP-3* and *MMP-13* gene expression as compared to the controls in response to IL-1. Following this, IL-1Ra–transfected cells, both normal and degenerated, were first labeled with a fluorescein-based dye that allowed their distinction and then injected into IVD explants in an ex vivo method. It was shown that 2 weeks following successful injection of transduced cells, IL-1Ra was still detectable at a statistically significant amount in the disc. IL-1Ra was thus shown in this study to be yet another gene of interest for gene therapy. Further studies are needed to see if this can be applied to in vivo applications as well.[10]

## CONCLUSIONS

Gene therapy for the IVD is an exciting and active line of continued research. Multiple anabolic and catabolic factors have been identified and are capable of being transferred through vectors to in vivo rabbit models, in vitro human IVD cells, and ex vivo disc explant models. These biologic factors have been shown to be effective in shifting the balance between anabolism and catabolism of the IVD structural matrix toward that of anabolism. It is hypothesized that this shift will be associated with the eventual regeneration of the IVD. Great strides have been made with regard to the possible avenues for therapeutic gene treatment, but there is much research remaining prior to successful implementation in in vivo human disc degeneration.

## FUTURE CONSIDERATIONS

The ultimate goal of gene therapy, the repair and restoration of the IVD, still must be reliably and reproducibly shown in a rabbit in vivo model prior to its application to humans. Along with this, the unique environment of the degenerated IVD must be evaluated with regard to transducibility and subsequent gene product production as well.

The length of activity that is necessary for chronic treatment must be delineated. The persistence of gene expression has not yet been defined in rabbit models, nor is the time course necessary for continued treatment known. It is still possible that host immune responses will eventually begin to detect and kill cells that have been transduced.

Safety of the adenoviral vectors is also a concern. The relative sequestration of IVD contents due to the avascular nature of the structure seems to be a natural defense against systemic effects of local injection. However, injections that miss the IVD or leak into surrounding tissues pose a safety hazard and must still be addressed. Research is also being undertaken in areas of inducible gene systems, such as tetracycline on/off systems. The ability to turn the transferred gene on or off based on the application of an external stimulus, such as an oral pharmaceutical, would be a great advantage, both as a safety feature and as a method to modify treatment.

Much more research is needed to answer these as well as many other questions about gene therapy for the IVD. With continued efforts by researchers around the world, the goal of a therapeutic gene-vector construct to lead to the repair and reconstruction of IVDD can be achieved.

## REFERENCES

1. Nishida K, et al: Modulation of the biologic activity of the rabbit intervertebral disc by gene therapy: An in vivo study of adenovirus-mediated transfer of the human transforming growth factor beta 1 encoding gene. Spine 24(23):2419–2425, 1999.
2. Wallach CJ, et al: Gene transfer of the catabolic inhibitor TIMP-1 increases measured proteoglycans in cells from degenerated human intervertebral discs. Spine 28(20):2331–2337, 2003.
3. An HS, et al: Intradiscal administration of osteogenic protein-1 increases intervertebral disc height and proteoglycan content in the nucleus pulposus in normal adolescent rabbits. Spine 30(1):25–31; discussion 31–32, 2005.
4. Kang JD, et al: Toward a biochemical understanding of human intervertebral disc degeneration and herniation: Contributions of nitric oxide, interleukins, prostaglandin E2, and matrix metalloproteinases. Spine 22(10):1065–1073, 1997.
5. Yoon ST, et al: ISSLS prize winner: LMP-1 upregulates intervertebral disc cell production of proteoglycans and BMPs in vitro and in vivo. Spine 29(23):2603–2611, 2004.

6. Paul R, et al: Potential use of Sox9 gene therapy for intervertebral degenerative disc disease. Spine 28(8):755–763, 2003.
7. Sobajima S, et al: Gene therapy for degenerative disc disease. Gene Ther 11(4):390–401, 2004.
8. Moon SH, et al: Human intervertebral disc cells are genetically modifiable by adenovirus-mediated gene transfer: Implications for the clinical management of intervertebral disc disorders. Spine 25 (20):2573–2579, 2000.
9. Kim DJ, et al: Bone morphogenetic protein-2 facilitates expression of chondrogenic, not osteogenic, phenotype of human intervertebral disc cells. Spine 28(24):2679–2684, 2003.
10. Le Maitre CL, Freemont AJ, Hoyland JA: A preliminary in vitro study into the use of IL-1Ra gene therapy for the inhibition of intervertebral disc degeneration. Int J Exp Pathol 87(1):17–28, 2006.

CHAPTER 87

# Autologous Disc Chondrocyte Transplant: Early Clinical Results

**Rudolf Bertagnoli**

## KEY POINTS

- Autologous disc chondrocyte transplant (ADCT) is a novel treatment option used in mild forms of degenerative disc disease in addition to removal of sequester from a disc herniation.
- The disc material is harvested and transferred to a cell culture in which chondrocytes are proliferated over several weeks along with the patient's own serum. There is no genetic manipulation of the cells.
- Around 3 months later, when the disc annulus is healed, this chondrocyte cell suspension is reinjected into the affected disc in a minimally invasive surgery to compensate for the lost disc material.
- The biologic reconstitution of the disc in delaying the degenerative process of the intervertebral disc is a promising treatment option as preliminary results show. Long-term data remain to be collected.

During recent years degenerative changes of the lumbar segments have become an enormous medical problem in industrial nations,[1,2] leading to increased progress in clinical medicine and the knowledge of the pathomechanisms of intradiscal degenerative processes.[3–7] Factors such as heredity traits are discussed in the literature.[8–11]

Disc herniation, generally caused by trauma and degeneration, and the resulting low back pain cannot be avoided and has to be treated. Besides conservative methods there are several surgical interventions for the treatment of chronic back pain resulting from disc herniation. At this point, however, no established clinical procedure or treatment option is available that slows down the progression of degeneration caused by the loss of disc tissue due to the herniation and sequestration following an intervertebral disc operation. The biologic reconstitution of degenerated discs is a big challenge for novel therapeutic methods to regain the functional state of the intervertebral disc and to prevent further deleterious changes of adjacent vertebrae as well as extensive surgeries in the future (Fig. 87–1).

The main goal of this new method was to show a slowing of the ongoing degeneration process involving the intervertebral disc following disc herniation.

## INDICATIONS AND CONTRAINDICATIONS

In a prospective, randomized study autologous disc chondrocyte transplant was indicated for patients between 18 and 60 years old with a body mass index (BMI) less than 28. Patients with monosegmental disc protrusion, disc prolapse, or sequester between L3 and S1 have been enrolled in the study. Exclusion criteria include prior surgery on the abovementioned segments, previous chemonucleolysis or other percutaneous discectomy procedures, ankylosing spondyloarthrosis, end plate edema or sclerosis, modic II or III changes, chronic facet syndrome, stenosis of the spinal canal, spondylolysthesis, severe motor deficits, and congenital abnormalities of the spinal nerves. Additionally, patients who suffered from diseases such as borreliosis, pancreatitis, diseases of the kidney, or traumatic neurologic disorders are excluded.

## OPERATIVE TECHNIQUES

### First Surgical Intervention

Operative access is accomplished through a microsurgical or endoscopic assisted posterior approach. The sequestrectomy itself follows the normal clinical routine under microscopic visualization and subsequent removal of the hernitated disc.

In cases with a smaller sequester an additional biopsy of nucleus material has to be added to harvest approximately 1.0 to 1.5 $cm^3$ of material.

### Second Surgical Intervention

Healing and stability of the posterior annulus and longitudinal ligament return about 3 months after the first surgical intervention. At this point the patients in the active treatment group are ready for the transplantation to take place.

The reinjection of the cells is performed using fluoroscopy for guidance and local anesthesia. A volume pressure measurement of the affected disc is then performed to proof the closure of the

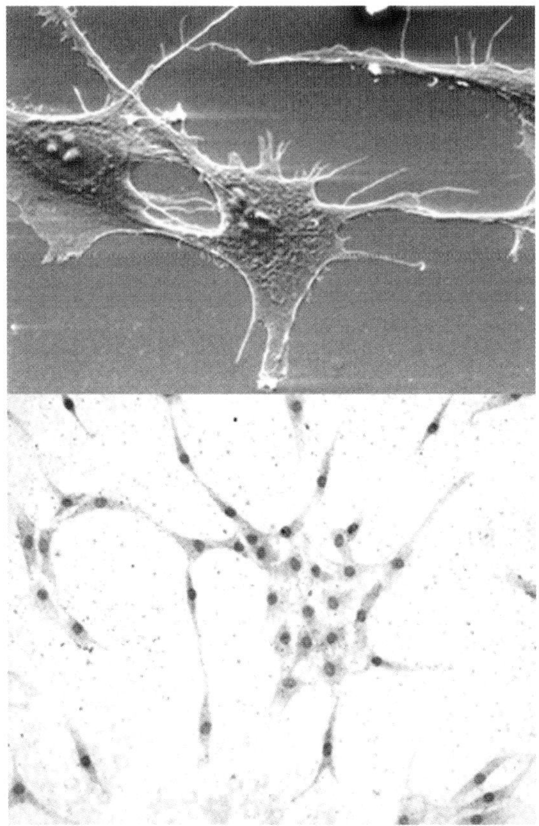

■ **FIGURE 87–1.** Monolayer of chondrocytes.

defect in the posterior annulus from the primary surgery. The suspension of the autologous disc-derived chondrocytes are transplanted into the affected intervertebral disc.

## POSTOPERATIVE CARE

Patients in the ADCT treatment group must remain in the hospital at least 24 hours. During the first 12 hours the patients are restricted to bed rest in the supine position with preferable angled legs. Standard bed rest is then prescribed for the remaining 12 hours of the first 24 hours after surgery. On the second day the patient's bed rest continues and the first isometric exercises can be performed. A dynamic lumbar orthosis is required to be worn for 4 weeks to avoid maximum motion excursions.

## CLINICAL PRESENTATION AND EVALUATION

The prospective and randomized trial was performed on 53 patients, divided into two groups: 27 patients within the treatment group and 26 patients within the control group. All patients participating in this trial received an eligible treatment for their complaints and were treated with a sequestrectomy, a well-known and widely used method to treat a lumbar disc herniation. The sequester obtained during the procedure was taken along with a defined volume of patient blood for culturing the chondrocytes for all patients. Patients in the control group underwent no additional surgical procedure while the treatment group received sequestrectomy plus ADCT. The disc biopsy and the human blood serum of these patients were forwarded to cell culture laboratory (co.don AG). Autologous disc–derived chondrocytes were then isolated from the disc biopsy. Each cell transplant was individually manufactured with each patient's own serum and own disc chondrocytes. The cultivation time of the cells varied between 2 and 4 weeks, depending on the growth habit of the cells. About 3 months after the index surgery the chondrotransplant was applied through a minimally invasive operative procedure.

Patient outcome was assessed using radiologic, physician, and patient self-assessment. The primary criterion used to evaluate the state of health of the patients was the Oswestry Low Back Pain Disability Questionnaire (according to Hudson-Cook) (OPDQ), and the Quebec Back Pain Disability Scale (QBPD), Prolo scale, the Visual Analog Score (VAS), and the SF-36 were used as secondary criteria. Magnetic resonance imaging (MRI) and x-ray studies were used for the radiologic evaluation for the treated and adjacent levels. Images were analyzed to evaluate morphologic changes such as the intervertebral disc height (affected intervertebral disc height was compared to the mean height of the two adjacent nonaffected discs), adjacent end plates, and deprivation of liquid. Adverse events/serious adverse events (AE/SAE) and all other complications following the surgical intervention have been documented with regard to their possible relationship to the surgery.

The control group showed a constant value up to 6 months and a slight decrease after 24 months for these parameters. In comparison, the ADCT-treated group showed a progressive significant decrease in the total sum score and disability index OPDQ. After 12 months the scores have been already decreased by more than 40% (Fig. 87–2).

As a secondary parameter the mean and median of the total sum score of the QBPD score showed a decrease of more than 50% after 1 year and more than 40% after 2 years compared to that of the control group (Fig. 87–3). The pain assessment via VAS showed an improvement of 60% after 1 year for the

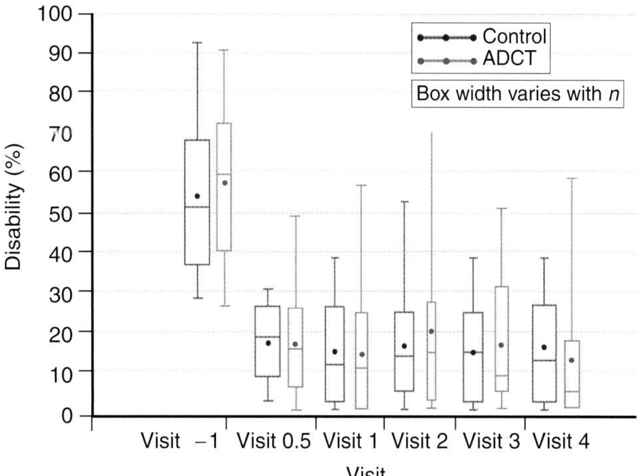


■ **FIGURE 87–2.** Disability index (%) of the Oswestry Low Back Pain Disability Questionnaire (OPDQ) based on patients with at least 2 years of visits. Visit −1: Sequestrectomy. Visit 0.5: ADCT/control. Visit 1: 3 months after ADCT/control visit 0.5. Visit 2: 6 months after ADCT/control visit 0.5. Visit 3: 12 months after ADCT/control visit 0.5. Visit 4: 24 months after ADCT/control visit 0.5. *(From co.don AG.)*

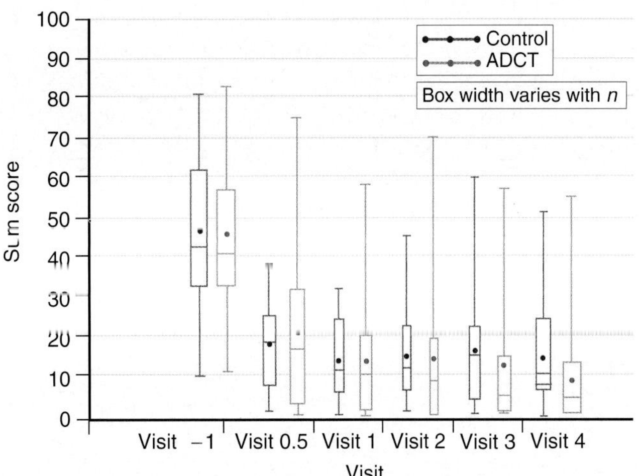


■ **FIGURE 87–3.** Total sum score of the Quebec Back Pain Disability Scale (QBPD) based on patients with at least 2 years of visits. Visit −1: Sequestrectomy. Visit 0.5: ADCT/control. Visit 1: 3 months after ADCT/control visit 0.5. Visit 2: 6 months after ADCT/control visit 0.5. Visit 3: 12 months after ADCT/control visit 0.5. Visit 4: 24 months after ADCT/control visit 0.5. *(From co.don AG.)*

ADCT-treated group, but the VAS for the control group showed nearly a constant level. According to the evaluation of disc height, the mean height of the affected discs was lower than that of the nonaffected discs. No difference between both groups was found in the mean intervertebral disc height of the affected discs. All these data confirm a significant clinical improvement of patients that received ADCT compared to the control group.

In total, 17 adverse events have been reported. Seven of these AEs were reported by four patients of the ADCT group and the other 10 AEs were reported by seven patients of the control group. In both groups the adverse events showed no relationship to the treatment.

## COMPLICATIONS AND AVOIDANCE

Risks involved with autologous disc chondrocyte transplant procedure include the normal problems that can occur during surgical interventions, such as hematoma, infections, neurologic deterioration, cerebrospinal fluid fistula, retroperitoneal lesions, column instability, and relapsing herniation. There are no additional risks for patient who undergo sequestrectomy and ADCT. No immune incompatibility reactions to autologous cell transplants have been reported in our patients and in the literature so far.

### CASE STUDY

A 33-year-old female patient had a multiyear history of low back pain with unsuccessful conservative treatment due to a disc herniation at L5-S1.

The patient received a sequestrectomy procedure and ADCT 3 months later. Postoperatively the patient was completely satisfied with the surgery and had no back pain. The VAS improved by 92% (from 6 points preoperative to 0.5 points 15 months after surgery) (Fig. 87–4). Radiographic and MRI evaluation showed a maintenance of disc height as well as nearly normal hydration of the operated disc.

## CONCLUSION

The regenerative capacity of autologous disc–derived cultured chondrocytes for the regeneration of damaged or degenerated discs was already shown in animal trials.

The aim of this prospective, randomized, assessment-blinded, controlled clinical study is to evaluate the clinical relevance of this biologic therapeutic method designed to delay or inhibit the progressive disc degeneration following disc herniation and sequestrectomy. The outcome has shown a significant therapeutic benefit of the ADCT group compared to the patient group having undergone sequestrectomy only. After transplantation of autologous disc cells, the progression of degenerative disc disease (DDD) was delayed or even inhibited by regeneration of the treated nucleus. All observed adverse events were not related to the transplant.

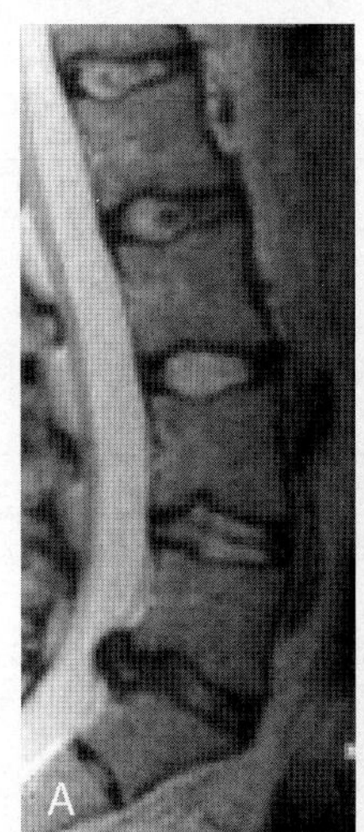

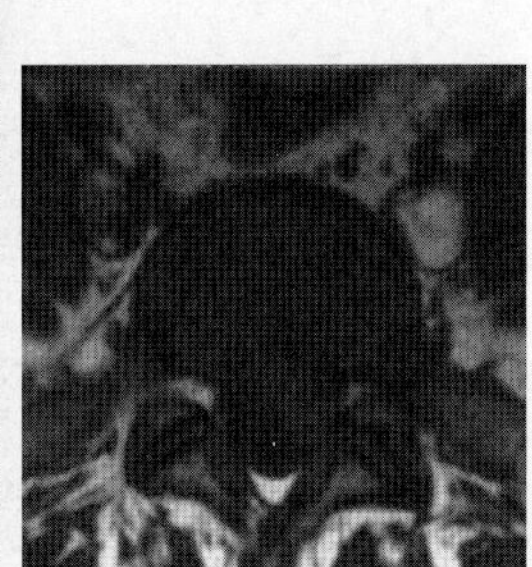
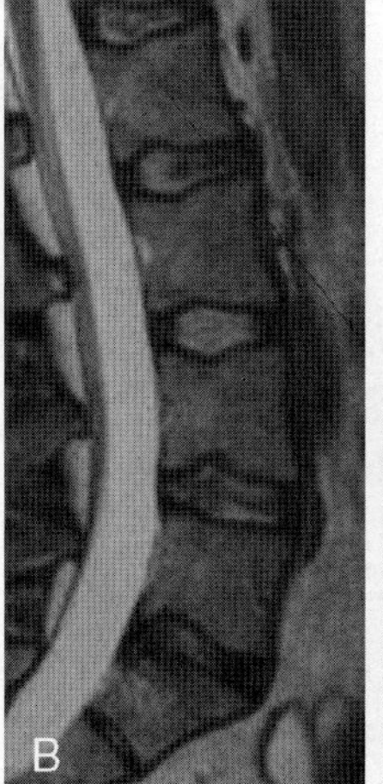

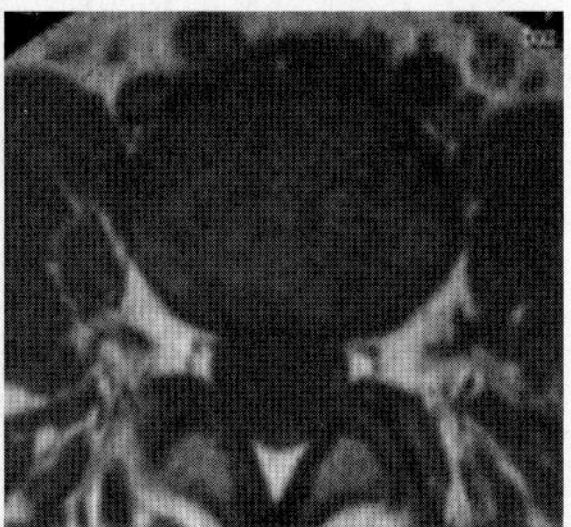

■ **FIGURE 87–4.** Magnetic resonance images before surgery **(A)** and 15 months after surgery **(B)**.

Even though the results of the study have been very promising, long-term follow-up data and a bigger cohort of patients are still necessary to establish this biologic solution as a standard treatment option for patients who suffer from low back pain caused by early disc herniation and maintenance of the nutrition barrier of the end plate.

## REFERENCES

1. Nachemson A: Recent advances in the treatment of low back pain. Int Orthop 9:1–10, 1985.
2. Kopec JA, Esdaile JM, Abrahamowicz M, et al: The Quebec Back Pain Disability Scale: Conceptualization and development. J Clin Epidemiol 49:151–161, 1996.
3. Kraemer J: Bandscheibenbedingte Erkrankungen, 4th ed. Stuttgart, Germany, Thieme, 1997.
4. MacIniosh JE, Bogduk N: The morphology of the lumbar erector spinae. Spine 12:658–668, 1987.
5. Parke WW, Watanabe R: Lumbosacral intersegmental epispinal axons and ectopic ventral nerve rootlets. J Neurosurg 67:269–277, 1987.
6. Rydevik R, Brown MD, Lundborg G: Pathoanatomy and pathophysiology of nerve root compression. Spine 9:7–15, 1984.
7. Watanabe R, Parke WW: Vascular and neural pathology of lumbosacral spinal stenosis. J Neurosurg 64:64–70, 1986.
8. Anders DG, Tannoury C: Molecular pathogenetic factors in symptomatic disc degeneration. Spine J 5:260S–266S, 2005.
9. Solovieva S, Lohiniva J, Leino-Arjas P, et al: COL9A3 gene polymorphism and obesity in intervertebral disc degeneration of the lumbar spine: Evidence of gene-environment interaction. Spine 27:2691–2696, 2002.
10. Sambrook PN, MacGregor AJ, Spector TD: Genetic influences on cervical and lumbar disc degeneration: A magnetic resonance imaging study in twins. Arthritis Rheum 42:1729–1735, 1999.
11. Annunen S, Paassilta P, et al: An allele of COL9A2 associated with intervertebral disc disease. Science 285(5426):409–412, 1999.

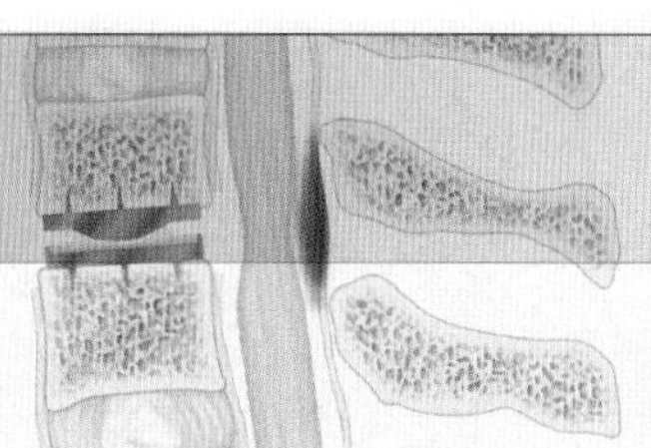

PART

# XII

# CONTROVERSIES

CHAPTER 88

# The Development of a Personalized Hybrid EMG-Assisted/Finite Element Biomechanical Model to Assess Surgical Options

**William S. Marras, Gregory G. Knapik,** and **Josue Gabriel**

## KEY POINTS

- A hybrid biodynamic EMG-assisted/finite element model has been developed that integrates the muscle recruitment benefits of biologically assisted models with finite element disc modeling.
- The model can incorporate patient specific anthropometry and spine geometry into the representation of the spine.
- Model mechanics have been validated in a series of laboratory studies.
- The model can be used to assess surgical options and understand the benefits and limitations of spine instrumentation through "virtual surgery."
- This approach will allow surgeons to appreciate the biomechanical consequences of surgical interventions for specific patients prior to surgery.

Biomechanical models of the human spine have evolved rapidly over the past two decades. With the dramatic increases in computing power and a large range of mechanical engineering software now available, we are at the point where powerful models can be created that represent the human spine and the surrounding structures in a system that functionally describes the physical capabilities and limitations of the spine.

In general, biomechanical models are nothing more than a mathematical representation of our knowledge regarding how the spine functions. However, biomechanical models are able to logically account for a large amount of information in a single system. In addition, models have the ability to consider the effects of various interactions among different mechanical properties that govern human function. Therefore, biomechanical models can be considered the "glue" that holds our logic together when we are trying to understand how complex physiologic functions influence the development of forces acting on the spine. A well-developed model can help us understand how exposure to environmental or occupational conditions can influence spine loading and the subsequent breakdown of the tissues. Ultimately, biomechanical models can not only quantitatively represent the current status of a specific subject's spine but will also be capable of predicting the impact of various potential surgical interventions so that the surgeon can make the best informed decision when considering surgical options. If the spine is accurately characterized with a model, then it is possible to assess the impact upon tissue loading of hardware interventions and compare these potential surgical procedures to a control condition such as conservative treatment options. In this manner, it can be possible to predict the degree of change in tissue stress that will occur with a surgical intervention and help establish reasonable expectations with the patient.

One of the characteristics of a useful biomechanical model is realism. Through a mathematical representation of the principles of physics applied to the spine structures we are attempting to characterize the essential features of the spine so that the various conditions can be simulated. The essential features of the spine that must be represented accurately in a model consist of both spine geometry as well as the functional loading of the spine tissues. Both of these essential features can be a challenge. Models capable of representing the spine geometry of different people and representing the severity of different spine disorders can be particularly difficult. In addition, spine loading is governed by the muscle recruitment pattern of an individual, and these patterns are dictated by the disease process as well as by the experiences and psychological state of the patient. Thus, these features determine how representative the model is of a given situation.

Although model realism is somewhat related to model complexity, complexity alone is not sufficient for a realistic model and can even detract from realism. More complex models are often difficult to validate and may not provide any more useful information than a more general model. One problem with a greater level of detail involves the consequences of any improperly modeled features. These features can interact with other model features and make the model predictions unreliable. Once the model becomes complex, it is difficult to identify these flaws. Thus, the rule of thumb for biomechanical modeling is to make the model only as complex and detailed as necessary to represent the function of interest.

## BASIC BIOMECHANICS

Biomechanical logic is generally concerned with a load-tolerance relationship of tissues. Traditionally this logic has been applied to physical tissue stress. Conceptually, the biomechanical model is used to quantify the loads imposed upon tissues due to an activity. These loads are then compared to a tolerance limit for the tissue. This tolerance limit is often derived from cadaver testing. Depending upon the relationship between the imposed load and the tissue tolerance, risk of tissue damage can be assessed.

Models must consider the contribution of both external and internal forces to functional tissue loading. *External forces* are those forces imposed upon the body by physical factors outside the body. For example, lifting a box subject to the forces of gravity imposes a load upon the body and can be defined by the weight of the object lifted multiplied by the distance of the object from the spine (defined as the external moment). Internal forces refer to the bodily reactions to those external forces (or external moments). Internal forces involve muscle responses, pressures, ligament reactions, and so on that occur within the body in response to the external force. However, because the mechanical advantage of the *internal forces* relative to the spine (internal moment) is much less than that typically associated with the external force, the internal forces are generally very large and play a major role in defining tissue load. Thus, the representation of the internal force generators within the model is critical to model accuracy. The representation of internal force generators represents a major functional loading component and is often considered one of the essential features of model construction.

A major difficulty with assessing internal force generation is that this assessment requires knowledge of the recruitment pattern of numerous muscles surrounding the spine in reaction to the external forces. Muscle recruitment patterns appear to be unique to an individual and are a function of the physical requirements of a task, the individual's genetic "programming," the experiences of the individual, and their strategy in coping with disorders and pain. If these muscles are recruited sequentially, the impact upon spine tissue loading is much different than if the muscles are recruited simultaneously in a coactive pattern. Because there are many power-producing muscles within the trunk, the muscle recruitment patterns are difficult to predict.

An important difference among spine models involves the way in which they consider the muscle recruitment activities within the model. Muscle recruitments are usually considered via one of the following methods: (1) muscle involvement assumptions, (2) inverse dynamics (based upon the body actions), (3) optimization-based muscle involvement, (4) stability-derived muscle activation, or (5) biologically derived muscle involvement. Although the first four methods have been shown to predict muscle activities under constrained conditions (e.g., steady-state static conditions), they have not been successful in predicting muscle coactivations under realistic dynamic movement of the torso, especially when back pathology is present.

For these reasons, our model is a biologically assisted model. Instead of trying to predict how the patient will recruit the trunk muscles, this model predicts activities based upon biologic signals from the muscle. Our model employs electromyography (EMG) recordings from the power-producing muscles of the trunk. In this manner, unique and specific muscle recruitment patterns associated with complex motions, patient experiences, and guarding behaviors (characteristic of low back pain patients) can be considered in the model.

The other essential feature of a model involves the representation of spine tissue geometry. Although the functional loading features of our model has been developed using a "generic" spine, recent advances have permitted us to import images of a patient's spine into the model so that the specific geometry of the individual is represented in the model. Thus, the representation of actual functional muscle activations along with specific spine geometry has permitted us to develop a model with a high level of realism.

## BASIC MODEL STRUCTURE

Over the past 24 years, our laboratory has been developing a dynamic biomechanical model that determines how the lumbar spine's vertebral joints and surrounding tissues experience loads under realistic environmental conditions.[1–6] The key to understanding tissue loading is to understand how the internal forces (primarily muscles) within the trunk respond to various activities. Our early studies have identified significant differences in trunk muscle recruitment (coactivation) patterns as a function of trunk kinematics[7] and emphasize the need for a biologically assisted approach to modeling. Trunk muscle coactivations have been attributed to physical requirements, and are also a function of the organizational or psychosocial environment, training, and individual characteristics.[8] Thus, the only way to accurately understand the trunk's coactivation response is to directly monitor the muscle activities. Biologically assisted models directly monitor the trunk muscle responses to physical loading conditions and use this information as input to a biomechanical model so that the effects of realistic muscle coactivation can be considered in defining tissue loading. Thus, biologically assisted models provide specific and precise information regarding muscle recruitments associated with a particular patient and a particular activity.

Our biologically assisted model is, specifically, an EMG-assisted model. The biodynamic EMG-assisted model is unique because it is *person-specific* in terms of anthropometry (muscle location and size), motion (inputs trunk as well as limb motion), and muscle activities. The model structure is multidimensional, and considers the dynamic response of the individual. Trunk moments and tissue loads are determined from dynamic muscle force vectors and internal trunk muscle moment arms. Our current EMG-assisted, free-dynamic lifting model employs 10 muscle equivalent vectors to approximate trunk anatomy and mechanics[9–12] (Fig. 88–1). Muscle fibers sampled by EMG were originally monitored via intramuscular electrodes[13] but are now sampled using surface electrodes.

The EMG derived from the muscles of interest is assumed to be representative of, and linearly related to, the net muscle force. Some authors[12,14–17] believe surface EMG is linearly related to voluntary isometric joint torque, whereas others[18–20] believe the relation is strictly nonlinear. Hof and van den Berg[21] explained this paradox by demonstrating that EMG is linearly related to muscle force, but is nonlinearly related to joint torque due to

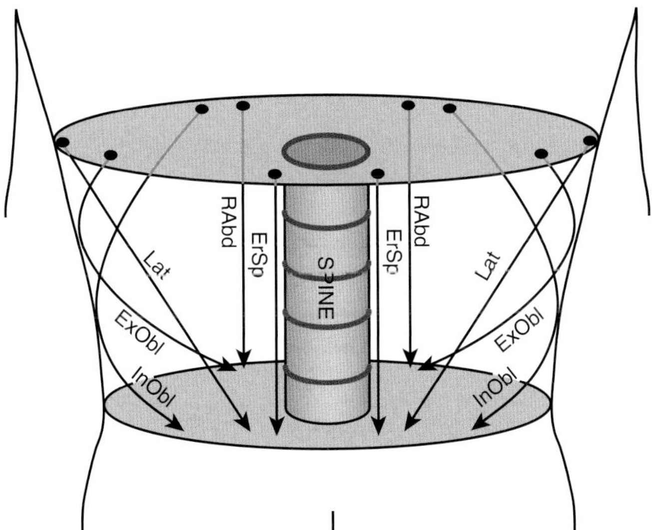


■ **FIGURE 88–1.** Trunk model underlying structure representation.

coactivity. Because EMG-assisted models account for muscle coactivity, a linear assumption is reasonable.

The model employs kinematic input (measured from the subject) and anthropometrically scaled musculoskeletal anatomy to determine the muscle vector directions. Processed EMG data and a calibrated muscle stress value (gain) are combined with muscle size, length, and contraction velocity to determine the force magnitudes. Multidimensional, dynamic trunk moments and spinal loads are computed from muscle force and moment arm vectors.

Our model is free-dynamic in that it permits each muscle orientation, length, and velocity to vary throughout the exertion, thus constantly updating muscle position, length, and velocity. Muscle origins are assigned a three-dimensional location relative to the spinal axis, coplanar with the iliac crest. Muscle insertions are located coplanar with the 12th rib. Muscle forces are represented as vector quantities between their two endpoints. The mechanics of this model can be visualized as two "plates" that move relative to one another (see Fig. 88–1). Dynamic motions of the trunk are recorded from the patient with a goniometer (lumbar motion monitor, or LMM) placed over the back and appropriately modeled via the relative dynamic orientations of the two mathematical planes or "plates." Thus, as the patient moves, the mechanical advantage of each muscle vector is adjusted so that the contribution to tissue loading is constantly updated. Specific vertebral body orientations are also instantaneously defined via the LMM position[22] (not shown in Fig. 88–1). Because the origins and insertions of the 10 trunk muscles are fixed on the surface of the thoracic and iliac "plates," dynamic motions of the trunk (measured by the LMM) generate three-dimensional motion in the muscle. Using this approach, muscle orientations and relative lengths are permitted to change throughout a movement, realistically representing each muscle's changing mechanical advantage during a task. Muscle vector directions, lengths, and velocities are continuously determined from the instantaneous positions and motions of the muscle endpoints. Loads imposed on the spine are assessed by continuously summing the force vectors in each direction.

Magnetic resonance imaging (MRI) is used to identify the geometric relationships between the power-producing muscles of the trunk. A recent study evaluated the torso architecture of 20 females and 10 males.[23,24]. The subjects were scanned at each vertebral level from T8 to S1. Muscle cross-sectional area and moment arm distances of the 10 trunk muscles used in the model were documented. Significant differences in *cross-sectional area* of the torso muscles were noted between males and females. Males muscle area was on average 60% larger than female muscle area, and significant differences were noted between the right and left sides of the body for four of the seven muscle pairs examined. This effort has also permitted us to document the *lines of action of the muscles* in terms of origins and insertions. These findings showed that there were significant differences in muscle mechanical advantage between males and females. The final contribution of this effort involved the development of a series of regression equations that has permitted us to estimate muscle area and location based upon physical anthropometry.[24,25] This effort has resulted in statistically significant equations for all muscles included in the model. These efforts resulted in about a 25% improvement in cross-sectional area and muscle moment arm prediction compared to previous efforts. The overall advantage of these efforts has been the realization of a "fine tuning" of the model.

The literature has suggested that different muscles in humans tend to have different values for muscle gains. However, currently, most biomechanical multiple muscle models employ a single muscle gain for all muscles. The inclusion of individual muscle gains would be expected to improve the precision of biologically assisted models. A linear optimization program was developed to predict the individual gains associated with each of the muscles in a biologically assisted trunk torso model. Data from three studies were selected based on their complexity of muscle recruitment to exercise the model. The model performance measure of average absolute error between measured and predicted moment was found to be statistically improved for the optimized model involving tasks that required most complex muscle recruitment. Thus, the OSU biologically assisted model that sets gains via the optimization function performs significantly better when complex tasks are assessed. Hence, a proper selection of model calibration tasks result in reasonable gain values for individual muscles.[26]

Spinal unit loads are calculated from the vector sum of the muscle forces. Muscle-generated moments about the spinal axis are predicted from the sum of vector products combining dynamic tensile forces, and moment arms of each muscle. Measured and predicted values of the trunk moments, as well as predicted compression, anterior shear, and lateral shear forces are stored for postmodeling analysis. The muscle gain (biomechanical muscle stress) correlation and root mean square (RMS) error between measured and predicted moment profiles are recorded for model performance evaluation.

These spine loadings have traditionally been compared to tolerance limits of the spine (derived from both cadaver studies and finite element models) to quantify the degree of biomechanical risk.

### Performance and Validation of Basic Model Structure

Measured and model-predicted trunk moments are compared and must agree if the model is correctly simulating trunk[23,24] mechanics. Statistical correlations between predicted and measured moment profiles serve to measure model performance and indicate how well the model accounts for the variability in the dynamic moment. Because there are no means by which one can measure spine loading in vivo, direct comparison of measured and modeled spinal load is impractical. However, we feel that since the model accurately predicts applied moments about the spine, then the predicted spinal load must also be reasonable.

The biodynamic EMG-assisted biodynamic model has been tested and validated in numerous studies. Three studies have evaluated model sensitivity in each of the primary planes of movement. Each experiment was intended to test model robustness, independently, in each of the cardinal planes of the body.

Three measures of performance and validity were used as criteria with which to evaluate model performance. First, for a model to be considered robust and accurate it must precisely represent the *changes* in trunk and spine loading over time. The measure of performance that relates to *changes* in trunk loading during these trials is the correlation between predicted and measured (via the force plate) trunk moment as a function of time. The $R^2$ statistic indicating the relationship between measured trunk moment (via the force plate) and predicted trunk moment (via the EMG assisted model) serves as an indication of the ability of the model to accurately assess the changes in dynamic trunk loading. This statistic is an indication of the robustness of the model and is sensitive to changes in shape of the trunk moment versus time curve generated by both the model and force plate during an experimental run.

Second, a well-developed biomechanical model must accurately estimate the *magnitude* of trunk load during a lifting trial. By comparing the measured and predicted *magnitude* of external load imposed about the spine (moment) we can evaluate the magnitude of the error inherent in the model. The statistic employed to indicate this quantity was the average absolute error (AAE) between the measured moment and the predicted trunk moment during a lifting trial.

Finally, a realistic biomechanical model should reflect biomechanical and physiologic plausibility. This plausibility is often reflected by comparing model predicted parameters to the limits described in the physiologic literature. Predicted muscle gain provides a good measure of this physiologic feasibility. The literature[27–29] suggests that muscle gain should be between 30 and 100 N/cm$^2$. Estimates of muscle gains above this limit would suggest an infeasible model.

Table 88–1 summarizes the experimental parameters and model validity performance measures for each of the three experiments. This summary indicates that the model has been thoroughly tested over a variety of physiologically relevant conditions.[30,31] The analysis also shows that the model performance is well within acceptable performance limits for accuracy as well as biomechanical plausibility.

As an example of the model sensitivity, Figure 88–2 shows spine loading in response to twisting velocity.[32] This figure shows that the model is sensitive to changes in spinal loading as a function of even small changes in trunk velocity. These changes in loading are directly traceable to changes in trunk muscle coactivation. As trunk twisting velocity increases the trunk muscles increase their coactivity which increases spine loading. Such changes would not be identified with evaluation systems that are not able to account for the coactive changes that occur with changes in trunk velocity. Similar changes in spinal loading were noted for tests in the other planes of the body.[33,34]

## MODEL REPEATABILITY AND VARIABILITY

Several types of variability are inherent in biomechanical assessments associated with trunk exertions. Variability may occur as a function of variations in spine loading due to either subject variations in motion profiles (kinematics) or biomechanical model performance. Variability may also be observed as a function of spine tolerance. A study was conducted to assess the sources of variability associated with the EMG-assisted model of spine loading. An experiment was performed that required a mix of 12 experienced and inexperienced subjects to perform 10 repeated lifts in which load weight, asymmetry, and velocity were varied. The experiment was replicated on a second day for each subject to determine whether the model performance varied from day to day. Three indicators of model performance indicated that variability was mainly a function of individual subject characteristics and subject experience and *not* a function of model inconsistencies.[35] These results imply that by properly calibrating the model it is reasonable to assume that the vast majority of variations observed in repeated exertions of a particular trial are due to kinematic and kinetic

TABLE 88–1. Summary of Trunk Loading Conditions and Model Validity Measures in the Three Cardinal Planes of the Body

| Motion Plane | Reference | No. of Subjects | No. of Trials | Loads Supported (kg) | Trunk Velocity (deg/sec) | $R^2$ (Avg) | AAE (Nm) | Gain (N/cm$^2$) |
|---|---|---|---|---|---|---|---|---|
| Forward bending (sagittal plane) | 34 | 10 | 703 | 0,18.2, 36.4 | 0, 30, 60, 90 + free dynamic | 0.89 | <15 | 47 |
| Lateral bending (frontal plane) | 33 | 12 | 574 | 13.6, 27.3 | 0, 15, 30, 45 | 0.91 | 6–10 | 64 |
| Twisting (transverse plane) | 32 | 12 | 320 | Max, 50% max | 0, 10, 20 | 0.80 | N/A | 35 |

AAE, average absolute error.

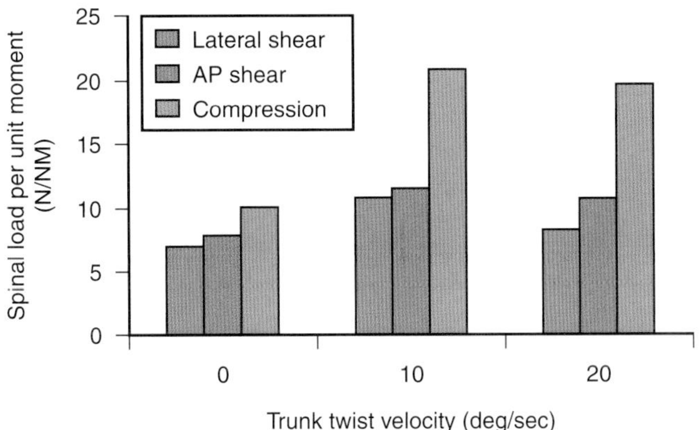


■ **FIGURE 88–2.** Spine compression and shear loading as a function of twisting velocity.

differences inherent in the muscle control system and are not a function of model randomness.

### Sensitivity to Nonphysical Stress

As an example of model sensitivity, we have been able to document biomechanical responses to psychosocial stress.[8] In a unique study, subjects were asked to perform precisely controlled physical exertions under conditions in which the subject was exposed to psychosocially stressful or nonstressful conditions. Although the physical requirements were exactly the same under both psychosocial conditions, some subjects experienced up to 27% more lateral shear under the stressful psychosocial conditions compared to the nonstressful psychosocial condition. The analyses showed that those who responded to the psychosocial stress were of particular personality types (introverts and intuitors) and coactivated their trunk muscles to a greater degree. This investigation clearly demonstrates the sensitivity and specificity of the model and its potential to identify the specific tissues that are subject to increased stress due to occupational requirements.

## PERSONALIZED HYBRID BIOLOGICALLY ASSISTED/FINITE ELEMENT MODEL

Over the past 2 years even more dramatic enhancements and improvements have been incorporated into the biodynamic EMG-assisted model. These enhancements build upon the fundamental underlying structure and model enhancements of recent years (just described), yet have expanded the analytic capabilities of the model as well as included the ability to further "personalize" the model to a particular patient.

Three significant improvements have occurred to the model. The first improvement involved switching to the MSC.ADAMS software environment (MSC.Software, Inc., Santa Ana, CA). MSC.ADAMS is a multibody dynamic analysis program that is used in conjunction with the LifeMod (Biomechanics Research Group, Inc., San Clemente, CA) biomechanical overlay. Using the existing EMG-assisted basic model structure as a starting point (see Fig. 88–1), MSC.ADAMS was employed to more comprehensively assess loads throughout the lumbar spine. In this effort each major body section is represented with rigid segments interconnected with simplified joints. Kinematics recorded directly from the subject drive the motion of each of the body segments. As is the case with the original underlying basic model structure, torso muscles are represented with force vectors using EMG to derive muscle force. In this embodiment of the model, the lumbar spine is represented in much greater detail than the rest of the body. The intervertebral discs are represented with flexible bodies. Spinal ligament forces are represented with nonlinear spring-dampers connected to adjacent vertebral bodies with stiffness and damping properties from literature values. These improvements retain the underlying model logic and enhancements yet greatly improve the mechanical sensitivity of the model as well as include specific anthropometric fidelity for a particular subject. This system representation allows one to consider the effects of full body movements (such as walking and carrying) on spine kinetics and facilitates modeling of each vertebra along the lumbar spine as well as all of the connective tissues (end plates, discs, ligaments, muscles, etc.) and bone contact forces at each level. Table 88–2 summarizes the tissue loads that can now be monitored through these measures. In addition, MSC.ADAMS provides a much improved visual presentation. The user interface provides a very accurate representation of the human body allowing immediate visual inspection of the modeled data. Figure 88–3 shows a skeletal representation of the model.

The second enhancement has integrated a *finite element analysis* into the model structure along with the EMG-assisted model. This yields a hybrid biologically assisted model so that the discs can be better represented. Intervertebral discs are modeled as flexible finite element bodies. The vertebral end plates are modeled as solid elements and the nucleus pulposus is modeled as essentially an incompressible fluid. The annulus fibrosus is modeled as a series of composite concentric bands. This accounts for the highly directional nature of the annular fibers as well as the interaction of the fibers and the ground substance. This hybrid representation permits better assessment of disc forces and has the potential to track remodeling of the tissue over the course of years of exposure to risk. Figure 88–4 visually displays the hybrid model with flexible intervertebral discs, facet contact forces (blue arrows), and muscle and ligament forces (red numbers).

The advantage of this hybrid model that incorporates biologic inputs along with finite element modeling is that the model now includes enough information to permit one to evaluate the effects of various interventions. Figure 88–5 shows a concept model that evaluates the biomechanical effects of a surgical intervention. In this model a simulation of a posterior-lateral fusion using pedicle screws and titanium rods was modeled. Because this is a biologically assisted model, it is possible to consider the effects of this type of fusion when the patient recruits her muscles in a natural fashion. Note the differences in the loadings of the adjacent discs in this figure compared to Figure 88–4 (nonfusion). Figure 88–6 shows a similar analysis, but in this model an

TABLE 88–2. Model Output Measures

| Muscle Tensions/Forces | Motion Segment Measures at Each Vertebral Level From L5/S1 to T12/L1 | Kinematic Spine Measurements |
|---|---|---|
| Right latissimus dorsi tension | Intervertebral disc stress/strain | Motion segment angular position, velocity, and acceleration |
| Left latissimus dorsi tension | Superior vertebral end plate compression | Motion segment relative translational position, velocity, and acceleration |
| Right erector spinae tension | Superior vertebral end plate AP shear | Muscle and ligament length, velocity, and acceleration |
| Left erector spinae tension | Superior vertebral end plate lateral shear | Facet contact location and contact depth |
| Right rectus abdominus tension | Inferior vertebral end plate compression | Intervertebral disc center of mass position, velocity, and acceleration |
| Left rectus abdominus tension | Inferior vertebral end plate AP shear | |
| Right external oblique tension | Inferior vertebral end plate lateral shear | |
| Left external oblique tension | Right facet compressive contact force | |
| Right internal oblique tension | Right facet lateral contact force | |
| Left internal oblique tension | Right facet AP contact force | |
| | Left facet compressive contact force | |
| | Left facet lateral contact force | |
| | Left facet AP contact force | |
| | Anterior longitudinal ligament tension | |
| | Posterior longitudinal ligament tension | |
| | Ligamentum flavum tension | |
| | Capsular ligament tension | |
| | Interspinous ligament tension | |
| | Supraspinous ligament tension | |
| | Intertransverse ligament tension | |

interbody fusion device has been added along with the pedicle screws and rods. Note the effects of this intervention on the bone contact forces in the adjacent vertebrae. These types of analyses may help explain the common observation of adjacent level disease in those who have had fusion surgery. In this manner it is possible to perform "virtual surgery" on patients and predict the effects of different surgical interventions on the tissues of interest. In addition, using a finite element model (FEM) analysis, it will

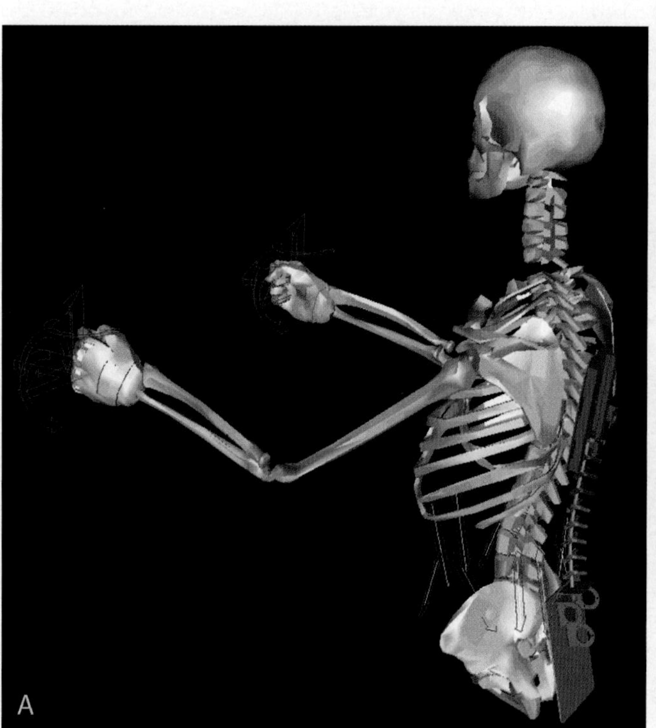


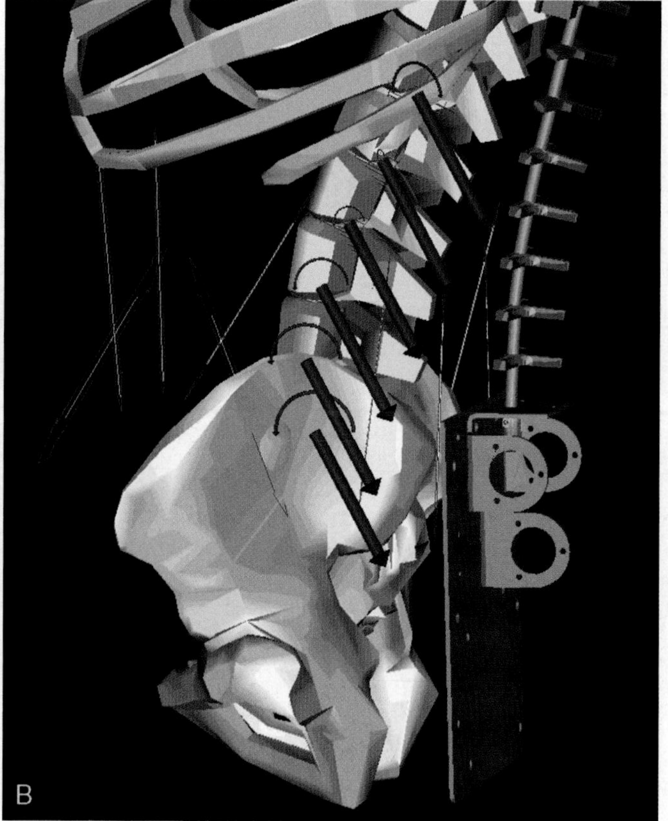


■ **FIGURE 88–3.** **A** Personalized model with subject anthropometric scaling considering hand loads, muscle activities, and spine kinematics (lumbar motion monitor is shown on the back that tracks vertebral motion). **B** Resultant force vectors and moments experienced at each lumbar vertebra.

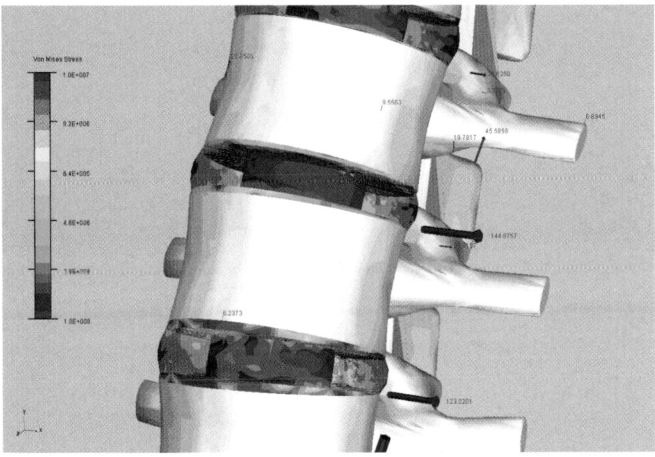

■ **FIGURE 88–4.** This incorporates both the EMG-assisted forces and flexible discs. End plate and disc forces, contact forces (blue arrows and numbers), and ligament forces (red arrows and numbers) are all shown graphically in the figure.

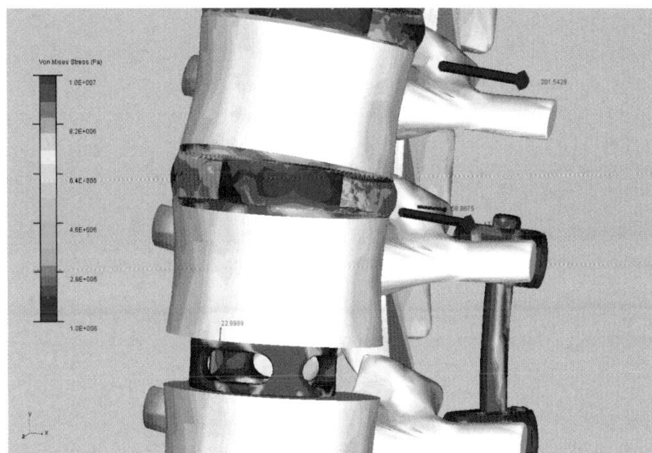

■ **FIGURE 88–6.** "Virtual surgery" that includes a fusion and an interbody fusion device. Note the difference in disc and contact forces at the superior disc in this figure compared to Figures 88–4 and 88–5.

eventually be possible to run the model in scaled time over the course of years or decades and predict the effects of the intervention in the future.

The final improvement of the model has permitted us to *import subject specific images (CT or MRI) of a patient's spine into the model* (Fig. 88–7) and use these images as a basis for the underlying mechanical structure of the spine. Subject-specific vertebral bodies generated from CT- and MRI-based geometry data are imported directly into the model. In addition, the disc's geometry is also generated from MRI-based data and used to create finite element bodies. In this manner, we are able to uniquely model a specific individual's spine tissue loads and consider how subject irregularities can influence tissue forces. This model permits us to uniquely and specifically model any individual while precisely and accurately evaluating loads on specific tissues.

This hybrid biodynamic EMG-assisted/finite element model will be effective at providing clinically relevant predictions. The model predictions will become increasingly relevant as it is applied to the design characteristics of current and future implants as well as in the design of motion preservation systems.

## CONCLUSIONS

This brief description of the hybrid biodynamic EMG-assisted/finite element model has shown that it is possible to develop patient-specific models that are able to test the impact of various surgical interventions upon the biomechanical functioning of a particular patient. The keys to developing realistic patient-specific models involve the ability to (1) capture the specific trunk muscle activities of a patient and use these signals to "drive" model mechanics, (2) accurately incorporate patient anthropometry and

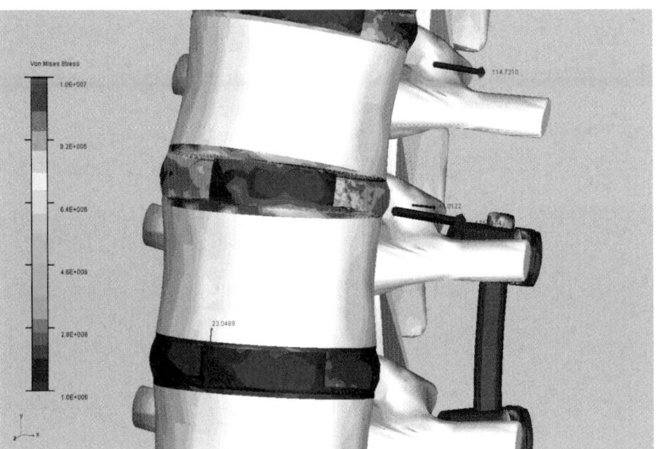

■ **FIGURE 88–5.** "Virtual surgery" included in the model. Here a posterior-lateral fusion is incorporated in the model. Note the increased loading incurred on the adjacent superior disc in this figure compared to the nonsurgical conditions shown in Figure 88–4.

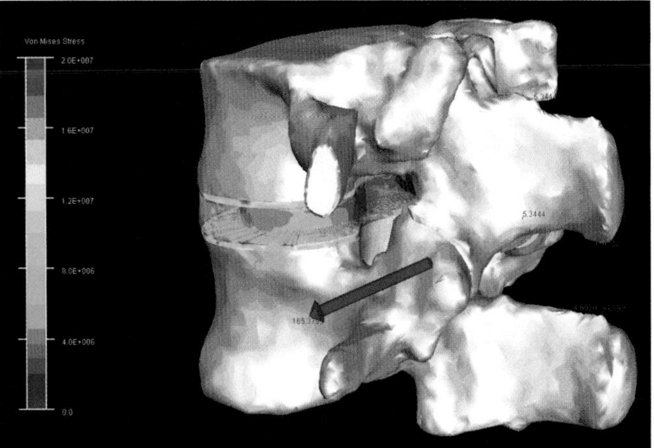

■ **FIGURE 88–7.** Finite element model of the disc shown embedded with spine imaging imported from a specific subject. Spine imaging was imported into the model so that the tissue loads unique to an individual could be assessed.

spine imaging into the model mechanics, and (3) use finite element modeling to understand disc deformation during spine loading. We expect that this model will be used to "virtually" assess the tradeoffs associated with different surgical instrumentation and allow surgeons to appreciate the biomechanical consequences of surgical interventions for specific patients prior to surgery.

## REFERENCES


1. Granata KP, Marras WS: An EMG-assisted model of loads on the lumbar spine during asymmetric trunk extensions. J Biomech 26(12):1429–1438, 1993.
2. Granata KP, Marras WS: An EMG-assisted model of trunk loading during free-dynamic lifting. J Biomech 28(11):1309–1317, 1995.
3. Marras WS, Ferguson SA, Burr D, et al: Spine loading in patients with low back pain during asymmetric lifting exertions. Spine J 4(1):64–75, 2004.
4. Marras WS, Granata KP: The development of an EMG-assisted model to assess spine loading during whole-body free-dynamic lifting. J Electromyogr Kinesiol 7(4):259–268, 1997.
5. Marras WS, Sommerich CM: A three-dimensional motion model of loads on the lumbar spine, I: Model structure. Hum Factors 33(2):123–137, 1991.
6. Reilly CH, Marras WS: Simulift: A simulation model of human trunk motion. Spine 14(1):5–11, 1989.
7. Marras WS, Reilly CH: Networks of internal trunk-loading activities under controlled trunk-motion conditions. Spine 13(6):661–667, 1988.
8. Marras WS, Davis KG, Heaney CA, et al: The influence of psychosocial stress, gender, and personality on mechanical loading of the lumbar spine. Spine 25(23):3045–3054, 2000.
9. Dumas GA, Poulin MJ, Roy B, et al: Orientation and moment arms of some trunk muscles. Spine 16(3):293–303, 1991.
10. McGill SM, Patt N, Norman RW: Measurement of the trunk musculature of active males using CT scan radiography: Implications for force and moment generating capacity about the L4/L5 joint. J Biomech 21(4):329–341, 1988.
11. Schultz AB, Andersson GB: Analysis of loads on the lumbar spine. Spine 6(1):76–82, 1981.
12. Yoo JH, Herring JM, Yu J: Power spectral changes of the vastus medialis electromyogram for graded isometric torques (I). Electromyogr Clin Neurophysiol 19(1–2):183–197, 1979.
13. Marras WS, King AI, Joynt RL: Measurement of loads on the lumbar spine under isometric and isokinetic conditions. Spine 9(2):176–187, 1984.
14. Lippold O: The relation between integrated action potentials in the human muscle and its isometric tension. J Physiol 117:492–499, 1952.
15. Lippold OC: Oscillation in the stretch reflex arc and the origin of the rhythmical, 8-12 C-S component of physiological tremor. J Physiol 206(2):359–382, 1970.
16. Moritani T, deVries HA: Reexamination of the relationship between the surface integrated electromyogram (IEMG) and force of isometric contraction. Am J Phys Med 57(6):263–277, 1978.
17. Moritani T, et al: Electrophysiology and kinesiology for health and disease. J Electromyogr Kinesiol 15(3):240–255, 2005.
18. Komi PV, Vitasalo JH: Signal characteristics of EMG at different levels of muscle tension. Acta Physiol Scand 96(2):267–276, 1976.
19. Vredenbregt J, Rau G: Surface electromyography in relation to force, muscle length and endurance. *In* New Developments in Electromyography and Clinical Neurophysiology. Basel, Krager, 1973.
20. Zuniga EN, Simons EG: Nonlinear relationship between averaged electromyogram potential and muscle tension in normal subjects. Arch Phys Med Rehabil 50(11):613–620, 1969.
21. Hof AL, van den Berg J: Linearity between the weighted sum of the EMGs of the human triceps surae and the total torque. J Biomech 10(9):529–539, 1977.
22. Splittstoesser RE: A simple method for predicting dynamic lumbar motion segment angles using measures of trunk angle and subject anthropometry. Columbus, Ohio State University, 2001, 63 leaves.
23. Jorgensen MJ, Marras WS, Granata KP, et al: MRI-derived moment-arms of the female and male spine loading muscles. Clin Biomech (Bristol, Avon) 16(3): 182–193, 2001.
24. Marras WS, Jorgensen MJ, Granata KP, et al: Female and male trunk geometry: Size and prediction of the spine loading trunk muscles derived from MRI. Clin Biomech (Bristol, Avon) 16(1):38–46, 2001.
25. Jorgensen MJ, Marras WS, Gupta P: Cross-sectional area of the lumbar back muscles as a function of torso flexion. Clin Biomech (Bristol, Avon) 18(4):280–286, 2003.
26. Prahbu J, Marras WS, Mount-Campbell C: An investigation on the use of optimization to determine the individual muscle gains in a multiple muscle model. Clin Biomech (Bristol, Avon) 2005 (in review).
27. McGill SM, Norman RW: Effects of an anatomically detailed erector spinae model on L4/L5 disc compression and shear. J Biomech 20(6):591–600, 1987.
28. Reid JG, Costigan PA: Trunk muscle balance and muscular force. Spine 12(8):783–786, 1987.
29. Weis-Fogh T, Alexander RM: The sustained power output from striated muscle. *In* Scale Effects in Animal Locomotion. London, Academic Press, 1977, pp 511–525.
30. Marras WS, Lavender SA, Leurgans SE, et al: Biomechanical risk factors for occupationally related low back disorders. Ergonomics 38(2):377–410, 1995.
31. Marras WS, Lavender SA, Leurgans SE, et al: The role of dynamic three-dimensional trunk motion in occupationally-related low back disorders: The effects of workplace factors, trunk position, and trunk motion characteristics on risk of injury. Spine 18(5):617–628, 1993.
32. Marras WS, Granata KP: A biomechanical assessment and model of axial twisting in the thoracolumbar spine. Spine 20(13):1440–1451, 1995.
33. Marras WS, Granata KP: Spine loading during trunk lateral bending motions. J Biomech 30(7):697–703, 1997.
34. Marras WS, Sommerich CM: A three-dimensional motion model of loads on the lumbar spine, II: Model validation. Hum Factors 33(2):139–149, 1991.
35. Marras WS, Granata KP, Davis KG: Variability in spine loading model performance. Clin Biomech (Bristol, Avon) 14(8):505–514, 1999.

CHAPTER 89

# Spinal Deformity and Motion-Sparing Technology

Paul C. McAfee

## KEY POINTS

- Four main comparative differences make lumbar disc replacements more unstable than cervical disc replacements: (1) the angle of influence of the facets, (2) the facet/end plate ratio, (3) the tensile strength of the capsular ligaments compared to the anterior longitudinal ligament, and (4) the uncovertebral joint's role as a stabilizing bony stop to rotation in the cervical spine.
- Total disc replacement accentuates scoliotic tendencies in the lumbar spine.
- The arc of influence for the cervical facets (153.6 degrees) is larger than that of the lumbar facet joints (98.0 degrees).
- Because the facet capsular ligaments are mechanically less effective with lower tensile strength in the lumbar spine, multiple-level arthroplasty tends to accentuate scoliotic tendencies—this tendency is independent of prosthetic design and surgical technique.
- The combined joint surface area of the cervical facets relative to the cervical disc cross-sectional area (0.519) is almost twice the magnitude of the same relationship in the lumbar spine (0.293). This greater surface area leads to greater inherent stability with anterior motion-preserving technology in the cervical spine compared to the lumbar spine.

The rotational stability of the lumbar and cervical spinal motion segment has become critically important with artificial disc replacement because the procedure requires sacrificing the anterior longitudinal ligament (ALL), posterior longitudinal ligament (PLL), and portions of the annulus fibrosis.[1–4] At first glance it is tempting to consider application of lumbar disc replacement to degenerated segments below previously fused scoliotic segments; however, this serves to increase the rotational deforming loads at the adjacent degenerated disc. The successful application of disc replacement technology requires an understanding of the normal constraints to axial rotation, which are both anatomic and biomechanical. At the current time the application of disc replacement in scoliosis is "off-label" with regard to approved FDA indications, and scoliosis greater than 11 degrees at the index level is one of the exclusion criterion for all four completed or ongoing lumbar disc arthroplasty FDA trials (Fig. 89–1). Rotational stability also becomes more critical with multilevel use and there are currently no disc replacements with approved labeling for multilevel implantation. Therefore, the importance of anatomic and physiologic constraints for rotation are highlighted with multilevel disc replacement and arthroplasty below long deformity constructs. At tertiary referral centers for motion preservation there are already alarming numbers of iatrogenic scoliosis deformities (Fig. 89–2) either caused or exacerbated by lumbar disc replacement, particularly with unconstrained devices.[5–7]

In contrast, the analogous unconstrained designs of cervical disc replacement do not seem to cause iatrogenic rotational instability, or "spinning out" of the motion segment in the cervical spine. The goals of this study are to isolate and examine the major constraints to axial rotation in the lumbar spine and to compare them to the cervical spine (Table 89–1). In addition, this study attempts to determine how this influences the rotational stability in a spine with scoliotic tendencies after disc replacement in both the cervical and lumbar spinal segments.

## SCIENTIFIC TESTING METHODS

This basic scientific investigation is in two parts. The anatomic measurements were performed on 60 randomly selected skeletons in the Hamann-Todd Osteological Collection. This collection, which is part of the Cleveland Museum of Natural History, comprises over 3,100 modern human and some 900 non-human primate skulls and skeletons, attracting researchers in the fields of anthropology and medicine from around the globe.

The biomechanical studies were performed on fresh cadaveric specimens with intact surrounding ligaments using a six degrees of freedom spine simulator, testing sequentially prepared surgical preparations relevant to lumbar and cervical disc replacement.

### Anatomic Measurements

The 60 human specimens from the Hamann-Todd Osteological Collection were randomly selected and photographed with size reference markers. The C6 vertebra and the L5 vertebra from the same skeleton were measured to control for variations in age, ethnicity, and gender.

The first objective was to determine the rotational arc of influence (AOI), which is the arc or angle formed from the center of axial rotation to the outermost lateral extent of the facet joints

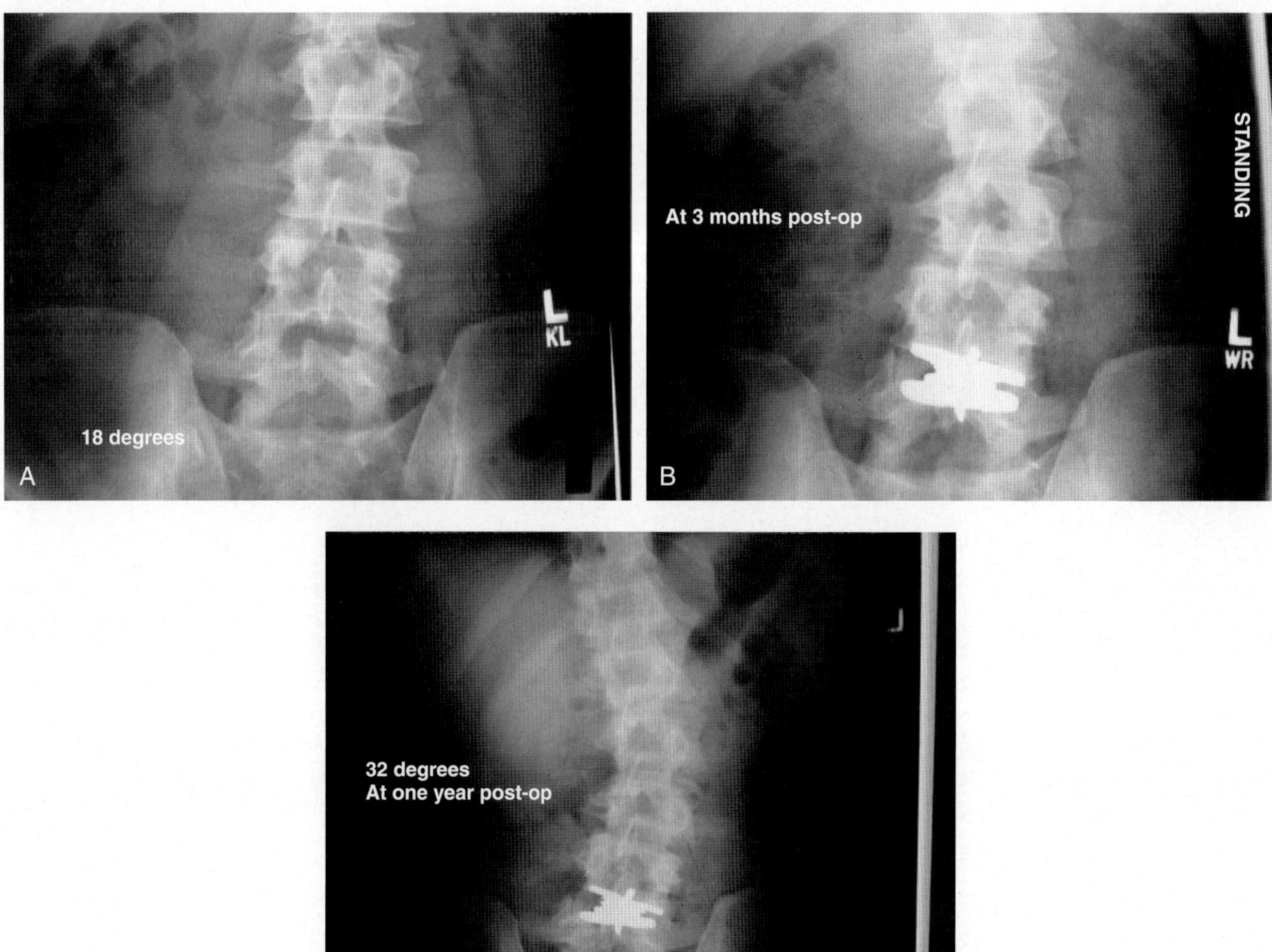


■ **FIGURE 89–1.** Progression of scoliosis with a keeled prosthesis. **A,** This AP radiograph of this patient demonstrates 18 degrees of lumbar scoliosis. He fit the inclusion criteria for lumbar disc arthroplasty in the US IDE study due to symptomatic discogenic pain at L4-L5. **B,** Within 3 months following an L4-L5 lumbar arthroplasty his scoliosis increased from 18 degrees to 25 degrees. **C,** By 1 year after surgery the scoliotic deformity had increased to 32 degrees in spite of the so-called "greater constraints" of a keeled prosthesis. This indicates that even with a keeled prosthesis some of the normal rotational constraints are compromised with lumbar arthroplasty.

(Fig. 89–3A). The center point of the angle is the center of rotation (COR) of the motion segment and was determined as the point on the midsagittal line two thirds from the front of the vertebral body and one third from the posterior margin (see Fig. 89–3B). It stands to reason that the facet's influence or effect on the restriction of vertebral rotation has to act within the anatomic pie-shaped structure of its location in relation to the center of vertebral axial rotation. The best mechanical advantage of the facets would occur if the facets surrounded the intervertebral disc in a 360-degree arc. The worst mechanical situation would occur if the facets overlapped each other and were straight, acting within a pie-shaped radius of only 1 degree. It is understood that the specific plane of the facet joint surface is a three-dimensional structure and that a sagittally oriented joint surface would resist rotational forces more efficiently than a coronal plane of orientation. The facet joints actually can change their plane of orientation from top to bottom, or they may even be curved. For this reason, this complex structure is best analyzed by showing the contained angle of influence that anatomically confines these two complex three-dimensional structures.

The second objective was to determine the relative anatomic size discrepancy between the zygoapophyseal facet joint contact surface area and the area of the corresponding intervertebral disc. Obviously, if the facet joints are large and the disc is small, then resecting or replacing the disc would have less of a mechanical effect on stability of the spinal column (Fig. 89–4A). For these measurement purposes the cross-sectional area of the disc was approximated as the cross-sectional area of the vertebral end plate on the skeleton. The combined joint surface areas of the left and right facets were added together and compared to the cross-sectional area of the intervertebral disc, yielding the facet/end plate ratio (FER) (see Fig. 89–4B).

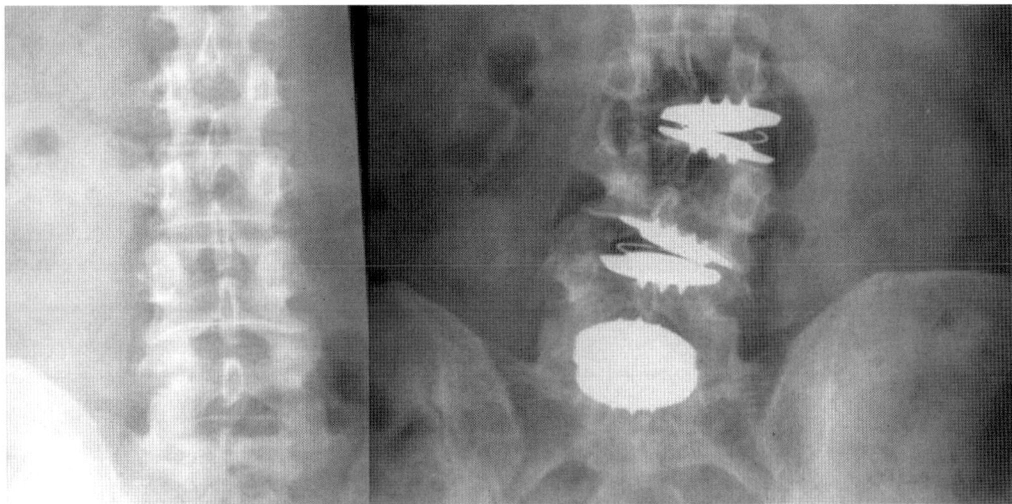

■ **FIGURE 89–2.** Three-level lumbar total disc replacement. These AP radiographs demonstrate progressive severe rotational instability from preoperative state to 18 months after three-level CHARITÉ lumbar disc replacement. The patient became even more disabled, with an Oswestry Functional Outcome over 60, and could not return to his job. The spine is now 2.0 cm out of balance at each disc at L4-L5, and L3-L4 has 18 degrees iatrogenic scoliotic deformity. This type of iatrogenic rotational deformity is an increasingly frequent presentation at tertiary referral centers, even originating from experienced surgical centers outside the U.S.

## Biomechanical Testing

Six degrees of freedom motion analysis compared the rotational stiffness of the cervical and lumbar spine ($n = 8$) intact, status post anterior discectomy, and after total disc replacement (TDR). Cunningham and associates have developed a pure moment biomechanical testing apparatus which is consistent with Panjabi's principles: (a) the uppermost vertebrae in the spinal column are not constrained and are free to move, (b) pure moments are applied, (c) an optoelectronic image analysis system (OptoTrak 3020, Northern Digital, Inc.) measures skeletal markers on each independent spinal segment with LEDs (light-emitting diodes), (d) there is a skeletal three-axis (x, y, and z) coordinate system skeletally attached to each cervical or lumbar vertebral level, and (e) there is conventional anchoring of the lowest (C7) cervical vertebra or the sacrum to a six-axis load cell. Multidirectional flexibility testing utilized the Panjabi Hybrid Testing protocol, which includes pure moments for the intact condition with the overall spinal motion replicated under displacement control for subsequent reconstructions. Unconstrained intact moments of ± 8 Nm were used for axial rotation in the lumbar spine and ± 3 Nm for the cervical spine, with quantification of the operative and adjacent level range of motion (ROM) and neutral zone (NZ). All data were normalized to the intact spine condition.

The lumbar disc replacement used in these biomechanical studies was the CHARITÉ Artificial Disc (DePuy Spine Inc., Raynham, MA) and the cervical disc replacement utilized was the Porous-Coated Motion (PCM) device (Cervitech, Inc., Rockaway, NJ)—in both an unconstrained design was used and the biomaterials for the bearing surface were cobalt-chrome and UHMWPE (ultra-high-molecular-weight polyethylene).

### Sequential Rotational Testing of Soft tissue Preparation for Disc Replacement

Fresh-frozen human cadaveric spines ($n = 6$, C5-C6; $n = 6$, L4-L5) were used for the biomechanical testing and underwent the following graded instability conditions:

1. Intact
2. Resection of ALL, annulus, disc, and PLL as if in a clinical setting simulating the preparation for a TDR
3. A more radical annulus resection
4. Entire 360-degree annular resection and insertion of the respective unconstrained type disc replacement

**TABLE 89–1. Major Constraints in Limiting Axial Rotation in the Lumbar and Cervical Motion Segment**

| Concept | Definition | Cervical | Lumbar | *P* value |
|---|---|---|---|---|
| 1. Arc of influence (AOI) (degrees) | The center of the arc of rotation is the COR of the motion segment. AOI is the arc or angle formed by the outermost edges of the facets. | 153.6 (8.9) | 98 (9.1) | $P<0.001$ |
| 2. Facet/end plate ratio (FER) | The combined joint surface contact area of the two facets divided by the cross-sectional area of the vertebral end plate. | 0.519 (0.112) | 0.283 (0.06) | $P<0.001$ |
| 3. CL/ALL ratio | The tensile strength of the facet capsular ligament (CL) divided by the tensile strength of the anterior longitudinal ligament (ALL). | 1.83 | 0.493 | |
| 4. Presence of a bony block to rotation in the anterior column | Uncovertebral joint | Yes | No | |

*Statistic analysis = t-test.

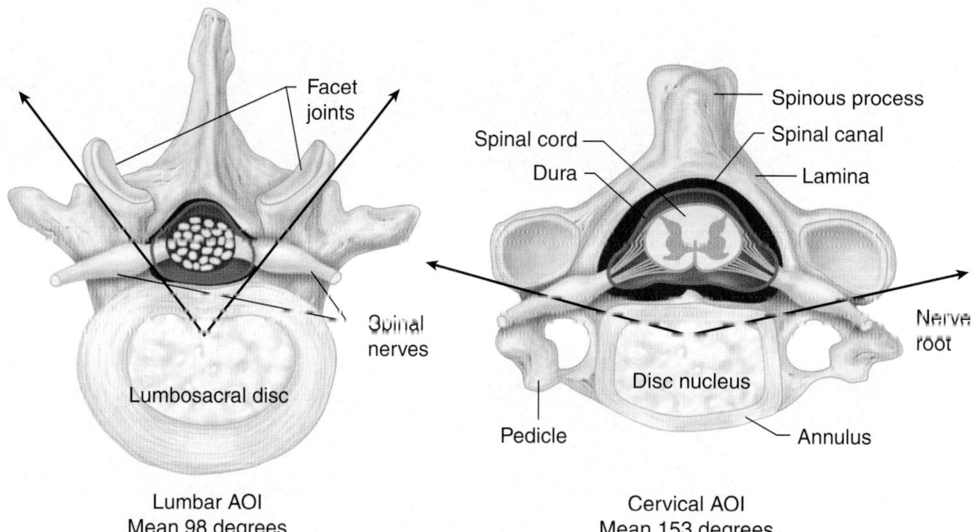


The arc or angle of influence (AOI) is much greater for cervical facet joints compared to the lumbar spinal facet joints.

A

DETERMINATION OF THE ANGLE OF INFLUENCE (AOI)

1) Establish Center of Rotation (COR).

2) Line that bisects the disk and COR.

3) Line from most anterior portion of facet to COR.

4) Measure angle

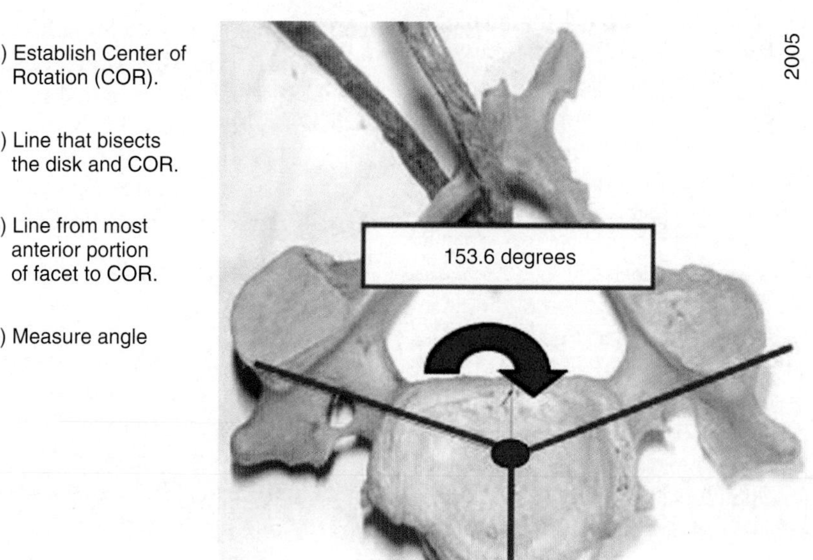


B

60 cervical and lumbar (same specimens measured)

■ **FIGURE 89–3. A,** Arc of influence (AOI). The illustration depicts the arc or angle of influence of the zygoapophyseal joints. The origin of angle is the center of rotation (COR) of the motion segment, along the midsagittal line of the vertebral body, two thirds from the anterior longitudinal ligament and one third from the posterior longitudinal ligament. The AOI is a measure of the stability of the motion segment to rotation; the most stable situation would be a pair of facet joints that circumferentially enclose the intervertebral disc. The lines of the pie-shaped angle extend to the outermost edge of the facet joints. The mean AOI of the cervical spine was 153 degrees versus 98 degrees for the lumbar vertebra from the same skeleton ($P < 0.001$). **B,** Determination of the arc (angle) of influence (AOI). This drawing shows the practical technique for measuring 60 randomly selected skeletons in the Hamann-Todd Osteological Collection. The AOI illustrated here is 153.6 degrees at C5-C6.

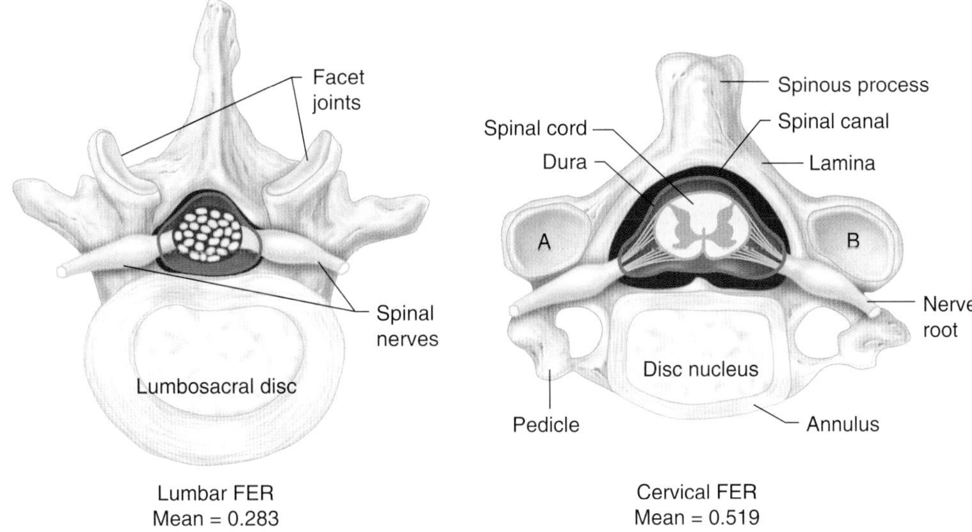


Facets are comparatively small in proportion to lumbar intervertebral disc.

A + B is larger proportion of disc area.

A

DETERMINATION OF THE FACET/END PLATE RATIO (FER)

1) Use size marker to calculate the facet Surface Area (SA).

- Multiply × 2

2) Calculate end plate SA.

3) Calculate ratio.

Facet SA/End Plate SA = (FER)

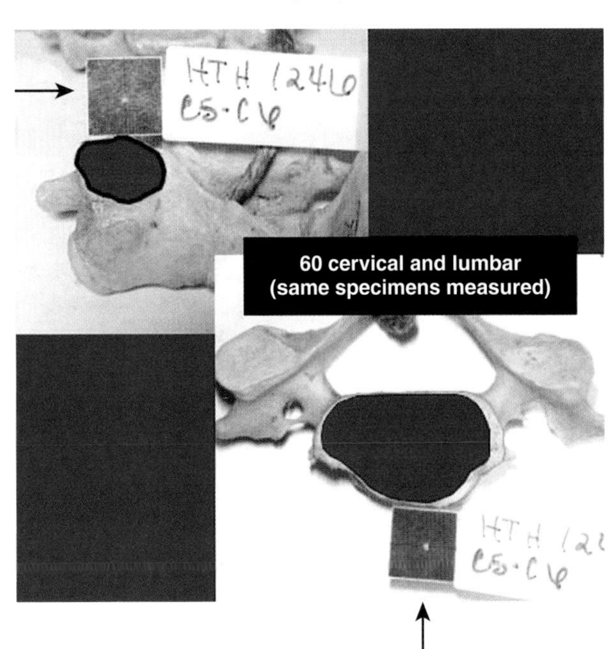


B

■ **FIGURE 89–4.** **A,** Facet/end plate ratio (FER). The FER is a measure of the relative size of the facet joints compared to the cross-sectional area of the intervertebral disc at the same level. The combined area of the left and right facet joints is divided by the cross-sectional area of the vertebral end plate. Note that the angle of influence can be measured on an axial CT slice but that the FER cannot, as this would require a three-dimensional reconstruction at the same angle as the facet joint surface. The mean FER of the cervical spine, 0.519, is almost twice that of the lumbar spine, 0.283. This means that the cervical facet joints and their surrounding capsular ligaments are much larger in proportion to the corresponding intervertebral disc and its surrounding annulus, compared to the lumbar spine. **B,** This practical demonstration on a skeleton shows how the areas were measured using photographs taken at a right angle to the joint surface, with a reference square of known dimensions in the field. The areas were digitally measured. A lumbar facet at L4-L5 is shown, and the cervical C5-C6 end plate area is outlined.

### Rotational Testing of Single-Level and Double-Level CHARITÉ Disc

This subset of in vitro biomechanical study was undertaken to compare the multidirectional flexibility kinematics of single versus multilevel lumbar CHARITÉ reconstructions. A total of seven ($n = 7$) human cadaveric lumbosacral spines (L1 to sacrum) were utilized to investigate and biomechanically evaluate the following L4-L5 reconstruction conditions:

1. Intact spine
2. Discectomy alone
3. CHARITÉ (L4-L5)
4. CHARITÉ + pedicle screws (L4-L5)
5. Two-level CHARITÉ (L4-S1)
6. Two-level CHARITÉ + pedicle screws (L4-S1)
7. CHARITÉ (L4-L5) with pedicle screws and femoral ring allograft (L5-S1)
8. Pedicle screws and femoral ring allograft (L4-S1)

### Uncovertebral Joint Analysis

Six fresh frozen human cadaveric cervical spines were used for the multidirectional flexibility testing and evaluated under the following C5-C6 reconstruction conditions: (1) intact C5-C6, (2) clinical discectomy, (3) radical discectomy to the lateral edge of the uncovertebral joint, (4) PCM Cervical Disc, (5) unilateral uncovertebral resection, (6) unilateral uncovertebral resection + PCM, (7) bilateral uncovertebral resection with discectomy, and (8) bilateral uncovertebral resection + PCM. Unconstrained pure moments of ± 3.0 Nm were used for axial rotation, flexion-extension, and lateral bending testing, with quantification of the C5-C6 operative level range of motion (ROM) and neutral zone (NZ) and with data normalized to the intact spine condition.

## RESULTS OF TESTING

### Anatomic Measurements

The mean arc of influence of rotational stability of the cervical spine (153.6 degrees) was significantly greater than that of the corresponding lumbar spine (98 degrees) ($P < 0.001$). The facet/end plate ratio was significantly greater for the cervical spine (0.519) than for the corresponding lumbar vertebra (0.283, $P < 0.001$).

### Biomechanical Testing

#### Sequential Rotational Testing of Soft tissue Preparation for Disc Replacement

Rotational testing for the neutral zone (NZ) for cervical spine showed the following:

a. Intact cervical spine = 4.63 degrees
b. Discectomy for TDR = 5.25 degrees
c. Radical discectomy = 5.82 degrees
d. Insertion of a PCM. TDR restored the NZ back to 3.76 degrees.

This is in great contrast to the lumbar spine where the intact NZ was 4.3 degrees, and after preparation for clinical lumbar TDR, the ROM more than doubled to 9.68 degrees. Implantation of the lumbar TDR never restored the motion segment back to the rotational stability of the intact segment achieving a range of 120% to 140% rotational ROM compared to the intact condition. This rotational instability proved to be additive, and a two-level lumbar TDR resulted in between 240% and 260% increase in rotational instability compared to the intact condition.

#### Rotational Testing of Single-Level and Double-Level CHARITÉ

The most significant finding is that in this acute instability type model, with resection of the structures required to insert the CHARITÉ prosthesis, the rotational stability of the CHARITÉ implanted spine never restored the neutral zone back to that of the intact condition. With two-level CHARITÉ implantation the rotational instability was additive, showing progressive rotational instability (Fig. 89–5).

Axial rotation loading produced the greatest differences in segmental range of motion at the operative and adjacent levels, particularly under two-level reconstructions. There were no differences observed at the L3-L4 level for any treatment group – single or two level ($P > 0.05$). The motion produced at L4-L5 following a single level discectomy, single-level CHARITÉ, or two-level CHARITÉ (L4-S1) was significantly greater than the intact condition, CHARITÉ combined with pedicle screws, and FRA combined with pedicle screws (single and two levels) ($P < 0.05$). The most pronounced changes in L4-L5 segmental motion were observed for the two-level CHARITÈ reconstruction and hybrid reconstruction: CHARITÈ (L4-L5) combined with pedicle screws and FRA (L5-S1). When compared to the intact condition, segmental motion at the L4-L5 level markedly increased from 160 ± 26% to 263 ± 65% with the implantation of the second CHARITÈ at L5-S1. Moreover, the addition of pedicle screws and FRA at L5-S1 further increased the motion at L4-L5 to 292 ± 71%, which was significantly greater than all other groups except the two-level CHARITÉ ($P < 0.05$). As expected, segmental motion at the inferior L5-S1 level was significantly greater following the single-level (L4-L5) discectomy condition, CHARITÉ alone, and CHARITÉ combined with pedicle screws compared to the two-level CHARITÈ and FRA—both augmented with pedicle screws ($P < 0.05$). The most interesting finding under this loading modality was that observed with the addition of a second CHARITÈ at L5-S1. While segmental motion at L4-L5 markedly increased, motion at L5-S1 significantly increased to 292 ± 71% over the intact condition, which was different from all other treatments ($P < 0.05$). There were no differences between the CHARITÉ augmented with pedicle screws or pedicle screws with femoral ring allograft ($P > 0.05$).

#### Uncovertebral Joint Analysis (Fig. 89–6)

Axial rotation loading for conditions of unilateral or bilateral uncovertebral joint resection demonstrated significant increases in range of motion compared to all other groups ($P < 0.05$). With the insertion of the PCM Cervical Disc, rotational stability of the unilateral resected uncovertebral joint was restored to the intact motion segment for both range of motion and neutral zone ($P > 0.05$). Bilateral uncovertebral joint resection combined with disc arthroplasty indicated significantly greater segmental motion than the intact spine ($P < 0.05$). Flexion-extension testing demonstrated a significant increase in range of motion for all groups with discectomy and uncovertebral joint resection when compared to the intact condition or those stabilized with the PCM arthroplasty ($P < 0.05$). PCM arthroplasty reconstruction following discectomy restored the flexion-extension neutral zone and range of motion to the intact condition ($P > 0.05$). Unilateral and bilateral uncovertebral joint resection demonstrated increased neutral zone values compared to all other treatments ($P < 0.05$). Neutral zone values for the unilateral and bilateral uncovertebral joint resection were significantly greater than all other treatments groups ($P < 0.05$); however, cervical arthroplasty restored neutral zone levels to the intact condition ($P > 0.05$).

## DISCUSSION

Because of the resection of ligaments and portions of the annulus fibrosis, the preparation for a TDR always destabilizes both the cervical and the lumbar spinal segments to some extent.[8,9] However, implanting an unconstrained cervical TDR restores the rotational stability back to the level of the intact condition, whereas inserting an unconstrained lumbar TDR remains rotationally more unstable. This study characterized four significant biomechanical differences, highlighting four biomechanical and anatomic factors for superior inherent rotational stability in cervical TDR versus lumbar TDR:

1. Cervical TDR has a larger arc of influence (153.6 degrees versus 98 degrees).
2. Cervical TDR had a greater facet/end plate area ratio (0.519 versus 0.283).
3. The tensile load of the major ligaments of the lumbar and cervical spines was quantitated by White and Panjabi. The rank order of ligament tensile strength from highest to lowest for the lumbar spine is ALL → PLL → LF → CL. For the cervical spine the rank order is quite different—CL → LF → ALL → PLL. This difference has important ramifications for arthroplasty stability because the ALL is always resected and the PLL is released or stretched. Whereas the ligamentum flavum (LF) and the capsular ligaments

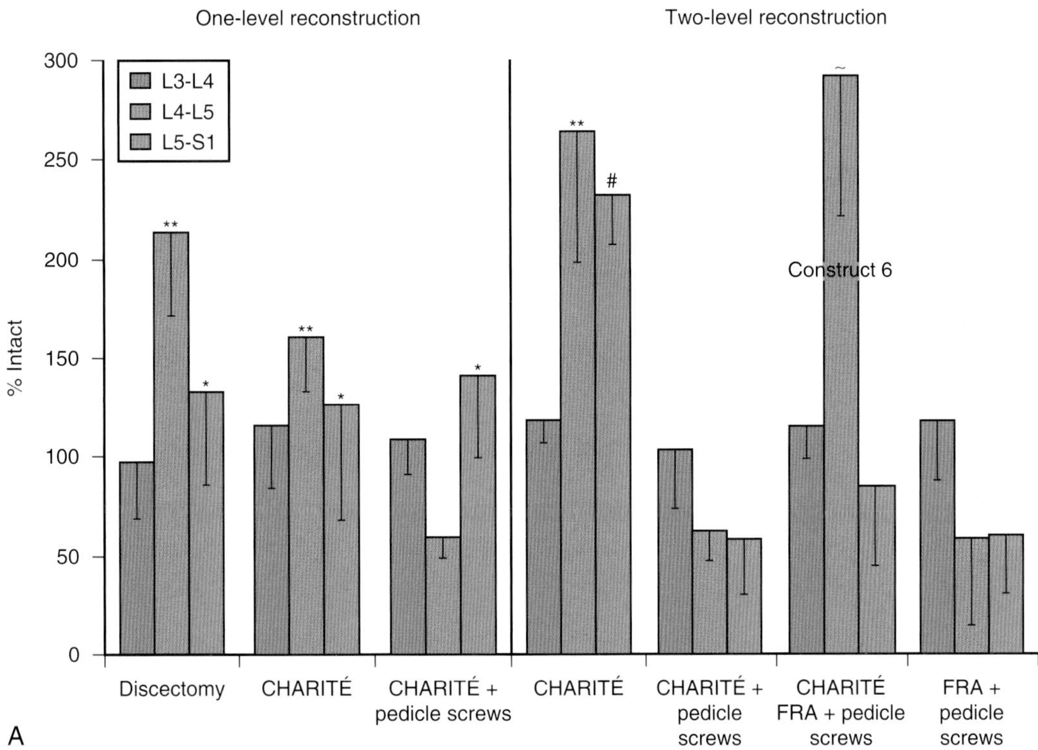


■ **FIGURE 89–5. A,** Rotational biomechanical testing of one-level and two-level CHARITÉ. Peak range of motion comparing the intact spine to seven methods of reconstruction highlighting changes in segmental motion at the L3-L4, L4-L5, and L5-S1 levels. The seven series of three bar graphs ($n = 7$) represent the peak range of motion (ROM) at three levels, L3–4, L4–5, and L5-S1, normalized to the intact lumbar cadaveric segment before treatment, with intact percentage designated as 100% on the graph. From left to right the seven treatments were (1) destabilized (discectomy preparation for lumbar total disc replacement) at L4-L5; (2) one-level CHARITÉ at L4-L5; (3) CHARITÉ and pedicle screws at L4-L5; (4) two-level CHARITÉ at L4-L5 and L5-S1; (5) CHARITÉ and pedicle screws at two levels; (6) CHARITÉ + FRA (femoral ring allograft) spacer and pedicle screws at two levels; and (7) FRA and pedicle screws at two levels. Notice that with one-level CHARITÉ at L4-L5 that the rotational stiffness is 160% (SD 26%), meaning that the acute rotational stability is not restored to the level of the intact segment.

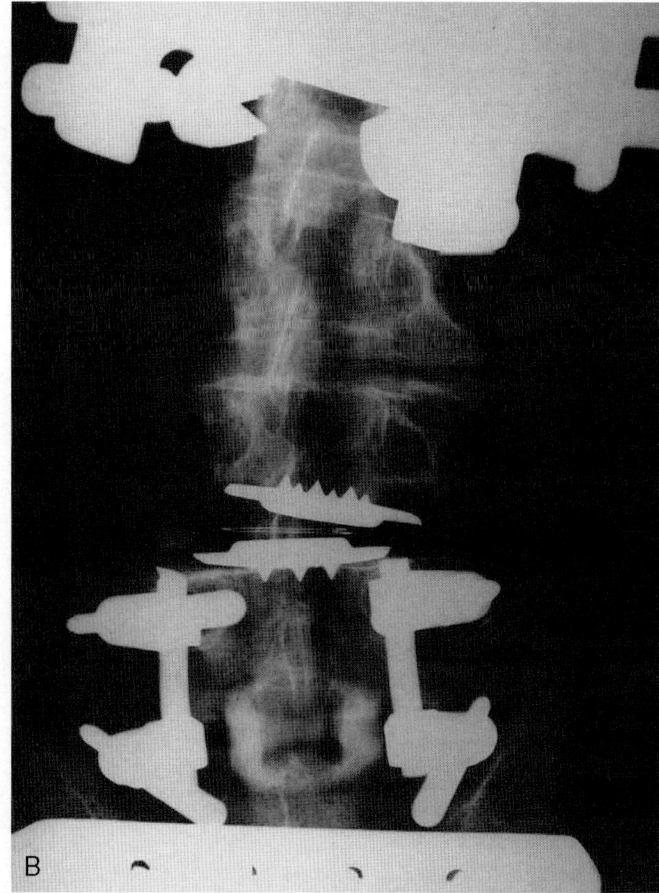


■ **FIGURE 89–5. Cont'd.** **B,** An AP radiograph of construct number 6 is shown in the fully rotated position on the spine simulator. The three levels are intact L3-L4, CHARITÉ at L4-L5, and 360 instrumentation at L5-S1 (femoral ring allograft + pedicle screws). The AP radiograph of the specimen looks very similar to the rotational deformity of the clinically failed CHARITÉ at L4-L5 shown in Figure 89–2. Notice the rotation of the spinous processes as well as the obliquity of the implant components. We can attest that the CHARITÉ was placed in midcenter of L4-L5 in the laboratory specimen. If the intact disc is taken as 100%, the CHARITÉ demonstrated 290%, whereas the 360-degree instrumentation demonstrated 85% rotation. In absolute degrees, the total rotational deformity of the hybrid construct was 10.86 degrees compared to an intact (unoperated) specimen of 3.31 degrees.

(CL) are, of course, preserved with arthroplasty. The ratio of CL/ALL tensile load for the cervical spine is 204/111 $n = 1.93$. The CL/ALL tensile load ratio is much smaller for the lumbar spine at 222/450 $n = 0.493$.

4. Depending on the amount of disc height distraction and lateral decompression with the cervical TDR, the uncovertebral joints contribute to rotational stability. We found with unilateral uncovertebral joint resection, however, that even an unconstrained cervical TDR restored the neutral zone of the intact condition.

The capsular ligaments and lateral masses clearly are the primary stabilizers of rotational stability in the cervical spine. The implications in the cervical spine for TDR clearly show that even for a radical discectomy and uncovertebral resection a TDR can safely restore the stability of the cervical spine back to the physiologic neutral zone. However, in the lumbar spine the annulus fibrosis, ALL, and PLL are the three most important primary stabilizers in rotation and all three are compromised in lumbar TDR. Even with normal preparation of the lumbar disc for TDR, the CHARITÉ does not return the rotational stability back to the physiologic neutral zone but results in 120% to 140% rotation compared to the intact condition. The multilevel TDR lumbar implantation has an additive destabilizing effect, as two-level annulus lumbar resection results in 240% to 260% rotation (with intact being normalized to 100%).

The findings in the present biomechanical investigation highlight a variety of important trends at the operative and adjacent

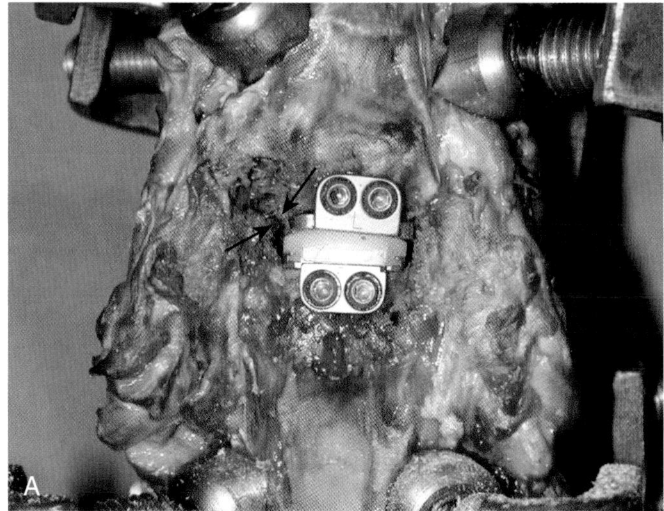

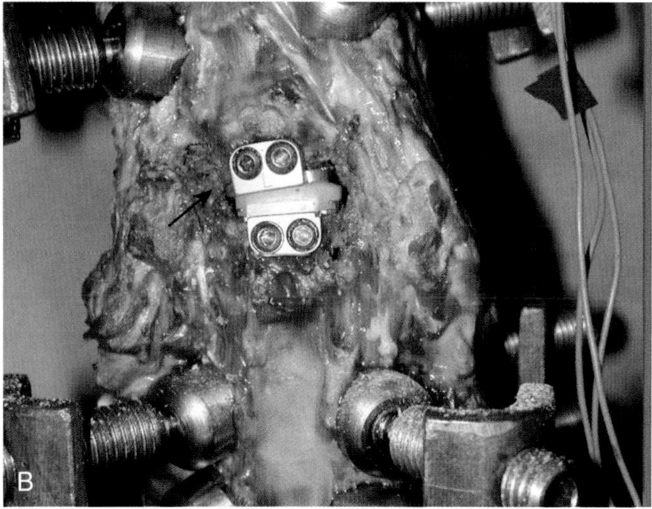


■ **FIGURE 89–6.** **A** and **B,** Uncovertebral joint restrains rotation. This is the benchtop rotational testing of stability to an axially rotated cervical segment with an unconstrained prosthesis implanted at C5-C6. The arrows designate the right uncovertebral joint. Notice that with axial rotation to the right side that the uncovertebral joint closes down, serving as a rotational bony block. An exact number or percentage of the contribution of the uncovertebral joint toward rotational stability is not possible—the contribution of the uncovertebral joint is extremely variable, depending on the amount of the uncus resected during the lateral extent of the cervical neural decompression, and the amount of disc space height restored during artificial disc implantation. Notice also that in the cervical spine coupled motions are much more important. As the specimen is rotated toward the right, the two vertebrae demonstrate right lateral bending with the vertebral end plates laterally bending toward each other. This also tends to close down the uncovertebral joint and also serves as a constraint toward cervical rotation.

levels. Axial rotation loading produced the greatest differences in segmental range of motion, particularly under two-level reconstructions. There were no differences observed at the L3-L4 level for any treatment group—single or two level. When compared to the intact condition, segmental motion at the L4-L5 level markedly increased from 160 ± 26% to 263 ± 65% with the implantation of the second CHARITÈ at L5-S1. Moreover, the addition of pedicle screws and FRA at L5-S1 further increased the motion at L4-L5 to 292 ± 71%, which was significantly greater than all other groups except the two-level CHARITÉ ($P < 0.05$). The most interesting finding under this loading modality was that observed with the addition of a second CHARITÈ at L5-S1. While segmental motion at L4-L5 markedly increased, motion at L5-S1 significantly increased to 263 ± 65% over the intact condition, which was different from all other treatments ($P < 0.05$). This suggests that a disc replacement adjacent to a 360-degree instrumentation can become unstable.

These benchtop biomechanical findings from the current study corroborate the clinical work of Sariali and associates[10] who investigated the in vivo kinematic response to single- and two-level CHARITÈ reconstructions. A comparative retrospective study of motion in axial rotation at L4-L5 level was carried out on 17 patients with the CHARITÈ device versus six healthy volunteers. Five patients had one prostheses at the L4-L5 level and 12 had two prosthesis at L4-L5 and L5-S1 levels. The follow-up ranged from 10.8 to 14.3 years (average 12.4 ± 1, median 12.6). Eleven (65%) patients had a normal mobility in torsion, identical to those of the volunteers and of the literature, whereas six (35%) had an abnormal increased mobility. According to Sariali and associates, if only one disc was replaced, mobility in torsion was identical to that of the volunteers. In the case of two replaced discs, 50% (6 of 12) of the patients had an abnormal increased mobility. Moreover, in the subgroup of increased mobility, the coupling was different with increased flexion (10 degrees) ($P < 0.001$). According to Sariali and associates, the implantation of one CHARITÈ device appears to restore kinematics close to that of the healthy volunteers. However, two adjacent prostheses produce a condition of abnormal kinematics in 50% of the cases.

There should be a *disclaimer*—a major shortcoming of this type of acute instability found in biomechanical testing cannot be emphasized enough. The major limitation of all phases of this investigation is the lack of consideration of the contribution of muscular forces, progressive biologic healing, heterotopic ossification, fibrosis, adhesions, and other processes that would be expected to contribute to long-term rotational stability following clinical surgical recovery.

## What About a More Constrained Prosthesis Design?

We did not study the effect of having a more constrained prosthesis design. Perhaps the effect might be more stress internal to the prosthesis with a higher incidence of lateral or scoliotic articulation of the components rather than more obvious obliquity of the vertebral bodies. For example, notice that the same anatomic and biomechanical forces are still relevant to the motion segment. This constrained device required revision due to asymmetric scoliotic collapse and unintended metal-on-metal contact of a nonarticular part of the prosthesis. The spinal malalignment is not as obvious by Cobb measurement, but the premature failure of the prosthesis is just as clinically significant. The removal of an ingrown keeled prosthesis due to premature biomaterial failure less than 12 months postoperatively is a supreme surgical challenge and one of the most difficult procedures in spinal surgery. The use of a more constrained prosthesis in the peripheral skeleton does not obviate problems, as a more constrained prosthesis increases the stresses at the metal-bone interface, increases the incidence of loosening, and can reduce the range of prosthetic motion.

## CONCLUSIONS

1. There are four main rotational stabilizing considerations in the functional spinal unit, and all four favor cervical versus lumbar rotational integrity.
2. Compared to the intact nonoperated motion segment, the preparation for both cervical and lumbar disc replacements compromises the axial rotational stability of both the cervical and lumbar spine—resection of the ALL, stretching or "release" of the PLL, increasing the disc space height which "unlocks" the posterior facet joints, and removal of portions of the uncovertebral joints in the cervical spine.
3. With an unconstrained prosthesis, the uncovertebral joint can be resected and the rotational stability of the intact cervical segment can be restored, but not with bilateral uncovertebral joint resection.
4. Implantation of an unconstrained lumbar disc replacement fails to restore the acute rotational stability of the lumbar spine. However, with an unconstrained prosthesis in the cervical spine, the rotational stability is restored within the neutral zone of the intact condition. With multilevel or successive lumbar artificial disc replacement, the instability is additive—what is lost in resecting the annulus, ALL, and PLL is not compensated for totally in the acute postoperative condition.

## REFERENCES


1. McAfee PC, Cunningham BW, Lee GA, et al: Revision strategies for salvaging or improving failed cylindrical cages. Spine 24:2147–2153, 1999.
2. McAfee PC, Cunningham BW, Hayes V, et al: Biomechanical analysis of rotational motions after disc arthroplasty: Implications for patients with adult deformities. Spine 31(19):S152–S160, 2006.
3. Blumenthal SL, McAfee PC, Guyer RD, et al: A prospective, randomized, multi-center FDA IDE Study of lumbar total disc replacement with the CHARITÉ™ Artificial Disc vs. lumbar fusion: Part I—Evaluation of clinical outcomes. Spine 2005 (in press).
4. McAfee PC, Cunningham BW, Holtsapple G, et al: A prospective, randomized, multi-center FDA IDE Study of lumbar total disc replacement with the CHARITÉ™ Artificial Disc vs. lumbar fusion: Part II—Evaluation of radiographic outcomes and correlation of surgical technique accuracy with clinical outcomes. Spine 2005 (in press).
5. Buttner-Janz K, Hochshuler SH, McAfee PC: The Artificial Disk. New York, Springer-Verlag, 2003.
6. McAfee PC: Artificial disc prosthesis: The link SB CHARITÉ. *In* Kaech DL, Jinkins JR (eds): Spinal Rehabilitation Procedures. St. Louis, Elsevier, 2002, pp 299–310.
7. McAfee PC, Cunningham BW, Orbegoso CM, et al: Analysis of porous ingrowth in intervertebral disc prostheses: A nonhuman primate model. Spine 28:332–340, 2003.
8. McAfee PC, Geisler FH, Saiedy SS, et al: Revisibility of the CHARITÉ Artificial Disc: Analysis of 688 patients enrolled in the US IDE Study of the Charite Artificial Disc. Spine 31(11):1217–1226, 2006.
9. McAfee PC, Geisler FH, Scott-Young M (eds): Roundtables in Spine Surgery: Complications and Revision Strategies in Lumbar Spine Arthroplasty. St. Louis, Quality Medical Publishing, 2005.
10. Sariali EH, Lemaire JP, Pascal-Mousselard H, et al: In vivo study of the kinematics in axial rotation of the lumbar spine after total intervertebral disc replacement: Long-term results: A 10-14 year follow-up evaluation. Eur Spine J 21:1–10, 2006.

CHAPTER 90

# Can Lumbar Disc Replacement Be Used Adjacent to a Scoliotic Deformity?

Thierry Marnay, Patrick Tropiano, James J. Yue, and Geneste Guilhaume

## KEY POINTS

- Lumbar disc replacement adjacent to pre-existing scoliosis is currently being evaluated.
- Scoliosis has recently been classified into four types.
- Use of semiconstrained ProDisc implant adjacent to scoliotic deformity or within scoliotic deformity may be achievable in select patients.
- Extensive preoperative evaluation is mandatory in this expanded indication patient group.

Although the use of total disc replacement (TDR) has been shown to be at least equally effective and in some studies superior to fusion of the spine,[1–6] the use of total disc replacement in the patient with a scoliotic deformity has not been examined in great detail. Most, if not all, prospective randomized studies have excluded patients with greater than 11 degrees of scoliosis in the frontal plane.[4,6]

In general and in broad terms, scoliosis in the pediatric population can be defined as being idiopathic, congenital, neuromuscular, and syndrome-related.[7] In the adult patient, scoliosis has been recently categorized by Aebi into four types[8]:

Type 1: Primary degenerative or de novo scoliosis resulting from disc degeneration or facet joint arthritis with or without signs of spinal stenosis.

Type 2: Idiopathic adolescent scoliosis of the thoracic or lumbar spine which progresses in adult life and is usually combined with secondary degeneration or imbalance. The patient who has had fusion of an adolescent curve and now has progression of a pre-existing curve or the formation of a new adjacent curve are categorized as 3a.

Type 3: Patients with secondary adult curves are subcategorized into Types 3a and 3b.

Type 3a: In the context of an oblique pelvis, for instance, due to a leg-length discrepancy or hip disease or as a secondary curve in idiopathic, neuromuscular, and congenital scoliosis, or asymmetric anomalies at the lumbosacral junction.

Type 3b: In the context of a metabolic bone disease (mostly osteoporosis) combined with asymmetric arthritic disease or vertebral fractures.

In Chapter 89, Paul McAfee discussed the formation of sagittal and frontal plane deformities at the level of total disc replacement in patients who had no pre-existing scoliosis. This chapter will evaluate the use of ADR surgery within a pre-existing curve in a degenerative/de novo scoliosis (Aebi Type I) or in a patient who has undergone previous spinal fusion for idiopathic adolescent scoliosis and has developed adjacent level changes to the prior curve. The solutions proposed as a surgical treatment for scoliosis has always been limited to a fusion with an instrumentation that tries to reduce the curve and maintain the reduction until the fusion has healed. With the capacity of the total disc replacement (ProDisc as a semiconstrained implant) to reduce a part of the deformity, stabilize the space, and maintain the motion, we present here a new approach to the scoliosis surgical treatment.

## CLINICAL BACKGROUND AND METHODS

Historically, the senior author (TM) designed the ProDisc[5] implant (Synthes, Paoli, PA) to be utilized not in patients with primary disc degeneration in a neutral spine. Rather, the ProDisc implant was designed to be utilized in those patients who had had prior scoliotic surgery and developed adjacent level degeneration. The ProDisc implant is a keeled implant and can resist sheer forces due to the fixed ball-and-socket design. The keel permits not only strong primary fixation but also permits for stabilization of reduction of deformity in the frontal plane in the presence of a lateral spondylolisthesis.

The senior author (TM) began a clinical trial in 2000, evaluating using the ProDisc semiconstrained lumbar total disc replacement in the treatment of adult patients either within a scoliotic deformity or adjacent to a scoliotic curve.[9] For evaluation purposes the patients were classified into Type 1 (TDR in the curve itself) and Type 2 (TDR below the curve) (Table 90–1). Type 1 patients were stratified into those patients with idiopathic scoliosis, (Type 1aI) and those patients with a

**TABLE 90–1. Classification Total Disc Replacement in Scoliotic Spinal Curve**

Type 1: Total disc replacement in the curve, 18 patients*
 Type 1a: Idiopathic scoliosis, 9 patients
 Type 1b: Degenerative scoliosis, 9 patients
Type 2: Total disc replacement below the curve, 24 patients†
 Type 2a: Already instrumented, 23 patients
 Type 2b: Not instrumented, 1 patient

*Six men, 12 women.
†Three men, 21 women.

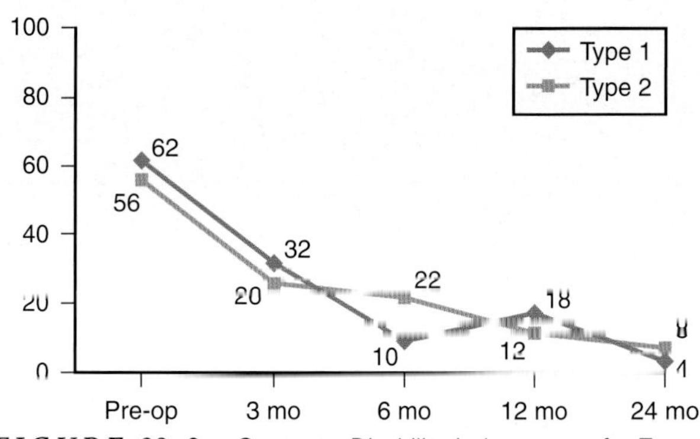


■ **FIGURE 90–2.** Oswestry Disability Index scores for Types 1 and 2.

degenerative curve (Type 1b). Type 2 patients were stratified into those patients that had prior scoliosis surgery (Type 2a) and those who had not had prior surgery (Type 2b). Average age of patients was 52 years old (range 32–69), the weight 64 kg (50–83 kg), and a height 167 cm (155–185 cm). Minimum follow-up period was 24 months. A total of 42 patients were enrolled in the study. Twelve patients had one-level surgery, 16 patients had bilevel surgery, 10 patients had trilevel surgery, and 4 had four-level surgery.

## RESULTS

Figures 90–1 and 90–2 show clinical outcome scores for Visual Analog Score (VAS) and Oswestry measurements. All groups showed excellent improvement with maintenance of this improvement at 2 years. The patients who needed a TDR in the curve (idiopathic or degenerative) presented a leg pain more important than the group who needed a surgery below the curve. It seemed that the radicular pain coming from the curve dislocation was less tolerated than the roots compression in the degenerated discs below the scoliosis. However, the results were the same after the surgery, regardless of the anatomic situation before surgery. Figure 90–3 illustrates pre- and postoperative radiographs of a type 1a patient with a pre-existing idiopathic scoliosis. Figures 90–4 and 90–5 illustrate the pre- and postoperative imaging studies of a Type 1b patient. The patient had a degenerative scoliosis and underwent 3 level ProDisc surgery with reduction of the L3-L4 lateral spondylolisthesis. The patient's 4-year follow-up VAS and Oswestry scrores were 1 and 5, respectively. Figures 90–6 to 90–9 illustrate the pre- and postoperative radiographs of Type 2b patients.

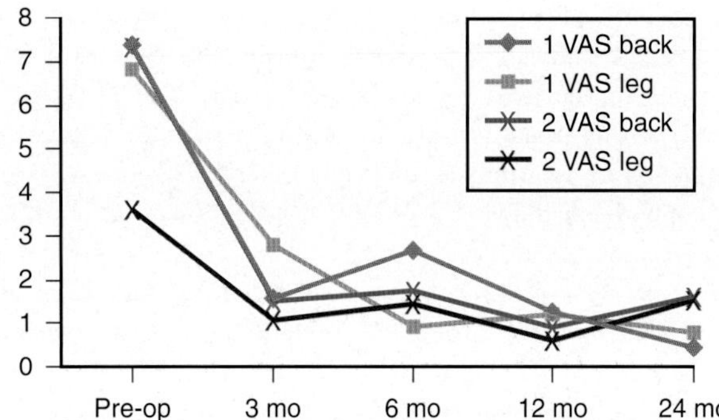


■ **FIGURE 90–1.** Visual Analog Scale (VAS) scores (from 0 to 10) for Type 1a, Type 1b, Type 2a, and Type 2b patient groups. There is a difference in the preoperative signs, with a lower level of leg (neurologic) pain in the group with a need of total disc replacement below the curve.

## DISCUSSION

The usage and indications of total disc replacement surgery continue to evolve. One of these expanded indications that is currently being evaluated is in the patient with either de novo degenerative scoliosis or who has had prior scoliosis surgery and now is suffering from adjacent level degeneration. As presented in other chapters in this text, great care must be taken to evaluate the patient for TDR surgery. The patient with scoliosis is no exception and must be even more carefully assessed for facet degeneration and segmental instability, osteoporosis, and other exclusionary criteria. As the age of the patient is on average 52 (10 years older than the patients with a current degenerative disc disease[6]) with a majority of females, the osteodensitometry limit for surgery is −1. The quality of the outcomes has to be unlighted, especially in the Type 2a, with the poor results of the extension of the fusion to the pelvis below a scoliosis with the complete ankylosis of the spine, and the mechanical complications of the pelvic fixation procedure. The capacity of the total disc replacement in scoliosis seems for the future to be able to modify the indications in scoliosis surgery, and could change our surgical behaviors—not to extend the fusion below L4, not to operate too early on the lumbar curves, decide to include hybrid constructs with fusions in the thoracolumbar area, and disc replacements below, as we have seen the capabilities we have to extend the TDR to L2-L3. The senior author's early study results appear to show positive value in the usage of TDR surgery in a select group of scoliotic surgery.

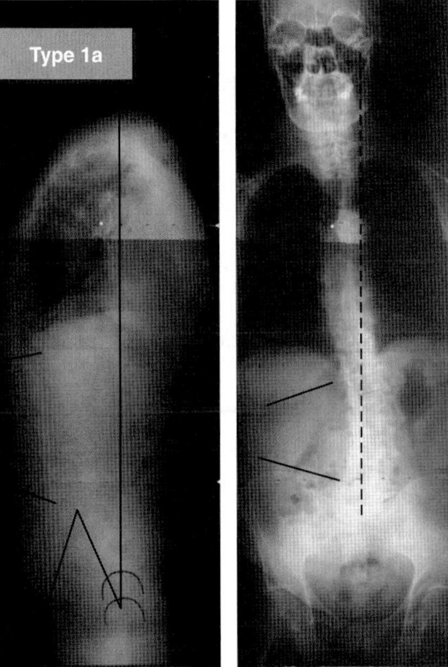


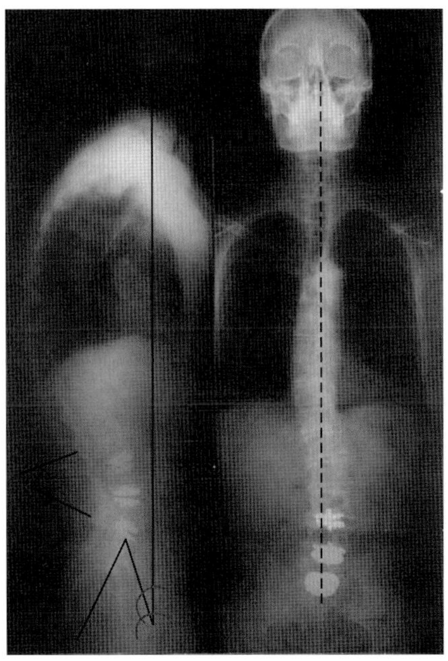

■ **FIGURE 90–3.** Preoperative and postoperative radiographs of Type 1a patient. The delordotic curve of the lumbar spine is associated with a retroversion of the pelvis. The capability of adaptation of the patient is limited with the stiff kyphotic curve of the thoracic spine. In the frontal plane, there are also no possibilities to balance the occipital axis preoperatively. We can see in postoperative films the capacity for the lumbar spine to reestablish a lordosis curve and so reduce the version angle. The design of the prothesis with an anchorage with a keel and a ball-and-socket as a joint that neutralizes the shear forces allows those changes.

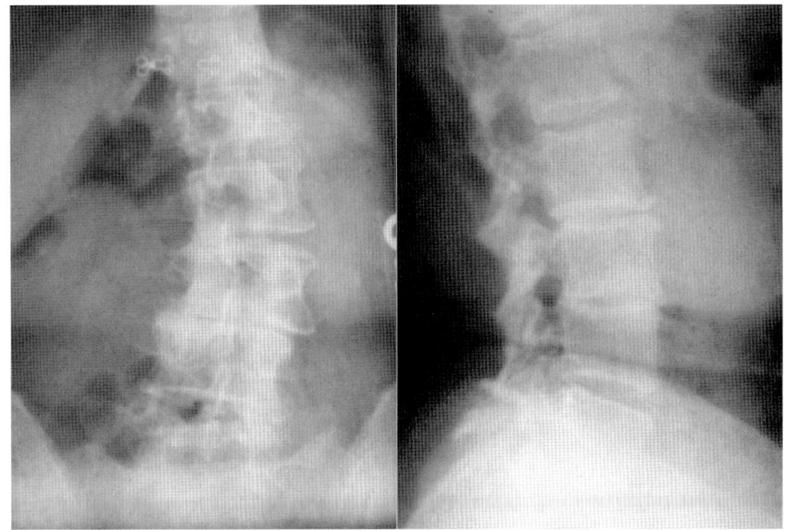

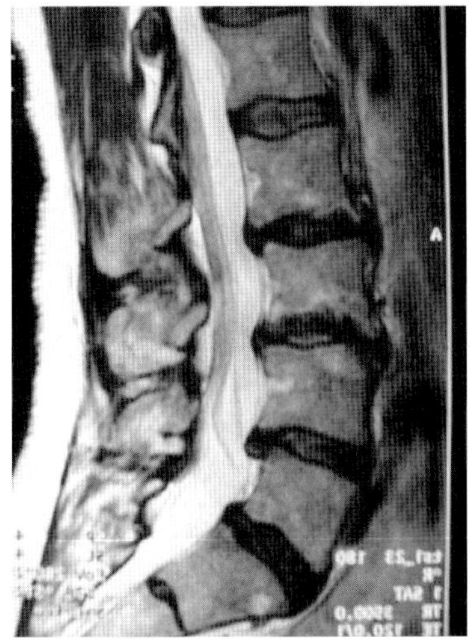

■ **FIGURE 90–4.** Preoperative radiographs of Type 1b patient. We can see the asymmetry of the frontal inclination of the L4-L5 disc and the dislocation of L3-L4.

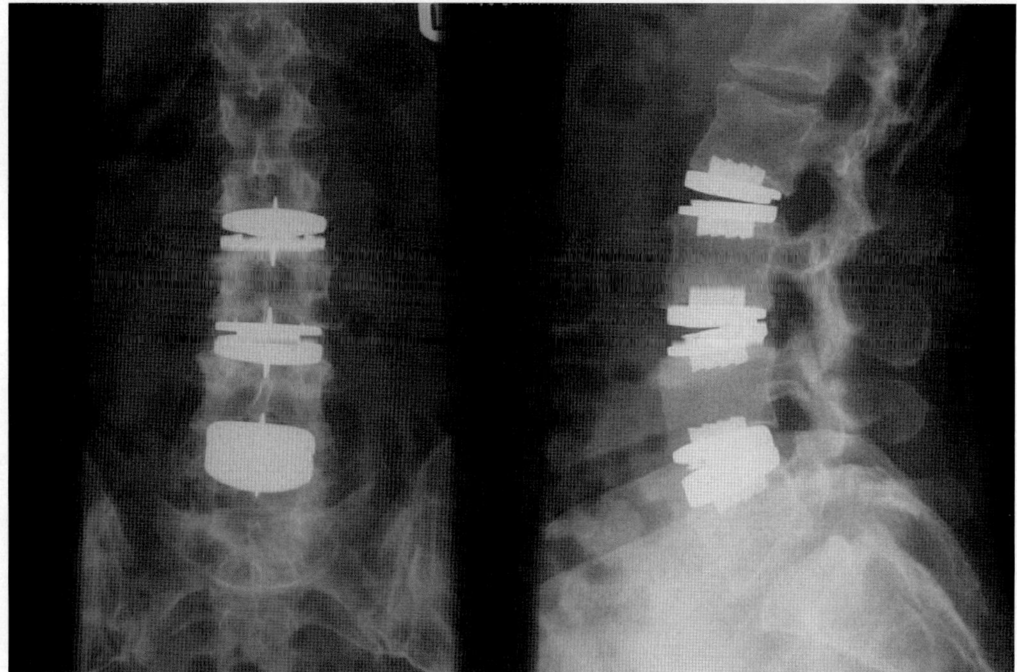

■ **FIGURE 90–5.** Postoperative radiographs of Type 1b patient. The quality of the realignment of the spine in the frontal view shows the capacity of reduction of curves with the release of the space and the semiconstrained prosthesis.

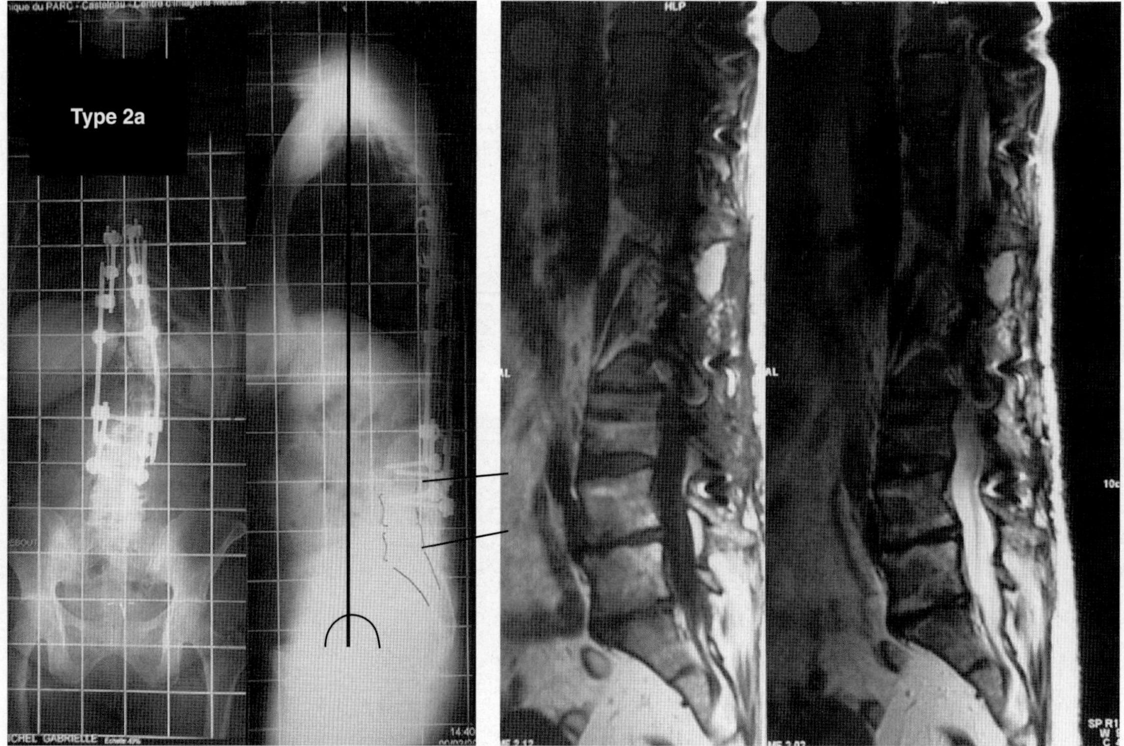


■ **FIGURE 90–6.** Preoperative radiographs of Type 2a patient. The kyphosis of the two lowest levels creates a retroversion of the pelvis and a sagittal unbalance.

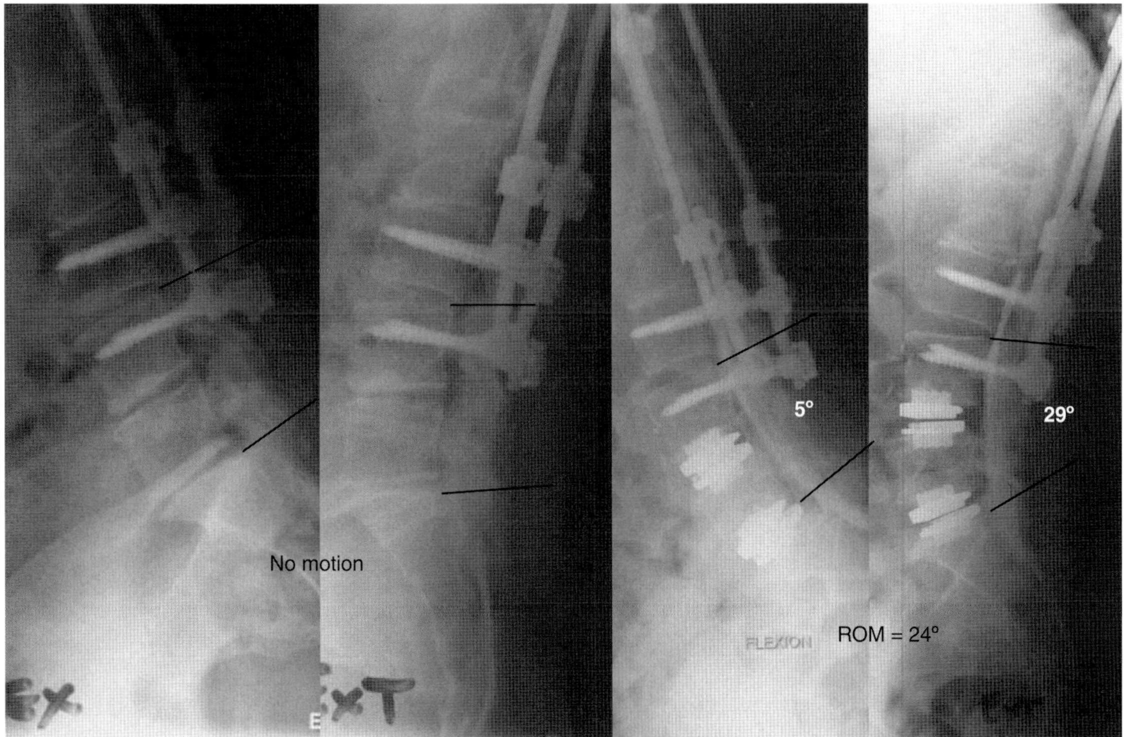


■ **FIGURE 90–7.** Postoperative radiographs of Type 2a patient. The 24 degrees of range of motion (ROM) and especially the restitution of a lumbar lordosis re-create the conditions for a better everyday life.

■ **FIGURE 90–8.** Preoperative radiographs of Type 2a patient. The degeneration of the discs below an instrumented idiopathic curve may be solved through a total disc replacement on the degenerated levels. The alternative of an extension of the fusion to the pelvis has never been a satisfactory procedure, with a high rate of pseudarthrosis and mechanical complications on the pelvic fixation, and the fair outcomes of the total spine fusions to the pelvis.

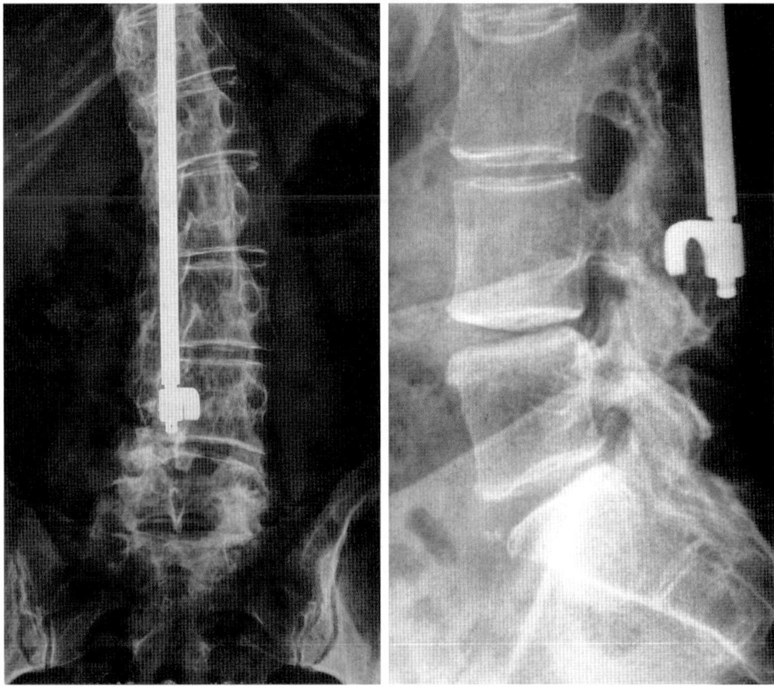

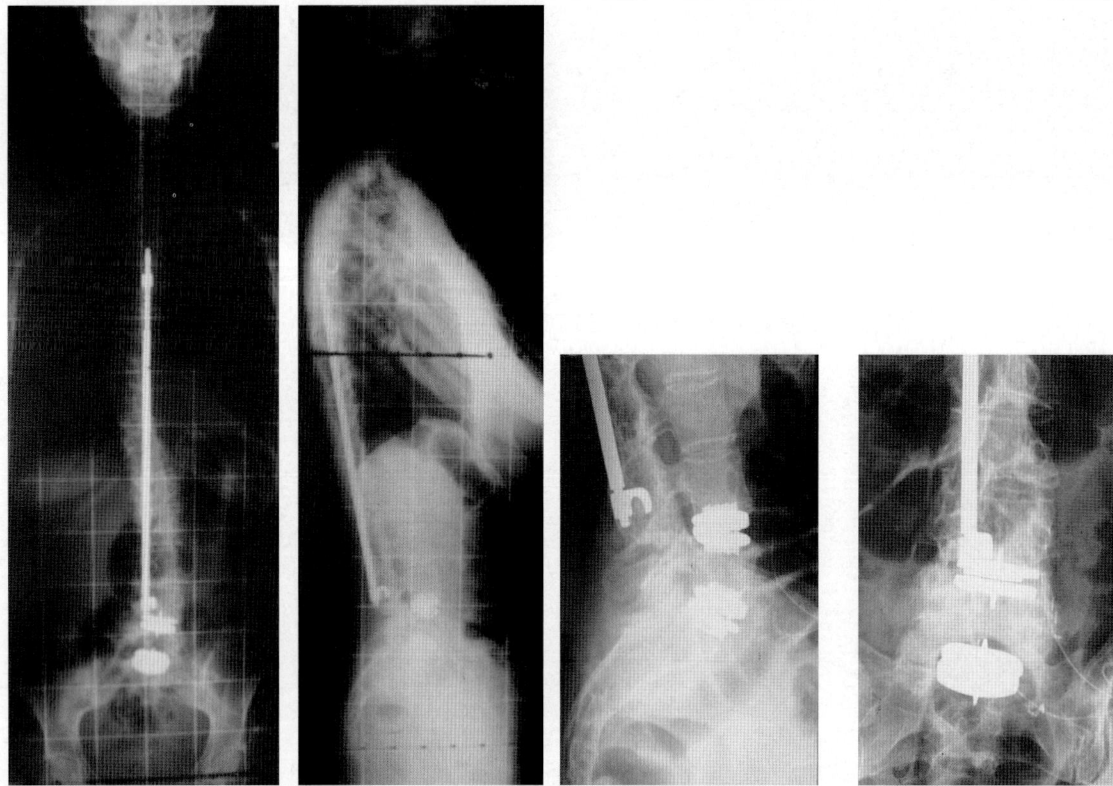

■ **FIGURE 90–9.** Postoperative radiographs of Type 2a patient. The ball-and-socket joint allows a frontal inclination of the implant without any risk of lateral dislocation, and is perfectly adapted to this type of pathologic anatomy.

## REFERENCES

1. Bertagnoli R, Yue JJ, Kershaw T, et al: Lumbar total disc arthroplasty utilizing the ProDisc prosthesis in smokers versus nonsmokers: A prospective study with 2-year minimum follow-up. Spine 31:992–997, 2006.
2. Bertagnoli R, Yue JJ, Shah RV, et al: The treatment of disabling multilevel lumbar discogenic low back pain with total disc arthroplasty utilizing the ProDisc prosthesis: A prospective study with 2-year minimum follow-up. Spine 30:2192–2199, 2005.
3. Bertagnoli R, Yue JJ, Shah RV, et al: The treatment of disabling single-level lumbar discogenic low back pain with total disc arthroplasty utilizing the Prodisc prosthesis: A prospective study with 2-year minimum follow-up. Spine 30:2230–2236, 2005.
4. Blumenthal S, McAfee PC, Guyer RD, et al: A prospective, randomized, multicenter Food and Drug Administration investigational device exemptions study of lumbar total disc replacement with the CHARITÉ artificial disc versus lumbar fusion, Part I: Evaluation of clinical outcomes. [erratum appears in Spine 30(20):2356, 2005]. Spine 30:1565–1575; discussion E1387–1591, 2005.
5. Tropiano P, Huang RC, Girardi FP: Lumbar total disc replacement, 7 to 11 years of follow up. J Bone Joint Surg Am 87:490–496, 2005.
6. Zigler J, Delamarter R, Spivak JM, et al: Results of the prospective, randomized, multicenter Food and Drug Administration investigational device exemption study of the ProDisc-L total disc replacement versus circumferential fusion for the treatment of 1-level degenerative disc disease. Spine 32:1155–1162; discussion 1163, 2007.
7. Newton PO, Wenger DR: Pediatric spinal deformity. Orthopaedic Knowlege Update. Spine 2:361–376, 2002.
8. Aebi M: The adult scoliosis. Eur Spine J 14:925–948, 2005.
9. Marnay T, Tropiano P, Geneste G, Blondel B: Scoliosis and TDR Classification of Indications and Preliminary Results. Presented at Spine Arthroplasty Society, Montreal, Canada, 2006.

CHAPTER 91

# Orthobiom: A Nonfusion Treatment for Pediatric Scoliosis

Charles H. Rivard, Christine Coillard, Souad Rhalmi, Marco Bérard, Robert T. Chomiak, and Gary L. Lowery

## KEY POINTS

- The Orthobiom is intended to treat pediatric patients suffering from scoliosis.
- The Orthobiom Spinal System is a pedicle screw system.
- The Orthobiom allows stabilization and correction of the curve.
- The primary difference between the Orthobiom and other pedicle screw systems is the incorporation of a mobile connector into the subject device.
- The Orthobiom has not yet been implanted in humans but has been implanted in minipigs.

Scoliosis is defined by the Scoliosis Research Society as a structural curve of the spine greater than 10 degrees.[1] The lateral spinal curvature along with the spinal rotation causes the trunk and the rib asymmetry (rib hump). Scoliosis is typically associated with subnormal thoracic kyphosis; hence, structural scoliosis is a three-dimensional deformity with significant cosmetic implications. Idiopathic scoliosis is the most common type of scoliosis. Onset of scoliosis may be in infancy (age 0–3 years) or childhood (age 4–10 years). The vast majority of patients who present with idiopathic scoliosis are diagnosed during adolescence, during the growth spurt of puberty. The etiology of adolescent idiopathic scoliosis is multifactorial and includes genetic, hormonal, neuromuscular, and growth factors.

The course of treatment for patients in different scoliosis age groups varies considerably and depends on a variety of factors including the extent of the curve at the time of diagnosis and during follow-up, the patient's stage of remaining bone growth, the amount of pain and deformity associated with the condition, and the patient's willingness and ability to withstand surgery should it be deemed necessary. Treatment options for the various types of scoliosis are categorized into observation, conservative, and surgical, depending on the individual case. Treatment selection is based on the measurement of the Cobb angle. Conservative treatment, such as bracing and casting, aim at preventing or slowing the curve progression and require flexibility and growth potential to be effective. As a consequence, congenital and adult scoliosis are usually nonresponsive to bracing. If the curve is at high risk of progression and is of significant magnitude, surgical correction may be indicated. For all patients with scoliosis, the goals of treatment are the same, which is to alleviate symptoms and to prevent curve progression.

The Orthobiom Spinal System (Paradigm Spine, GmbH, Wurmlingen, Germany) is a posterior pedicle screw system indicated for the treatment of pediatric scoliosis by (1) correction, (2) stabilization, (3) adjustment, and (4) fixation of the scoliotic spine. The Orthobiom Spinal System fuses the apical level to better stabilize and maintain the curve similar to the currently cleared scoliosis-specific pedicle screw systems while allowing the possibility of longitudinal adjustment.

## DESCRIPTION OF THE DEVICE

The Orthobiom Spinal System is a pedicle screw scoliosis system consisting of pedicle screws, rods, fixed and mobile connectors, and cross connectors designed to correct and stabilize the scoliotic spine (Fig. 91–1).

The pedicle screws, rods, and fixed connectors behave identically to other pedicle screw systems such as the ISOLA (DePuy Spine, Inc., Raynham, MA), CD Horizon (Medtronic Sofamor Danek, Memphis, TN), and TSRH Spinal Systems (Medtronic Sofamor Danek, Memphis, TN), (with the exception that the polyaxial screw head does not lock). These components rigidly fix the spine and allow for fusion at one or more levels. The mobile connector is similar to the fixed connector except it allows the connector to slide axially on the rod at levels superior and inferior to the fusion site. Therefore, the mobile connector still allows correction of the spine in flexion/extension and lateral bending, but do not axially fix the spine at these levels. This characteristic allows the levels above and below the fused level(s) to potentially continue natural spinal growth (adjustment without repeat operations) but maintain stabilization of the corrected scoliotic curve.

The Orthobiom Spinal System is made of three different materials:

1. Nitrogen-strengthened steel (BioDur 108): rods, pedicle screws, and cross connector

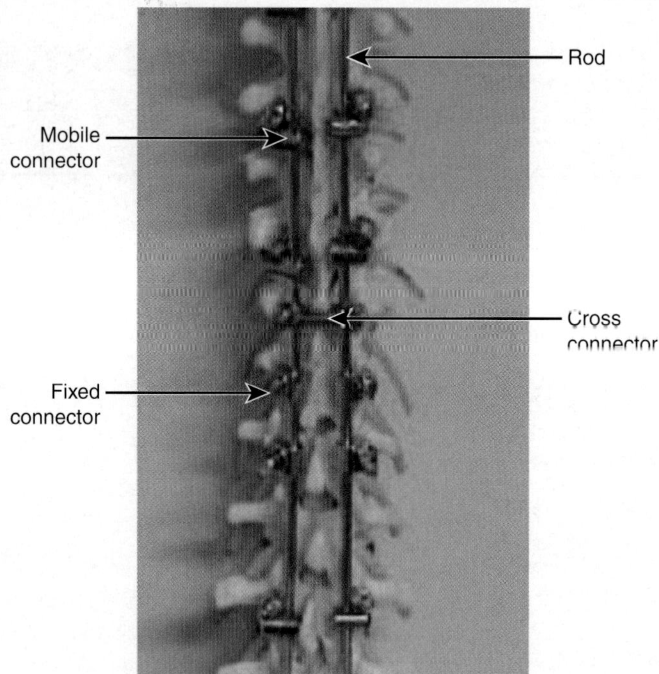


■ **FIGURE 91–1.** Orthobiom Spinal System.

2. Standard stainless steel (316LS-type): fixed and mobile connectors
3. UHMWPE (ultra-high-molecular-weight polyethylene): roller inside mobile connector.

The Orthobiom Spinal System can be described by its five main components: rod, pedicle screws, fixed connectors, mobile connectors, and cross connector.

## INDICATIONS

The indications for the Orthobiom are stated as follows: "The Orthobiom Spinal System is a posterior pedicle screw system indicated to treat pediatric scoliosis by (1) correction, (2) stabilization, (3) adjustment and (4) fixation of the scoliotic spine. Also, the Orthobiom Spinal System should be used with bone graft around the fixed connectors only."*

## CONTRAINDICATIONS

The following are the specific exclusion criteria for the Orthobiom:

1. Patient had a previous spinal surgery with fusion.
2. Patient's Risser sign is greater than 3 or there is a nonflexible curve.
3. Patient has a neuromuscular disorder.
4. Patient has a pathologic spinal malformation, such as spondylolisthesis.
5. Patient has a previous history of systemic infection or infection at the site of surgery.
6. Patient has previous history of osteopenia, osteoporosis, or osteomalacia to a degree that spinal instrumentation would be contraindicated.
7. Patient has a previous history of disease of bone metabolism.
8. Patient has a previous history of allergy to any component of the Orthobiom Spinal System.
9. Patient has a previous history of severe allergy or anaphylaxis.
10. Patient has a previous history of malignancy.
11. Patient is pregnant.

*Paradigm Spine, LLC.

## SCIENTIFIC TESTING

Because Orthobiom is a dynamic system, normal load-controlled corpectomy testing as described in ASTM F1717 could not be performed. Each screw allows for some degree of rotation and movement and some of the interconnections are not fixed; therefore, the test blocks touch under any amount of load. Since acquisition of Orthobiom by Paradigm Spine, LLC (New York, NY), new test setups and data were generated. Paradigm is committed to characterizing each potential failure mode and each loading scenario; therefore, multiple static and dynamic tests have been designed. Testing is under way, with some of the tests completed while others are still in the preparation stage. Testing that has been completed is described here, but ongoing tests and those in the design phase will not be reported.

There are two primary types of components of the Orthobiom Spinal System: the fixed segments and the mobile segments. In order to adequately correct and maintain the scoliotic spine, high bending strength is required initially for the construct to sustain flexion/extension forces caused by daily activities, and medial/lateral forces induced by the realignment of the scoliotic spinal segment. Under this scenario, the construct will mainly apply (or resist) three-point bending forces to (or from) the spine. This variation in the load-sharing/load-bearing requirements imposed to the new construct implies that minimum axial and torsional forces are withstood by the longitudinal elements. There is a potential for wear because some of the components of the Orthobiom articulate or telescope. Therefore, wear resistance is a requisite at the various sliding interfaces of the mobile connectors as well as in the links between those connectors and the pedicle screws.

### Component Testing

#### Static Torsion Bending (Screw and Rod)

Static torsion bending testing was performed on the screw/rod interconnection in accordance with ASTM F1798. The static test was performed due to quasi-static correction moment. The purpose of this test was to evaluate the rod/clamp interface under a torsional load. The rod was stabilized while the distal end of the screw was loaded, which placed a torsional load on the interconnection of the fixed connector. The average load on the screw was 5.7 Nm of torque.

#### Static Torsion Bending (Cross Connector and Rod)

Static torsion binding testing was performed on the screw/rod interconnection to evaluate torsion moments on the clamp. This test was performed in accordance with ASTM F1798. Only static testing was performed owing to the quasi-static correction moment. A load was placed on the opposite side of the cross connector, which placed a torsional load on the rod interconnection of the cross connector. The mean load measured on the connector/rod interconnection was 6 Nm of torque.

### Axial Loading of Fixed Connector

The static strength of this interconnection in the longitudinal direction was measured because the fixed connector needs to secure the rod in position against frictional forces and gravity to provide stability for fusion. An axial load was placed on the fixed connector while the rod was fixed. This test is currently ongoing.

### Mobile Connector Against Rod

One potential cause for wear generation is between the rod and the mobile connector. As the patient moves, flexes, extends, and bends side to side, the mobile connectors will slide on the rods. Therefore, in order to mimic the worst-case loading scenario that the Orthobiom Spinal System and mobile connector would experience, a lateral load (72 N) was placed on the rod and connector. The mobile connector was then articulated up and down on the rod 5 mm (±2.5 mm) with the simultaneous lateral load. This loading scenario was performed out to 10 million cycles, and all wear debris was collected and analyzed.

The results of the mobile connector wear testing demonstrated very little wear of the mobile connector (UHMWPE roller). After 10 million cycles, only 0.001 mg of wear was seen per 1 million cycles. This correlates to only 10 μg of wear.

### Cross Connector Wear

As the patient moves, micromotion on the cross connector parts will take place while quasi-static correction forces will be applied. Wear is assumed to occur between sleeve and bolt, and between sleeve/bolt and clamp/locking screw. The objectives of the test are to quantify the amount of metal-on-metal wear generated as a function of the motion cycles and to evaluate the bearing surfaces for changes. A characterization of the size distribution and shape of the particles generated will be performed.

The specimens are mounted on two rods and subjected to cyclic linear motion. During testing, a constant torsional preload of 3 Nm is applied to the rods. After the cross connector was attached to the rods, the rods were moved axially 2 mm (±1 mm). This distance was thought to represent a worst-case scenario because the cross connector is only to be applied between the fixed pedicle screws and, therefore, will see only minimal micromotion. The tests are carried out in newborn calf serum.

The testing will run out to 10 million cycles at a frequency below 5 Hz. Wear indicators such as weight loss, wear tracks, scratching, and burnishing were measured and analyzed. Visual surface characterization was performed at the end of the test. Frictional forces were monitored throughout the duration of the test and any changes reported. This testing is still ongoing.

## Construct Testing

### Static Axial Compression Bending

A modified ASTM F1717 test was used to measure the static and dynamic axial compression of the Orthobiom VI Spinal System because it includes mobile connectors which cannot transfer longitudinal forces. Once the screws reach their highest range of motion and the rods and screw/rod connection are being loaded, the gauge length of the test setup is representative of what is described in ASTM F1717, which is 76 mm. All other parameters are identical to that described in ASTM F1717. The smallest rod and screw were both used to represent worst-case setup. This test is still under development. Any differences from ASTM F1717 will be justified, and the loading scenario will have a physiologic justification.

### Dynamic Axial Compression Bending

The dynamic test was performed with the same parameters out to 5 million cycles. This test is expected to have at least two samples run-out at 100 N for 5 million cycles. This resulting load will be the same as several other pedicle screw systems out to 5 million cycles. This test was only run out to 5 million cycles because it is evaluating the effect of the fixed connectors on the rods. The fixed connectors hold the rod in place so fusion can occur, allowing a comparison to other systems on the strength of the Orthobiom at the fusion level. This load is much higher than the anticipated loads expected by a child. Therefore, the Orthobiom VI will withstand the physiologic loading by the patient.

### Static Corpectomy Lateral Bending

This test was developed to study the effects of lateral bending on the construct. The experimental setup used for the flexion/lateral bending tests of the implant assembly is based on the principles proposed by ASTM F1717 for testing spinal constructs in a corpectomy model. Three PE (polyethylene) blocks, instead of two, simulating the vertebrae are used for setting up a three-point bending test.

The implant is assembled using three UHMWPE blocks to simulate the vertebrae. The use of UHMWPE eliminates the effects of the variability of native bone properties. The supports of the PE blocks are positioned so that a horizontal distance of 76 mm between the screw axes is achieved.

The fixed and mobile connectors are attached to the polyaxial pins of the pedicle screws by self-breaking nuts, which are tightened until breakage of the nut occurs. Per implant assembly tested, four mobile connectors, two fixed connectors, and one cross-link are used. The two fixed connectors attached to the middle PE block prevent the rods from moving along the rod axis.

At a distance of 2 to 3 mm from the fixed connectors, one cross-link is attached to both rods. The position of the cross-link is adapted so that the distance of the rod axes (which is variable due to the polyaxial pins of the pedicle screws) is 18 mm. The outer PE blocks are rigidly attached to the test frame, but a linear bearing is used to enable the middle block to move in the horizontal direction.

All connectors, screws, and rods were the smallest in size, representing the worst-case scenario. The maximum load that was measured before any component failed was 1,000 N and the yield load was 800 N. The method of failure was yielding of the rods.

### Dynamic Corpectomy Lateral Bending

The same test set-up was used and tested out to 10 million cycles. During the dynamic testing a sinusoidal compression load is applied at a rate of 5 Hz. The test is carried out at room temperature (20°C) in ambient air. This test setup mimics the physiologic loading of the device when the patient bends side to side. With this test setup, the Orthobiom ran out to 10 million cycles with a load of 250 N. This is much higher than any expected lateral load on the spine by a child. The method of failure was screw and rod breakage. Another failure observed was the screw twisting out of UHMWPE block under loads above the fatigue strength. This result demonstrates how the device is able to correct and maintain the scoliotic spine.

### Static Corpectomy Flexion/Extension

A similar test setup was used as presented in the static and dynamic corpectomy lateral bending test. Instead of the lateral three-point bending load placed on the construct, an anterior load was placed on the construct. All connectors, screws, and rods were the smallest in size, representing the worst-case scenario. This mimics the patient bending forward. Testing the three-level corpectomy model in a flexion/extension scenario resulted in a maximum load of 1,200 N with a yield load of 900 N.

### Dynamic Corpectomy Flexion/Extension

Dynamic testing was performed using the same test setup. This test was performed to evaluate how the device behaves when a cyclic load was placed on it, mimicking a patient bending over. The test was run out to 10 million cycles. The results demonstrated that when a flexion/extension load is placed on the Orthobiom, it can run out to 10 million cycles at a load of 250 N. The method of failure was rod breakage.

### Static Torsion

A static torsion test was performed in close accordance with ASTM F1717. Owing to the technical characteristics of the Orthobiom Spinal System, the standard was modified slightly. A static load was applied to the construct and the failure load and yield load were measured. This test is still under development.

## FUNCTIONAL ANIMAL STUDY

### Minipigs

The Orthobiom IV was studied in a minipig model to evaluate the effect on the intervertebral joints by allowing intervertebral micromotion as compared to the effect of rigid fixation on the biologic changes in the intervertebral joints incorporated within the instrumented (nonmobile) segments. Twenty minipigs with scoliosis-induced spines were studied according to the following distribution:

Rigid fixation ($n$ = 6)
Mobile fixation with Orthobiom ($n$ = 11)
Control group, no surgery ($n$ = 3)

Minipigs in the rigid fixation group were evaluated at 12 and 18 months. Those in the Orthobiom group were evaluated at 6, 12, 18, and 24 months postoperatively. The Orthobiom group included 2 minipigs with implants removed at 12 months, then were followed for an additional 12 months. Evaluations included anteroposterior (AP) and lateral radiographs (Fig. 91–2), CT scans on select minipigs, and histologic examination. The results demonstrated that the mobile fixation permitted by the Orthobiom preserves the intervertebral joints while providing the stability and correction necessary for a scoliotic spine.

### Rabbit Particulate Study

A particulate injection study was performed in the lumbar spine of New Zealand rabbits to study the local and systemic effects of UHMWPE.[2] Macroscopic and histopathologic evaluations were conducted on the nerve structures and lymph nodes. The purpose of the study was to determine if UHMWPE is a suitable material for components of the Orthobiom Spinal System. Medical grade UHMWPE powder was commercially obtained in a mix of the following sizes: 90% 60- to 250-μm; 5% below 60 μm; and 5% above 250 μm (Ticona, NJ). This particle size distribution was selected because it is representative of the observed wear particles collected following wear testing of the rollers. Eighteen New Zealand white female rabbits weighing 2.5 to 3 kg were allocated into the following three groups:

UHMWPE with Orthobiom ($n$ = 12)
Control group, no treatment ($n$ = 3)
Sham procedure, without wear particle injection ($n$ = 3)

The quantity of the particles implanted per site ranged from 10 to 15 mg, which is equivalent to $5.5 \times 10^3 - 8 \times 10^3$ particles per site. Each of the 15 rabbits operated on survived the operation with no remarkable events or complications. Four test rabbits, one control rabbit, and one sham rabbit were used per evaluation period at 1 week, 4 weeks, and 12 weeks.

The biologic response of the test rabbit spinal cords (UHMWPE implantation) was evaluated macroscopically in comparison with the spinal cords of the control and sham rabbits. The spinal cord appearance of the control rabbits, at 12 weeks after observation, was identical to the spinal cord of the control rabbits at 1 and 4 weeks after observation as well as to the spinal cord appearance of the sham rabbits at 1, 4, and 12 weeks after surgery. No adverse reactions such as necrosis developed secondary to particle implantation.

Inflammation was observed in the UHMWPE group at 12 weeks but was limited to the connective tissue close to the dura mater and had subsided when compared to 1 week and 4 weeks after implantation. This is considered a normal, acute immunologic response to foreign material.

The reactions to UHMWPE particles in the spinal cord tissue from test rabbits were evaluated histologically in comparison with

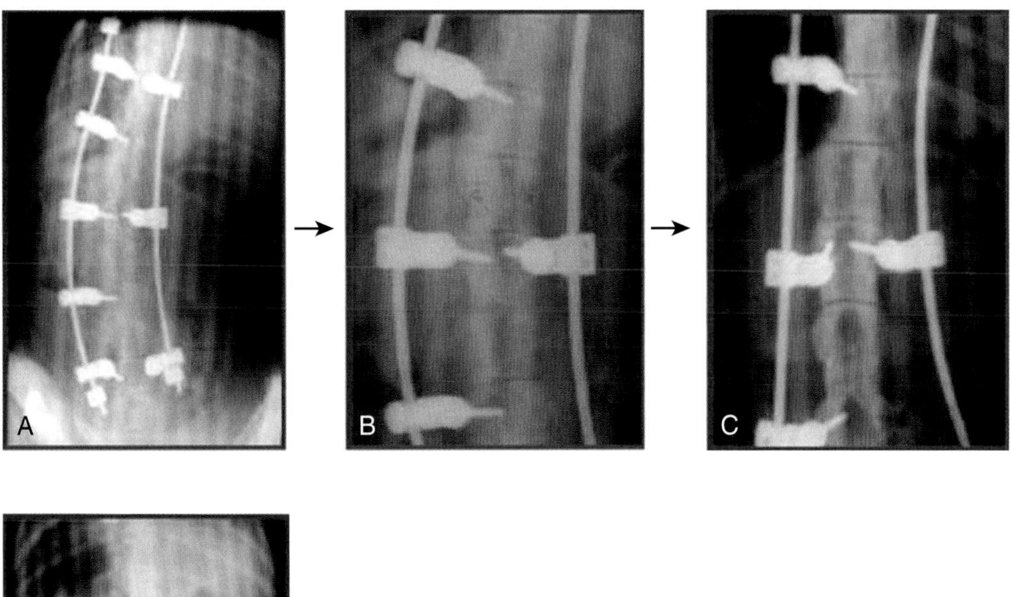

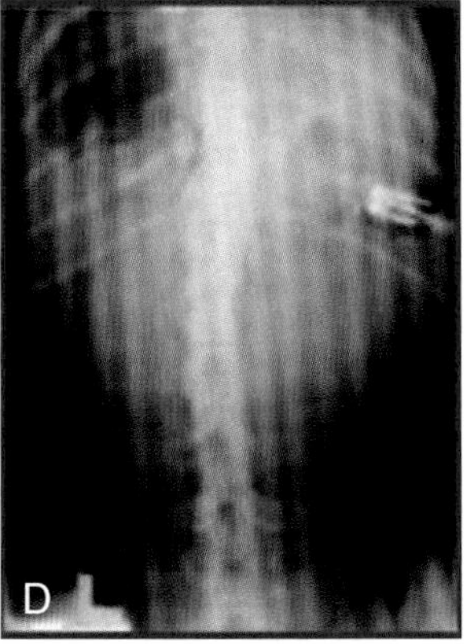

■ **FIGURE 91–2.** Posteroanterior radiographs of a minipig instrumented with a mobile fixation, Orthobiom Spinal System. **A,** Immediately after surgery; Cobb angle of 20 degrees. **B,** High magnification of A showing thoracolumbar region. Note the disc thickness. **C,** At 12 months follow-up: high magnification of the thoracolumbar region. Note the disc thickness that is similar to B; Cobb angle of 15 degrees. **D,** Immediately after implant retrieval, minipig survival, 12 months follow-up.

the spinal cords of the control and sham rabbits. UHMWPE particles were found in the histologic sections of the implantation sites. Polarized microscopy was used to show the particles present in all the test rabbits. The histology analysis showed normal spinal cord tissue with normal cells and dura mater and normal nerve roots.

At 4 weeks and 12 weeks after implantation, the mass of particles at the implantation sites were more adhered to the dura mater than at 1 week after implantation. The embedded mass of particles, with a vascularized lattice of connective tissue and without any appearance of necrosis or swelling, is therefore an evident sign of the material tolerance by the living tissue. The dura mater vascularization and the spinal cord appearance adjacent to the implantation sites appear identical to that of the control and sham rabbits.

These results demonstrate that UHMWPE is a suitable material for the Orthobiom System.

## OPERATIVE TECHNIQUE

### Positioning

The patient is lying supine with the hips and the knees extended. Both arms should be flexed on each side of the head.

### Incision

The skin and the soft cutaneous tissue will be opened, going down to the supraspinous ligament by a midline incision usually centered on the proximal and distal spinous process. Orthobiom Spinal System requires a different approach around the spinous process. Because fusion is not wanted, it is important to not go subperiosteal. It means that the surgeon must open the supraspinous ligament approximately 2 mm lateral from the tip of the spinous process; it is very easy to find a plane of soft tissue between the muscle and the insertion of the small muscle at the level of the spinous process. It is easy to develop a complete dissection plane to displace laterally the mass of the two muscles without touching the periosteum at the level of the spinous process. What is important is also not to touch the periosteum at the level of the laminae or the articular facet.

### Screw Insertion

This instrumentation will be used with pedicular screws in the lumbar and thoracic regions. The pedicular screw link incorporates a ball and socket that permits easy insertion of the rod and connector. In the lumbar region, screws of 5 or 6 mm can be used.

A hole is perforated with a 3.2-mm drill bit for the 5-mm screw and 4.5-mm for the 6-mm screw. The entry point of the pedicular screw should be at the intersection of the longitudinal transverse process midline and the interarticular facet line.

The superior articular facet of the inferior vertebrae must not be altered; it must be preserved to ensure some movement and normal articulation during adult life. After the point of entry has been chosen, we will aim at a 150-degree medial angle toward the corpus of the vertebrae. In the thoracic region, screws of 4.5 or 5 mm in diameter can be used. The entry point will be at the intersection of the vertical midline of the inferior articular process of the superior vertebra and a line tangent to the lower point of the same inferior articular process. When the hole has been made in the lumbar or thoracic region, its depth is measured after probing the pedicle on the medial side, the inferior side, the lateral side, and the upper side. This probing of the pedicle hole is very important to ensure that bone is present at the medial and inferior portion of the hole to prevent any damage to the dura mater and for the lateral and upper part of the pedicle to ensure a good grip on the bone. On the concave side of the deformation, it is recommended to use a segmental fixation at every level or at least at every possible level. On the convex side of the deformation, fewer pedicular screws are required and are normally 60% of the number placed on the concave side. As a first step, the pedicular screws are only partially inserted. Once this is complete, AP and lateral radiographs are taken to define the placement and the angle of the screws. If each screw angle is correct, the screws can be inserted to the normal position. If a screw does not have a proper position or angle, it must be corrected and then inserted to the normal position.

### Curve Correction

As with any other scoliosis instrumentation the rod is bent and cut to the proper length to correct the three-dimensional deformation. The mobile and fixed connectors are then slid onto the rod in the proper sequence. All connectors are positioned on the corresponding pedicular screw link. The derotation maneuver of the rod is performed to induce the translation of the spine and then the two fixed connectors are tightened to stabilize the rods and prevent derotation.

### Completion of Surgery

A wake-up test is performed along with evoked potentials. The achieved correction is evaluated through an x-ray examination (AP and lateral) and it can be determined if readjustment of the instrumentation is required. As with any other fusion instrumentation, the surgeon needs to close the muscle aponeurosis, the subcutaneous tissue, and the skin with different separated stitches, and therefore, closure is done in multiple layers. Normal dressing is then performed.

## POSTOPERATIVE CARE

The surgeon must inform the patient regarding the level of activity that he/she can do. This list of activities gives only a general progression of the allowed postoperative activities for the patient. As for any other surgeries, general postoperative instructions unrelated to the Orthobiom Spinal System should also be provided by the surgeon.

## COMPLICATIONS

The risks associated with the use of the Orthobiom Spinal System include those related to any surgery, those related to any instrumentation of the spine for scoliosis correction, and finally, the risks directly associated with the use of the Orthobiom Spinal System.

### Risks Associated with any Type of Surgery

There is a risk of death associated with any surgery. There are also risks any time a person receives a general anesthetic. These risks include reactions to the anesthetic, blood clots that may move through the blood vessels and damage major organs, pneumonia, abnormal heartbeats, or heart attack. Anesthesia is planned before the surgery and is controlled during the surgery by a qualified anesthetist. At the end of the surgery the wakening of the patient progresses under a close supervision from the hospital staff members who follow a protocol specific to each medical center. The second major risk is related to the blood transfusion, which is controlled by autologous blood donation before surgery. The third major risk is associated with infection that is minimized using prophylactic antibiotic therapy during and following the surgery. The patient may also develop a hematoma, a wound that will not heal properly, bleeding, or a vessel tear at a surgical opening. The close postoperative follow-up during the hospitalization period helps to detect and react properly to these events.

### Risks Associated with any Instrumentation of the Spine

The major risk associated with any instrumentation of the spine is temporary or permanent neurologic deficits for the patient. This is controlled by recording the sensory and motor evoked potentials during the surgery and by doing a wake-up test at the end of the instrumentation procedure. There are also risks related to material breakage, malfunction, or vertebral fracture that could result in a loss of scoliosis curvature correction or injuries to adjacent tissues. The nonfusion of vertebral segments also limits the efficacy of the conventional implants. However, nonfusion does not represent a failure for the Orthobiom Spinal System, because this characteristic is anticipated. In all cases, these possibilities are closely followed by periodic clinical and radiologic examinations. If such an event occurs, a revision of the system may be planned. Additional complications may occur as a result of having a foreign object implanted. This could cause infection and allergic reactions.

### Risks Associated with the Orthobiom Spinal System

The risks associated with the Orthobiom Spinal System include those already described. Two different features specific to the implant itself could also be sources of risks. First, because some parts of the Orthobiom Spinal System are made of polyethylene, a material that has not been previously used for a spinal corrective implant, biocompatibility could be a concern. However, this material has been used extensively for many other types of orthopaedic implants[3–5] for many years and the results of the cytotoxicity tests done by the sponsor before this study showed no negative effects on tissues surrounding the spine. Second, some components of the Orthobiom Spinal System are free to move to a certain extent. This feature adds some degree of risk, because the implant could be exposed to greater stresses, which could cause breakage of certain parts. However, results from exhaustive finite element analysis and mechanical tests support the strength of the implant over a long period of time because only micromotion is anticipated.

The mobility of the implant could also affect the spinal system in different ways. It could reduce its ability to maintain the spinal correction or it could increase the loading on the pedicles and induce changes on their bony structure. The close follow-up of the patients recruited for this study allows the clinician to quickly detect the problem. The fusion solution could then be applied and represents a second surgery comparable to a system revision for a conventional implant. On the other hand, fusion could occur, even if not induced during the surgery. This event should not change the result of the spinal correction, but the patient will experience the loss of some potential benefits associated with the use of the Orthobiom Spinal System. Risk is then associated with the uncertainty of the Orthobiom Spinal System effectiveness. The mobility of its components has been designed to take into account the mobility of the spine and to overcome the problems associated with the nonfusion of the spine. There still is a possibility that this available mobility limits the quality of the correction or its progression in time. Based on the same principles, it is unclear whether at maturity, when the Orthobiom Spinal System is removed, the complete spinal correction will persist. However, the neuromuscular system should have adapted and a new equilibrium should have developed. Furthermore, the growth of the patient has ended. If scoliosis curves progress at maturity, a conventional instrumentation with fusion could be carried out. The risks associated with the use of the Orthobiom Spinal System will be minimized by giving intensive training to the investigator/surgeon responsible for performing the surgery with the instrumentation. This consists of theoretical training sessions and instrumentation on animal or cadaver models. In any case, the consequences of the described adverse events will be controlled by a close follow-up of the patients with clinical and radiologic evaluations and appropriate recording of the patient's condition.

## DISCUSSION

Arthrodesis is an effective means of eliminating disease and providing a permanent structural stability for disease processes that involve mobile joints in both the extremities and the axial skeleton. However, being essentially irreversible and at best nonphysiologic, it is also accused of many undesirable long-term side effects.

During the last couple of decades, there has been a definite trend in the field of orthopaedic surgery toward preservation of the mobile joint for a more physiologic functional restoration. Controlling the spine without an arthrodesis is not new. It has a much longer history than spinal arthrodesis techniques. External spinal immobilization by plaster of Paris cast and braces before the instrumentation era and spinal instrumentation without fusion,[6] rod-long-fuse-short method for the treatment of unstable fractures,[7] and use of subcutaneous rods and growing rods for pediatric deformities all fall into this category.[8]

Despite the definite theoretical advantages they offer, such as permitting spinal growth before definite fusion, reduction of the fusion level, or eliminating the need of arthrodesis altogether, these procedures are not very popular except for external immobilization. This is due to their limited indications, uncertainty of the result, and the high rate of mechanical and biologic failure.[9,10] Because instrumentation without fusion procedures rely heavily on the spontaneous acquisition of spinal stability either by healing of the destabilizing lesion or anatomic alteration by growth, the spinal implant will have to withstand stress much longer than those used with fusion, making them more vulnerable to mechanical failures.

Spontaneous fusion is the most common and important reason for biologic failure that compromises the result of the instrumentation without fusion, as the goal of the surgery is preservation of the motion segments. It also greatly compromises the ability of the vertebral column to reacquire intrinsic stability by limiting the growth-determined alteration of the vertebral shape and also by alteration of the force acting on the unfused segments.

Degenerative changes in the intervertebral disc, facet joint articular cartilage, and intervertebral joint ankylosis are biologic failures that affect the long-term result mainly after the removal of the instrument and cause pain, stiffness, or hypermobility and precocious degenerative changes. They occur mainly in the instrumented area but also may occur in the motion segments neighboring the instrumentation due to the stress concentration caused by abrupt change in mobility.

Disturbance in the intervertebral disc and facet joint articular cartilage nutrient transport mechanism by rigid fixation seriously compromises the biologic function of the cartilage/disc cells and results in degenerative changes, which may lead to total disappearance of the articular cartilage and bony fusion of the joint in extreme instances. Our experimental results show that the viability of the joint cartilage and the intervertebral disc may be maintained, not only by allowing a normal full range of motion but also by micromotion of the intervertebral joint just sufficient for loading/unloading of the avascular connective tissues. In the rigid fixation group (Fig. 91–3), one animal was sacrificed at 12 months and five animals at 18 months after surgery. Despite significant growth of the animals from 32±5.14 kg to 62.7±14.8 kg, the length of the instrumented segment measured by the distance between the uppermost and the lowermost screws remained unchanged. Initial scoliosis of 31±5 degrees created by rod rotation was maintained at 27±8 degrees at the time of euthanasia with no significant change in the curve magnitude ($P = 0.37$, paired t-test), therefore showing an acceptable maintenance of fixation (Table 91–1).

In the mobile fixation (Fig. 91–4), one animal was sacrificed at 6 months, three animals at 12 months, three at 18 months, and two at 24 months. In the observation period, the animals demonstrated significant growth from 29.9 to 67.2 kg. The length of the instrumented segment changed from 25.3±2.0 cm to 30.0±1.5 cm showing a growth of 4.7±1.4 cm ($P = 0.0004$, paired t-test). Despite three minor fixation failures detected on the final

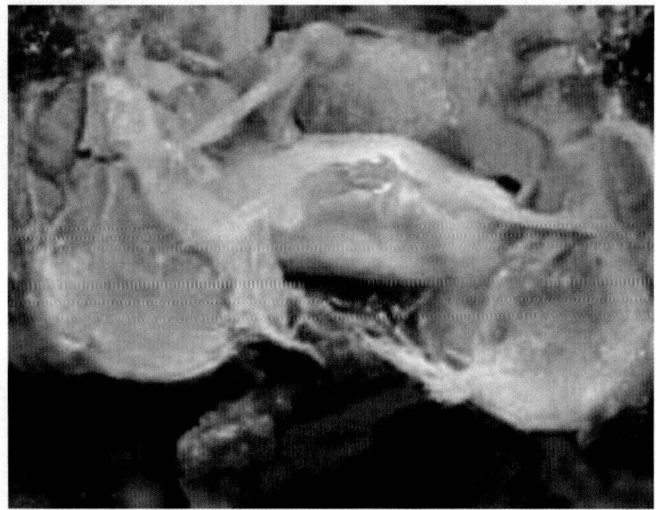

■ **FIGURE 91–3.** Minipig at 12 months follow-up with a rigid fixation (Colorado). A disc from the instrumented segment shows loss of the nucleus pulposus and degenerative changes in the annulus fibrosus and the end plate cartilage.

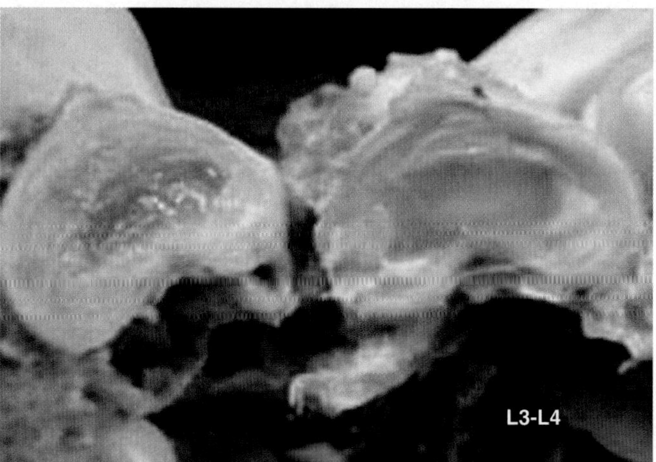


■ **FIGURE 91–4.** Minipig instrumented with a mobile fixation Orthobiom System, disc L3-L4. Nucleus pulposus and annulus fibrosus are well preserved.

x-ray examinations before euthanasia (two pigs with one broken screw, one pig with two broken screws), the experimental scoliotic curve of 19 ± 4 degrees was maintained at 17± 5 degrees, showing a reasonable maintenance of fixation with no statistically significant alteration of the curve magnitude ($P$ =0.21, paired t-test) (Table 91–2).

In fact, with the immunohistochemistry, we realized that the presence of collagen X in the rigid fixation group was far more predominant than in the mobile fixation group (Orthobiom). However, the comparison of the samples between the mobile fixation (Orthobiom) group and the rigid fixation (Colorado and TSRH) group revealed that the presence of collagen X was statistically far more significant in the intervertebral discs of the rigid fixation (Colorado and TSRH). For the rigid fixation, the collagen X represents 92.84% of the field and the background up to 6.42% of the field with the remainder of the total percentage belonging to other types of collagen. For the mobile fixation (Orthobiom) samples, the normal collagen represented 62.96% of the field and for the mean the collagen X represented 7.84% of the background 14.81%; the remainder of the total percentage belongs to other types of collagen. The ANOVA (analysis of variance) statistical analysis for the comparison between the Orthobiom and Colorado system had a $P$ value of 0.00094.

Failure to grow and heal as desired forms the third category of biologic failures and would eventually necessitate a definite restoration of spinal stability by fusion. This may be due to spontaneous fusion, degeneration of the intervertebral and the articular cartilage, and inappropriate mechanical forces hindering the growth in the desired direction.[9] Though it is difficult to conclude at this moment, this may be controlled by appropriate combination of rigid and mobile fixations in the same construct.

This experiment of comparing the biologic response of the unfused intervertebral joint to the rigidity of spinal fixation was part of our attempt to develop an instrumentation system to be used in nonfusion treatment of pediatric spinal deformities. In younger patients with large deformities, unlike in adults and patients near the end of growth, the bone growth has to be considered in the treatment of the spinal deformities. The remaining growth in the spinal column and the extremities in young children act both as a negative and a positive factor in the treatment of spinal deformities. It is negative in the sense that a lengthy fusion of the spine would result in trunk shortening compared to the extremities, and that fear of such shortening often leads to an inappropriately short fusion, resulting in failure of the deformity control. The positive aspect is that the growth, with an appropriate force application system, may be exploited to restore the intrinsic mechanical stability of the vertebral column, reversing the destabilizing anatomic alteration in the vertebral body. Our goal was to

**TABLE 91–1. Results of Group 1: Rigid Fixation**

| Measurements | Immediate Postoperative | 18 Months | $P$* |
|---|---|---|---|
| Scoliosis (degrees) | 31 ± 5 | 27 ± 8 | 0.37 |
| Instrumented section (mm)† | 276 ± 25 | 283 ± 29 | 0.10 |
| Minipig growth (kg) | 32 ± 5.14 | 62.7 ± 14.8 | — |

*Paired t-test.
†Corrected for magnification, using the length of the longitudinal members.

**TABLE 91–2. Results of Group 2: Mobile Fixation**

| Measurement | Immediate Postoperative | 18 Months | $P$* |
|---|---|---|---|
| Scoliosis (degrees) | 19 ± 4 | 17±5 | 0.21 |
| Instrumented section (mm)† | 253 ± 20 | 300±15 | 0.0004 |
| Minipig growth (kg) | 29.9 | 67.2 | — |

*Paired t-test.
†Corrected for magnification, using the length of the longitudinal members.

avoid the negative effects of lengthy fusion while taking advantage of the positive effects of the remaining growth to restore stability. For an adequate function, the instrumentation system needed to offer a reliable fixation of the vertebral column to exert the desired mechanical force and at same time allow some motion in the incorporated intervertebral joints to maintain the viability and translation on the rods for longitudinal growth.

This experiment was performed to determine the balance point in the rigidity/flexibility of the implant that permits both the control of the vertebral column and the maintenance of the joint viability, and to test the hypothesis that micromotion of the joint is sufficient to maintain the viability of the intervertebral disc and the articular cartilage. The concept of the micromotion of the joint was particularly important because mechanical fixation failures are the most common mode of failure of the instrumentation without fusion. This could only be overcome by narrowing the difference in the flexibility between the vertebral column and the implant. The difference may be reduced either by making the spinal column stiffer by increasing the fixation rigidity or by reducing the stiffness of the spinal implant construct through modification of the components. However, because the prime goal of the instrumentation surgery is maintenance of the corrective force on the spine, the balance had to be on the side of making the spine significantly stiffer than the uninstrumented spine, leaving little other alternative than controlled micromotion.

The implant-bone interface forms the grip on the vertebral body and determines the strength of the vertebral stabilization effected through the instrumentation. Failure here, though heavily influenced by the overall stiffness of the implant construct, may be also influenced by the biomechanical characteristics of the anchoring member, namely the pedicle screws.

The characteristic of the longitudinal member determines the overall gross stiffness of the implant construct, but not necessarily the intersegmental motion, as the lever arm of the intersegmental motion is very small compared to the length of the entire implant. A failure here is mainly due to the difference in stiffness of the implant and the vertebral column. A smaller diameter (5-mm) rod was initially created using a titanium alloy to permit 15% elastic deformation of the rods under physiologic loads to reduce the stiffness of the implant. The rods are now made of polished stainless steel, which provides minimal wear debris at the rod-polyethylene roller junction.

The connecting mechanism that forms the implant construct determines the stability between the implant members and is the main site determining the intersegmental and the translational motion. Two types of connecting mechanisms were designed, one called the fixed connector, which locks the interface and offers control of the rods (e.g., prevent slippage and rotation), and the mobile connectors which allow 6 degrees of freedom to allow unconstrained linking between the anchoring and the longitudinal member. By combining two types of connection mechanisms on the same rod, the desired mechanical forces could be exerted on the motion segments incorporated within the instrumented segments.

## CONCLUSION

Pediatric scoliosis can severely affect a large population of children if not treated properly and immediately. The best-case scenario is to treat and arrest the progression of the curve with bracing. However, if progression of the curve continues, other options should be considered, such as the Orthobiom Spinal System.

## REFERENCES

1. Rogala EJ, Drummond DS, Gurr J: Scoliosis: Incidence and natural history: A prospective epidemiological study. J Bone Joint Surg Am 60(2):173–176, 1978.
2. Rivard CH, Rhalmi S, Coillard C: In vivo biocompatibility testing of peek polymer for a spinal implant system: A study in rabbits. J Biomed Materials Res 62(4):488–498, 2002.
3. McGloughlin TM, Kavanagh AG: Wear of ultra-high molecular weight polyethylene (UHMWPE) in total knee prostheses: A review of key influences. Proc Inst Mech Eng [H] 214(4):349–359, 2000.
4. Edidin AA, Kurtz SM: Influence of mechanical behavior on the wear of 4 clinically relevant polymeric biomaterials in a hip simulator. J Arthroplasty 15(3):321–331, 2000.
5. Bavaresco VP, de Carvalho Zavaglia CA, de Carvalho Reis M, Malmonge SM: Devices for use as an artificial articular surface in joint prostheses or in the repair of osteochondral defects. Artif Organs 24(3):202–205, 2000.
6. Soucacos PN, Zacharis K, Gelalis J, et al: Assessment of curve progression in idiopathic scoliosis. Eur Spine J 7(4):270–277, 1998.
7. Kane WJ: Scoliosis prevalence: A call for a statement of terms. Clin Orthop 126:43–46, 1977.
8. Lonstein JE, Carlson JM: The prediction of curve progression in untreated idiopathic scoliosis during growth. J Bone Joint Surg Am 66(7):1061–1071, 1984.
9. Cobb JR: Outline for the study of scoliosis. Instructional Course Lectures, American Academy of Orthopaedic Surgeons, Vol 5. Ann Arbor, MI, JW Edwards, 1948.
10. Labelle H, Dansereau J: Orthotic treatment of pediatric spinal disorders and diseases. *In* Spine: State of the Art Reviews, Vol 4, No 1. Philadelphia, Hanley & Belfus, 1990.

CHAPTER 92

# Considerations for Spinal Arthroplasty in Elderly and Osteoporotic Patients

**James J. Yue**

**KEY POINTS**

- Comprehensive history and physical examination are mandatory prior to considering motion-sparing technology in elderly patients and in those with osteoporotic bone.
- Lumbar total disc replacement results in an overall lordosis of the lumbar spine. Therefore, circumferential spinal stenosis should be considered a relative contraindication to lumbar disc replacement.
- Dynamic posterior stabilization procedures require careful analysis of coronal and sagittal instability prior to implementation.
- The adjunctive use of bone augmentation such as PMMA (polymethyl/methacrylate) or Cortoss may permit limited use of motion-sparing technologies in the osteoporotic patient.

The use of motion-sparing technologies such as total disc arthroplasty, nucleus replacement, and posterior dynamic stabilization has been shown to be safe and effective in patients who are 18 to 60 years old.[1–4] Except for interspinous spacers, the use of nonfusion technologies has not been evaluated to any great degree in the elderly.[5–8] A number of considerations such as, but not limited to, the presence, degree, and location of spinal stenosis, degenerative facet disease, bone density, and vascular status should be carefully evaluated in all patients, especially those older than 60, before proceeding with a nonfusion surgical technique. Because of the increase in potential medical complications, this patient population requires careful general medical evaluation prior to undergoing any surgical procedure.

## CONSIDERATIONS FOR DISC ARTHROPLASTY

Although most patients over 60 years old are not ideal candidates for total disc replacement (TDR), TDR can be performed successfully in a select subset of carefully chosen patients in this age group.[9] As with all patients being considered for TDR, a detailed history and physical examination are required. Patients with a history of neurogenic claudication secondary to circumferential stenosis as demonstrated on magnetic resonance imaging (MRI) are not ideal candidates for lumbar TDR (Fig. 92–1). The overall effect of a lumbar TDR is to place the spine in a lordotic position. If there is subarticular/foraminal or central canal stenosis, compression of the neural elements may occur and lead to neurologic deficit (Fig. 92–2).[10,11] Physical examination should assesss for the presence of abdominal pulsatile masses indicative of an abdominal aortic aneurysm. Pulses should be evaluated for vascular insufficiency. Unilateral low back pain on extension and lateral bending should prompt an evaluation of facet integrity as well as sacroiliac (SI) joint disease. "Hip" pain should prompt careful assessment of intra-articular femoral-acetabular disease.

Radiographically, all patients should undergo plain x-rays, MRI, computed tomography (CT), and bone density evaluation. Standing radiographs should be assessed for scoliotic deformity, dynamic degenerative spondylolisthesis, aortic calcification, and osteopenia. MRI evaluation should include careful evaluation for other "red flag" findings such as infection and tumor. In addition, significant facet disease, facet cysts, and osteoporotic compression fractures should be assessed. One of the most significant contraindications, as already mentioned, is circumferential spinal stenosis. The degree and location of foraminal stenosis should be evaluated carefully. CT scans should be obtained to assess for facet degeneration, pars defects, and SI joint disease. Lastly, but equally as important, a DEXA (dual-emission x-ray absorptiometry) scan should be obtained in all patients. A T-score less than −1.0 should be considered a contraindication in this patient population.

## POSTERIOR DYNAMIC LUMBAR STABILIZATION

The indications for posterior dynamic stabilization of the lumbar spine are evolving and are currently undergoing formal randomized testing.[12–16] The majority of these devices are pedicle screw based and, therefore, depend on adequate bone quality to assure appropriate bone fixation. Few of these devices, other than the total posterior arthroplasty systems such as the Total Facet Arthroplasty System (TFAS) (Archus Orthopedics, Redmond, WA) or the TOPS device (Impliant Spine, Princeton, NJ), are able to adequately control for sagittal or coronal instability.[17,18] Therefore,

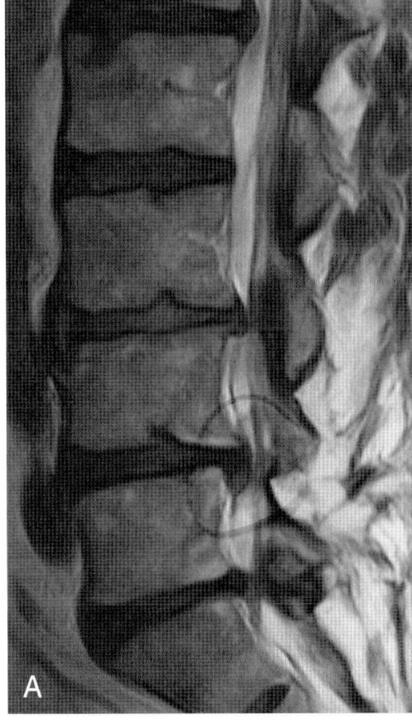


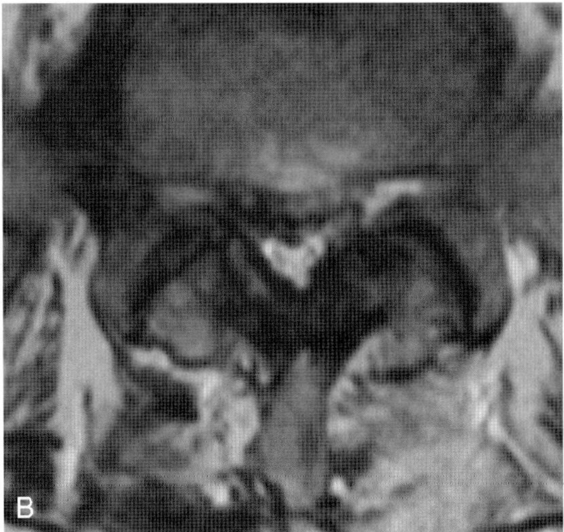


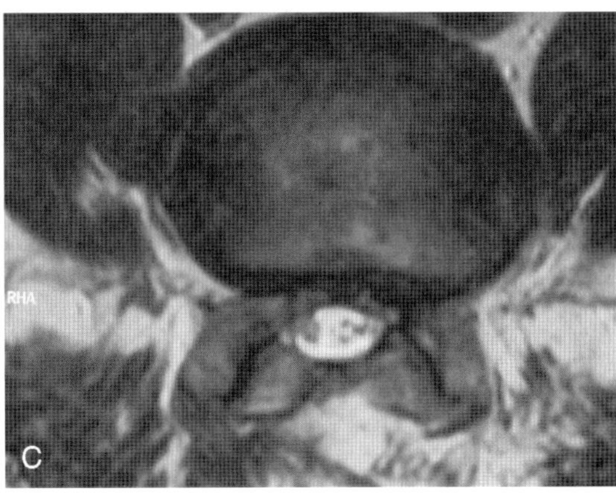


■ **FIGURE 92–1.** Circumferential lumbar spinal stenosis.

careful assessment for excessive spinal motion (e.g., greater than Grade 1 dynamic spondylolisthesis) in either the coronal or sagittal plane should be made. Patients with excessive spinal motion should be considered for fusion.

Of all of the motion-sparing devices available to date, the interspinous spacer devices have been examined most critically in the elderly population.[5–8] Advantages include limited spinal exposure, minimal blood loss, and the potential for the use of local anesthesia. The device is highly dependent on the structural integrity of the two immediately adjacent spinous processes. Patients with severe spinal stenosis and concomitant cauda equine syndrome should not be considered for this type of intervention. These patients should undergo formal decompression with or without fusion. Patients with poor bone quality defined as T-scores less than −2.5 should also be considered for alternative therapies.

## CONSIDERATIONS FOR THE OSTEOPOROTIC PATIENT

Subsidence has been reported to occur in 9% of patients when T-scores are less than −1.5[9] (Fig. 92–3). Vertebral bony augmentation using adjunctive bone fillers such as PMMA or Cortoss (Orthovita, Malvern, PA) is currently being evaluated under controlled studies. Cortoss is a bioactive glass ceramic polymer composite that has a high radiodensity, low exothermic reaction, and low viscosity[19] (Fig. 92–4). The polymer induces a local alkaline environment that induces the deposition of calcium phosphate and bone deposition. Yue and associates have presented non-randomized data evaluating the use of Cortoss to augment vertebral body strength in osteoporotic patients undergoing lumbar total disc replacement surgery.[20] They evaluated 33 patients with an average T-score of −2.5 (range −1.5 to −4.4). Thirty-three

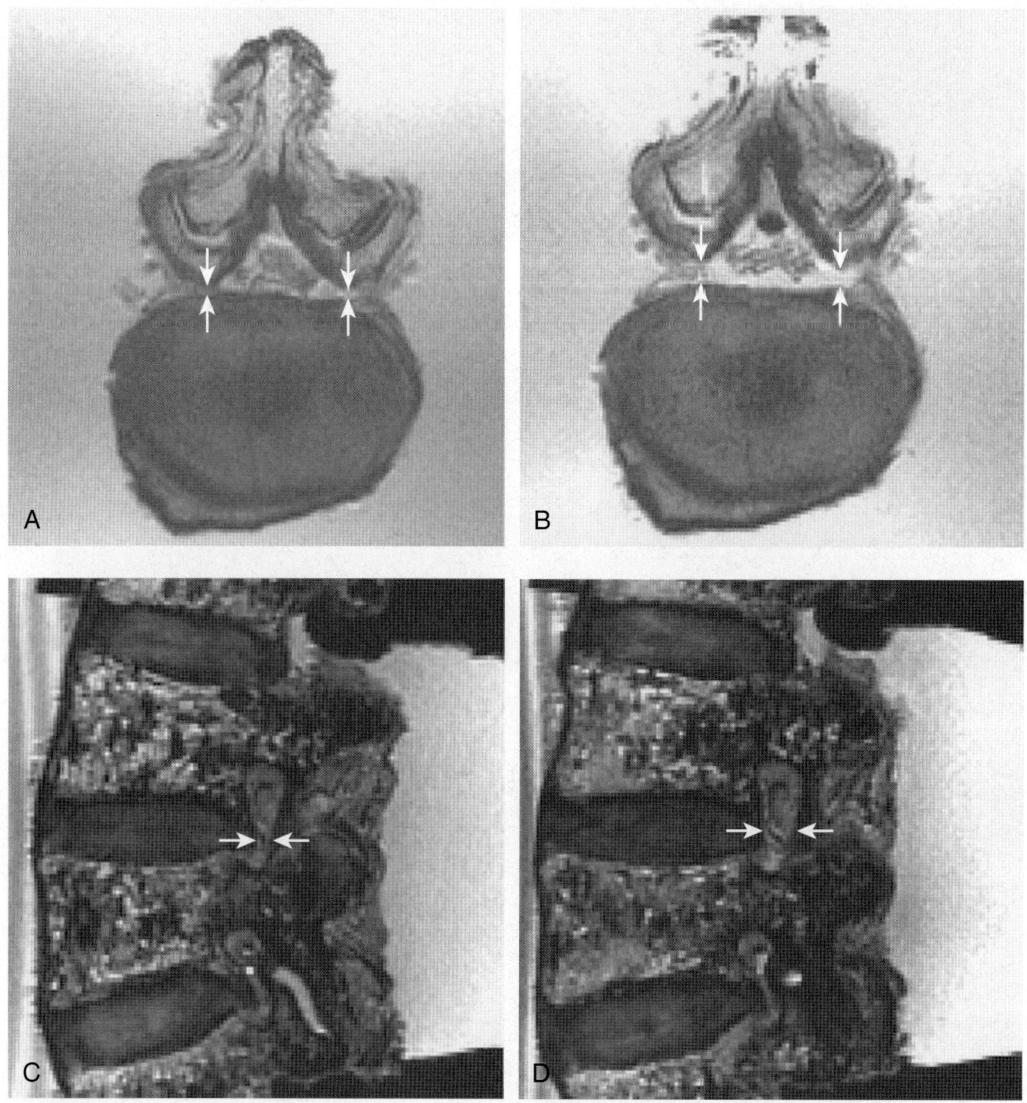


■ **FIGURE 92–2.** Decrease in central and foraminal area with lordosis of spine **(A** and **C).** Increase in central and foraminal area with flexion of spine **(B** and **D).** *(From Richards JC, Majumdar S, Lindsey DP, et al: The treatment mechanism of an interspinous process implant for lumbar neurogenic intermittent claudication. Spine 30:744–749, 2005; Siddiqui M, Karadimas E, Nicol M, et al: Influence of X STOP on neural foramina and spinal canal area in spinal stenosis. Spine 31:2958–2962, 2006.)*

percent were smokers. Subsidence rates decreased from 9% to 0% after the use of Cortoss placed anteriorly after implantation of the TDR device. No adverse events occurred in these patients over an average follow-up period of 35 months.

## SUMMARY

Careful clinical evaluation including a comprehensive history and physical examination and radiographic analysis is essential prior to considering the elderly or osteoporotic patient. Spinal stenosis and neurogenic claudication should be considered relative contraindications to lumbar TDR surgery. Patients with risk factors for osteoporosis should be carefully screened to ensure adequate bone strength. The use of adjunctive bone fillers such as PMMA and Cortoss may increase the relative bone strength and permit the limited use of motion-sparing technologies in this patient population. Further studies are warranted prior to utilizing these adjunctive technologies in all osteoporotic patients.

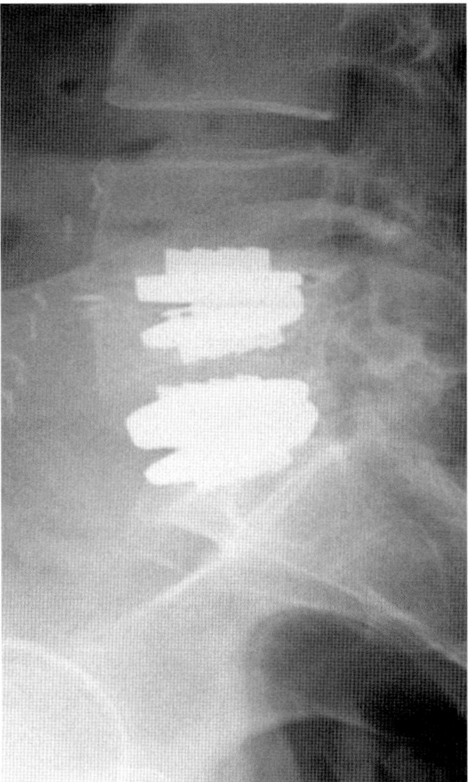

■ **FIGURE 92–3.** Example of subsidence.

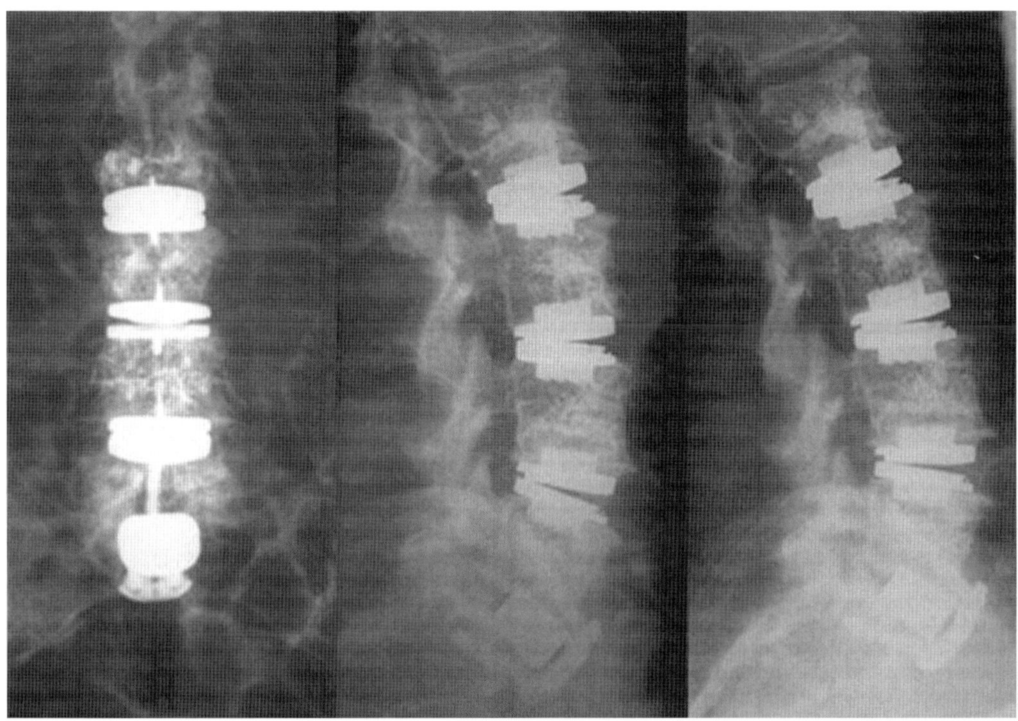

■ **FIGURE 92–4.** Use of Cortoss in multilevel total disc replacement surgery. *(Photograph courtesy of R. Bertagnoli.)*

## REFERENCES


1. Bertagnoli R, Yue JJ, Fenk-Mayer A, et al: Treatment of symptomatic adjacent-segment degeneration after lumbar fusion with total disc arthroplasty by using the Prodisc prosthesis: A prospective study with 2-year minimum follow-up. J Neurosurg Spine 4:91–97, 2006.
2. Bertagnoli R, Yue JJ, Kershaw T, et al: Lumbar total disc arthroplasty utilizing the ProDisc prosthesis in smokers versus nonsmokers: A prospective study with 2-year minimum follow-up. Spine 31:992–997, 2006.
3. Bertagnoli R, Yue JJ, Shah RV, et al: The treatment of disabling single-level lumbar discogenic low back pain with total disc arthroplasty utilizing the Prodisc prosthesis: A prospective study with 2-year minimum follow-up. Spine 30:2230–2236, 2005.
4. Bertagnoli R, Yue JJ, Shah RV, et al: The treatment of disabling multilevel lumbar discogenic low back pain with total disc arthroplasty utilizing the ProDisc prosthesis: A prospective study with 2-year minimum follow-up. Spine 30:2192–2199, 2005.
5. Anderson PA, Tribus CB, Kitchel SH: Treatment of neurogenic claudication by interspinous decompression: Application of the X STOP device in patients with lumbar degenerative spondylolisthesis. J Neurosurg Spine 4:463–471, 2006.
6. Chiu JC: Interspinous process decompression (IPD) system (X-STOP) for the treatment of lumbar spinal stenosis. Surg Technol Int 15:265–275, 2006.
7. Hsu KY, Zucherman JF, Hartjen CA, et al: Quality of life of lumbar stenosis-treated patients in whom the X STOP interspinous device was implanted. J Neurosurg Spine 5:500–507, 2006.
8. Kondrashov DG, Hannibal M, Hsu KY, et al: Interspinous process decompression with the X-STOP device for lumbar spinal stenosis: A 4-year follow-up study. J Spinal Disord Tech 19:323–327, 2006.
9. Bertagnoli R, Yue JJ, Nanieva R, et al: Lumbar total disc arthroplasty in patients older than 60 years of age: A prospective study of the ProDisc prosthesis with 2-year minimum follow-up period. J Neurosurg Spine 4:85–90, 2006.
10. Richards JC, Majumdar S, Lindsey DP, et al: The treatment mechanism of an interspinous process implant for lumbar neurogenic intermittent claudication. Spine 30:744–749, 2005.
11. Siddiqui M, Karadimas E, Nicol M, et al: Influence of X Stop on neural foramina and spinal canal area in spinal stenosis. Spine 31:2958–2962, 2006.
12. Beastall J, Karadimas E, Siddiqui M, et al: The Dynesys lumbar spinal stabilization system: A preliminary report on positional magnetic resonance imaging findings. Spine 32:685–690, 2007.
13. Cakir B, Richter M, Huch K, et al: Dynamic stabilization of the lumbar spine. Orthopade [illegible]
14. Nockels RP: Dynamic stabilization in the surgical management of painful lumbar spinal disorders. Spine 30:S68–S72, 2005.
15. Schwarzenbach O, Berlemann U, Stoll TM, et al: Posterior dynamic stabilization systems: DYNESYS. Orthop Clin North Am 36:363–372, 2005.
16. Yue JJ, Timm JP, Panjabi M, et al: Clinical application of the Panjabi Neutral Zone Hypothesis: The Stabilimax NZTM Posterior Lumbar Dynamic Stabilization System. Neurosurg Focus 22:E12, 2007.
17. Wilke HJ, Schmidt H, Werner K, et al: Biomechanical evaluation of a new total posterior-element replacement system. Spine 31:2790–2796; discussion 2797, 2006.
18. Zhu Q, Larson CR, Sjovold SG, et al: Biomechanical evaluation of the Total Facet Arthroplasty System: 3-dimensional kinematics. Spine 32:55–62, 2007.
19. Gheduzzi S, Webb JJ, Miles AW: Mechanical characterisation of three percutaneous vertebroplasty biomaterials. J Mater Sci Mater Med 17:421–426, 2006.
20. Yue JJ, Bertagnoli R, Lee R, Kirk J: A prospective, non-randomized analysis of the adjunctive use of Cortoss vertebroplasty in lumbar disc arthroplasty utilizing the Prodisc prosthesis. Presented at the Spine Arthroplasty Society Meeting, New York, NY, 2006.

CHAPTER 93

# Multilevel Lumbar Disc Arthroplasty

Rudolf Bertagnoli

## KEY POINTS

- For the generation of multilevel disc degeneration, a variety of intrinsic and extrinsic factors are discussed. The treatment of the consequently arising pain scenarios requires at some stage spinal arthroplasty when it is favorable to use motion-sparing devices instead of fusion procedures.
- If the disc (and not posterior structures) is identified as the pain generator, the use of total disc replacement appears to be beneficial. The use of multilevel motion-preserving devices appears to be superior to multilevel fusion procedures because the overall segmental stability is maintained.
- These procedures require critical patient selection and great surgical experience and precision.
- Multilevel fusion procedures will remain the option in treating conditions unrelated to degenerative disc disease such as scoliosis and long degenerations.

Degenerative multilevel lumbar disc disease (MLDD) is one of the most frequent reasons for chronic and disabling low back pain. This pain has an extensive impact on the social, economic, and psychological situation of the affected individual. The patient's history often includes repetitive external trauma. In most cases these patients received discectomies for disabling radicular symptoms and have also developed low back pain at the affected as well as the adjacent levels. Several risk factors also have to be taken into account when looking for the reasons of MLDD: Heredity factors (discussed in the literature[1–4]), smoking habits, obesity, and poor physical conditioning all influence the pathogenesis of MLDD. Typically, all nonsurgical options should be exhausted and disability and pain should still be present before operative intervention is considered. Different forms of spinal arthrodesis such as posterior, posterolateral fusion, anterior interbody fusion with or without instrumentation, and combined anterior/posterior fusion for the treatment of single- and bisegmental chronic discogenic low back pain have been investigated and experiences have been described.[5] Factors such as age, workers' compensation, and smoking status were considered. In prospective studies, direct correlation in patient satisfaction rates and fusion success could not be demonstrated.[6] There are also some disadvantages of spinal arthrodesis which are not negligible, for example, adjacent-level degeneration (36.1% at 10 years) of discs and facet joints as well as symptomatic pseudarthrosis, graft site morbidity, and pain due to reaction to instrumentation.[7]

## PATIENT SELECTION

The right indication, proper patient selection, and an optimally placed device are the key factors for successful treatment in total disc arthroplasty (TDA) in general and especially in multilevel TDA. Therefore, a thorough preoperative assessment is essential in which the commonly used diagnostic steps and tools for evaluating degenerative disc disease (DDD) should be applied to identify exactly the pain generator. The factors evaluated are age, gender, pain history and presence, prior conservative treatment, prior surgeries (spinal and abdominal), application for workers' compensation, and social and psychological factors. Furthermore, measurements and scores, such as the Oswestry Disability Index (ODI), SF-36, and Visual Analog Scale (VAS), and clinical investigation are employed for assessment.

Noninvasive radiographic evaluation (e.g., x-ray, magnetic resonance imaging [MRI], computed tomography [CT] studies) is mandatory to understand pathologic changes and static considerations.

Of great importance, however, is also the direct detection of the pain generators because in multilevel diseased situations often the pathologically changed areas are not the pain generators. In these situations only the invasive methods (e.g., nerve root blocks, facet blocks, discograms, myelography, technetium bone scan) can identify the pain generators. Discograms are very helpful in determining painful discs, and fluoroscopic or CT-guided facet or root blocks can help to detect pain generators in that area.

Additionally, osteodensiometries to understand the bone quality should be performed on a regular basis on patients over age 40 to reduce the risk of undetected subsidence in multilevel cases. Three-dimensional (3-D) angiography-CT can help in preoperative planning of the anterior approach.

Videofluoroscopy (moving radiograph) is useful for understanding the motion pattern of spinal areas.

In summary, only a multimodal investigational pattern can help in finding the objective diagnostic status.

## INDICATIONS

If in general the disc can be identified as the main pain generator in patients with low back pain, this is a good indication for TDA. If the posterior structures (e.g., facet joints) are the main cause for low back pain, TDA is not the choice of treatment. Also, patients with spinal deformities such as degenerative scoliosis are considered to be a critical group to be treated with TDA.

According to the Clinical Success Related Classification (C3RC),[8] the prime indication for TDA is monosegmental lumbar symptomatic DDD with or without herniation or large central herniations. The patient should not have had previous surgery at the affected level. Good indications are seen in failed disc surgery syndromes without laminectomy or severe facet alterations as well as bisegmental lumbar symptomatic DDD. Expanded indications are both fusion adjacent-level instabilities, cases with more than two-level DDD, degenerative scoliosis up to 25 degrees Cobb angle, and degenerative, self-reducible spondylolisthesis without mature canal stenosis (M I-II).

## CONTRAINDICATIONS

Contraindications for TDA in general are bone disorders such as osteoporosis, osteopathies, severe canal stenosis, hypertrophic spondyarthrosis, isolated radiculopathy, spinal deformities (spondylolisthesis), infections, tumors, and predominantly psychosocial factors. Significant facet joint arthritis, severe end plate irregularities, hemangiomas, metal allergies, pregnancy, and body mass index greater than 35 are also contraindicated.

## DESCRIPTION OF THE DEVICE

In the clinical application, unconstrained prostheses have been discovered as unsuitable in the use for multilevel disc replacement. In contrast, prosthesis with a semiconstrained kinematics in terms of controlling flexion and extension and left/right lateral bending in the given radius of the ball-and-socket concept proved to be suitable for the multilevel disc replacement in the coupled motion of the lumbar spine. It does not restrict randomized movements (Fig. 93–1).

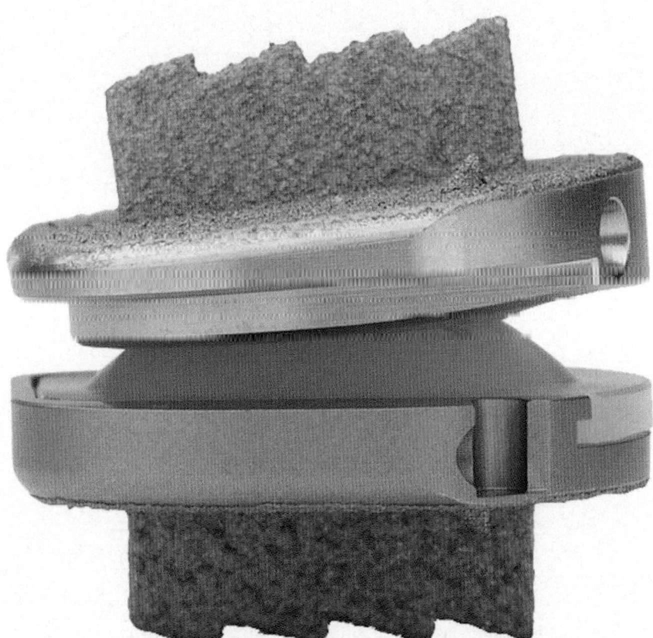

■ **FIGURE 93–1.** Modular design of the ProDisc-L implant.

In our clinical experience, the use of ProDisc-L (Synthes, Inc., Paoli, PA) (see Fig. 93–1) has been demonstrated to be a successful device in treatment of DDD patients.

## OPERATIVE TECHNIQUES

For the surgical approach, the patient is positioned in the da Vinci position on a radiolucent imaging table with arms and legs abducted. The surgeon is working between the patient's legs to get a better view of both sides of the disc and to have a better perspective view when applying the prosthesis perpendicular into the prepared disc space. To determine the level, the obliquity of the diseased disc, and an orthograde postion of the patient fluoroscopic imaging in the lateral and anteroposterior (AP) positions is conducted before skin incision. In multilevel procedures a paramedian left side longitudinal incision is recommended. A self-retaining retractor system such as the SynFrame (Synthes, Inc.) anterior spinal retractor is very useful for generation of a secure and stable retroperitoneal approach of the anterior aspect of the spine. The affected levels are approached segment by segment starting from the lowest level. As an exemption, the upper levels (L1-L2 and L2-L3) should be exposed first due to their cephalad orientation of the discal corridor line in the cranial portion of the lumbar lordosis. A complete release is essential to allow proper function of the device. Therefore, after a complete discectomy in cases with a disc height below 40% of the normal height, the resection of the posterior longitudinal ligament (PLL) as well as the intraforaminal annulus portion is necessary.

A moderate end plate remodeling for a better fit of the prosthesis is often necessary.

Generally, the largest possible footprint and the smallest possible disc height should be used to obtain an optimal load transmission onto the vertebrae and to avoid overdistraction of multiple segments.

Especially in multilevel procedures, a secure primary fixation is essential to avoid postoperative migration of the devices into an unfavorable kinematics of the coupled motion of the lumbar spine. Keel prosthesis like the ProDisc-L offers large benefits in this regard.

A precise positioning of the artificial disc and a precise matching of the centers of rotation are mandatory to allow a harmonic function in the treated areas. The more levels replaced by artificial discs, the greater the importance of these parameters.

## POSTOPERATIVE CARE

Remobilization can begin on the first postoperative day. Especially in multilevel treatment with collapsed discs, a significant increase of overall height leads to significant tension to ligaments, capsules of joints, and muscles. This might be the cause of "distention pain" that may occur after surgery. According to the Straubing Rehabilitation Index (SRI),[9] we recommend a dynamic orthesis for 6 weeks and no sports activity during this period. Multilevel patients should get physiotherapeutic treatment, but not before 6 weeks, and should avoid sports activities for at least 3 months.

## MATERIALS AND METHODS

Prospective data of all multilevel ProDisc-L procedures at our institution were collected for a minimum of 5 years. A complete radiographic assessment including AP, lateral, flexion, and extension imaging was performed before surgery as well as MRI and discography and optional CT scans. To reduce the amount of intraoperative variables (positioning of the patient, the approach or application technique, etc.) all the procedures were performed by the author at a single institution. The data were collected, compiled, and analyzed by independent examiners. Patients were assessed before surgery and after surgery at 3, 6, 12, 24, 36, and 48 months. The results were analyzed before and after surgery. Clinical scores and assessment parameters such as Oswestry Disability Index (ODI), Visual Analog Scale (VAS), patient satisfaction, back pain, radicular pain, medication usage, and complications have been investigated.

Radiographically disc heights affected and adjacent levels as well as the range of motion, flexion, and extension were obtained. All adverse outcomes related to the index procedure were recorded.

In the study 249 patients (139 male and 110 female patients) with multilevel lumbar ProDisc-L total disc arthroplasty have been included. The median age of all patients was 46 years (23–69 years); 120 patients were treated in two levels, 45 patients in three levels, 1 patient in four levels, and 1 patient in five levels.

## CLINICAL OUTCOMES

The ODI score was reduced from 49% before surgery to 27% after the 1-year follow-up, 27% after 2 years, 26% after the 3-year and 4-year follow-up periods.

The VAS score decreased from 7.2 preoperatively to 4.1 at the 1-year follow-up, 3.2 after 2 years, 3.8 after 3 years, and 3.8 after 4 years.

Eighty-seven percent of the patients reported to be completely satisfied or satisfied with the surgery 1 year postoperatively and 94% were satisfied 2, 3, and 4 years postoperatively. While all patients complained about continuous back pain preoperatively, 60% could be reported to have no back pain after surgery, 37% had moderate pain, and 3% had less back pain 2 years postoperatively. This improvement did not change at 4 years of follow-up.

## COMPLICATIONS

In eight cases device- or approach-related complications occurred, resulting in an overall complication rate of 3.2%.

### Device-Related Complications

Five cases of partial implant subsidence (2%) (Fig. 93–2A, B) and one case of polyethylene inlay extrusion (0.4%) have been observed. No other cases of loosening, migration, allergic rejection/reaction, visceral or neurologic injuries were caused by the device components or infection.

### Approach-Related Complications

One case of subcutaneous hematoma (0.4%) was identified that required reintervention as well as one case of retrograde ejaculation (0.4%). No cases of vascular injury, ureteral, or neurologic injury occurred.

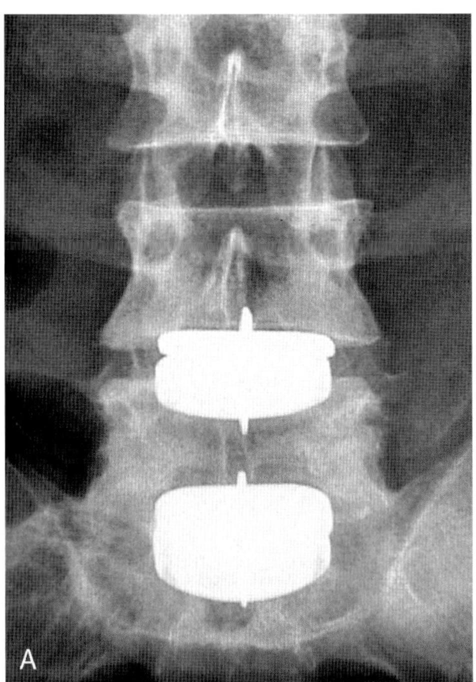


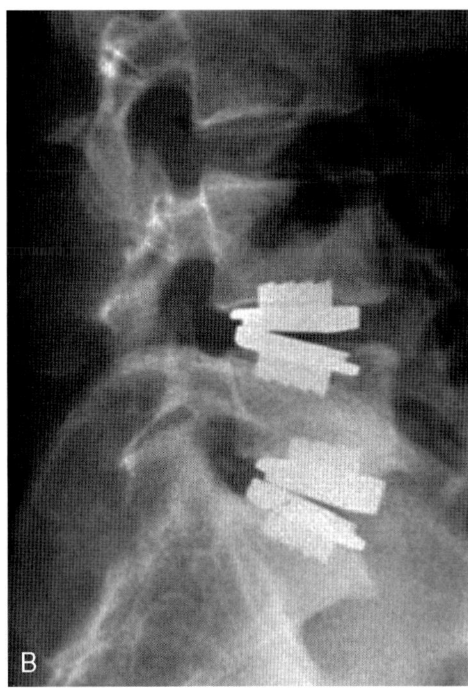


■ **FIGURE 93–2.** Anteroposterior **(A)** and lateral **(B)** postoperative radiographs showing subsidence.

## CASE STUDIES

### Case 1 (Two Levels)

A 61-year-old man with a multiyear history of low back pain remained resistant to conservative therapy. He had developed vertical segmental instabilities at levels L3-L4 and L4-L5 as well as FDS at level L4-L5 (Fig. 93–3A, B). Surgical treatment was multilevel total disc arthroplasty (two levels) with ProDisc-L at levels L3 to L5. Postoperative radiographs show good maintenance of mobility of the segments (see Fig. 93–3C to E).

### Case 2 (Three Levels)

A 42-year-old man was suffering from pseudoradicular lower back pain accompanied by leg pain resisting conservative treatment for years. Surgical treatment of the diagnosed symptomatic disc disease at levels L3-S1 was a three-level total disc replacement with ProDisc-L. X-ray studies showed proper vertebral alignment (Fig. 93–4A to C).

### Case 3 (Four Levels)

A 52-year-old man suffered several years from low back pain. All conservative treatment options failed. Radiographic and MRI revealed vertical segmental instabilities from L1 to S1 and herniations from L1 to L4 (Fig. 93–5A, B). Surgical treatment was multilevel total disc arthroplasty (four levels) with ProDisc-L at levels L1 to L5 and vertebroplasty. Postoperative radiographs showed correct positioning of the devices and a good restoration of disc height (see Fig. 93–5C, D).

### Case 4 (Five Levels)

A 50-year-old man with low back pain for years that failed nonsurgical treatment revealed on radiographic and MRI scans a symptomatic degenerative disc disease. This extended from L1 to S1 with a hyperlordosis and imbalanced lumbar spine. Surgical treatment was a multilevel total disc replacement (five levels) with ProDisc-L prosthesis, which was combined with a vertebroplasty to stabilize the bone (Fig. 93–6A to D). Postoperative imaging showed correct positioning and good restoration of disc heights and a rebalanced spine.

## CONCLUSION

The reason for MLDD seems to be a multifactoral combination of genetic, traumatic, social (tobacco use), physical (obesity), and age (senescence) factors.[10] Also, two different radiographic appearances of MLDD can be distinguished on MRI: In one, all affected levels seem to be more or less in the same status of degeneration; in another, different levels can be affected in different stages randomly. In patterns with more severe changes at the caudal level, this level (so-called "proximate disc") obviously is influencing subsequently the adjacent level degeneration.[11] Mostly, this proximate disc is situated more caudally. This type of MLDD is termed "proximate MLDD" (Fig. 93–7A, B). We have found extraordinary positive results in patients from this group, which makes this group the ideal group of patients for multilevel lumbar disc arthroplasty. Multilevel ProDisc lumbar surgery appears to ensure instantaneous implant stability and functional mobility, which allows a rapid reintegration in daily life and return to work. This applies for primary surgical procedures as well as for patients with prior posterior decompressive procedures.

Multilevel treatment with motion-sparing devices shows a more obvious benefit in maintenance of the segmental stability in the overall function of the patient than patients with multilevel fusion procedures. But these procedures require a high level of technical precision and surgical experience. Careful patient selection is essential for best surgical outcomes.

Also, motion-sparing technologies seem to be very beneficial for patients and do have a lot of advantages to multilevel fusion procedures in DDD patients; severe mechanical instabilities (e.g., fractures), tumors, spondylolisthesis, long deformities (e.g., scoliosis, kyphosis, stenosis, long degenerations), severe facet changes, and degenerative scoliosis will still remain for spinal fusion procedures.

Therefore, these procedures are not competitive with fusion procedures and allow the surgeon to be more selective in terms of treatment. Long-term data will be necessary to understand the real long-term value of multilevel motion-preserving procedures.

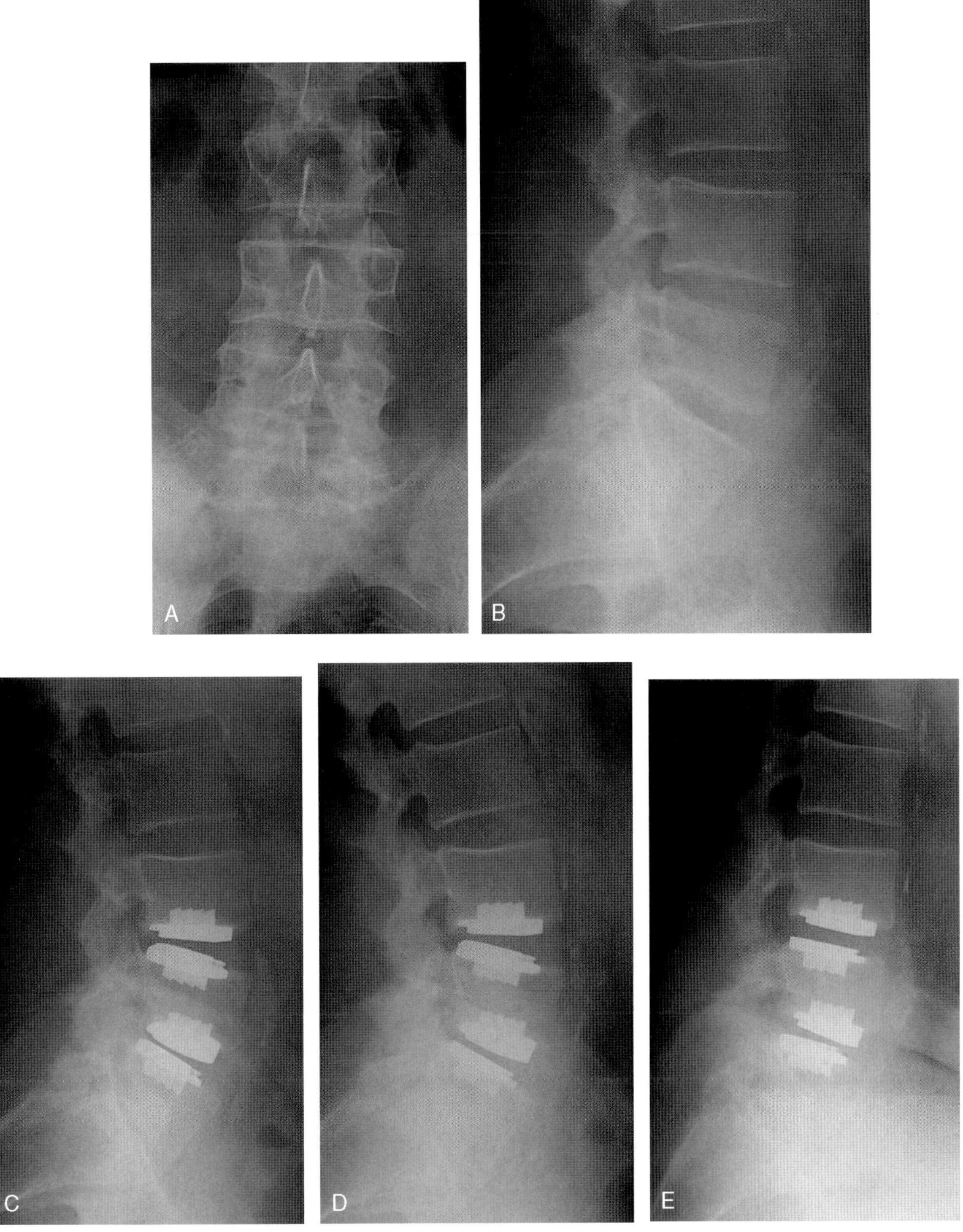

■ FIGURE 93–3. **A, B,** Preoperative radiographs: anteroposterior, lateral (from left to right). **C–E,** Postoperative radiographs: lateral, extension, flexion (from left to right).

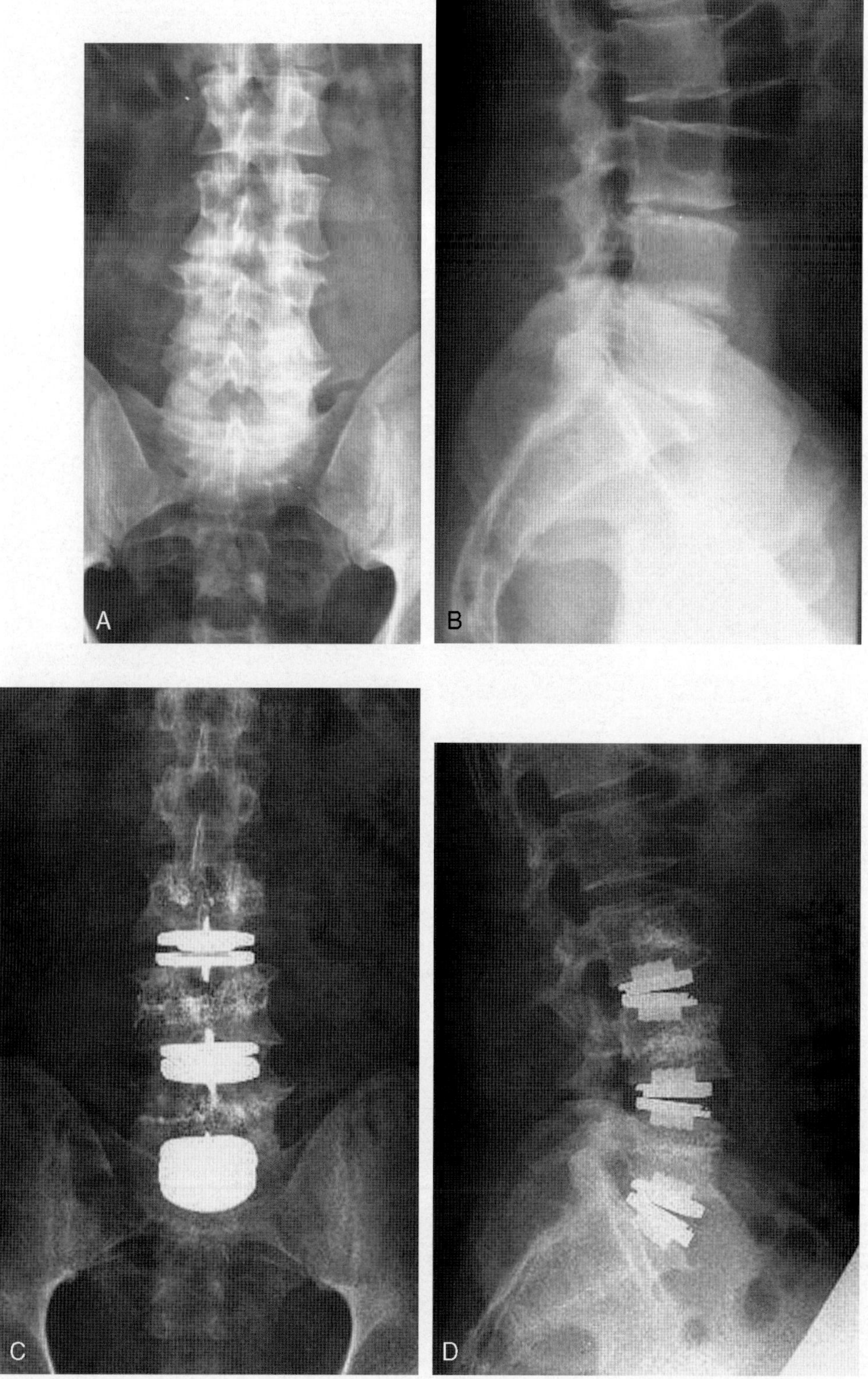


■ **FIGURE 93–4. A–D,** Pre- and postoperative radiographs: anteroposterior, lateral.

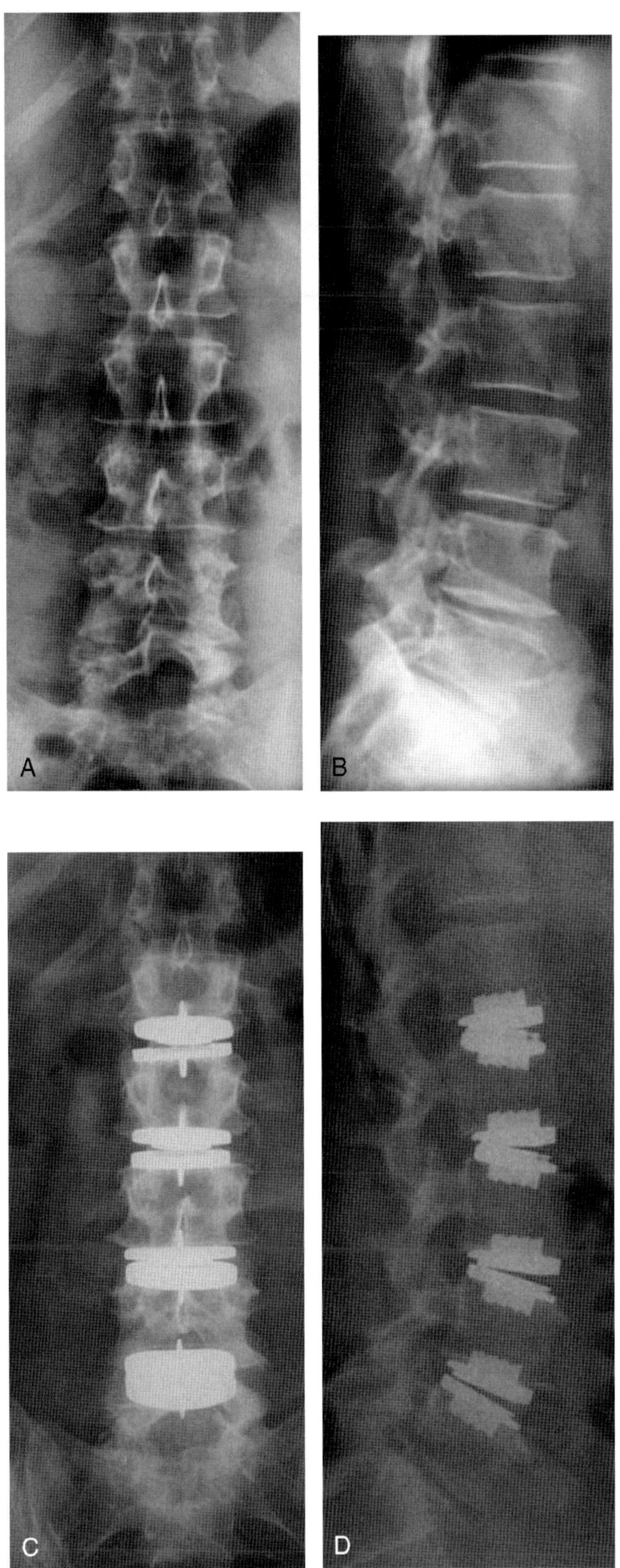


■ **FIGURE 93–5. A–D,** Pre- and postoperative radiographs: anteroposterior, lateral.

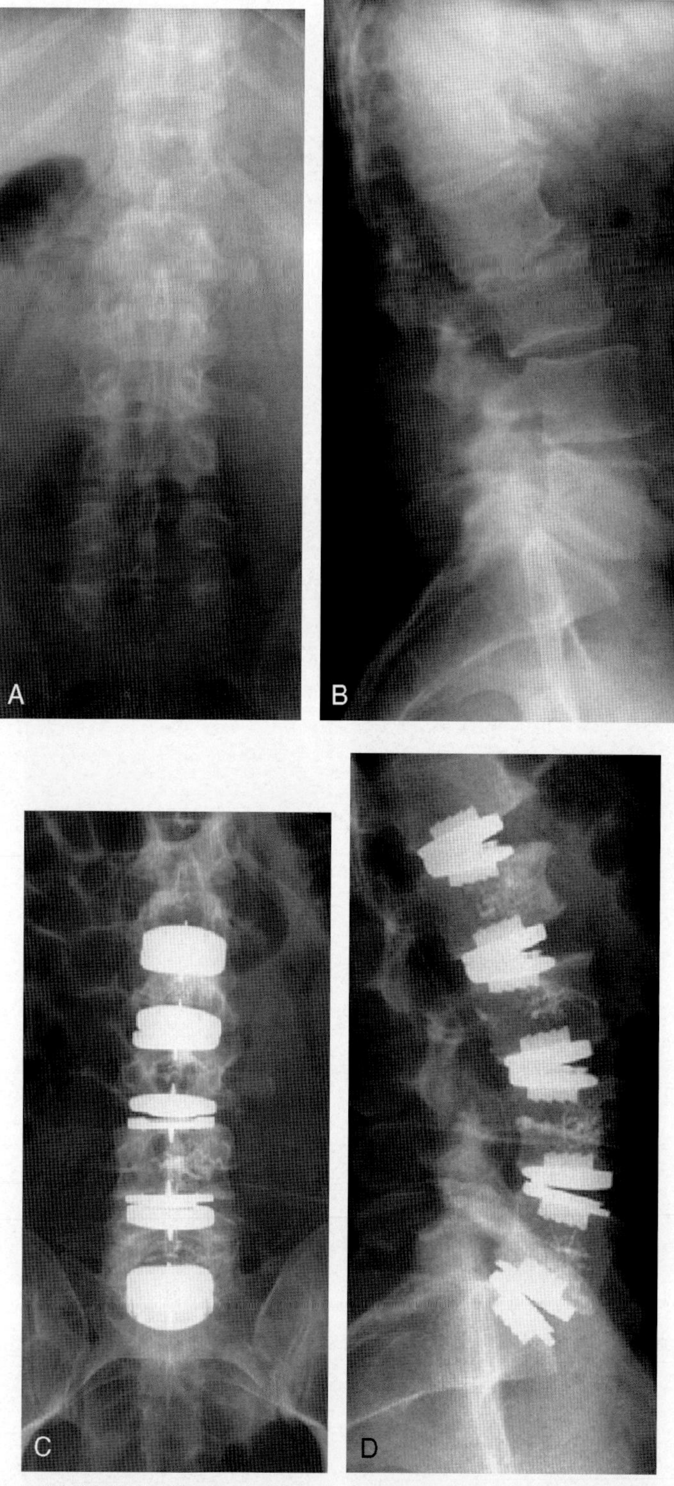


■ **FIGURE 93–6.** **A–D,** Pre- and postoperative radiographs: anteroposterior, lateral.

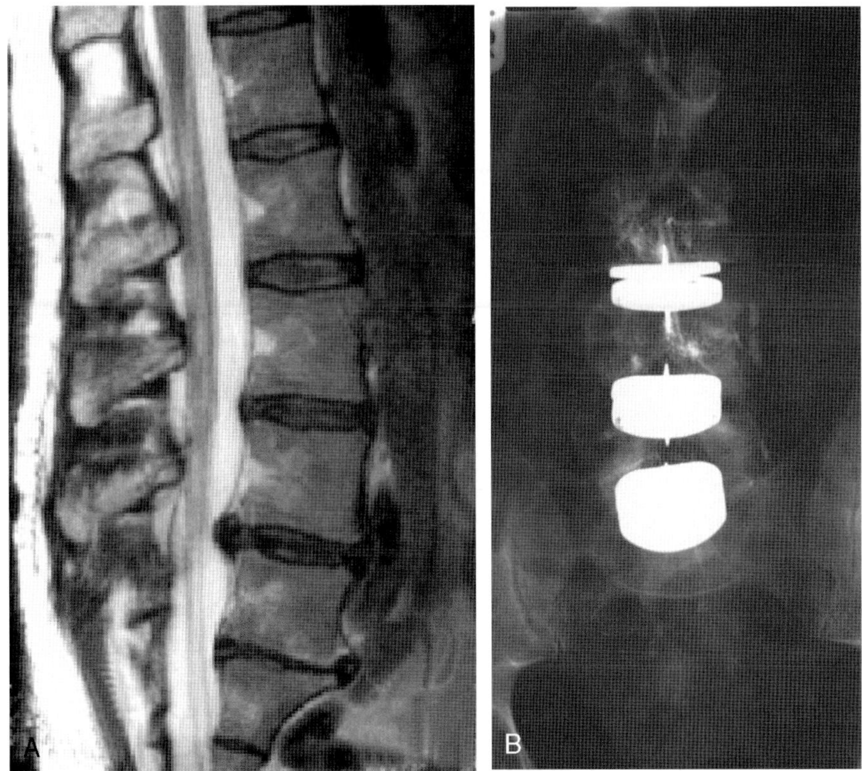


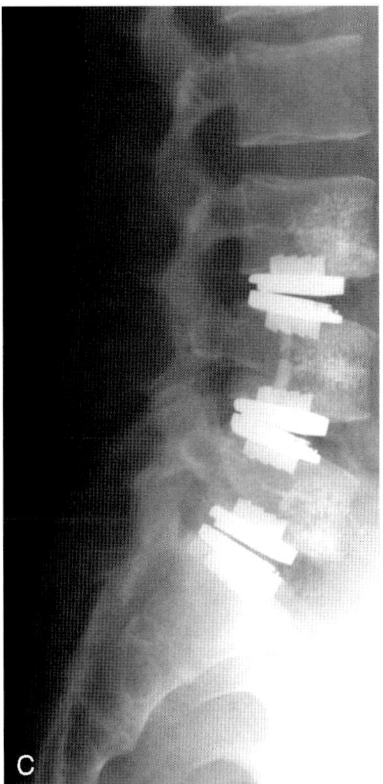


■ FIGURE 93–7. **A–C,** Proximate multilevel lumbar disc disease: example of cascade appearance.

## REFERENCES


1. Anderson DG, Tannoury C: Molecular pathogenetic factors in symptomatic disc degeneration. Spine J 5(6):260S–266S, 2005.
2. Solovieva S, Lohiniva J, Leino-Arjas P, et al: COL9A3 gene polymorphism and obesity in intervertebral disc degeneration of the lumbar spine: Evidence of gene-environment interaction. Spine 27:2691–2696, 2002.
3. Sambrook PN, MacGregor AJ, Spector TD: Genetic influences on cervical and lumbar disc degeneration: A magnetic resonance imaging study in twins. Arthritis Rheum 42:1729–1735, 1999.
4. Annunen S, Paassilta P, et al: An allele of COL9A2 associated with intervertebral disc disease. Science 285:409–412, 1999.
5. O'Brien JP: The role of fusion for chronic low back pain. Orthop Clin North Am 14:639–647, 1983.
6. Gibson A, Grant I, Waddel LG: The Cochrane review of surgery for lumbar disc prolapse and degenerative lumbar spondylosis. Spine 24:1820–1832, 1999.
7. Ghiselli GWJ, NN, Hsu WK, et al: Adjacent segment degeneration in the lumbar spine. J Bone Joint Surg Am 86:1497–1503, 2004.
8. Bhatia Bertagnoli R: Indications for total lumbar disc replacement. *In* Kim DH, Cammisa FP, Fessler RG (eds): Dynamic Reconstruction of the Spine (in process citation).
9. Bertagnoli R, Pfeiffer F: The Straubing Rehabilitation Index (SRI) as a guideline in postop treatment after ProDisc implantation. In process citation.
10. Savitz MH CJ, Yeung AT: The Practice of Minimally Invasive Spinal Technique. 2000, pp 149–165.
11. Bertagnoli R, Yue JJ, Shah RV, et al: The treatment of disabling multilevel lumbar discogenic low back pain with total disc arthroplasty utilizing the ProDisc prosthesis. Spine 30(19):2192–2199, 2005.

CHAPTER 94

# Posterior Lumbar Arthroplasty

**Manoj Krishna**

**KEY POINTS**

- Posterior lumbar arthroplasty has advantages over anterior arthroplasty in being easy to revise, dealing with disc/facet/nerve disease, having an easy approach, and being applicable to the vast majority of patients with lumbar pathology.
- A paired disc and posterior dynamic stabilizer (PDS) is a concept that is being developed.
- The instantaneous axis of rotation (IAR) of the disc and PDS needs to be matched for the system to function.
- The PDS on its own needs to offer shear stability, angular motion, and variable motion and must match the IAR of the disc to deliver the best results.
- The PDS may significantly reduce the need for posterolateral fusion.

Anterior lumbar arthroplasty is well established as a surgical option in the treatment of discogenic low back pain. Its clinical use has highlighted several problems with this technology including a difficulty in revision, continued facet pain, use of an unfamiliar approach, and its limited use in patients with facet or neural pain.

In response to these issues, surgeons started exploring the concept of posterior lumbar arthroplasty. Its main potential advantages are that it uses a familiar approach, deals with all the pain generators in a motion segment, and can be easily revised through an anterior lumbar interbody fusion (ALIF).

This chapter explores the concepts and challenges in the development of posterior lumbar arthroplasty.

## HISTORY

The history of anterior lumbar arthroplasty is well documented elsewhere in this book, from its origins in the Charité Hospital in Berlin.

The rationale for arthroplasty is to reduce disc degeneration adjacent to a fused lumbar segment and provide more physiologic kinetics and load transmission across the disc.

The evidence that it actually does so is emerging from various studies but is by no means conclusive at this stage.

If one excludes the PDN and other nucleus replacement devices, there have been few posteriorly inserted arthroplasty devices which replace the disc and allow motion. Globus Medical (Audubon, PA) has developed a posteriorly inserted paired disc replacement that needs to have parallel insertion into the disc space.

A number of dynamic stabilization devices that are pedicle-based allow some motion, usually less than 3 degrees. The GRAF ligament system (Neoligaments, Leeds, U.K.), the Dynesys (Zimmer Spine, Inc., Warsaw, IN), Isobar (Scient'x, Aylesbury, U.K.), Agile (Medtronic Sofamor Danek, Memphis, TN), and various PEEK (polyetheretherketone) and metal rods with some give in them are part of this group. Their aim is more stability than motion; any motion provided is designed mainly to prevent breakage of the device under repetitive loading rather than restore normal kinematics to the motion segment.

Facet replacement devices form a third group of posteriorly inserted motion devices. The Total Facet Arthroplasty System (TFAS) from Archus Orthopedics Inc. (Redmond, WA) is currently undergoing clinical trials. It is a pedicle-based system that requires the pedicle screws/bolts to be cemented in. This is a concern to some surgeons. Facet Solutions (Logan, UT) has developed the Anatomic Facet Replacement System (AFRS), a pedicle-anchored facet replacement system that is undergoing clinical evaluation. Impliant Spine (Princeton, NJ) has developed the TOPS system, a pedicle-based system that replaces the posterior facets and spinous processes and requires removal of the midline for insertion. This is also undergoing clinical evaluation.

The indications for these dynamic stabilization and facet replacement devices are mainly spinal stenosis with instability or following decompression requiring significant facet joint removal. These techniques may obviate the need for fusion and may have advantages in reducing operative time, morbidity, and length of hospital stay and in providing a faster recovery.

No system currently exists that combines a posteriorly inserted disc replacement with a coordinated posterior dynamic stabilizer. Disc Motion Technologies (Boca Raton, FL) is developing such a system. It will be a true total disc replacement (TDR) system and inserted through the posterior route, with all its inherent advantages.

## ANATOMIC CONSIDERATIONS

There are several aspects of the anatomy of the motion segment that influence the design and surgical technique in relation to posterior lumbar arthroplasty (PLA) surgery.

The aim of PLA is to deal with all the pain generators in a motion segment, which comprises the disc anteriorly, the two facet joints posteriorly, and the neural structures.

It is important to consider the disc and facets as part of one motion segment.

Fujiwara and associates[1] studied the radiologic relationship between disc and facet degeneration. They concluded that disc degeneration precedes facet degeneration.

Gries and associates[2] studied the histologic relationship between disc and facet degeneration. They found that microscopic changes of degeneration could be seen in the disc and facet at an early age and can be quite marked before 40 years of age, but there was no clear correlation between the two.

Butler and associates[3] found that discs degenerate earlier than facets. Anterior disc arthroplasty has been suggested in patients with no facet degeneration. If the anterior disc replacement does not restore synchronous movement to the facet, either through overdistraction or a mismatched instantaneous axis of rotation (IAR), it is probable that the facet may experience accelerated degeneration. Over a period of time, facet joints will degenerate and likely become pain generators. PLA has a theoretical advantage in being able to deal with the facet joint and the discs at the same time.

Tanaka and associates[4] studied the relationship between disc degeneration and mobility in cadaveric motion segments. Grades 1 through 4 degeneration was associated with more movement in the segment and Grade 5 with reduced movement.

The end plates are thickest at the rim laterally and thinnest centrally. To avoid subsidence problems, devices will need to be placed as laterally as possible. In order to place a device laterally, the lateralmost annulus will need to be removed. This is difficult because it is a solid structure and not routinely accessible to the shavers that go into the space occupied by the nucleus. Placing a device laterally implies that it is more likely to be angled slightly medially, as there is not enough room in the lateral disc to accept a 25-mm long device.

If paired bilateral devices are used, then they need to be parallel to each other or must be able to function as one device in a non-parallel insertion. The end plates of the disc in the anteroposterior (AP) view are not parallel to each other but slope laterally toward each other. The extent of this slope varies. It is greater in advanced degeneration and lower levels. This has implications in the design of the disc prosthesis. If one wants to place these devices laterally for maximum end plate strength, then the devices need to be anatomically adapted to the lateral disc space and the implants need to follow the end plate contour. If this is not done, as the device height increases, they will need to be placed more medially.

The degree of osteoporosis in the vertebra adjacent to the disc has implications for subsidence. After 55 years of age, a bone density scan needs to be done, and disc replacements avoided in patients with bone density more than 2 standard deviations below the norm.

Conjoined nerve roots are seen in approximately 4% of patients. One needs to keep that in mind during surgery and have a technique which excludes a conjoined nerve root before using the cautery to stop bleeding. If a conjoined nerve root is found and retraction is stretching the nerve, then no implant should be placed on that side and one may need to revise the procedure to a fusion.

Epidural veins can cause significant bleeding during surgery, as they cover the disc. Care must be taken to reduce the abdominal pressure. Careful bipolar cautery of the veins needs to be done, but avoid cautery in areas which are close to the nerve (e.g., the foramen or next to the exiting nerve above the disc). The main epidural vein is present just above the lower pedicle.

The triangle formed between the traversing nerve and the exiting nerve is the area where the disc can be accessed safely, without needing to retract the traversing nerve root. The course of the exiting nerve above the disc varies. In some cases it can be quite vertical, crossing the disc more medially than normal. Its distance from the upper disc border also varies. In some cases, particularly where the disc height is reduced, it can appear perilously close to the disc and needs careful retraction.

## BIOMECHANICAL CONSIDERATIONS

There are various causes of back pain. We will focus here on the patient with discogenic back pain who has failed conservative measures and is being considered for surgery. These patients typically present with a history of exacerbations and remissions of their symptoms, pain increased on sitting, a catch on extension from the flexed position, a history of instability, and tenderness often localized to the painful segment.

Though there are many theories for the cause of axial back pain, clinical and experimental data suggest pain is caused by axial loading of an inflamed disc. This may explain the pain on axial loading and the intermittent flare-ups and remissions. This may also explain the success of interbody stabilization in relieving this pain. Lotz and associates[5] studied pathologic disc degeneration via animal studies and suggested a similar theory.

The goal of successful surgery for axial low back pain is to address the biomechanics of the painful segment by removing the pain generator (the disc) and restoring axial loading across the disc space. Anterior lumbar arthroplasty, anterior lumbar interbody fusion, and PLIF/TLIF with cages all remove the painful disc and restore loading across the disc. The PLIF/TLIF procedure in addition removes the painful facets and decompresses the neural structures. The goals of posterior lumbar arthroplasty are outlined in Table 94–1.

The question arises whether we need to replace just the disc posteriorly or both the disc and facet. Replacing the disc alone would need at least 50% of the facets to be preserved, thus requiring significant dural retraction to insert the discs. There would be a concern that the discs may back out without a posterior tension band. If one were going to replace the disc alone, there would be a good

**TABLE 94–1. Goals of Posterior Lumbar Arthroplasty**

1. Remove painful disc
2. Restore normal loading across the disc
3. Decompress neural structures
4. Remove painful facets if needed
5. Restore motion to the painful disc
6. Allow segment to assume a physiologic position in sitting and standing
7. Match instantaneous axis of rotation of disc and posterior dynamic stabilizing device
8. Preserve normal loading of adjacent discs

argument to do this anteriorly. Adding a posterior dynamic stabilizer allows a generous removal of as much facet as required, a better decompression of the neural structures, and avoidance of the problem of overdistraction of the facet joint capsule (if the facet is removed). My opinion is that the disc and posterior dynamic stabilizer (PDS) should be used in conjunction to start with, and as clinical experience grows, some surgeons may try the posterior disc on its own.

If the PDS and the disc are used together, then for any movement to occur, their centers of rotation must be matched (Fig. 94–1). In Figure 94–1 the arc of the posterior dynamic stabilizer (Truedyne) and the posterior prosthetic disc (Truedisc) are matched.

Asynchronous movement will result in strains on the adjacent segment. Matching the centers of rotation is not an easy task as the IAR keeps changing during motion and is not in a predictable place in degenerative discs in any case.

Rousseau and associates[6] highlighted this in their paper on the IAR at the L5-S1 disc.

The PDS device will need to provide shear stability throughout its range of movement. The typical lumbar segment moves through an arc in flexion and extension, and the term *angular motion* is one way of describing it. The disc/PDS combination also needs to restore angular motion to the segment. This is different from devices that allow only rotation around a ball and socket or translation.

How much motion needs to be restored to the operated lumbar segment? One has to remember that a diseased disc has less motion than a normal disc in most cases, except in the instability phase of degeneration. The aim is not to restore motion to normal but only to the extent that the disc above or below does not get excessive load transmitted to it or move in an asynchronous manner. Flexion-extension is the main movement to restore, with some lateral bending and rotation. How much motion is then ideal? Finite element analysis (FEA) is probably the best way to address this question.

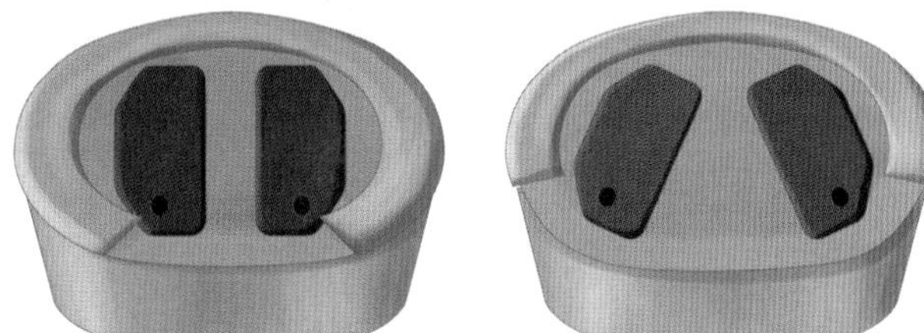

■ **FIGURE 94–2.** FEM pictures of a posterior lumbar disc prosthesis (TrueDisc) inserted in a parallel and in a nonparallel manner.

The loading on the end plate will be an important consideration in PLA. The contact surface area of a paired disc, placed on either side of the dura, is less than that of an anteriorly placed disc, and so point loading through the end plates will be higher. Careful placement of the discs laterally under the thickest part of the end plate will be important to avoid subsidence.

If placed laterally, the discs will probably angle toward the midline. Getting a paired posteriorly placed disc that is not parallel to allow the segment to move synchronously will be challenging, and a simple ball-and-socket design may not work in this situation. Figure 94–2 illustrates discs placed parallel and nonparallel in the disc space. Figure 94–3 illustrates the movement of the disc prosthesis developed by Disc Motion Technologies, when placed in a parallel and in a nonparallel manner, as seen in Figure 94–2.

Figure 94–4 illustrates a posterior disc replacement system from Disc Motion Technologies, comprising a paired posteriorly inserted disc combined with a paired posterior dynamic stabilizer. The technique of insertion is similar to a bilateral TLIF.

The posterior dynamic stabilizer can be used on its own as well, and the indications for this are discussed later. Matching the IAR of the motion segment during movement is important even when it is used on its own; otherwise, this will probably result in asynchronous movement in the disc above.

The need to minimize wear is an important factor in material selection for the disc. Cobalt-chrome has a history of being used successfully in lumbar discs (e.g., Maverick disc [Medtronic Sofamor Danek, Memphis, TN]). It is not, however, MRI (magnetic

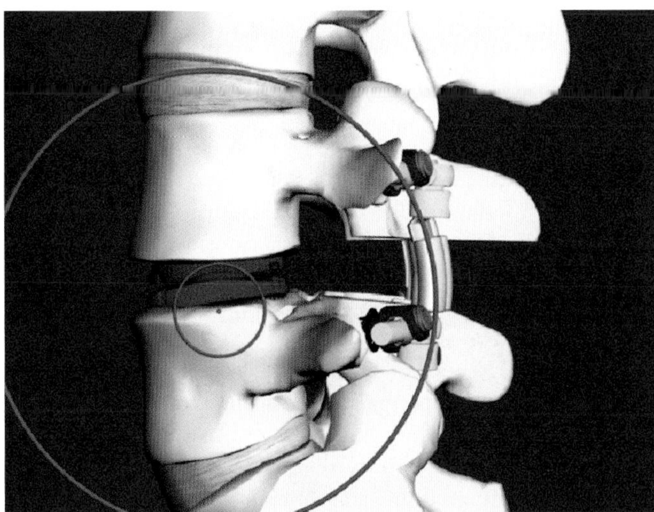

■ **FIGURE 94–1.** This model demonstrates the importance of matching the IAR (instantaneous axis of rotation) of the posterior disc and a posterior dynamic stabilizer.

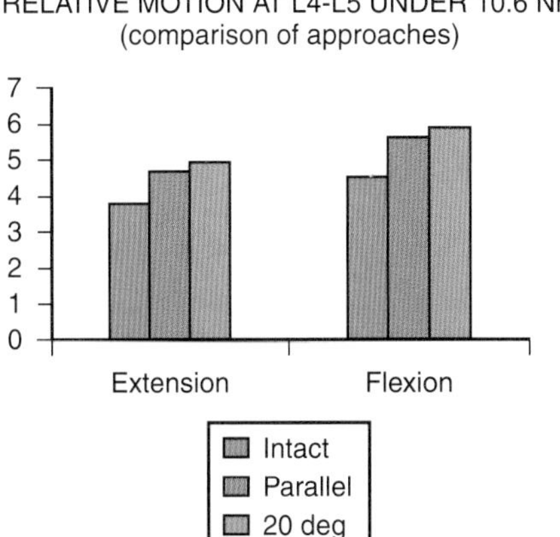


■ **FIGURE 94–3.** Graph illustrating the relative motion of the L4-L5 motion segment before and after the insertion of a posterior lumbar disc and posterior dynamic stabilizer, with the discs inserted parallel and nonparallel. It shows that the Truedisc allows similar motion whether placed parallel or nonparallel.

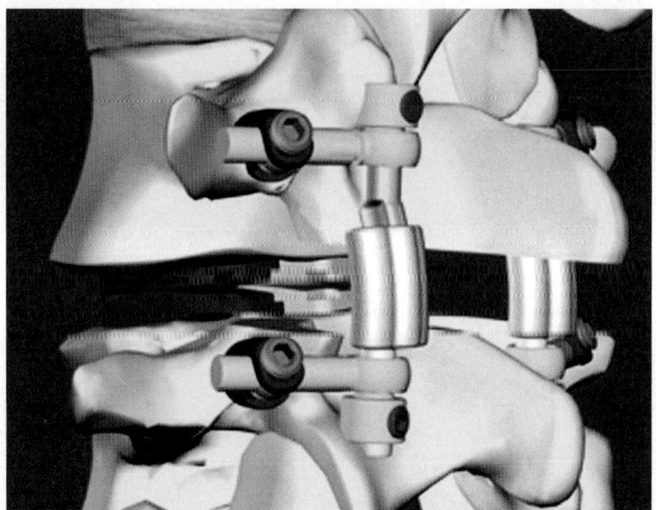

■ **FIGURE 94–4.** The Disc Motion Technologies Total Spinal Motion Segment (TSMS) replacement system comprising the paired Truedisc posterior lumbar disc and the paired Truedyne posterior dynamic stabilizer (PDS). The lateral connectors ensure a parallel placement of the Truedyne PDS devices and also house a ball-and-socket connector allowing for fine tuning of changes in the instantaneous axis of rotation during motion.

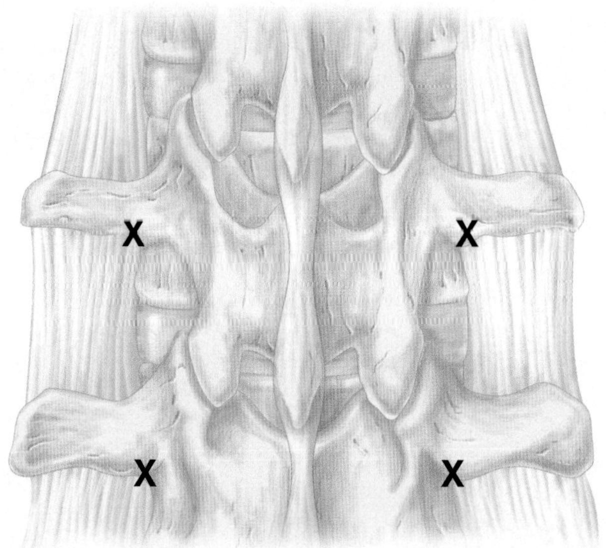
X
X
X
X
The xs mark the pedicle screw insertion points.
Do not expose TP's.

■ **FIGURE 94–5.** Features of the surgical technique of posterior lumbar arthroplasty. The xs mark the pedicle screw insertion points. Do not expose the transverse processes.

resonance imaging) compatible, which is a disadvantage. New materials which will have good wear characteristics and be MRI compatible are being tested (e.g., titanium-ceramics), but it will take time before they can be fully studied and introduced into clinical use.

As far as the PDS device is concerned, a similar rationale applies. Cobalt-chrome will be preferable for its excellent wear characteristics if there are components that are subject to wear during motion (e.g., the Truedyne from DMT).

## OPERATIVE TECHNIQUE

Posterior lumbar arthroplasty (PLA) is very similar to the bilateral TLIF approach, but there are some special considerations that need to be kept in mind. These, along with other general advice, are discussed in this section.

The use of a good xenon 300-watt headlamp and loupes (×2.5 magnification) adds to the safety and speed of this procedure and is routine in many practices.

A bloodless field is desirable for this surgery. Careful patient positioning to avoid any pressure on the belly reduces venous pressure and bleeding. Hypotensive anesthesia is useful at reducing intraoperative venous bleeding. A skilled anesthetist can have a significant impact on blood loss. Understanding the anatomy of the epidural venous plexus is important so the veins can be cauterized before the bleeding starts. Bipolar cautery is used. There are usually large veins going around each pedicle and also coursing along the nerve roots and fanning across the disc space laterally. Gelfoam and Flowseal used intraoperatively help to stop any bleeding that cannot be controlled with a cautery. With these techniques, bleeding can be reduced to about 150 mL for a one-level procedure.

The surgical approach is illustrated in Figure 94–5. A midline approach, sparing the interspinous ligament, is used. A 6-cm incision is usually enough for a one-level procedure. Exposure is only necessary to the edge of the facet joint. Exposing the transverse process is not needed. If the patent is obese, the pedicle screws are inserted through stab incisions lateral to the midline incision in order to get the proper medial angulation of the screws without having to enlarge the midline incision and overretract the soft tissues. Correct medial angulation is especially important at S1 where the L5 nerve root is at risk as it crosses over the ala of the sacrum. This does not require elaborate percutaneous instrumentation and can be done under direct vision.

Correct pedicle screw placement is crucial to PLA. We advocate the use of an image intensifier to check that the screws are placed in the center of the pedicle. An off-center placement of the screw can result in early loosening or screw breakout. A visual and mechanical check of the medial pedicle wall after screw placement is important, as the pedicle probe is not foolproof. Some surgeons like to insert the screws after doing the decompression, so the pedicle can be visualized during insertion.

A bilateral TLIF type approach allows access to the disc between the traversing and exiting nerve roots and avoids the need to retract the dura. The quickest way is to ostetomize the inferior facet first, the horizontal cut being at the level of the pars. The second cut is through the superior facet, just above the pedicle. With a Kerrison rongeur, bone is removed up to the pedicle above and below the disc, and the traversing and exiting nerve roots are deroofed. Care is taken to decompress the exiting nerve root above the disc. This also allows a manual inspection of the medial pedicle wall.

Before cauterizing the epidural veins, check for conjoined nerve roots, which occur in 4% of patients. The disc is then incised. This should be done bilaterally before sequential spreaders are used. It is very important to cut the lateralmost part of the disc, as it can form a lateral tether preventing disc distraction and, worse, destruction of the end plate with the use of aggressive shavers. This is illustrated in Figure 94–6.

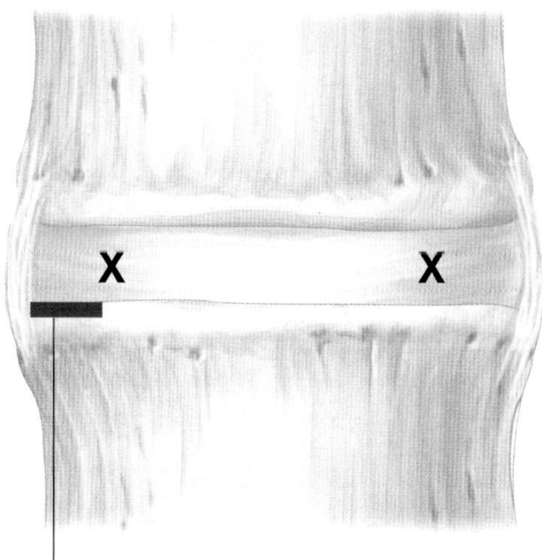
X
X
Osteotomize lateral annulus to release lateral tether.

■ **FIGURE 94–6.** When incising a disc, it is important to cut the lateralmost annulus to release a possible lateral tether.

End plate damage can lead to subsidence of the implant. The lateralmost disc is best cut using an osteotome, just above the pedicle below, taking care to protect the exiting nerve root.

Shavers should not be used till the disc is opened to the required height, and even then they are used sparingly and carefully. A down-biting curette is also useful to remove the disc material.

It is important to remove the lateralmost part of the annulus. One test of this is a clear view of the empty disc space, lateral to the traversing nerve root, without any retraction.

A common problem is not enough room for the disc. To get around this use a disc trial. This creates the space the disc will occupy, and if it is not going in easily, one may need to remove more of the annulus from under the lateral edge of the dura.

One should remember that the anterior annulus may have been torn during distraction, and so there is a risk to the anterior major vessels and also a chance that the disc can be inserted too far anteriorly and out into the retroperitoneal space.

If a conjoined nerve root is found on one side, then the disc replacement is not possible, and one needs to convert this procedure to a fusion.

The Disc Motion TrueDisc has a unique rail system, which makes the insertion of the spreaders and disc easy.

The sizing of the disc is different from the way one sizes a cage. For the disc to move, we need to avoid overdistraction. If one is able to open the disc space to, say, 11 mm using spreaders, then a 10-mm disc prosthesis should be used, whereas an 11-mm fusion cage would probably be appropriate if one were doing a fusion.

One must try to place the discs as parallel as possible and as laterally as possible. The discs must also be placed at the same depth from the posterior vertebral wall. Always make more room for the nerves by decompressing them, as they do swell after surgery due to handling, and relative stenosis may cause leg pain.

Surgeons may prefer to take the midline out, only do a partial facetectomy, and place the discs more medially, as in the traditional PLIF approach, but the end plate strength is maximal laterally, rather than medially.

Along with the disc, a posterior dynamic stabilizer (PDS) will be necessary to control motion of the discs and provide shear stability. The placement of this is important. The pedicle screws are placed in the usual manner. The PDS device needs to be lined up so its IAR will match that of the disc.

## CHALLENGES

Posterior lumbar arthroplasty is a new concept and there are a few disc systems in development. Clinical studies will begin in 2008. There are some challenges we can foresee and others that will emerge only after clinical use.

Just as ALIF evolved into anterior lumbar arthroplasty, it is anticipated that the PLIF/TLIF procedure will evolve into posterior lumbar arthroplasty. The surgical approaches and techniques are familiar and well established for PLIF/TLIF procedures and the same will be applied to PLA.

Matching the IAR of the disc and the posterior dynamic stabilizer will be a challenge for many reasons. Our understanding of the IAR in degenerative discs is incomplete, and there are variations between different degenerate segments. The IAR also changes in motion, and the system will need to adapt to that.

Preventing subsidence through the end plate will be important. Strategies that may help here will include placing the discs laterally under the strongest part of the end plate, using the widest discs that can be safely inserted, and avoiding surgery in patients with osteoporosis.

Disc retropulsion into the spinal canal is a potential problem. Features will need to be built into the disc to resist this. The PDS will help reduce this risk by controlling the movement of the disc and avoiding hyperflexion posteriorly.

Putting the implants in with the disc slightly distracted to create appropriate tension will also help to avoid retropulsion. How much tension one needs to create is difficult to quantify at this stage. Too much distraction will result in a loss of movement, so the amount of distraction needs careful calibration, but there are no clear guidelines at this stage.

The width of the discs will need to be balanced between the need to provide maximum end plate coverage and the ability to insert the disc past the neural structures without undue retraction.

If paired discs are used, placing them parallel will be important. If placed laterally to take advantage of the strong end plate, they will invariably end up being angled medially. In this case, getting the discs to move, even when placed in a nonparallel manner, will require innovations in disc design.

If the PDS system that is used in conjunction with the disc is anchored to the pedicle, then pedicle screw loosening will be an issue. This is because there will be torsion forces transmitted to the screw during motion. Mechanisms in the screw will need to be designed to counter this.

How much movement in the motion segment should we aim for in PLA? Too little movement will cause additional stresses on the adjacent level. Too much movement will result in possibly more pain from the neural structures, loosening of the components, and wear issues. These questions need further study.

## DISCUSSION

Posterior lumbar arthroplasty represents a natural evolution of lumbar arthroplasty, after anterior lumbar arthroplasty has become established as a clinical procedure. It aims to deal with the obvious clinical problems we have encountered with anterior arthroplasty.

The posterior disc replacement, along with a dynamic stabilizer, aims to restore kinematics of the spine to near normal. There are many clinical questions being raised as total lumbar disc replacement continues to emerge in clinical practice. Many variables, such as effects on adjacent level degeneration, will take years to define. Finite element analysis allows for evaluation of motion and load changes which can be anticipated and help predict potential effects of clinical scenarios.

The posterior lumbar discs need to function even when placed in a nonparallel manner. This simulates their insertion from a far lateral TLIF type approach, where the midline is spared and the facet removed to place the discs. This approach has additional advantages in that the neural structures need minimal retraction and there is a thorough decompression of the exiting nerve roots. Placing discs exactly parallel to each other is very difficult, as MRI scans of postoperative patients with implanted PLIF cages have shown, in clinical practice. Posterior lumbar arthroplasty is a true TDR and has several possible advantages to anterior lumbar arthroplasty. These are summarized in Table 94–2.

The finite element analysis of the posterior disc and PDS system from Disc Motion Technologies (DMT, Inc., Boca Raton FL) shows that it is possible to design a system whereby the disc and PDS are matched as far as their center of rotation is concerned and that this results in near-normal motion at the implanted level, with no additional movement at the adjacent level. This was explained in detail by Goel and associates in their paper.[7] It has also been corroborated by cadaver kinematic studies.

Restoring angular motion with shear stability is one of the goals of PLA. Two separate meta-analyses of the literature[8,9] suggest that PLIF gives better clinical results than ALIF. This may be because the PLIF deals with more pain generators. It is postulated these results may be similar for posterior lumbar arthroplasty, as compared to anterior arthroplasty, but clinical studies will be needed to confirm this.

The term posterior lumbar arthroplasty could be extended to include the dynamic stabilization devices such as Isobar (Scient'x), Agile and Dynesys. The aim of these devices is to provide stability, and the slight movement they offer results in the device absorbing the loads and not breaking. This will avoid the need for posterolateral fusion. Other devices in this group (e.g., the Truedyne) allow the desired range of movement to be dialed into the device from 0 to 8 mm.

**TABLE 94–2. Comparison of Posterior and Anterior Lumbar Arthroplasty**

| Posterior Lumbar Arthroplasty | Anterior Lumbar Arthroplasty |
|---|---|
| Deals with all three pain generators—disc, nerve, and facet joint | Deals only with disc |
| Can be easily revised via an anterior lumbar interbody fusion | Revision is difficult and hazardous |
| Approach familiar to all surgeons | Often needs a separate approach surgeon |
| Fewer contraindications than anterior arthroplasty | Applicable to only approximately 5% of patients |
| Can be done even with facet degeneration and neural impingement | Facet degeneration and neural impingement a contraindication; postoperative facet pain a possibility |

**TABLE 94–3. Uses of Posterior Dynamic Stabilizers**

1. For micromovement, which enhances a posterolateral fusion
2. To stabilize, after decompression in spinal stenosis
3. To protect a segment above a fusion
4. In conjunction with a posterior disc replacement
5. For the treatment of low back pain
6. Stabilization of degenerative scoliosis.

These devices have multiple uses, as outlined in Table 94–3. These are the clinical scenarios in which surgeons are either using these devices already or contemplating their use. The clinical evidence for their use in these situations is being collected but has not yet been published. Each indication will require a different range of movement in the device, with minimal movement for the fusion indication (0–2 mm), 2 to 3 mm after decompression for spinal stenosis, 3 to 5 mm to protect a segment adjacent to a fusion, and 6 to 8 mm when used in conjunction with a posterior disc replacement. These figures are a clinical estimate at this stage, and further research is needed to quantify these more accurately. The aim should be not only to stabilize the segment without the need for a fusion but to allow enough movement in the device to avoid excessive adjacent segment movement and subsequent accelerated degeneration at that level. Allowing motion while preserving shear stability and matching the IAR of the motion segment is the challenge in designing these devices.

The ideal surgical candidate for this procedure will be similar to that for a PLIF/TLIF procedure. To start with, however, it is recommended that the PLA be avoided in cases with a complete collapse of the disc with osteophytes. This is because once the disc height is restored in this group, movement in the segment will be limited.

A potential problem is subsidence of the discs, as the end plate contact area is less than for anteriorly placed discs. This will be minimized with the lateral placement of the discs, where the end plate is strongest. The widest discs that can be accommodated will need to be placed in the discs. Other potential problems are similar to those seen with the PLIF/TLIF procedure, including neural irritation.

## CONCLUSION

Posterior lumbar arthroplasty represents the next generation of lumbar arthroplasty devices, with several advantages over anteriorly placed discs. These advantages include a familiar approach, ease of revision, few contraindications, dealing with neural compression and facet degeneration in addition to disc degeneration, and applicability in a larger group of patients.

It is important that the posterior disc be matched with a posterior dynamic stabilizer and that they both have a matched center of rotation.

Posterior dynamic stabilizers are another group of posterior arthroplasty devices which can be used on their own or in conjunction with a posteriorly placed paired lumbar disc. They are used on their own in posterolateral fusion to stabilize a segment after a spinal fusion and to protect a segment above a fused level. Allowing the motion needed for the indication it is used for, preserving shear stability, and matching the IAR of the motion segment are desirable qualities in a PDS device.

## REFERENCES


1. Fujiwara A, Tamai K, An HS, et al: The relationship between disc degeneration, facet joint osteoarthritis, and stability of the degenerative lumbar spine. J Spinal Disord 13(5):444–450, 2000.
2. Gries NC, Berlemann U, Moore RJ, Vernon-Roberts B: Early histologic changes in lower lumbar discs and facet joints and their correlation. Eur Spine J 9(1):23–29, 2000.
3. Butler D, Trafimow JH, Andersson GB, et al: Discs degenerate before facets. Spine 15(2):111–113, 1990.
4. Tanaka N, An HS, Lim TH, et al: The relationship between disc degeneration and flexibility of the lumbar spine. Spine J 1(1):47–56, 2001.
5. Lotz JC, Ulrich JA: Innervation, inflammation, and hypermobility may characterize pathologic disc degeneration: Review of animal model data. J Bone Joint Surg Am 88(2):76–82, 2006 (review).
6. Rousseau MA, Bradford DS, Hadi TM, et al: The instant axis of rotation influences facet forces at L5/S1 during flexion/extension and lateral bending. Eur Spine J 15(3):299–307, 2006 (epub Sept 20, 2005).
7. Goel V, Kiapour A, Faizan A, et al: Finite element study of matched paired posterior disc implant and dynamic stabilizer (360° motion preservation system). SAS J 1:55–62, 2007.
8. Boos N, Webb JK: Pedicle screw fixation in spinal disorders: A European view. Eur Spine J 6(1):2–18, 1997 (review).
9. Turner JA, Herron L, Deyo RA: Meta-analysis of the results of lumbar spine fusion. Acta Orthop Scand Suppl 251:120–122, 1993.

CHAPTER 95

# Cervical Arthroplasty with Myelopathy

**Jonathon R. Ball** and **Lali H.S. Sekhon**

**KEY POINTS**

- The natural history of cervical spondylotic myelopathy is unclear.
- Surgery for cervical spondylotic myelopathy is of unproven benefit.
- Cervical arthroplasty is an alternative to fusion after anterior cervical decompression.
- Cervical arthroplasty may be beneficial in selected patients with cervical spondylotic myelopathy as long as careful patient selection is undertaken.
- Patient selection should be guided by an understanding of the pathophysiology of cervical spondylotic myelopathy and the benefits and limitations of cervical arthroplasty.

Surgery for cervical myelopathy has been performed for over 50 years. The natural history of myelopathy is still unclear and the effects of our interventions sometimes unclear. Significant variations in surgical approaches to cervical disease, including cervical myelopathy, have been demonstrated in surveys of spine surgeons.[1] The strategies to manage cervical myelopathy are manifold and include nonoperative management and surgical treatment using anterior and posterior approaches. Cervical arthroplasty introduces a new dimension into the management armamentarium, promising retained motion and decreased adjacent segment degeneration. The application of cervical arthroplasty to the treatment of cervical myelopathy is relatively new, and the long-term consequences are not entirely clear.

This chapter will review the clinical and pathologic features of cervical myelopathy as well as more recent management strategies and finally the role of cervical arthroplasty in the surgical management of myelopathy.

## CERVICAL MYELOPATHY

### Presentation

Cervical myelopathy refers to a symptom complex caused by compromise of the cervical spinal cord. Cervical spondylosis that leads to canal stenosis and cord compression is the most commonly encountered cause. The first clear delineation of this syndrome from other cervical diseases is attributed to Brain and associates in 1952 who stressed the distinction between the presentations of radiculopathy and myelopathy and highlighted the difference between acute disc protrusions and chronic degenerative changes in the cervical spine.[2] The symptoms and signs exhibited by patients are variable and were grouped by Crandall and Batzdorf into five categories that covered the spectrum of spinal cord syndromes. It has been reported that gait abnormalities are among the earliest noticeable changes. More recent electrophysiologic studies have found that abnormalities of motor and somatosensory evoked potentials precede the development of clinically noticeable signs.[3]

### Pathophysiology

The pathophysiology of cervical spondylotic myelopathy (CSM) remains incompletely understood. Current thinking is that static compressive elements cause dynamic effects with cervical motion. The forces developed in the cord substance together with potential vascular compromise combine to cause neural injury. Subcellular mechanisms of neural injury, similar to those elucidated in acute spinal cord injury, continue to be investigated. Presumably there is a point that is reached in terms of degree and severity of compression where cell death occurs, affecting both neurons and supporting elements. Consequent gliosis and scarring may contribute to a poor outcome after decompression.

Cervical spondylosis is accompanied by structural changes that can lead to canal stenosis. A congenitally narrow cervical spinal canal is a predisposing factor for the development of CSM. The degree of stenosis has been quantified in a number of ways by different authors. The sagittal developmental diameter of the spinal canal is measured at the level of the midvertebral body to avoid inaccuracy by disease at the level of the disc space. In normal subjects, the diameter at levels from C3 and C7 is around 17 to 19 mm.[4–6] Decreased developmental canal diameters are observed in patients with CSM. Some authors have proposed the use of ratios to evaluate spinal canal stenosis to account for variations that may occur with race, gender, or body size and radiographic distortion. The Torg/Pavlov ratio describes the relationship of the sagittal diameter of the spinal canal to the sagittal diameter of the vertebral body. Lower ratios have been found in patients with CSM.[7]

The degenerative process of cervical spondylosis produces anatomic changes that decrease the canal volume from all directions.

Anterior compression from disc space disease rises as a result of disc herniation, osteophyte formation, and PLL (posterior longitudinal ligament) calcification while uncovertebral osteophytes can lead to anterolateral compromise. Synovial hypertrophy or osteophyte formation affecting the facet joints may cause lateral narrowing, and the ligamentum flavum can encroach on the canal posteriorly.

Static compressive elements do not act alone in the pathophysiology of CSM. Dynamic changes that occur with cervical motion are believed to be an important contributor. In flexion, the cord is "draped" over anterior compressive elements and the cord is stretched. In extension, cord shortening leads to thickening of the spinal cord that combines with buckling of the ligamentum flavum to exacerbate posterior compression. Dynamic changes may exacerbate the vascular compromise that has been proposed to contribute to the development of CSM. Putative mechanisms include radicular feeder compromise with foraminal stenosis, anterior spinal artery compression in flexion, elongation of transversely directed terminal arteries, and compromise of venous drainage.

Aside from a vascular cause, mounting evidence from experimental models suggests important biomechanical factors in CSM pathophysiology.[8] Spondylotic changes deform and tether the cord. With movement, stretching of the cord causes increased intramedullary strain and shear forces that injure axons. Further subcellular mechanisms of neural injury have been proposed to include apoptosis, excitotoxicity, free radical formation, and cationic mediated injury.[9,10]

## Natural History and Conservative Management

The true natural history of untreated cervical myelopathy is not well established because all series are subject to bias from retrospective data collection, selection of patients for treatment, the use of nonoperative treatments, and the failure to use a validated clinical scale. These limitations mean that series purporting to describe the natural history may be able to describe the patterns of progression but will fail to estimate the true rates of progression in a patient population. The 1956 paper by Clarke and Robinson, often quoted as describing natural history, was based on the prodromal history of 120 patients before treatment and included a prospective cohort of 26 selected patients who received no treatment.[11] They described three patterns of disease history—episodic deterioration, slow progressive deterioration, and prolonged stability/eventual deterioration—leading to the conclusion that the ultimate prognosis in most cases was poor. Lees and Turner in 1963 reported on 44 patients with myelopathy of whom 22 were followed for more than 10 years.[12] The initial development of symptoms was often followed by a period of clinical stability or improvement. In those with longer follow-up, exacerbations of disease occurred with intervening periods of nonprogressive disability. A pattern of steady deterioration was rarely seen. The authors called for "reflection about the question of operation." A 1966 paper by Roberts described spondylotic cervical myelopathy as a benign condition noting motor improvement in about a third of patients. However, a similar proportion deteriorated in the same time frame. Phillips rallied against this prevailing notion of cervical spondylotic myelopathy as a benign condition in his 1973 paper.[13] He criticized the methodology of earlier papers and, based on his good experience with anterior cervical decompression, recommended early surgery for the best results. Such advocacy of early surgery was often based on a theory that surgical delay may lead to permanent neurologic injury. Opponents claimed that surgical successes reflected patients who would have improved or stabilized without surgery if given enough time.

## Surgical Management

Surgery has been proposed for CSM since its earliest definition. Generally speaking, surgery is utilized for those with severe or progressive symptoms.[14] Numerous surgical techniques have been developed since, each purporting unique benefits. There is, however, little consensus between surgeons about the best approach. There is no class I evidence to support the superiority of surgical management.[15] The only randomized controlled trial, reported by Kadanka and associates in 2000, randomized 48 patients with mild-to-moderate CSM (mJOA $>$ 12) to conservative therapy or surgical management.[16] The surgeries predominantly employed anterior approaches. At 2 years, no substantial difference in outcome was seen between groups.[16] An analysis of an expanded series with longer follow-up attempted to identify predictors of good outcome through univariate analysis.[17,18] Older age, wider canals, and normal central motor conduction time were predictive of response to conservative therapy. The degree of canal stenosis and worse preoperative function were more prevalent in surgical responders. On behalf of the Cervical Spine Research Society, Sampath published the results of a prospective, non-randomized, multicenter study of patients undergoing medical or surgical management for CSM.[19] The treatment allocation was at the discretion of the participating surgeon. Despite having a poorer clinical status at baseline, surgical patients had improved outcome at follow-up.

## Surgical Approaches

Surgical options in CSM involve both anterior and posterior approaches and have been developed to address both the static and dynamic causative components.

### Posterior Approaches

The initial description of spondylotic cervical myelopathy by Brain and associates[2] included a description of a surgical series by Northfield. At that time, the operation performed was a posterior decompression by laminectomy with section of the dentate ligaments. This approach was based on the rationale that posterior decompression alone would not always allow sufficient relief of cord compression from anterior disease. Section of the dentate ligaments allowed further displacement of the cord away from compressive elements. Although dentate ligament section is no longer routine, it is now widely recognized that posterior decompression alone is not sufficient in all situations, particularly in the presence of significant anterior disease or kyphosis that drapes the cord over anterior compressive elements. Of a series of 100 patients with cervical spondylotic myelopathy reported by Ebersold in 1995, 51 underwent a laminectomy.[20] Improvement was noted in about 70% of patients at early follow-up; however, 10%

of patients suffered a delayed deterioration. Several causes of deterioration after laminectomy have been proposed and include spinal instability, accelerated spondylotic changes, extradural scarring, and tethering. The incidence of postlaminectomy kyphosis was reported to be 21% in a study by Kaptain and associates and noted to be higher in patients with a preoperative loss of cervical lordosis.[21] For this reason, it has been proposed that posterior decompression be accompanied by posterior fixation and fusion to prevent the development of deformity. The use of fusion techniques can also allow a wider decompression to be performed without chancing instability. This approach, involving wide laminectomy and lateral mass fixation, has been reported by Sekhon for patients with circumferential stenosis. In a report of this technique in 50 patients, he reported radiographic evidence of adequate decompression in all patients and a decrease in Nurick grade in the majority of patients. Progression of deformity was seen in only two patients.[22]

Another form of posterior decompression, laminoplasty, was pioneered by several Japanese groups. Various methods have been described but most involve detaching the laminae and repositioning them in an orientation that increases the diameter of the canal. These approaches purport to maintain spinal motion by preserving facet joints, prevent kyphosis through preservation of the posterior elements, and protect the dura from tethering to muscle. Kawaguchi and associates reported an impressive case series of lamininoplasty in 133 patients.[23] Of the 84 patients who were alive and available for follow-up after a minimum of 10 years, 35 had their initial surgery for CSM. Improvement in clinical status, measured by the Japanese Orthopaedic Association (JOA) myelopathy score, was noted in 55.1% of subjects at last follow-up. The average preoperative score of 9.1 improved to 13.7 at 1 year and was maintained at 13.4 at last follow-up. A North American group has reported the results of cervical laminoplasty in 204 patients with CSM at an average follow-up period of 16 months.[24] They reported a decrease in Nurick grade in 62% of patients. Radiographic progression of kyphosis was seen in two patients.

Other variations on the posterior approach include a dorsolateral operation that involves the exposure and removal of one hemilamina and skip laminectomy where decompression is performed at discontinuous levels with preservation of muscle attachment at other levels.[25,26] These procedures both aim to limit the disruption of spinal extensor musculature and decrease the risk of deformity. However, they are limited to CSM related to predominant posterior compression.

### Anterior Approaches

As noted earlier, it is widely accepted that the use of posterior decompressive techniques is not appropriate in all situations of CSM. This is particularly so when significant ventral disease exists or kyphotic deformity allows the spinal cord to be draped over anterior compressive elements. In fact, most surgeons embrace anterior techniques ahead of any posterior procedure, particularly for disease affecting fewer than three levels. Methods of anterior cervical spine surgery were initially described by Bailey and Badgley, Smith and Robinson, and Cloward.[27–29] Historically, anterior approaches in the cervical spine have included anterior cervical discectomy alone (ACD), anterior cervical discectomy with fusion (ACDF), and ACDF with anterior plating. These can be performed at single or multiple levels. For more extensive disease, including disease behind the vertebral bodies inaccessible through the disc space, cervical corpectomy and fusion can be performed. The substrate for fusion has included autograft, often from the iliac crest, human or animal allograft, or more recently bone graft substitutes and osteogenic factors. Intervertebral cages have been developed for graft containment and structural support, and the proliferation of different design in anterior cervical plates has necessitated the development of a classification scheme. Emery and associates reported the results of anterior cervical surgery in 108 patients with CSM at a minimum follow-up of 2 years.[30] Operative treatment consisted of anterior discectomy, partial corpectomy, or subtotal corpectomy at one level or more, followed by placement of autogenous bone graft from the iliac crest or the fibula; 92% of subjects with motor weakness, 89% of subjects with sensory deficit, and 86% of those with gait abnormality showed some improvement postoperatively. One patient had marked neurologic deterioration after surgery and myelopathy recurred in five patients.

## CERVICAL ARTHROPLASTY

Clear guidelines for the use of cervical arthroplasty surgery are lacking. The earliest clinical reports on cervical arthroplasty devices were dominated by patients with spondylotic myelopathy,[31] but modern devices are recommended cautiously in this setting by manufacturers.

Without consensus on best current management, the benefit of a new technology is difficult to assess and its introduction carries the risk of inappropriate use. However, a firm understanding of the pathophysiology of the disease, as already outlined, married with an appreciation of the principles of the technology, allows the formulation of a framework to guide the appropriate use of cervical arthroplasty in patients with spondylotic cervical myelopathy.

### Theoretical Considerations

As with all surgical therapies for CSM, decompression of neural elements is the primary aim in cervical arthroplasty for myelopathy. Compressive elements can be anterior, posterior, or lateral and may occur in the context of a congenitally narrow canal. Significant compression by ventral disease accessible through the disc space approach is most suitable. The presence of ventral disease that extends behind the vertebral body and is inaccessible through the disc space may not be appropriate. Dorsal compressive elements cannot be removed through an anterior approach (Fig. 95–1). The constricting nature of a congenitally narrow canal is not addressed by anterior discectomy. The critical nature of adequate decompression must be emphasized. Given the role of dynamic effects in CSM, the presence of any residual compressive elements will be unacceptable. Such elements may be allowed in a fusion situation, when movement that causes dynamic compression is eliminated. If motion is preserved, such elements may impinge on the cord with movement and cause further neural injury. The unconstrained nature of many cervical disc prostheses limits their use in the presence of cervical

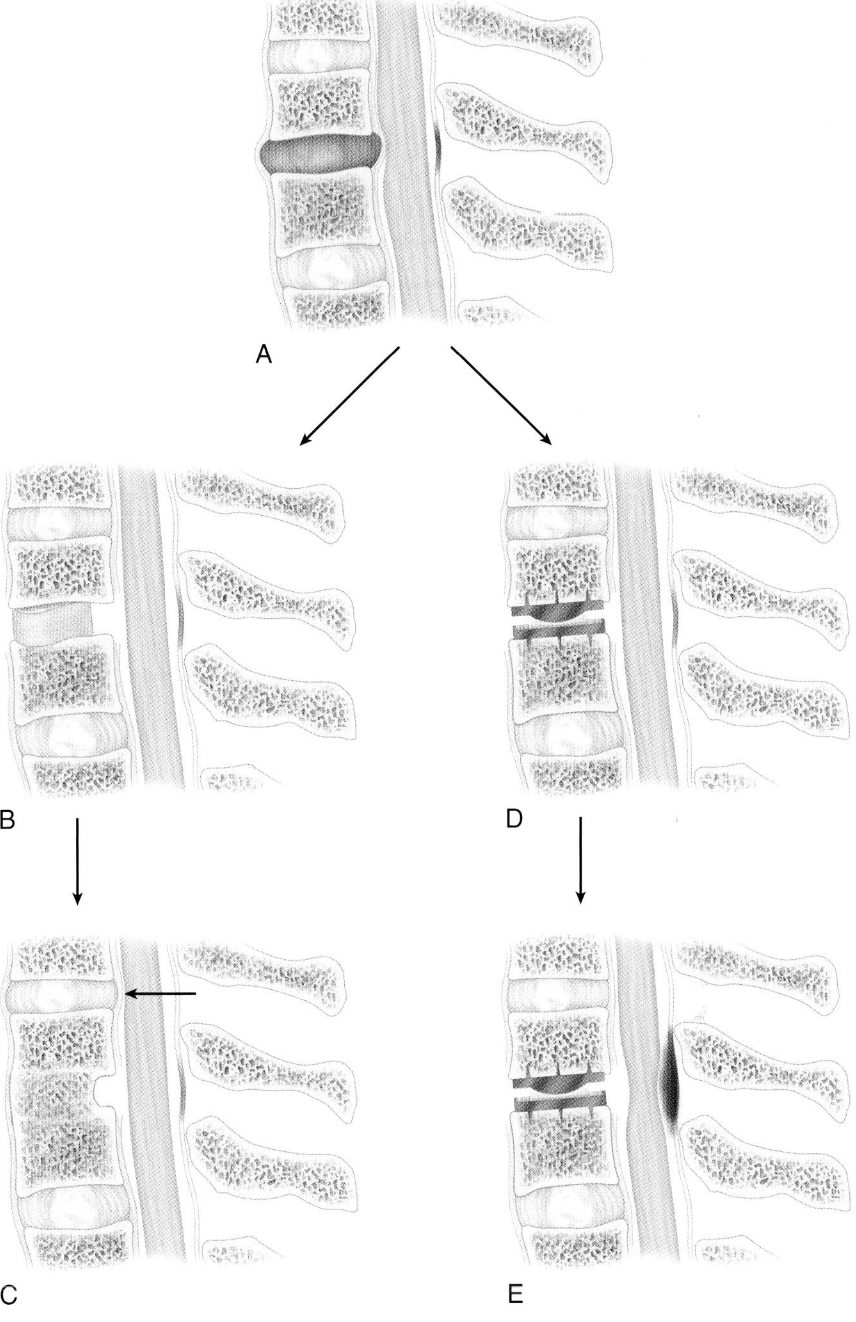


■ **FIGURE 95–1.** Typical patient with cervical stenosis and potential outcomes from anterior fusion surgery and anterior cervical decompression and arthroplasty. In the fusion situation, over time, degenerative changes may develop at the adjacent level, whereas in the arthroplasty scenario possible posterior ligamentous thickening may worsen over time and cause recurrent stenosis. **A,** A hypothetical situation with predominantly ventral cord compression in a patient with some posterior ligamentous thickening as well. The two treatment algorithms are shown in **(B)** and **(D)** with either an arthroplasty or a fusion being performed. The hypothetical future situation is shown below this. In **(C)** the fusion is solid, no recurrent stenosis has occurred but there is some adjacent degeneration at the level above. In part **(E)** the arthroplasty is moving and unchanged. The adjacent level is intact. Note, however, that the posterior ligaments at the operated levels have thickened because of retained motion and recurrent stenosis is occurring. This scenario could also potentially cause foraminal stenosis with facet osteophytosis occurring over time.

deformity and instability, although correction of deformity may be an option with newer devices.

Figure 95–2 illustrates a situation inappropriate for arthroplasty. A 44-year-old man with myelopathy had a congenitally narrow canal with significant dorsal and some ventral compression at multiple levels. Loss of lordosis is seen in the upper cervical spine. Arthroplasty would have addressed the ventral compression, but the combination of residual dorsal compression and a narrow canal may continue to cause compression, particularly in the presence of preserved motion. A posterior decompression and lateral mass fusion was performed from C3 to C6.

Figure 95–3 illustrates another situation in which arthroplasty may be unsuitable. This 76-year-old woman presented with myelopathy due to disc-osteophyte compression predominantly at C5-C6 and C6-C7. This was associated with a kyphotic deformity that draped the spinal cord over the compressive elements. Adequate decompression may have been difficult through the disc space, and the unconstrained nature of many disc prostheses would not enable the restoration of cervical lordosis. Anterior decompression with multilevel corpectomy and local autografting into a PEEK (polyetheretherketone) cage was performed with anterior plating.

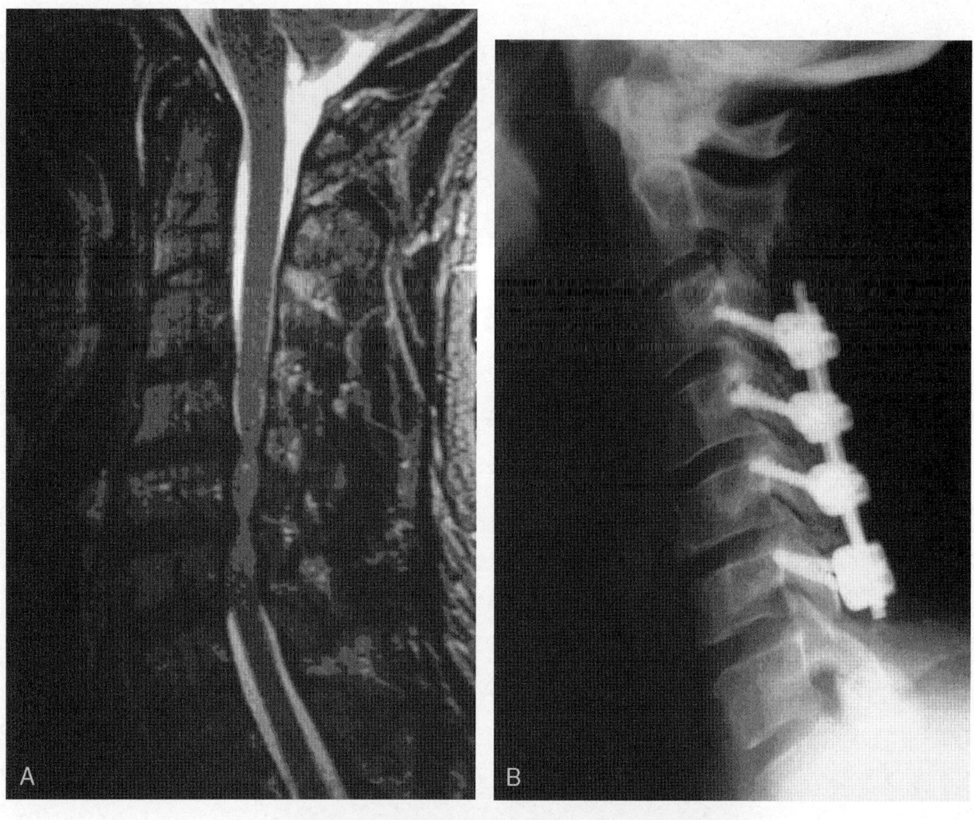


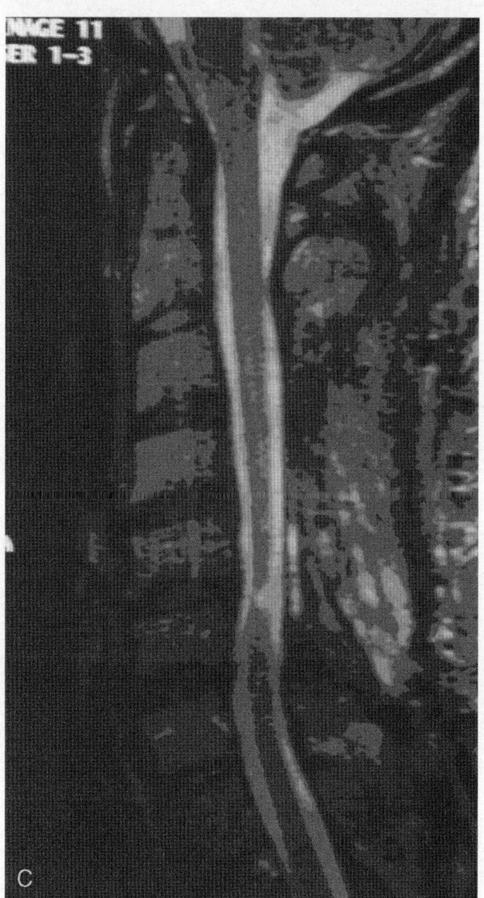


■ **FIGURE 95–2.** This 44-year-old man presented with clinical cervical myelopathy, a congenitally narrow canal, and anterior and posterior compressive disease **(A).** In this scenario wide posterior laminectomy and fusion **(B)** lead to a successful decompression of the spinal cord **(C)**.

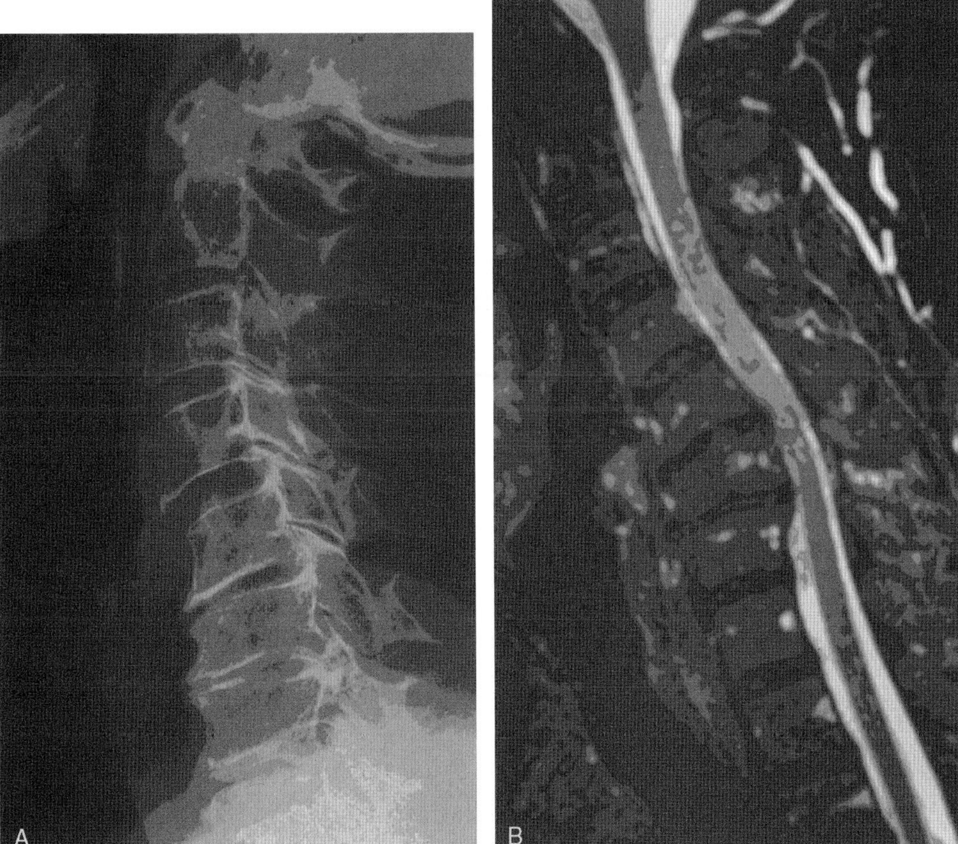


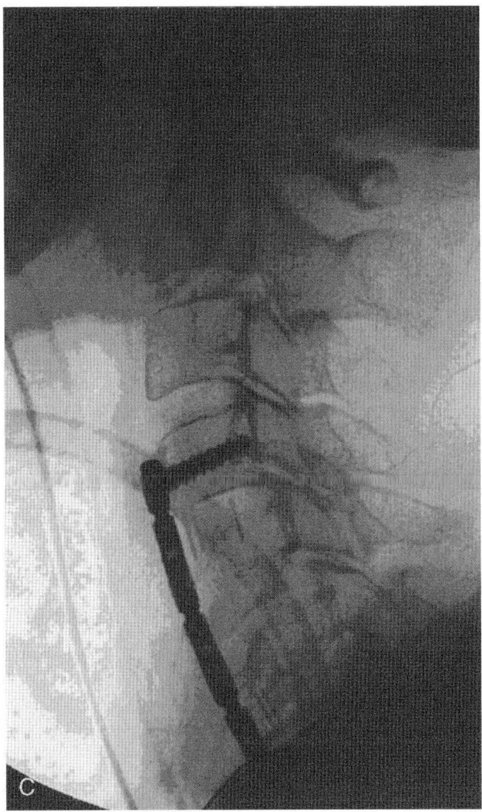


■ **FIGURE 95–3.** This 76-year-old woman presented with a progressive myelopathy, a focal radiologic kyphosis **(A),** and evidence of cord compression on magnetic resonance imaging **(B).** Three-level anterior corpectomy was effected with reduction of the kyphosis using a PEEK (polyetheretherketone) cage, local autograft, and plating **(C).** Subsequent posterior fixation was also performed. Again, this is not a case suitable to current arthroplasty technologies.

Figure 95–4 illustrates a situation in which arthroplasty was used. This 45-year-old woman presented with a clinical myelopathy due to anterior disc compression at C4-C5 and C5-C6. The canal was relatively capacious, and there was no significant dorsal compression. The degree of loss of lordosis was considered acceptable. Cervical disc arthroplasty was performed at two levels with good results.

## Clinical Studies

It has been proposed that the ideal patient for insertion of an artificial disc prosthesis has a soft disc herniation causing neurologic symptoms or signs, motion at the involved segment with no evidence of instability or hypermobility, and an absence of osteoporosis or infection. Normal sagittal alignment with the absence of focal or global kyphosis is desirable. To date, the published clinical series of cervical disc arthroplasty has predominantly included patients with radiculopathy and myelopathy, secondary to acute disc herniations or degenerative spondylotic change. The initial series describing the Cummins/Bristol disc (produced in the hospital workshop at Frenchay Hospital, Bristol) included 16 patients with myelopathy, 3 with radiculopathy, and 1 with severe neck pain.[31] In reporting the initial use of the Bryan disc (Medtronic, Memphis, TN), Goffin described results in 53 patients with radiculopathy and 7 with myelopathy.[32] Goffin and associates reported an expanded series of 146 patients including 43 two-level cases.[33] They further reported 6-, 12-, and 24-month success rates of 90% (83/92), 86% (76/89), and 90% (44/49) for single-level surgery. Duggal and associates examined outcomes in 26 patients implanted with Bryan discs who had myelopathy or radiculopathy, most of which were favorable.[34] Pimenta and associates reported their experience with the PCM (Cervitech, Inc., Rockaway, NJ) prosthesis in 40 patients with radiculopathy and 13 with myelopathy.[35] This series yielded good or excellent outcomes greater than 90% at 3, 6, and 12 months. A study analyzing the use of ProDisc-C (Synthes, West Chester PA), reported results in 16 patients with "symptomatic cervical spondylosis."[33] It included 4 patients with severe axial neck pain and 12 with established radiculopathies or myelopathies. Significant postoperative decreases in neck and arm pain intensity and frequency were noted. A similar decrease was recorded in the Oswestry Disability Index.

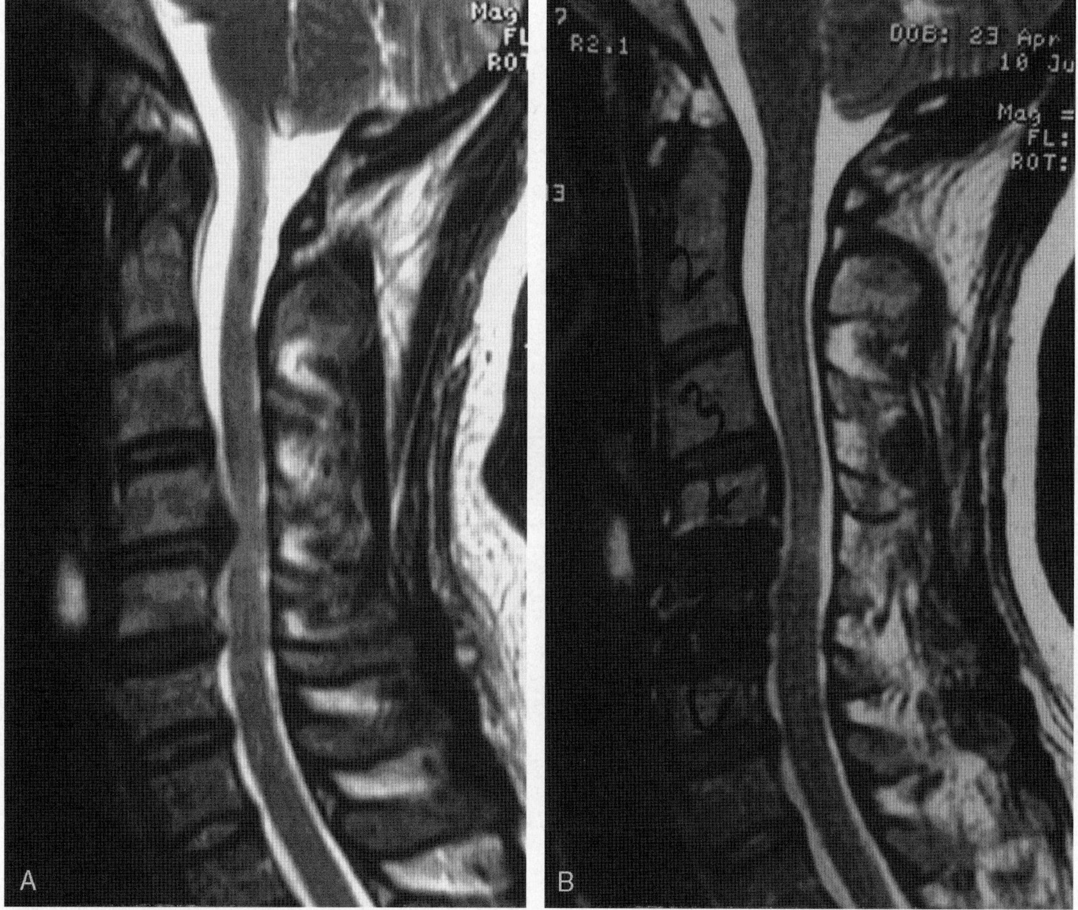

■ **FIGURE 95–4.** This 45-year-old woman presented with bilateral arm weakness and a clinical picture of cervical spondylotic myelopathy. The preoperative magnetic resonance (MR) scan showed evidence of predominantly C4-C5 cord compression with a smaller disc at C5-C6 **(A).** The patient underwent uneventful two-level cervical arthroplasty at these levels with good decompression of the spinal cord on postoperative MR scanning **(B).**

**TABLE 95–1. Results of Cervical Arthroplasty in 11 Patients with Spondylotic Myelopathy Showing Good Initial Outcomes**

| Patient | Preop Nurick | Postop Nurick | Levels | Follow-up (mos) | Preop Curvature | Postop Curvature |
|---|---|---|---|---|---|---|
| 1 | II | I | C5-C6 | 31.9 | Loss of lordosis | Loss of lordosis |
| 2 | I | I | C5-C6 | 29.3 | Loss of lordosis | Loss of lordosis |
| 3 | I | I | C6-C7 | 24.6 | Loss of lordosis | Loss of lordosis |
| 4 | III | I | C6-C7 | 18.0 | Loss of lordosis | Loss of lordosis |
| 5 | I | I | C5-C6, C6-C7 | 17.2 | Loss of lordosis | Lordosis |
| 6 | I | II | C6-C7 | 13.7 | Lordosis | Lordosis |
| 7 | III | I | C4-C5, C6-C7 | 15.9 | Kyphosis | Kyphosis |
| 8 | III | I | C3-C4 | 11.8 | Lordosis | Lordosis |
| 9 | III | I | C4-C5 | 11.7 | Lordosis | Loss of lordosis |
| 10 | I | I | C4-C5, C5-C6 | 10.4 | Lordosis | Kyphosis |
| 11 | III | I | C5-C6, C6-C7 | 18.0 | Lordosis | Lordosis |

From Sekhon LH: Cervical arthroplasty in the management of spondylotic myelopathy: 18-month results. Neurosurg Focus 17(3):E8, 2004.

The use of Bryan disc arthroplasty exclusively in patients with cervical spondylotic myelopathy was reported in a series reported by Sekhon.[36] Eleven patients with MRI-confirmed spinal cord compression or had a clinically confirmed myelopathy were included. A coexistent radiculopathy was present in eight subjects. Six patients had high signal in the spinal cord on $T_2$-weighted imaging. Exclusion criteria included the presence of kyphotic deformity, severe multilevel spondylotic disc degeneration, spinal cord injury with possible instability, or pure radiculopathy secondary to posterolateral disc protrusion or foraminal stenosis. Average follow-up was 18.4 months, ranging from 10 to 32 months. Ten of the 11 (91%) patients had a good or excellent outcome and a statistically significant decrease in Nurick myelopathy scores. Further details of this cohort are presented in Table 95–1.

## Recomendations

Cervical arthroplasty represents an exciting alternative to current strategies for the management of cervical myelopathy. Born out of trying to develop a solution to the shortcomings of cervical fusion surgery, cervical arthroplasty is itself presenting new challenges, some anticipated, others not, and others yet to be seen. Careful patient selection with, at this stage, avoidance of its application in situations of deformity, congenital stenosis, or multilevel disease is prudent, as is the long-term radiologic and clinical follow-up of these patients. Its ultimate role remains to be seen.

## REFERENCES


1. Pickett GE, Van Soelen J, Duggal N: Controversies in cervical discectomy and fusion: Practice patterns among Canadian surgeons. Can J Neurol Sci 31(4):478–483, 2004.
2. Brain WR, Northfield D, Wilkinson M: The neurological manifestations of cervical spondylosis. Brain 75(2):187–225, 1952.
3. Crandall PH, Batzdorf U: Cervical spondylotic myelopathy. J Neurosurg 25(1):57–66, 1966.
4. Payne EE, Spillane JD: The cervical spine: An anatomico-pathological study of 70 specimens (using a special technique) with particular reference to the problem of cervical spondylosis. Brain 80(4):571–596, 1957.
5. Adams CB, Logue V: Studies in cervical spondylotic myelopathy, II: The movement and contour of the spine in relation to the neural complications of cervical spondylosis. Brain 94(3):568–586, 1971.
6. Edwards WC, LaRocca H: The developmental segmental sagittal diameter of the cervical spinal canal in patients with cervical spondylosis. Spine 8(1):20–27, 1983.
7. Yue WM, Tan SB, Tan MH, et al: The Torg-Pavlov ratio in cervical spondylotic myelopathy: A comparative study between patients with cervical spondylotic myelopathy and a nonspondylotic, nonmyelopathic population. Spine 26(16):1760–1764, 2001.
8. Henderson FC, Geddes JF, Vaccaro AR, et al: Stretch-associated injury in cervical spondylotic myelopathy: New concept and review. Neurosurgery 56(5):1101–1113; discussion 1113, 2005.
9. Fehlings MG, Skaf G: A review of the pathophysiology of cervical spondylotic myelopathy with insights for potential novel mechanisms drawn from traumatic spinal cord injury. Spine 23(24):2730–2737, 1998.
10. Kim DH, Vaccaro AR, Henderson FC, Benzel EC: Molecular biology of cervical myelopathy and spinal cord injury: role of oligodendrocyte apoptosis. Spine J 3(6):510–519, 2003.
11. Clarke E, Robinson PK: Cervical myelopathy: A complication of cervical spondylosis. Brain 79(3):483–510, 1956.
12. Lees F, Turner JW: Natural history and prognosis of cervical spondylosis. Br Med J 5373:1607–1610, 1963.
13. Phillips DG: Surgical treatment of myelopathy with cervical spondylosis. J Neurol Neurosurg Psychiatry 36(5):879–884, 1973.
14. Edwards CC 2nd, Riew KD, Anderson PA, et al: Cervical myelopathy: Current diagnostic and treatment strategies. Spine J 3(1):68–81, 2003.
15. Fouyas IP, Statham PF, Sandercock PA: Cochrane review on the role of surgery in cervical spondylotic radiculomyelopathy. Spine 27 (7):736–747, 2002.
16. Kadanka Z, Bednarik J, Vohanka S, et al: Conservative treatment versus surgery in spondylotic cervical myelopathy: A prospective randomised study. Eur Spine J 9(6):538–544, 2000.
17. Kadanka Z, Mares M, Bednarik J, et al: Predictive factors for spondylotic cervical myelopathy treated conservatively or surgically. Eur J Neurol 12(1):55–63, 2005.
18. Kadanka Z, Mares M, Bednarik J, et al: Predictive factors for mild forms of spondylotic cervical myelopathy treated conservatively or surgically. Eur J Neurol 12(1):16–24, 2005.
19. Sampath P, Bendebba M, Davis JD, Ducker TB: Outcome of patients treated for cervical myelopathy: A prospective, multicenter study with independent clinical review. Spine 25(6):670–676, 2000.
20. Ebersold MJ, Pare MC, Quast LM: Surgical treatment for cervical spondylitic myelopathy. J Neurosurg 82(5):745–751, 1995.
21. Kaptain GJ, Simmons NE, Replogle RE, Pobereskin L: Incidence and outcome of kyphotic deformity following laminectomy for cervical spondylotic myelopathy. J Neurosurg 93(2):199–204, 2000.
22. Sekhon LH: Posterior cervical decompression and fusion for circumferential spondylotic cervical stenosis: Review of 50 consecutive cases. J Clin Neurosci 13(1):23–30, 2006.
23. Kawaguchi Y, Kanamori M, Ishihara H, et al: Minimum 10-year follow-up after en bloc cervical laminoplasty. Clin Orthop Relat Res 411:129–139, 2003.
24. Wang MY, Shah S, Green BA: Clinical outcomes following cervical laminoplasty for 204 patients with cervical spondylotic myelopathy. Surg Neurol 62(6):487–492; discussion 492–493, 2004.

25. Hidai Y, Ebara S, Kamimura M, et al: Treatment of cervical compressive myelopathy with a new dorsolateral decompressive procedure. J Neurosurg 90(2):178–185, 1999.
26. Shiraishi T: Skip laminectomy—A new treatment for cervical spondylotic myelopathy, preserving bilateral muscular attachments to the spinous processes: A preliminary report. Spine J 2(2):108–115, 2002.
27. Bailey RW, Badgley CE: Stabilization of the cervical spine by anterior fusion. J Bone Joint Surg Am 42-A:565–594, 1960.
28. Smith GW, Robinson RA: The treatment of certain cervical-spine disorders by anterior removal of the intervertebral disc and interbody fusion. J Bone Joint Surg Am 40-A(3):607–624, 1958.
29. Cloward RB: The anterior approach for removal of ruptured cervical disks. J Neurosurg 15(6):602–617, 1958.
30. Emery SE, Bohlman HH, Bolesta MJ, Jones PK: Anterior cervical decompression and arthrodesis for the treatment of cervical spondylotic myelopathy: Two- to seventeen-year follow-up. J Bone Joint Surg Am 80(7):941–951, 1998.
31. Cummins BH, Robertson JT, Gill SS: Surgical experience with an implanted artificial cervical joint. J Neurosurg 88(6):943–948, 1998.
32. Goffin J, Casey A, Kehr P, et al: Preliminary clinical experience with the Bryan Cervical Disc Prosthesis. Neurosurgery 51(3):840–845, 2002.
33. Goffin J, Van Calenbergh F, van Loon J, et al: Intermediate follow-up after treatment of degenerative disc disease with the Bryan Cervical Disc Prosthesis: Single-level and bi-level. Spine 28(24):2673–2678, 2003.
34. Duggal N, Pickett GE, Mitsis DK, Keller JL: Early clinical and biomechanical results following cervical arthroplasty. Neurosurg Focus 17(3):E9, 2004.
35. Bertagnoli R, Yue JJ, Pfeiffer F, et al: Early results after ProDisc-C cervical disc replacement. J Neurosurg Spine 2(4):403–410, 2005.
36. Sekhon LH: Cervical arthroplasty in the management of spondylotic myelopathy: 18-month results. Neurosurg Focus 17(3):E8, 2004.

CHAPTER 96

# Cervical Arthroplasty Adjacent to Fusion, Multiple-Level Cases, and Hybrid Applications

**Paul C. McAfee, Matthew Scott-Young,** and **Rudolf Bertagnoli**

## KEY POINTS

- Cervical arthroplasty can be safely inserted in combination with or adjacent to anterior cervical discectomy and fusion (ACDF).
- Cervical arthroplasty can reduce the compensatory hypermobility found at cervical levels above ACDF.
- The outcomes of cervical arthroplasty adjacent to ACDF are comparable to virgin arthroplasty but clearly superior to multi-level cervical fusions.
- A hybrid procedure could be performed at two adjacent cervical levels if one level presented with translational instability. This level should be stabilized with fusion if there is 3.5 mm or greater translational instability.
- With progressively more and more vertebral levels of ACDF, the outcomes diminish and the complications increase—pseudarthrosis, instrumentation failure, reduced clinical success. This diminishing trend is not seen with progressive numbers of adjacent cervical arthroplasties.

The use of cervical arthroplasty devices in patients with symptomatic radiculopathy or myelopathy adjacent to a prior anterior cervical decompression and fusion (ACDF) is an attractive reconstructive option, obviating the need for a multilevel fusion surgery. This chapter reports a comparison of outcomes from patients with and without previous ACDF enrolled by five centers in a U.S. Food and Drug Administration (FDA) Investigative Device Exemption (IDE) clinical trial of the Porous-Coated Motion (PCM) artificial cervical disc (Cervitech, Inc., Rockaway, NJ) and PCM experience in Australia and Brazil.

Retrospective reviews of ACDF have described the appearance of new degenerative disc disease (DDD) at levels adjacent to fused segments. Hilibrand[1] has reported that adjacent motion segment disease occurred in 2.9% of patients annually. They found up to 25% of patients developed DDD at adjacent levels within 10 years of the initial surgery and that 7% to 15% of these patients required reoperation. In a recent study, Robertson and associates[2] assessed the incidence of adjacent motion segment disease in patients treated with cervical fusion and arthroplasty. They found the incidence of new symptomatic DDD in the fusion group at 24 months was 13.9% (6.9% annually). In the arthroplasty group, the incidence of adjacent motion segment disease was 1.3% (0.65% annually). The authors demonstrated that maintaining motion, rather than fusion, will prevent symptomatic adjacent disc disease and a reduction in the adjacent level radiologic indicators of disease at a 24-month postoperative interval.

Gore[3] studied lateral radiographic findings in asymptomatic persons with a 10-year follow-up to reveal that degenerative changes progress with age. He found 34% of asymptomatic patients with normal findings on the baseline cervical spine lateral x-rays developed degenerative disc disease 10 years later. He stated that 97% of patients with pre-existent disc degeneration showed progression over 10 years. Adjacent motion segment disease is defined as the development of a new radiculopathy or myelopathy or symptoms referable to a segment adjacent to a previously fused level in the cervical spine. It is thought to arise as a result of the biomechanical alterations and biologic changes that occur in the cervical spine subsequent to treatment.

Schwab and associates[4] found that motion compensation following arthrodesis was distributed through the unfused segments, with significant compensation at the segments adjacent to the fusion. They found significant differences occurring at the level above the fusion site for C3-C4 and C4-C5 in both flexion and extension. When the lower levels were fused, a significant amount of increased motion was observed at the levels immediately above and below the fusion. However, greater compensation occurred at the caudal segments than the cephalad segments for the lower level fusions (C5-C6 and C6-C7).

This chapter focuses on the clinical incidence of adjacent motion segment degeneration and disease in the cervical spine adjacent to a cervical fusion. Hilibrand and associates[1] published a report of 374 patients who had a total of 409 anterior cervical arthrodeses for the treatment of cervical spondylosis. They reported an average annual incidence of the development of adjacent level disease as 2.9%. Survivorship analysis predicted that 25% of the patients (95% confidence interval) who undergo ACDF would have new disease in an adjacent level within 10 years of the operation. They also found that the incidence of new disease at an adjacent level was significantly lower following a multilevel arthrodesis, than it was following a single-level arthrodesis. The concept of the multifocal nature of cervical spondylosis was also introduced.

Ishihara and associates[5] followed 112 patients, clinically and radiologically, for 2 years. The incidence of adjacent motion segment disease/degeneration was 19% and they applied a Kaplan-Meyers Survivorship Analysis to follow the disease-free survivorship in the entire series of patients. They found an 84% incidence at 10 years. They also concluded that adjacent motion segment disease was more common in those who showed asymptomatic disc degeneration preoperatively.

## MATERIALS AND METHODS

For the U.S. study on adjacent segment PCM, patients were enrolled into the initial non-randomized "training" and subsequent randomized investigational device arms of the multicenter clinical trial comparing PCM arthroplasty with ACDF. Inclusion and exclusion criteria specified patients between the ages of 18 and 65 with symptomatic cervical radiculopathy or myelopathy at one level, unresponsive to at least 6 weeks of nonsurgical therapy, or experiencing progressive neurologic symptoms. Of 103 patients enrolled in the IDE study at these sites, 19 patients had previous ACDF at a single adjacent level, and 84 patients had the PCM as a primary intervention. The Neck Disability Index (NDI), neck and arm Visual Analog Scale (VAS) scores, and recorded complications and adverse events for both groups were compared. There was a minimum of 12 months follow-up, the average follow-up being 26 months (range 46–12 months).

Fifty-one patients (31 female and 20 male) were included in the international study group. Entry into the study group required symptomatic evidence of adjacent motion segment disease that required surgical intervention. The primary diagnosis of radiculopathy occurred in 36 patients and myelopathy in 15 patients; 36 patients had a prior one-level fusion, 9 had a prior two-level fusion, and 6 had a prior three-level fusion.

Surgeons from Brazil, Australia, and the United States participated in this study. Each surgeon was asked to participate in the treatment of adjacent motion segment degeneration with total disc replacement (TDR), provided the indications were appropriate. FDA regulations restricted patient selection and the treatment options in the United States. The surgeons in Australia and Brazil were able to treat extensive and complex disease and perform one or more TDRs at adjacent levels, as indicated. Thirty-six one-level PCMs were performed adjacent to fusions (20 from the United States, 11 from Brazil, and 5 from Australia). Nine two-level PCMs were performed (7 in Brazil and 2 in Australia). Six three-level PCMs were performed (4 in Brazil and 2 in Australia). The outcome measures that were utilized included the NDI, VAS, SF-36, and neurologic status. Scores were recorded preoperatively and at 3 months, 6 months, 1 year, and 2 years after surgery where applicable. Cervical lordosis was measured from the posterior surface of the body of C2 in a line parallel to the posterior surface of the body of C7. The postoperative lordosis was measured at the postoperative intervals and the change in lordosis was determined.

Radiographic outcomes included flexion and extension and lateral bending range of motion. Disc space height restoration was measured, the presence of heterotopic ossification was noted, and the translational and rotational stability was assessed.

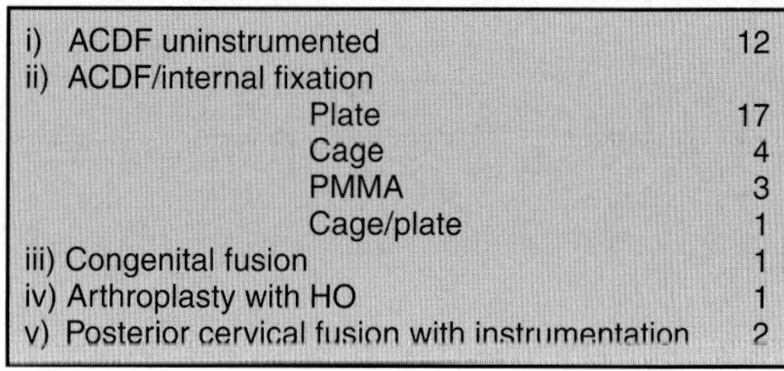

| | |
|---|---|
| i) ACDF uninstrumented | 12 |
| ii) ACDF/internal fixation | |
| Plate | 17 |
| Cage | 4 |
| PMMA | 3 |
| Cage/plate | 1 |
| iii) Congenital fusion | 1 |
| iv) Arthroplasty with HO | 1 |
| v) Posterior cervical fusion with instrumentation | 2 |

**FIGURE 96–1.** Types of prior fusion mechanisms, listing prior instrumented as well as uninstrumented anterior cervical discectomy and fusion (ACDF) procedures

The prior fusion mechanism is illustrated in Figure 96–1; 60% of patients had an ACDF with a form of internal fixation, 30% had an uninstrumented fusion, and 10% had either a posterior spinal cervical fusion, congenital fusion, or a spontaneous fusion around a previous TDR.

Figure 96–2 shows the number of levels fused, compared to the number of levels replaced. As expected, the majority of the fusions involved C4 to C7. Sixty-two levels had undergone arthrodesis at some stage in the past. Fifty-nine prostheses were inserted in the distribution shown in Figure 96–2 and represent treatment of symptomatic discs adjacent to a fusion.

## RESULTS

### U.S. Prospective Randomized Study

Among the 19 patients in the U.S. study with previous "adjacent" fusion, there were 6 males and 13 females with a mean age of 49.1 years. There were 50 males and 34 females with a mean age of 47.0 years comprising the "primary" patients. There were no significant differences in age, height, weight, or body mass index (BMI). Average time of surgery was 97 minutes in the primary group, and 91 minutes in the adjacent to fusion group ($P > 0.1$). Estimated blood loss was 79 mL and 76 mL in the primary and adjacent to fusion groups, respectively ($P > 0.1$). Follow-up at 6 months was reached by 68 primary patients and 15 adjacent patients, and at 12 months by 41 primary patients and 11 adjacent patients. Clinical outcomes were similar between groups at all time points.

Revision for subsidence, misalignment, or device migration occurred in 2 of 84 patients in the primary group, and in 2 of 19 patients in the adjacent to fusion group. One device migration not requiring revision occurred in the adjacent to fusion group. Other reported complications including dysphagia and postoperative neck or arm symptoms were comparable in both groups (Table 96–1).

### International Study

For the international study, the average length of the procedure was 91 minutes. The estimated blood loss was 56 mL on average. The average length of stay was 1.65 days. The mean preoperative cervical lordosis was 2.65 degrees (−32 to 25 degrees). The mean postoperative lordosis was 12.3 degrees (−17 to 30 degrees).

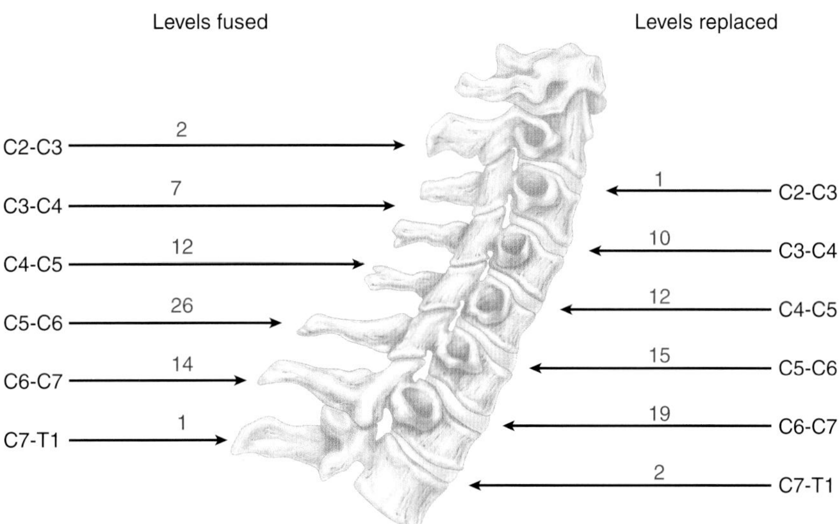


■ **FIGURE 96–2.** A comparison of the number of levels fused with the number of vertebral levels replaced with a Porous-Coated Motion device in the international study.

The mean improvement was 9.4 degrees of cervical lordosis (−15 to 23 degrees). The clinical follow-up period varied from 12 to 46 months, the average follow-up time being 26 months.

There was one revision case that occurred in Australia where the patient had a two-level PCM inserted above a previously uninstrumented C5-C6 fusion. Six weeks postoperatively, the patient was involved in a rear-end motor vehicle accident, sustaining a whiplash injury. Radiographs were taken that showed an anterior lip fracture of the superior surface of C5 with no migration of the inferior end plate of the prosthesis anteriorly. The patient was advised to have a reduction of the fracture to prevent any late mechanical instability. In the operating theater, the end plate was found to be securely fixed to the device. This required removal of the device in order to reduce the fracture and then a new prosthesis was inserted with an inferior flange and two screws. The patient has had an excellent result.

In this international multicenter study, a mean improvement in the VAS of 60.9% was recorded (Fig. 96–3). In terms of the specific regional results, the VAS improvement in Australia was 79.6% (Fig. 96–4). The mean improvement in VAS in the United States was 80%. The mean improvement in VAS in Brazil was 51%.

In this study, the average mean improvement in the NDI was 54% (Fig. 96–3). In regards to regional variations, the mean improvement in NDI in Australia was 53% (Fig. 96–5). The mean improvement in NDI in the United States was 81%. The mean improvement in Brazil was 45%.

The range of flexion and extension motion at the level of prosthesis was a mean of 8.5 degrees (4 to 20 degrees). There was no evidence of translational or rotational instability. All patients were neurologically intact at the conclusion of the study. The disc heights were restored to the heights of the implant (6.5 mm, 7.2 mm, and 8.5 mm). There was no loss of disc height or subsidence noted.

The mean SF-36 physical component summary (PCS) increased to 70% from 38%, representing an 86% improvement. The mean SF-36 mental component summary (MCS) increased to 66% from 43%, representing a 34% improvement. In relation to the significant improvements that were seen in both the physical and mental scores in the SF-36 data, significant improvements occurred within the first 3 months. Between 3 and 6 months, there was no statistical improvement, and between 6 and 12 months, there was a moderate

**TABLE 96–1. Outcomes after PCM Arthroplasty***

| Time | NDI (Primary/ Adjacent) | Neck VAS (Primary/ Adjacent) | Arm VAS (Primary/ Adjacent) |
|---|---|---|---|
| Baseline | 27/27 | 67/73 | 69/78 |
| 6 weeks | 14/14 | 25/31 | 21/28 |
| 12 weeks | 12/11 | 24/30 | 23/21 |
| 26 weeks | 11/11 | 24/33 | 23/26 |
| 52 weeks | 10/11 | 23/24 | 26/25 |

*United States study only.
NDI, Neck Disability Index; PCM, Porous-Coated Motion; VAS, Visual Analog Scale.

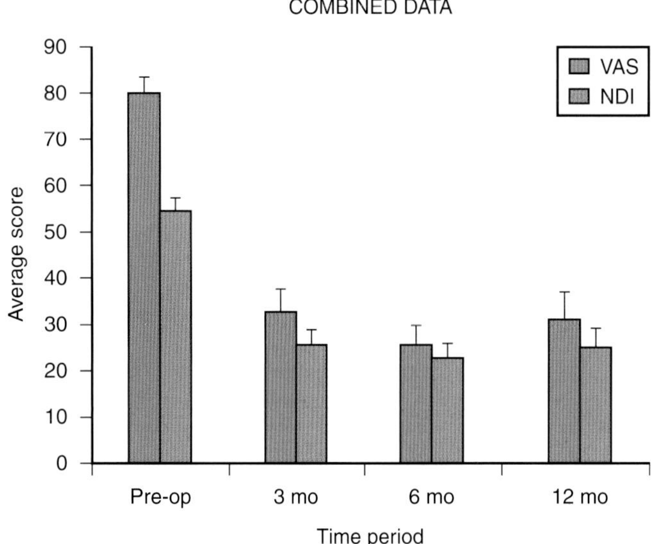


■ **FIGURE 96–3.** The combined Neck Disability Index (NDI) and Visual Analog Scale (VAS) clinical outcomes in the international study.

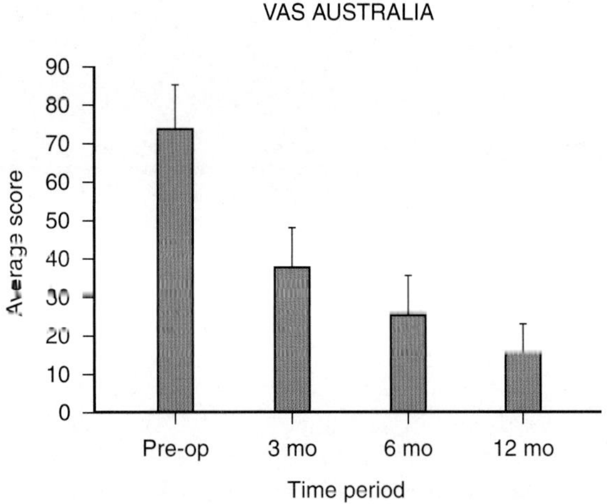


■ **FIGURE 96–4.** Visual Analog Scale (VAS) scores for the patients in Australia. Notice that the speed of improvement is not quite as rapid as for virgin-level cervical arthroplasties, even from the same surgeon's experience.

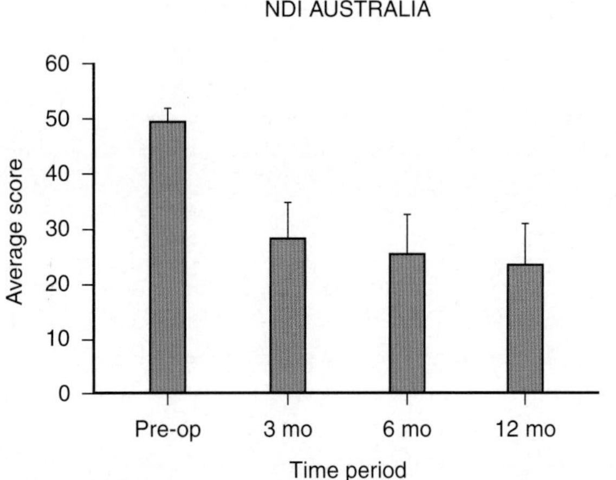


■ **FIGURE 96–5.** The Neck Disability Index (NDI) results of the patients with adjacent level fusions in Australia.

improvement, once again. The data, combined with the NDI data and VAS data, highlight the concept that the patient's pain is initially reduced fairly dramatically but that it takes some time to adjust their functional impairments. There is often a lag between the two. It also highlights the importance of a functional rehabilitation program following surgery. Long-term follow-up is also essential to determine whether the results deteriorate with time.

## DISCUSSION

Cervical arthroplasty adjacent to a previous cervical fusion, as an alternative to multilevel fusion, is an attractive clinical option.[6–8] Although the level adjacent to a prior cervical fusion is subject to altered biomechanical forces, the PCM arthroplasty was well tolerated at these levels. The initial clinical results of PCM arthroplasty adjacent to a prior fusion were excellent and comparable to the outcomes after primary PCM surgery.

Wigfield[9] reported the results of a 2-year pilot study where the new Frenchay Artificial Cervical Joint was inserted in 15 patients. This was a clinically prospective cohort study. All patients had a previous adjacent level surgical fusion or congenital spinal fusion or radiologic evidence of adjacent level degenerative disc disease. Improvements in the VAS scores showed a 45% improvement, NDI a 31% improvement, and SF-36 PCS quotient 14% improvement. The conclusions from the study were that the prosthesis maintains physiologic motion, that the device maintained its position, and the improvements in the functional scores were acceptable.

Tu and associates[10] recently reported the treatment of adjacent motion segment degeneration with the ProDisc-C (Synthes, West Chester, PA) TDR in a prospective study with a minimum of 2 years follow-up and which included 15 patients (Fig. 96–6). They concluded that the results were inferior to historical control subjects. The study showed that the application of a ProDisc-C device for the treatment of adjacent motion segment degeneration only achieved 80% of what a ProDisc-C device achieved in the management of a one-level cervical DDD.

The treatment of adjacent motion segment disease above a fusion has a variety of solutions. A cervical TDR serves to replace a symptomatic degenerative disc, restore the functional biomechanical properties of the motion segment, and protect the neurologic structures. Treatment of adjacent motion segment degeneration with cervical arthroplasty is a very challenging environment, for many reasons (Fig. 96–7). First, these patients are physically and emotionally distraught as they are faced with further surgery that they in all probability did not expect. Second, the patient, by definition, has had a history of prior surgery. As a general rule, all patients with prior spine operations have reduced clinical outcomes compared to patients with virgin procedures. This is why every U.S. prospective randomized clinical arthroplasty trial with the exception of the PCM excludes patients with even one prior cervical arthrodesis. The prior surgery leads to scarring, both externally and internally, which then increases the complication rate. Third, these patients often have internal fixation devices, such as plates, that will need to be removed before the insertion of a prosthesis. This may require a larger dissection than an approach to one level. Often the previously fused level has been inappropriately fixed in a kyphotic position (Fig. 96–8) and the end plates can be damaged by malpositioned screws.

The mechanism of the prior fusion methods in this study is described in Figure 96–1. The variety of instrumentation used increases the complexity of the surgery. As can be seen from the preoperative lordotic angles, considerable kyphosis made these cases extremely challenging, and despite the complicated presenting disease, PCM prostheses successfully restored some element of the cervical lordosis. It also restored stability to the cervical segments, based on the flexion and extension and rotation shown radiologically. It also preserved 8.9 degrees of flexion and extension mobility.

Despite the complexity of the revision cases, the PCM device and its modularity appeared to achieve the goals of the hypothesis of this study. There was also a lower incidence of dysphagia and soft tissue retraction in the cervical arthroplasty cases compared to the ACDF with instrumentation procedures (Fig. 96–9).

The PCM international study is the largest study, to date, investigating prospectively the value of arthroplasty in adjacent motion segment disease. The overall results are encouraging

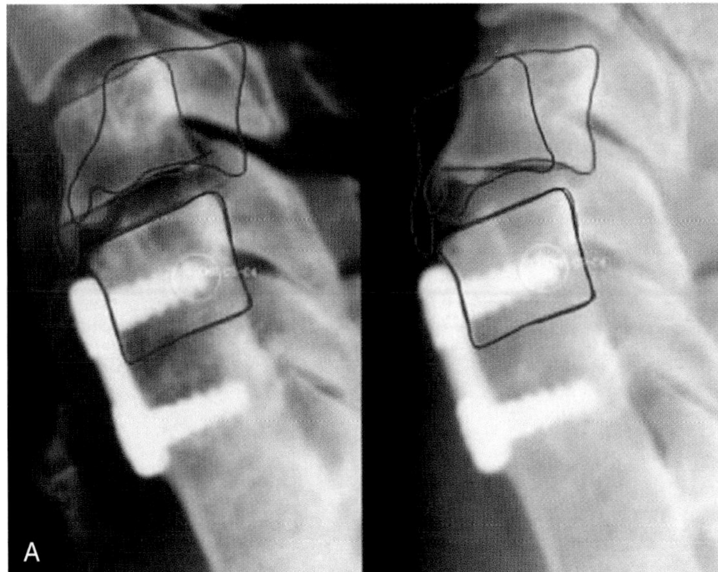


19.7 degrees
pre-op motion

Adjacent level is challenging

1. Excessive motion
2. Previous surgery
3. Prior instrumentation
4. Disc height collapse
5. Localized kyphosis

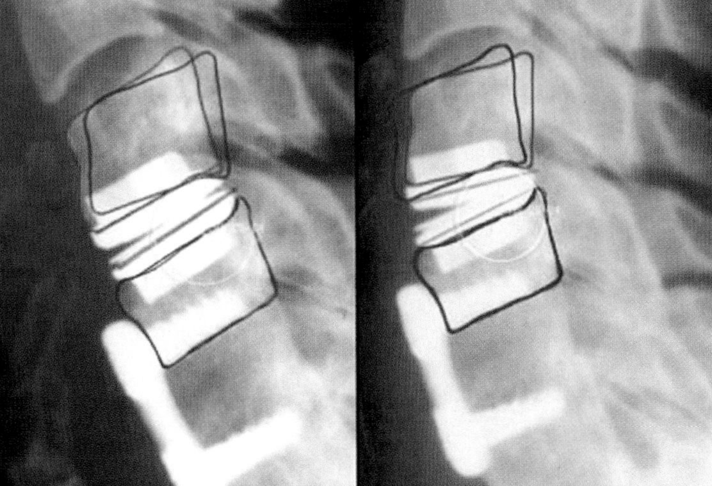


10.0 degrees
post-op motion

Prosthesis has to ratchet down or restrict the mobility

■ **FIGURE 96–6.** This patient had excessive motion at C4-C5 measuring 19.7 degrees on flexion-extension. **A,** Hypermobility is seen adjacent to a prior two-level arthrodesis, instrumented at C5-C6 and uninstrumented at C6-C7. The adjacent level problems include excessive compensatory motion, previous surgery, prior instrumentation, disc height collapse, and localized kyphosis. **B,** The purpose of a cervical arthroplasty is not necessarily to increase motion but rather to make the motion more physiologic within the neutral zone. The C4-C5 level was successfully replaced with a ProDisc-C cervical arthroplasty. Now the postoperative flexion-extension motion is more physiologic at 10.1 degrees, and the patient is clinically much improved.

and discussion is essential in relation to the regional variations in the results. In terms of the American results, these show significant improvements in VAS and NDI and are as good as the historical control results for one-level cervical TDR with the PCM device. It should be noted that, from an FDA perspective, the IDE criteria for the American patients had to be met in that they needed to present with radiculopathy and corresponding neurologic deficit, confirmed by an MRI compressive lesion. The Brazilian and Australian cases were not constrained by the IDE criteria and, as a result, more complex disease was included at these two sites.

Based on the biomechanical data, the clinical studies indicating adjacent motion segment degeneration/disease, and the various solutions to the problem that the surgeons had at their disposal, a study was performed to assess the safety and efficacy of the PCM prosthesis in the treatment of adjacent motion segment disease. In this study of 51 cervical arthroplasty procedures, there was one revision, following a trauma, resulting in one device-related complication, and no approach-related complications. No adjacent motion segment disease had developed adjacent to cervical TDR. There were no cases of heterotopic ossification, and there was no evidence of any neurologic deterioration. Considering the degree

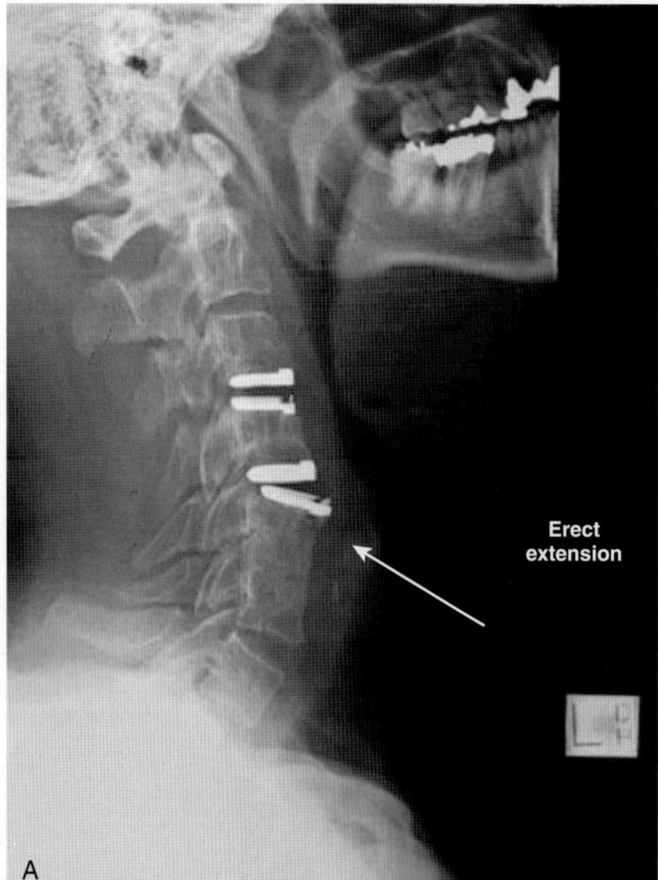


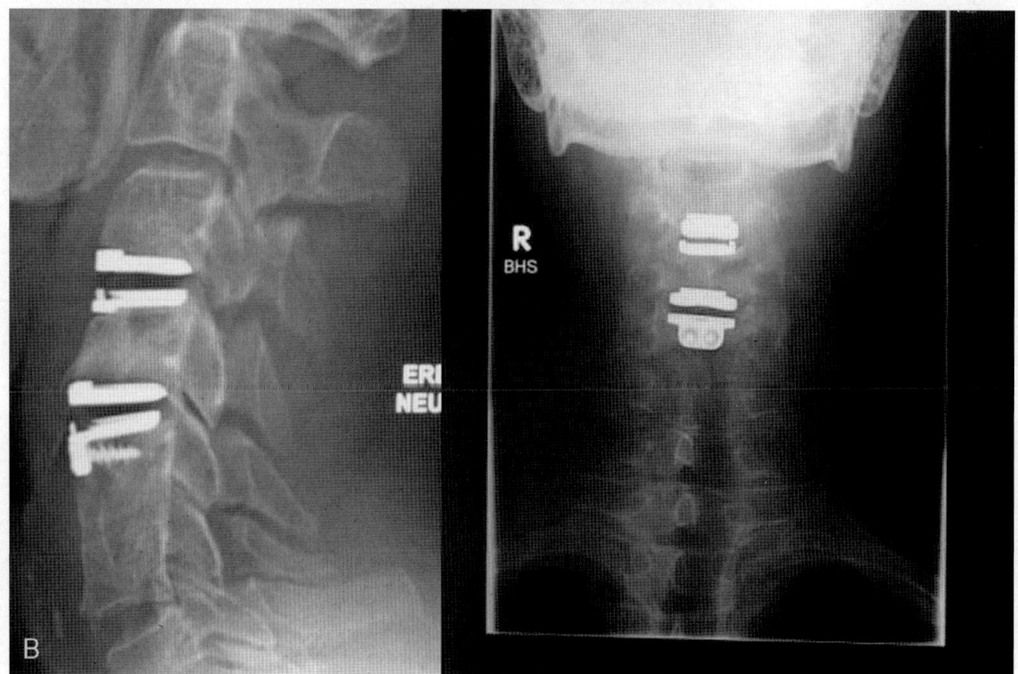


■ **FIGURE 96–7.** This 57-year-old man from Australia had a prior adjacent level fusion at C5-C6. **A,** Five months after a two-level Porous-Coated Motion (PCM) device arthroplasty at C3-C4 and C4-C5, he was involved in a head-on motor vehicular accident and fractured the cephalad C5 vertebral end plate. **B,** The loose prosthesis and C5 fracture were successfully treated by inserting a flanged version of the PCM prosthesis with fixation with two screws. One year later he had preserved cervical motion and was asymptomatic.

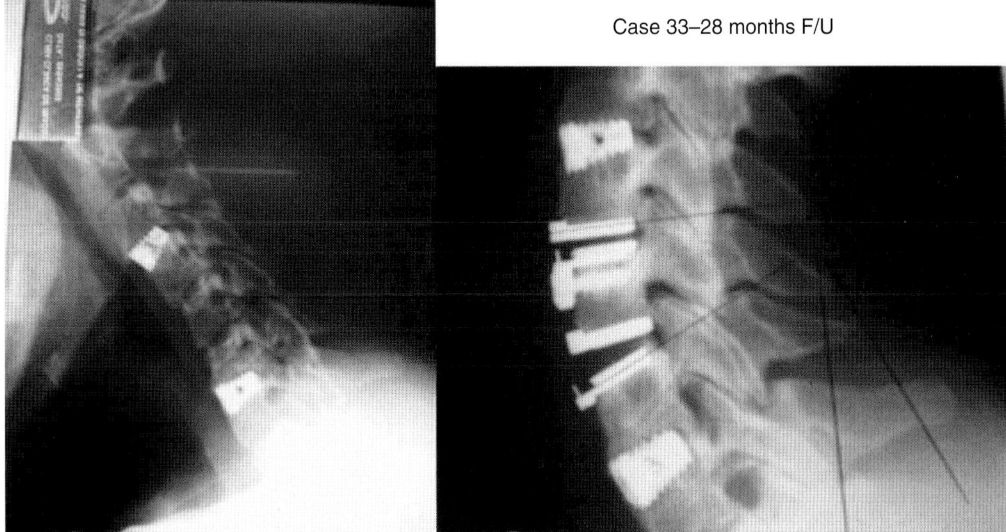


■ **FIGURE 96–8.** This 39-year-old woman had prior lordotic "cages" at C3-C4 and C6-C7 and presented with severe myelopathy and cervical kyphosis. Two-level cervical decompressison and Porous-Coated Motion (PCM) arthroplasties at C4-C5 and C5-C6 successfully corrected 30 degrees of kyphosis and restored 27 degrees of flexion-extension motion. Overall, the 51 patients in the international study improved from a mean of 2.65 degrees of kyphosis to 12.3 degrees of kyphosis. This patient is clinically neurologically intact at 28 months' follow-up.

of difficulty of this group of patients, the clinical success rate, the complication rate, and the revision rate, the author's consensus is that the PCM is a device that is safe and effective for use in patients with adjacent motion segment degeneration in the cervical spine.

The hypothesis was verified showing a significant improvement in functional scores and a reduction in pain scores. In terms of the American results, the results are as good as historical control results when using the PCM prostheses. Yue and associates reported that treating adjacent motion segment degeneration with ProDisc-C prostheses, the results were only 80% of historical controls.[10] This highlights the versatility of the PCM prosthesis in catering for the variety of anatomic and pathologic configurations

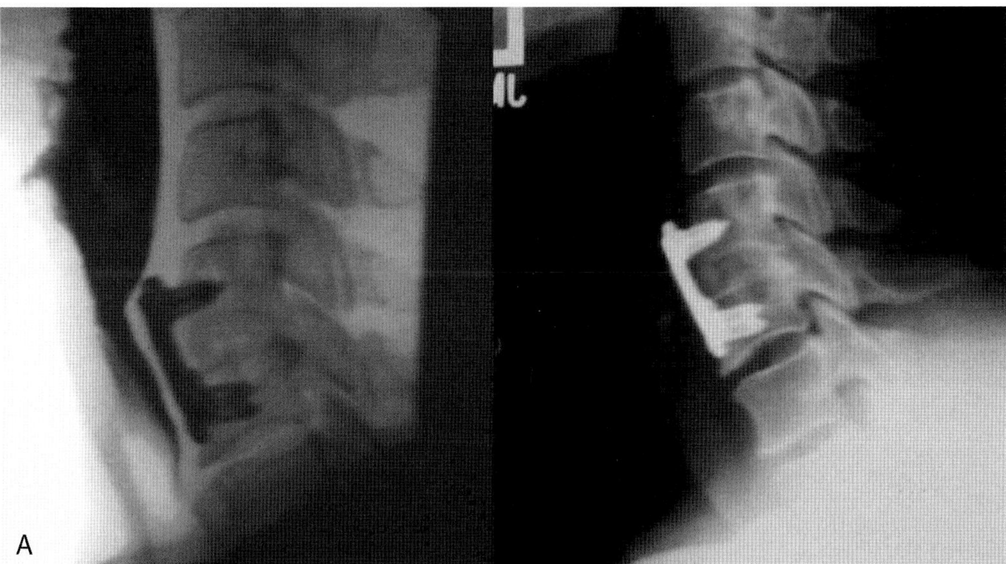


■ **FIGURE 96–9.** Lower incidence of dysphagia with total disc replacement versus anterior cervical discectomy and fusion (ACDF). **A,** This 45-year-old man presented with dysphagia for the last 9 months following ACDF with a poorly placed anterior plate. He could only swallow by leaning forward. His Gastrografin swallow on the left demonstrates the location of esophageal compression from the upper margin of the cervical plate.

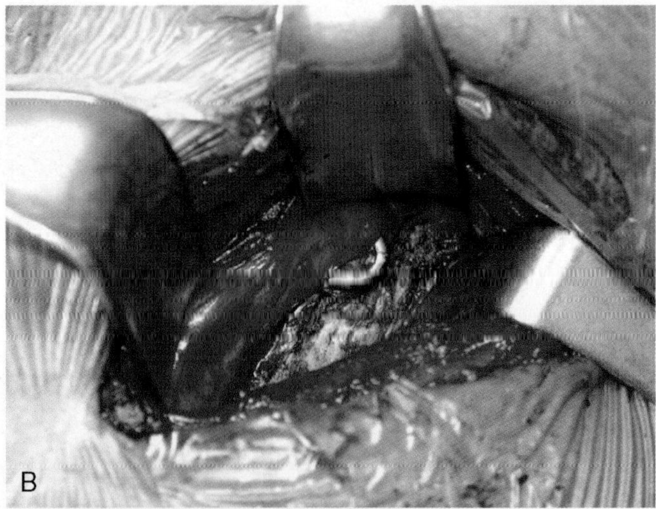

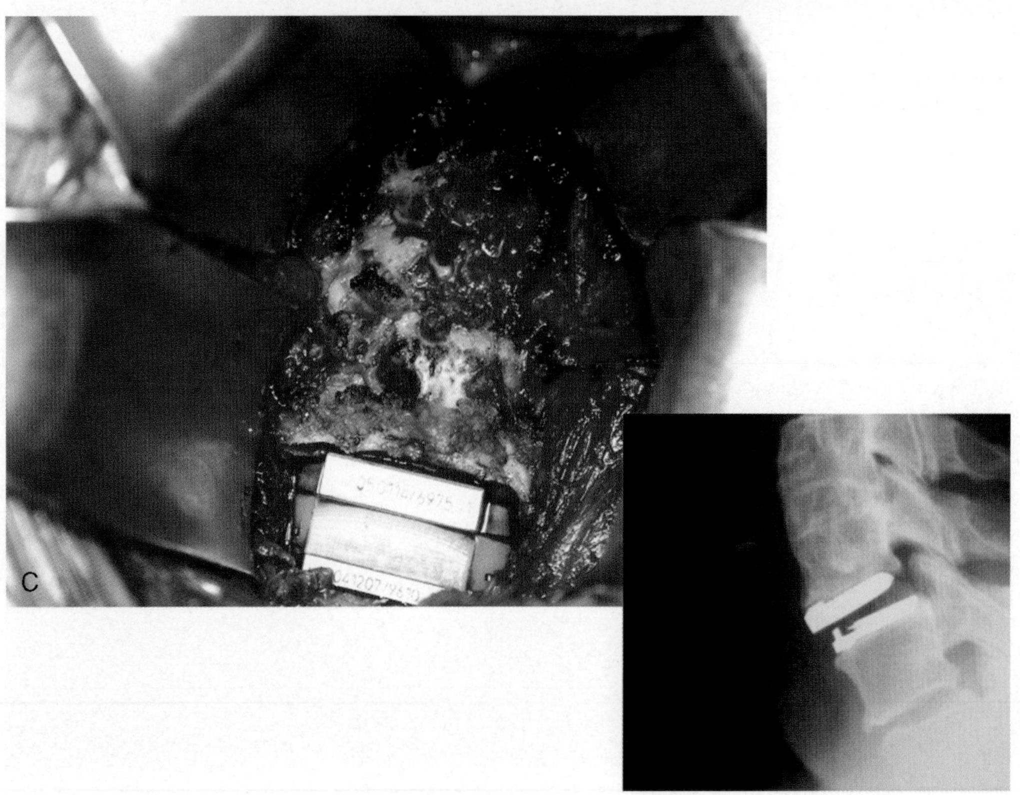

■ **FIGURE 96–9. Cont'd** Lower incidence of dysphagia with total disc replacement versus anterior cervical discectomy and fusion (ACDF). **B,** The patient presented with C6-C7 HNP, and at surgery the esophageal compression was visualized and required a difficult dissection off the hardware. **C,** After removal of the cervical plate and successful C6-C7 cervical discectomy and Porous-Coated Motion (PCM) arthroplasty, not only was the patient's right arm radiculopathy relieved but his dysphagia completely resolved. The PCM device has no anterior profile compared to anterior cervical plates and screws. The severity of dysphagia has been found to correlate with the thickness of the anterior cervical plate instrumentation.

that may be present in an adjacent motion segment that is degenerate and painful.

In terms of the Australian results in comparison to historical control findings within one author's (MSY's) practice, the VAS scores and NDI scores at 12 months of follow-up were exactly the same. However, it appears that the patients treated for adjacent motion segment degeneration took longer to recover following the surgery than the historical control subjects. In terms of the Brazilian data, this also illustrates the fact that multilevel total disc replacements often do better than single-level disc replacements.

In regard to the 51 patients within this international study of PCM applied to adjacent levels, the complexity of the preoperative surgery and the complexities of the preoperative diagnosis tend to lower the results below the historical control results.

## CONCLUSIONS

It is clear that cervical adjacent motion segment degeneration represents a hostile environment for the revision surgeon, first, because of prior surgery and, second, because of the altered mechanics. This is a multicenter prospective descriptive study that showed a mean improvement of 60.9% in VAS and a mean improvement of 54% in NDI.

The safety and efficacy of the device in this biomechanically challenging situation have been proved. Nevertheless, long-term follow-up of these devices is essential.

## REFERENCES


1. Hilibrand AS, Carlson GD, Palumbo MA, et al: Radiculopathy and myelopathy at segments adjacent to the site of a previous anterior cervical arthrodesis. J Bone Joint Surg Am 81(14):519–528, 1999.
2. Robertson JT, Papadopoulos SM, Traynelis VC: Assessment of adjacent segment disease in patients treated with cervical fusion or arthroplasty: A prospective 2-year study. J Neurosurg Spine 3:417–423, 2005.
3. Gore DR: Roentgenographic findings in the cervical spine in asymptomatic persons: A ten-year follow-up. Spine 26(22):2463–2466, 2001.
4. Schwab JS, DiAngelo DJ, Foley KT: Motion compensation associated with single-level cervical fusion: Where does the lost motion go? Spine 31(21):2439–2448, 2006.
5. Ishihara H, Kanamori M, Kawaguchi Y, et al: Adjacent segment disease after anterior cervical interbody fusion. Spine J 4(6):624–628, 2004.
6. McAfee PC, Cunningham BW, Hayes V, et al: Biomechanical analysis of rotational motions after disc arthroplasty. implications for patients with adult deformities. Spine 31(19):S152–S160, 2006.
7. McAfee PC, Geisler FH, Saiedy SS, et al: Revisibility of the Charite Artificial Disc: Analysis of 688 patients enrolled in the US IDE Study of the Charite Artificial Disc. Spine 31(11):1217–1226, 2006.
8. McAfee PC, Geisler FH, Scott-Young M (eds): Roundtables in Spine Surgery: Complications and Revision Strategies in Lumbar Spine Arthroplasty. St. Louis, MO, Quality Medical Publishing, 2005.
9. Wigfield CC, Gill SS, Nelson RJ, et al: The new Frenchay Artificial Cervical Joint: Results from a two-year pilot study. Spine 15:27 (22):2446–2452, 2002.
10. Yue J, Bertagnoli R, Fenk-Mayer A, et al: The treatment of symptomatic adjacent segment degeneration after cervical fusion with total disc arthroplasty utilising the ProDisc-C Prosthesis: A prospective study with 2 year minimum follow-up. Spine J 6:1S–161S, 2006. Proceedings of the NASS 21st Annual Meeting, Seattle, WA, Sept. 28, 2006.

CHAPTER 97

# The Future of Motion Preservation

**Stephen H. Hochschuler** and **Donna D. Ohnmeiss**

## KEY POINTS

- We are already seeing new design concepts for total disc replacements, and nucleus replacements are being evaluated.
- One of the next phases of motion preservation will be combining existing technologies such as anterior and posterior dynamic stabilization.
- Treatment will be improved through increased understanding of pain origins, disc biochemistry, and mechanical function of the spine.
- While spine technology grows, its development and acceptance will have to be founded in critical cost-effectiveness studies, and the key may be identifying specific subgroups of patients who are the best candidates for specific treatments rather than large-scale use of any emerging technology.
- Many metal implants and surgeries may eventually become obsolete and be replaced by biologic and pharmacologic therapies.

## OVERVIEW

Achieving the goal of providing the best care for patients with back and neck pain requires advancements in many areas. These advancements include a better understanding of the pain generators, more reliable diagnostic evaluations (preferably noninvasive), comprehensive understanding of the physiologic effects of various treatment alternatives, and, of course, the treatments themselves. As demonstrated in the various chapters of this book, there are a myriad of emerging treatment options for patients with low back or neck pain. Total disc replacement (TDR) is becoming a commonly used alternative to fusion in patients with symptomatic disc degeneration. There are already new concepts for disc designs being evaluated. Completely new treatment alternatives are also under investigation. There are and will likely continue to be, however, many challenges in the ongoing development and acceptance of these new treatments. In this chapter, we will present ongoing developments in spine technology, including those in the near future as well as those that may emerge years in the future. In addition, challenges to the development and use of these technologies will be discussed.

## NEW KNOWLEDGE

One of the venues by which care may be improved is through advances in our understanding of the spine and pain. This area includes understanding the tissues involved, the chemistry and biomechanics of pain mechanisms, the physiologic effect of various treatments, and the influence of behavioral and psychological factors on pain. Through increased knowledge in each of these areas, more comprehensive and accurate diagnostic evaluations and treatment plans can be derived. The expanding number of treatment options will drive the need for better diagnostics to maximally match the treatment to the individual patient's problem. Fully accomplishing the goal of providing the best possible treatment for each patient will require many years of careful data documentation to assess and reassess indications and outcomes for subgroups of patients undergoing various motion-preserving treatments.

Without a doubt, as knowledge of disc tissue increases so will the treatment options. Not all disc problems are created equal. Much too often in the literature and clinical reports, too many terms are used interchangeably when in actuality there are distinct differences in the various disc diseases. It is likely that true disc degeneration is a normal part of aging. However, disc herniation, disruption, and other problems, which are more typically associated with clinical pain, should not be considered a part of the natural aging process.

## PAIN MECHANISMS

Traditionally, the exact mechanisms of back pain have been poorly understood and often without definitive diagnostic evaluation. One of the reasons for the spine patient being so difficult to treat is that there are many possible origins for pain in the same body region. For example, pain in the buttock region may be related to disc, facets, sacroiliac joints, hips, nerve roots, pyriformis muscle, or any combination of these structures. Noninvasive clinical evaluations with high specificity and sensitivity have yet to be developed to identify pain origin in many patients. Most typically, combinations of clinical signs and symptoms, imaging, and injections are used to confirm some pain origins and rule out others. However, it is likely that in many patients some problems go undiagnosed or the diagnosis is delayed until after treatment for one problem and symptoms persist and further diagnostics are pursued. On the other hand, it is not practical to expose the majority of patients to extensive and expensive injections to fully evaluate every possible source of symptoms. More research is needed in the area of creating inexpensive diagnostic evaluations with high rates of sensitivity and specificity for the various possible origins of back pain. These advances will enhance the matching of treatment with problems, reduce the potential for treating a structural problem not related to symptoms, accelerate the patient's treatment plan, decrease costs, and potentially reduce the chances of patients developing chronic back pain behaviors.

Ongoing research is leading to enhanced understanding of spine-related pain. Discussed here are some of the newer studies that are enhancing our understanding of the tissue and biochemistry of disc-related pain. Not only are some of these studies providing information on discal tissue and pain generators but these results may also have important implications in the development of motion-preserving technologies. This may be particularly true for therapies targeting tissue regeneration, in that the cellular and structural changes that take place within the disc may limit or at least affect the performance of these emerging treatments. Some of the biologic therapies have been investigated in ideal laboratory conditions or in animals with normal discs, but not in models with the type of ruptures and degenerative changes that are being identified in anatomic and biochemical studies of painful discs encountered clinically.

Several inflammatory mediators have been identified in relation to back and radicular pain. Among them are substance P, prostaglandin $E_2$, nitric oxide, TNF-$\alpha$, and interleukins 1, 6, and 8. The exact role of these agents in producing back and leg pain is the topic of much investigation, but a more specific understanding of these inflammatory mediators and their role in different pain situations is developing. For example, Burke and associates found that disc tissue removed from patients with discogenic pain had greater expression of prostaglandin $E_2$, and interleukins 1, 6, and 8.[1]

In addition to enhanced understanding of back pain–related inflammatory mediators, a greater knowledge concerning specific tissue-related changes that occur in an injured disc is being developed. Coppes and associates reported that in discs that were positive on discography, compared to normal discs, there was more extensive innervation in the disc.[2] In particular, these nerve fibers were substance P immunoreactive. In a similar study of discographically positive discs, Freemont and associates found nerve fibers passing into the inner annulus and into the nucleus of some specimens. These fibers expressed substance P. No nerve fibers were found in the control discs.[3] Further investigation in this area involved analyzing disc tissue removed during surgery from patients with positive discograms, aging patients undergoing surgery for stenosis, and control tissue from cadavers.[4] The authors found that a zone of vascularized granulation tissue had formed along the painful disc tears passing from the nucleus to the outer annulus. Nerve growth was noted along the granulation tissue. Substance P, neurofilament, and vasoactive-intestinal peptide immunoreactive nerve fibers in the painful discs were more extensive than in the control discs. The same investigators differentiated asymptomatic degenerated discs, painful discs, and normal discs by comparing the expressions of basic fibroblast growth and its receptor and transforming growth factor-$\beta$1 and its receptor using immunohistochemistry methods.[5] The primary differences were that along the granulation tissue of the painful discs, there were strong expressions of basic fibroblast growth factor, transforming growth factor-$\beta$1, and their receptors, as well as proliferating cell nuclear antigen. These were only weakly noted in the nonpainful discs and in tissue from areas without granulation tissue in the painful disc. There was no expression of these agents in the control discs. Also, differentiating the painful discs was the large number of macrophages and mast cells. Along with these investigations of disc degeneration, results from an animal model found an association between disc degeneration and calcification of the end plate.[6] Such calcification may interfere with the diffusion of nutrients to the disc and be related to degeneration or reduced healing potential after an intradiscal injury.

All of these studies provide an increased understanding of painful disc degeneration. Their findings may provide insight as to challenges that are likely to be encountered when trying to develop tissue engineering based therapies.

## PAIN IMAGING

One emerging area of research that has the potential to greatly impact all types of pain-related treatment, including those in the spine, is pain imaging of the brain. This application was developed in the 1990s and was based on PET (positron emission tomography) and SPECT (single photon emission computed tomography) imaging. Now it is possible to use functional MRI (magnetic resonance imaging) to perform imaging of the brain to investigate patterns associated with changes in pain. This technology has application in pharmacologic studies.[7] It is anticipated that fMRI will become a valuable tool in evaluating responses to various spinal treatment interventions, both nonoperative and operative. This evaluation should compliment emerging back pain therapies such as inhibitors for TNF-$\alpha$ and other inflammatory mediators that have been implicated in chronic back pain.

## BIOMECHANICS

Traditionally in the spine, a biomechanical relationship has been the primary explanation sought for many of the types of back pain. However, there remains a chasm between biomechanical concepts and information that can be applied during the treatment of an individual patient. The concept of the neutral zone has been widely accepted. However, in terms of treating an individual, no clinically executable definition has been developed. In relation to total disc replacement, there has been discussion of the center of rotation of various implants as well as the merits of constrained, semi-constrained, and unconstrained devices. However, there has been no compelling evidence provided concerning how these concepts influence patient outcomes. A stronger relationship between biomechanical knowledge, theory, and the clinical situation needs to be developed.

New implants such as the Theken disc open the door for exploration into the loads on the disc in everyday use. This device is an artificial disc with electronics that allows monitoring of the loads and movement of the implant. The data are read with an external unit. There will likely be important information gained on the influence of implant position within the disc space and the load-bearing capability demanded from it. Implants such as this, incorporating microelectronics, will allow the collection of "real life" data on how spines function. This type of information may have a significant impact in improving computerized models used for spine research as well as changing the biomechanical testing protocols for spinal implants due to the more direct information gained on the demands on the disc in everyday life. This device has been implanted in a few patients outside the United States and data are currently being collected on the functioning of the implant.

## CURRENT TECHNOLOGIES

### Total Disc Replacement

Total disc replacement may no longer qualify as a "new technology." It was first used clinically in the 1980s. There are long-term data available from Europe supporting that these implants are safe and effective following more than 10 years of use.[8] All the current designs to date depend on the basic concept of motion through the articulation of curved surfaces. However, the next generation is being introduced that is made of materials with properties that more closely mimic the properties of the natural disc. This concept was described years ago by Lee and associates[9] and is currently coming to fruition with clinical trials being initiated. Rather than allowing motion through sliding surfaces, these new devices allow motion through the compression of the materials making up the disc.

### Nucleus Replacement

Nucleus replacements can be divided into three basic types: injectable, soft implants, and hard implants. The very first nuclear implant was the stainless steel ball described by Fernstrom. These were implanted into the disc space after discectomy, and they reportedly produced results superior to discectomy alone, although in some patients, they eventually subsided into the vertebral bodies. The first modern-day nucleus replacement to undergo widespread use, and now clinical trials, is based on a hydrogel as first described as a discal implant by Ray and called the PDN (prosthetic disc nucleus; Raymedica, Inc., Minneapolis, MN).[10,11] Initially there were problems with displacement, but changes in the implant design should address this problem. Just as the CHARITÉ total disc replacement (DePuy Spine, Raynham, MA) was based on studies of the motion of the natural disc, the PDN was based on the hydrostatic properties of the disc nucleus. Several nucleus replacements exist that are based on hydrogel technologies. These implants should absorb water after being implanted into the nuclear cavity and subsequently mimic the natural disc nucleus.

In addition to hydrogels and other "elastic" materials that allow motion through compression of the implanted device, one mechanical nucleus replacement has been introduced. The NeuDisc (Replication Medical, Cranbury, NJ) is similar in concept to the current total disc replacements by allowing motion through sliding articulation between concave and convex surfaces.

One concern with nuclear implants is that most require the implant to pass through the disc annulus. There is concern that this may possibly initiate degeneration of the annulus. However, if the artificial nucleus can reduce the load on the annulus, this may not be of clinical relevance. This potential problem may be avoided altogether with the tran-S1 technique of approaching the disc space through the sacrum and thus not violating any of the annular layers while providing access to the nucleus.

### Posterior Dynamic Stabilization

In addition to the disc replacements, there have been numerous dynamic posterior stabilization devices developed in recent years. Many of these have incorporated adaptations from existing pedicle screw technology with flexible rods and screws. The primary mechanical goal of these implants is to allow controlled motion. Pedicle anchoring has also been used for new devices such as the TFAS (Archus Orthopedics, Redmond, WA), TOPS (Impliant Spine, Princeton, NJ), and Anatomic Facet Replacement System (Facet Solutions, Logan, UT). One additional posterior dynamic device is the M-Brace (Advanced Spinal Technologies, Boca Raton, FL), which is designed to be implanted using a minimally invasive technique. These new technologies are currently being evaluated in clinical trials. The future will undoubtedly bring more variations of pedicle screw dynamic devices such as that being developed by Innovative Spinal Technologies (IST, Mansfield, MA).

### Interspinous Spacers

Another type of dynamic posterior instrumentation is the interspinous spacer. These devices are designed to be minimally invasive and provide distraction. The first of these devices to receive FDA approval for sale in the United States was the X-STOP (Kyphon, Inc., Sunnyvale, CA). This device was investigated for the treatment of spinal stenosis and favorable results were achieved.[12] It provides symptomatic relief by distracting the foramen and decreasing the potential for nerve root compression. Currently, several other types of spinous process spacers are undergoing formal clinical evaluation, including the Wallis (Abbot Spine, Austin, TX), Diam (Medtronic Sofamor Danek, Memphis, TN), and coflex (Paradigm Spine LLC, New York, NY). Some of these devices will be investigated to determine their effectiveness in the treatment of symptomatic disc degeneration by unloading the disc. The concept of this type of technology, decreased cost (compared to open decompression or fusion), minimally invasive surgical approaches, and possible applications in patients who are not good candidates for the alternative treatment (such as multilevel decompression or fusion in elderly patients for treating stenosis) may set a new standard for emerging implant technologies.

### Spinous Process Plate

In the arena on minimally invasive implants, an interspinous plate has been described.[13,14] The goal of the device is to provide the same degree of stability to the lumbar spine as pedicle screws and rod systems, but to achieve this using a minimally invasive surgical technique. The plate appears to be simpler to implant than percutaneous pedicle screws. A biomechanical study found that the plate provides stability very similar to bilateral pedicle screws and rods.[14] Results of a clinical study found that the plate could be implanted in significantly less time and with less blood loss compared to pedicle screw placement through an open approach or a technique using a tubular retractor.[13] Additionally, the implant did not result in an increased rate of pseudoarthrosis of the anterior interbody fusion graft.

### Percutaneous Osteoporotic Fracture Treatment

One of the advances in recent years has been the methods for treating osteoporotic spinal fractures. However, there is potential for improvement in these treatments that will likely be addressed in the near future. Two issues are the density of the PMMA (polymethyl/methacrylate) that is currently used for the treatment and the possibility for the material to leak through fractures in the vertebrae. A strong, less dense injectate is desirable due to the potential for fracture of the adjacent vertebrae when the dense PMMA is injected. It may be possible to use materials similar to existing bone graft supplements to inject into the fractured body. This should help to reduce the problem of adjacent vertebral body fracture. Also emerging in the treatment arena for spinal fractures are technologies to re-establish the vertebral body height such as the systems from Crosstrees Medical (Boulder, CO) and Spine-Wave Inc. (Shelton, CT).

### Combined Motion-Preserving Technologies

Just as there became a role for combined anterior/posterior fusion, there will likely be a role of combined anterior/posterior dynamic stabilization. A biomechanical study investigating such a combination has already been undertaken.[15] A CHARITÉ device combined with the TOPS device posteriorly was compared to the intact spine. This combined construct provided good results. No clinical application of combined motion retaining technologies, however, has been found.

Development and evaluation of combined disc and posterior arthroplasty systems are under way such as the Total Spinal Motion Segment system (Disc Motion Technologies, Boca Raton, FL), the flexible spine segment replacement system being developed by Flexuspine, Inc. (Tyler, TX).

## EMERGING NEW THERAPIES

One of the most exciting areas for the treatment of back pain is the possibility of treating back pain using pharmacologic or biologic agents. As discussed earlier in this chapter, a better understanding of the disc and its role in pain is continually developing. From this knowledge, biologic and pharmacologic therapies may be possible. This area holds the promise of directly addressing chemically mediated pain as well as regenerating deteriorating disc tissue. This technology well may make many of the metallic implants obsolete. In the pharmacologic arena, therapies targeting pain caused by inflammatory mediators may be used. Some investigation in this area has already been undertaken for disc herniation. Clinical investigation using a TNF-α inhibitor originally yielded favorable results; however, results of a randomized trial found it provided no benefit over placebo.[16,17] A study with a small series has been published on the perispinal injection of etanercept, a TNF-α inhibitor, with very favorable results.[18] However, it should be noted that the authors included favorable response as an inclusion criteria for the study reported and therefore the number of patients in whom the injection was beneficial versus not beneficial cannot be determined.

Painful disc ruptures are associated with neovascularization in a zone of granulation tissue that forms along annular tears.[4] Based on this finding, combined with the reported neurotropic effect of methylene blue, investigators conducted a prospective clinical trial to determine if it could be used to treat painful disc disruption. A series of 24 patients with chronic back pain but no radicular symptoms, and for whom interbody fusion was considered to be indicated based on positive discography, underwent methylene blue intradiscal injection. The authors reported significant improvement after the injections that was sustained during a minimum 12-month follow-up. There were no complications in the series. Further investigation in a large series of patients is needed to verify these encouraging findings.

The intradiscal injection of steroids has also been investigated.[20] The results of the randomized trial found that this treatment yielded no significant benefit. Other approaches have been described for the injection therapy of disc-related pain. Some of the effects of disc injury and degeneration are dehydration of the disc and reduced proteoglycans. To treat these effects, the injection of glucosamine and chondroitin sulfate combined with hypertonic dextrose and dimethyl sulfoxide (DMSO) has been investigated.[21] This analysis was undertaken in a series of 30 patients who had a positive discogram. At a mean follow-up of 12 months, the overall group improved significantly based on pain and function questionnaires. However, the authors noted that 43% of patients had little or no improvement and the remaining 57% of patients had very good outcomes. Factors related to the poor outcomes were failed surgery, stenosis, and long-term disability. The authors also noted that patients had moderate to severe pain 48 to 72 hours following the injections.

### Biologics and Tissue Engineering

A host of studies has discussed various potential ways to restore disc tissue. Some of these methods are based on the concept of preventing, or at least slowing the rate of, disc degeneration. Other possible treatments have the goal of either replacing or regenerating disc tissue. The following is an overview of some of the most recent reports related to the biologic therapy of the intervertebral disc.

BMP has been shown to increase bony fusion rates in interbody fusion procedures. There is also a potential for BMP to result in enhanced disc tissue growth. In a recent study, apoptosis was induced by TNF-α or hydrogen peroxide in disc cells removed during surgery.[22] The authors found among the cells that were pretreated with BMP, apoptosis was retarded, which may help guard against degeneration. There is interest in determining if osteogenic protein-1 (OP-1) can be used to regenerate disc tissue. In a bovine study, it was found that OP-1 significantly increased the proteoglycan content of cells from the disc nucleus, inner annulus, and outer annulus.[23]

Another strategy emerging for discal repair is providing a scaffold to guide and encourage restorative cell growth. This type of tissue restorative therapy was recently described in a study using a rabbit model.[24] The authors found that using atelocollagen scaffolds, disc nucleus cells were responsive to growth factors.

This type of work lays the groundwork for further development of tissue engineering using scaffolds. Wilke and associates performed a biomechanical study to determine the feasibility of using a scaffold consisting of a collagen matrix seeded with cells to be placed into the nuclear cavity.[25] They found that the implant restored disc space height, although there was a significant problem with device extrusion. The authors indicated that overcoming extrusion of implanted devices is one of the primary biomechanical challenges that must be overcome in order for the scaffold-based therapies to be optimized. They suggested that a means by which to seal the annulus may help reduce the problem of extrusion.

One strategy for addressing painful disc degeneration following disc injury is to treat patients very early after rupture of the disc annulus. To investigate one such possible treatment, disc injury was induced in an ovine model.[26] PMMA microspheres and collagen were then injected along the tear. Sacrifice of the animals revealed that the microspheres maintained their position and were encapsulated. The tear was healed with the growth of the new collagen and without severe inflammatory response. There was no evidence of neovascularization along the tear. While the treated discs went on to heal, the control disc showed signs of progressive degeneration. The authors concluded that the injection slowed or prevented the degeneration that typically occurs after disc injury and suggested that further investigation for early disc therapy was warranted.

Based on the potential of stem cells to grow various tissue types, there has been an interest in spine applications. In a small clinical trial of 10 patients with discogenic pain, Haufe and Mork injected hematopoietic stem cells obtained from the patient's pelvis into the disc.[27] The authors reported that this treatment was ineffective in reducing pain.

Another therapy that has been evaluated in a clinical series is disc chondrocyte transplantation.[28] Following success in animal studies, this treatment was undertaken in humans. Patients were randomized to discectomy alone versus discectomy combined with autologous disc chondrocyte transplantation into the disc. The transplantation required an injection performed after the chondrocytes were expended for 12 weeks. The patients were followed for 2 years. The authors reported that the pain relief was greater in the chondrocyte treated group compared to the discectomy only group. Also, disc hydration was maintained in the chondrocyte group, unlike the control group in which it decreased over time. The authors concluded that the treatment was feasible and prevented ongoing degeneration following discectomy.

Another possible intradiscal therapy is the injection of growth factor into the disc. This has been studied using a rabbit model with favorable results reported.[29] The authors found that an injection of OP-1 restored the biomechanical properties of the intervertebral disc.

A very good update and review of potential molecular therapies for disc degeneration was recently published by Yoon and Patel.[30] The authors described four categories of molecules currently being investigated for possible therapeutic application in intradiscal therapy. These included anticatabolic, mitogens, morphogen, and intracellular regulators. As the authors noted, in vitro data are available for these molecules, although few have been evaluated in animal models evaluating their potential as a treatment for disc problems.

As seen in other chapters in this book, there are promising new technologies for regeneration of disc tissue. Exactly which of these biologics will emerge as the best for painful disc disruption will require much investigation. It may be that some of the biologics will be combined with mechanical annular repair devices or even the interspinous devices. Such combined therapies would allow unloading of the disc, creating an environment that may maximize the chances for tissue regeneration.

### Unloading the Disc

One well-accepted contributor to disc injury and degeneration has been the mechanical load put upon the disc. Although the disc is dependent upon load to stimulate the diffusion of nutrients into the disc, there is a point at which the disc may become overloaded, resulting in injury. It has long been known that during periods of load bearing the disc loses hydration, while during periods of rest, or unloading, the disc rehydrates and its height increases. The effect of loading and unloading the disc has been studied in animal models using external fixation to compress and unload the disc.[31] The investigators found that distraction of the disc space resulted in rehydration, stimulated extracellular matrix gene expression, and increased in the number of protein-expressing cells. These data support that there may be a role for mechanical disc unloading in conjunction with cell-based intervertebral disc therapies to help create an environment favorable for stimulating cell growth. As previously discussed, some of the interspinous spacers may play a role in reducing the load on the intervertebral disc.

Data concerning the unloading of the disc with dynamic stabilization devices are starting to emerge. Putzier and associates reported that Dynesys (Zimmer Spine, Inc., Warsaw, IN) had a protective effect on the disc following nucleotomy.[32] It cannot be clearly determined if the benefit was related to disc unloading, controlled motion, or a combination of the two.

## CHALLENGES

Small-scale early investigations of various potential therapeutics, as discussed earlier, are starting to provide insight into possible new treatments for back pain. However, the results need to be interpreted with care. For several of these studies, the patients undergoing treatment are very select and the results may not be achieved with less homogeneous patients. With medication as well as BMP applications for spinal fusions, the dosing may have a significant impact on the effectiveness of the treatments investigated. Much more research will be needed to determine which emerging therapies are beneficial and to refine the dosing.

Like all technologies, biologics face many challenges. While the results from many studies conducted in laboratories using only cell cultures in extremely controlled conditions yield promising results, which one will emerge as effective in adult patients? What are the long-term safety concerns of some of the proposed gene-based therapies?

There may also be a lot of work required to determine the window of opportunity with respect to timing the intervention in relation to pain onset. As described by Peng and associates,[4,5,33,34] as the disc is injured and the degenerative process progresses, there are changes in the composition of the disc tissue. These changes include neovascularization and the formation of granulation tissue along the tears in the annulus. The long-term influence of these structural changes within the disc on efforts to regenerate disc tissue or for nuclear repair remains to be seen. Also, as attempts are made to encourage the disc to regenerate tissue, a question arises as to the quality of the tissue that will be regenerated. As described by Roberts and associates,[35] some disc cells demonstrate senescence. This occurred much more frequently in herniated discs than in normal discs or discs related to discogenic pain. While this finding provides new insight into cell biology, as the authors discussed, it also has very important implications in tissue engineering and intradiscal gene therapy in that if such cells are used, the desired regeneration may not occur. This consequence is particularly important considering that the highest rate of senescence was found in herniated discs. It has been suggested that disc tissue removed surgically to relieve back pain could be used for tissue engineering; however, these findings suggest that such tissue may be less than optimal for therapeutic interventions.

Getting cells to grow in ideal laboratory conditions is a first step, but the real question remains: Which will grow within the human body to an extent that will provide favorable clinical results? There are also many environmental factors to consider in attempting to regenerate disc tissue in back pain patients and relieve pain:

Considering that the end plates are the conduit for nutrition to the disc, what is the role of end plate assessment, such as Modic changes, in determining if the environment will support new cell growth? If the end plates became too dense, either leading to degeneration in the first place or as a result of degeneration, can enough nutrition be transferred to the disc to sustain regenerative cell growth?

What is the ideal biomechanical environment for new cells to grow within the disc? Too much load may compromise cell life, but some load is needed to stimulate tissue growth.

Can the load within the disc be manipulated by devices such as intraspinous spacers or other implants to create the ideal biomechanical environment for new cell growth?

In the future, is there a potential role for microelectromechanical systems (MEMS) to assess the load in the disc space to provide information concerning if the ideal environment has been achieved and maintained?

If therapy involves regeneration of the existing disc tissue, is there a potential problem in that the factors that originally led to deterioration in the first place will result in the failure of the regenerated tissue as well?

Will changes that take place following disc injury, such as neovascularization and the formation of granulation tissue, lead to failed attempts to regenerate healthy tissue and diminish the patient's pain? Or once these changes in the disc have occurred, is it too late to use biologics to treat disc-related symptoms?

## CURRENTLY EMERGING HIGH-TECH TREATMENTS

Over the past several years, image-guided systems and robotics have been adapted to spine applications. A few articles have been published on the development of image-guided and robotic systems.[36–40] This technology was primarily introduced in routine spine surgery for pedicle screw placement, but potential applications for disc arthroplasty are being investigated. The image-guided systems have not yet gained widespread acceptance. One concern is the accuracy of the registration systems. Even slight misalignment has the potential to create significant malpositioning of the instrumentation. As with any electronic technology, each advance in development provides significant improvement over its predecessor. A remaining question is addressing the potential variation introduced by the patient positioning required for surgery on the accuracy of the registration when based on images with the patient lying supine in a scanner or when the relationship of the vertebral bodies has been altered during the surgical procedures, as occurs with distraction of the disc space. Perhaps the greatest challenge for these devices will be addressing the cost-effectiveness of their utilization. If a specific image scanning protocol has to be employed to generate the images to be used with the registry system, this also increases the overall cost of these systems. The data needed will be related to demonstrating if the benefits gained by more accurate device placement potentially achieved by this technology can overcome its costs.

### Electronics and Other Downstream Technologies

We are already seeing the incorporation of electronics into spinal devices such as the Theken disc. This type of microtechnology may be incorporated into other implants to provide valuable information related to the load demands and function of various implants. The next phase of electronics in spinal implants may be those that actually respond to changes in their environment or play a role in stimulating tissue or dispensing pharmacologic agents. These microelectronics and possibly nanotechnology may be programmed in such a way as to sense changes in their environment and respond to such. For example, a device may be programmed to sense an acute increase in neurotoxic agents being released from the disc and respond by releasing a predetermined dosage of anti-inflammatory medication. Other devices may also be programmed to respond to acute changes in load, that is, to trigger the implant to provide more resistance during activities that place greater loads on the spinal column and then become less rigid during rest times. Perhaps one of the applications of nanotechnology in the spine is for an extremely small device to be programmed to detect neurotoxic agents and destroy them.

Microelectromechanical systems (MEMS) are extremely small "smart" devices. That is, they can be programmed to respond to changes in their environment, usually triggered by chemical or mechanical alterations. The devices include a circuit board and may incorporate motors, sensors, gears, pumps, and other items needed to perform the desired task.

Several applications of MEMS technology in the spine have been described. These included measuring load or pressure within a bone graft or fusion cage.[41] This information may provide insight into the biomechanics of bone healing and modeling in a fusion mass. Devices utilizing MEMS technology may also act on the information they collect. For example, if the device senses a pattern or trigger for pseudoarthrosis in a fusion mass, it may be programmed to release BMP at a certain point to maximize the chances of achieving a bony union without any other surgical intervention.

Aebersold described the design of a MEMS device to be used with posterior internal fixation combined with posterior fusion.[42] The device incorporates a telemetry unit that records stresses on the fusion rods. The theory is that reduced stress on the rod is indicative of fusion mass incorporation. Such a device could provide a noninvasive means to assess fusion that is more reliable than currently used radiographs.

Perhaps one of the most important potential applications of MEMS and nanotechnology is in the area of spinal cord injury. The knowledge base is increasing dramatically in the area of understanding the function and growth patterns of the spinal cord. It may be possible to use MEMS to stimulate and guide the growth of neural tissue in such a way as to repair or replace damaged tissue, thus restoring function to a person with a devastating spinal cord injury.

Some of the potential challenges in the process of incorporating MEMS technology in medical applications have been discussed.[41] The human body is a harsh environment for many materials, including those used in the design of MEMS devices. The humidity is high and the body often mounts a response, including inflammation and scarring, that may compromise the performance of these implants.

## Patient Selection

Although there is great excitement over developing new technologies, old facts must be considered. As always, patient selection is vital for good clinical outcome for any spine surgery, including motion-preserving technologies. As our diagnostic evaluations improve and more knowledge is gained concerning the role of chemical irritation of neural tissue, the role of facet and sacroiliac joints, as well as the disc itself, clinical outcomes will likely improve as well. One well-documented component of clinical outcome in spinal surgery is the strong role of psychological factors.[43] Preoperative screening has been shown to be helpful in differentiating patients who do well following surgery from those who do not.[44] Even with TDR, it has recently been found that the single factor most strongly related to the extremes of total disc replacement was the length of time off work prior to surgery. Factors that were not related were device placement, age, gender, level operated, body mass index, previous discectomy, as well as preoperative pain and function scores. More extensive understanding and evaluation of psychosocial factors should improve the chances of the full potential of new treatment technologies to be reached. Some of the less invasive biologic and pharmacologic interventions may have the added benefit of being administered early after pain onset. This timing may help to improve results by providing treatment before the patient lapses into a pattern of chronic pain behavior.

## As Technology Changes, so Do Patients

Not only is technology changing the treatments available to back pain patients, it is changing our patients themselves. The ready access to the Internet has created a new generation of patients. Many are much better educated than patients in the past. They now have access to the same abstracts, meeting proceedings, and often literature that previously had primarily been limited to care providers. The Internet also provides many sources of information on various web pages that provide good quality information on anatomy, various diagnoses, and treatment options. But for all the benefits, the Internet also provides the opportunity for misinformation and biased communication. There is no regulation for quality control on the web. This situation can have detrimental effects for patients seeking information upon which to make their decisions about treatment options. In addition, there is the potential for sales of unfounded therapies touted by "experts" and numerous testimonials. One responsibility care providers should take on is to help patients locate unbiased web pages. This assistance should help patients become better educated on their spine-related problem and the care options available to them. Computers have also made it possible to provide patients much better education in the office than what was previously available. In our clinic, for example, we have created several interactive Power Point educational programs with voice overlay. Such materials require time to produce but provide patients with visual as well as audio explanations that are easy to understand. The materials can also be produced in handouts or CDs for patients to take home to review the content or to share with their family members.

## Limiting Factors

Although the future of spine technology is exciting, there are also factors potentially limiting its fruition. Perhaps the greatest factors are cost, safety, and proven effectiveness. It is clear that new "add-on technologies" such as image guidance combined with existing pedicle screw or TDR add cost to the procedures. The outstanding question remains: Is the new technology cost-effective? It is possible that such technology is cost-effective in subgroups of patients but not if used for all cases. The key will be to identify the subgroups in which it is cost-effective and avoid its routine use unless proven to be cost-effective for all cases.

We can learn much from the history of other spine technologies. In the report by Bono and Lee, despite the enthusiasm over pedicle screws, there are not much data to support that they resulted in a significantly improved clinical outcome.[46] Although the implants inevitably add to the cost of the surgery, the technology might not be to blame. As discussed here, responsible use and employment of well-defined selection criteria will be key for the benefit of the new treatments to be realized.

In the past, FDA approval was typically enough for insurance approval for a procedure. Presently, however, the standards seem to have been raised with unclear guidance for the type and amount of data needed to gain widespread acceptance from insurers for reimbursement of new technologies. To address this problem as well as concerns over the rising cost of health care in general, there will be a new responsibility for manufacturers to investigate the cost-effectiveness of new technologies. Although it is expeditious for manufacturers to get 510(k) approval from the U.S. Food and Drug Administration (FDA) to market their new implants, this leaves them without adequate data to demonstrate the effectiveness of their new products. The use of registries for new product use after FDA approval will likely continue to increase.

Another important arena will be the precise matching of technology to patients. We have seen numerous times the very successful results of FDA-regulated or other initial studies of devices, only to be followed several years later by reports of failures or results no better than those reported prior to the new technology. This result is likely based on not following the stringent inclusion/exclusion criteria used in the early studies or the users of the technology not being as well trained as needed to be as successful as the early users. The keys to success for any of the emerging technologies will be physician training and employment of appropriate selection criteria.

There are already growing concerns over the rapidly rising cost of health care. No palatable end to this trend is foreseeable. Considering the high cost of back pain, there is a tremendous need to control the cost of spine care. This appears to almost be in conflict with the inevitable costs associated with developing new technology. In spinal care, we are already seeing the emergence of quality assurance programs such as that being established by the NCQA (National Committee for Quality Assurance). This same group has already launched similar programs for cardiology and diabetes. Spine care providers are also becoming familiar with the concepts and terminology related to Pay-for-Performance. These new initiatives may help to drive what is needed to fully evaluate new technologies, that is, comprehensive data collection. This process will also be facilitated by the increasing use of electronic medical records and other computerized data capture systems. Regardless of how good a treatment is, a single one will not emerge as best due to the various origins of back pain. The real key to optimizing treatment will be the matching of the best treatment for a particular well-defined spinal problem. This goal is also the key to maximizing cost-effectiveness, which may be one of the greatest challenges facing the ongoing incorporation of new technologies into everyday spine practice. However, achieving the optimal matching of treatment to pain generators will require developing not only new treatments but also better diagnostics to more accurately identify the source(s) of each patient's symptoms.

### Responsible Use

Although these are exciting times in spine surgery, technology must be embraced responsibly by all involved. The primary responsibility is with physicians, but manufacturers also play a significant role in responsibly introducing technology for clinical use. Physician users of technologies must be trained appropriately in technique as well as patient selection.

With new initiatives being introduced, such as quality assurance programs for spine care providers, patient case registries for all providers, electronic patient data capture, and electronic medical records, there will be greater opportunity for care providers to monitor and report results, both successful and not successful, to other care providers. Through the use of registries and comprehensive data capture, it is likely that greater insight will be gained into indications and contraindications, complications, and the results of off-label use.

We have seen the high rates of fusion reported for BMP which has been approved by the FDA to be marketed for use in tapered interbody fusion cages. However, as a result of its success, many have been tempted to use it off-label for other applications. In the cervical spine, its use has been associated with several reports of increased incidence of difficulties swallowing in up to 42% of patients and consequently other complications.[47,48] Naraghi and associates reported that the incidence of complications was significantly less when the dosage was reduced.[47] They also suggested that fibrin glue used anteriorly and posteriorly may reduce the incidence of complications. As these physicians did, all physicians using devices off-label need to document and share their experiences, both good and bad, to improve patient care and to reduce the risk to patients when using materials for which the application has not been previously investigated. Physicians using new technologies also have a responsibility to report less than desirable results and problems encountered with its use. Only through this system of open reporting can problems be identified and addressed and, most importantly, patient safety optimized. Using the BMP and fusion experience again, there are now reports of problems in the lumbar spine that were not identified in the early studies using this graft material.[49] Bone resorption defects in the vertebral bodies next to the intervertebral space where BMP was used were noted in 69% of the study group. Just as this problem, as well as those discussed concerning the use of BMP in the cervical spine, is emerging as use of this new technology expands, there is no doubt that as we move into an age of new implant materials and pharmacologic and biologic spinal therapies, they too will create unanticipated problems or events that did not occur in the clinical trials. Only through vigilant data collection by users and open and honest reporting can such problems be identified and addressed.

As has been seen in recent years, there will be more effort to address concerns related to finances and the relationship between manufacturers, investors, and physicians. Cessation of these relationships will lead to slower development and acceptance of technologies. However, with the increasing number of reported ethics violations, the concern is certainly legitimate and needs to be addressed.

The Internet has brought with it great capabilities for information exchange and education. However, it has also brought with it the possibility for patients to get erroneous information or develop unrealistic expectations based on the enthusiasm for new technologies. We have already seen this with patients interested in TDR. In their desperation to find relief, patients do not understand the finer details of selection criteria for new technology. Instead, they just want relief and have seen something about a new breakthrough in spine care. Only by making quality, unbiased educational material available to patients can we help them become better consumers. For years, web sites such as spine-health.com and spineuniverse.com have provided quality information to the public. Professional societies such as the North American Spine Society (NASS), American Academy of Orthopaedic Surgeons (AAOS), and Spine Arthroplasty Society (SAS) are increasingly making materials available to the public.

## CLOSING

This is a time of great changes in spine surgery. Technology is growing rapidly with many promising treatments on the horizon in an environment of changing health care ethics and reimbursement requirements. Patients are becoming more educated concerning their treatment options than ever before. The new technologies hold the promise of further developing minimally invasive surgery, motion-retaining devices, the repair or regeneration of degenerated tissue, and microelectronics that can monitor and respond to changing conditions in the spinal microenvironment. As with all exciting prospects, not all of the individual devices and treatments will evolve into successful therapies for clinical use. Some will fail biomechanical tests, and for others the promising results seen in ideal laboratory conditions will not be realized in humans. Also, enthusiasm for new treatments must be tempered with responsibility. The bar will be raised for the acceptance of new technologies. Some manufacturers will have to expand their clinical trials to not only prove the new technology not inferior to currently accepted care but also to prove its superiority. Also, cost-effectiveness must be addressed. This may mean that the spine market will be less attractive to investors, as the cost-effectiveness may require a lesser return on investment than what may be earned in other investment arenas. Physicians using the new technologies must also take on the responsibility of monitoring their results, particularly when using new treatments off-label, and reporting any complications or undesirable events related to the use of such technologies. Issues related to the financing of new technology development and relationships between industry and physicians will have to be addressed to ensure as much impartiality as possible, while allowing fair sharing of profits from intellectual properties. Although there are biologic and social challenges to overcome, the future of spine medicine is bright with many emerging options that should offer reduced treatment-related morbidity, yield good results, and offer earlier effective interventions for patients.

## REFERENCES


1. Burke JG, Watson RW, McCormack D, et al: Intervertebral discs which cause low back pain secrete high levels of proinflammatory mediators. J Bone Joint Surg Br 84:196–201, 2002.
2. Coppes MH, Marani E, Thomeer RT, et al: Innervation of "painful" lumbar discs. Spine 22:2342–2349, 1997.
3. Freemont AJ, Peacock TE, Goupille P, et al: Nerve ingrowth into diseased intervertebral disc in chronic back pain. Lancet 350:178–181, 1997.
4. Peng B, Wu W, Hou S, et al: The pathogenesis of discogenic low back pain. J Bone Joint Surg Br 87:62–67, 2005.
5. Peng B, Hao J, Hou S, et al: Possible pathogenesis of painful intervertebral disc degeneration. Spine 31:560–566, 2006.
6. Peng B, Hou S, Shi Q, et al: The relationship between cartilage endplate calcification and disc degeneration: An experimental study. Chin Med J (Engl) 114:308–312, 2001.
7. Borras MC, Becerra L, Ploghaus A, et al: fMRI measurement of CNS responses to naloxone infusion and subsequent mild noxious thermal stimuli in healthy volunteers. J Neurophysiol 91:2723–2733, 2004.
8. Lemaire JP, Carrier H, Sariali el H, et al: Clinical and radiological outcomes with the CHARITÉ artificial disc: A 10-year minimum follow-up. J Spinal Disord Tech 18:353–359, 2005.
9. Lee CK, Langrana NA, Parsons JR, et al: Development of a prosthetic intervertebral disc. Spine 16:S253–S255, 1991.
10. Klara PM, Ray CD: Artificial nucleus replacement: Clinical experience. Spine 27:1374–1377, 2002.
11. Ray CD: The PDN prosthetic disc-nucleus device. Eur Spine J 11 (2):S137–142, 2002.
12. Zucherman JF, Hsu KY, Hartjen CA, et al: A multicenter, prospective, randomized trial evaluating the X STOP interspinous process decompression system for the treatment of neurogenic intermittent claudication: Two-year follow-up results. Spine 30:1351–1358, 2005.
13. Wang JC, Haid RW Jr, Miller JS, et al: Comparison of CD HORIZON SPIRE spinous process plate stabilization and pedicle screw fixation after anterior lumbar interbody fusion. Invited submission from the Joint Section Meeting on Disorders of the Spine and Peripheral Nerves, March 2005. J Neurosurg Spine 4:132–136, 2006.
14. Wang JC, Spenciner D, Robinson JC: SPIRE spinous process stabilization plate: Biomechanical evaluation of a novel technology. Invited submission from the Joint Section Meeting on Disorders of the Spine and Peripheral Nerves, March 2005. J Neurosurg Spine 4:160–164, 2006.
15. Cunningham BC, Hu N, Beatson H, et al: Biomechanical evaluation of a posterior dynamic stabilization system combined with total disc replacement. International Meeting on Advance Spine Technologies. Athens, Greece, 2006.
16. Korhonen T, Karppinen J, Malmivaara A, et al: Efficacy of infliximab for disc herniation-induced sciatica: One-year follow-up. Spine 29:2115–2119, 2004.
17. Korhonen T, Karppinen J, Paimela L, et al: The treatment of disc herniation-induced sciatica with infliximab: Results of a randomized, controlled, 3-month follow-up study. Spine 30:2724–2728, 2005.
18. Tobinick EL, Britschgi-Davoodifar S: Perispinal TNF-alpha inhibition for discogenic pain. Swiss Med Wkly 133:170–177, 2003.
19. Peng B, Zhang Y, Hou S, et al: Intradiscal methylene blue injection for the treatment of chronic discogenic low back pain. Eur Spine J 16:33–38, 2007.
20. Simmons JW, McMillin JN, Emery SF, et al: Intradiscal steroids: A prospective double-blind clinical trial. Spine 17:S172–S175, 1992.
21. Klein RG, Eek BC, O'Neill CW, et al: Biochemical injection treatment for discogenic low back pain: A pilot study. Spine J 3:220–226, 2003.
22. Wei A, Chung S, Brisby H, et al: Bone morphogenic protein rescues human intervertebral disc cells in vitro from apoptosis. Spine Arthroplasty Society. Montreal, Canada, 2006.
23. Zhang Y, An HS, Song S, et al: Growth factor osteogenic protein-1: Differing effects on cells from three distinct zones in the bovine intervertebral disc. Am J Phys Med Rehabil 83:515–521, 2004.
24. Lee K-I, Moon E-S, Kim H, et al: Tissue engineering of the intervertebral disc with cultured nucleus pulposus cells using atelocollagen scaffold and growth factors. Spine Arthroplasty Society. Montreal, Canada, 2006.
25. Wilke HJ, Heuer F, Neidlinger-Wilke C, et al: Is a collagen scaffold for a tissue engineered nucleus replacement capable of restoring disc height and stability in an animal model? Eur Spine J 15(15):433–438, 2006.
26. Taylor W, Ozgur B: Biologic collagen agent repairs mid annular defects and prohibits early stage disc degeneration in the ovine model. Spine Arthroplasty Society. Montreal, Canada, 2006.
27. Haufe SM, Mork AR: Intradiscal injection of hematopoietic stem cells in an attempt to rejuvenate the intervertebral discs. Stem Cells Dev 15:136–137, 2006.
28. Meisel HJ, Siodla V, Ganey T, et al: Clinical experience in cell-based therapeutics: Disc chondrocyte transplantation: A treatment for degenerated or damaged intervertebral disc. Biomol Eng 24:5–21, 2007.
29. Miyamoto K, Masuda K, Kim J, et al: Intradiscal injections of osteogenic protein-1 restore the viscoelastic properties of degenerated intervertebral discs. North American Spine Society. Seattle, WA, 2006.

30. Yoon ST, Patel NM: Molecular therapy of the intervertebral disc. Eur Spine J 15(15):379–388, 2006.
31. Guehring T, Omlor GW, Lorenz H, et al: Disc distraction shows evidence of regenerative potential in degenerated intervertebral discs as evaluated by protein expression, magnetic resonance imaging, and messenger ribonucleic acid expression analysis. Spine 31:1658–1665, 2006.
32. Putzier M, Schneider SV, Funk JF, et al: The surgical treatment of the lumbar disc prolapse: Nucleotomy with additional transpedicular dynamic stabilization versus nucleotomy alone. Spine 30:E109–114, 2005.
33. Peng B, Hou S, Wu W, et al: The pathogenesis and clinical significance of a high-intensity zone (HIZ) of lumbar intervertebral disc on MR imaging in the patient with discogenic low back pain. Eur Spine J 15:583–587, 2006.
34. Peng B, Wu W, Li Z, et al: Chemical radiculitis. Pain 127:11–16, 2007.
35. Roberts S, Evans EH, Kletsas D, et al: Senescence in human intervertebral discs. Eur Spine J 15(15):312–316, 2006.
36. Holly LT, Bloch O, Johnson JP: Evaluation of registration techniques for spinal image guidance. J Neurosurg Spine 4:323–328, 2006.
37. Lieberman IH, Togawa D, Kayanja MM, et al: Bone-mounted miniature robotic guidance for pedicle screw and translaminar facet screw placement, Part I: Technical development and a test case result. Neurosurgery 59:641–650, 2006.
38. Richards PJ, Kurta IC, Jasani V, et al: Assessment of CAOS as a training model in spinal surgery: A randomised study. Eur Spine J 16:239–244, 2007.
39. Thomale UW, Kneissler M, Hein A, et al: A spine frame for intra-operative fixation to increase accuracy in spinal navigation and robotics. Comput Aided Surg 10:151–155, 2005.
40. Wolf A, Shoham M, Michael S, et al: Feasibility study of a mini, bone-attached, robotic system for spinal operations: Analysis and experiments. Spine 29:220–228, 2004.
41. Benzel E, Ferrara L, Roy S, et al: Micromachines in spine surgery. Spine 29:601–606, 2004.
42. Aebersold JMW: Design and development of a MEMS-based capacitive bending strain sensor and a biocompatible housing for a telemetric strain monitoring system. Department of Mechanical Engineering. Louisville, KY, University of Louisville, 2005.
43. Block AR, Gatchel RJ, Deardoff WW, et al: The Psychology of Spine Surgery. Washington, DC, American Psychological Association, 2003.
44. Block AR, Ohnmeiss DD, Guyer RD, et al: The use of presurgical psychological screening to predict the outcome of spine surgery. Spine J 1:274–282, 2001.
45. Siddiqui S, Guyer RD, Zigler JE, et al: Factors related to the 20 best and 20 worst 24-month outcomes of total disc replacement in prospective FDA-regulated trials. North American Spine Society. Seattle, WA, 2006.
46. Bono CM, Lee CK: Critical analysis of trends in fusion for degenerative disc disease over the past 20 years: Influence of technique on fusion rate and clinical outcome. Spine 29:455–463, 2004.
47. Naraghi F, Wolfer L, Lewis M, et al: BMP-2 dose correlates with increased postoperative edema and swallowing complications after cervical fusion. North American Spine Society. Seattle, WA, 2006.
48. Shields LB, Raque GH, Glassman SD, et al: Adverse effects associated with high-dose recombinant human bone morphogenetic protein-2 use in anterior cervical spine fusion. Spine 31:542–547, 2006.
49. McClellan JW, Mulconrey DS, Forbes RJ, et al: Vertebral bone resorption after transforaminal lumbar interbody fusion with bone morphogenetic protein (rhBMP-2). J Spinal Disord Tech 19:483–486, 2006.

# Index

Note: Page numbers followed by *f* indicate figures; *t* indicate tables; *b* indicate boxes.

## B

## C

## E



## F

## G

## H



## I

## J



## K

## M

## N



## O

## P

## Q



## R



## S

## T

## U



## V



## W



## X

## Y



## Z